# Core Curriculum
*for* Primary Care
Pediatric
Nurse Practitioners

This
self

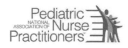
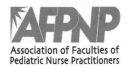

Association of Faculties of
Pediatric Nurse Practitioners

# Core Curriculum *for* Primary Care Pediatric Nurse Practitioners

*Volume Editor*

NANCY A. RYAN-WENGER, PhD, RN, CPNP, FAAN
Professor
College of Nursing
The Ohio State University
Columbus, Ohio

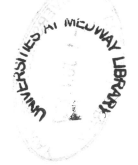

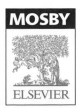

MOSBY
ELSEVIER

# MOSBY
ELSEVIER

11830 Westline Industrial Drive
St. Louis, Missouri 63146

CORE CURRICULUM FOR PRIMARY CARE PEDIATRIC
NURSE PRACTITIONERS

ISBN-13: 978-0-323-02756-4
ISBN-10: 0-323-02756-3

---

### Notice

Knowledge and best practice in this field are constantly changing. As new research and experience broaden our knowledge, changes in practice, treatment and drug therapy may become necessary or appropriate. Readers are advised to check the most current information provided (i) on procedures featured or (ii) by the manufacturer of each product to be administered, to verify the recommended dose or formula, the method and duration of administration, and contraindications. It is the responsibility of the practitioner, relying on their own experience and knowledge of the patient, to make diagnoses, to determine dosages and the best treatment for each individual patient, and to take all appropriate safety precautions. To the fullest extent of the law, neither the Publisher nor the Editors or Authors assume any liability for any injury and/or damage to persons or property arising out of or related to any use of the material contained in this book.

**The Publisher**

---

ISBN-13: 978-0-323-02756-4
ISBN-10: 0-323-02756-3

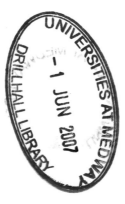

*Acquisitions Editor:* Barbara Nelson Cullen
*Managing Editor:* Robin Levin Richman
*Publishing Services Manager:* Jeff Patterson
*Design Direction:* Amy Buxton

Printed in the United States of America

Last digit is the print number: 9 8 7 6 5 4 3 2 1

### Working together to grow libraries in developing countries

www.elsevier.com | www.bookaid.org | www.sabre.org

ELSEVIER    BOOK AID International    Sabre Foundation

# Acknowledgments

I am sincerely grateful to Jill F. Kilanowski, PhD, RN, CPNP, my "Editorial Assistant Extraordinaire," whose attention to detail and perseverance made this book possible. I am deeply indebted to the authors of each chapter for their patience with the process of developing this book, and for sharing their primary care expertise in so many different age groups, body systems, and childhood disorders.

Thank you to my husband, Samuel Wenger, for his unqualified support and encouragement throughout this process.

I dedicate this book in memory of my sister, Carole J. Frames, and in celebration of my granddaughter, Ailionora Ryan McQuigg.

*Nancy A. Ryan-Wenger*

# Contributors

**Annette Baker,** MSN, RN, PNP
Preventive Cardiology Pediatric Nurse
    Practitioner
Cardiology Program
Boston Children's Hospital
Boston, Massachusetts

**Janet M. Banks,** PHD, RN, CPNP
Associate Professor
College of Nursing and Health
    Sciences
Texas A&M University Corpus Christi
Corpus Christi, Texas

**Lisa Marie Bernardo,** PHD, MPH, RN
Associate Professor
School of Nursing
Director of Continuing Education
Department of Health & Community
    Systems
University of Pittsburgh
Pittsburgh, Pennsylvania

**Stephanie Bonney,** MS, RN, CPNP
Pediatric Nurse Practitioner
St. Mary's Hospital for Children
Bayside, New York

**Terry A. Buford,** RN, PHD, CPNP
Clinical Associate Professor
University of Missouri-Kansas City
School of Nursing
Kansas City, Missouri

**Marianne Buzby,** RN, MSN, CRNP
Nurse Practitioner
Department of Endocrinology
Diabetes Center for Children
Children's Hospital of Philadelphia
Lecturer, School of Nursing
University of Pennsylvania
Philadelphia, Pennsylvania

**Barbara Cardinal-Busse,** MSN, CRNP
Clinical Assistant Professor of Pediatrics
Division of Adolescent Medicine
Children's Hospital of Pittsburgh
Pittsburgh, Pennsylvania

**Maria S. Chico,** RN, CPNP
Pediatric Nurse Practitioner
Pediatric Neurology
Medical College of Wisconsin
Children's Hospital of Wisconsin
Milwaukee, Wisconsin

**Charlene Cowley,** MS, RN, CPNP
Nurse Program Coordinator, Pain
    Management
Phoenix Children's Hospital
Phoenix, Arizona

**Kari L. Crawford,** MS, APRN, BC, PNP-AC
Pediatric Heart Center
Program Coordinator, Mended Hearts
    Support Group
Brenner Children's Hospital
Wake Forest University Baptist Medical
    Center
Winston-Salem, North Carolina

**Cynthia Danford,** PHD, RN, APRN, BC
Assistant Professor, College of Nursing
PNP Program Coordinator
Wayne State University
Detroit, Michigan

**Leslie Dieterich,** MSN, CNP
Pediatric Nurse Practitioner
Licking Memorial Pediatrics
Newark, Ohio

**Sharron L. Docherty, PHD, CPNP-AC**
Assistant Professor, School of Nursing
Director, Pediatric Acute/Chronic Care
  Advanced Practice Specialty
Duke University
Pediatric Nurse Practitioner, Valvano Day
  Hospital
Duke University Medical Center
Durham, North Carolina

**Karen Duderstadt, MS, RN, CPNP**
Associate Clinical Professor
Department of Family Health Care Nursing
School of Nursing
University of California San Francisco
San Francisco, California

**Sandra L. Elvik, MS, RN, CPNP**
Associate Professor of Pediatrics
UCLA School of Medicine
Assistant Medical Director
Child Abuse Crisis Center
Harbor-UCLA Medical Center
Torrance, CA

**Juli-anne K. Evangelista, MS, APRN, BC, PNP**
Heart Transplant Pediatric Nurse
  Practitioner
Cardiovascular Program
Boston Children's Hospital
Boston, Massachusetts

**Dawn Lee Garzon, PHD, APRN, BC, CPNP**
Assistant Professor
College of Nursing
University of Missouri-St. Louis
St. Louis, Missouri

**Nan M. Gaylord, PHD, RN, CPNP**
Assistant Professor
College of Nursing
University of Tennessee
Knoxville, Tennessee

**Mary Margaret Gottesman, PHD, RN, CPNP, FAAN**
Associate Professor, College of Nursing
Director, Pediatric Nurse Practitioner
  Program
The Ohio State University
Columbus, Ohio

**Mary Enzman Hagedorn, RN, PHD, HNC, CNS, CPNP**
Professor of Nursing
Beth-El College of Nursing and Health
  Sciences
University of Colorado at Colorado Springs
Colorado Springs, Colorado

**Kimberly Handrock, RN, MS, CPNP**
Pediatric Pulmonology Nurse
  Practitioner
St. Vincent Hospital and Health Services
Indianapolis, Indiana

**Susan M. Heighway, MS, APRN, BC-PNP, APNP**
Clinical Professor and Nurse Practitioner
Waisman Center, University Center for
  Excellence in Developmental
  Disabilities
Faculty Associate, School of Nursing
University of Wisconsin-Madison
Madison, Wisconsin

**Gail Hornor, RNC, MS, CPNP**
Center for Child and Family Advocacy
Children's Hospital
Columbus, Ohio

**Jean B. Ivey, DSN, CRNP**
Associate Professor, School of Nursing
Coordinator of Pediatric Graduate
  Options
University of Alabama at Birmingham
Birmingham, Alabama

**Ritamarie John, RN, DrNP, PNP**
Assistant Professor of Clinical
  Nursing
Columbia University
School of Nursing
New York, New York

**Nicole M. Joshi, MSN, RN, CPNP**
Pediatric Nurse Practitioner
Mount Laurel, New Jersey

**Jo Ellen Lee, MS, RN, CPNP**
Pediatric Nurse Practitioner
Neurology Clinic
Columbus Children's Hospital
Columbus, Ohio

**Deborah G. Loman,** PHD, MSN, CPNP
Assistant Professor
School of Nursing
Saint Louis University
St. Louis, Missouri

**Valerie Marburger,** MS, RN, CPNP, NNP
Clinical Instructor
College of Nursing
The Ohio State University
Neonatal Nurse Practitioner
Mount Carmel Hospital, St. Ann's Hospital
Columbus, Ohio

**Riza V. Mauricio,** MSN, RN, CCRN, CPNP
Pediatric Nurse Practitioner
M. D. Anderson Cancer Center
University of Texas
Houston, Texas

**Bernadette Mazurek Melnyk,** PHD,
RN, CPNP/NPP, FAAN, FNAP
Dean and Distinguished Foundation
    Professor in Nursing
College of Nursing
Arizona State University
Tempe, Arizona

**Zendi Moldenhauer,** PHD, RN-CS,
PNP/NPP
Pediatric & Psychiatric Nurse Practitioner
Private Practice
and
COPE for HOPE
Rochester, New York

**Wendy M. Nehring,** PHD, RN, FAAN
Associate Dean for Academic Affairs
College of Nursing
Rutgers, The State University of New
Jersey
Newark, New Jersey

**Victoria Page Niederhauser,** DRPH,
APRN-BC, PNP
Assistant Professor
Coordinator Advanced Practice Nursing
Nurse Practitioner Option Director
Caring for Vulnerable Children in
    Communities PNP Program
School of Nursing & Dental Hygiene
University of Hawaii
Honolulu, Hawaii 96822

**Julie Novak,** DNSC, RN, MA, CPNP,
FAANP
Professor and Head, Purdue School of
    Nursing
Associate Dean, College of Pharmacy,
    Nursing, and Health Sciences
Purdue University
West Lafayette, Indiana

**MiChelle Passamaneck,** RN, MSN,
CPNP, CUNP
Pediatric and Urology Nurse
    Practitioner
The Childrens Hospital
Faculty Instructor
University of Colorado Denver Health
    Sciences Center
Denver, Colorado

**Judy Pitts,** MSN, RN, CPNP
Clinical Instructor, College of Nursing
The Ohio State University
Pediatric Nurse Practitioner-Pulmonary
Children's Hospital
Columbus, Ohio

**Nancy A. Ryan-Wenger,** PHD, RN,
CPNP, FAAN
Professor
College of Nursing
The Ohio State University
Columbus, Ohio

**Sheila Judge Santacroce,** PHD,
APRN, CPNP
Associate Professor, School of Nursing
Yale University
New Haven, Connecticut

**Barbara Hoyer Schaffner,** PHD, RN,
CPNP
Professor, Department of Nursing
Otterbein College
Westerville, Ohio

**Janice Selekman,** DNSC, RN
Professor
School of Nursing
University of Delaware
Newark, Delaware

**Naomi A. Schapiro**, RN, MS, CPNP
Associate Clinical Professor
Department of Family Health Care Nursing
UCSF School of Nursing
San Francisco, California

**Vicki W. Sharrer**, MS, RN, CPNP
Professor, Department of Nursing
Ohio University-Zanesville
Zanesville, Ohio

**Theresa Skybo**, PhD, RN, CPNP
Assistant Professor, College of Nursing
The Ohio State University
Columbus, Ohio

**Leigh Small**, PhD, RN, CPNP
Assistant Professor, College of Nursing
Coordinator, Care of Children
Specialty Graduate Program
Arizona State University
Tempe, Arizona

**Janalee Taylor**, RN, MSN, CNS
Associate Clinical Director
Clinical Nurse Specialist
William S. Rowe Division of Rheumatology
Cincinnati Children's Hospital Medical
    Center
Cincinnati, Ohio

**Mary Tedesco-Schneck**, RN, MS, CPNP
Assistant Professor
Husson College
Pediatric Nurse Practitioner
Penobscot Pediatrics
Bangor, Maine

**Stacy Teicher**, MS, RN-CS, CNS, CPNP
Pediatric Nurse Practitioner
Lucille Packard Children's Hospital
Stanford University Medical Center
Palo Alto, California

**Debbie Terry**, CNRN, MS, CNP
Pediatric Nurse Practitioner
Department of Neurology
Columbus Children's Hospital
Columbus, Ohio

**Tener Goodwin Veenema**, PhD,
MPH, MS, CPNP
Assistant Professor
University of Rochester School of Nursing
    and School of Medicine & Dentistry
Rochester, New York

**Julee Waldrop**, MS, FNP, PNP
Clinical Associate Professor
School of Nursing
Pediatric Department, School of Medicine
The University of North Carolina
Chapel Hill, North Carolina

**Michelle Walsh**, PhD, RN, CPNP
Pediatric Nurse Practitioner
Pulmonary Clinic
Children's Hospital
Columbus, Ohio

**Jeanne Weiland**, MS, CPNP
Cystic Fibrosis Center
Cincinnati Children's Hospital Medical
    Center
Cincinnati, Ohio

**Victoria Weill**, MSN, RN, CPNP, APRN
Clinical Coordinator
School of Nursing
University of Pennsylvania
Philadelphia, Pennsylvania

**Kiersten A. M. Wells**, MS, CPNP, RN
Certified Pediatric Nurse Practitioner
Pediatric Cardiology
Lucille Salter Packard Children's Hospital
Palo Alto, California

**Barbara Vollenhover Wise**, PhD, RN,
CPNP
Pediatric Nurse Practitioner
Pediatric Oncology Branch
Center for Cancer Research
National Cancer Institute
National Institutes of Health
Bethesda, Maryland

# Reviewers

**Patricia Amerson,** MSN, RN, CPNP
University of Texas Health Science Center
   at San Antonio
San Antonio, Texas

**Heather Bastardi,** MSN, RN, PNP, CCRN,
AANC
Children's Hospital, Boston
Boston, Massachusetts

**Margaret Brady,** PHD, RN, CPNP
Past President NAPNAP
Professor, Department of Nursing
California State University—Long Beach
Nursing Department
Long Beach, CA

**Kimberly Demchak,** MSN, RN,
C-PNP, CNS, BC
Phoenix Children's Hospital
Phoenix, Arizona

**Vicki M. Lofquist,** MS, RN, CPNP
San Ramon Regional Medical Center,
   Pediatric Clinical Nurse Specialist/
   Nurse Manager
San Ramon, California
Adjunct Clinical Instructor
Samuel Merritt College, Graduate Division
Family Nurse Practitioner
Oakland, California

**Karen McKearney,** MSN, CPNP
Columbia University School of Nursing
New York, New York

**Carol Ann Okuhara,** BSN, MN, FNP-C
Childrens Hospital Los Angeles - USC
   affiliate
Los Angeles, California

**Roberta (Bobbie) Salveson,** MS, RN,
CPNP
St. Mary's/Duluth Clinic Health System
Duluth, Minnesota

**Patricia Ann Schlosser,** MS, APN, CNS,
CPNP
University of Wisconsin Children's
   Hospital—Madison
Madison, Wisconsin

**Janet Somlyay,** MSN, RN, CNS, CPNP
Fay W. Whitney School of Nursing
University of Wyoming
Laramie, Wyoming

**Jill Stites,** MN, RN, FNP, CPON
Children's Hospital of Orange County
Orange, California

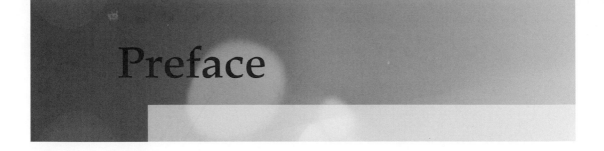

# Preface

Publication of *Core Curriculum for Primary Care Pediatric Nurse Practitioners* is the result of a joint effort between the National Association of Pediatric Nurse Practitioners (NAPNAP) and the Association of Faculties of Pediatric Nurse Practitioners (AFPNP). This publication can guide the development of pediatric nurse practitioner curricula and function as a means of monitoring and evaluating the comprehensiveness of the educational program for both pediatric and family nurse practitioner specialties. The outline format functions as a framework for building curriculum and as well as a review guide for students preparing for certification examination.

The *Core Curriculum for Primary Care Pediatric Nurse Practitioners* provides structured outlines for content on the role of the pediatric nurse practitioner, physical assessment, health assessment, health promotion, evaluation of common signs and symptoms in children and adolescents, and management of common acute illness and chronic physical and mental conditions. Each of these chapters is current, with excellent summary or review tables, and well referenced. Unique contributions are the chapters on diagnostic testing methods, emergencies in primary pediatrics, and pharmacologic management of common infective conditions, skin lesions, pain, and complementary and alternative therapies and nonpharmacologic treatments.

Solidly within the nursing model, *Core Curriculum for Primary Care Pediatric Nurse Practitioners* is a welcome addition to the resources available for faculty, students, and practitioners. The authors, clinicians, and faculty, and the editor, Dr. Nancy Ryan-Wenger, must be commended for the creation of this current and very useful curriculum guide for pediatric primary care providers.

**Patricia Clinton, PhD, RN, ARNP, FAANP**
President, National Association of Pediatric
Nurse Practitioners (NAPNAP)

**Patricia Jackson Allen, MS, RN, PNP, FAAN**
President, Association of Faculties of Pediatric
Nurse Practitioners (AFPNP)

# Contents

# Role of the Pediatric Nurse Practitioner

# Evolution of the Pediatric Nurse Practitioner Role

JULIE NOVAK, DNSc, RN, MA, CPNP, FAANP

1. Creation of the pediatric nurse practitioner (PNP) and formation of the National Association of Pediatric Nurse Associates and Practitioners
   a. Dr. Loretta Ford (1994, 1997, 1999) and Dr. Henry K. Silver established the first PNP program at the University of Colorado in 1965
      i. To meet a need for extension of child health care services
      ii. Taught registered nurses to do physical examinations, diagnose and treat patients, and assist in family counseling
   b. Other programs developed, but there was no standardization of programs or titles
      i. Some were post–RN certification programs for nurses with diplomas, associate degrees, or baccalaureate degrees
      ii. Some were master's degree programs
   c. Titles included pediatric nurse associates, pediatric nurse clinicians, and pediatric nurse practitioners.
   d. By 1992 all PNP programs were master's degree or post-master's certification to meet the requirement of a minimum of a master's degree to sit for certification examination by the National Certification Board of PNPs (see Section 3)
   e. 1990s—83 PNP programs
   f. 2005—more than 100 PNP programs
   g. In May 1973, PNP leaders in education and clinical practice met in Columbus, Ohio, to form the National Association of Pediatric Nurse Associates and Practitioners (NAPNAP)
   h. With the support of the partner organizations and individuals like Ann McRedmond of Ross Laboratories, the first national and organizational meeting was held in conjunction with the American Academy of Pediatrics (AAP) meeting on October 23, 1973, in Chicago at the Palmer House
   i. The 400 attendees included PNPs and Pediatric Nurse Associates from across the United States, AAP executive board members and representatives from the newly formed American Nurses Association PNP Council
   j. NAPNAP is the first-ever nurse practitioner (NP) membership organization
   k. The early goals of NAPNAP reflect goals that are still relevant (Clinton & Novak, 2001; Hobbie, 1998):
      i. To provide continuing education relevant to PNP needs
      ii. To provide standards for PNP education and practice
      iii. To support legislation to improve the health of children and adolescents

l. In February 1980, NAPNAP's first nursing conference on pediatric primary care was held in Washington, D.C.

m. In 1983, the 10th anniversary celebration of the organization (and 18th anniversary of the first program) was held in Chicago

n. The 1998 strategic plan defined NAPNAP mission as a "professional organization that advocates for infants, children, and adolescents and provides leadership for PNPs who deliver primary care in a variety of settings"

o. In 2000, a new integrated strategic planning model was developed that included:
   i. Research
   ii. Collaboration
   iii. Health policy
   iv. Practice
   v. Education
   vi. All based on a foundation of leadership development

p. In 2001, the Health Policy focus was further strengthened with regular visits to Capitol Hill, meetings with President Bush's Deputy Health Advisor, attendance at Nurse in Washington Internship (NIWI), annual legislator awards, and collaboration with our Washington Advisors at Arent Fox
   i. A new Research Chair board position was created

q. In 2001 the organization name changed to National Association of Pediatric Nurse Practitioners ("Associates" removed because this title is no longer used)

r. Growth of the NAPNAP membership from 1973 to present is shown in Box 1-1

s. NAPNAP presidents from 1973 to present are listed in Box 1-2

2. Association of Faculties of Pediatric Nurse Practitioners (AFPNP) (Pulcini & Wagner, 2002)

a. Standards for curricula of PNP programs were first developed by a group of PNP faculty at the University of Connecticut in 1972

■ **BOX 1-1**
■ **GROWTH IN NAPNAP MEMBERSHIP FROM 1973 TO PRESENT**

| YEAR | NUMBER |
|------|--------|
| 1973 | 400 |
| 1974 | 650 |
| 1975 | 800 |
| 1977 | 958 |
| 1980 | 2200 |
| 1982 | 2470 |
| 1985 | 2500 |
| 1988 | 2800 |
| 1991 | 3200 |
| 1992 | 3500 |
| 1993 | 4000 |
| 1994 | 4500 |
| 1995 | 5000 |
| 1996 | 5300 |
| 1998 | 5500 |
| 2000 | 5788 |
| 2005 | 7000 |

■ **BOX 1-2**
■ **NAPNAP PRESIDENTS FROM 1973 TO PRESENT**

| | |
|---|---|
| Jan McCleery | 1973–1974 |
| Phillis Cunningham | 1974–1978 |
| Barbara Dunn | 1975–1978 |
| Margaret Hicks | 1978–1980 |
| Karen Fond | 1980–1981 |
| Janet Nystrom | 1981–1982 |
| Sally Walsh | 1982–1983 |
| Carol Rudy | 1983–1985 |
| Beatrice Gaunder | 1985–1986 |
| Linda Jonides | 1986–1987 |
| Linda Gilman | 1987–1988 |
| Cynthia Hobbie | 1988–1989 |
| Virginia Millonig | 1989–1990 |
| Ruth Mullins | 1990–1991 |
| Ellen Rudy Clore | 1991–1992 |
| Margaret Grey | 1992–1993 |
| Catherine Burns | 1993–1994 |
| Joan Greene | 1994–1995 |
| Ardy Dunn | 1995–1996 |
| Renee McLeod | 1996–1997 |
| Patricia Franklin | 1997–1998 |
| Beth Richardson | 1998–1999 |
| Barbara Kelly | 1999–2000 |
| Barbara DeLoian | 2000–2001 |
| Julie C. Novak | 2001–2002 |
| Mary Margaret Gottesman | 2002–2003 |
| Margaret Brady | 2003–2004 |
| Ric Ricciardi | 2004–2005 |
| Jo Ann Serota | 2005–2006 |
| Patricia Clinton | 2006–2007 |

    **b.** In 1978, the AFPNP was formally established in Iowa City, Iowa
    **c.** The AFPNP has been responsible for two documents that guide education and practice
        **i.** *Philosophy, Conceptual Model and Terminal Competencies for the Education of Pediatric Nurse Practitioners*
        **ii.** NAPNAP *Scope and Standards of Practice* first developed in 2000
        **iii.** In 2004, the NAPNAP *Scope and Standards of Practice* document revised to recognize the expanded role of the PNP across settings and with children who are well, at risk, and have chronic and acute health conditions (NAPNAP, 2004)
**3.** Development of a PNP certification board
    **a.** As the NP movement began to grow, the National Council of State Boards of Nursing and other nursing organizations raised concerns about evaluation of NP clinical competency
    **b.** In 1975, the National Certification Board of Pediatric Nurse Practitioners and Associates (NCBPNP/A) was established as an entity separate from NAPNAP
        **i.** Goal: To develop a certification process that incorporated the high quality standards of excellence in PNP education and clinical practice

      **ii.** Board members included representatives from:
        (a) NAPNAP
          (1) One NAPNAP Executive Board member—called the NAPNAP certification chair
          (2) One NAPNAP presidential appointee—to focus on PNP practice trends
        (b) Association of Faculties of PNP programs (AFPNP)
        (c) American Academy of Pediatrics (AAP)

  **c.** NAPNAP recognized the importance of national certification and actively encouraged its members to become certified through the NCBPNP/A

  **d.** One of the hallmarks of the developing collaborative partnership was the Pediatric Nurse Practitioner Educational Program review
      **i.** Determines the eligibility of graduates of PNP programs to sit for NCB-PNP/A certification
      **ii.** As of April, 2006, PNP primary care programs have been approved in 94 colleges and universities (PNCB, 2005)

  **e.** In 1990, the name was changed to National Certification Board for Nurse Practitioners and Nurses (NCBPNP/N) to reflect the addition of a general pediatric nursing certification exam (PNCB, 2005)

  **f.** In 1995–1996, the National Council of State Boards of Nursing announced plans to require a second licensure for NPs, but NAPNAP and other NP organizations and certifying bodies strongly objected

  **g.** NAPNAP reaffirmed the NCBPNP/N examination as a model for national-certification for graduates of programs that meet:
      **i.** Rigorous program review
      **ii.** Minimum faculty/student ratios
      **iii.** Precepted clinical hour requirements
      **iv.** Program director certification requirements

  **h.** NCBPNP/N was the first nursing certifying body to meet the rigorous accreditation standards of the U.S. Department of Education–approved National Commission on Certifying Agencies (NCCA)

  **i.** 1992—A minimum of a master's degree, or completion of the PNP courses within a doctoral program, was required to sit for PNP certification exam (PNCB, 2005)

  **j.** 2003—Name changed to Pediatric Nursing Certification Board (PNCB, 2005)

  **k.** Certified PNPs use the credential CPNP

  **l.** An alternative to PNCB certification for PNPs is available from the American Nurses Credentialing Center, 2006
      **i.** The American Nurses Association, Inc. (ANA) established the ANA Certification Program in 1973 to "provide tangible recognition of professional achievement in a defined functional or clinical area of nursing"
      **ii.** The American Nurses Credentialing Center (ANCC) was established as a separately incorporated center to promote and enhance public health by certifying nurses that meet nationally recognized standards
      **iii.** Two levels of credentialing and their acronyms are available:
        (a) Board Certified (BC)
        (b) Certified (RN, C)

**4.** Government initiatives that influenced PNP education and practice
  **a.** The 1981 Graduate Medical Education National Advisory Committee
      **i.** Charged with the task of advising the Secretary of the Department of Health and Human Services on overall strategies on the present and

        future supply and requirements of physicians by specialty and geographic location

    **ii.** Indicated that the perceived shortage of physicians was really the result of physician misdistribution and an overabundance of specialists

    **iii.** Reflected a positive view of NPs as primary care providers

  **b.** 1990s—Several states passed legislation that provided third-party reimbursement and prescriptive authority for NPs

  **c.** Landmark federal legislation in 1990 allowed PNPs to obtain direct reimbursement under Medicaid for services provided to individuals and families covered under the Federal Employee Health Benefits Program

  **d.** U.S. Congress passed legislation to provide direct Medicare reimbursement to NPs

**5.** NAPNAP initiatives that influenced PNP education and practice

  **a.** McNeil Grant-in-Aid scholarships to attend NAPNAP meetings began in 1981

  **b.** NAPNAP revised the PNP Scope of Practice statement to change physicians' relationship with PNPs from "supervisory" to "collegial"

    **i.** The AAP executive committee was concerned about this expansion of the PNP role

    **ii.** PNPs rallied and gained grassroots support for the new language from pediatricians who worked with PNPs

    **iii.** As a result, the AAP renewed their positive working relationship with NAPNAP

  **c.** The first NAPNAP director of government relations, Jacquelyn Ryberg, was appointed in 1983

  **d.** Recognizing the increased independence in clinical decision making by PNPs, Johnson & Johnson Consumer Products Company began sponsoring travel fellowships to the annual conference

  **e.** NAPNAP selected a lobbyist, Debra Hardy-Havens of Capitol Associates to represent NAPNAP in Washington, D.C. to:

    **i.** Advocate for programs for children and young people

    **ii.** Remove barriers to practice for PNPs

    **iii.** Negotiate the complexities of the health care system, in the areas of reimbursement and later, managed care

  **f.** Nurse in Washington Internship (NIWI) program was started in 1986

  **g.** NAPNAP began appointing task force committees to study and make recommendations about important issues such as liability/malpractice, human immunodeficiency virus (HIV) testing in health care workers, and lactation education

  **h.** NAPNAP's official journal was changed from *Pediatric Nursing* to the new *Journal of Pediatric Health Care*, published by Mosby and later, by Elsevier

  **i.** NAPNAP began releasing public service announcements regarding topics of concern to children, parents, and providers

  **j.** NAPNAP began publishing information booklets such as "Take Time for Your Child's Health" and "Medicine Cabinet Essentials for Your Child's Health" (Hobbie, 1998)

  **k.** NAPNAP joined the Pediatric AIDS Coalition and published a pediatric HIV/AIDS professional review

  **l.** NAPNAP's new focus on health care reform led to an invitation to participate with First Lady Hillary Rodham Clinton in describing the potential role of nursing in a reformed health care system in 1993

  **m.** Capitol Associates began publishing the NAPNAP *Legislative Update* in 1993

n. NAPNAP successfully competed for a contract from the Office of Health Promotion and Disease Prevention to evaluate the implementation of the "Put Prevention into Practice" initiative
   i. This was NAPNAP's first external funding for such a project
   ii. The project was successfully concluded in 1996
o. NAPNAP position, policy and practice statements are continually developed, revised and reaffirmed (NAPNAP, 2006b)
p. A second edition of a *Nurse Practitioner Career Resource Guide* was released by the NAPNAP Professional Issues Committee in 2005 to provide career counseling to new and experienced NPs in a variety of settings
q. ASTRA USA provided funds to support NAPNAP members' research on pain
r. NAPNAP's logo of an infant sleeping in a prone position was eliminated to support current practice recommendations that infants sleep on their back to prevent sudden infant death syndrome (SIDS)
s. NAPNAP Keep Your Child/Yourself Safe and Secure (KySS) campaign was launched to "promote the mental health of children and adolescents through the integration of mental health promotion, screening, and early evidence-based interventions" (KySS, 2006)
   i. After analysis of the fall 2001 data collection, Dr. Bernadette Melnyk, KySS principal investigator, Chapter KySS campaign coordinators, and the KySS management task force met to plan the intervention phase of the project
   ii. An educational grant was funded by the MCH Bureau for support of a Summit of Experts held at the University of Rochester, led by PI Dr. Bernadette Melnyk and co-project directors, Drs. Julie Novak and Dolores Jones
   iii. The KySS Summit further informed the development of KySS interventions
   iv. In 2005, the KySS Program Work Group refined the strategic direction for the campaign to include:
      (a) Promoting mental health in children and teens
      (b) Raising public awareness
      (c) Disseminating information about and implementing effective screening
      (d) Educating healthcare professionals and others
      (e) Affecting change in public policies
      (f) Developing effective partnerships
t. In 2002 NAPNAP launched a collaborative effort with iVillage to produce *Baby Steps*, a magazine for new parents
u. To increase recognition and marketing of PNPs, NAPNAP developed and published:
   i. "The PNP Advantage"
   ii. "Why a PNP Is Right for Your Child"
   iii. "Educational Preparation and Role Delineation of PNPs"
v. Creation of the Legislative Listserv to allow rapid dissemination of information regarding legislative issues that are critical to PNP practice
   i. A plan was initiated to identify a legislative liaison in each of 12 regions of the United States
w. In 2002, Health Policy Chair Karen Duderstadt developed a draft statement regarding the critical nature of alarming rates of obesity in the U.S. and requested that NAPNAP develop a clinical focus area targeting this issue
   i. The Healthy Eating and Activity Together (HEAT) Initiative was launched in 2003 by NAPNAP (HEAT, 2006)

          ii. Dr. Mary Margaret Gottesman is the National Chair of the HEAT Initiative

          iii. The primary focus is on prevention, identification of those at risk, cultural relevance and advocacy

          iv. In 2005, the strategic plan was refined to include a focus on national leadership, implementation, evaluation and research of an evidence-based HEAT Clinical Practice Guideline

          v. The HEAT Guideline includes recommendations for practice, education, dissemination, advocacy and collaboration

          vi. The HEAT Guideline was released to all NAPNAP members in March, 2006

     x. NAPNAP's Executive Board voted to adopt a new logo design on December 4, 2003

          i. The process involved Executive Board members, NAPNAP Past Presidents, Chapter Presidents, industry partners and ultimately, NAPNAP members

     y. A new NAPNAP website design was launched in April 2005 (NAPNAP, 2006a)

          i. Guided by the Communications Technology Work Group of NAPNAP led by Dr. Linda Lindeke

          ii. The website represents NAPNAP's commitment to service, community and growth

     z. In December 2005, NAPNAP Executive Board approved a new Strategic Direction, mission and vision for the organization emphasizing NAPNAP's commitment to "promoting optimal health for children through leadership, practice, advocacy, education and research"

---

# REFERENCES

American Nurses Credentialing Center (ANCC). (2005). ANCC certification for professional nurses—certifying excellence in nursing practice. Retrieved on March 7, 2006 at http://nursingworld.org/ancc/inside.html.

Clinton, P., & Novak, J. C. (2001). NAPNAP and NCBPNP: A history intertwined. *PNP Newsletter, 12*(6), 1-2.

Ford, L. C. (1994). Nurse practitioners: myths and misconceptions. An article excerpted from "Myths and misconceptions regarding the nurse practitioner" in "Critical issues in American nursing in the twentieth century," (1994), published by the Foundation of the New York State Nurses Association, Inc. *Pulse, 32*(4), 9-10.

Ford, L. C. (1997). A voice from the past: 30 fascinating years as a nurse practitioner. *Clin Ex Nurse Pract, 1*(1), 3-6.

Ford, L. C. (1999). NP 2000. Thoughts for the 21st century. *Nurse Pract: Am J Prim Health Care, 24*(5), 17.

HEAT (2006). "Healthy eating and activity together" initiative. Retrieved on March 8, 2006 at http://www.napnap.org/index. cfm?page=198&sec=220

Hobbie, C. (1998). NAPNAP: The first 25 years. *J Pediatr Health Care, 28*(5), part 2, S3-S8.

KySS (2006). "Keep your children/yourself safe and secure" program Retrieved on March 8, 2006 from http://www.napnap. org/index. cfm?page=198&sec=221

National Association of Pediatric Nurse Practitioners Annual Reports 1973–74 to 2002-2003.

National Association of Pediatric Nurse Practitioners. (2004). *Scope and standards of practice*. Cherry Hill, NJ: NAPNAP.

National Association of Pediatric Nurse Practitioners. (2006a). About NAPNAP. Retrieved on March 8, 2006 from www.napnap.org/index.cfm?page=9

National Association of Pediatric Nurse Practitioners. (2006b). Position statements. Retrieved on March 8, 2006 from http://www.napnap.org/index.cfm?page=10&sec=54

Pediatric Nurses Certification Board (PNCB). (2005). Personal communication with executive director Jan Wyatt on June 29, 2005. See also the website at www.pncb.org/ptistore/control/index

Pulcini, J., & Wagner, M. (2002). Nurse practitioner education in the United States: A success story. *Clin Ex Nurse Pract, 6*(2), 51-56.

## ACKNOWLEDGMENT

Joe Casey, NAPNAP director of Marketing and Communications

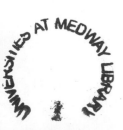

# 2

**■■■**

# Essential Elements of the Advanced Practice Role for Pediatric Nurse Practitioners

NAN M. GAYLORD, PhD, RN, CPNP

## LEGAL AND PROFESSIONAL CREDENTIALING IN THE ADVANCED PRACTICE ROLE FOR THE PEDIATRIC NURSE PRACTITIONER (PNP)

1. Licensure for advanced practice nursing (Pearson, 2006a, 2006b; Phillips, 2006)
   a. Few states require an advanced practice nursing license
   b. 41 states require an additional registration/state certificate to practice as a PNP
   c. Board of nursing has sole authority in PNP scope of practice in 46 states
   d. Board of nursing and board of medicine authorize the scope of practice in 5 states
   e. No requirements for physician involvement, i.e., collaboration, authorization, delegation, supervision, or direction of activities in 23 states
   f. Physician involvement with written documentation required in 24 states
   g. Physician involvement with no written documentation required in 4 states
   h. The Advanced Practice Registered Nurse (APRN) Compact is an agreement between selected states for mutual recognition of RN and APRN licenses to practice (National Council of State Boards of Nursing, 2006)
      i. In 2005, Utah and Iowa agreed to mutually recognize APRN licenses
      ii. No date has been set for wider implementation of the APRN Compact
   i. NAPNAP strongly supports national certification of PNPs (NAPNAP, 2001b)
2. Prescriptive privilege
   a. An annual update on nurse practitioner prescriptive privilege status in each state is published in a leading nurse practitioner journal
   b. Levels of prescriptive authority vary by state (Pearson, 2006a)
      i. Prescribe (including controlled substances) independent of physician involvement: 10 states
      ii. Prescribe (including controlled substances) with some degree of physician involvement or delegation of prescription writing with written documentation: 39 states, and without written documentation: 1 state
      iii. Prescribe (excluding controlled substances) with some degree of physician involvement or delegation of prescription writing: 4 states

   c. All PNPs may receive and/or dispense drug samples according to their state authorized scope of practice

   d. Information about states in which midlevel practitioners (e.g., NP, PA) are authorized to prescribe controlled substances is provided on the Drug Enforcement Agency (DEA) website (DEA, 2006b)

   e. For PNPs able to prescribe controlled substances, a DEA number is required. The DEA Form 224 application is available from the website (DEA, 2006a)

   f. NPs must have physician collaboration to prescribe controlled substances III–IV in the state of Washington, and for Schedule II–III in Maine and Utah (Pearson, 2005)

      i. Several barriers to meeting patient needs for Schedule II–IV drugs were identified by 976 Washington NPs in a survey (Kaplan & Brown, 2004)

        (a) Physician concerns about liability

        (b) Physician chooses different drug than NP selects

        (c) Physician reluctant to prescribe drug selected by NP

        (d) NP does not feel comfortable/competent prescribing scheduled drugs

        (e) Pharmacist does not take verbal orders from NP

        (f) Employer prohibits use of standing orders or protocols for Schedule II–IV drugs

   g. NAPNAP (2003b) "advocates that nurse practitioners have unlimited prescriptive authority and dispensing privileges within their scope of practice"

3. Liability insurance for clinical practice

   a. The PNP role has increased autonomy but also has increased accountability and liability

   b. The PNP is a member of a profession with the potential to have lawsuits filed against its members and needs the protection of liability insurance (Guido, 2006)

   c. Professional behaviors that decrease lawsuits include (Guido, 2006):

      i. Communicating clearly and openly with patients and families

      ii. Ensuring valid and informed consent before proceeding to care for a patient

     iii. Informing the patient/guardians that you are a PNP

      iv. Seeking assistance from other specialists and physicians when circumstances exceed the PNP's scope of practice

      v. Maintaining current skills

      vi. Documenting carefully and accurately

   d. All professional liability policies include:

      i. Payment for an attorney to represent the nurse in the event of a claim

      ii. Payment for settlements or jury awards

     iii. Specific limits of legal liability

   e. Other inclusions may be:

      i. Deductibles—Some policies deduct the amount paid for the PNP's legal defense from the total limits of liability

      ii. Exclusions—Activities that will prevent coverage, such as:

        (a) Criminal actions

        (b) Incidents occurring while the insured was under the influence of alcohol or drugs

        (c) Actions that violate state nursing practice acts

   f. Three types of professional liability coverage exist (Guido, 2001)

      i. Individual policy

        (a) Specific to the individual

(b) Insures the PNP 24 hours/day 7 days/week for paid and volunteer services

   ii. Group policy

     (a) A group of similarly licensed professionals are insured by one company

     (b) All practice in the same facility

     (c) All have very similar job descriptions

   iii. Employer policy

     (a) The employer only insures the PNP for the services provided to that employer

     (b) Requires that PNPs practice within the scope of their employment as well as the scope of professional nursing practice

     (c) Favored by institutions as the coverage is written specifically for the business and its major concerns

     (d) Health care facilities may not be able to protect the individual PNP's best interests; i.e., the facility may settle out of court but the nurse's best interest would be served through a court hearing

     (e) PNPs are encouraged to purchase supplemental individual policies to cover nursing activities performed beyond the scope of employment, such as volunteer work, emergencies, or simply responding as a nurse (NAPNAP, 2004c)

  g. Within these types, three levels of coverage are available (ASRT, 2006)

   i. "Claims made" policy protects PNP against incidents that arise from treatment provided after the policy's retroactive date and are reported while the policy is in force

   ii. "Tail" coverage is optional protection that allows PNP to report claims after a "Claims made" policy has ended for alleged injuries that occurred while that policy was in force

   iii. "Occurrence" policy protects PNP against incidents that occur while the policy is in force, regardless of when the claim is reported

**4.** Continuing education

  **a.** NAPNAP believes that continuing education is essential for PNPs to acquire and enhance the knowledge and skills necessary to ensure optimal patient care and professional development (NAPNAP, 2000)

  **b.** Required for maintenance of the professional nursing license in some states

  **c.** Required for maintenance of PNP national certification

   **i.** PNCB certification (PNCB, 2006)

     (a) Valid for 6 years

     (b) Requires participation in a specified cycle of continuing education options

   **ii.** ANCC certification (ANCC, 2006)

     (a) Valid for 5 years

     (b) Requires documentation at the end of 5 years of 1500 clinical practice hours in pediatric primary care and various options for continuing education

**5.** Hospital privileging and credentialing

  **a.** Initiated after the *Darling vs Charleston Community Memorial Hospital* case (Jones, 2002)

   **i.** Found that hospitals were liable for the quality of medical care delivered and for ensuring the clinical competence of their practitioners

  **b.** Credentialing

   **i.** Performed by the institution upon employment of the PNP

        **ii.** An administrative process of collecting, assessing, and validating:
           (a) Professional licensure
           (b) Clinical experience
           (c) Educational preparation
           (d) Certification for specialty practice
           (e) References
           (f) Professional activity

  **c.** Privileging is the process through which a health care organization grants a practitioner specific authority to perform designated clinical activities in the facility
        **i.** Individually based
        **ii.** Specific to the granting institution
        **iii.** Designated in the job description and in the institution's policies

  **d.** For PNPs not employed by the institution, both credentialing and privileging is through the medical staff department similar to that of physicians

  **e.** NAPNAP's position statement on credentialing and privileging supports these regulatory actions, including continuous monitoring, and fair, cost-effective and uniform disciplinary processes (NAPNAP, 2003a)

**6.** Reimbursement for services
  **a.** Payment for PNP services is connected to the reimbursement for services in Medicare
  **b.** Medicare will compensate NPs 85% of the physician fee schedule
  **c.** Medicaid fees and billing are based on the Medicare program
  **d.** Therefore the PNP must apply for an individual Medicare personal identification number (PIN) through the Health Care Financing Administration (Abood & Keepnews, 2000a)
  **e.** Once the PIN number is obtained, the PNP must apply for reimbursement as a health care provider through individual patient insurance companies
  **f.** PNPs may bill under the name of the physician, called *incident*-to or indirect billing (Abood & Keepnews, 2002a; 2002b)
        **i.** If the PNP is an employee of the physician
        **ii.** Only if the physician is on the premises
        **iii.** The service is then billed at 100% of the physician's fee
  **g.** Current procedural terminology (CPT) coding is the term used to document the health care services provided
        **i.** American Medical Association (2006) publishes the CPT manual
        **ii.** Coding is the responsibility of the health care provider at the time of service
        **iii.** CPT codes are listed on the bill generated to the patient and insurers for the services rendered (Jones, 2002)
        **iv.** Billing and reimbursement depend on the level of care provided
        **v.** Level of care is determined by the health history, physical examination, and the complexity of medical decision making
        **vi.** Of the six categories of CPT codes, Evaluation and Management (E&M) is the most common code used in pediatrics
        **vii.** The health history ranges from lowest to highest level:
           (a) Problem focus—brief history of the chief complaint
           (b) Expanded problem focus—brief history of the chief complaint and review of other pertinent systems
           (c) Detailed problem focus—extended history of the chief complaint, extended review of systems, and pertinent past, family, or social history

(d) Comprehensive problem focus—extended history of the chief complaint, extended review of systems, complete past medical history, and complete family and social history

viii. The physical examination ranges from lowest to highest level:
(a) Problem focus—examination of one system
(b) Expanded problem focus—examination of affected system and related systems
(c) Detailed problem focus—examination of affected system and related systems
(d) Comprehensive problem focus—complete single system and specialty examination or a multisystem examination

ix. The complexity of medical decision making ranges from lowest to highest level:
(a) Straightforward—minimal number of diagnoses, minimal complexity of data, minimal risk of complications
(b) Low complexity—limited number of diagnoses
(c) Moderate complexity—multiple diagnoses
(d) High complexity—extensive number of diagnoses, extensive complexity of data and high risk of complications

x. Other codes are available for complete physical examinations at every age

xi. In addition to the CPT code, which describes the service performed, a diagnostic code is identified
(a) The *International Classification of Diseases, 9th Edition, Clinical Modification* (ICD-9-CM) is the official system of assigning codes to diseases (National Center for Health Statistics, 2005)

h. NAPNAP (2004b) asserts that "NPs should be reimbursed directly and on par with physicians for the health care services they provide"
i. *The Nurse Practitioner Career Resource Guide* available from NAPNAP (2005) provides advice on preparing a resume, interviewing, and negotiating a contract
ii. Sample contracts for primary care and specialty care can be found in the Guide

## LEADERSHIP SKILLS AND PROFESSIONAL SERVICE RELATED TO LEGAL AND PROFESSIONAL CREDENTIALING

1. Professional responsibilities
   a. Maintain membership in professional organizations
      i. Ensure that PNPs have a voice in the maintenance of professional standards
      ii. The National Association of Pediatric Nurses and Practitioners (NAPNAP, 2006a) is the specialty organization for PNPs
   b. Attend continuing education programs
   c. Maintain liability insurance coverage
   d. Provide continuing education to peers through presentations and clinical articles as requested
   e. Negotiate with managed care organizations and insurers to ensure PNPs are designated primary care providers in available health plans and paid at same rate as physicians for the same services

# PNP CLINICAL EXPERTISE

1. Scope of practice and general standards of care
   a. The National Association of Pediatric Nurse Practitioners
      i. Scope: PNP provides health care to children from birth through 21 years of age, and in specific situations, to individuals older than the age of 21 years
      ii. *Scope and Standards of Practice* document outlines the definition, education, practice parameters, and professional accountability of the PNP (NAPNAP, 2004c)
      iii. The NAPNAP (2006c) website has a Frequently Asked Questions section that may be useful to both new and experienced PNPs
   b. The American Nurses Association
      i. *Scope and Standards of Advanced Practice Registered Nursing* (American Nurses Association, 1996)
      ii. Defines advanced practice registered nursing
      iii. Describes both standards of care and professional performance expectations
      iv. Discusses roles, settings, education, certification, regulation, and ethics of advanced practice nursing with input from more than 25 nursing organizations.
2. Core competencies of PNPs
   a. Developed by the Association of Faculties for Pediatric Nurse Practitioners (AFPNP, 1996) and fully supported by NAPNAP
      i. Systematically collect and evaluate health assessment data to determine the health status of children
      ii. Provide primary health care for the child
      iii. Provide the child with opportunities to engage in positive health care practices
      iv. Assess and promote growth and development of children from birth through adolescence
      v. Assess, diagnose, and manage pediatric problems, illness, and chronic conditions
      vi. Exemplify accountability for professional nursing practice
      vii. Advance the role of the PNP in the health care system
3. Clinical practice guidelines and standards of care
   a. Evidence-based medicine (nursing)
      i. "The conscientious, explicit, and judicious use of current best evidence in making decisions about the care of individual patients" (Sackett, 1996)
      ii. The integration of the best research evidence with clinical expertise and patient values
   b. Evidence is derived from systematic reviews of the research literature
      i. Randomized controlled clinical trials are the gold standard
      ii. The quality of other studies is also considered
      iii. Examples of such reports can be located at:
         (a) Agency for Healthcare Research and Quality (AHRQ, 2006b; 2006c)
         (b) The Cochrane Collaboration (2006)
         (c) Professional journals, including on-line journals (e.g., Bandolier, 2006)
   c. The clinician makes a conscientious and explicit but judicious use of these summaries based on individual patients' desires, values, and unique biology

   **d.** Clinical practice guidelines

      **i.** Protocols of care for specific problems or disease entities based on the best evidence

      **ii.** Once published and distributed these standards are the measures of the quality of care provided to a patient

      **iii.** Examples of clinical practice guidelines for the PNP:

         (a) Protocol books (Boynton et al., 2003)

         (b) PNP texts (Burns et al., 2004)

         (c) Professional organizations (NAPNAP, 2006a; American Academy of Pediatrics, 2006a)

         (d) Government agencies (AHRQ, 2006a)

   **e.** Professional organization policy or position statements

      **i.** Organizational principles to guide and define the child health care system and/or improve the health of all children

      **ii.** Policy statements written by professional organizations are applicable to the PNP's administrative role, e.g. National Association of Pediatric Nurse Practitioners (NAPNAP, 2006b), American Academy of Pediatrics, American Nurses Association, AHRQ (2004d)

**4.** Provide culturally competent care

   **a.** Culture—a society's way of life, derived from their particular worldview, that evolves over time (Green-Hernandez et al., 2004)

   **b.** The National Organization of Nurse Practitioner Faculties (NONPF, 2000) agrees that the NP demonstrates *cultural competence* when she or he:

      **i.** Shows respect for the inherent dignity of all human beings, whatever their characteristics

      **ii.** Accepts the rights of individuals to choose their health care provider, participate in care, and refuse care

      **iii.** Acknowledges own personal biases and prevents them from interfering with care

      **iv.** Recognizes cultural issues and interacts with patients in culturally sensitive ways

      **v.** Develops patient-appropriate educational materials that address the language and cultural beliefs of the patient

      **vi.** Accesses culturally appropriate resources to deliver care

      **vii.** Assists patient to access quality care within a dominant culture

   **c.** Strategies that NPs can use in their care to increase cultural competence with diverse patients

      **i.** Become familiar with sources of information about health, health care disparities, and key health indicators in children

         (a) Children's Defense Fund (2006): Mission—"To Leave No Child Behind and to ensure every child a Health Start, a Head Start, a Fair Start, a Safe Start, and a Moral Start in life and successful passage to adulthood with the help of caring families and communities"

         (b) Annie E. Casey Foundation (2006): Annual *KIDS COUNT Data Book* provides a state-by-state statistical portrait of the educational, health, and economic conditions of American children

         (c) Centers for Disease Control and Prevention, Office of Minority Health (2006)

            (1) With the goal of eliminating health disparities in six major areas by 2010, CDC has embarked on work that will result in:

               a) New knowledge about the causes of health disparities

               b) Enhanced disease prevention programs for all individuals

        c) Innovative methods of promoting health

        d) Delivery of culturally competent and linguistically specific preventive and clinical services

  ii. Learn important phrases in the languages most common in your practice (Leininger, 2001)

        (a) e.g., "How are you today? How can I help you? What is your child's name? What a sweet baby!"

        (b) These efforts are interpreted as a desire to connect, lower communication barriers, and invite trust

  iii. Develop knowledge about the culture, its worldview, and common beliefs and practices, e.g., *The Spirit Catches You and You Fall Down* (Fadiman, 1997).

  iv. Develop a relationship with someone from that culture to help interpret meanings and context

  d. Strategies that NPs can use to enhance competency in working with other disciplines who often have a culture, language, and beliefs of their own

    i. Engage in interdisciplinary role-playing or role reversals

    ii. Use media programs on interdisciplinary communication

    iii. Share critical incidents and discuss how each discipline handled it from its perspective

    iv. Clinic retreats with shared agendas

## COLLABORATION AND REFERRAL IN CLINICAL PRACTICE

1. The PNP is an integral part of the pediatric health care team
2. Most states require formal collaborative practice agreements that stipulate terms of agreement between PNPs and collaborators (see Box 2-1 for a sample collaborative agreement) (See also NAPNAP, 2005)
3. Collaboration means working together with other health care professionals to benefit the pediatric patient
4. Other members may be physicians, physician assistants, dietitians, nurses, social workers
5. The PNP refers pediatric patients who require services beyond the PNP's expertise or scope of practice to other specialists (e.g., MD, PT)

## TEACHING IN CLINICAL PRACTICE

1. Teaching staff and peers in the clinical setting is an important PNP role that enhances quality of care
2. A significant component of clinical practice is teaching parents how to care for their children and teaching children about choices for healthy lifestyles
3. People learn in many different ways, therefore PNPs should become familiar with various theories of teaching and learning (Boyd, 1998)
4. Assessment of the learner is an important component of teaching
   a. Learner's knowledge of the subject
   b. Previous experience with the subject
   c. Learner's preference for learning (e.g., visual, auditory, perceptual, demonstration-return demonstration, group learning)

■ **BOX 2-1**
■ **COLLABORATIVE PRACTICE AGREEMENT**

■ It is the intent of this document to authorize the nurse practitioner(s) at the _____ _____ clinic(s) to practice under these protocols without direct supervision, as specified in the Nurse (Medical) Practice Act, xx State Civil Statutes, Article xxx, section xx(d)(5) and (6). This document sets forth guidelines for collaboration between the supervising physician(s) and the nurse practitioner(s).

**DEVELOPMENT, REVISION, AND REVIEW**
■ By whom
■ How often revised
■ How often reviewed

**APPROVAL**
■ Annual approval
■ Signed by all parties listed in the agreement

**SETTING**
■ The nurse practitioners will operate under these protocols at the (Name of Institution) clinics listed below:
Clinic 1: (name and address)
Clinic 2: (name and address)

**SUPERVISION**
■ The nurse practitioners are authorized to practice under the protocols established in this document without the direct (onsite) supervision or approval of the supervising physicians. Consultation with the supervising physicians or their designated back-up, is available at all times, either on-site or by telephone when consultation is needed for any reason.

**CONSULTATION**
■ NPs will provide health promotion, screening, safety instructions, management of acute episodic illness, and stable chronic diseases
■ Referrals and consultations will be specifically noted on patient's medical record
■ Referrals will be made, as needed to other health care providers
■ Physician consultation will be sought for all of the following situations and any others deemed appropriate
  ■ Whenever situations arise that go beyond the intent of the protocols or the competence, scope of practice, or experience of the nurse practitioners
  ■ Whenever the patient's condition fails to respond to the management plan within an appropriate time frame, based on the provider's clinical judgment
  ■ For any uncommon, unfamiliar, or unstable patient condition
  ■ For any patient condition that does not fit the commonly accepted diagnostic pattern for a disease/condition
  ■ For any unexplained physical examination or historical finding or abnormal diagnostic finding
  ■ Whenever a patient requests
  ■ For all emergency situations after initial stabilizing care has been initiated

**MEDICAL RECORDS**
■ The nurse practitioners are responsible for the complete, **legible** documentation of all patient encounters using an xxx format.

**EDUCATION AND TRAINING**
■ The nurse practitioners must possess a valid (State) license as a Registered Nurse and be recognized by the (State) Board of Nursing (Medicine) as a Nurse Practitioner.

*Continued*

■ **BOX 2-1**
■ **COLLABORATIVE PRACTICE AGREEMENT—cont'd**

**EVALUATION OF CLINICAL CARE**
- A minimum of a monthly review by the supervising physicians of a minimum of 10% of patient charts (a written record of the review is to be kept)
- Annual evaluation by the supervising physicians based on written criteria
- Informal evaluation during consultations and case review

**PRACTICE GUIDELINES**
- The nurse practitioners are authorized to diagnose and treat common medical conditions under the following current guidelines (including, but not limited to):
  - [cite guidelines used in practice]
- and other published, accepted sources of medical information, as agreed upon by the collaborating parties and /or identified below:
  - OSHA guidelines
  - CDC guidelines for immunizations

**DRUG PRESCRIPTIONS**
- Cite source of authorization (state rules, regulations)
- Cite limitations of prescriptive privileges

**CITE ACCEPTED REFERENCES FOR PRESCRIPTIONS (E.G., *PHYSICIANS' DESK REFERENCE*, APPROVED FORMULARY**

**COLLABORATING PARTIES: STATEMENT OF APPROVAL**
- We, the undersigned, agree to the terms of this Collaborative Practice Agreement as set forth in this document.
  _____ Medical Director
  _____ Supervising Physician
  _____ Supervising Physician
  _____ Supervising Physician
  _____ Nurse Practitioner
  _____ Nurse Practitioner
  _____ Nurse Practitioner
Approval Date _____
Renewal Date _____
Renewal Date _____

**d.** Variables that influence learning
  **i.** Health status
  **ii.** Stress level
  **iii.** Ability to understand
  **iv.** Health values
  **v.** Learning environment
  **vi.** Relationship of the learner to the teacher
  **vii.** Affect and enthusiasm of the teacher
  **viii.** Organization and presentation of the material

# ETHICAL ISSUES IN CLINICAL PRACTICE

1. No easy answers to ethical concerns involving children in clinical practice (Fleischman & Collogan, 2004)
2. Develop an ethical decision framework
   a. Discuss the dilemma with all involved parties
   b. Determine the possible options
   c. Act on one option
   d. Evaluate the decision and process
3. The bioethical principles that assist in discussing ethical dilemmas include (American Nurses Association, 2002; Guido, 2006):
   a. Autonomy—the right to self-governance and moral independence
   b. Beneficence—doing good
   c. Nonmalfeasance—avoiding harm
   d. Veracity—truthfulness, accuracy
   e. Fidelity—faithfulness to an obligation, trust, or duty
   f. Justice—impartial, fair, conformity to truth, fact, or reason
   g. Respect for others regardless of age, sex, race, ethnic group, disease, etc.
4. Other bioethical perspectives
   a. Ethics of caring
   b. Feminist perspectives
   c. Deontologic theory—study of moral obligation
   d. Utilitarian arguments—"right" is what leads to the greatest good for the greatest number
5. Some common ethical concerns in pediatric primary care include:
   a. How "informed" are parents who sign informed consents?
      i. e.g., How much information is required before consenting to immunizations?
   b. Child assent
      i. Child's agreement to participate in the care
      ii. How old must a child be to provide assent?
      iii. Should assent be verbal, written, or both?
      iv. State laws may dictate the following limits:
         (a) Age that assent should be obtained (age 7 to 9 years, typically)
         (b) Age that a minor have a choice in the care
         (c) Age that a minor should *not* have a choice in the care
   c. Child consent
      i. Consent means child has a legal right to agree to participate in care
      ii. State laws may dictate the legal age of consent for children
      iii. Legal age of consent may also vary according to the services requested, e.g., family planning, STD treatment, pregnancy care, abortion, treatment for strep throat
      iv. Know the policies established at each health facility
   d. How much autonomy should the parents have in determining the health needs of the child?
   e. How much intervention should health professionals pursue in the conflict between the autonomy of the parents and the welfare of the child?
6. See NAPNAP (2004a) position statement on PNP's role in the protection of children involved in research studies

## OPPORTUNITIES FOR LEADERSHIP SKILLS AND PROFESSIONAL SERVICE

1. Seek committee positions in professional organizations and local agencies
   a. Boards of nursing, credentialing committees, certification boards
   b. Legal boards and institutional committees
   c. Collaborative professional organizations
   d. Health facility ethics committees and institutional review committees
2. Become involved in research activities in the health care setting
   a. NAPNAP (2004a) strongly supports practitioners' participation in research in order to develop the evidence for quality pediatric care, e.g.:
      i. Critically analyze the results of research studies on both direct pediatric care and health policy applicable to clinical practice (American Association of Colleges of Nursing (AACN, 1996, 2006)
      ii. Utilize research findings for the care of patients in the health care setting
      iii. Implement changes in practice based on research findings
      iv. Evaluate present care policies based on more recent research findings
      v. Identify clinical issues, problems and questions that need to be studied (AACN, 1996, 2006)
      vi. Collaborate with nurse researchers to generate studies on clinical issues, problems and concerns (AACN, 1996, 2006)
      vii. Participate as a member of the research team (AACN, 1996, 2006)
3. Volunteer to be a PNP student preceptor and mentor for new PNPs
4. Respond to requests in the community for health care presentations
5. Develop skill as a test writer for nursing boards in pediatrics and the advanced practice certification board
6. Advocate for children's access to care
   a. NAPNAP (2001a) "believes that primary health care services provide a way of ensuring a comprehensive array of support services to children and families and that all children need access to these services"
   b. NAPNAP (2002b) believes that all children should have a "health care home" where they can receive high quality comprehensive health care services by pediatric health care providers
   c. The PNP is qualified to coordinate this care, provide direct care, advocate for the child, and make appropriate referrals when needed (NAPNAP, 2002b)
   d. Your state, and every state in the nation, has a health insurance program for infants, children, and teens (Centers for Medicare and Medicaid Services-CMS, 2004; USHHS, 2006)
   e. State Children's Health Insurance Program (SCHIP) insurance is available to children in working families, including some immigrant families (CMS, 2006)
      i. For details, select your state at www.cms.hhs.gov/schip/statemap.asp
      ii. Or select your state on www.insurekidsnow.gov
      iii. Or make a free call to 1–877-KIDS-NOW (543–7669)
   f. For little or no cost, this insurance pays for doctor visits, prescription medicines, hospitalizations, and much more
   g. Eligibility
      i. The states have different eligibility rules, but in most states…
         (a) Children who do not currently have health insurance are likely to be eligible, even if parent is working
         (b) Children 18 years old and younger

(c) Children whose families earn up to $34,100 a year (for a family of four) are eligible

h. NAPNAP (2004d) supports the use of PNPs in school based health centers to eliminate access to care barriers for children by providing comprehensive primary care and linking these services with other community resources

## HEALTHCARE FACILITY ACCREDITATION REQUIREMENTS

1. Joint Commission on Accreditation of Healthcare Organizations (JCAHO, 2004)
   a. JCAHO is the performance measurement used by health care organizations to demonstrate accountability to the public
   b. Provides a comprehensive evaluation of the quality of care
   c. PNPs assist with the documentation required for JCAHO accreditation
2. Clinical Laboratory Improvement Amendments (CLIA, 2006)
   a. CLIA establishes quality standards for all laboratory testing to ensure the accuracy, reliability, and timeliness of patient test results (Centers for Medicare & Medicaid Services, 2003)
      i. A laboratory is defined as any facility that performs testing on specimens derived from humans for the purpose of providing information for the diagnosis, prevention, treatment of disease, or impairment or assessment of health
      ii. Regulations are based on the complexity of the test method
         (a) Waived (e.g., quick strep tests, urine dipsticks)
         (b) Moderate complexity (e.g., provider-performed microscopy)
         (c) High complexity (CBC, electrolyte assays)
   b. CLIA specifies quality standards for:
      i. Proficiency testing
      ii. Patient test management
      iii. Quality control
      iv. Personnel qualifications
      v. Quality assurance for laboratories performing moderate and/or high complexity tests
3. Occupational Safety and Health Administration (OSHA, 2006a)
   a. OSHA is a division of the U.S. Department of Labor
   b. Employers are required by law to provide a safe and healthy work environment and to protect the employee against job hazards
   c. OSHA's Occupational Exposure to Bloodborne Pathogen Standards are required policies for all health facilities to protect the health care worker from bloodborne pathogens (OSHA, 2006b)
4. Health Insurance Portability and Accountability Act (HIPAA)
   a. Implemented and enforced by the Department of Health and Human Services, Office for Civil Rights
      i. A set of national standards based on the Privacy Rule, i.e., Standards for Privacy of Individually Identifiable Health Information
      ii. Addresses the use and disclosure of individual's "protected health information"
   b. This regulation affects the PNP's practice by regulating:
      i. How patients are called into the examination room
      ii. Who may accompany a child to the facility
      iii. Who can receive information (without formal written consent) about a child

    iv. How information about a child is released
    v. How a medical record is stored
    vi. Where a child's medical record is located while a child is in the facility
5. National Committee on Quality Assurance (NCQA, 2006)
    a. A private nonprofit organization committed to the assessment of the quality of managed health care plans
    b. PNPs are important contributors to the quality of health care delivery
    c. NCQA accreditation goes to health plans that meet the following standards:
        i. Access to service
        ii. Qualified providers
        iii. Goals of the plan include staying healthy, getting better and living with illness
    d. Accreditation by NCQA is labeled:
        i. Excellent
        ii. Commendable
        iii. Accredited
        iv. Provisional
        v. Denied
    e. Once accredited, health care plans are required to report the following results:
        i. The Health Care Employer Data and Information Set (HEDIS) is a comprehensive set of standardized measures of all health plans' performance in such significant public health issues as cancer, heart disease, smoking, asthma, and diabetes
        ii. Consumer Assessment of Health Plans Survey (CAHPS) is a standardized survey of consumers' experiences that evaluates plan performance in area such as members' satisfaction, access to care, and claims processing

---

# REFERENCES

Abood, S., & Keepnews, D. (2000a). *Understanding payment for advanced practice nursing services, Volume 1: Medicare reimbursement.* Washington DC: American Nurses Publishing.

Abood, S., & Keepnews, D. (2000b). *Understanding payment for advanced practice nursing services, Volume 2: Fraud and abuse.* Washington DC: American Nurses Publishing.

Agency for Health Care Research and Quality. (2006a). Clinical practice guidelines, 1992–1996. Retrieved March 10, 2006, from www.ahrq.gov/clinic/cpgsix.htm.

Agency for Healthcare Research and Quality (2006b) Evidence-based practice centers. Retrieved March 10, 2006, from www.ahrq.gov/clinic/epc.

Agency for Healthcare Research and Quality. (2006c). Evidence report topics and technical reviews. Retrieved March 10, 2006, from www.ahrq.gov/clinic/epcix.htm.

Agency for Healthcare Research and Quality. (2006d). State and local policy makers. Retrieved March 10, 2006, from www.ahrq.gov/news/ulpix.htm.

American Academy of Pediatrics. (2006a). Clinical practice guidelines. Retrieved March 10, 2006, from http://aappolicy.aappublications.org./practice_guidelines/index.dtl.

American Academy of Pediatrics. (2006b). Policy statements. Retrieved March 10, 2006, from http://aappolicy.aappublications.org/policy_statement/index.dtl.

American Association of Colleges of Nursing (1996). *The essentials of master's education for advanced practice nursing.* Washington DC: American Association of Colleges of Nursing Publishing.

American Association of Colleges of Nursing. (2006). Position statement on nursing research. Retrieved April 20, 2006, from www.aacn.nche.edu/Publications/positions/rscposst.htm.

American Medical Association. (2006). *Current procedural terminology: CPT 2006: Professional edition*. Chicago: American Medical Association.

American Nurses Association. (1996). *Scope and standards of advanced practice registered nursing*. Washington DC: American Nurses Publishing.

American Nurses Association. (2002). *Code of ethics for nurses, with interpretive statements*. Washington DC: American Nurses Publishing.

American Nurses Association. (2006). Position statements. Retrieved March 10, 2006, from www.nursingworld.org/readroom/position.

American Nurses Credentialing Center. (2006). Homepage. Retrieved March 10, 2006, from www.nursingworld.org/ancc.

Annie E. Casey Foundation. (2006). Kids count. Retrieved March 10, 2006, from www.aecf.org/kidscount.

Association of Faculties of Pediatric Nurse Practitioner Programs (AFPNP). (1996). *Philosophy, conceptual model, terminal competencies for the education of pediatric nurse practitioners*. Cherry Hill, NJ: AFPNP/NAPNAP.

Bandolier Journal. (2006). Home page [Electronic journal]. Retrieved March 10, 2006, from www.jr2.ox.ac.uk/bandolier/aboutus.html

Boyd, M. D. (1998) *Health teaching in nursing practice: A professional model* (3rd ed.). Stamford, CT: Appleton Lange.

Boynton, R. W., Dunn, E. S, Stephens, G. R., & Pulcini, J. (2003). *Manual of ambulatory pediatrics* (5th ed.) Philadelphia: Lippincott Williams & Wilkins.

Burns, C.E., Brady, M. A., Dunn, A. M., et al. (2004). *Pediatric primary care: A handbook for nurse practitioners* (3rd ed.). Philadelphia: Elsevier Science.

Centers for Disease Control and Prevention. (2006). Office of Minority Health. *Reports and publications*. Retrieved March 10, 2006, from www.cdc.gov/omh/reportspubs.htm.

Centers for Medicare and Medicaid Services. (2003, January 24). Clinical laboratory improvement program. Retrieved March 10, 2006, from www.cms.hhs.gov/clia.

Centers for Medicare and Medicaid Services. (2006). State Children's Health Insurance Programs. Retrieved on March 10, 2006, from www.cms.hhs.gov/schip.

Children's Defense Fund. (2006). Mission of the Children's Defense Fund. Retrieved on March 10, 2006, from www.childrensdefense.org.

Clinical Laboratory Improvement Amendments. (2006). Home page. Retrieved on March 10, 2006 at http://www.phppo.cdc.gov/clia/default.aspx

[The] Cochrane Collaboration (2006). Cochrane reviews: abstracts and full-text access. Retrieved November 8, 2004, from www.cochrane.org/reviews/index.htm.

Department of Health and Human Services Office for Civil Rights (2006) HIPAA medical privacy—national standards to protect the privacy of personal health information. Retrieved on March 10, 2006, from www.hhs.gov/ocr/hipaa.

Drug Enforcement Agency. (2006a). *Drug registration applications*. Retrieved on March 10, 2006, from www.deadiversion.usdoj.gov/drugreg/index.html.

Drug Enforcement Agency. (2006b). Mid-level practitioners authorization by state. Retrieved on March 10, 2006, from www.deadiversion.usdoj.gov/drugreg/practioners/index.html.

Fadiman, A. (1997). *The spirit catches you and then you fall down*. New York: Farrar, Straus & Giroux.

Fleischman, A. R., & Collogan, L. K. (2004). Addressing ethical issues in everyday practice. *Pediatr Ann, 33*(11), 740-745.

Green-Hernandez, C., Quinn, A. A., Denman-Vitale, S., et al. (2004). Making primary care culturally competent. *Nurse Pract, 29*(6), 49-55.

Guido, G. W. (2006). *Legal and ethical issues in nursing*. (4th ed.). Upper Saddle River, NJ: Prentice Hall.

Joint Commission on Accreditation of Healthcare Organizations. (2006). How to become accredited. Retrieved on March 10, 2006, from www.jcaho.org/htba/index.htm.

Jones, D. (2002). Reimbursement, privileging and credentialing for pediatric nurse practitioner. Paper presented at the National Association of Pediatric Nurse Associates and Practitioners 23rd Annual Nursing Conference for Pediatric Primary Care, April 10–13, 2002, Reno, Nevada. Retrieved October 15, 2004, from www.medscape.com/viewarticle/433372.

Kaplan, L., & Brown, M-A. (2004). Prescriptive authority and barriers to practice. *Nurse Pract, 29*(3), 28-35.

Leininger, M. M. (2001). *Cultural care diversity and universality: A theory of nursing*. Sudbury, MA: Jones and Bartlett.

National Association of Pediatric Nurse Practitioners. (2000). *Continuing Education*. Retrieved January 6, 2006 from http://www.napnap.org/index.cfm?page=10&sec=54&ssec=61

National Association of Pediatric Nurse Practitioners. (2001a). *Access to care*. Retrieved January 6, 2006 from http://www.napnap.org/index.cfm?page=10&sec=54&ssec=55

National Association of Pediatric Nurse Practitioners. (2001b). *Certification*. Retrieved January 6, 2006 from http://www.napnap.org/index.cfm?page=10&sec=54&ssec=58

National Association of Pediatric Nurse Practitioners. (2002a). *Age parameters for pediatric nurse practitioner practice*. Retrieved January 6, 2006 from http://www.napnap.org/index.cfm?page=10&sec=54&ssec=170

National Association of Pediatric Nurse Practitioners. (2002b). *Pediatric health care home*. Retrieved January 6, 2006 from http://www.napnap.org/index.cfm?page=10&sec=54&ssec=68

National Association of Pediatric Nurse Practitioners. (2003a). *Credentialing and privileging for pediatric nurse practitioners*. Retrieved January 6, 2006 from http://www.napnap.org/index.cfm?page=10&sec=54&ssec=63

National Association of Pediatric Nurse Practitioners. (2003b). *PNP prescriptive privilege*. Retrieved January 6, 2006 from http://www.napnap.org/Docs/pos_prescriptive.pdf

National Association of Pediatric Nurse Practitioners. (2004a). *Protection of children involved in research studies*. Retrieved January 6, 2006 from http://www.napnap.org/Docs/pos-child-research.pdf

National Association of Pediatric Nurse Practitioners (2004b). *Reimbursement for nurse practitioner services*. Retrieved January 6, 2006 from http://www.napnap.org/Docs/ps-reimbursement.pdf

National Association of Pediatric Nurse Practitioners (2004c). *Scope and standards of practice: Pediatric nurse practitioner (PNP)*. Retrieved January 6, 2006 from http://www.napnap.org/Docs/FinalScope2–25.pdf

National Association of Pediatric Nurse Practitioners (2004d). *School-based and school-linked centers*. Retrieved January 6, 2006 from http://www.napnap.org/index.cfm? page=10& sec=54&ssec=74

National Association of Pediatric Nurse Practitioners. (2005). *Nurse practitioner career resource guide*. Retrieved on January 6, 2006 http://www.napnap.org/index.cfm?page=10&sec=463

National Association of Pediatric Nurse Practitioners. (2006a). Home page. Retrieved January 8, 2006 from http://www.napnap.org

National Association of Pediatric Nurse Practitioners. (2006b). *Position statements*. Retrieved January 8, 2006 from http://www.napnap.org/practice/positions/

National Association of Pediatric Nurse Practitioners (2006c). *Practice Issues: Frequently Asked Questions*. Retrieved January 6, 2006 from http://www.napnap.org/index.cfm?page=10&sec=390

National Center for Health Statistics. (2005). International classification of diseases, 9th revision, clinical modification (ICD-9-CM) (6th ed.). Retrieved March 10, 2006, from www.cdc.gov/nchs/about/otheract/icd9/abticd9.htm

National Committee for Quality Assurance. (2006). NCQA programs. Retrieved March 10, 2006, from www.ncqa.org/ index.htm.

National Council of State Boards of Nursing. (2006). Nurse Licensure Compact: Advanced Practice Model Legislative Language. Retrieved on March 10, 2006 from www.ncsbn.org/nlc/aprncompact.asp.

National Organization of Nurse Practitioner Faculties (NONPF). (2000). *Cultural guidelines. Washington, DC: NONPF*.

National Organization of Nurse Practitioner Faculties (NONPF). (2006). Sample collaborative agreement. Retrieved March 10, 2006, from www.nonpf.com/fpcollabagreesample.htm.

Occupational Safety and Health Administration (OSHA). (2006). Bloodborne pathogens and needlestick prevention. Retrieved March 10, 2006, from www.osha.gov/SLTC/bloodbornepathogens/index.html.

Pearson, L. J. (2006a) A national overview of nurse practitioner legislation and health-care issues. *Amer J Nurse Pract, 10*(1), 15-84.

Pearson, L. J. (2006b) A national overview of nurse practitioner legislation and health-care issues. *Amer J Nurse Pract, 10*(2), 13-84.

Pediatric Nursing Certification Board (PNCB). (2006). Retrieved March 10, 2006, from www.pncb.org/ptistore/control/index.

Phillips, S. J. (2006). Eighteenth annual legislative update. *Nurse Pract, 31*(1), 6-38.

Sackett, D. L., Rosenberg, W. M. C., Muir, J. A., et al. (1996). Evidence based medicine: What it is and what it isn't. *BMJ, 312,* 71-72.

United States Department of Health and Human Services (HHS). 2006. Insure kids now! Linking the nation's children to health insurance. Retrieved March 10, 2006, from www.insurekidsnow.gov.

# Clinical Reasoning and Clinical Decision Making

MARIANNE BUZBY, RN, MSN, CRNP

## OVERVIEW

1. Clinical reasoning by advanced practice nurses is a complex cognitive process that involves critical thinking about and synthesis of previous knowledge, advanced knowledge, and advanced clinical experience leading to a clinical decision
2. Clinical decision making is learned through a variety of teaching and learning methods
3. Components of the clinical decision making process (Box 3-1)

## CRITICAL THINKING

1. Definition of critical thinking
   a. Dynamic creative process and a skill that can be learned
   b. The foundation of advanced practice nursing (Barnsteiner et al., 1993)
   c. An experiential, cognitive and affective process that combines the art of reason and logic with reflection, feeling, and values in order to challenge assumptions, acknowledge the unknown or unexpected, and make decisions based on sound rationale that lead to action (Thompson, Kershbaumer, & Krisman-Scott, 2001)
2. Cognitive dimension
   a. Allows nurses to reason and make clinical judgments about patients in their care
   b. The rational investigation of ideas, inferences, assumptions, principles, arguments, conclusions, issues, beliefs, and actions
   c. The cognitive component of nursing process (assess, plan, implement, evaluate) and the scientific method (observe, group data, draw logical conclusions, form and test hypotheses)
   d. Entails purposeful, outcomes-directed thinking; is driven by patient, family, and community needs (Alfaro-LeFevre, 2004)
   e. Guided by professional standards and code of ethics
   f. Requires strategies that make the most of human potential and compensate for problems created by human nature (Alfaro-LeFevre, 2004)
   g. Is constantly reevaluating, self-correcting, and striving to improve (Alfaro-LeFevre, 2004)

■ **BOX 3-1**
■ **CLINICAL REASONING: CRITICAL THINKING IN THE CLINICAL SETTING**

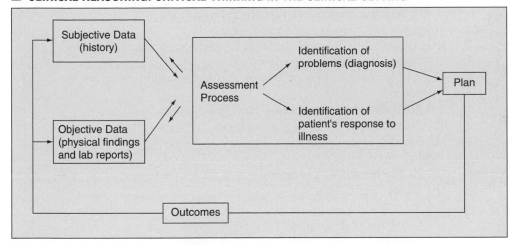

Adapted with permission from Bickley & Szilagyi, 2003

3. Affective dimension
   a. Critical thinking requires a strong affective dimension
   b. Critical reflection is a critical examination of one's own practice and under-standing of the situation
   c. Requires willingness to think and be responsible for the outcomes of that think-ing (Thompson et al., 2001))
   d. Affective attitudes of critical thinking include intellectual humility, intellectual courage, intellectual empathy, intellectual integrity, intellectual perseverance, faith in reason, intellectual sense of justice
   e. Tools for reflection (Logsdon & Merkt, 2000)
      i. Time
      ii. Motivation to learn
      iii. Probing questions and an expert to facilitate discussion
      iv. Practice
4. *Clinical reasoning* is critical thinking in clinical situations (Alfaro-LeFevre, 2004)
   a. Dexter and colleagues (1997) developed operational definitions of the cognitive skills required for clinical reasoning
      i. Interpretation
         (a) Understand
         (b) Comprehend or decipher written materials
         (c) Identify nursing problems
         (d) Identify themes
         (e) Avoid reading into data
         (f) Recognize
         (g) Consider alternative explanations
      ii. Analysis
         (a) Prioritize
         (b) Identify implications and possible consequences
         (c) Examine ideas
         (d) Identify and analyze arguments
         (e) Problem solve

      iii. Evaluation
         (a) Assess claims and arguments
         (b) Assess the credibility of information sources
         (c) Assess the strength of conclusions
         (d) Assess relevance and significance of information and rationales
         (e) Assess bias and stereotypes
         (f) Apply criteria appropriately in a given situation
      iv. Inference
         (a) Formulate hypotheses and draw conclusions
         (b) Demonstrate the principles of logic
         (c) Identify knowledge gaps
      v. Explanation
         (a) Justify reasoning processes
         (b) Make conclusions
      vi. Self-regulation
         (a) Continually question one's own thinking
         (b) Reconsider interpretation and judgments
         (c) Examine the influence of personal biases
         (d) Demonstrate the attributes of a critical thinker

5. Attributes of critical thinkers (Alfaro-LeFevre, 2004)
    a. Self-aware
    b. Genuine
    c. Self-disciplined
    d. Autonomous and responsible
    e. Careful and prudent
    f. Confident and resilient
    g. Honest and upright
    h. Curious and inquisitive
    i. Truth seeking
    j. Alert to context
    k. Analytic and insightful
    l. Logical and systematic
    m. Intuitive
    n. Open and fair-minded
    o. Mature
    p. Sensitive to diversity
    q. Creative
    r. Realistic and self-corrective
    s. Proactive
    t. Courageous
    u. Patient and persistent
    v. Flexible
    w. Empathic
    x. Improvement-oriented (self, patients, systems)
6. Strategies to promote critical thinking (Alfaro-LeFevre, 2004)
    a. Awareness of personal style
      i. Learning style preference (visual, auditory, interactive)
      ii. Thinking style (e.g., Myers-Briggs Type Inventory, available at http://www.myersbriggs.org/)
      iii. Cultural influences

    **b.** Example: Covey's *7 Habits of Highly Effective People*
    **c.** Expand theoretical, empirical, and experiential knowledge
    **d.** Develop interpersonal skills
    **e.** Practice technical skills

## CLINICAL DECISION MAKING

**1.** Phases of clinical decision making
    **a.** Collection and analysis of situation-specific data relevant to the issue
    **b.** Consideration of alternative approaches and the consequences of each approach
    **c.** Make the best decision
**2.** Approaches to clinical decision making (Burman et al., 2002; Steiner & Burman, 2000)
    **a.** Hypothetico-deductive: propose hypotheses, then test them against the data
    **b.** Schematic
        **i.** Pattern recognition and matching
        **ii.** Data clustering
        **iii.** Search for red flags
    **c.** An iterative and spiral process
    **d.** Arborization—branching out of thought processes; can be diagrammed
**3.** Components of clinical decision making (Webber, 2000)
    **a.** Knowledge—discipline-specific knowledge
        **i.** What you know
            (a) Not all knowledge can be obtained through clinical experience
            (b) Less common conditions may not present themselves
            (c) "Book knowledge" is essential
            (d) If you don't *know* about a particular diagnosis, you will not recognize it, diagnose it or properly treat it
        **ii.** What you understand
        **iii.** How you apply it in clinical situations
    **b.** Skills
        **i.** Types
            (a) Intellectual
            (b) Psychomotor
            (c) Interpersonal
        **ii.** Integration of skills into practice involves transition of discipline specific knowledge, values, meanings, and experiences into intentional acts and activities
        **iii.** Experiential knowledge is learned over time
        **iv.** The clinical situation significantly influences clinical reasoning and critical thinking abilities (Benner 1984, 1994; Lipman & Deatrick, 1997)
    **c.** Values that establish moral boundaries of right and wrong
        **i.** Beliefs
        **ii.** Attributes
        **iii.** Virtues
        **iv.** Ideals
    **d.** Meanings
        **i.** Expanded meaning of words that exist in the nursing profession based on:
            (a) Knowledge
            (b) Skills

(c) Values

(d) Experiences—active process of integrating knowledge, skills, values, and meaning used in clinical reasoning in clinical situations over time

    ii. Challenge is to incorporate these meanings into advanced nursing practice

4. Cognitive skills involved in clinical decision making (Alfaro-LeFevre, 2004; Flagler, 2000)

    a. Searching—what is known and what needs to be known

        i. Use references to enhance experiential knowledge

        ii. Follow policies, procedures, and standards of care and learn the reasoning that supports them

        iii. Understand the rationale for and the risks of procedures before performing them

        iv. Use appropriate evidence-based guidelines (e.g., AHRQ, AAP, NAPNAP, CDC, Cochrane Database)

        v. Aim of evidence-based practice is to integrate clinical experience with the best available research evidence in order to make the best decisions in conjunction with patients and their families (Logan & Gilbert, 2000; Melnyk & Fineout-Overholt, 2004)

        (a) Evidence is basis for logical thinking

        (b) Needed to support opinions and recommendations for care

        (c) Outcome-focused, data-driven, evidence-based care is key to critical thinking (Alfaro-LeFevre, 2004)

    b. Recalling—accessing long-term memory, clinical resources, and history, physical and lab data to guide searching and to develop the plan of care

    c. Judging value—determining the relevance of data from patient and efficacy of diagnostic tests or treatment plans

        i. Levels of data—primary, secondary, tertiary

        ii. Sensitivity, specificity, predictive value

    d. Assessing the patient

        i. Apply the nursing process to make comprehensive patient assessments and make judgments based on evidence

        ii. Develop a systematic and comprehensive approach to patient assessment

        iii. Learn to prioritize what needs to be done

        iv. Recognize relationships and patterns—cognitive connection between different aspects of the situation

        v. Do the data collected match diagnostic patterns from textbooks or clinical variations observed in practice?

        vi. Collaborate with more experienced nurses and health care professionals

        vii. Practice with new technology before using it in patient care

        viii. Focus on patient-centered care

        ix. Allow time for direct and indirect patient care activities

        x. Challenge your reasoning with "what if" questions

    e. Evaluating cost versus benefit to decide if more data need to be collected

        i. Costs include time, risk, discomfort, and money

        ii. Consider diagnostic certainty

        iii. Consider utility—consequences of missed diagnosis and availability of effective treatment

    f. Prioritizing

        i. Identifying the order of importance of possible diagnoses

        ii. Also need to prioritize pertinent data to efficiently focus history and physical examination

    **g.** Sorting—strategies for organizing data
        **i.** Normal versus abnormal
        **ii.** Body system
        **iii.** Pathologic process
        **iv.** Sorting data to match up with hypotheses
    **h.** Hypothesizing—generating plausible explanations for what is going on with the patient
        **i.** Differential diagnosis—several possible explanations
            (a) Limiting the possible explanations to the 3 to 5 most likely diagnoses; helps with structure for what data need to be collected
            (b) Consider probability of the diagnosis and prevalence of the diagnosis
                (1) Common conditions occur commonly, and rare conditions occur rarely
                (2) Therefore, "If you hear hoof beats in the street, don't look for zebras"
            (c) However, there are 4 reasons why practitioners must be aware of rare conditions (McKusick, 1967):
                (1) Rare disorders can teach us much about the normal or about more common disorders
                (2) Rare manifestations are sometimes valuable clues to the existence of grave internal disease
                (3) People have them
                (4) They are a break in the routine and "keep [the practitioner's] powers of observation from undergoing atrophy"
            (d) Consider the consequences of a missed diagnosis
        **ii.** Drawing conclusions involves hypothesizing, recalling, sorting and matching to patterns
    **i.** Using intuition
        **i.** "Knowing" without evidence
        **ii.** Guides search for evidence
        **iii.** Based on depth of experiential knowledge
        **iv.** Blended with logical thinking, it is typically evident in expert nurses' thinking
    **j.** Reflecting—thinking about your thinking
  **5.** Attributes of good decision makers (Thompson et al., 2001)
    **a.** Personal attributes
        **i.** Common sense
        **ii.** Humility
        **iii.** Human sensitivity
        **iv.** Pervasive calmness
        **v.** Willingness to make decisions
        **vi.** Accountability for the outcomes
    **b.** Essential knowledge
        **i.** Knowledge of self
        **ii.** Access to pertinent information
        **iii.** Understanding the health condition
        **iv.** Professional knowledge
        **v.** Knowing what you know and what you don't know
    **c.** Environmental attributes
        **i.** Time
        **ii.** Mutual trust
        **iii.** Commitment to maintaining patient confidentiality

        **iv.** Supportive environment for mistakes

        **v.** Clear boundaries of safety

**6.** Challenges to clinical reasoning and clinical decision making

  **a.** Limitations

      **i.** Novice to expert phenomenon (Benner, 1984, 1994)

        **(a)** The practice of a novice nurse practitioner (NP) is guided primarily by theoretical scientific evidence until the NP is comfortable with integrating experiential knowledge into decision making (Alfaro-LeFevre, 2004; Webber, 2000)

        **(b)** Linear thinking—characteristic of new nurse practitioners; identifies primary concepts and unidirectional conceptual relationships (Webber, 2000)

      **ii.** Personal unwillingness to think and to reflect on thinking before taking action

      **iii.** Time (emergency situations)

  **b.** Risks

      **i.** Time it takes to think and decide

      **ii.** Emotional investment in understanding self and others

      **iii.** Willingness to listen to alternative approaches

      **iv.** Decision may be unpopular

## OUTCOMES OF CLINICAL DECISION MAKING

**1.** Working diagnosis

  **a.** Diagnoses are not always crystal clear

  **b.** Evaluate your level of certainty with which each diagnosis is made

  **c.** Evaluate the outcome of your treatment based on the diagnosis

**2.** Treatment trials

  **a.** A treatment is based on a working diagnosis, then evaluated for effectiveness

  **b.** If ineffective, a new working diagnosis and new treatment is recommended

**3.** DATA, DATA, DATA

  **a.** Practitioners should keep spreadsheets of data from their practice, including:

      **i.** Time required for a visit

      **ii.** Diagnostic tests conducted or ordered

      **iii.** Treatments instituted in the office

      **iv.** Diagnoses made

        **(a)** Use CPT Codes

        **(b)** Code level of diagnostic certainty, e.g., 1 to 10

      **v.** Treatments recommended

      **vi.** Effectiveness or failure of the treatment

      **vii.** Changes in diagnoses and treatment and evaluation of these changes

  **b.** Analysis of these data provide objective evidence about:

      **i.** The quality of one's practice

      **ii.** Contributions of one's practice to the agency or group

      **iii.** Changes over time in the quality of one's diagnostic and treatment skill

## METHODS OF TEACHING CRITICAL THINKING AND CLINICAL DECISION MAKING

**1.** Modeling

  **a.** Faculty

  **b.** Preceptors (Myrick & Yonge, 2002)

2. Guided imagery—promotes reflection; illustrates the affective dimensions or traits of critical thinking (Thompson et al., 2001)
3. Case studies
    a. Most effective when students are encouraged to consider alternate solutions and go beyond the obvious (Thompson et al., 2001)
    b. Should be brief, provide progressive steps in thinking through the problem, center on real problems, and provide clear directions that focus on the objective of the assignment
    c. Allows students to link new knowledge to previous knowledge and relate that to clinical experiences, which enhances the learning (DeToma, 2000; Dumas, 2000; & Lee and Ryan-Wenger, 2000)
    d. Types of case studies—problem based, inquiry based, clinical reasoning
4. Guided questioning: "Think Aloud" (Abegglen & Conger, 1997; Lee & Ryan-Wenger, 2000)
    a. In case presentations, students ask questions about the case and state their rationale for asking the questions, i.e., what were they thinking?
    b. Provides opportunity for a variety of management options to be discussed and supported using different rationales
    c. Most effective technique to foster critical thinking is questions that guide students to think about issues and solutions in different ways
    d. The students' thought processes are demonstrated in the discussion
5. Written assignments
    a. Log of self-reflection (Logsdon & Merkt, 2000)
    b. Student portfolio
    c. Written case analyses
    d. Think Aloud written case studies (Lee & Ryan-Wenger, 2000)
6. Socratic method (Thompson et al., 2001)
    a. Teaching by asking questions of the learner
    b. Fosters thinking, reflection, risk taking, decision making
7. Debate (Candela, Michael, & Mitchell, 2003)
    a. Promotes organizing and applying evidence-based research to development and support of a stance on a particular issue
    b. A variation is to have students support one side of an issue, then switch and support the other side
8. "Puzzle patients"—use of a child's puzzle to illustrate critical thinking skills in assessment process (Rosner, 2002)
9. Concept mapping (King & Shell, 2002)
    a. Visual representation of thinking
    b. Assessment data are grouped in diagram format and relationships between the data are drawn with arrows and other symbols
    c. Faculty-guided discussion enhances understanding of relationship between data groups and promotes clinical judgment
10. Seminar (Gray, 2003)
    a. Specific roles assigned to each student: leader, participant, evaluator
    b. Each role has specific responsibilities that foster reflective thinking beyond the clinical content presented in the discussion
11. Web-based modules (Bonnel, 2000)
    a. Accommodate different learning styles
    b. Engage students in the content
    c. Types of activities
        i. Case study
        ii. Quiz

      iii. Application exercises

      iv. Website reviews

12. Grand rounds (Lee & Ryan-Wenger, 2000)
    a. Formal forum for discussion of clinical and professional issues
    b. May promote interdisciplinary communication about alternate approaches to care

13. Apprenticeship (Lee & Ryan-Wenger, 2000; Myrick & Yonge, 2002)
    a. Opportunity for experiential learning
    b. Students use preceptors as models to compare their clinical decision making

14. Algorithms and practice guidelines (Alfaro-LeFevre, 20004; Cabana et al., 2001; Lee & Ryan-Wenger, 2000)
    a. Guide the practitioner through the assessment process toward a diagnosis and sometimes, treatment decisions
    b. Purpose is to improve quality of care, not replace clinical judgment and the individual nuances of a patient
    c. Most are based on a review of the literature; however, when evidence does not exist, the recommendations of expert professionals in the specific area are used

15. Computer-based simulations (Lee & Ryan-Wenger, 2000)
    a. Allows all students to have access to the same "patient" experience
    b. Provides a safe environment to consider alternative solutions and risk making mistakes

16. Standardized patients (Lee & Ryan-Wenger, 2000)
    a. Trained "actors" simulate the history associated with specific health conditions.
    b. Provides some of the same benefits as computer-based simulations, but better simulates the clinical setting

---

## REFERENCES

Abegglen, J., & Conger, C. O. (1997). Critical thinking in nursing: Classroom tactics that work. *J Nurs Educ, 36*(10), 452-458.

Alfaro-LeFevre, R. (2004). *Critical thinking and clinical judgment: A practical approach* (3rd ed.). St. Louis: Saunders.

Barnsteiner, J., Deatrick, J., Grey, M., et al. (1993). Future of pediatric advanced nursing practice. *Pediatr Nurs, 19*(2), 196-197.

Benner, P. (1984). *From novice to expert.* Menlo Park, CA: Addison-Wesley. (Reprinted in 2001)

Benner, P. (1994). The role of articulation in understanding practice and experience as sources of knowledge in clinical nursing. In J. Tully, & D. M. Weinstock, Eds., *Philosophy in an age of pluralism: the philosophy of Charles Taylor in question.* Cambridge, NY: Cambridge University Press.

Bickley, L.S., & Szilagyi, P. G. (Eds.) (2003). *Bates' guide to physical assessment and history taking* (8th ed.). Philadelphia: J. B. Lippincott.

Bonnel, W. B. (2000). Adding the detail for clinical decision making: Web-based modules as classroom adjunct. In M. K. Crabtree (Ed.). *Teaching clinical decision making in advanced practice nursing* (pp. 75-81). Washington, DC: NONPF.

Burman, M. E., Stepans, M. B., Jansa, N., & Steiner, S. (2002). How do NPs make clinical decisions? *Nurse Pract, 27*(5), 59-64.

Cabana, M. D., Medzihradsky, O. F., Rubin, H. R., & Freed, G. L. (2001). Applying clinical guidelines to pediatric practice. *Pediatr Ann, 30*(5), 274-282.

Candela, L., Michael, S. R., & Mitchell, S. (2003). Ethical debates: Enhancing critical thinking in nursing students. *Nurse Educ, 28*(1), 37-39.

DeToma, H. R. (2000). Clinical decision making: A student perspective on problem-based learning. In M. K. Crabtree (Ed.). *Teaching clinical decision making in advanced practice nursing* (pp. 91-96). Washington, DC: NONPF.

Dexter, P., Applegate, M., Backer, J., et al. (1997). A proposed framework for teaching and evaluating critical thinking in nursing. *J Prof Nurs, 13*(3), 160-167.

Dumas, M. A. (2000). Problem based learning: Using case studies and elaboration to teach clinical decision making. In M. K. Crabtree (Ed.). *Teaching clinical decision making in advanced practice nursing* (pp. 97-119). Washington, DC: NONPF.

Flagler, S. (2000). Recognizing the thinking processes behind clinical decision making. In M. K. Crabtree (Ed.). *Teaching clinical decision making in advanced practice nursing* (pp. 7-16). Washington, DC: NONPF.

Gray, M. T. (2003). Beyond content: Generating critical thinking in the classroom. *Nurse Educ, 28*(3), 136-140.

King, M., & Shell, R. (2002). Critical thinking strategies: Teaching and evaluating critical thinking with concept maps. *Nurse Educ, 27*(5), 214-216.

Lee, J. E. & Ryan-Wenger, N. (2000). Standard methods of teaching clinical decision making: Strengths, limitations, and enhancements. In M. K. Crabtree (Ed.). *Teaching clinical decision making in advanced practice nursing* (pp. 47-54). Washington, DC: NONPF.

Lipman, T. H., & Deatrick, J. A. (1997). Preparing advanced practice nurses for clinical decision making in specialty practice. *Nurse Educ, 22*(2), 47-50.

Logan, S. & Gilbert, R. (2000). Framing questions. In V. A. Moyer, E. J. Elliott, R. L.

Logsdon, M. C., & Merkt, J. T. (2000). Reflection: An aid to clinical decision making. In M. K. Crabtree (Ed.). *Teaching clinical decision making in advanced practice nursing* (pp. 83-89). Washington, DC: NONPF.

Melnyk, B. M., & Fineout-Overholt, E. (2004). Evidence-based practice in nursing and healthcare. Philadelphia: Lippincott, Williams & Wilkins.

McKusick, K.A. (1967). Foreword. In W.B. Bean, *Rare diseases and lesions: Their contributions to clinical medicine.* Springfield, IL: Thomas. Editor's note: a rare book in itself, but the message is important.

Myrick, F., & Yonge, O. (2002). Preceptor behaviors integral to the promotion of student critical thinking. *J Nurs Staff Dev, 18*(3), 127-135.

Rosner, A. M. (2002). Teaching tools: "Puzzle patients" and critical thinking. *Nurse Educ, 27*(4), 155-156.

Steiner, S. H., & Burman, M. E. (2000). Integrating clinical decision making and advanced assessment. In M. K. Crabtree (Ed.). *Teaching clinical decision making in advanced practice nursing* (pp. 55-67). Washington, DC: NONPF.

Thompson, J. E., Kershbaumer, R. M., & Krisman-Scott, M. A. (2001). *Educating advanced practice nurses and midwives: From practice to teaching.* New York: Springer.

Webber, P. B. (2000). Clinical decision making: Components, processes, and outcomes. In M. K. Crabtree (Ed.). *Teaching clinical decision making in advanced practice nursing* (pp. 17-25). Washington, DC: NONPF.

# Health Assessment and Physical Examination

# Measures of Child Growth and Development

THERESA SKYBO, PhD, RN, CPNP

## PHYSICAL GROWTH

1. Growth charts
   a. Standardization of growth charts (CDC, 2006d)
      i. Charts can be downloaded at www.cdc.gov/growthcharts
      ii. Revised to extend growth percentiles to age 20; also reflect secular changes (CDC, 2002; Roberts & Dallal, 2001)
      iii. Data for revised charts derived from both formula- and breast-fed infants
      iv. Growth percentiles range from 3 to 97% for age and gender
      v. Desirable weight, height, head circumference for age and gender is more than 5% and less than 95%
      vi. Greater than 85% indicates at risk for nutritional problems (CDC, 2006d)
   b. Selection of growth charts (CDC, 2006d)
      i. Growth charts are selected considering:
         (a) Gender
         (b) Age
            (1) Birth to 2 years
            (2) 2 to 20 years
      ii. Growth parameter percentile is determined by the intersection of the child's age and:
         (a) Weight
         (b) Height
         (c) Head circumference
         (d) Body mass index (BMI)
      iii. See Figure 4-1 for example of girls' stature-for-age and weight-for-age percentiles
      iv. Plot measurements according to the premature infant's *corrected* age until 2 years of age; i.e., the age of an infant from birth, minus the number of weeks premature (CDC, 2006e)
      v. For infants weighing less than 1000 g at birth, corrected age is used until 3 years of age
      vi. If the premature infant's growth catches up before 3 years of age, chronologic age is used instead of the corrected age (Maternal and Child Health Bureau, 2006)

## CDC Growth Charts: United States

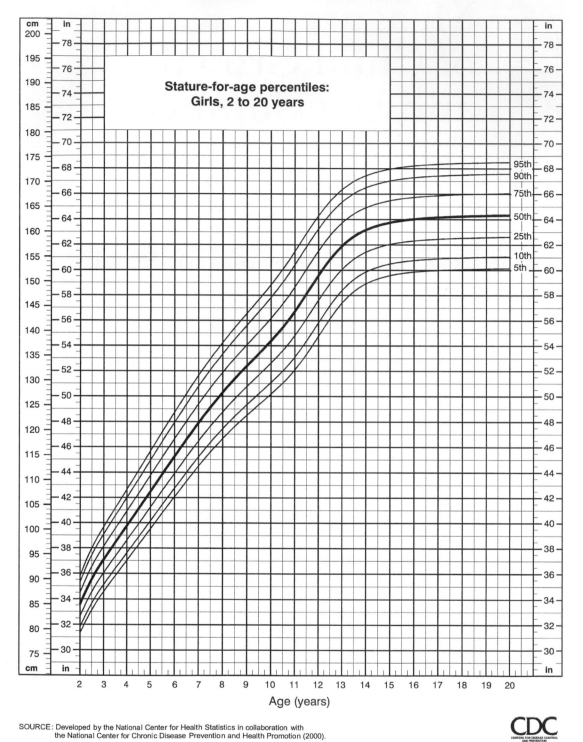

SOURCE: Developed by the National Center for Health Statistics in collaboration with
the National Center for Chronic Disease Prevention and Health Promotion (2000).

**CDC**
CENTERS FOR DISEASE CONTROL
AND PREVENTION

FIGURE 4-1 ■ Two to 20 years: Girls stature-for-age and weight-for-age percentiles. (From Centers for Disease Control and Prevention, www.cdc.gov/growthcharts.)

**CDC Growth Charts: United States**

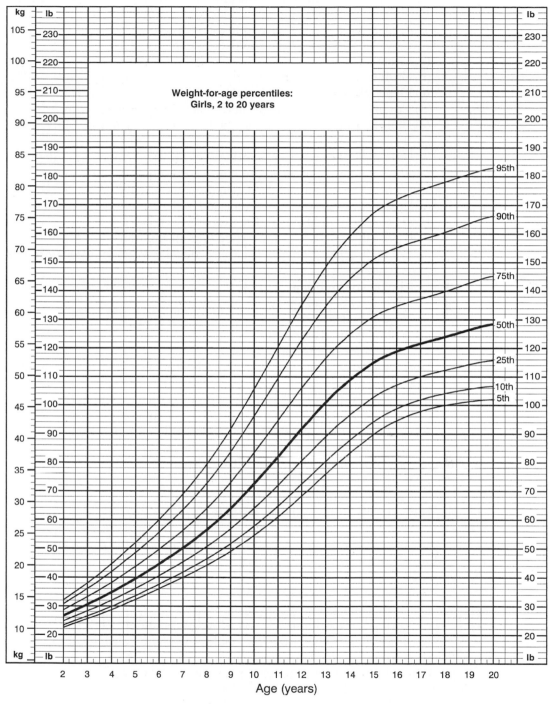

Weight-for-age percentiles:
Girls, 2 to 20 years

Age (years)

SOURCE: Developed by the National Center for Health Statistics in collaboration with the National Center for Chronic Disease Prevention and Health Promotion (2000).

CDC
CENTERS FOR DISEASE CONTROL
AND PREVENTION

FIGURE 4-1 ■ (*Continued*)

  **c.** Accuracy of the growth charts
   **i.** One measurement plotted on the growth chart may be used to screen for children at risk for nutritional problems
   **ii.** Serial measurements are needed to establish growth patterns or to evaluate growth patterns that are affected by such factors as:
    (a) Gestational age
    (b) Birth weight
    (c) Genetic influence and genetic disorders
    (d) Environmental influences—nutrients, socioeconomic status
    (e) Biologic influences—disease, medications, impaired mobility (CDC, 2006e)
   **iii.** Typically, infants gain more weight between birth and 7 months than between 7 and 12 months. A single measurement between birth and 7 months may falsely indicate excessive weight gain (Roberts & Dallal, 2001)
   **iv.** Adolescent growth spurt is not reflected in the growth charts because this spurt is an individual experience (Roberts & Dallal, 2001)
   **v.** CDC growth charts are recommended for all children
    (a) Some clinicians prefer to use charts developed for children with special needs
     (1) Down syndrome
     (2) Turner's syndrome
     (3) Achondroplasia
     (4) Prader-Willi syndrome
     (5) Marfan syndrome
   **vi.** Limitations of special needs charts (Maternal & Child Health Bureau, 2006)
    (a) Developed from small samples with unknown nutritional status
    (b) Do not reflect racial, ethnic, or geographic diversity
    (c) Secondary medical conditions, which influence growth, are not considered in the development of these charts
  **d.** Components of accurate measuring (CDC, 2006a)
   **i.** Technique—standardized
   **ii.** Equipment—calibrated, accurate
   **iii.** Trained measurers—reliable, accurate
**2.** Weight
 **a.** Weight is the force exerted on a body by the gravity of the earth; an indirect measure of body mass
 **b.** Types of scales
  **i.** Beam-balanced or electronic scales
   (a) Infant table scale (2 years of age and less)
   (b) Upright/platform scale (3 years of age and older)
   (c) Practitioner's choice of either table or upright scale (ages 2 to 3 years)
  **ii.** Sling scale
  **iii.** Wheelchair/chair scale for children with special needs
 **c.** Measurement technique (CDC, 2006a; 2006c)
  **i.** Balance the scale before use by verifying that the beam balances or that the electronic scale is set at zero
  **ii.** Ideally, weigh the child before feeding (breakfast)
  **iii.** Weigh the child at the same time each day with the same amount of clothing on child (Zemel, Riley, & Stallings, 1997)
  **iv.** Infants should be weighed nude or with a clean diaper, taking the weight of the diaper into account (CDC, 2006a; Zemel et al., 1997)

    **v.** Toddlers to 5 years are weighed wearing only a clean diaper or underwear (CDC, 2006a; Engel, 1997)

    **vi.** Older children (more than 5 years) should be weighed without heavy clothing or shoes

    **vii.** Infants weighed supine or sitting on table scale

    **viii.** Older children's feet are placed together in the center of the platform of an upright scale

    **ix.** Safety considerations—nurse should place a hand near infant or child to prevent falling off the scale

    **x.** Movement will interfere with the accuracy

    **xi.** Uncooperative children or children who cannot stand can be held by the parent and weighed. To obtain the child's weight, subtract the weight of the parent from the weight of the parent and child (CDC, 2006e)

    **xii.** Read the measurement to the nearest quarter pound (CDC, 2006a)

**3.** Recumbent length

    **a.** Recumbent length, a measure of child's length lying down, is used for children Younger Than 2 Years Of Age (CDC, 2006a, 2006c; Goldbloom, 2003; Zemel et al., 1997)

    **b.** Measurement technique

        **i.** Use a measuring board for recumbent length and for children unable to stand (Maternal and Child Health, 2006)

            (a) Place the child's head at the top of the measuring board

            (b) Fully extend the child's body

            (c) Hold the child's head midline and fully extend the legs against the back of the measuring board

            (d) Feet are perpendicular to the horizontal footboard

            (e) Length is measured from the tape measure that is mounted on the base of the measuring board (CDC, 2006) (Figure 4-2)

            (f) Measure to the nearest ⅛ inch

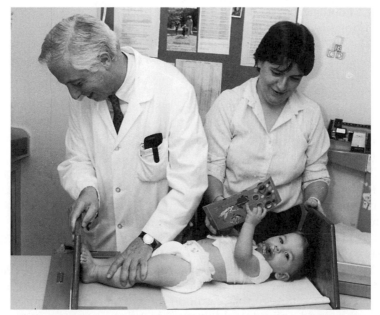

FIGURE 4-2 ■ Measuring recumbent length. (From Goldbloom, R. [1997]. *Pediatric clinical skills* (2nd ed.). New York: Churchill Livingstone.)

  **c.** Common, but inaccurate, measurement techniques

    **i.** Marking examination paper on which child is lying to determine location of the child's head and feet, then removing the child and measuring between the two marks

    **ii.** Laying child on examination paper and placing a tape measure next to child

**4.** Height

  **a.** Height is a measurement of a child standing upright

  **b.** Measurement technique

    **i.** Use a stable, accurate, fixed device for measurement (Goldbloom, 2003), e.g., a standing height board or stadiometer for cooperative children who are able to stand

    **ii.** Head, back, buttocks, and heels should touch the vertical surface of the stadiometer while the child maintains a natural stance (CDC, 2006a; 2006c)

      **(a)** For children who are unable to maintain this stance, a minimum of two contact points is needed—either head and buttock or buttock and heels

    **iii.** The head should be placed in the Frankfort plane

      **(a)** Imaginary line is drawn from the child's lower margin of the eye to the tragus (CDC, 2006d)

      **(b)** This line is horizontal to the headpiece

      **(c)** Perpendicular to the measuring rod

    **iv.** The headpiece is lowered until it touches the crown of the head at a right angle

    **v.** Read the measurement to the nearest ⅛ inch (Figure 4-3)

    **vi.** Height is less in the afternoon due to gravity and compression of vertebrae

  **c.** Alternative height measurements may be used for children with special needs

    **i.** Crown-rump length (Maternal & Child Health, 2006)

      **(a)** Position head at top of recumbent board

      **(b)** Legs are raised

      **(c)** Thighs are at a 90-degree angle to board

      **(d)** Footboard is placed against the buttock

    **ii.** Sitting height (Maternal & Child Health Bureau, 2006)

      **(a)** Child is seated on a stool in front of a wall-mounted stadiometer

      **(b)** Child's buttock, shoulders, and head are in contact with the stadiometer

      **(c)** Height is measured

      **(d)** Height of the stool is subtracted from the total height

    **iii.** Arm span

    **iv.** Upper arm length

    **v.** Lower leg length (Maternal & Child Health, 2006)

    **vi.** These measurements can be plotted on the CDC growth charts for length-for-age. Despite no standards for crown-rump length, growth patterns can be assessed over time

**5.** Head circumference

  **a.** Serial head circumference measurements provide a pattern of brain growth

  **b.** Measurement technique

    **i.** Measure head circumference for all children younger than 2 years of age

      **(a)** The child may be sitting in the parent's lap (CDC, 2006a)

      **(b)** Wrap the tape measure around the most prominent parts of the forehead and occiput (Goldbloom, 2003)

        **(1)** Tape measure should be above the eyebrows and pinna (Figure 4-4)

        (c) Read the measurement to the nearest 0.1 cm (CDC, 2006a)

        (d) Record the measurement on the gender-specific head circumference-for-age chart

  **c.** Accuracy (Goldbloom, 2003)

     **i.** Use a paper tape measure because a cloth tape measure may stretch

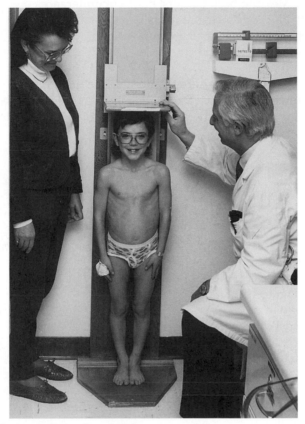

FIGURE 4-3 ■ Measuring standing height.

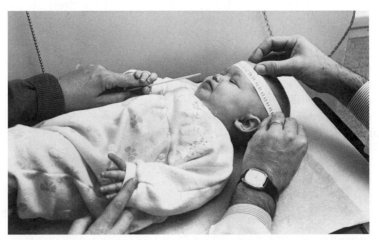

FIGURE 4-4 ■ Measuring head circumference in an infant. (From Goldbloom, R. [1997]. *Pediatric clinical skills* (2nd ed.). New York: Churchill Livingstone.)

   **ii.** Shape of the head may affect the measurement; therefore a second measurement may be needed

   **iii.** Variations in head circumference

   **iv.** Unusually large head in an otherwise normal infant/child may be hereditary (benign familial megalencephaly)

   (a) If the child's head circumference is 2 SD above the mean:

   (1) Measure both parents' head circumferences

   (2) Plot their measurements (Goldbloom, 2003)

   **v.** Larger than normal head circumference may indicate:

   (a) Hydrocephalus

   (b) Brain tumor

   **vi.** Below-normal head circumference may be due to:

   (a) Premature fusion of the cranial sutures (premature synostosis)

   (b) Being born to mothers who abuse cocaine or alcohol

6. Body mass index (BMI)
   a. Screening tool
      **i.** Indirect measure of body fat
      **ii.** Not diagnostic
   b. Measurement technique
      **i.** BMI is calculated by weight (kg) divided by height in meters squared (CDC, 2006b)
      **ii.** For ease of calculation, BMI tables are provided by the CDC for ages 2 to 20 (2006b)
      **iii.** BMI is plotted on the gender specific, body mass index-for-age percentile chart (Figure 4-5)
   c. Risk association
      **i.** Elevated BMI for older than 2 years of age is strongly associated with adolescent and adult obesity
      **ii.** BMI greater than 85% increased significantly from 1986 to 1998 among Blacks and Hispanics and increased, but not at a significant level, among Whites (Strauss & Pollack, 2001)
   d. Used for children who are at risk for weight problems
   e. Benefits of BMI
      **i.** Weight-for-stature and BMI are equally valuable as screening tools for children 3 to 5 years of age. After age 6, BMI is slightly better (CDC, 2006b)
      **ii.** BMI can be plotted on the growth charts for children up to 20 years of age; whereas weight-for-stature is available on charts for children less than 12 years of age (CDC, 2006b)
      **iii.** BMI screening criteria (CDC, 2006)
      (a) Overweight: greater than or equal to 95th percentile
      (b) Risk of overweight: 85th to less than 95th percentile
      (c) Normal weight: 5th to less than 85th percentile
      (d) Underweight: less than 5th percentile
   f. Accuracy
      **i.** BMI may be inaccurate due to:
      (a) Edema
      (b) Excess fat or muscle
      (c) Large or small stature
      (d) Varying weight and height distributions associated with puberty (Zemel et al., 1997)
      **ii.** Children diagnosed with trisomy 21, spina bifida, and cerebral palsy have varying measurement issues as compared to the average child

**CDC Growth Charts: United States**

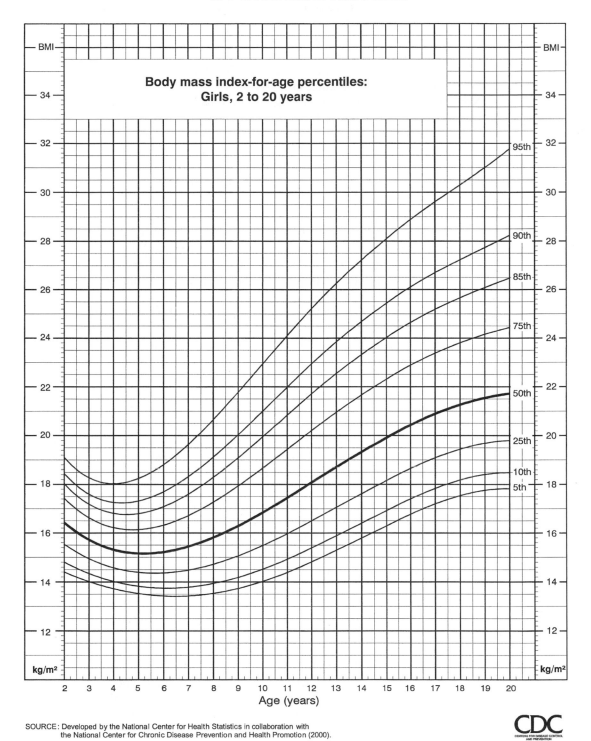

**Body mass index-for-age percentiles:
Girls, 2 to 20 years**

SOURCE: Developed by the National Center for Health Statistics in collaboration with
the National Center for Chronic Disease Prevention and Health Promotion (2000).

CDC
CENTERS FOR DISEASE CONTROL
AND PREVENTION

FIGURE 4-5 ■ Two to 20 years: Girls body mass index-for-age percentiles. (From Centers for
Disease Control and Prevention, http://www.cdc.gov/growthcharts.)

(a) Weight gain and weight-related problems in children with reduced linear growth are similar to typically growing children (Maternal and Child Health Bureau, 2006)

(b) Reference data in growth charts may be unreliable in these children because of differences in bone size and fat and muscle distribution (Maternal and Child Health Bureau, 2006)

7. Body fat–bioelectrical impedance analysis (BIA)
   a. Not a required screening test, but useful in mass screening situations
   b. Desirable body fat range is 14% to 20% (males) and 17% to 24% (females)
      i. According to a recent study, body fat percentages of school-age children range from 11% to 44 % (males) and 17% to 46% (females) (Skybo & Ryan-Wenger, 2003)
      ii. Another study found that the body fat of females 9 to 19 years of age ranged from 22% to 35% (Morrison et al., 2001)
   c. Measurement technique
      i. BIA passes a low frequency of electrical current through the body and measures the electrical impedance of this current in the body tissues
         (a) This impedance is proportional to the total body water
         (b) Limited resistance is found in lean tissue, which contains intracellular fluid and electrolytes
         (c) Fat tissue has limited fluid content and thus a high resistance to electrical current
         (d) Electrical current is not perceptible or dangerous to the child
      ii. BIA is measured in children 8 years of age and older (National Health and Nutrition Examination Survey, 2000)
      iii. BIA is measured via a portable scale that includes four electrodes in the form of steel footpads (anterior portion and heel of both feet) on top of the scale platform (Utter et al., 2001)
         (a) Electrical current is applied via the anterior portion of the footpad and drops across the heel electrode, which is then measured
         (b) Leg-to-leg impedance and body mass are calculated by the scale (Utter et al., 2001)
         (c) The scale provides the child's weight and body fat percentage
      iv. Accuracy of BIA
         (a) Body fat percentages should be measured in the evening because electrical resistance decreases when the body is active
         (b) Measurements taken at other times throughout the day may not have the same absolute value; these readings are accurate for determining the percentage of change in body fat from day to day (Tanita, 1996)
         (c) Dehydration overestimates body fat percentage (Utter et al., 2001)
8. Body fat—skin calipers
   a. Noninvasive method of measuring body fat
   b. Body fat is distributed subcutaneously
      i. The thicker the skinfold, the greater the amount of fat (Talbot & Lister, 1995)
      ii. Average tricep skinfold measurements in 8- to 9-year-old children are 13mm (males) and 15mm (females) (Robinson et al., 2001; Skybo & Ryan-Wenger, 2003)
      iii. In early childhood, subcutaneous fat decreases as muscle mass increases (AAP, 1993)
   c. Measurement technique (Talbot & Lister, 1995)
      i. Children should wear loose-fitting clothes

    ii. Sites are located and measured in millimeters, added together, and compared to composition profile charts

    iii. Anatomic sites for girls are the triceps, suprailium, and thigh skinfolds

    iv. Anatomic sites for boys are the chest, abdominal, and thigh skinfolds

    v. Skinfold is grasped between thumb and index finger. Gently shake to exclude the underlying muscle

    vi. Place the calipers 1 cm below the finger grasp. Read result to nearest 0.5 mm

    vii. Release skinfold grasp. Repeat procedure and average the readings

    viii. Measurements more than 90% for age and gender are considered overweight (AAP, 1993)

  **d.** Accuracy of skin calipers

    i. Separating the subcutaneous tissue from the underlying muscle may be difficult in muscular or obese children, thus leading to inaccurate readings

    ii. Unreliable readings may result from improper placement of the calipers or faulty equipment

    iii. Skin calipers measure subcutaneous fat but not internal fat, whereas the BIA method provides an overall measurement of body fat (Morrison et al., 2001)

    iv. Measuring body fat by skinfold measurements correlates with the BIA method ($r = 0.425\text{-}0.79$, $p > 0.01$) (Skybo & Ryan-Wenger, 2003; Morrison et al., 2001; Utter et al., 2001)

    v. For children with special needs, skinfold measurements should not be compared to reference data but used to monitor changes

**9.** Short stature

  **a.** Defined as height less than third percentile (U. S. Department of Health and Human Services [HHS], 2003a)

  **b.** Causes

    i. Familial short stature (FSS)

      (a) Occurs when a child's height is below the third percentile due to a genetic tendency for short stature

      (b) Children reach adult height consistent with their family background

    ii. Constitutional growth delay (CGD) (HHS, 2003a)

      (a) Occurs when a child is shorter than expected based on family genetic background

      (b) No medical cause for short stature is found

      (c) Children experience a delayed onset of puberty

      (d) Generally attain normal or near normal adult height

    iii. Medical causes of short stature

      (a) Decreased growth hormone

      (b) Diminished response to growth hormone

      (c) Hypothyroidism

      (d) Cushing disease

      (e) Genetic disorders

        (1) Chromosomal

        (2) Metabolic

        (3) Single gene disorders

        (4) Skeletal dysplasias involving formation and growth of the long bones or spine (HHS, 2003a)

10. Failure to thrive (FTT)
    a. Defined as a weight below the third percentile or less than 75% of median weight-for-height for children younger than 2 years of age. There should be no underlying medical disorder and growth failure should be expected to persist for 12 months (HHS, 2003b)
    b. Significant susceptibility to acute and chronic infection (HHS, 2003b)
    c. More likely than well-nourished children to exhibit negative affect
        i. During feeding
        ii. Insecure attachment to a caregiver
        iii. Poor psychologic developmental
        iv. More family problems
        v. Decreased cognitive development (HHS, 2003b)

## DEVELOPMENTAL ASSESSMENT

1. Developmental, motor, and cognitive milestones
    a. *Bright Futures* provides health supervision guidelines based on infancy, early childhood, middle childhood, and adolescence (Green & Palfrey, 2002). The following are included in each section:
        i. An overview of developmental changes for each age-group focusing on physical, cognitive, social, emotional, and health behaviors
        ii. A developmental chart provides lists of developmental achievements, tasks for the child to complete, and health supervision outcomes
        iii. Family preparation for health supervision contributes suggestions for preparing the family for health visits such as a history form and injury prevention survey
        iv. Lists of strengths and issues of the child, family, and community
        v. Health supervision interviews are structured around issues raised by the parents
        vi. Developmental surveillance and milestones assess a child's abilities over time
        vii. Observation of parent-child interaction identifies strengths, issues, and risk factors within the family
        viii. A list of additional screening procedures (hearing, vision, and lead) is provided to warrant areas that require further assessment
        ix. Immunizations due for each age-group are provided
        x. Anticipatory guidance provides information on the current and next developmental phase
    b. Denver II (Denver Developmental Materials, 1999)
        i. Professionals and paraprofessionals must be trained in the administration, scoring, and interpretation of the findings
        ii. Used to identify children at risk for developmental delays
        iii. This tool is not diagnostic for developmental delays
        iv. Screens children from birth to 6 years of age for personal-social, fine motor, gross motor, and language skills
    c. Ages and Stages Questionnaire (Bricker & Squires, 1999)
        i. Scoring should be completed by a healthcare professional
        ii. Completed by parents, caretakers, or nurses
        iii. Used to identify children with potential developmental problems
        iv. This tool is not diagnostic for developmental delays
        v. Screens children from 4 months to 5 years for communication, gross motor, fine motor, problem solving, and personal-social skills

    **d.** Nursing Child Assessment Satellite Training (NCAST) and parent-child interaction (PCI)

        **i.** Assessment techniques that provide observable behaviors that describe the mother-infant interaction, infant behavior, and maternal behavior (NCAST Programs, 2003; Sumner & Spietz, 1994)

            (a) Birth to 12 months for assessment during feedings

            (b) Birth to 36 months for assessment during a teaching interaction concerning feeding

            (c) Parental subscales include sensitivity to cues, response to distress, social-emotional growth fostering, and cognitive growth fostering

            (d) Child subscales include clarity of cues and responsiveness to caregiver

        **ii.** The nurse practitioner must complete a training course before using these techniques.

        **iii.** Scores correlate with cognitive abilities

    **e.** Children's drawings

        **i.** Coincide with stages of motor and cognitive development (Ryan-Wenger, 2001)

            (a) Drawings progress from scribbles (2 to 3 years of age)

            (b) Circles and other shapes (3 to 4 years)

            (c) First attempts of drawing a human figure appear at 3 years of age

            (d) Progressions in the human figure drawing (HFD) are seen until age 12 years

        **ii.** Human figure drawings (HFD)

            (a) HFD are completed by giving a child an 8½ × 11-inch blank piece of paper and a #2 pencil

            (b) Instructed to "draw one whole person. You can draw any kind of person you want to draw, but not a stick figure" (Koppitz, 1984, p. 10)

            (c) No time limit is given; however, most children finish their picture within 10 minutes

            (d) The structure of the HFD provides a measure of cognitive maturity and the style projects the child's attitude and emotions (Koppitz, 1984)

            (e) The HFD is analyzed for the presence or absence of emotional indicators such as large hands or legs pressed together (Koppitz, 1968)

            (f) Scoring criteria are available in Ryan-Wenger, 2001

**2.** Speech development

    **a.** Denver Articulation Screening Examination (DASE) (Denver Developmental Materials, 1973)

        **i.** 5-minute test

        **ii.** Screens children 2½ to 17 years of age

        **iii.** Identifies articulation disorders by having the child repeat words provided by the examiner

            (a) Words pronounced correctly provide a raw score

            (b) These scores are compared to the child's age, and a percentile rank is determined

            (c) If an abnormal percentile rank is achieved, the child is rescreened within 2 weeks

            (d) Children who maintain an abnormal percentile rank are referred for a speech evaluation

   **b.** Cognitive Adaptive Test/Clinical Linguistic and Auditory Milestone Scale (CAT/CLAMS) (Accardo & Capute, 2005)
      **i.** Neurodevelopmental tool for the cognitive assessment of children younger than 36 months
      **ii.** Assesses visual-motor functioning and expressive and receptive language development
      **iii.** Correlates with the Bayley Scales of Infant Development (r=0.89, p<.01) (Kube et al., 2000)
      **iv.** Sensitivity (81%) and specificity (85%) for detecting overall cognitive impairment (Kube et al., 2000)
      **v.** Administered by general practitioners or specialists (speech pathologists or occupational therapists)
   **c.** Fluharty 2 screening test
      **i.** Tests articulation and language performance in children 3 to 6 years of age
      **ii.** Children are tested on their ability to identify, articulate, and comprehend, and on repetition by repeating words and sentences, responding to directions, and describing actions (AGS, 2003)
      **iii.** Children who fail any part of examination are referred for a speech and language evaluation

## REFERENCES

Accardo, P. & Capute, A. (2005). *The Capute Scales: Cognitive Adaptive Test and Clinical Linguistic and Auditory Milestone Scale (CAT/CLAMS)*. Baltimore: Brookes.

AGS Publishing (2004). Fluharty2: Fluharty preschool speech and language screening test. Retrieved March 11, 2006 from www.agsnet.com/Group.asp?nMarketInfoID=42&nCategoryInfoID=2668&nGroupInfoID=a11390.

American Academy of Pediatrics, Committee on Nutrition. (2004). *Pediatric nutrition handbook* (5th ed.). Elk Grove Village, IL: American Academy of Pediatrics.

Bricker, D. & Squires, J. (1999). *Ages and Stages Questionnaires: A parent-completed, child-monitoring system (2nd ed)*. Baltimore: Brookes.

Centers for Disease Control and Prevention. (2002). National health and nutrition examination survey: Overweight among U.S. children and adolescents. Retrieved March 11, 2006, from www.cdc.gov/nchs/data/nhanes/databriefs/overwght.pdf.

Centers for Disease Control and Prevention. (2006a). Accurately weighing and measuring. Module 1: Equipment; Module 2: Technique. Retrieved March 11, 2006, from http://depts.washington.edu/growth.

Centers for Disease Control and Prevention. (2006b). CDC table for calculated body mass index values for selected heights and weights for ages 2 to 20 years. Retrieved March 11, 2006, from www.cdc.gov/nccd-php/dnpa/bmi/00binaries/bmi-tables.pdf.

Centers for Disease Control and Prevention. (2006c). Growth chart training. Retrieved March 11, 2006, from http://depts.washington.edu/growth.

Centers for Disease Control and Prevention. (2006d). Overview of the CDC growth charts. Retrieved March 11, 2006 from www.cdc.gov/nccdphp/dnpa/growthcharts/training/modules/module2/text/page1a.htm.

Centers for Disease Control and Prevention. (2006e). The CDC growth charts for children with special health care needs. Retrieved March 11, 2006, from http://depts.washington.edu/growth/cshcn/text/page1a.htm.

Denver Developmental Materials, Inc. (1999). Denver II. Retrieved March 11, 2006, from www.denverii.com/DenverII.html.

Denver Developmental Materials, Inc. (1973). Denver Articulation Screening Exam (DASE). Retrieved March 11, 2006, from www.denverii.com/DASE.html.

Goldbloom, R. (2003). Assessment of physical growth. In R. Goldbloom (Ed.). *Pediatric clinical skills* (3rd ed., pp. 23–48). New York: Churchill Livingstone.

Green, M. & Palfrey, J. S. (Ed.). (2002). *Bright futures: Guidelines for health supervision of infants, children, and adolescents.* (3rd ed.). Arlington, VA: National Center for Education in Maternal and Child Health.

Koppitz, E. (1984). *Psychological evaluation of human figure drawings by middle school pupils.* Orlando, FL: Grune & Stratton, Inc.

Koppitz, E. (1968). *Psychological evaluation of children's human figure drawings.* New York: Grune & Stratton.

Kube, D., Wilson, W., Peterssen, M., & Palmer, F. (2000). CAT/CLAMS: its use in detecting early childhood cognitive impairment. *Pediatric Neurology, 23,* 208–215.

Maternal and Child Health Bureau. (2006). Identifying poor growth in infants and toddlers. Retrieved March 11, 2006, from http://depts.washington.edu/growth/poorgrowth/text/intro.htm

Morrison, J., Barton, B. Obarzanek, E. et al. (2001). Racial differences in the sums of skinfolds and percentage of body fat estimated from impedance in black and white girls, 9 to 19 years of age: The National Heart, Lung, and Blood Institute Growth and Health Study. *Obesity Res, 9,* 297.

National Health and Nutrition Examination Survey. (2002). *Anthropometry procedures manual.* Retrieved March 11, 2006 from www.cdc.gov/nchs/data/nhanes/nhanes_01_02/body_measures_year_3.pdf.

National Health and Nutrition Examination Survey (2000). *Body composition procedures manual.* Retrieved March 11, 2006 from www.cdc.gov/nchs/data/nhanes/bc.pdf.

NCAST AVENUW. (2004). *NCAST Programs, University of Washington.* Retrieved March 11, 2006 , from www.ncast.org.

Roberts, S. & Dallal, G. (2001). The new childhood growth charts. *Nutr Rev, 59,* 31.

Robinson, T., Kiernan, M., Matheson, D. M., & Haydelet, K. F. (2001). Is parental control over children's eating associated with childhood obesity? Results from a population-based sample of third graders. *Obesity Res, 9,* 306.

Ryan-Wenger, N. (2001). Use of children's drawings for measurement of developmental level and emotional status. *J Child Family Nurs, 4,* 139.

Skybo, T., & Ryan-Wenger, N. (2003). Measures of overweight status in school-age children. *J School Nurs, 19,* 172.

Strauss, R., & Pollack, H. (2001). Epidemic increase in childhood overweight: 1986–1998. *JAMA, 286,* 2845.

Sumner, G., & Spietz, G. (1994). *NCAST caregiver/parent-child interaction feeding manual.* Seattle: NCAST Publications, University of Washington, School of Nursing.

Talbot, L., & Lister, Z. (1995). Assessing body composition. *AAOHN, 43,* 605.

Tanita. (2003). Tanita: FatCheck. Retrieved March 11, 2006, from www.fatcheck.com/home.html.

U. S. Department of Health and Human Services. (2003a). *Criteria for determining disability in infants and children: Short stature.* (AHRQ Publication No. 03-E025). Rockville, MD: Author. Retrieved March 13, 2006 from www.ahrq.gov/clinic/epcsums/shorts.htm

U. S. Department of Health and Human Services. (2003b). *Criteria for determining disability in infants and children: Failure to thrive.* (AHRQ Publication No. 03-E019). Rockville, MD: Author. Retrieved March 13, 2006 from www.ahrq.gov/clinic/epcsums/fthrivesum.htm

Utter, A., Scott, J., Oppliger, R., et al. (2001). A comparison of leg-to-leg bioelectrical impedance and skinfolds in assessing body fat in collegiate wrestlers. *J Strength Condition Res, 15,* 157.

Zemel, B., Riley, E., & Stallings, V. (1997). Evaluation of methodology for nutritional assessment in children: Anthropometry, body composition, and energy expenditure. *Ann Rev Nutr, 17,* 211.

# Assessment of the Head, Eyes, Ears, Nose, and Throat

JULEE WALDROP, MS, FNP, PNP

## FETAL DEVELOPMENT

1. Embryology, structure, and function of the head, eyes, ears, nose and throat (Larsen, 2001; Moore & Persaud, 2003)
   a. Six branchial arches, separated by branchial grooves, are evident in the human embryo by about 28 days
      i. Arch #1 forms the face, specifically, the:
         (a) Mandible
         (b) Malleus and incus bones of the inner ear
      ii. Arch #2 forms the stapes bone of the middle ear, lesser cornu, upper portion of hyoid bone, styloid process of temporal bone
      iii. Arch #3 forms the greater cornu, lower portion of hyoid bone
      iv. Arches #4, 5, and 6 form the laryngeal cartilages, including thyroid
   b. Pharyngeal pouches
      i. Pouch #1 produces the eustachian tube
      ii. Pouch #2 forms the tonsils and lymph nodules
      iii. Pouch #3 forms the thymus and inferior part of parathyroid gland
      iv. Pouch #4 forms the thyroid gland and superior part of the parathyroid gland
   c. Between the 4th and 14th weeks, the structures of the face develop
   d. The palate develops during weeks 6 through 12
   e. See Chapter 41, Section 1 for details on development of the nose, lips and hard and soft palate

## FOCUSED HISTORY

1. Focused history
   a. See Table 5-1 for relevant history items for focused assessment of the head, eyes, ears, nose (includes sinuses), and throat (includes oral cavity and teeth)
   b. See Table 5-2 for visual development milestones
   c. See Table 5-3 for receptive and expressive language development milestones

■ **TABLE 5-1**
■ ■ **Relevant History Related to Focused Assessment of Head, Eyes, Ears, Nose, Mouth, Teeth, and Throat**

| | Head | Eyes | Ears | Nose | Mouth, Teeth, Throat |
|---|---|---|---|---|---|
| Prenatal | Medications, drugs, alcohol<br>Medical problems during pregnancy<br>Hypertension<br>Diabetes<br>Failure to progress<br>Dystocia<br>Cesarean delivery<br>Forceps delivery<br>Hypoxia | | | | Maternal exposure to tetracycline |
| Neonatal | LGA: large for gestational age<br>SGA: small for gestational age<br>Intracranial hemorrhage<br>Apgar scores<br>Resuscitation<br>Myelomeningocele<br>Encephalocele<br>Microcephaly<br>Hydrocephaly | Prematurity<br>Oxygenation/ ventilation<br>Retinopathy<br>Cerebral palsy | Newborn hearing screen<br>Skin tags<br>Pits or fistulas<br>Gentamicin (ototoxic) | Dislocation of septum or triangular cartilage | Natal teeth<br>Cleft lip and/or palate<br><br>Attached frenulum |
| Past and/or current medical | Medications<br>Immunizations<br>Head trauma<br>Falls<br>Motor vehicle accidents (MVAs)<br>Subdural hematomas<br>Fractures<br>Loss of consciousness<br>Seizure disorders<br>Lumbar punctures<br>Radiation therapy<br>Surgery<br>Headache<br>Syncope<br>Dizziness | Strabismus<br>Corrective lenses | Hearing loss<br>Allergies<br>Otitis<br>Allergies<br>Trauma | Trauma<br>Surgery<br>Epistaxis | Infections<br>Tonsillectomy<br>Adenoidectomy<br>Malocclusion<br>Braces<br>Dental caries<br>Dental restorations |
| Developmental | Cognitive milestones<br>School performance<br>Behavior | See Table 5-2 for visual development milestones | See Table 5-3 for language development milestones | | Primary, secondary teeth |
| Family | | Retinoblastoma<br>Color blindness<br>Cataracts | Hearing loss<br>Allergies<br>Otitis | Allergies<br>Sinus infections | Malocclusion<br>Dental caries |

*Continued*

■ **TABLE 5-1**
■ ■ **Relevant History Related to Focused Assessment of Head, Eyes, Ears, Nose, Mouth, Teeth, and Throat—cont'd**

| | Head | Eyes | Ears | Nose | Mouth, Teeth, Throat |
|---|---|---|---|---|---|
| Family (cont'd) | | Macular degeneration<br>Altered visual acuity<br>Nearsighted<br>Farsighted<br>Strabismus<br>Amblyopia | | | |
| Social/ Environment | Stress<br>Sports<br>Drinking and driving | Protective lenses for risky sports | Exposure to loud noises<br>Exposure to smoke, allergens<br>Helmets<br>Seatbelts | Exposure to smoke, allergens<br>Cocaine | Exposure to smoke, allergens |
| Current medical | Medications | Visual acuity<br>Blurred vision<br>Pain<br>Photophobia<br>Change in eye appearance | Pain<br>Discharge<br>Tinnitus<br>Vertigo | Change in sense of smell<br>Obstruction<br>Epistaxis<br>Postnasal discharge<br>Sinus pain | Toothbrushing<br>Flossing<br>Dental caries<br>Dental restorations<br>Bleeding or swelling gums<br>Tooth eruptions, trauma, infection<br>Mouth ulcers<br>Speech<br>Hoarseness<br>Sore throat |

■ **TABLE 5-2**
■ ■ **Visual Development Assessment**

| Age | Developmental Abilities |
|---|---|
| Birth/neonatal | Awareness of light and dark; closes eyes to bright light; fixation on near objects |
| 2 to 4 weeks | Brief monocular fixation, can follow large discrete objects |
| 6 to 8 weeks | Begins and improves binocular fixation and convergence |
| 12 weeks | Follows objects with head and eyes, convergence improving, beginning depth perception |
| 16 weeks | Inspects own hands, immediate fixation on interesting objects; visual acuity 20/300 to 20/200 |
| 20 to 24 weeks | Follows dropped toy; voluntary fixation; accommodative convergence; can attend to object >3 feet away |
| 28 weeks | Binocular vision established |
| 40 weeks | Fixates on tiny objects; vision 20/200 |
| 1 year | Discriminates simple geometric forms; vision 20/180 |
| 12 to 18 months | Distance vision and depth perception still underdeveloped |
| 2 years | Accommodation well developed; vision 20/30 |
| 6 to 7 years | Vision 20/20 |

Adapted from Seidel, H. M., Ball, J. W., Dains, J. E., & Benedict, G. W. (2003). *Mosby's guide to physical examination* (5th ed.). St. Louis: Mosby, p. 282.

■ **TABLE 5-3**
■ ■ **Receptive and Expressive Language Development Milestones**

| Age | Receptive Language | Expressive Language |
|-----|--------------------|--------------------|
| 0 to 4 weeks | Responds to sound (bell) by startling or blinking if in quiet state; by quieting if in active state | Cries |
| 2 months | Increases vocalization when spoken to | Coos<br>Makes single vowel sounds ("ah," "uh") |
| 3 months | | Chuckles |
| 4 months | Increases vocalizations to toys and people | Laughs out loud<br>Shows excitement with voice inflection and breathing |
| 5 months | Lateralizes to sound | Growls<br>Two-syllable vocalizations |
| 6 months | | Babbling increases<br>Expresses displeasure without crying |
| 7 months | Imitates sounds (e.g., cough, "raspberry")<br><br>Plays peek-a-boo | Beginning to make consonant sounds ("da," "ba," "ga")<br>Says "mum-mum" when crying |
| 8 months | Responds to name by turning<br>Understands "no" when strongly spoken | |
| 9 months | Responds to no regardless of tone | Says "Mama" "Dada" nonspecifically |
| 10 months | Performs one action with verbal command only (e.g., wave bye-bye) | Says one word with meaning (often "Dada") |
| 11 to 12 months | Performs three actions with verbal command only | Says two words with meaning |
| 15 months | | Four or five words<br>Uses gestures to seek help and indicate wants |
| 18 months | Follows simple directional commands ("give it to Mommy")<br>Points to one to four body parts | |
| 21 months | Follows associative commands ("put the ball on the table")<br>Points to pictures on request<br>Points to four to six body parts | 20 to 50 words<br>Combines two words<br>Repeats words<br>Names one picture in book |
| 24 months | Fills in missing word in songs or nursery rhymes<br>Points to seven body parts | At least 50 words<br>Three-word sentences<br>Uses personal pronouns (me, you, I)<br>Names one body part |
| 30 months | Points to pictures of object according to their use ("Show me what you eat with") | Multiple-word sentences<br>Carries a tune<br>Refers to self as "I"<br>Uses plurals<br>Names many objects and body parts |
| 36 months | Understands action agents ("What flies?") | Gives first and last name<br>Recites nursery rhyme or song |
| 48 months | Answers comprehension questions ("What do you do when you're cold?") | Understands prepositions<br>Names opposites<br>Counts three objects correctly |
| 5 years | Points to colors on request<br>Points to objects according to characteristics of widest, center, etc. | Asks questions<br>Defines words by their use |

*Continued*

■ **TABLE 5-3**
■ ■ **Receptive and Expressive Language Development Milestones—cont'd**

| | |
|---|---|
| 6 years | Sentences usually grammatically correct |
| | Few articulation errors |
| | Defines words by category, composition, use |
| | States differences between objects |
| 7 to 8 years | States similarities and differences between objects |
| | Defines concrete words |
| 9 years | Understands absurdities in sentences |
| 10 years | Understands abstract words (grief, surprise) |

Derived from Goldbloom, R. B. (2003). *Pediatric clinical skills* (3rd ed.). Philadelphia: Saunders, pp. 93-98.

## FOCUSED EXAMINATION

1. Focused examination (Seidel, et al., 2003)
   a. Measurement (Colyar, 2003; Goldbloom, 2003)
      i. Head
         (a) Head circumference (if ≤2 years of age or indicated)
            (1) See Section 5 on physical growth, for measurement technique
            (2) Occipitofrontal circumference
            (3) Plot on growth chart (percentile)
            (4) Larger than chest circumference at birth; equal to chest circumference at 6 to 24 months of age (Colyar, 2003)
         (b) Fontanelle size measurement (Moses, 2005)
            (1) Obtain anteroposterior (AP) diameter
            (2) Obtain transverse (T) diameter
            (3) Size = (AP + T) / 2
               a) Anterior fontanelle—mean newborn size: 2.1 cm (larger in Black infants)
               b) Posterior fontanelle—mean newborn size: 0.5 to 0.7 cm
      ii. Eyes
         (a) See Table 5-2 for visual development milestones
         (b) Visual acuity screening (Curnyn & Kaufman, 2003)
            (1) Snellen alphabet chart for children in second grade or higher
               a) Child stands 10 feet away from chart on wall
               b) Start with right eye occluded and have child read letters on the 20/50 line and proceed downward
               c) If child misses a letter on 20/50 line, proceed upward
               d) To receive credit for lines 20/40 and higher all letters must be correct
               e) On 20/20 and 20/30 lines, child may miss two letters and still receive credit
               f) Child's visual acuity is the smallest line the child reads correctly
               g) Repeat with left eye occluded
               h) Rescreen (check poorer eye first) children with 20/40 or worse in one or both eyes
               i) Refer to ophthalmologist:
                  i) Children with 20/40 or worse in one or both eyes

          ii) If two line difference between eyes even if both are within passing range

      (2) The U.S. Preventive Services Task Force (2004) recommends screening of children *younger than age 5* for visual impairment

        a) Snellen Tumbling E chart

        b) Allen Object Recognition chart contains pictures of familiar objects

        c) HTOV chart contains only the letters H, T, O, and V

        d) These three charts are used similarly to the Snellen alphabet chart

        e) Photoscreening is more accurate, requires little cooperation other than fixating on an object, but requires special equipment to perform (AAP, 2003)

   **iii.** Ears

     (a) Hearing assessment—infant (Cunningham & Cox, 2003)

       (1) Moro reflex—startle reflex seen in infants only; disappears at 3 to 4 months

       (2) Responds to voice or sound

       (3) Results of newborn hearing screening

     (b) Hearing assessment—older infants and children (Kenna, 2003)

       (1) Audiometry—begin at age 5 to 6 years; age 4 years according to AAP (2003)

       (2) Whisper test—child can repeat words whispered behind his or her back

       (3) Weber test—test of lateralization

         a) Place vibrating tuning fork on top of head or upper forehead

         b) Ask child if sound is heard in one or both ears

       (4) Rinne test—test of bone versus air conduction of sound

         a) Place vibrating tuning fork on mastoid process

         b) Ask child to say when he or she no longer hears the hum or feels the vibration; note number of seconds

         c) Then place the tuning fork by the ear

         d) Ask child when he or she can no longer hear the vibrations; note number of seconds

         e) Air conduction should be twice as long as bone conduction

  **iv.** Nose—not applicable

  **v.** Oral cavity and teeth—not applicable

  **vi.** Throat—not applicable

**b.** Inspection (Colyar, 2003; Goldbloom, 2003)

   **i.** Head

     (a) Shape

       (1) If unusual, inquire about similarity to a parent's head shape

       (2) Bony abnormalities (craniosynostosis, hydrocephalus)

       (3) Soft tissue abnormalities/newborn (craniotabes, caput succedaneum, cephalhematoma)

       (4) Flat occiput

         a) Prematurity

         b) Sleeping on back

       (5) Frontal bossing—prominent forehead; may be due to large browline or rare syndromes

       (6) Hydrocephalus (increased intracranial pressure)

     (b) Hair

       (1) Color, abnormal pigmentation

       (2) Distribution—v-shaped peak at top of hairline; bald spots

   (3) Texture—soft, coarse

   (4) Whorls—hair growth in a swirl pattern from the scalp

  (c) Scalp

   (1) Smooth

   (2) Scaly, lesions

   (3) Prominent veins

 ii. Eyes

  (a) Periorbital area

   (1) Allergic shiner—dark areas on skin under eyes related to allergies

   (2) Dennie's lines—creases on skin under eyes related to allergies

  (b) Papillary reflex—darkened room, light shining in eye causes pupil to constrict; removal of light causes pupil to dilate

  (c) Cover-uncover test—screens for strabismus ("crossed eyes"), esotropia, exotropia

   (1) Examiner covers child's right eye

   (2) Child focuses on an object with left eye

   (3) Examiner observes left eye for movement indicating fixation

   (4) Examiner removes the cover and observes right eye for evidence of deviation of eye to right, left or upward

   (5) Procedure continues with alternating cover and uncover to detect deviation of eyes during fixation

  (d) Corneal light reflex—screens for strabismus

   (1) Hirschberg test—symmetric placement of the corneal light reflex

   (2) Strabismus—asymmetric corneal light reflexes

   (3) Pseudostrabismus—eyes appear to be strabismic, but corneal reflexes are symmetric; results from a flat nasal bridge, wide epicanthal folds, and closely placed eyes

  (e) Red reflex—Brückner test; screens for abnormalities of the back of the eye and for cataracts and retinoblastoma (AAP, 2002); test eyes separately or simultaneously

   (1) Set ophthalmoscope at +4.00 diopter, and illuminate both pupils simultaneously from a distance of 12 to 18 inches.

   (2) Normal: reflections of the two eyes are equivalent in color, intensity, and clarity and there are no opacities or white spots

  (f) Funduscopy—i.e., ophthalmoscopy; use of the ophthalmoscope to observe structures in back of the eye

   (1) Procedure requires hours of practice to become proficient

   (2) Goals are to observe:

    a) Clarity of cornea, lens, and vitreous

    b) Blood vessels in each quadrant of fundus for obvious abnormalities (veins are large and dark red, veins are small and pale red)

    c) Optic disc for color, margins and evidence of a physiologic cup

    d) Foveal reflex—point of light in front of the retina moves in the opposite direction to the direction the ophthalmoscope is moved

    e) Hemorrhage (evidence of trauma)

  (g) Ocular mobility

   (1) Cardinal fields of gaze—superior rectus, inferior oblique, medial rectus, superior oblique, inferior rectus, lateral rectus

   (2) Reveals evidence of nystagmus

       (h) Structures—symmetry, normal variations, abnormalities
          (1) Lids—lashes, epicanthal folds, ptosis (drooping)
          (2) Globes—prominence
          (3) Conjunctiva—injection (color), discharge, tearing
          (4) Sclera—color, vessels
          (5) Cornea—clarity

  **iii.** Ears
     (a) External ear
        (1) Shape—size, symmetry, normal variations, abnormalities
        (2) Presence of dimples, nodules, skin tags
        (3) Position—should be along an even plane with outer canthus of eyes; note if low-set
     (b) Internal ear
        (1) Method
           a) Hold otoscope upright or upside down, with some part of your hand on child's head to stabilize otoscope
           b) Maneuver pinna to straighten the canal and improve visualization of the tympanic membrane
        (2) Canal
           a) Cerumen—note amount, color
           b) Note if foreign body, signs of inflammation, drainage
     (c) Tympanic membrane (TM)
        (1) Landmarks—note visibility of malleus, borders of TM, light reflex
        (2) General appearance, color
        (3) Mobility—pneumatic otoscopy used to insert a puff of air into canal and observe for movement of the TM
        (4) Presence of tympanostomy tubes, perforations
        (5) Behind the TM, presence of fluid/air demarcations, pus (yellow, opaque fluid)

  **iv.** Nose
     (a) External nose
        (1) Symmetry, size, normal variations, abnormalities
        (2) Discharge
        (3) Flaring
        (4) Allergic crease across nose where nasal bone ends—also called nasal pleat; result of child pushing up nose with palm of hand (an "allergic salute")
     (b) Internal nose
        (1) Septum—central, deviated, intact
        (2) Nares—patency
        (3) Mucosal edema, erythema, bleeding, discharge

  **v.** Oral cavity and teeth
     (a) Lips
        (1) Moistness
        (2) Symmetry
        (3) Color
        (4) Lesions
        (5) Mouth breathing
        (6) Shape of philtrum (groove between bottom of nose and top of lip)
     (b) Buccal mucosa (inside of cheek)
        (1) Color
        (2) Lesions

    (c) Gums
        (1) Color
        (2) Swelling
        (3) Bleeding
    (d) Tongue
        (1) Size
        (2) Color
        (3) Mobility
        (4) Lesions
        (5) Frenulum
            a) Upper frenulum between upper lip and maxillary gingiva; attaches midway between tip of tongue and attachment of tongue to mucosa
            b) Lower frenulum under the tongue
            c) Check mobility of lips and tongue; shortened frenula may inhibit speech and feeding
    (e) Palate
        (1) Color
        (2) Symmetry, closure
        (3) Hard palate—between premaxillary, maxillary and palatine bones
        (4) Soft palate—behind hard palate, ends in uvula
    (f) Tonsils (Colyar, 2003)
        (1) Normal to see large tonsils in toddlers, preschoolers, and school-aged children
        (2) Grade size of tonsils as 1+ (visible), 2+ (halfway between tonsillar pillars and uvula), 3+ (touching uvula), 4+ (touching each other)
    (g) Pillars—located lateral, and anterior as well as posterior to the tonsils
    (h) Pharynx—posterior, at back of throat
        (1) Color
        (2) Edema: "cobblestone" typical of allergies
        (3) Exudates: note color and consistency, e.g., patches, film
        (4) Petechiae
    (i) Epiglottis
        (1) Normally, epiglottis is not visible in children
        (2) Located at base of posterior tongue and posterior pharynx
        (3) Note color, edema
        (4) NOTE: If red and edematous, stop the exam and refer to emergency department
        (5) NOTE: If child is symptomatic, call 911; may need intubation at any time
    (j) Adenoids
        (1) Mass of lymphoid tissue in the roof of the nasopharynx
        (2) Present in infants and children; regress during adolescence
        (3) Note color, edema
    (k) Uvula
        (1) Note if bifid (normal variation), erythematous or edematous
        (2) Have child say "ah"; uvula should deviate upward; abnormal if deviates sideways
    (l) Parotid glands—located in front of ear
        (1) Stensen's ducts of the parotid located below the second upper molar

(2) Look like dimples

(3) Note color, edema, exudates

   (m) Submandibular glands—located in mandibular area between chin and ear

     (1) Wharton's ducts located under tongue on each side of frenulum

     (2) Look like raised dimples

     (3) Note color, edema

   (n) Sublingual gland—located at base of tongue

     (1) Sublingual ducts located under tongue at most lateral edges

   (o) Teeth (AAP, 2003; Colyar, 2003)

     (1) Primary dentition—temporary teeth erupt between 6 and 24 months

     (2) Secondary dentition—permanent teeth erupt between ages 6 and 13—earlier in girls than boys, and earlier in Black than white children

     (3) Quantity/number compared with expected number

       a) All 20 temporary teeth expected by age 2½

       b) 28 permanent teeth expected by age 13

       c) Third molars (wisdom teeth) erupt between ages 17 and 25

     (4) Occlusion/malocclusion—note obvious misalignment of teeth and jaws

     (5) Discolorations

     (6) Caries

   (p) Gag reflex

**c.** Palpation

  **i.** Head

   (a) Palpate fontanelles with infant sitting upright quietly

     (1) Soft

     (2) Not sunken or bulging

     (3) Anterior fontanelle

       a) Junction of coronal suture and sagittal suture

       b) Diamond shape

       c) Closes between 4 to 26 months (median 13.8 months)

     (4) Posterior fontanelle

       a) Junction of lambdoidal suture and sagittal suture

       b) Triangular shape

       c) Closes by 2 months

   (b) Suture lines should not be palpable

   (c) Mastoid area for lumps

   (d) Sinuses—tenderness, swelling

     (1) Ethmoid—present at birth

     (2) Maxillary—present at birth

     (3) Sphenoid—present by age 5, fully developed by adolescence

     (4) Frontal—present by ages 7 to 8, fully developed by adolescence

  **ii.** Eyes

   (a) Palpate lacrimal duct for discharge

  **iii.** Ears

   (a) Palpate external ear for tenderness

   (b) Palpate pre- and postauricular nodes for swelling

   (c) Traction on tragus should not be painful except with external otitis

  **iv.** Nose—not applicable

  **v.** Oral cavity and teeth—palpate palate and strength of suck in infant

  **vi.** Thyroid gland (Colyar, 2003)

(a) Newborn
  (1) Place hand under scapulae and raise shoulders so that head falls back gently to rest on table or mother's lap
  (2) Palpate thyroid area with second and third fingers of other hand
  (3) Note: thyroid is normally not palpable in newborn
(b) Infants, toddlers, and preschoolers
  (1) Place fingers on front of trachea by the cricoid and palpate for lumps
(c) School-age children and adolescents
  (1) From *behind*, place fingers on front of trachea by the cricoid
  (2) Ask child to swallow and feel for lumps in thyroid as trachea rises
  (3) Move the trachea right and left and palpate the thyroid on opposite side

**d.** Auscultation and percussion
  **i.** Head (Moses, 2005)
  (a) Auscultate fontanelles for bruit; suggests AV malformation
  (b) Percuss fontanelle at junction of frontal, temporal and parietal bones for Macewen's sign—dull "cracked pot" sound; suggests increased intracranial pressure
  **ii.** Eyes—bell of the stethoscope can be applied to the closed orbit or temple to detect an intracranial bruit
  **iii.** Ears—not applicable
  **iv.** Nose—not applicable
  **v.** Oral cavity and teeth—not applicable
  **vi.** Throat—auscultate over carotid arteries for bruit (vibration due to constricted flow)

---

## REFERENCES

American Academy of Pediatrics. (2003). Oral health risk assessment timing and establishment of the dental home. *Pediatrics, 111*(5), 1113-1116.

American Academy of Pediatrics, Committee on Practice and Ambulatory Medicine and Section on Ophthalmology. (2002). Use of photoscreening for children's vision screening. *Pediatrics, 109*(3), 524-525.

American Academy of Pediatrics. (2003). Hearing assessment in infants and children: Recommendations beyond neonatal screening. *Pediatrics, 111*(2), 436-440.

Colyar, M. R. (2003). *Well-child assessment for primary care providers.* Philadelphia: F. A. Davis.

Cunningham, M., Cox, E. O. (2003). American Academy of Pediatrics Committee on Practice and Ambulatory Medicine and the Section on Otolaryngology and Bronchoesophagology. Hearing assessment in infants and children: Recommendations beyond neonatal screening. *Pediatrics, 111*(2), 436-440.

Curnyn, K. M., & Kaufman, L. M. (2003). The eye examination in the pediatrician's office, *Pediatr Clin North Am, 50*(1), 25-40.

Goldbloom, R. B. (2003). *Pediatric clinical skills* (3rd ed.). Philadelphia: Saunders.

Larsen, W. J. (2001). *Human embryology.* New York: Churchill Livingstone.

Moore, K. L., & Persaud, T V. N. (2003). *The developing human: Clinically oriented embryology.* Philadelphia: Saunders.

Moses, S. (2005). Fontanelle. Retrieved from the *Family Practice Notebook* August 8, 2005, at www.fpnotebook.com/NIC25.htm.

Seidel, H. M., Ball, J. W., Dains, J. E., & Benedict, G. W. (2003). *Mosby's guide to physical examination* (5th ed.). St. Louis: Mosby.

U.S. Preventive Services Task Force. *Screening for visual impairment in children younger than age 5 years: recommendation statement.* May 2004. Agency for Healthcare Research and Quality, Rockville, MD. Retrieved August 8, 2005, from www.ahrq.gov/clinic/3rduspstf/visionscr/vischrs.htm.

# 6 Assessment of the Pulmonary System

JULEE WALDROP, MS, FNP, PNP

## FETAL DEVELOPMENT

1. Embryology, structure, and function of the pulmonary system (CATS, 2003; Larsen, 2001; Moore & Persaud, 2003)
   a. Lungs begin as a small anterior bud off of the foregut tube
      i. The bud elongates and branches into two buds
      ii. Each new bud becomes the mainstem bronchus of each lung (carina)
      iii. Each mainstem bronchus lengthens and branches into two lungs
      iv. Fissures separate the lobes of each lung
         (a) Right lung has three lobes: upper, middle, and lower
         (b) Left lung has only two lobes: upper and lower
      v. The mesenchyme, a mass of primitive cells within the bronchus and lung tissue differentiates into muscle, nerves, and blood vessels of the lungs
      vi. Alveoli, the functional units of gas exchange, arise as clusters (sacs) at the ends of the terminal branches of the foregut tube
         (a) Alveoli are lined by type I cells, which are flat, specialized epithelial cells
         (b) For every nine type I cells there is one type II cell that produces a lipid detergent molecule called surfactant
         (c) Surfactant helps keep the alveoli from collapsing at low lumenal pressures (as at the end of exhalation)
      vii. Airways are lined by a protective epithelium that begins at the vocal cords
         (a) Epithelium is ciliated, columnar, and pseudostratified
         (b) Mucus secreting goblet cells appear among the columnar cells
         (c) When the airway is only millimeters in diameter, goblet cells are replaced by clara cells that secrete a thin watery fluid instead of mucus
      viii. Macrophages migrate over all epithelial surfaces of the lung and engulf particulate material
         (a) With the help of cilia in the larger airways, macrophages move inhaled material up and out of the airways
      ix. The most important functions of the upper respiratory tract are warming, moisturizing, and cleaning

# FOCUSED HISTORY

1. Focused history (Colyar, 2003; Goldbloom, 2003; Seidel et al., 2003)
   a. Prenatal history
      i. Maternal smoking
   b. Neonatal history
      i. Prematurity
      ii. Low birth weight
      iii. Apgar scores
      iv. Oxygen use
      v. Resuscitation
      vi. Ventilation
      vii. Chronic lung disease of prematurity (bronchopulmonary dysplasia)
   c. Medical history
      i. Pertussis
      ii. Asthma
      iii. Cystic fibrosis
      iv. Tuberculosis
      v. Pneumonia
      vi. Foreign body aspiration
   d. Current medical history
      i. Sore throat
      ii. Cough
      iii. Difficulty swallowing
      iv. Feeding difficulties
      v. Dyspnea
      vi. Chest pain
      vii. Cyanosis
      viii. Wheezing
      ix. Symptoms related to exercise and activity
      x. Apnea
      xi. Medications
   e. Immunizations
      i. Diphtheria
      ii. Pertussis
      iii. *Haemophilus influenzae* Type B (HIB)
      iv. *Streptococcus pneumoniae*
   f. Family history
      i. Allergies
      ii. Asthma
      iii. Cystic fibrosis
   g. Social or environmental history
      i. Number of people in home
      ii. Exposure to passive smoke
      iii. Exposure to carbon monoxide
      iv. Smoking
      v. Occupational exposures
      vi. Exposure to illness
      vii. School absences
      viii. Pets
      ix. Allergens, dust, dirt

    **x.** Travel

    **xi.** Institutional living (e.g., dormitory, homeless shelter)

## FOCUSED PHYSICAL EXAMINATION

1. Focused examination (Colyar, 2003; Goldbloom, 2003; Seidel et al., 2003)
   a. Measurement
      i. Chest circumference (if indicated by suspicion of growth problem) (Colyar, 2003)
         (a) Measure at nipple line; measure three times and take average
         (b) Newborn—chest circumference slightly less than head circumference
         (c) 6 to 24 months—chest circumference = head circumference
      ii. A/P diameter—anteroposterior diameter of chest
      iii. Respiratory rate (Table 6-1)
      iv. Pulmonary function measurements
      v. Peak expiratory flow rate
         (a) Via peak flowmeter when able
         (b) Average and 95th percentile boundaries for boys and girls based on their height (Figure 6-1)
   b. Inspection
      i. Chest wall shape (Dorland's Illustrated Medical Dictionary, 2003)
         (a) Symmetry
         (b) Barrel chest—a rounded, bulging chest with abnormal increase in the anteroposterior diameter, showing little movement on respiration
         (c) Pectus excavatum—funnel chest; deep indentation of sternum
         (d) Pectus carinatum—pigeon breast
      ii. Chest wall expansion
         (a) Symmetry
         (b) Depth
         (c) Rhythm
            (1) Newborns
               a) Irregular rate and rhythm is normal
               b) Note if periodic breathing, paradoxical breathing or apnea
      iii. Oxygen perfusion
         (a) Skin color: pink, pale, cyanotic, cherry red
         (b) Nail beds: capillary refill
         (c) Fingers: clubbing

■ **TABLE 6-1**
■ ■ **Normal Range of Respiratory Rates in Children**

| Age | Breaths per Minute |
| --- | --- |
| Newborn | 30-80 |
| 1 year | 20-40 |
| 3 years | 20-30 |
| 6 years | 16-22 |
| 10 years | 16-20 |
| 17 years | 12-20 |

Adapted from: Seidel et al. (2003). *Mosby's guide to physical examination* (5th ed.). St. Louis: Mosby, p. 394.

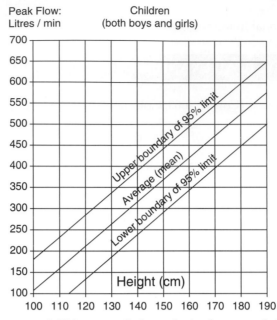

FIGURE 6-1 ■ Average and 95th percentile boundaries for normal children's peak flow values. (Reprinted with permission from Asthma and Allergy Information and Research [3/24/2003]. Asthma: What should my child's peak flow be? Retrieved August 8, 2005, from www.users.globalnet.co.uk/~aair/asthma_PEFCH.htm.)

       **iv.** Work of breathing
          **(a)** Nasal flaring
          **(b)** Use of accessory muscles
          **(c)** Sternal retraction
          **(d)** Grunting
          **(e)** Expiratory phase greater than inspiratory phase
       **v.** Sputum—color, consistency
   **c.** Palpation
       **i.** Symmetry of chest expansion
       **ii.** Central position of trachea
       **iii.** Fremitus (vibration during speech) in older children and adolescents
       **iv.** Crepitus—subcutaneous emphysema
          **(a)** Crackling sensation from air within the tissues
   **d.** Percussion
       **i.** Systematically percuss lung fields and note quality of tone (Fig. 6-2)
          **(a)** Resonance: normal
          **(b)** Hyperresonance: pneumothorax
          **(c)** Dullness: pleural effusion or pneumonia
       **ii.** Note if bilateral equality of tone
       **iii.** Diaphragmatic excursion
          **(a)** Find the level of the diaphragmatic dullness on both sides
          **(b)** Ask the patient to inspire deeply
          **(c)** The level of dullness (diaphragmatic excursion) should go down 3 to 5 cm symmetrically
  **e.** Auscultation
       **i.** Use diaphragm of stethoscope to hear high-pitched sounds
       **ii.** Systematically auscultate lung fields (see Figure 6-2)

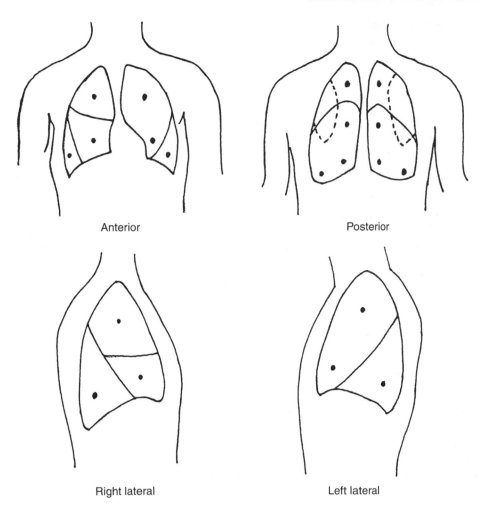

Anterior

Posterior

Right lateral

Left lateral

● — Suggested auscultation sites

FIGURE 6-2 ■ Location of lung fields for percussion and auscultation. (Reprinted with permission from Goldbloom, R. B. [2003]. *Pediatric clinical skills* [3rd ed.]. Philadelphia: Saunders, p. 163.)

    **iii.** Symmetry of normal breath sounds
    **iv.** Normal breath sounds (RNCeus, 2004)
       (a) Tracheal
         (1) Heard over the trachea
         (2) Sounds are harsh, like air blowing through a pipe
       (b) Bronchovesicular
         (1) Heard in the posterior chest between the scapulas and in the center part of the anterior chest
         (2) Softer than bronchial sounds, but have a tubular quality
         (3) Sounds are about equal during inspiration and expiration
       (c) Vesicular
         (1) Normally heard throughout most of the lung fields
         (2) Sounds are soft, blowing, or rustling
         (3) Normally heard throughout inspiration, continue without pause through expiration, and then fade away about one third of the way through expiration

    (d) Bronchial

        (1) Heard over the large airways in the anterior chest near the second and third intercostal spaces

        (2) Loud and high pitched with a short pause between inspiration and expiration

        (3) Expiratory sounds last longer than inspiratory sounds

  **v.** Adventitious and other abnormal sounds

    (a) Crackles—short, crackling, nonmusical sounds

    (b) Wheezes—continuous musical sounds, usually expiratory

    (c) Friction rub—harsh grating sound with respirations

    (d) Stridor—continuous, harsh inspiratory sound

    (e) Grunting—episodic, short expiratory sound

  **vi.** Vocal resonance

    (a) Whispered pectoriloquy—increased quality and loudness of whispers that are heard with a stethoscope over an area of lung consolidation

    (b) Bronchophony (Dorland's Illustrated Medical Dictionary, 2002)

        (1) Normal voice sounds heard over a healthy large bronchus

        (2) Abnormal voice sounds heard over the lung, with the voice transmitted unusually clearly and with a high pitch

---

## REFERENCES

Asthma and Allergy Information and Research. (3/24/2003). Asthma: What should my child's peak flow be? Retrieved August 8, 2005, from www.users.global-net.co.uk/~aair/asthma_PEFCH.htm.

CATS—*Computer assisted teaching system.* University of Vermont College of Medicine. Retrieved August 8, 2005, from http://cats.med.uvm.edu.

Colyar, M. R. (2003). *Well-child assessment for primary care providers.* Philadelphia: F. A. Davis.

Dorland's illustrated medical dictionary. (2002). Philadelphia: Saunders. Retrieved August 8, 2005, from www.Mercksource.com.

Goldbloom, R. B. (2003). *Pediatric clinical skills* (3rd ed.). Philadelphia: Saunders.

Larsen, W. J. (2001). *Human embryology.* New York: Churchill Livingstone.

Moore, K. L., & Persaud, T. V. N. (2003). *The developing human: Clinically oriented embryology.* Philadelphia: Saunders.

RNCeus. (2004). Normal breath sounds. Retrieved August 8, 2005, from www.rnceus.com/resp/respnorm.html.

Seidel, H. M., Ball, J. W., Dains, J. E., & Benedict, G. W. (2003). *Mosby's guide to physical examination* (5th ed.). St. Louis: Mosby.

# Assessment of the Cardiovascular System

NICOLE M. JOSHI, MSN, RN, CPNP

## FETAL DEVELOPMENT

1. Fetal development of the cardiovascular system (Larsen, 2001; Moore & Persaud, 2003)
   a. Cardiovascular tissues arise from the mesoderm
   b. Blood vessel formation evident
      i. On yolk sac at day 17
      ii. In embryonic disk at day 18
   c. Umbilical arteries develop in the connective stalk by week 4
   d. Five pairs of arteries called *aortic arches* arise from the aortic sac
      i. At week 4, the dorsal aortic arch artery gives rise to vessels for the gastro-intestinal (GI) tract
      ii. At days 26 to 29, aortic arch arteries 2, 3, 4, and 6 give rise to vessels for the head, neck, and upper thorax
   e. Development of the heart
      i. Week 3—a pair of endothelial strands appear
      ii. Canalization leads to endothelial heart tubes that then fuse to form a single heart tube
      iii. Week 4—three paired veins drain into heart tube
      iv. Days 21 to 22—heart begins to contract
      v. Weeks 4 to 5—primitive atrium and ventricle develop
      vi. By 8 weeks, heart has four chambers

## FOCUSED HISTORY

1. Birth
2. Prenatal
   a. Maternal illness or infection
      i. Exposure to teratogens
         (a) Rubella in first trimester may cause congenital heart defect (patent ductus arteriosus [PDA], pulmonary artery stenosis)
         (b) Alcohol
         (c) Hydantoins
      ii. Diabetes

3. Neonatal
   a. Birth date
   b. Birth weight
      i. Apgar scores
      ii. Delivery room intervention
      iii. Feeding problems
         (a) Noninterest, ineffective, slow eater
         (b) Tachypnea, diaphoresis (Pelech, 1999)
      iv. Presence of murmur noted
   c. Presence of a congenital syndrome
      i. Down syndrome associated with cardiac defects in 40% of cases
      ii. Fetal alcohol syndrome associated with atrial or ventricular septal defects
      iii. Marfan syndrome associated with serious aortic defects
      iv. Noonan's syndrome associated with many cardiac defects and cardio-myopathy
   d. Gender
      i. Certain cardiac malformations maintain a sex predilection
4. Past medical history
   a. Growth patterns and developmental milestones
      i. Delay in weight increase more than height increase
      ii. Fatigue or exercise intolerance
      iii. Developmental milestones requiring muscle strength may be delayed (Johnson & Moller, 2001)
   b. Previous illness and/or hospitalizations
   c. Respiratory illness, especially pneumonia
4. Current health status
   a. Activity level and tolerance
   b. Airway issue
      i. Stridor or dysphagia with food
      ii. Work of breathing, cough, tachypnea, dyspnea
   c. Cardiovascular issues—cyanosis, tachycardia, arrhythmia
   d. Age—some cardiac murmurs or symptoms become evident at different ages
      i. Neonatal—congenital aortic stenosis and pulmonary stenosis
      ii. 4 to 6 weeks—ventricular septal defect
      iii. Preschool—atrial septal defect
   e. Risk factors for cardiovascular disease that may manifest in adolescence or adulthood
      i. Tobacco use
      ii. Hypercholesterolemia
      iii. Obesity
      iv. Poor nutrition
      v. Minimal exercise
      vi. Family history
5. Family history
   a. Siblings and other family members with:
      i. Genetic or congenital syndromes
      ii. Cardiac lesions
      iii. Sudden death
      iv. Hearing loss (Pelech, 1999)
   b. Compare growth and development data from siblings, parents, and grandparents (Johnson & Moller, 2001)

# FOCUSED PHYSICAL EXAMINATION

1. Normative values
   a. Vital signs
      i. Blood pressure (BP)
         (a) National High Blood Pressure Education Program Working Group on High Blood Pressure in Children and Adolescents (NHBPEP, 2004)
            (1) Published the *Fourth Report on the Diagnosis, Evaluation and Treatment of High Blood Pressure in Children and Adolescents*
            (2) Provides guidelines for detection, evaluation, and management of hypertension in children and adolescents
            (3) Updated BP tables for children and adolescents available on the Internet at www.nhlbi.nih.gov/guidelines/hypertension/child_tbl.htm
               a) Based on revised child height percentiles on new growth charts from Centers for Disease Control and Prevention (CDC)
               b) Includes BP data from the 1999–2000 NHANES study
               c) 50th, 90th, 95th, and 99th percentiles for systolic blood pressure (SBP) and diastolic blood pressure (DBP) according to height, sex, and age are given for boys and girls
            (4) Abnormal values
               a) Hypertension
                  i) ≥3 occasions of average systolic and/or diastolic BP that is ≥95th percentile for gender, age, and height
               b) Prehypertension
                  i) ≥90th but <95th percentiles
                  ii) Adolescents with BP levels ≥120/80 mm Hg
                  iii) Recheck in 6 months
               c) See Chapter 29 for information on management of hypertension
      ii. Pulse volume (pressure) (Roy, 2003)
         (a) The difference of the systolic and diastolic pressures
         (b) If pulse volume is increased:
            (1) Hyperkinetic circulation
            (2) Aortic insufficiency
            (3) Patent ductus arteriosus
      iii. Pulse
         (a) Note rate, rhythm, and quality
         (b) See Table 7-1 for normal pulse rates in children at rest
      iv. Respiratory rate and effort
         (a) See Chapter 6
2. Inspection (Allen, et al., 2001; Barkauskas, et al., 2003)
   a. Examine child's general physical characteristics for indication of syndromes
      i. Fetal alcohol syndrome
      ii. Down syndrome
      iii. Marfan syndrome
      iv. Noonan's syndrome
   b. Color
      i. Pink versus cyanotic
         (a) Lips
         (b) Nail beds

■ **TABLE 7-1**
■ ■ **Normal Pulse Rates in Children at Rest**

| Age | Resting (Awake) | Resting (Asleep) | Exercise and Fever |
|---|---|---|---|
| Birth | 100-180 | 80-160 | Up to 220 |
| 1-3 months | 100-220 | 80-180 | Up to 220 |
| 3-48 months | 80-150 | 70-120 | Up to 200 |
| 2-10 years | 70-110 | 60-100 | Up to 180 |
| greater than 10 years | 55-90 | 50-90 | Up to 180 |

From Engel, J. (2002). *Pocket guide to pediatric assessment.* St. Louis: Mosby, p. 81.

    **c.** Clubbing of fingers
      **i.** Nail root—skin angle is flattened
      **ii.** Tip of finger is shiny
      **iii.** Best seen with the digit in the lateral projection (Bernstein, 2004)
    **d.** Mucous membranes
    **e.** Poor perfusion, mottling
    **f.** Breathing
      **i.** Comfortable
      **ii.** Observe for respiratory distress
        (a) Tachypnea
        (b) Retractions
        (c) Diaphoresis
    **g.** Edema
      **i.** Facial
      **ii.** Extremities
    **h.** Chest
      **i.** Symmetry
      **ii.** Cardiac hyperdynamics; abnormally increased muscular activity
      **iii.** Apical pulse (Bickley & Szilagyi, 2004)
      **iv.** Look for precordial bulge
**3.** Palpation (Allen, et al., 2001; Barkauskas, et al., 2003; Seidel, et al., 2003; Roy, 2003)
    **a.** Point of maximal impulse (PMI)
      **i.** Infants and children less than age 4—fourth intercostal space at midclavicular line
      **ii.** At 7 years, fifth intercostal space at the midclavicular line
      **iii.** Location (left vs right)
      **iv.** Impulse quality (Bickley & Szilagyi, 2004; Engel, 2002)
        (a) 0 Not palpable
        (b) +1 Thready, difficult to find, easy to obliterate
        (c) +2 Difficult to find, pressure may obliterate
        (d) +3 Normal; easy to find, difficult to obliterate
        (e) +4 Bounding, strong, cannot be obliterated
      **v.** Rate (see Table 7-1)
    **b.** Thrills (Johnson & Moller, 2001)
      **i.** Use palmar surfaces of the metacarpophalangeal and proximal interphalangeal joints to assess

       **ii.** Coarse, low-frequency vibrations

       **iii.** Occur in same area as maximum sound of a murmur

   **c.** Heaves

       **i.** Forceful outward movements

       **ii.** Indicate ventricular hypertrophy

   **d.** Peripheral pulses

       **i.** Technique

          (a) Use first and second digits of dominant hand

          (b) Check both extremities

          (c) Note presence and quality of pulses (Pelech, 1999)

             (1) Strength

             (2) Regularity

             (3) Rate

       **ii.** Start with brachial pulses

          (a) Closest to heart

          (b) Truer in quality

          (c) Palpate just above the antecubital fossa

          (d) Older children—support the child's right arm with your left, and palpate

       **iii.** Ulnar

       **iv.** Femoral

       **v.** Posterior tibial

       **vi.** Palpate radial and femoral pulses simultaneously

          (a) Should be in synchrony

          (b) Delay of the femoral pulse suggests coarctation of the aorta (Hoffman, 2002)

   **e.** Abdomen

       **i.** Palpate liver edge

          (a) Enlargement

          (b) Signs of congestive heart failure

   **f.** Capillary refill (Hoffman, 2002)

       **i.** Should not be greater than 3 seconds

       **ii.** Time increases with heart failure and shock

**4.** Auscultation (Allen, et al., 2001; Barkauskas, et al., 2003; Seidel, et al., 2003; Roy, 2003)

   **a.** Decide best time to auscultate

       **i.** A quiet child and quiet environment are needed

       **ii.** Auscultate first if infant is sleeping

       **iii.** Auscultate last if toddler is apprehensive and needs time to "warm up" to examiner

   **b.** Position

       **i.** Ages 1 to 3 years best in parent's lap

       **ii.** Older children in sitting position

   **c.** Technique

       **i.** Stethoscope

          (a) Warmed stethoscope

          (b) Best size in pediatrics is ¾-inch bell and 1-inch diaphragm

          (c) Place diaphragm with moderate pressure to hear

             (1) High-pitched murmurs

             (2) First and second heart sounds

          (d) Place bell with light pressure, just enough to make contact to hear

(1) Low-pitched murmurs
(2) Third heart sound
ii. Systematic, orderly manner with bell and diaphragm
    (a) Anatomic location of heart sounds (Figure 7-1)
    (b) Area where value closure is best heard (Bickley & Szilagyi, 2004)
        (1) Mitral—apex, fifth left intercostal space at midclavicular line
        (2) Triscupid—left sternal border at fourth left intercostal space
        (3) Pulmonic—second left intercostal space at sternal border
        (4) Aortic—second right intercostal space at sternal border
    (c) Note quality and clarity of $S_1$, $S_2$
    (d) Presence and sound of any murmur
    (e) Rate and rhythm
        (1) All areas of valve closure
        (2) Axilla
        (3) Back (Bickley & Szaligyi, 2004)
iii. First heart sound ($S_1$)
    (a) Sound of the closure of the mitral and tricuspid valves
    (b) Marks beginning of systole (ventricular contraction) (Bickley & Szilagyi, 2004)
    (c) Best auscultated at the apex
    (d) Usually single
    (e) Loud $S_1$ heard with:
        (1) Mitral stenosis
        (2) Shortened P-R interval, such as tachycardia (Hoffman, 2002)
iv. Second heart sound ($S_2$)
    (a) Comprised of two sounds occurring in close proximity to each other
    (b) Marks beginning of diastole (atrial contraction)
        (1) Closure
            a) Aortic valve ($A_2$)
            b) Pulmonic valve ($P_2$)
    (c) $A_2$ is normally louder than $P_2$
        (1) Higher pressures in the aortic circuit than the pulmonary circuit

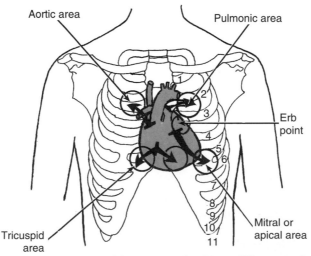

FIGURE 7-1 ■ Anatomic location of heart sounds. (From Wong, et al., 1999. *Whaley & Wong's nursing care of infants and children* [6th ed.]. St. Louis: Mosby, Figure 7-40.)

(d) Auscultate for the splitting of $A_2$ and $P_2$ ("lub d-dub")
- (1) Best accomplished on the left second or third intercostal space (Bickley & Szilagyi, 2004)
- (2) Heard in most infants and children
- (3) Widens with inspiration

(e) Widened split of $S_2$
- (1) Atrial septal defect
- (2) Pulmonic stenosis

(f) Absence of any split
- (1) Atresia
- (2) Severe stenosis of aortic or pulmonic valves (Hoffman, 2003)

v. Third heart sound ($S_3$) (Johnson & Moller, 2001)
- (a) Normally present in one third to one half of children
- (b) Accentuated in pathologic conditions
- (c) Heard early in diastole
- (d) Origin is transition from rapid to slow filling phase

d. Murmur—turbulent blood flow that causes cardiac structures and vasculature to vibrate
- i. When assessing murmurs, note:
  - (a) Timing—location in cardiac cycle
    - (1) Systolic
    - (2) Diastolic
    - (3) Continuous
  - (b) Thorax location of murmur
  - (c) Radiation of murmur
  - (d) Loudness—graded I to VI out of VI
    - (1) I is very soft and heard only with very careful listening
    - (2) IV is accompanied by a thrill
    - (3) VI is very loud and heard with stethoscope held off the chest
  - (e) Pitch
    - (1) Low
    - (2) Medium
    - (3) High
  - (f) Character
- ii. Innocent murmurs are defined as normal turbulence and not indicative of any heart disease (Hoffman, 2003)
  - (a) Certain characteristics
  - (b) Grade I or II in volume
  - (c) Vibratory in nature
  - (d) Change with position of child
  - (e) Never harsh
  - (f) No radiation
  - (g) Never in diastole
    - (1) Still's murmur
      - a) Most common 2 to 6 years
      - b) Musical/vibratory quality
      - c) Systolic ejection murmur
      - d) Low in pitch
      - e) Located generally left lower sternal border
      - f) Loudest when supine
      - g) Many theories to its etiology, none proven

      (2) Venous hum
         a) Continuous, low-pitched sound heard above or below the clavicles
         b) Originates in the internal jugular vein
         c) Most common 2 to 8 years
         d) Right upper sternal edge
         e) Best heard when child sits
         f) Altered with:
            i) Turning head to side
            ii) Child lying down
         g) Continuous murmur—attributed to blood draining down the jugular veins (Hoffman, 2003)
      (3) Carotid bruit
         a) Quiet systolic ejection murmur
         b) Heard over carotids on neck
         c) Decreases in volume as auscultation proceeds closer to the aortic and pulmonic areas
      (4) Peripheral pulmonic stenosis
         a) Most common in infants up to 6 months
         b) Loudest
            i) Left upper sternal border
            ii) Axillae
         c) Blowing in nature
         d) Relatively high in pitch
            i) Due to the small size of the pulmonary arteries
            ii) And the acute angles coming off of the larger main pulmonary artery (Hoffman, 2003)
   iii. Note that some functional murmurs resolve when the underlying condition resolves, e.g. anemia, fever
   iv. Refer to a pediatric cardiologist
      (a) Murmurs that do not fit the innocent murmur patterns (see Chapter 29)
      (b) Other abnormalities in the cardiovascular exam
      (c) A potential pathologic condition is suspected
   v. Blood pressure (BP) (Arafat & Mattoo, 1999; NHBPEP, 2004)
      (a) Children older than age 3 who are seen in a medical setting should have their BP measured
      (b) Children younger than age 3 with special circumstances should have their BP measured (Box 7-1)
      (c) Equipment
         (1) See Table 7-2 for cuff sizes
         (2) The inflatable bladder in the cuff must be able to encircle the arm by at least 80%
         (3) Mercury manometers pose a biohazard and should be removed from clinics and offices
         (4) Aneroid manometers are accurate if calibrated semiannually
      (d) Methods
         (1) Manual
            a) Auscultation—BP tables are based on auscultation method
            b) Flush method
            c) Palpation
         (2) Automated
            a) Preferred method for newborns and young infants
            b) If BP is greater than 90th percentile, repeat by auscultation

■ **BOX 7-1**
■ **CONDITIONS UNDER WHICH CHILDREN YOUNGER THAN 3 YEARS OLD SHOULD HAVE BP MEASURED**

- History of prematurity, very low birth weight, or other neonatal complication requiring intensive care
- Congenital heart disease (repaired or nonrepaired)
- Recurrent urinary tract infections, hematuria, or proteinuria
- Known renal disease or urologic malformations
- Family history of congenital renal disease
- Solid-organ transplant
- Malignancy or bone marrow transplant
- Treatment with drugs known to raise BP
- Other systemic illnesses associated with hypertension (neurofibromatosis, tuberous sclerosis, etc)
- Evidence of elevated intracranial pressure

From the National High Blood Pressure Education Program (NHBPEP) working group on high blood pressure in children and adolescents (2004). Fourth report on the diagnosis, evaluation and treatment of high blood pressure in children and adolescents. *Pediatrics, 114*(2), 555-576.

 

   (3) Ambulatory BP monitor
      a) Requires staff who are trained in its use and interpretation
      b) Used for "white coat hypertension"—BP levels greater than 95th percentile in office, but normotensive at home
      c) Use a portable device that monitors BP for 24-hour period for diagnosis
  **e. Lungs**
    **i.** Lungs often have compensatory findings due to increased cardiac work or failure
      (a) Auscultate all lung fields (see Chapter 6 for detail)
      (b) Lung sounds
      (c) Quality
      (d) Respiratory effort (Bickley & Szilagyi, 2004)

 

■ **TABLE 7-2**
■ ■ **Recommended Dimensions for BP Cuff Bladders**

| Age Range | Width (cm) | Length (cm) | Maximum Arm Circumference (cm) |
|---|---|---|---|
| Newborn | 4 | 8 | 10 |
| Infant | 6 | 12 | 15 |
| Child | 9 | 18 | 22 |
| Small adult | 10 | 24 | 26 |
| Adult | 13 | 30 | 34 |
| Large adult | 16 | 38 | 44 |
| Thigh | 20 | 42 | 52 |

From the National High Blood Pressure Education Program (NHBPEP) working group on high blood pressure in children and adolescents (2004). Fourth report on the diagnosis, evaluation and treatment of high blood pressure in children and adolescents. *Pediatrics, 114*(2), 555-576.

# REFERENCES

Allen, H., Phillips, J., Chan, D. (2001). History and physical examination. In H. Allen, H. Gutgesell, E. Clark, & D. Driscoll (Eds.). *Moss and Adams' heart disease in infants, children, and adolescents, volume 1* (6th ed.). Philadelphia: Lippincott Williams & Wilkins.

Arafat, M., & Mattoo, T. (1999). Measurement of blood pressure in children: Recommendations and perceptions on cuff selection, *Pediatrics, 104,* 30-34.

Barkauskas, V., Baumann, L. & Darling-Fisher, C. (2002). *Health and physical assessment* (3rd ed.). Philadelphia: Elsevier.

Bernstein, D. (2004). Evaluation of the cardiovascular system. In R. Behrman, R. Kliegman, & H. Jenson (Eds.). *Nelson textbook of pediatrics* (17th ed.). Philadelphia: Saunders, pp. 1481-1498.

Bickley, L., & Szilagyi. P. (2004). *Bates' guide to physical examination & history taking* (8th ed.). Philadelphia: Lippincott.

Engel, J. (2002). *Pocket guide to pediatric assessment*. St. Louis: Mosby.

Hoffman, J. (2003). The circulatory system. In A. M. Rudolph & C. D. Rudolph (Eds.). *Rudolph's pediatrics* (21st ed.). New York: McGraw-Hill, pp. 1745-1904.

Johnson, W., & Moller, J. (2001). *Pediatric cardiology*. Philadelphia: Lippincott Williams & Wilkins.

Larsen, W. J. (2001). *Human embryology*. New York: Churchill Livingstone.

Moore, K. L., & Persaud, T V. N. (2003). *The developing human: Clinically oriented embryology*. Philadelphia: Saunders.

National High Blood Pressure Education Program (NHBPEP) working group on high blood pressure in children and adolescents (2004). Fourth report on the diagnosis, evaluation and treatment of high blood pressure in children and adolescents. *Pediatrics, 114*(2), 555-576.

Pelech, A. N. (1999). Evaluation of the pediatric patient with a cardiac murmur. *Pediatr Clin North Am, 46,* 167-188.

Roy, D. (2003). Cardiovascular assessment of infants and children. In R. Goldbloom (Ed.). *Pediatric clinical skills* (3rd ed.). Philadelphia: Saunders, pp. 169-190.

Seidel, H., Ball, J., Dains, J. & Benedict, G. (2003). Mosby's guide to physical examination (5th ed.). St. Louis: Mosby.

# Assessment of the Gastrointestinal System

LEIGH SMALL, PhD, RN, CPNP

## FETAL DEVELOPMENT

1. Embryology, structure, and function of the gastrointestinal system (Larsen, 2001; Moore & Persaud, 2003)
   a. Week 4—head, tail, and lateral folds incorporate the dorsal part of the yolk sac into the embryo to form the primitive gut, which has three significant areas:
      i. Foregut
         (a) Develops into the primitive pharynx, oral cavity, and upper respiratory system
         (b) Development of the tracheoesophageal septum causes esophagus to separate from the pharynx; completed by week 7
         (c) Esophagus has striated muscle in top one third, and smooth muscle in lower one third, both innervated by vagus nerve (cranial nerve X)
         (d) Stomach derives from the caudal end of the foregut, forming a convex curvature, and rotating around its longitudinal axis by end of week 7
         (e) Liver, gallbladder, and pancreas form from caudal end of foregut
         (f) Duodenum forms a C-shaped loop from the caudal end of foregut and cranial end of midgut
      ii. Midgut
         (a) End of week 5, small intestine herniates into the umbilical cord due to lack of space (liver and kidneys are very large)
         (b) During week 10, liver and kidneys decrease in relative size so that intestines can return to the midgut
         (c) Ascending colon, descending colon, cecum, and appendix lengthen and fixate in the midgut
      iii. Hindgut
         (a) Urorectal septum separates the urinary bladder from the rectum by end of week 6

## FOCUSED HISTORY

1. Focused history (Burns, et al., 2004; Fox, 2003; Schwartz, 2003)
   a. Birth history

       **i.** Weeks of gestation
      **ii.** Apgar
     **iii.** Length of newborn hospital stay
     **iv.** Pattern of weight gain
      **v.** Neonatal nutrition
         (a) Nasogastric
         (b) Orogastric feedings
         (c) Total parenteral nutrition
         (d) Breast-fed or type of formula
         (e) Spitting up/vomiting
            (1) Amount
            (2) Frequency
            (3) Duration
      **vi.** Episodes of apnea
     **vii.** History of bowel movements shortly after birth
         (a) Passage of meconium plug
         (b) Color, consistency, frequency of stools
  **b.** Child or family health history
       **i.** Place of family origin
      **ii.** Stomach problems
         (a) Pyloric stenosis
         (b) Ulcers
         (c) Gastroesophageal reflux
     **iii.** Intestinal problems
         (a) Melena—black, tarry, foul-smelling stools
         (b) Hematochezia—red or maroon stools
         (c) Pain before, during, or after bowel movement
         (d) Irritable bowel syndrome—functional GI disease; pain and altered bowel habits
         (e) Inflammatory bowel disease, e.g., Crohn's disease, ulcerative colitis
         (f) Intussusception—portion of the bowel telescopes into adjacent portion of bowel
         (g) Appendicitis
         (h) Diverticulosis (outpouching of bowel); diverticulitis (inflammation of pouch)
         (i) Intestinal cancer
         (j) Celiac disease—genetic autoimmune disorder; gluten proteins damage small intestine
         (k) Familial polyposis
            (1) Gardener's syndrome—rare, hereditary disorder involving multiple polyps in the colon; patients also develop bone and soft tissue tumors
            (2) Peutz-Jeghers syndrome—autosomal dominant hereditary disorder characterized by brown or black spots on the lips and inside the mouth; small percentage of patients develop cancer of the gut, breasts, or ovaries
      **iv.** Liver problems
         (a) Hepatitis
         (b) Wilson's disease—genetic disorder that results in excessive accumulation of copper in many parts of the body, particularly the liver and the brain; can be fatal if not treated
         (c) Gilbert's disease—multifactorial inherited disorder that affects the way bilirubin is processed by the liver and causes inconsequential, fluctuating low levels of jaundice

      (d) Hemochromatosis—an inherited disorder that causes the body to absorb and store too much iron. The extra iron builds up in organs and damages them. Without treatment, the disease can cause these organs to fail

      (e) Cirrhosis

      (f) Transplant

   v. Pancreatic problems

      (a) Pancreatitis

      (b) Diabetes, type 1, type 2 and Cystic Fibrosis Related Diabetes (CFRD)

      (c) Cystic fibrosis

  vi. Gallbladder problems

      (a) Cholecystitis

      (b) Cholelithiasis

  vii. Inborn errors of metabolism

 viii. Allergy

      (a) Food allergy

      (b) Asthma

      (c) Eczema

      (d) Hay fever

  ix. Intolerance

      (a) Carbohydrate intolerance/sensitivity

      (b) Lactose intolerance

   x. Abdominal surgery

      (a) Request surgical reports

c. Child's current medical history and symptoms

   i. Bowel status—all ages

      (a) Frequency

      (b) Color

      (c) Consistency

        (1) Obstipation—hard stools every 3 to 5 days

        (2) Constipation—difficulty passing hard, dry stools

      (d) Tenesmus—straining to pass stools

      (e) Diarrhea

      (f) Urgency

      (g) Flatulence, distention

      (h) Change in bowel pattern

      (i) Use of laxatives

  ii. Feeding issues—all ages

      (a) Change in appetite

      (b) Indigestion

      (c) Nausea

      (d) Vomiting

      (e) Anorexia

      (f) Polyphagia

      (g) Eructation (belching)

      (h) Dehydration

      (i) Recent or longitudinal weight loss or gain

      (j) Food avoidance

      (k) Family dietary practices

  iii. Past and current use of medications—prescription, over-the-counter, herbal supplements

  iv. Immunization history—all ages

      (a) Hepatitis A and B status

      (b) Status of other immunizations

     **v.** Social history
        (a) Recent travel
        (b) Recent moves
        (c) Exposure to polluted drinking water, source of drinking water
        (d) Sanitation problems
        (e) Family stressors or family changes
            (1) New or changed parental relationship
            (2) Newly diagnosed illness or death of a relative
            (3) Death of a pet
        (f) Personal or academic stressors
        (g) Change in social relationships
    **vi.** Neonatal period
        (a) Request results from required newborn screening tests
        (b) Hyperbilirubinemia
        (c) Necrotizing enterocolitis
        (d) Gastroesophageal reflux
        (e) Hirschsprung's disease
        (f) Total parenteral nutrition therapy
   **vii.** Infancy
        (a) Colic, irritability
        (b) Pyloric stenosis
        (c) Growth patterns
        (d) Failure to thrive
        (e) Gastroesophageal reflux
  **viii.** Childhood, adolescence
        (a) Abdominal pain
        (b) Hemorrhoids
        (c) Encopresis
        (d) Blood disorders
            (1) Anemia
            (2) Hepatitis
            (3) Elevated lead levels
        (e) Alcohol or substance abuse/dependence or treatment
        (f) Migraines
        (g) Anxiety or other mood disorders
        (h) Heart disease
        (i) Diabetes
        (j) Thyroid disease

## FOCUSED EXAMINATION

**1.** Focused examination (Bickley & Szilagyi, 2003; Boynton, et al., 2003; Colyar, 2003; Goldbloom, 2003)
  **a.** Measurement
    **i.** Anthropometric measures—record and note patterns of change
        (a) Height/length and percentiles
        (b) Weight and percentiles
        (c) Weight for height/length and percentiles
        (d) Head circumference and percentiles
        (e) Body mass index (BMI) and percentiles
        (f) Waist circumference
        (g) Skinfold measurement (special training required)

    ii. Complete nutritional assessment
       (a) Breast and/or formula—amount, calories per day
       (b) Intake of major food groups
         (1) Compare with minimum daily requirements for age
       (c) Frequency of meals
       (d) Nutritional supplements
 **b.** Inspection
    **i.** Appearance
       (a) Underweight, average, overweight, obese
       (b) Color
         (1) Jaundice (i.e., icterus); scleral, skin
         (2) Spider nevi on face, neck, upper trunk
         (3) Palmar erythema
       (c) Hydration
       (d) Comfort
    **ii.** Systematic inspection
       (a) Patient's head toward the examiner's dominant hand
       (b) Legs flexed at a 45-degree angle
       (c) Divide abdomen into four quadrants
       (d) Proceed with a consistent systematic assessment pattern (i.e., clockwise, counterclockwise)
       (e) Visualize underlying organs (Table 8-1)
    **iii.** View abdomen at two angles to aid inspection
       (a) Facing the child's abdomen
         (1) Observe overlying skin
           a) Asymmetric venous patterns
           b) Hair growth

### ■ TABLE 8-1
### ■ ■ Location of Abdominal Organs by Quadrant

| Location/Quadrant | Organ |
| --- | --- |
| Right upper quadrant | Liver and gallbladder |
| | Duodenum and part of the ascending and transverse colon |
| | Head of the pancreas |
| | Right kidney |
| Left upper quadrant | Stomach |
| | Spleen |
| | Left lobe of the liver |
| | Body of the pancreas |
| | Left kidney |
| | Part of the transverse and descending colon |
| Right lower quadrant | Right ureter |
| | Right ovary |
| | Right spermatic cord |
| Left lower quadrant | Left ureter |
| | Left ovary |
| | Left spermatic cord |
| | Part of the descending colon |
| | Sigmoid colon |
| Midline | Aorta |
| | Uterus |
| | Bladder |
| | Umbilicus |

         (2) Note pulsations—common in thin children

         (3) Masses

         (4) Umbilicus

            a) Contour

            b) Location

            c) Signs of inflammation

            d) Herniation

      (b) A parallel viewing position

         (1) Contour of abdomen

            a) Flat

            b) Protuberant—common in toddlers

            c) Scaphoid, i.e., sunken, hollowed out

            d) Obese

         (2) Landmarks

            a) Xyphoid process

            b) Rib margins

            c) Ileac crests

            d) Pubic bone

            e) Umbilicus

      (c) Observe for:

         (1) Pulsations—common in thin children

         (2) Peristaltic waves

         (3) Abdominal breathing—common in children younger than 6 or 7 years of age

         (4) Absence of movement requires further investigation

         (5) Striae

         (6) Rashes, lesions

         (7) Scars

         (8) Diastasis recti—bulge between rectus muscles

         (9) Epigastric hernia

    **iv.** Notable skin manifestations

      (a) Jaundice

      (b) Pallor

      (c) Diaphoresis

      (d) Capillary hemangiomas (infants)

      (e) Skin rashes or nodules

  **c.** Auscultation

    **i.** General information

      (a) Use diaphragm of stethoscope

      (b) Proceed systematically (i.e., clockwise) to every quadrant

    **ii.** Listen for bowel sounds

      (a) Location

         (1) In all four quadrants (see Table 8-1)

         (2) Epigastrium

      (b) Normal bowel sounds occur 5 to 34 times each minute

      (c) Describe

         (1) Location

         (2) Pattern of sounds

         (3) Pitch

      (d) Specific types

         (1) Borborygmi—Loud bowel sounds

         (2) Hyperperistalsis—May be normal but may also be abnormal

   (3) High-pitched, frequent bowel sounds may indicate:
    a) Early peritonitis
    b) Gastroenteritis
    c) Intestinal obstruction
   (4) Absence of bowel sounds for greater than 3 minutes of continuous auscultation may indicate:
    a) Peritonitis
    b) Intestinal obstruction
   (5) Example of findings: high-pitched bowel sounds occurring less than every 2 seconds in all four quadrants
  **iii.** Listen for audible heart sounds in the four quadrants
   (a) Not normally audible unless the patient has a scaphoid abdomen
   (b) Murmurs or bruits near the renal, iliac, or abdominal aortic arteries are not normal
   (c) Listen over solid organs (i.e., liver and spleen) when indicated
   (d) Listen for friction rubs
  **iv.** Auscultation of the liver
   (a) Technique
    (1) Place stethoscope below the xyphoid
    (2) Begin "scratching" the overlying skin in the lower left quadrant of the abdomen
    (3) Move toward the chest
   (b) Usual finding—There will be a change in the sound generated from the scratching as the examiner passes over the intestinal area and progresses over the liver
   (c) Unusual finding—Hepatomegaly (see following discussion under *Palpation of the Liver*)
 **d.** Palpation
  **i.** General information
   (a) Proceed systematically (i.e., clockwise) to every quadrant
   (b) Light touch to deep touch
   (c) Repeat systematic assessment pattern (i.e., clockwise)
   (d) Use child's hand under yours if abdomen is sensitive
  **ii.** Light palpation in all four quadrants
   (a) ½- to 1-inch depressions pressing down and releasing slowly and then pressing down and releasing quickly
   (b) Purpose
    (1) Appreciate the temperature and pulsations
    (2) Identify muscular rigidity
    (3) Voluntary
    (4) Involuntary guarding
  **iii.** Repeat the pattern of assessment with deep palpation
   (a) 1- to 2-inch depressions pressing down and releasing slowly and then pressing down and releasing quickly
   (b) Purpose
    (1) Note areas that produce complaints of pain
    (2) Palpate painful areas with and without muscle flexion
    (3) New area of pain or chronic pain
    (4) Delineate painful areas
   (c) Unusual findings
    (1) McBurney's point—most tender area of the abdomen
    (2) CVAT—costovertebral angle tenderness

            (3) Muscular rigidity

            (4) Fluid waves

            (5) Masses

            (6) Rebound tenderness

  **iv.** Palpation of the liver

     (a) Technique

        (1) Support the liver by holding left hand behind the 11th and 12th ribs ("floating ribs")

        (2) Press down at the midclavicular line parallel to the umbilicus, and:

           a) Gently press down and toward the head

           b) Reposition right hand 2 to 3 cm toward the head

           c) Repeat procedure until the liver edge is felt

           d) Note size of liver in centimeters (Table 8-2)

     (b) Usual findings with palpation:

        (1) Firm, sharp, smooth liver edge 1 to 2 cm below the right costal margin

        (2) Infant's liver may be normally palpated 2 to 3 cm below the right costal margin

        (3) It is normal to **not** feel the liver edge or to only perceive fullness

     (c) Atypical findings

        (1) Hepatomegaly

           a) Liver edge greater than 2 cm below the right costal margin

           b) Round, firm liver edge

  **v.** Palpation of the spleen

     (a) Technique

        (1) Similar to the liver

        (2) Place left hand across patient over the left costovertebral angle

        (3) Press upward to lift the spleen toward anterior abdominal wall

        (4) Palpate with fingers of right hand as patient takes a deep breath

        (5) Feel for the edge of spleen, beginning below the left costal margin

     (b) Usual findings with palpation—normally only palpated in the first years of life

     (c) Atypical findings

        (1) Splenomegaly

        (2) Spleen is felt when it had not been palpated before

  **vi.** Rectal examination (only if indicated by history and symptoms)

     (a) Explain the procedure to the child

     (b) Gently insert gloved, lubricated finger into anal opening

     (c) Rectum is normally empty of stool

     (d) Feel for impacted stool or mass, sphincter tone, length of anal sphincter, anal fissures, hemorrhoids

---

■ **TABLE 8-2**
■ ■ **Normal Liver Size in Children**

| Age | Liver Span |
| --- | --- |
| 6 months | 2 cm |
| 3 years | 4 cm |
| 10 years | 6 cm |
| Adult | 8 cm |

      **vii.** Skin

        (a) Capillary refill

        (b) Skin turgor

  **e.** Percussion

    **i.** Generalized tympanic sound of free air in the abdomen

      (a) Normal

    **ii.** Generalized dullness

      (a) Suspect ascites

    **iii.** Gastric bubble

      (a) Location—left lower anterior ribs

      (b) Usual sound with percussion is tympani

    **iv.** Spleen

      (a) Tympani should be elicited in the last rib space (before the 10th rib) in the left anterior axillary line

      (b) A large inhaled breath by the patient causes splenic displacement

      (c) Continue to percuss at the same space during inspiration

      (d) Usual sound with percussion—continued tympani

      (e) Atypical findings—a shift to dull sounds with inspiration indicates splenic enlargement

    **v.** Liver

      (a) Begin at the right midclavicular line below the level of the umbilicus where there is tympani and percuss toward the head to find the lower border of the liver (dull sound)

      (b) Next start at the midclavicular line in the lung fields and percuss toward the feet to find the superior liver border (dull sound)

      (c) Space between these two measures is the liver height or vertical span

      (d) This process of outlining the liver may be repeated at the midsternal line if the size appears abnormal

---

## REFERENCES

Bickley, L. S., & Szilagyi, P.G. (2003). *Bates' guide to physical examination and history taking* (8th ed.). New York: Lippincott Williams & Wilkins.

Boynton, R.W., Dunn, E. S., Stephens, G. R., & Pulcini, J. (2003). *Manual of ambulatory pediatrics* (5th ed.). New York: Lippincott Williams & Wilkins.

Burns, C. E., Brady, M. A., Blosser, C., et al. (2004). *Pediatric primary care: A handbook for nurse practitioners* (3rd ed.). New York: Saunders.

Colyar, M. R. (2003). *Well-child assessment for primary care providers.* Philadelphia: F. A. Davis.

Fox, J. A. (2003). *Primary health care of infants, children, & adolescents* (2nd ed.). St. Louis: Mosby.

Goldbloom, R. B. (2003). *Pediatric clinical skills* (3rd ed.). Philadelphia: Saunders.

Larsen, W. J. (2001). *Human embryology.* New York: Churchill Livingstone.

Moore, K. L., & Persaud, T. V. N. (2003). *The developing human: Clinically oriented embryology.* Philadelphia: Saunders.

Schwartz, M. W. (2003). *Clinical handbook of pediatrics* (3rd ed.). New York: Lippincott Williams & Wilkins.

# Assessment of the Reproductive and Urologic Systems

GAIL HORNOR, RNC, MS, CPNP

## FETAL DEVELOPMENT (MOORE & PERSAUD, 2003)

1. Urinary structures arise from intermediate mesoderm
   a. 24 days to 16 weeks of gestation—differentiation into ureters and kidneys
   b. 6 to 9 weeks—kidneys ascend to lumbar area
   c. 10 to 12 weeks—nephrons become functional when they connect to the collecting ducts
   d. 14 weeks—urogenital folds enclose the urethra within penis (male) or remain separate to form labia minora (female)
   e. 32 to 38 weeks—collecting duct system matures
2. Genital structures arise from primordial germ cells that migrate from yolk sac to posterior body wall
   a. 5 to 6 weeks—germ cells form genital ridges
   b. SRY (sex determining region of Y chromosome) is expressed in sex cord cells of male and causes a developmental cascade of male characteristics
   c. Absence of SRY causes a developmental cascade of female characteristics
   d. 7 to 13 weeks—follicle cells and bulbourethral glands, uterus and vagina form
   e. 10 to 13 weeks—prostate, seminal vesicles develop; testes are in inguinal canal
   f. 7 to 9 months—testes descend into scrotum

## FOCUSED HISTORY

1. Birth
   a. Abnormalities noted at birth, e.g., genitourinary, ears, heart (see Chapters 31 and 40)
   b. Urination difficulties in first 24 hours
2. Past medical
   a. Present or past history of genitourinary problems (see Chapter 31)
3. Current health
   a. Current medications
   b. Vital signs
   c. Height/weight/BMI

4. Family
   a. History of congenital anomalies in any close relative
   b. Urologic disease—hydronephrosis, polycystic kidney disease, urethral reflux, neuroblastoma, etc
   c. Reproductive disease—cancer, ovarian cysts, infertility, endometriosis, etc.
5. Social history and habits
   a. Toilet training
      i. Age initiated and completed
      ii. Enuresis—daytime, nocturnal, frequency, methods used to control enuresis
      iii. Any unusual behaviors associated with urination—purposefully urinating in inappropriate places or refusing to urinate in the toilet
   b. Sexuality and sexual behaviors
      i. Sexual abuse—any sexual act, including pornography, involving a child who is unable to give consent
      ii. Questions that elicit information about sexual abuse
         (a) Do you have parts of your body that no one is supposed to look at, touch, kiss, or tickle?
         (b) What do you call those body parts?
         (c) Has anyone ever touched, tickled, kissed, or hurt those body parts?
      iii. Prepubertal (Box 9-1)
         (a) Common, normal sexual behaviors
         (b) Sexually acting out behaviors that raise the index of suspicion for sexual abuse or psychologic disorder (Hornor, 2002)
      iv. Pubertal
         (a) Consensual sexual activity—age of sexual partners, number of partners, gender of partner, use of "safe sex" practices, and birth control
   c. Genital care practices (Box 9-2) (Hornor & Ryan-Wenger, 1999)
      i. Questions to elicit information about genital care practices
      ii. Evaluate whether the practices are age appropriate or indicate unnecessary emphasis on genital care

## ■ BOX 9-1
## ■ NORMAL AND ABNORMAL SEXUAL BEHAVIORS IN CHILDREN

**COMMON, NORMAL SEXUAL BEHAVIORS IN PREPUBERTAL CHILDREN**
Masturbation
Touching own genitals
Touching mother's breasts
Sex play (touching and looking at genitals) between age-mates (<4 years' age difference)

**SEXUAL BEHAVIORS THAT RAISE THE INDEX OF SUSPICION FOR SEXUAL ABUSE OR PSYCHOLOGIC DISORDER**
Object insertion into own vagina or anus
Sex play involving one or more of the following:
   Four years or greater age difference between children
   Oral-genital contact
   Anal-genital contact
   Genital-genital contact
   Digital penetration of vagina/anus
   Object penetration of vagina/anus
   Use of force, threat, or bribe
Age-inappropriate sexual knowledge

■ **BOX 9-2**
■ **QUESTIONS THAT ELICIT INFORMATION ABOUT GENITAL CARE PRACTICES**

> ■ Is your child able to wipe himself or herself after toileting without help, or are you involved in some aspects of his or her care related to toileting needs?
> ■ Does your child bathe himself or herself entirely, or do you regularly perform some aspects of care during the child's bath or shower?
> ■ Describe how you bathe your child's genitalia.
> ■ Do you ever feel the need to inspect your child's genitals? Why?
> ■ Describe how the inspection of your child's genitals is done.
> ■ Do you ever use medications or creams on your child's genital or anal area? If so, how frequently do you use medications? Do you consult with a doctor or nurse before using creams or medications?

   d. Male circumcision (Alanis & Lucidi, 2004; Shoen et al., 2000)
      i. Cultural beliefs (Miller, 2002)
         (a) Circumcision is a cultural/religious tradition for Jews and Muslims
         (b) Circumcision has become a societal tradition in the United States (60% of males are circumcised at birth)
      ii. Research evidence on the advisability of circumcision (See Chapter 18, Section 12)
   e. Menarche—age of onset, regularity, duration, amount of flow, dysmenorrhea
   f. Female genital mutilation
      i. Female circumcision practiced in 26 African countries, in the Middle East, and Muslim populations of Indonesia and Malaysia
      ii. Approximately 80 to 110 million females affected
      iii. Usually performed between 4 and 10 years of age without anesthesia
      iv. Procedures vary from removal of part or all of clitoris and labia minora; labia majora is reapproximated to cover the urethra and introitus, leaving a small opening for passage of urine and menstrual blood
      v. Legs of the girl are bound from ankle to hip for up to 40 days to allow scar tissue to form
      vi. Surgical revision necessary prior to intercourse

## FOCUSED EXAMINATION

1. Preparation of the patient and family for the examination
   a. Explain genital exam to patient and family
   b. Anticipate adolescent embarrassment and apprehension (Elford & Spence, 2002)
   c. Remind younger children about when it is okay and not okay to allow someone to touch their genital area
   d. Maintain a calm, matter-of-fact attitude
   e. Allow parent or guardian in exam room with younger child
   f. Allow older child or adolescent to decide if parent is wanted in exam room
   g. Allow older child or adolescent to choose the gender of the examiner if possible
   h. Position patient in supine position on exam table or semireclining position in parent's lap
   i. A frog-leg position may be used for a younger child
   j. Universal precautions: wear gloves for genital exam

■ **BOX 9-3**
■ **CONGENITAL ANOMALIES AND INDICATIONS FOR REFERRAL**

- Exstrophy of bladder—eversion of posterior wall of the bladder; immediate referral to surgery or urology
- Ambiguous genitalia—abnormal sexual; a medical emergency; involves endocrine, genetics, urology, and surgery
- Hypospadias—urethra opens on ventral surface of penis or anywhere on penile shaft; refer to urology
- Epispadias—anterior urethra terminates on the dorsum of the penis; refer to urology
- Hydrocele—peritoneal fluid between the parietal and visceral layers of the tunica vaginalis, anterior to the testicle; if communicating form, amount of fluid fluctuates; refer to physician for surgical repair if no spontaneous resolution by 1 year
- Cryptorchidism—undescended testicles; refer to urology if bilateral and nonpalpable anywhere in canal; if unilateral refer to urology by 6 months (Kolon, 2006)
- Inguinal hernia—swelling in scrotal or inguinal area; processus vaginalis fails to obliterate; refer to surgery
- Chordee—downward concave curvature of penis; refer to urology

2. Inspection
  a. Congenital abnormalities and indications for referral (Box 9-3)
  b. Note the appearance of the male genitalia (Figure 9-1)
       i. Inspect the penis for bruising, swelling, erythema, lesions, rashes, or other irregularities
      ii. In infants and young children the foreskin is normally tight and not retracted during physical exam until approximately 6 years of age
     iii. Gently retract uncircumcised foreskin or prepuce if child is more than 6 years old

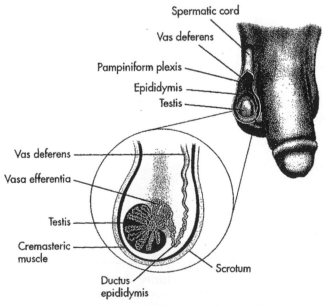

FIGURE 9-1 ■ Male external genitalia.

      **iv.** Never forcefully retract foreskin; doing so may damage tissue and cause adhesions between the foreskin and the glans

      **v.** Examine the urethral meatus for location and presence of discharge

      **vi.** Observe strength and direction of urinary stream if possible

      **vii.** Inspect the size and position of the scrotum and testicles

      **viii.** Note the Sexual Maturity Rating (Tanner stage) of male external genitalia (Figure 9-2)

          **(a)** Inspect the amount and distribution of pubic hair, size of the penis, and development of the testicles and scrotum

          **(b)** Typically, testicles and scrotum begin growing, then pubic hair develops, and finally the penis enlarges

  **c.** Male genital abnormalities that require referral to urology (see Chapter 31)

      **i.** Testicular torsion—twisting of the testicle on its spermatic cord, causing sudden onset of acute unilateral scrotal pain; immediate referral

      **ii.** Phimosis—tightening of foreskin that prevents its retraction over the glans penis; if severe may require circumcision

      **iii.** Penile mass or nodule

      **iv.** Ballooning of foreskin with urine during urination

  **d.** Note the appearance of the female external genitalia (Figure 9-3)

      **i.** Inspect the mons pubis and labia for color, size, symmetry, bruises, lesions, and rashes

      **ii.** Separate labia majora; use traction to pull toward examiner to reveal clitoris, labia minora, posterior fourchette, urethral meatus, hymen, and vaginal orifice (Box 9-4)

      **iii.** Use penlight or otoscope light to provide illumination

      **iv.** Note normal anatomic variations of prepubertal hymen and common benign congenital abnormalities of the hymen

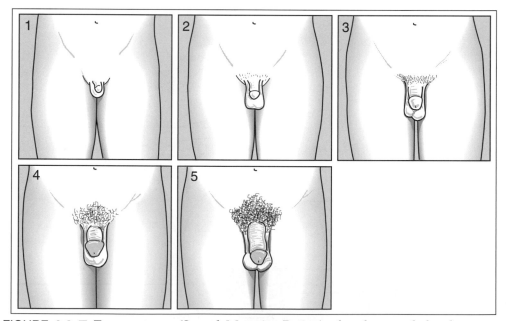

**FIGURE 9-2** ■ Tanner stages (Sexual Maturity Rating) of male sexual development. (From Berkowitz, C. D. [2000]. *Pediatrics: A primary care approach.* Philadelphia: Saunders, Fig. 21-3.)

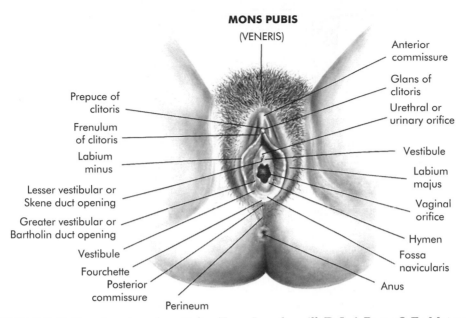

**MONS PUBIS**
(VENERIS)

Anterior commissure

Glans of clitoris

Urethral or urinary orifice

Prepuce of clitoris

Frenulum of clitoris

Labium minus

Vestibule

Labium majus

Lesser vestibular or Skene duct opening

Vaginal orifice

Greater vestibular or Bartholin duct opening

Hymen

Vestibule

Fossa navicularis

Fourchette

Posterior commissure

Anus

Perineum

FIGURE 9-3 ■ Female external genitalia. (From Lowdermilk D. L. & Perry, S. E.: *Maternity Nursing*, ed. 6, 2006, St. Louis: Mosby.)

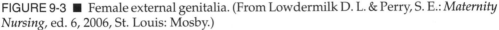

■ **BOX 9-4**
■ **TECHNIQUES FOR INSPECTING THE HYMEN**

- When inspecting the external female genitalia it may be difficult to view the hymenal orifice
- Gently apply traction on labia pulling toward the examiner
- Flush area with a small amount of water or saline using a syringe or angiocatheter attached to a syringe
- Place child in knee-chest position for the best view of the hymen; can place in a frog leg position if child is unable to cooperate with knee-chest position
- Prepubertal hymen is very sensitive to touch; avoid touching with an applicator
- Pubertal hymen may be palpated with a cotton-tipped applicator to aide in visualizing the hymen and the hymenal opening

   **v.** Note normal changes that occur to the hymen with puberty due to estrogen thickening, redundancy, moisture, and dull color or pallor

  **vi.** Imperforate hymen (no visible opening); a simple hymenotomy is required at the time of diagnosis; refer to gynecology

 **vii.** Microperforate, cribriform, and septate hymen; a hymenotomy is required before tampon use or sexual intercourse; refer to gynecology

**viii.** Note inability to view structures in the vestibule due to labial adhesions

  **ix.** Inspect the vestibule and the structures within for lesions

   **x.** Note characteristics of any vaginal/urethral discharge or bleeding

  **xi.** Note the Sexual Maturity Rating (Tanner stage) of female external genitalia (Figure 9-4)

    (a) Initially no pubic hair

    (b) Soft downy hair, straight, or slightly curly along the labia majora indicates puberty is beginning

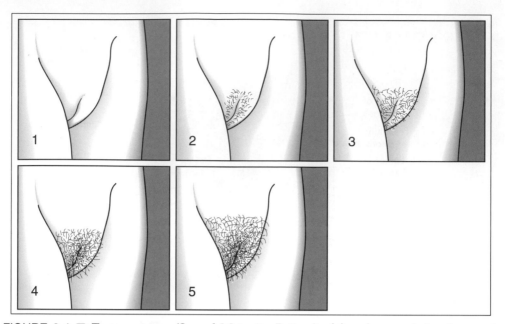

FIGURE 9-4 ■ Tanner stages (Sexual Maturity Raings) of female sexual development. (From Berkowitz, C. D. (2000). *Pediatrics: A primary care approach.* Philadelphia: Saunders, Fig. 21-1.)

        (c) Pubic hair becomes progressively coarser, darker, and curlier and spreads to mons pubis and then to the medial thighs as sexual maturity progresses

    **xii.** Note presence and extent of female genital mutilation

  **e.** Either gender: note urethral prolapse—urethral mucosa protrudes beyond the urethral meatus; refer to urology if persistent (Shurtleff & Barone, 2002)

  **f.** Inspect the inguinal area in both males and females for change in contour and symmetry

    **i.** Females—small bulging over the femoral canal may indicate a femoral hernia

    **ii.** Males—bulging in inguinal area may indicate an inguinal hernia

**3.** Palpation

  **a.** Palpate the inguinal area in males and females for lymph nodes and other masses

    **i.** Tenderness, heat, or inflammation in palpated lymph nodes could be due to a localized infection

  **b.** Palpation of the kidney is difficult due to its deep position within the abdominal cavity

  **c.** In infants and young children the bladder may be palpated slightly above the pubic symphysis

  **d.** Palpation of the male genitalia

    **i.** Palpate the penile shaft for nodules or masses

    **ii.** Palpate the scrotum for the presence of testicles (Box 9-5)

    **iii.** Palpate the spermatic cord for tenderness, masses, or swelling

  **e.** Palpation of the female genitalia – palpate labia for nodules, lumps

**4.** Pelvic exam

  **a.** Indications (see Chapter 31)

    **i.** Typically performed only on adolescents

■ **BOX 9-5**
■ **TECHNIQUES FOR PALPATING THE TESTICLES**

- Warm your hands
- Cremasteric reflex (retraction of the testes into the abdomen) is stimulated by cold, touch, emotional excitement, or exercise
- Place index finger and thumb over the upper part of the scrotal sac along the inguinal canal
- Note testicle size and shape
- Testicles are normally smooth and equal in size
- If the testicle is not palpated in the scrotum, palpate the inguinal canal for a soft mass (testicle)
- Attempt to move the testicle to the scrotum (descendable testicle)
- If the testicle cannot be moved into the scrotum or cannot be palpated in the inguinal canal, it is an undescended testicle

    ii. Irregular vaginal bleeding
    iii. Complaints of unexplained abdominal or pelvic pain
    iv. Severe dysmenorrhea
    v. Consensually sexually active adolescent with vaginal discharge
    vi. Sexually transmitted infections (STI)—chlamydia, gonorrhea
    vii Wet prep positive for trichomonas, bacterial vaginosis, and candida
    viii. Amenorrhea
    ix. Sexual assault/sexual abuse in an adolescent giving history of genital to genital contact

**b.** Timing
    i. Nonsexually active adolescents should begin routine pelvic exams at 18 years of age
    ii. Sexually active adolescent should have a pelvic exam, Pap smear, and testing for STIs annually
    iii. More frequently when the adolescent changes sexual partners, experiences vaginal symptoms, is exposed to or has a history of STI, or engages in high risk sexual behaviors

**c.** Contraindications for speculum examination
    i. Always perform the least invasive examination that will answer the clinical question
    ii. Nonsexually active adolescent with a vaginal discharge—obtain cultures by touching vagina with a cotton-tipped applicator without the use of a speculum
    iii. Primary amenorrhea—a cotton-tipped applicator can be used to determine vaginal length, followed by one-finger vaginal-abdominal exam

**d.** Cultural aspects
    i. Some parents and adolescents fear that the speculum will alter virginity
    ii. Reassure patients and families that speculum exams are not associated with changes in the hymen

**e.** Procedure
    i. Explain pelvic exam procedure to patient using a diagram and showing the speculum if patient desires
       (a) Huffman speculum ($\frac{1}{2} \times 4\frac{1}{2}$ inches) is used if hymenal opening is small
       (b) For a sexually active adolescent, a Pedersen speculum ($\frac{7}{8} \times 4\frac{1}{2}$ inches) or occasionally a Graves speculum ($1\frac{3}{8} \times 3\frac{3}{4}$ inches) is appropriate
       (c) A plastic speculum with an attached light source may be used

■ **BOX 9-6**
■ **SEXUAL ABUSE REPORTING**

- PNPs are legally mandated to report suspicion of child abuse to the appropriate child protective service (CPS) agency
- If a child gives history of sexual abuse, a report to CPS is essential
- If on physical examination of the child, the PNP notes a physical finding associated with sexual abuse, a report to CPS is essential
- If a prepubertal child or a nonconsensually sexually active adolescent has a positive culture for GC, chlamydia, a wet prep positive for trichomonas, or presents with lesions that clinically appear to be herpes, a report to CPS is essential
- In instances in which the PNP is uncertain about the interpretation of a physical finding or lab result, a clinician with expertise in child abuse should be consulted

    **ii.** Patient in lithotomy position with feet in stirrups
    **iii.** External genitalia inspected first
        (a) Inspect pubic hair for pediculosis pubis if itching is present
        (b) Sexually active adolescent may have a hymen without any obvious changes, a narrow hymenal rim or myrtiform caruncles (small bumps of residual hymen along lower edge)
    **iv.** Warm the speculum
        (a) Place one gloved finger on hymenal rim at 6 o'clock position and tell the adolescent to relax in this area
    **v.** Insert the speculum posteriorly with a downward direction
    **vi.** Open the speculum to reveal the cervix
    **vii.** Note any discharge, color, consistency, and odor
    **viii.** Cervix is usually dull pink; however, many adolescents may have an erythematous area surrounding the os
        (a) Note, size, shape, color, and mobility of cervix
        (b) Note presence and characteristics of any discharge
        (c) Small pinpoint hemorrhagic spots on the cervix; "strawberry cervix" may be due to *Trichomonas*
        (d) Samples for Pap smear, cultures, and wet prep are obtained with speculum in place
    **ix.** After visualization of vagina and cervix, the speculum is removed
    **x.** Next the uterus and adnexa are carefully palpated
        (a) One or two gloved fingers with lubricant gel are inserted into the vagina and the other hand is on the abdomen
        (b) Normal ovaries are <3 cm long and are rubbery
        (c) Adolescent may complain of discomfort with palpation
        (d) Urine or serum HCG should be completed if indicated
**5.** Suspicion of sexual abuse (see also Chapter 31)
    **a.** Sexual abuse reporting (Box 9-6)
    **b.** From 70% to 95% of children who give history of sexual abuse, including penile penetration of the vagina and/or anus, will have a normal genital exam (Adams, 1996; Heger et al., 2002; Johnson, 2002)

# REFERENCES

Adams, J. A. (1996). Genital findings in adolescent girls referred for suspected sexual abuse. *Arch Pediatr Adolesc Med, 150,* 850-856.

Alanis, M. C., & Lucidi, R. S. (2004). Neonatal circumcision: A review of the world's oldest and most controversial operation. *Obstet Gynecol Surv, 59* (5), 379-395.

Berkowitz, C. D. (2000) *Pediatrics: A primary care approach.* Philadelphia: Saunders.

Elford, K. J., & Spence, J. E. H. (2002). The forgotten female: Pediatric and adolescent gynecological concerns and their reproductive consequences. *J Pediatr Adolesc Gynecol, 15,* 65-77.

Heger, A. H., Tieson, L., Guerra, L., et al. (2002). Appearance of the genitalia in girls selected for non-abuse: Review of hymenal morphology and nonspecific findings. *J Pediatr Adolesc Gynecol, 15,* 27-35.

Hornor, G. (2002). Child sexual abuse: Psychological risk factors. *J Pediatr Health Care, 16,* 187-192.

Hornor, G., & Ryan-Wenger, N. (1999). Aberrant genital care practices: An unrecognized form of child sexual abuse. *J Pediatr Health Care, 13,* 12-17.

Hymel, K. P., & Jenny, C. (1996). Child sexual abuse. *Pediatr Rev, 17,* 236-249.

Johnson, C. F. (2002). Child maltreatment 2002: Recognition, reporting and risk. *Pediatr Int, 44,* 554-560.

Kolon, T. F. (2006). Cryptorchidism. Retrieved on March 13, 2006 from http://www.emedicine. com/med/topic2707.htm

Miller, G. P. (2002). Circumcision: Cultural-legal analysis. *Virginia J Soc Policy & Law, 9,* 497-985.

Schoen, E., Wiswell, T., & Moses, S. (2000). New policy on circumcision: Cause for concern. *Pediatrics, 105,* 620-623.

# Assessment of the Integumentary System

JANET M. BANKS, PhD, RN, CPNP

## FETAL DEVELOPMENT

1. Embryology, structure, and function of the integumentary system (McCance & Heuther, 2002; Moore & Persaud, 2003)
   a. Skin (Figure 10-1)
      i. Epidermis—top layer
         (a) Derived from the ectoderm during first and second trimesters
         (b) 0.2 to 0.3 mm thick
         (c) Avascular, cornified cells, keratinocytes
         (d) Two layers
            (1) Stratum germinativum forms new skin cells
               a) Complete by 11 weeks
               b) Forms permanent epidermal ridges on hands and feet by 17th week
                  i) Shape of ridges influenced by developing afferent nerve fibers
                  ii) Distinctive patterns associated with some genetic syndromes
               c) Melanocytes account for skin and hair tones by 7th week
            (2) Strateum corneum or horny cell layer
               a) Begins to develop at 21st week
               b) Nourished by underlying dermis layer
               c) Sheds, with complete turnover in cells every 3 to 4 weeks
               d) Appendages include hair, nails, sweat glands, sebaceous glands
      ii. Dermis—middle layer derived from the mesoderm
         (a) Nerves
         (b) Sensory receptors
         (c) Lymph vessels
         (d) Capillary blood vessels begin to develop at 5th week
         (e) Hair follicles
         (f) Sebaceous glands
            (1) Arise from hair follicle
            (2) On all parts of body except palms and soles
            (3) Produce sebum for lubrication of epidermis
            (4) Sebum mixes with desquamated cells to form vernix caseosa
         (g) Sweat glands
            (1) Eccrine

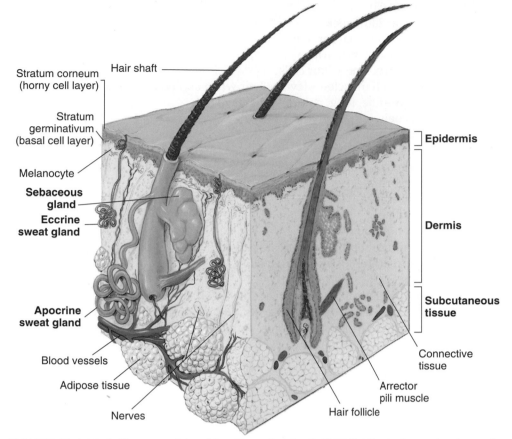

**FIGURE 10-1** ■ A diagram of the skin. (From Jarvis, C. [2004]. *Physical examination and health assessment* [4th ed.]. Philadelphia: Saunders, p. 222.)

       a) Sweat is a dilute saline solution
       b) Wide distribution, including palms and soles
     (2) Apocrine
       a) Sweat is a milky viscid solution
       b) Excreted from hair follicles
       c) When contaminated by bacteria
         i) Sweat decomposes
         ii) Causes body odor
       d) Located in genital, axillary, and areolar areas
       e) Begins functioning at puberty
  **iii.** Subcutaneous—innermost layer
     (a) Fat cells
       (1) Provide temperature control and insulation
       (2) Cushion underlying tissues
       (3) Store fat for energy
  **iv.** Other functions of skin
     (a) Barrier
     (b) Racial identifier
     (c) Communication tool (blanching and blushing)
     (d) Production of vitamin D
     (e) Adsorption and secretion

    **b.** Hair (Alaiti, 2005)

        **i.** Visible at 20th week

        **ii.** Shaft—visible part of hair

        **iii.** Root—below the surface

        **iv.** Bulb matrix—new hair cells

        **v.** Errector pili muscle—elevates hair when chilled or fearful

        **vi.** Lanugo—fine, long, colorless neonatal hair

        **vii.** Vellus hair—fine body hair

        **viii.** Terminal hair

            (a) Darkly pigmented

            (b) Long and thick hair primarily on scalp and face of males

            (c) Eyebrows

            (d) Pubic area

            (e) Axillae

        **ix.** Sebaceous glands

            (a) Produce sebum to lubricate skin and hair

            (b) Slow water losses through skin

    **c.** Nails (Jarvis, 2004)

        **i.** Fingernails begin to develop at 10th week, toenails at 14th week

        **ii.** Nails reach fingertips at 32 weeks, and toe tips by 36 weeks

        **iii.** Lateral and posterior nail folds—cuticles

        **iv.** Lunula—"half moon" area above the posterior nail fold

        **v.** Nail matrix

            (a) Extends beneath the cuticle and lunula

            (b) New keratinized cells form here

        **vi.** Nail plate—visible part of nail, consists of clear keratin

        **vii.** Changes in shape, texture, length of nail may indicate systemic illnesses

## FOCUSED HISTORY

**1.** Focused history (Bickley & Szilagyi, 2004)

    **a.** Relevant to all ages

        **i.** Identification of racial or ethnic group

        **ii.** Congenital nevus (nevi) or other birthmarks

            (a) Location on body

            (b) Size

            (c) Change in size, color, shape

        **iii.** Changes in skin appearance and texture

            (a) Dryness

            (b) Lesions, drainage

            (c) Itching, scratching, and rubbing

            (d) Excessive bruising

            (e) Tattoo, piercing

        **iv.** Allergies or rashes

        **v.** Food reactions

            (a) Eggs

            (b) Chocolate

            (c) Nuts

            (d) Other

        **vi.** Skin care

            (a) Bathing schedule

            (b) Duration in tub or shower

      (c) Soaps

      (d) Bubble bath

      (e) Skin care products (moisturizers, lotions, oils, sunscreen)

  vii. Hair

      (a) Grooming and styling

      (b) Shampoos

      (c) Conditioners, gels, etc.

      (d) Hair loss or bald spots

      (e) Hats

 viii. Nails

      (a) Nail bed shape and length

      (b) Thin

      (c) Soft

      (d) Brittle

      (e) Change in appearance or texture

      (f) Biting

   ix. Jewelry – metal composition, i.e. nickel allergy

    x. Changes in hair

      (a) Loss

      (b) New growth patterns

      (c) Texture

      (d) Color

   xi. Recent medications or treatments

      (a) Oral or topical

      (b) Including herbals

  xii. Recent insect bite

 xiii. Home environment

      (a) Average temperature in house

      (b) Humidity inside

  xiv. External environment

      (a) Seasonal variations in skin appearance and texture

      (b) Clothing worn when outside

      (c) Humidity outside

      (d) Exposure to sun

      (e) Use of sunscreen

      (f) Hats for sun protection

  xv. Environmental contact

      (a) Grasses

      (b) Leaves

      (c) Plants

      (d) Dust

      (e) Carpet

      (f) Pets

      (g) Cleaning solutions

      (h) Solvents

  xvi. Play equipment

      (a) Sandboxes

      (b) Playground soil

      (c) Wading/swimming pools (chlorine)

 xvii. Change in environment

      (a) New environmental exposures (new school, home)

      (b) Remodeling

      (c) New play areas

       **xviii.** Exposure to illness or lesions on others
          (a) Family members
          (b) Relatives
          (c) Daycare attendees
          (d) Friends of the family
          (e) Family pets with or without skin lesions
       **xix.** Family history
          (a) Skin, hair, or nail conditions
          (b) Allergies
          (c) Hair loss
          (d) Skin malignancies
       **xx.** Social history
          (a) Travel
          (b) Play or sports activities and sites
          (c) Part-time job or work
          (d) Recent travel or family outing
       **xxi.** Environment and exposure to hazardous materials
          (a) Home
          (b) Daycare
          (c) School
          (d) Child/adolescent workplace
          (e) Parental workplace
   **b.** Unique to birth through infancy (Furdon & Clark, 2003)
       **i.** Changes in skin color after birth
          (a) Pallor
          (b) Redness
          (c) Mottling
          (d) Cyanosis
          (e) Yellowing
       **ii.** Feeding patterns
          (a) Type of formula and/or breast-feeding
          (b) Type and order of new food introduction
      **iii.** Elimination patterns
          (a) Diaper changes
             (1) Number of diaper changes each day
             (2) Cleansing agents or wipes
             (3) Creams applied
             (4) Brand or type of diapers used
          (b) Diarrhea
       **iv.** Laundry methods
          (a) Soap or detergent for clothing and bedding
          (b) Separation of infant bedding and clothing from family laundry
          (c) Water temperature
          (d) Use of fabric softener sheets in dryer
   **c.** Unique to older children through young adults
       **i.** Individual or group sports participation and special equipment
          (a) Padding
          (b) Helmets
          (c) Gloves
          (d) Goggles
          (e) Shoes
       **ii.** Cosmetic use

       **iii.** Hair
         (a) Coloring
         (b) Gels
         (c) Dyes
       **iv.** Acne
         (a) Onset
         (b) Treatment
       **v.** Workplace
         (a) Exposures
         (b) Chemicals
         (c) Uniforms
         (d) Goggles
      **vi.** Bathing habits
         (a) Home
         (b) School locker rooms
         (c) Gyms
         (d) Attention to:
           (1) Soaps
           (2) Community towels
           (3) Skin care products
     **vii.** Sexual activity
         (a) Condom use; latex allergy
         (b) Spermicidal foam, gel
         (c) Exposure to sexually transmitted infections, pubic lice, scabies
    **viii.** Sunlight exposure
         (a) Deliberate tanning
         (b) Tanning salons
         (c) Vacations
         (d) Occupational
         (e) Sunscreen use
       **ix.** Nails
         (a) Fake nails
         (b) Manicures
         (c) Pedicures
         (d) Nail biting
         (e) Cuticle picking
       **x.** Body image related to skin, scars, birthmarks, etc.
**d.** Past medical history
       **i.** Childhood diseases
      **ii.** Chronic conditions
     **iii.** Allergies
      **iv.** Skin sensitivities
       **v.** Thyroid conditions
      **vi.** Respiratory conditions
     **vii.** Injuries
    **viii.** Surgeries
      **ix.** Medications
         (a) Current
         (b) Previous
         (c) Skin reactions
**e.** Current health status
       **i.** Immunization status

  **ii.** Growth—undernourished, failure to thrive or overweight
  **iii.** Recurrent illnesses
  **iv.** Current skin condition
   (a) Skin
   (b) Hair
   (c) Nails

## FOCUSED EXAMINATION

**1.** Focused examination (Bickley & Szilagyi, 2004)
 **a.** Equipment
  **i.** Extra drapes to facilitate clothing removal
  **ii.** Penlight/flashlight; transilluminator
  **iii.** Measuring tape in centimeters
  **iv.** Good light source
  **v.** Wood's lamp
  **vi.** Scalpel blades for scrapings
  **vii.** Magnifying glass
  **viii.** Gloves
 **b.** Inspection
  **i.** Overall health status
  **ii.** Appearance
  **iii.** Color and skin tone
   (a) Note racial or ethnic origin (Engel, 2002)
    (1) Black—bluish tinge on gums, tongue, and nail borders
    (2) Asian—yellow skin tones
    (3) Mediterranean—bluish tinge on lips
   (b) If jaundice suspected
    (1) Use natural daylight
    (2) Blanch skin with glass slide to provide contrast
  **iv.** Thyroid enlargement
  **v.** Acne
  **vi.** Acanthosis nigricans—skin darkening and thickening around neck, axillae, waist, groin
  **vii.** Sweating
  **viii.** Odor
  **ix.** Striae
  **x.** Bruises—predicting the age of bruises is unreliable (Sibert, 2004)
  **xi.** Patterns of hair loss
  **xii.** May use Wood's lamp
  **xiii.** Attend to specific body locations
   (a) Axillae
   (b) Back of neck
   (c) Abdomen
   (d) Between fingers and toes
   (e) Between buttocks
   (f) Genitalia
   (g) Skinfolds
   (h) Raise hair to check for lesions
  **xiv.** Hair
   (a) Color
   (b) Amount

(1) Sparse

(2) Excessive

(3) Direction of growth

    a) Whorls

    b) Hairline

(c) Appropriate for age

    (1) Newborn hair growth and patterning (Furdon & Clark, 2003)

        a) Associated with development of the central nervous system

        b) Note abnormalities in color, quantity, texture, pattern

    (2) Axillary

    (3) Sexual Maturity Rating (Tanner stage) for pubic hair (See Chapter 9 Figures 9-2 and 9-4)

(d) Nits, larvae in hair

  **xv.** Nails

    (a) Shape of nail

    (b) Color of nail and surrounding nail bed

    (c) Nail angle

        (1) 160 degrees is normal

        (2) Less than 160 degrees indicates curving

        (3) Flat, ≥180 degrees indicates clubbing

    (d) Nail biting or cuticle picking

**c.** Palpation

  **i.** Skin

    (a) Temperature

    (b) Texture

    (c) Moisture

    (d) Turgor

    (e) Edema

    (f) Skin lesions (with gloves)

    (g) Birthmarks

  **ii.** Hair texture

  **iii.** Nail plate

    (a) Smooth consistency

    (b) Anchored in nail bed

    (c) Capillary refill ≤2 seconds (American Heart Association, 2002)

  **iv.** Thyroid

**d.** Description of skin lesions (Table 10-1 and Figures 10-2 to 10-8)

**e.** Configuration of skin lesions (Figure 10-9)

  **i.** Annular—complete circular lesion with discrete clear center and peripheral border

  **ii.** Arcuate—arc-shaped lesion

  **iii.** Circinate—incomplete circular lesion

  **iv.** Confluent—lesions run together

  **v.** Discoid—lesion clusters with a distinct border

  **vi.** Eczematoid—scaling, crusting flaking lesions

  **vii.** Grouped—lesion clusters appearing in same body location

  **viii.** Iris—pink macules with central purple papules

  **ix.** Keratotic—hypertrophic tissue formation (wart)

  **x.** Linear—in a line

  **xi.** Reticulated—netlike or lacy pattern

  **xii.** Serpiginous—Snakelike or wavy

  **xiii.** Telangiectasia—dilated blood vessels that blanch

  **xiv.** Zosteriform—follows a nerve tract on the body

■ **TABLE 10-1**
■ ■ **Names, Characteristics, and Examples of Primary Skin Lesions**

| Lesion | Characteristics | Examples |
|---|---|---|
| **PRIMARY SKIN LESIONS** | | |
| Nonpalpable, flat | | |
| Macule | <1 cm | Freckles, moles |
| Patch | >1 cm | Vitiligo, café-au-lait spots |
| Palpable, solid mass | | |
| Papule | <1 cm | Neoplasms |
| Nodule | 1-2 cm | Nevus, wart |
| Tumor | >2 cm | Neoplasms |
| Plaque | Flat, elevated, superficial papule with surface area greater than height | Psoriasis, seborrheic keratosis |
| Wheal | Superficial area of cutaneous edema | Hives, insect bites |
| Palpable, fluid filled | | |
| Vesicle | >1 cm; filled with serous fluid | Blister, herpes simplex |
| Bulla | >1 cm; filled with serous fluid | Blister, pemphigus vulgaris |
| Pustule | Similar to vesicle; filled with pus | Acne, impetigo |
| **SPECIAL PRIMARY SKIN LESIONS** | | |
| Comedo | Plugged opening of sebaceous gland | Blackhead |
| Burrow | <10 mm, raised tunnel | Scabies |
| Cyst | Palpable lesion filled with semiliquid material or fluid | Sebaceous cyst |
| Abscess | Localized accumulation of purulent material in dermis or subcutis; if deep, accumulation may not be visible | |
| Furuncle | Necrotizing form of inflammation of a hair follicle | |
| Carbuncle | Coalescence of several furuncles | |
| Milia | Tiny, keratin-filled cysts in the distal portion of the sweat gland | |
| **SECONDARY SKIN LESIONS BELOW THE SKIN PLANE** | | |
| Erosion | Loss of part or all of epidermis; surface is moist | Rupture of a vesicle |
| Ulcer | Loss of epidermis and dermis; may bleed | Stasis ulcer, chancre |
| Fissure | Linear crack from epidermis into dermis | Cheilitis, athlete's foot |
| Excoriation | Superficial linear or "dugout" traumatized area, usually self-induced | Abrasion, scratch mark |
| Atrophy | Thinning of skin with loss of skin markings | Striae |
| Sclerosis | Diffuse or circumscribed hardening of skin | |
| **SECONDARY SKIN LESIONS ABOVE THE SKIN PLANE** | | |
| Scaling | Heaped-up keratinized cells, exfoliated epidermis | Dandruff, psoriasis |
| Crusting | Dried residue of pus, serum or blood | Scabs, impetigo |

*Continued*

■ **TABLE 10-1**
■ ■ **Names, Characteristics, and Examples of Primary Skin Lesions—cont'd**

| Lesion | Characteristics | Examples |
| --- | --- | --- |
| **VASCULAR SKIN LESIONS** | | |
| Erythema | Pink or red blanchable discoloration of skin secondary to dilatation of blood vessels | |
| Petechiae | Reddish purple, nonblanching, <0.5 cm | Intravascular defects |
| Purpura | Reddish purple, nonblanching, >0.5 cm | Intravascular defects |
| Ecchymosis | Reddish purple, nonblanching, variable size | Trauma, vasculitis |
| Telangiectasia | Fine, irregular dilated blood vessels | Dilation of capillaries |
| Spider angioma | Central red body with radiating spider-like arms that blanch with pressure to the central area | Liver disease, estrogens |
| **MISCELLANEOUS SKIN LESIONS** | | |
| Scar | Replacement of destroyed dermis by fibrous tissue; may be atrophic or hyperplastic | Healed wound |
| Keloid | Elevated, enlarging scar growing beyond boundaries of wound | Burn scars |
| Lichenification | Roughening and thickening of epidermis; accentuated skin markings | Atopic dermatitis |

Adapted from Swartz, M. H. (2004). *Textbook of physical diagnosis, history and examination* (4th ed.). Philadelphia: Elsevier, pp. 135-139.

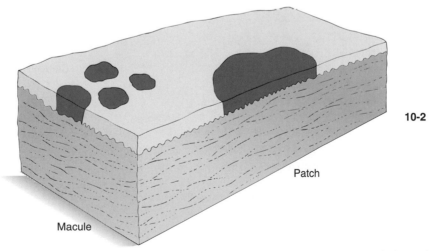

10-2

Patch

Macule

FIGURES 10-2 TO 10-8 ■ Skin lesions. (From Swartz, M. H. [2004]. *Textbook of physical diagnosis, history and examination* [4th ed.]. Philadelphia: Elsevier, pp. 135–139.)

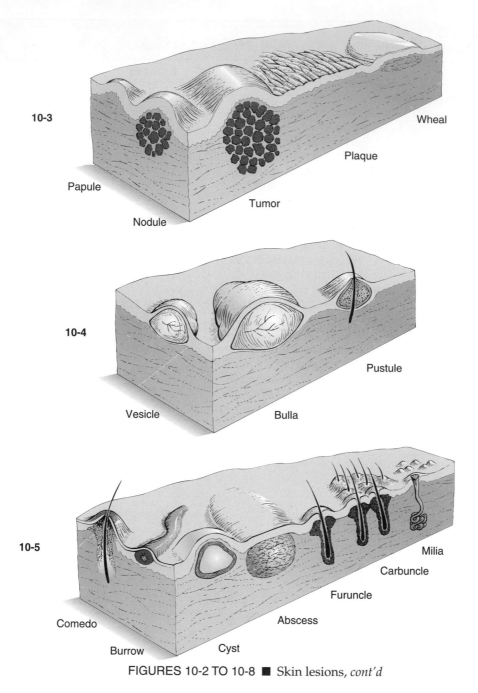

FIGURES 10-2 TO 10-8 ■ Skin lesions, *cont'd*

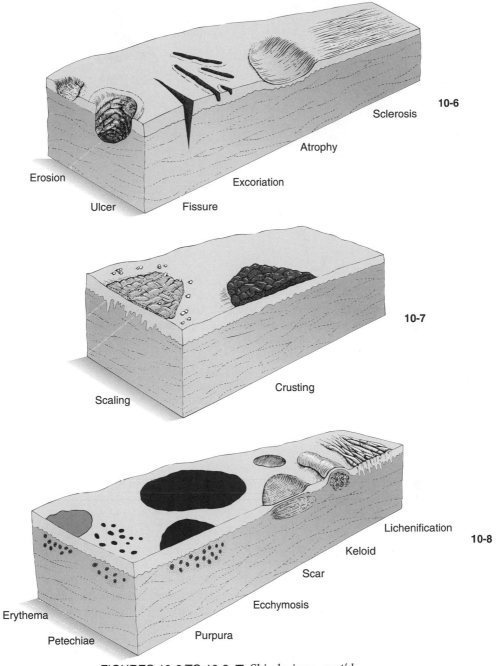

FIGURES 10-2 TO 10-8 ■ Skin lesions, *cont'd*

**f.** Documentation of findings
  **i.** Relevant history
  **ii.** Lesions
   (a) Type
   (b) Color
   (c) Distribution
   (d) Pattern
   (e) Measurements in cm or mm
  **iii.** Use of Wood's lamp

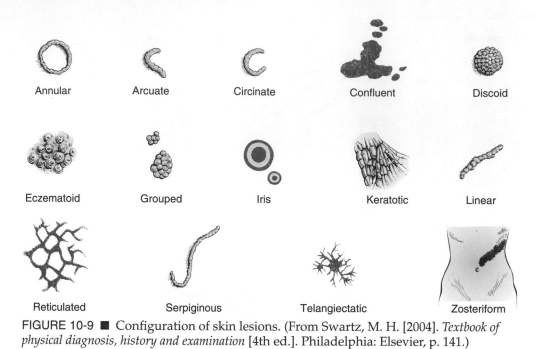

FIGURE 10-9 ■ Configuration of skin lesions. (From Swartz, M. H. [2004]. *Textbook of physical diagnosis, history and examination* [4th ed.]. Philadelphia: Elsevier, p. 141.)

    **iv.** Scrapings
        (a) Source of specimen
        (b) Method of analysis (e.g., KOH, culture)
        (c) Result
**5.** Diagnostic tests
  **a.** KOH test of scrapings
  **b.** Culture of exudates
See also Chapter 32 for common illnesses related to the integumentary system.

## REFERENCES

Alaiti, S. (2005). Hair growth. Retrieved from eMedicine on March 13, 2006 at http://www.emedicine.com/ent/topic16.htm

American Heart Association. (2002). *Pediatric advanced life support provider manual.* Dallas: American Heart Association.

Bickley, L. S., & Szilagyi, P.G. (2004). *Bates guide to physical examination and history taking* (8th ed.) Philadelphia: Lippincott Williams & Wilkins.

Engel, J. (2002). *Mosby's pocket guide series: Pediatric assessment* (4th ed.). St. Louis: Mosby.

Furdon, S. A., & Clark, D. A. (2003). Scalp hair characteristics in the newborn infant. *Advances in Neonatal Care, 3* (6), 286-296.

Jarvis, C. (2004). *Physical examination and health assessment* (4th ed.). Philadelphia: Elsevier.

McCance, K. L., & Heuther, S. C. (2002). Structure, function, and disorders of the integument. In K. L. McCance, & S. C. Heuther, *Pathophysiology: The biologic basis for disease in adults and children* (4th ed.). St. Louis: Mosby, pp. 1434-1468.

Moore, K. L., & Persaud, T. V. N. (2003). *The developing human: Clinically oriented embryology* (7th ed.). Philadelphia: Saunders.

Sibert, J. (2004). Bruising, coagulation disorder, and physical child abuse. *Blood coagulation and fibrinolysis: An international journal in haemostasis and thrombosis, 15*(Suppl. 1), S33-S39.

Swartz, M. H. (2004). *Textbook of physical diagnosis, history and examination* (4th ed.). Philadelphia: Elsevier.

# Assessment of the Hematologic and Lymphatic Systems

SHEILA JUDGE SANTACROCE, PhD, APRN, CPNP

## FETAL DEVELOPMENT OF THE HEMATOLOGIC SYSTEM

1. Embryology of the hematologic system (Moore & Persaud, 2003)
   a. During the third week of gestation blood vessels begin to develop
      i. In the yolk sac, connecting stalk and chorion
      ii. In the developing endothelial cells of the embryo
   b. During the fifth week, blood cells develop in the embryonic mesenchyme in liver, and later in spleen, bone marrow, and lymph nodes
   c. Hemoglobin
      i. Fetal hemoglobin (hemoglobin F)
         (a) Combination of two alpha globin chains and two gamma globin chains
         (b) Has a higher affinity for oxygen than hemoglobin A
      ii. Adult hemoglobin (hemoglobin A)
         (a) Combination of two alpha globin chains and two beta globin chains
         (b) At about 20 weeks, the percentage of gamma chains starts to drop, and percentage of beta chains increases
      iii. At 2 weeks, hemoglobin F is about 65% of hemoglobin
      iv. At 6 months, hemoglobin F is at a normal level (≤2%)
2. Anatomy and physiology
   a. Major components of the hematologic system (McCance & Huether, 2002)
      i. Fluid elements (plasma)—55% of blood volume
         (a) About 90% water
         (b) 10% solutes—depends on diet, vitamins, hormonal levels, metabolic needs
            (1) Albumin
               a) Essential to maintain osmotic and oncotic pressure
               b) Regulates fluid and solids to the capillaries
            (2) Electrolytes
            (3) Proteins
               a) Clotting factors
               b) Globulins
               c) Fibrinogen
               d) Circulating antibodies

   **ii.** Formed elements (blood cells)—45% of blood volume
- (a) Erythrocytes (red blood cells, or RBCs)
  - (1) Small biconcave disks that transport hemoglobin (Hgb)
    - a) Hgb binds to oxygen in the lungs and carries it throughout the body
    - b) Production is regulated by erythropoietin that is produced by the kidney in response to tissue hypoxia
    - c) Live for 100 to 120 days in the circulation
    - d) Then RBCs break down into their basic elements:
      - i) Iron, which is reused in the production of new RBCs
      - ii) Bilirubin, which is excreted by the liver in the bile
  - (2) Blood type
    - a) Determined by presence or absence of agglutinins on the surface of the RBC and in plasma
    - b) Agglutinins destroy "foreign" RBCs
      - i) Type O: no agglutinins on RBC, a and b agglutinins in plasma
      - ii) Type A: A agglutinins on RBC, b agglutinins in plasma
      - iii) Type B: B agglutinins on RBC, a agglutinins in plasma
      - iv) Type AB: A and B agglutinins on RBC, no agglutinins in plasma
  - (3) Rh factor—protein on surface of RBC in 85% of population
  - (4) Reticulocytes
    - a) Immature RBCs
    - b) Characterized by filaments and granules that are the remains of the nucleus
- (b) Leukocytes (white blood cells, or WBCs)
  - (1) Immune and inflammatory functions
  - (2) Consist of granulocytes, monocytes, and lymphocytes
  - (3) Granulocytes are phagocytes that include:
    - a) Neutrophils (polymorphonuclear leukocytes; polys, or PMNs)
      - i) Contain enzymes and oxidizing agents that can destroy foreign substances
      - ii) Play a major role in host defenses against infectious organisms and mediating inflammation
      - iii) Mature neutrophils have a segmented nucleus (segs)
      - iv) Those that are less mature have a band-shaped nucleus (bands)
    - b) Eosinophils
      - i) Selectively destroy parasites
      - ii) Release profibrinolysin that when activated:
        - *a)* Help dissolve a clot
        - *b)* Function in anaphylactic hypersensitivity reactions
        - *c)* Basophils
          - *i)* Called mast cells when they exit the blood vessels and enter tissue
        - *d)* Responsible for histamine release
          - *i)* Increases the permeability of blood vessels
          - *ii)* Allows WBCs to exit vessels and travel to where they are needed
  - (4) Monocytes
    - a) Called macrophages when they are in the tissues
    - b) Phagocytize large amounts of foreign material

        c) Present antigen to T cells to activate immune response

        d) Participate in chronic inflammatory processes

   (5) Lymphocytes have major immune functions (see The Lymphatic System section, following)

   (6) Thrombocytes (platelets) (King, 2005)

        a) Control bleeding after a vessel wall injury by:

           i) Adhering to the endothelium to form a plug

           ii) Releasing substances that attract other platelets to the site

           iii) Releasing serotonin, which causes vasoconstriction

        b) Coagulation cascades converge to form a fibrin clot (American Association of Clinical Chemistry, 2004; King, 2005)

           i) Extrinsic coagulation cascade

               *a)* A complex response to tissue injury

               *b)* Stimulated by exposure of collagen to a vessel surface and release of tissue factor (factor III)

               *c)* Requires factor II, VII, X

               *d)* Evaluated by prothrombin time (PT)

           ii) Intrinsic coagulation cascade

               *a)* A complex response to an abnormal vessel wall in the absence of tissue injury

               *b)* Requires clotting factors VIII, IX, X, XI, XII

               *c)* Evaluated by partial thromboplastin time (PTT)

           iii) Convergence of extrinsic and intrinsic coagulation cascade

               *a)* Factor Xa activates prothrombin (factor II) to thrombin (factor IIa), which in turn:

                   *i)* Activates factors XI, VIII, and V

                   *ii)* Activates factors XIII to XIIIa

                   *iii)* Converts fibrinogen to fibrin, and a clot forms

**iii.** Blood cell precursors

  (a) Located in the bone marrow

  (b) Pluripotent hematopoietic stem cells with lifelong potential for self-renewal and proliferation

  (c) Differentiated progenitor (parent) cells for each cell type

  (d) Functional mature blood cells of each type

**iv.** Blood-forming (hematopoietic) organs

  (a) Bone marrow (myeloid tissue)

  (b) Lymphatic tissues (see the Lymphatic System, following)

  (c) Liver and spleen play roles in hematopoiesis and blood cell waste removal

  (d) Pelvis, long bones, sternum, and skull

     (1) Contain most of the body's bone marrow reserve

     (2) Radiation to one or more of these areas will compromise hematopoiesis

  (e) Hematopoiesis

     (1) In part regulated by colony-stimulating factors (CSFs)

        a) A type of cytokine or glycoprotein that acts on blood cell precursors in the bone marrow

        b) Lineage-specific CSFs (e.g., granulocyte colony–stimulating factor or G-CSFs) act on differentiated cells

        c) Nonspecific cytokines (e.g., interleukin-3, or I-3) act on blood cell progenitors earlier in the hematopoietic process than lineage specific growth factors

          (2) Hematopoiesis can be accelerated by use of recombinant growth factors in conditions such as:

            a) Neutropenia after chemotherapy in cancer treatment

            b) Anemia of chronic renal failure

## FOCUSED HISTORY

1. Focused history (Bickley & Szilagyi, 2003)
   a. Birth history
      i. Abnormal bleeding at the separation of the umbilical cord
      ii. Abnormal bleeding with circumcision or heel sticks
      iii. Hyperbilirubinemia (jaundice)
      iv. ABO or Rh incompatibility
   b. Past medical history
      i. Fever: if yes, pattern, including time of day
      ii. Frequent infection: if yes, location, treatment and effects
      iii. Abnormal bleeding
         (a) At immunization sites
         (b) During eruption of teeth
         (c) With nosebleeds
         (d) With minor cuts or surgical procedures, and wound healing
   c. Ethnic background
   d. Current health status
   e. Energy level
   f. Dietary iron, including quantity of milk intake
   g. History of pica
   h. Cognitive and behavioral changes
   i. Family history
      i. Easy bleeding or bleeding disorder
      ii. Menorrhagia
      iii. Any type of anemia
      iv. Thyroid or immune disorders
      v. Early cerebrovascular accident
      vi. Myocardial infarction
      vii. Thrombosis
   j. Social history
      i. Quality and age of family housing for possible lead exposure
      ii. Other sources of lead, e.g. pottery, toys, Mexican candy
   k. Medications
      i. Use of over-the-counter, prescription medications, and complementary therapies:
         (a) Some may potentially prolong bleeding (e.g., penicillins, sulfon-amides, anticonvulsants)
         (b) Others are associated with thrombus formation (e.g., oral contraceptives)
      ii. Medications associated with G6PD deficiency and hemolysis of RBCs
2. Focused examination (Bickley & Szilagyi, 2003)
   a. Inspection
      i. Inspect skin on each part of the body for:
         (a) Pallor—gums and soft palate
         (b) Petechiae
            (1) Gums and soft palate

(2) Note location and pattern

(c) Bruises—note location, color, pattern, and reported source of injury

**b.** Auscultation

**i.** Check for systolic ejection murmur

**c.** Gentle palpation followed by percussion

  **i.** Right upper abdomen for the liver

  (a) Hepatic tenderness can be assessed by the child's response to examination

  (b) The liver edge is usually sharp and can be easily moved when pushed from below during inspiration

  (c) A liver edge that extends more than 2 cm beyond the right costal margin or is tender requires consultation and investigation into potential causes

  **ii.** Left upper abdomen for spleen tip

  (a) Normally 1 to 2 cm below left costal margin in infants and children

  (b) The normal spleen tip is nontender and soft with a sharp edge

  (c) A spleen tip that extends more than 2 cm should be considered abnormal and requires consultation and investigation into potential causes

  **iii.** Doubt about whether a palpable abdominal mass is spleen, liver, or tumor requires consultation and further investigation

**3.** Diagnostic tests (Corbett, 2004)

  **a.** Complete blood count (CBC)

  **i.** Red blood cells (RBCs)

  (a) RBC reference value for children is 4.6 to 4.8 million per mm$^3$, and varies with age

  (b) Elevations in RBCs—polycythemia

  (1) Seen in children who live at high altitude

  (2) Seen in diseases that cause chronic hypoxia

  a) Congenital heart disease

  b) Hyperproliferate bone marrow

  (3) Some tumors can lead to hypersecretion of erythropoietin, leading to polycythemia

  (4) At risk for venous thrombi formation

  (5) Optimal hydration should be determined and maintained

  (c) Decreased RBCs—anemia

  (1) Blood loss

  (2) Destruction of RBC

  (3) Lack of elements or hormones necessary for RBC production

  (4) Bone marrow suppression

  (d) Increase reticulocytes is a response to some anemias

  (e) Red cell distribution width (RDW)—measure of variability in size of RBCs

  (1) Increase in iron deficiency anemia

  (f) Hypochromic RBC is important in some diagnoses

  **ii.** White blood cells (WBCs)

  (a) WBC reference value for children varies with age

  (b) Infants and toddlers normally have higher WBC than older children

  (c) Differential (diff) determines the proportion of each WBC type relative to total percentage of WBCs

  (d) Absolute neutrophil count (ANC) provides the actual number of neutrophils

  (1) ANC = (segs % + bands %) × WBCs

        (e) Increased total WBCs and percent neutrophils for age suggests:
           (1) Bacterial infection
           (2) Physiologic stress
           (3) Tissue necrosis
        (f) Increase in percent bands, called a *shift to the left*, reflects release of bands into the bloodstream as a response to a demand for neutrophils in bacterial infection
        (g) Decrease in neutrophil count suggests:
           (1) Viral infection
           (2) Effect of some medications
           (3) Sepsis
               a) Especially in newborns in which sepsis causes a depletion of bone marrow reserves
        (h) The presence of abnormal lymphocytes or lymphoproliferation requires further investigation
    iii. Platelets (plts)
        (a) Platelet reference range is 150,000 to 300,000 per mm$^3$ after age 6 months
        (b) Low platelet levels suggest:
           (1) Decreased production, or
           (2) Increased consumption from:
               a) Primary platelet disorder
               b) Secondary to systemic disease
               c) Immune response
        (c) Normal platelet levels but abnormal function suggests abnormal morphology of platelets
        (d) Prothrombin time (PT)
           (1) PT tests clot formation from fibrinogen
           (2) Detects deficiencies in clotting factors II, V, VII, X, and fibrinogen
        (e) Partial thromboplastin time (PTT)
           (1) Detects congenital deficiencies of clotting factors II, V, VIII, IX, X, XI, XII
               a) II, VII, IX, X are vitamin K dependent
           (2) Detects hemophilia A and B
           (3) Detects lupus
    iv. Hemoglobin (Hgb) content of the blood
        (a) Hgb reference range depends on child's age
           (1) Infants have very high Hgb at birth, but Hgb breaks down quickly
           (2) Physiologic nadir for Hgb is 8 to 12 weeks when lower range is 9.5 g/dL
           (3) Normally lower in children ages 2 through 24 months than for others
        (b) Low Hgb can be seen in RBCs with abnormal types of Hgb
        (c) Hgb levels are considered in classification of anemia (see Chapter 33) and hemoglobinopathies (see Chapter 47)
    v. Hematocrit (Hct)—volume of cells in 100 mL of blood
    vi. Mean corpuscular volume (MCV)—mean size of red cells
    vii. Mean corpuscular hemoglobin concentration (MCHC)—concentration of hemoglobin in the red blood cells
    viii. Mean cell hemoglobin (MCH)—red cell mass
  b. Hemoglobin electrophoresis

    c. Blood type and screen
        i. ABO and Rh status
        ii. Presence of most common antibodies
    d. CT scan of enlarged lymph nodes
4. When to refer to a pediatric hematologist/oncologist (Nathan, 2003)
    a. When the CBC reveals unexplained anemia, neutropenia or thrombocytopenia, abnormal cells, primitive cells (blasts), or pancytopenia (severely low levels of all types of blood cells)
    b. When an evaluation and possible examination of bone marrow function are indicated

# FETAL DEVELOPMENT OF THE LYMPHATIC SYSTEM

1. Embryology of the lymphatic system (Moore & Persaud, 2003)
    a. By the end of the fifth week of gestation, the lymphatic system begins to develop
    b. Six primary lymph sacs develop from the neck to the iliac area of the embryo along the major veins
    c. Lymph sacs become future lymph nodes
    d. Lymphocytes develop from primitive stem cells in the yolk sac mesenchyme and later from liver and spleen
2. Anatomy and physiology (McCance & Huether, 2002)
    a. The lymphatic system consists of:
        i. Central lymphoid organs where lymphocyte precursors arise and develop
            (a) Bone marrow
            (b) Thymus
        ii. Peripheral lymphoid organs where lymphocytes mature and function
            (a) Lymph nodes
                (1) Usually occur in chains or clusters
                (2) Central lymph nodes usually smaller than peripheral lymph nodes
                (3) Amount of lymphatic tissue peaks in middle childhood
                (4) Amount of lymphatic tissue decreases during adolescence to adult level of 2% to 3% of total body weight (Figure 11-1)
                (5) Filter lymph to remove infectious and other matter
                (6) Present foreign matter to lymphocytes to stimulate immune responses
            (b) Spleen
                (1) Largest "lymph node" in the body
                (2) Consists of lymphoid and reticuloendothelial cells lying within a smooth muscle capsule
                (3) Enlarges from birth through adolescence
                (4) Diminishes during adulthood
                (5) Functions
                    a) Removes circulating bacteria from the body
                    b) Presents antigens to stimulate antibody production
                    c) Removes aged or abnormal cells from the blood
                    d) Acts as a reservoir for platelets and plasma proteins
            (c) Mucosa-associated lymphoid tissues (MALT) (Grethlein & Perez, 2005)
                (1) Protect the body from numerous antigens
                (2) Scattered along mucosal linings, e.g.

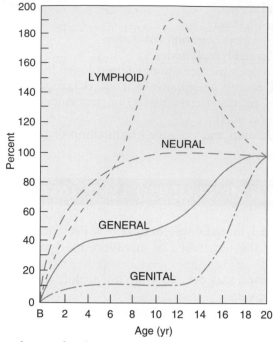

FIGURE 11-1 ■ Growth rates for three types of tissues. (From Wong, D. L., Hocken-berry-Eaton, M., Wilson, D., et al. [2001]. *Wong's essentials of pediatric nursing.* St. Louis: Mosby, p. 96.)

      a) Gut-associated lymphoid tissue (GALT)
         i) Peyer patches within the small intestine
         ii) Vermiform appendix
         iii) Accessory organs of the digestive tract
      b) Bronchus-associated lymphoid tissue (BALT), e.g., tonsils
         i) Tonsils
      c) Nose-associated lymphoid tissue (NALT)
      d) Vulvovaginal-associated lymphoid tissue (VALT)
      e) Parotid gland
  **iii.** Lymph is a blood ultrafiltrate that is collected by lymphatic capillaries located in all body organs except the heart and brain
  **iv.** Lymphatic vessels connect lymphoid organs to circulate lymphocytes and lymph through distinct regions of the body
  **v.** Lymphatic capillaries link to form ever larger lymphatic vessels that:
      (a) Carry lymph to regional lymph nodes
      (b) Drain lymph from distinct regions of the body into the venous system
  **vi.** Lymphocytes
      (a) Lymphoid stem cells arise from pluripotent hematopoietic stem cells in the bone marrow
      (b) B lymphocytes
         (1) Mature in the bone marrow
         (2) Provide humoral immunity by synthesizing and secreting antibodies
         (3) Make IgM antibodies at *initial* antigen exposure
         (4) Evolve into memory B cells that make IgG, IgA, or IgE antibodies at *reexposure* to an antigen
      (c) T lymphocytes that have circulated through the thymus
         (1) Signal B lymphocytes to produce antibodies

(2) Regulate humoral immunity
(3) Kill tumor and virus-containing cells
(d) Natural killer (NK) lymphocytes
(1) Secrete compounds that help B lymphocytes destroy foreign proteins
(e) Cytokines are hormone-like glycoproteins that are activated by T lymphocytes to:
(1) Mediate inflammation
(2) Support hematopoiesis
(3) Foster communication among lymphocytes and other cells

## FOCUSED HISTORY

1. Focused history (Bickley & Szilagyi, 2003)
   a. Recent contact with people with infectious diseases
   b. Fever; if yes, pattern including time of day
   c. Frequent infection; if yes, location, treatment, and effects
   d. History of enlarged lymph nodes
      i. History of regional swelling, tenderness, red streaks
      ii. If enlarged nodes located in the supraclavicular region, and,
         (a) History of cough, wheezing, difficulty breathing, or neck and facial swelling
         (b) May be indicative of mediastinal lymphadenopathy
   e. Exposure to cat, dogs, fleas, and ticks
   f. Sexual history
   g. Tobacco, drug, and alcohol use
   h. Family history of malignant and immune disorders

## FOCUSED EXAMINATION

1. Focused examination (Bickley & Szilagyi, 2003)
   a. See Figure 11-2 for location of lymph nodes and vessels
   b. Inspection
      i. Inspect area extending proximal from obvious nodes for tender red streaks
         (a) Red streaks can be a sign of infection, usually caused by *Staphylococcus aureus* or group A streptococci
         (b) Requires further investigation and treatment with antibiotics
      ii. Inspect skin in each area of the body as it is being examined for benign dilated lymph vessel masses (cystic hygroma) that often occur in the neck and less commonly in other areas
      iii. Inspect throat for tonsil size, color, lesions, and exudates
         (a) White exudate and a fetid odor suggests infection and requires further investigation
         (b) Peritonsillar abscess requires emergency referral to physician
   c. Palpation
      i. Palpate each area of the body for lymph nodes as it is being inspected
      ii. Lymph node size
         (a) Usually small
         (b) Nodes are not palpable in the newborn

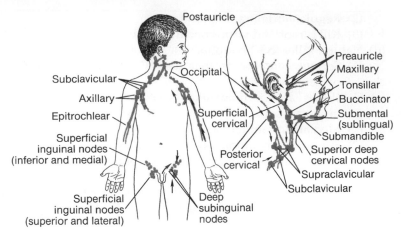

FIGURE 11-2 ■ Location of lymph nodes and direction of lymph flow. (From Engel, J. [2002]. *Mosby's pocket guide series. Pediatric assessment* [4th ed.]. St. Louis: Mosby, Fig. 18-1, p. 213.)

      (c) Measure enlarged nodes in centimeters

      (d) Size increases with exposure to antigens during childhood

      (e) Considered enlarged when cervical or axillary nodes exceed 1 cm in diameter, and inguinal nodes exceed 1.5 cm

   **iii.** Presence of enlarged mediastinal and abdominal nodes is considered abnormal and requires further investigation

   **iv.** Bilateral hilar adenopathy may be seen with cystic fibrosis

    **v.** Unilateral hilar adenopathy may seen with tuberculosis

   **vi.** Abdominal lymphadenopathy may be seen with the lymphomas and ulcerative colitis

      (a) Clinically associated with lower back pain, constipation, and urinary frequency

  **vii.** Gently palpate left upper abdomen for spleen tip

      (a) Note absent/present and distance in cm beyond the left costal margin

      (b) Normal spleen tip is nontender and soft with a sharp edge

      (c) A spleen tip that extends more than 1 to 2 cm should be considered abnormal and requires consultation and further investigation

      (d) Any doubt about whether a palpable mass in the abdomen is spleen, liver or tumor requires consultation and further investigation

 **viii.** Palpate extremities for edema that could be due to enlarged lymphatic tissue

      (a) Note absent/present and symmetry, nature (pitting/nonpitting)

      (b) Note skin texture and pigmentation

**2.** When to refer (Nathan, 2003)

  **a.** Refer to a physician as an emergency

     **i.** Peritonsillar abscess—one tonsil erythematous, enlarged, and protrudes toward the midline and forward

    **ii.** Generalized lymphadenopathy

      (a) Enlargement in two or more noncontiguous lymph node regions

      (b) Suggests systemic disease

      (c) Other symptoms are often present, most commonly hepatosplenomegaly

      (d) Consultation and further studies are necessary even when there are no symptoms

**b.** Refer to a pediatric oncologist
   **i.** If enlarged nodes fail to decrease in size after 10 to 14 days of antibiotics
   **ii.** If evidence of bacterial infection in the node or its drainage region
   **iii.** Rubbery, nontender, and matted lymph node, i.e., loss of individual characteristics (implies malignancy)
   **iv.** Fixed enlarged lymph node (implies malignancy)
   **v.** See Chapter 33, Common Illnesses related to the Hematologic and Lymphatic Systems

## REFERENCES

American Association for Clinical Chemistry. (2004). The coagulation cascade. Retrieved April 22, 2006, from www.labtestsonline. org/understanding/analytes/coag_cascade/coagulation_cascade.html.

Bickley, L., & Szilagyi, P. G. (Eds.) (2003). *Bates' guide to physical examination and history taking* (8th ed.). Philadelphia: Lippincott Williams & Wilkins.

Corbett, J. V. (2004). *Laboratory tests and diagnostic procedures with nursing diagnoses* (6th ed.). Upper Saddle River, NJ: Pearson/Prentice Hall.

Engel, J. (2002). *Mosby's pocket guide series: Pediatric assessment* (4th ed.). St. Louis: Mosby.

Grethlein, S., & Perez Jr. J. A. (2005). Mucosa-associated lymphoid tissue (MALT). Retrieved April 22, 2006, from www.emedicine.com/med/topic3204.htm (updated March 24, 2005).

King, M. W. (2005). Medical biochemistry: Blood coagulation. Retrieved April 22, 2006, from http://web.indstate.edu/thcme/mwking/ blood-coagulation.html.

McCance, K. L., & Heuther, S. C. (2002). *Pathophysiology: The biologic basis for disease in adults and children* (4th ed.). St. Louis: Mosby.

Moore, K. L., & Persaud, T. V. N. (2003). *The developing human: Clinically oriented embryology* (7th ed.). Philadelphia: Saunders.

Nathan, D. G., Orkin, S. H., Look, A. T., & Ginsburg, D. (2003). *Nathan and Oski's hematology of infancy and childhood* (6th ed.). Philadelphia: Saunders.

Wong, D. L., Hockenberry-Eaton, M., Wilson, D., et al. (2001). *Wong's essentials of pediatric nursing*. St. Louis: Mosby, p. 96.

# Assessment of the Musculoskeletal System

KAREN DUDERSTADT, MS, RN, CPNP AND NAOMI A. SCHAPIRO, RN, MS, CPNP

## FETAL DEVELOPMENT

1. Embryology, structure and function of the musculoskeletal system (Larsen, 2001; Moore & Persaud, 2003; U. S. National Cancer Institute, 2005)
   a. Muscular system
      i. Muscles develop from the mesoderm (except muscles for the iris of the eye, which come from ectoderm)
      ii. Nuclei and cell bodies from the mesenchyme (connective tissue) differentiate into myoblasts
      iii. Skeletal muscle
         (a) Myoblasts fuse to become myotubes
         (b) Myofilaments develop in the cytoplasm of the myotubes, and a laminar layer separates them from the connective tissue
         (c) Most skeletal muscle develops before birth
         (d) Remaining skeletal muscles develop by end of first year
         (e) Muscle size increases when formation of myofilaments increases the diameter of the fibers
      iv. Smooth muscle
         (a) Myoblasts develop filamentous contractile elements and a laminar layer separates them from the connective tissue
         (b) Smooth muscle fibers develop into sheets or bundles, and lay down collagenous, elastic and reticular fibers
   b. Skeletal system
      i. By 28 days, the upper and lower limb buds begin to develop
      ii. By 32 days, the upper limb buds are paddle shaped and lower limb buds are flipper shaped
      iii. By 48 days, the arm is elongated and the fingers begin to separate; the toes are separated by 56 days
      iv. The skeleton consists of membranes of connective tissue and hyaline cartilage; then ossification begins
      v. Intramembranous ossification
         (a) Osteoblasts migrate to the connective tissue membranes
         (b) Osteoblasts produce a bony matrix around themselves and become osteocytes
         (c) Some flat bones of the skull and irregular bones
         (d) Results in changes in bone width and strength

    **vi.** Endochondral ossification
        (a) Perichondrium around the hyaline cartilage becomes infiltrated with blood vessels and osteoblasts and changes into periosteum
        (b) Osteoblasts move in and ossify the matrix to form bone
        (c) Cartilage in the epiphyses grows to increase bone length until ages 20 to 25
    **vii.** Intramembranous ossification
        (a) New bone builds on newly formed bone in long shaft
        (b) Changes and models the skeletal system from childhood through adolescence
    **viii.** Factors influencing bone growth
        (a) Nutritional factors
            (1) Adequate protein in diet
            (2) Calcium intake
            (3) Vitamin D intake (especially breast-feeding infants)
        (b) Genetic factors
        (c) Hormonal factors
            (1) Growth hormone from the anterior pituitary gland
            (2) Sex hormones from the ovaries and testes
        (d) Environmental insults (exposure to toxins, radiographs)

## FOCUSED HISTORY

**1.** Focused history (Colyar, 2003)
    **a.** Family history
        **i.** Congenital anomalies
        **ii.** Skeletal deformities
        **iii.** Frequent fractures
        **iv.** Developmental delay
    **b.** Past medical history of mother and neonate
        **i.** Maternal prenatal history has greatest effect on child during first 2 years of life
        (a) Maternal, paternal age
        (b) Month prenatal care started
        (c) Planned or unplanned pregnancy
        (d) Length of pregnancy
        (e) Maternal nutrition
        (f) Maternal health before/during pregnancy
            (1) Substance use or abuse, including tobacco
            (2) Prescription or over-the-counter drug use
            (3) Injuries or exposure to abuse
            (4) Hypertension
            (5) Maternal infection while in utero including TB and HIV
        **ii.** Birth history of neonate
        (a) Has greatest effect on child during first 2 years of life
        (b) Length, complications of labor
        (c) Delivery
            (1) Cesarean or vaginal
            (2) Unusual presentation
                a) Vertex
                b) Breech
                c) Shoulder

(3) Trauma sustained at birth
(4) Forceps or vacuum
(d) Condition at birth
  (1) Initial assessment
    a) Length, head, chest circumference
  (2) Birth trauma, e.g., fractured clavicle
  (3) Apgar score
  (4) Need for ventilation or resuscitation
  (5) Problems during hospital stay
    a) Feeding
    b) Elimination
    c) Irritability
    d) Length of stay
iii. Preterm infant
  (a) Reason for prematurity
  (b) Hypoxia in early neonatal period
  (c) Intraventricular insult
  (d) Maternal alcohol or substance use
iv. Developmental history
  (a) Gross motor milestones
  (b) Fine motor milestones
v. Children and adolescents (Neinstein, 2002)
  (a) Injuries
  (b) Involvement in organized or competitive sports
  (c) Daily physical activity
    (1) Important in developing strength and agility
    (2) Lack of exercise may contribute to increased body mass index (BMI), which increases strain on growing joints
  (d) Any limited range of motion of the joints; joint stiffness or swelling
  (e) Any pain when walking or running or pain awakening child at night
  (f) History of limp or abnormal gait
  (g) Habitual slouching or other postural abnormalities
  (h) Weight of backpack for school
  (i) Age at menarche and frequency of menses (girls reach adult height approximately 2 years after menarche)
  (j) History of prolonged corticosteroid use with chronic conditions

# FOCUSED EXAMINATION

1. Focused physical examination (Colyar, 2003)
  a. Preparation and definition of terms
    i. Equipment needed
      (a) Tape measure
      (b) Reflex hammer
      (c) Stadiometer—a device to measure standing height
      (d) Scoliometer—a device that measures the angle of rotation of the spine
    ii. Preparation for the examination
      (a) Infants undressed except diaper
      (b) Young children barefoot and undressed except underwear
      (c) Modesty issues for adolescents

(1) Need full view of spine, hips, shoulders

(2) Gown, underwear for maturing female

(3) Gym shorts or gown, underwear for maturing males

iii. Inspection

(a) Apparent state of health

(b) Appearance of comfort or pain

(c) Nutritional status

(d) In each skeletal area, examine the skin for:

(1) Color, temperature

(2) Bruising, scars, unusual pigmentation or lesions

(3) Swelling or erythema

(4) Nodules

(5) Café-au-lait spots, axillary freckles (>5 spots or axillary freckles suggest neurofibromatosis)

(e) Evaluating Sexual Maturity Rating (Tanner stage) is key to determining skeletal maturity (see Chapter 9, Figures 9-2 and 9-4)

(f) Conduct the "2-minute orthopedic examination" (Table 12-1)

iv. Palpation—in each skeletal area, examine:

(a) Bone or joint tenderness

(b) Joints—swelling, erythema, tenderness, temperature changes

(c) Unusual prominences, nodules, thickening, or indentations in bones

(d) Muscular development and symmetry

### ■ TABLE 12-1
### ■ ■ Two-Minute Orthopedic Examination

| Instructions | Observations |
|---|---|
| Stand facing examiner | Acromioclavicular joints, general habitus |
| Look at ceiling, floor, over both shoulders, touch ears to shoulders | Cervical spine motion |
| Shrug shoulders while examiner provides resistance | Trapezius strength |
| Abduct shoulders 90 degrees while examiner resists at 90 degrees | Deltoid strength |
| Full external rotation of arms | Shoulder motion |
| Flex and extend elbows | Elbow motion |
| Arms at sides, elbows 90 degrees flexed, pronate and supinate wrists | Elbow and wrist motion |
| Spread fingers, make a fist | Hand and finger motion and deformities |
| Tighten (contract) quadriceps, relax quadriceps | Symmetry and knee effusion; ankle effusion |
| "Duck walk" four steps away from examiner with buttocks on heels | Hip, knee, and ankle motion |
| Back to examiner | Shoulder symmetry, scoliosis |
| Knees straight, touch toes | Scoliosis, hop motion, hamstring tightness |
| Raise up on toes, raise heels | Calf symmetry, leg strength |

From Goldbloom, R. B. (2003). *Pediatric clinical skills* (3rd ed.). Philadelphia: Saunders, p. 312.

    **v.** Range of motion (ROM)—conduct ROM for each skeletal area as appropriate
- (a) Flexion—a decrease in the angle of the resting joint in the upper or lower extremities
- (b) Extension—an increase in the joint angle
- (c) Hyperextension—an increase in the angle of the joint beyond the usual arc
- (d) Abduction—movement away from the midline
- (e) Adduction—movement toward the midline
- (f) Rotation—movement around a central axis
- (g) Circumduction—rotation or circular movement of the limbs
- (h) Dorsiflexion—rotation backward
- (i) Supination—turning palm upward
- (j) Pronation—turning palm downward

**b.** Assessment of muscles (Note: This section was contributed by Debbie Terry, RN, MS, PNP)

    **i.** Muscle bulk
- (a) Palpate muscles as a subjective estimate of muscle volume
- (b) Visually observe for muscle wasting

    **ii.** Muscle tone
- (a) Hypotonicity
  - (1) Decreased muscle tone
  - (2) No resistance to passive stretch
  - (3) Muscle feels flabby and soft
  - (4) When held out from the body, a flaccid limb falls quickly due to gravity
  - (5) Signs of hypotonia in infants
    - a) "Frog leg" posture when supine
    - b) "Scarf sign"—elbow can be pulled past the chin when arm is pulled across the body
    - c) "Traction response"—head lags significantly behind the trunk when pulled from infant from supine to sitting by the arms
    - d) Ventral suspension—when held upright under the arms, the infant slips through the examiner's hands, indicating poor truncal tone
    - e) Horizontal suspension—when held prone with the examiner's hand supporting the chest and abdomen, the infant drapes over the examiner's hand
    - f) Bearing weight—when held vertically and feet placed on a surface, the 4- to 5-month-old infant is unable to bear weight on its legs even temporarily
- (b) Hypertonicity
  - (1) Increased muscle tone
  - (2) Spasticity
  - (3) Increase in muscle tension during passive stretching, especially during rapid or forced stretching of muscles
  - (4) Toe walking in a child may indicate increased tone in legs and ankles
  - (5) Signs of increased tone in infants
    - a) When held vertically, infant's legs are held in an extensor posture and may cross or scissor
    - b) Continual or increased fisting of hands; hands remain tightly clenched at rest

        c) Thrusting backward when sitting or pulled from supine

        d) Tends to stand on toes when supported in a standing position

  **iii.** Muscle strength

      (a) Evaluate muscle strength in proximal and distal muscle groups in all extremities using a grading scale

      (b) Power should be graded according to the maximum power attained, no matter how briefly it is maintained

        (1) 5/5, normal—complete range of motion against gravity and full resistance

        (2) 4/5, good—complete range of motion against gravity and moderate resistance

        (3) 3/5, fair—complete range of motion against gravity only

        (4) 2/5, poor—complete range of motion possible only if extremity supported by the examiner to eliminate the force of gravity

        (5) 1/5, trace—muscle contraction is detectable but insufficient to move the joint

        (6) 0/5, none—complete absence of visible and palpable muscle contraction

      (c) Compare strength of muscle groups on one side to the other, and proximal to distal muscle groups

      (d) Observe symmetry of movements in infants and younger children who cannot cooperate with formal muscle testing

  **iv.** Gower sign

      (a) Inability to rise from a sitting to a standing position without using the arms to "climb up the legs," which may indicate:

        (1) Lower extremity proximal muscle weakness

        (2) More specifically Duchenne muscular dystrophy

**c.** Assessment of the upper extremities and clavicle and age-specific observations

  **i.** Infants

      (a) Full ROM of upper extremities, including elbows and wrists, to identify birth trauma to shoulder

      (b) Palpate clavicle to detect fracture secondary to traumatic delivery

      (c) Localized tenderness right after birth

      (d) Palpable bony prominence as fracture heals (Ganel, Dudkiewicz, & Grogan, 2003)

      (e) Erb's palsy—injury to fifth, sixth cervical nerves

        (1) No spontaneous abduction of shoulder muscles or flexion of elbow

        (2) Arm adducted, internally rotated, normal grip in ipsilateral hand

  **ii.** Toddlers

      (a) Shoulder dislocation possible in this age-group

        (1) Pain, swelling

        (2) Limp arm

  **iii.** Older children/adolescents

      (a) Trauma to upper extremities common

        (1) Strenuous activity, falls, motor vehicle accidents or pedestrian injuries, competitive sports

        (2) Sprains, strains, fractures, dislocation

      (b) Overuse injuries to shoulder common

**d.** Assessment of the legs

  **i.** Evaluate legs with child sitting and legs hanging freely

      (a) Flexion/extension

      (b) Adduction/abduction

(c) Internal/external rotation

(d) Evaluate leg length

   (1) Position: infant/child supine, knee and hip joints extended and legs aligned

   (2) Discrepancy or asymmetric appearance may indicate abnormality in hips, long bones, or knees

   (3) Asymmetry of leg creases in supine or prone position

ii. Galeazzi or Allis sign related to symmetry of knee height (Table 12-2)

iii. Inspect for torsion; half of all infants and toddlers have some degree of torsion (Goldbloom, 2003)

   (a) Malleoli

      (1) Medial malleolus at distal end of tibia (medial ankle)

      (2) Lateral malleolus at distal end of fibula (lateral ankle)

   (b) Place a thumb and forefinger on the lateral and medial malleoli, knee facing forward

      (1) Forefoot and hindfoot should be in line with the knees

      (2) Only the anterior edge of the lateral malleolus should be in the midline

      (3) Change in position with age

         a) Infants—medial and lateral malleoli parallel when supine

         b) Rotation of up to 20 degrees in lateral malleolus during growth

         c) By school age, lateral malleolus is posterior to medial malleolus

   (c) Genu varum (bowleg)

      (1) Related to fetal positioning

      (2) Normal until 2½ to 3 years of age

      (3) Most common cause of toeing-in in children

      (4) May be related to nutritional deficiencies

---

■ **TABLE 12-2**
■ ■ **Age-Related Musculoskeletal Screening Techniques**

| Age | Technique | Results That Require Referral to Specialist |
|---|---|---|
| Newborn and infant | Ortolani sign | Presence of a clunk on abduction of hips |
| | Barlow test | Any instability of hip joints |
| | Galeazzi or Allis sign | When flexed, the knees are unequal in height |
| | Foot alignment | Rigid foot with limited range of motion |
| | | Rigid in-turning, inability of the foot to assume a normal angle to leg |
| Toddler and preschooler | Trendelenburg sign | When child bears weight, note any asymmetry in the level of the iliac crests. With one leg lifted, the iliac crest drops, indicating weak hip abductor muscles on the weight-bearing side |
| School age and adolescent | Forward bend test | Asymmetric elevation of the scapula or rib hump. Unequal shoulders or iliac crests, uneven waistline. A rotation of 5 to 7 degrees requires further evaluation or referral |
| Newborn to adolescent | Nuchal rigidity | Resistance or pain when neck is flexed when lying supine |
| | Brudzinski sign | Involuntary flexion of the knees or legs when neck is flexed when lying supine |
| | Kernig sign | Resistance or pain to straightening knees or legs from flexed position when lying supine |

(5) Evaluate gait from behind, check effect on motor development, performance

(6) Significant bowing after age 2 warrants referral to rule out pathologic conditions

(d) Tibial torsion, a curvature or inward twisting of tibia/fibula

(1) Used to describe bowlegs after age 3 or 4

(2) Generally resolves with growth

(3) Parental reassurance required

(e) Genu valgum (knock knee)

(1) Medial malleoli are more than an inch apart and the knees are touching

(2) Normal until age 7 years when the rotational development of the lower extremities is nearly complete

e. Assessment of the feet and age-specific observations

  i. Infants

(a) Plantar creases

(b) Position and alignment of forefoot and heels (see Table 12-2)

(c) Range of motion of ankle and plantar arch

(d) Inspect thigh-foot angle while supine with knees flexed to 9 degrees, evaluate any adduction of forefoot past midline

(e) Abnormalities in newborns require immediate orthopedic referral

(1) Limited dorsiflexion

(2) Fixed position of hindfoot

(3) Adduction of the forefoot

(4) Decreased ROM in general and pain with motion

(f) Clubfoot—rigidity and inability to move foot from fixed medial position

(1) Talipes equinovarus—inversion of forefoot, plantar flexion, and heel inversion

(2) Talipes calcaneovalgus—eversion and dorsiflexion of forefoot

(3) Metatarsus adductus—varus abnormality of forefoot at tarsometatarsal junction

    a) Ankle and hindfoot normal

    b) Lateral border of forefoot curved in "kidney bean" shape

    c) Line drawn medially from heel intersects third toe

(4) Mild deformity with flexible foot treated with passive stretching

    a) Support heel at right angle to leg

    b) Rotate and stretch forefoot laterally

(5) Metatarsus adductus treated with manipulation and serial casting

(6) Goal of correction—supple foot at normal angle to tibia

  ii. Toddlers/older children

(a) Longitudinal arch develops second or third year of life

(b) Flat feet in toddler normal, often accentuated by fat pad on ventral surface

(c) Lack of development of longitudinal arch in preschooler may indicate generalized ligamentous laxity; assess muscle tone

(d) Pes planus, in school-age child is a flattening of longitudinal arch of foot, standing erect with full weight bearing

(1) Arch is present when on tiptoes or standing, but flat sitting

f. Assessment of the hip (AAP, 2000)

  i. Newborn and infant examination technique—remove diaper

(a) Ortolani sign

(1) Position supine with knees flexed bilaterally

(2) Support hip with thumb forefinger

(3) Place pad of second finger on bony prominence of greater trochanter, thumb near lesser trochanter

(4) With abduction of thighs, pressure to greater trochanter causes unstable hip to move from unreduced to reduced position

(5) Clunk during maneuver = positive Ortolani sign

(b) Barlow sign

(1) Infant supine, knees flexed

(2) Thigh grasped, adducted while applying downward pressure

(3) Dislocation of femoral head = positive Barlow test

(4) Clicks during maneuvers considered to be benign

(c) Symmetry

(1) Supine with knees flexed to 90 degrees—asymmetry may indicate subluxed or dislocated hip

(2) Prone, inspecting thigh folds—less sensitive (Ganel, Dudkiewicz, & Grogan, 2003)

(d) Trendelenburg test for asymmetry of hips (see Table 12-2)

(e) Developmental dysplasia of the hip

(1) Femoral head has abnormal relation to acetabulum, unstable, subluxated or dislocated (AAP, 2000)

ii. Older children/adolescents

(a) Femoral anteversion—increased forward rotation of femoral head in relation to knee

(b) Exacerbated by child sitting in "W" position on floor

(c) Common cause of toeing-in after age 3

(d) Evaluate child undressed and lying prone; internal rotation of hip with slightly medial alignment of knees

(e) Resolves for many children after age 7

g. Assessment of the knee

i. Check symmetry and range of motion in knee

ii. Kernig sign (see Table 12-2)

iii. Infants

(a) Galeazzi or Allis sign (see Table 12-2)

(b) Congenital dislocation of the patella rare; manifests as limited knee motion in newborn

iv. Older children and adolescents

(a) Common site for overuse and traumatic injury in athletes, especially adolescent females

h. Assessment of the spine

i. Inspect and palpate, looking for congenital abnormalities that could indicate spinal abnormalities:

(a) Hair tufts

(b) Dimples

(c) Sacral sinus

(d) Hemangiomas

ii. Nuchal rigidity (see Table 12-2)

iii. Brudzinski sign (see Table 12-2)

iv. Infants/toddlers

(a) Normal lordosis (inward curve) of neck and lumbar region, kyphosis (outward curve) of thorax

(b) Exaggerated lordosis is normal in this age-group

v. Older children and adolescents

(a) Child standing, facing away from examiner

(b) View from the side to check alignment and posture
   (1) Contour of back
   (2) Symmetry of shoulders
   (3) Shape or prominence of scapula and ribs
   (4) Symmetry of waistline and iliac crests
   (5) Alignment of head with respect to sacrum; deviation may indicate spinal deformity (Taft & Francis, 2003)
(c) Idiopathic scoliosis—lateral bending of the spine and associated rotation of vertebral bodies (Taft & Francis, 2003)
   (1) Evaluate range of motion, with child bending to side, flexion, extension and hyperextension
   (2) Adams forward bend test (test for scoliosis)
      a) Child bends forward and touches toes if possible with hands dangling or in a diving position
      b) Observe for alignment of spine, any curvature, asymmetry, or rib hump from the rear and the sides
   (3) Scoliometer
      a) Use level ruler or scoliometer to assess degree of asymmetry/rotation
      b) Place the scoliometer over the spine, gently move down the length of the spine, making sure to note readings at the peak of curvature
      c) Readings of 5 to 7 degrees or more merit further evaluation by radiographic examination; the examiner should request measurement of the Cobb angle. (Chin, Price, & Zimbler 2001)
      d) Lateral curvature of more than 10 degrees indicates scoliosis
   (4) A scoliometer reading of 7 degrees may correlate with up to a 20-degree radiologic curve
4. Preparticipation sports examination—musculoskeletal system (AAP, 2001; Metzl, 2001a, 2001b; Patel, et al., 2001)
   a. Purpose of musculoskeletal portion of the examination
      i. Exclude or restrict athletes with medical contraindications to sports
         (a) Musculoskeletal laxity or weakness
         (b) Sequelae of injury
            (1) Overuse
            (2) Sprain/strain/tear/fracture
      ii. Match athlete's skills/conditioning/size/maturity to appropriate sport
         (a) Sexual Maturity Rating (SMR, Tanner stage)
            (1) Rapid growth during SMR (Tanner) III (female) and IV (male) weakens growth plates (physes) and increases injury potential
            (2) Relative muscle strength and cartilaginous physes of SMR (Tanner) III increases risk of physeal fractures
            (3) Controversy about matching SMR (Tanner) II with SMR (Tanner) IV or V during contact sports; unclear who is at increased risk of injury
         (b) Female adolescent athlete triad (amenorrhea, disordered eating, osteopenia)
      iii. Injury prevention: appropriate strengthening exercises, stretching
         (a) Classification of sports by contact level (Table 12-3)
         (b) High contact/collision sports lead to acute injury, macrotrauma
         (c) Low contact/collision sports lead to overuse injury, microtrauma
      iv. Often the only opportunity for health care maintenance; teens least likely age-group to access medical care

■ **TABLE 12-3**
■ ■ **Classification of Sports by Contact Level**

| Contact/Collision Sports | Limited-Contact Sports | Noncontact Sports |
|---|---|---|
| Basketball | Baseball | Archery |
| Boxing | Bicycling | Badminton |
| Diving | Cheerleading | Bodybuilding |
| Field hockey | Canoeing/kayaking (white water) | Canoeing/kayaking (flat water) |
| Football, flag or tackle | Fencing | Crew/rowing |
| Ice hockey | Field events: high jump, pole vault | Curling |
| Lacrosse | Floor hockey | Dancing |
| Martial arts | Gymnastics | Field events: discus, javelin, shotput |
| Rodeo | Handball | Golf |
| Rugby | Horseback riding | Orienteering |
| Ski jumping | Racquetball | Power lifting |
| Soccer | Skating: ice, inline, roller | Race walking |
| Team handball | Skiing: cross-country, downhill, water | Riflery |
| Water polo | Softball | Rope jumping |
| Wrestling | Squash | Running |
| | Ultimate Frisbee | Sailing |
| | Volleyball | Scuba diving |
| | Windsurfing/surfing | Strength training |
| | | Swimming |
| | | Table tennis |
| | | Tennis |
| | | Track |
| | | Weight lifting |

American Academy of Pediatrics, Committee on Sports Medicine and Fitness. (1994). Medical conditions affecting sports participation. *Pediatrics, 94*, 757-760.

    **b.** Focused history for preparticipation sports examination
        **i.** Reason for sports physical
            (a) Ask about the sport the youth intends to play, including position
                (1) Some overuse injuries more common in specific positions (e.g., shoulder/elbow for pitcher, knee problems for catcher)
                (2) New sport? Any previous complaints/injuries when playing sport?
                (3) Requirements for team (e.g., running a timed mile, weight loss or gain)
                (4) Weight class for wrestling/boxing
                    a) Last year's weight class
                (5) Planned preseason training, conditioning
                (6) Any current complaints related to training/conditioning?
    **c.** Musculoskeletal symptoms related to preparticipation examination
        **i.** Musculoskeletal—instability of joints (especially shoulder, knee, ankle), leg or foot pain with exercise, swelling of joints, any weakness
        **ii.** History of contact (macrotrauma) injuries
        **iii.** History of overuse (microtrauma) injuries
        **iv.** Muscle weakness, difficulties with balance or gait
    **d.** Dietary history related to musculoskeletal system
        **i.** Milk or calcium intake
        **ii.** Supplements for muscle gain

    **e.** Use of steroids for muscle gain

    **f.** 2-minute musculoskeletal examination (see Table 12-1)

    **g.** Plan with respect to musculoskeletal system

        **i.** Cleared for sports

        **ii.** Reasons for exclusion (or referral to specialist for clearance)

            (a) Musculoskeletal problems

            (b) Acute or overuse injury

            (c) Atlantoaxial instability

        **iii.** Restrictions or cautions

        **iv.** Positive recommendations

            (a) Stretching, muscle strengthening

            (b) Equipment, shoes, arch supports if indicated

            (c) Wear properly fitted safety equipment

# REFERENCES

American Academy of Pediatrics, Committee on Quality Improvement (2000). Clinical practice guideline: Early detection of developmental dysplasia of the hip. *Pediatrics, 105*(4), 896-904.

American Academy of Pediatrics, Committee on Sports Medicine and Fitness (2001). Medical conditions affecting sports participation. *Pediatrics, 107*, 1205-1209.

Chin, K. R., Price, J .S., & Zimbler, S. (2001). A guide to early detection of scoliosis. *Contemp Pediatr, 18*(9), 77-103.

Colyar, M. R. (2003). *Well-child assessment for primary care providers.* Philadelphia: F. A. Davis.

Goldbloom, R. B. (2003). *Pediatric clinical skills* (3rd ed.). Philadelphia: Saunders.

Ganel, A., Dudkiewicz, I, & Grogan, D. P. (2003). Pediatric orthopedic physical examination of the infant: A 5–minute assessment. *J Pediatr Health Care, 17*(1), 39-41.

Metzl, J. D. (2001a). Preparticipation examination of the adolescent athlete: Part 1. *Pediatr Rev, 22*, 199-204.

Metzl, J. D. (2001b). Preparticipation examination of the adolescent athlete: Part 2. *Pediatr Rev, 22*, 227-239.

Neinstein, L. S. (2002). *Adolescent health care: A practical guide* (4th ed.) Baltimore: Williams & Wilkins.

Patel, D. R., Greydanus, D. E., & Pratt, H. D. (2001). Youth sports: More than sprains and strains. *Contemp Pediatr, 18*(3), 45-72.

Taft, E., & Francis, R. (2003). Evaluation and management of scoliosis. *J Pediatr Health Care, 17*(1), 42-44.

U.S. National Cancer Institute's Surveillance, Epidemiology and End Results (SEER) Program. Bone development and growth. Retrieved April 22, 2006, from http://training.seer.cancer.gov/module_anatomy/unit3_3_bone_growth.html.

# Assessment of the Neurologic System

DEBBIE TERRY, CNRN, MS, PNP

## FETAL DEVELOPMENT

1.  Embryology, structure, and function of the neurologic system (Larsen, 2001; Moore & Persaud, 2003; Miyan, 2005)
    a.  The inner cell mass of a blastocyst differentiates into endoderm, mesoderm, and ectoderm
        i.  Mesoderm, also called the primitive streak; on about day 16 it folds to form the notochord, a rodlike structure that much later becomes the vertebral column
        ii.  Notochord releases chemicals that stimulate the ectoderm to divide rapidly, thicken, and form a neural plate
        iii.  Neural plate folds to form a crease called the neural groove by about day 22; this is the precursor of the nervous system
        iv.  Neural groove folds over and closes to become the neural tube
            (a)  Top third of neural tube becomes the brain
            (b)  Lower two thirds of neural tube become the spinal cord
    b.  Brain—the neural tube swells at the top to form three fluid-filled lobes by day 23
        i.  Forebrain—responsible for senses, memory, thinking, reasoning, problem solving
        ii.  Midbrain—coordinates relay of messages to appropriate organs
        iii.  Hindbrain—regulates heart, breathing, and muscle movements
    c.  Nerve cell migration
        i.  Neural crest cells from both sides of the midline migrate peripherally to form peripheral nerves, roots, and ganglion cells
        ii.  Nerve cells produce extensions of two types
            (a)  Dendrites—multiple branches extend from the nerve cell body and increase the surface area for synaptic terminals
            (b)  Axons—connect to other neurons with projections of variable lengths; some may need to reach from the foot to the brain
    d.  Nerve cell maturation
        i.  Myelin sheath—deposit of a fatty substance around most of the axons of the cerebral cortex

    ii. Allows conduction of nerve impulses to occur from 10 to 100 times faster than would occur along a nonmyelinated axon

  e. Synapse formation—begins at 20 to 28 weeks gestation

    i. Method by which neurons, dendritic branches, and projective axons communicate

    ii. Neurotrasmitter chemicals are released at the synapses, cross the gap, and carry the neuronal message to the next synapse

    iii. Development of synapses is at its highest rate during the first 6 to 8 years of postnatal life, then plateaus and begins to decrease with onset of puberty

    iv. The more synaptic connections, the more opportunities for cognitive activity

  f. Dermatomes and myotomes

    i. Spinal nerves have motor fibers that innervate muscles, and sensory fibers innervate the skin

    ii. Dermotome—skin area innervated by the sensory fibers of a single nerve root

      (a) Named according to the spinal nerve that supplies the sensory fibers, e.g., C4, L1

      (b) Overlap of dermatomes minimizes loss of sensation due to trauma

      (c) A "map" of dermatomes can be seen at: www.emedicinehealth.com/etools/dermatomes.asp

    iii. Myotome

      (a) A group of muscles primarily innervated by the motor fibers of a single nerve root

      (b) Specific nerves or reflexes and their associated muscles are described below

## FOCUSED HISTORY

1. Focused history (Colyar, 2003; Goldbloom, 2003)

  a. Prenatal

    i. Infections or illnesses

    ii. Drug and/or alcohol use

    iii. Prescription and over-the-counter drug use

    iv. Complications of pregnancy

    v. Fetal movement

  b. Labor and delivery

    i. Gestational age

    ii. Vaginal or cesarean delivery, reason for cesarean

    iii. Complications

    iv. Apgar scores

    v. Weight

  c. Postnatal

    i. Length of hospitalization for infant

    ii. Feeding or breathing problems

    iii. Neonatal illness

  d. Past medical history

    i. Illnesses

      (a) Central nervous system infections

      (b) Recent infections or illnesses before onset of symptoms

      (c) History of seizures

      **ii.** Injuries
        (a) Head injury
        (b) Spinal injury
      **iii.** Febrile seizures
        (a) Immunizations
  **e.** Current health status
      **i.** Sleep
      **ii.** Diet
      **iii.** Fluid intake
      **iv.** Caffeine intake
      **v.** Drug/alcohol use
      **vi.** Tobacco use
      **vii.** Menstrual history
      **viii.** Exercise
  **f.** Developmental history
      **i.** Attainment of developmental milestones
      **ii.** Infant/child and parent interaction patterns
      **iii.** Loss or regression of previously learned skills
      **iv.** Previous or current treatment with physical, occupational, or speech therapy
      **v.** School
        (a) Grade in school
        (b) Years held back
        (c) Usual grades earned in school
        (d) Special education services used
        (e) Strong and weak academic subjects
        (f) Previous educational or neuropsychologic evaluations and their results
      **vi.** Family history
        (a) Congenital defects or infant deaths
        (b) Headaches
        (c) Seizures
        (d) Tics
        (e) Stroke
        (f) Tremor
        (g) Chorea
        (h) Ataxia
        (i) Neuromuscular disease
        (j) Rheumatic disease
        (k) Liver disease
        (l) Mental health disorder
        (m) Behavior disorder
        (n) Learning disabilities
        (o) Diabetes
        (p) Parental consanguinity
      **vii.** Social history
        (a) Recreational activities/hobbies
        (b) Relationships with peers/friends
        (c) Parents' marital status
        (d) Custody issues
        (e) Who lives in home
        (f) Exposure to toxic chemicals, pollutants, lead
        (g) Sexual activity/contraception

      **viii.** Current and past medications including:
- (a) Antidepressants
- (b) Antianxiety medications
- (c) Anticonvulsants
- (d) Narcotics
- (e) Neuroleptics

**g.** Review of systems
- **i.** Headache
- **ii.** Seizures
- **iii.** Cognitive changes or change in school performance
- **iv.** Visual problems
- **v.** Problems with sucking, swallowing, eating, or talking
- **vi.** Sleep disturbances
- **vii.** Sensory changes
- **viii.** Bowel or bladder problems
- **ix.** Tics
- **x.** Problems with coordination
- **xi.** Muscle weakness
- **xii.** Joint pain
- **xiii.** Skin lesions and birthmarks
- **xiv.** Behavior problems and/or changes

## FOCUSED EXAMINATION

**1.** Focused examination (Fily, et al., 2003; Fuller, 2004; Hobdell, 2001)

**a.** Measurements
- **i.** Height, weight, and head circumference measured and plotted
  - (a) See Chapter 5 for details on head circumference and fontanelle size measurement
- **ii.** Blood pressure and heart rate
  - (a) Sitting
  - (b) Standing
- **iii.** Developmental assessment (see Chapter 4)

**b.** Inspection
- **i.** Overall appearance
- **ii.** Head circumference compared with:
  - (a) Height and weight
  - (b) Parents' head circumference if micro- or macrocephalic
- **iii.** Dysmorphic features
- **iv.** Head shape
- **v.** Hair quality, thin or coarse
- **vi.** Inspection of back for sacral dimpling
- **vii.** Inspection of skin:
  - (a) Café-au-lait spots
  - (b) Hypopigmented areas
  - (c) Axillary and inguinal freckling
- **viii.** Muscle wasting
- **ix.** Skeletal abnormalities such as scoliosis
- **x.** Behavior
- **xi.** Level of consciousness
- **xii.** Speech and language
- **xiii.** Affect

      xiv. Eye contact
      xv. Social interaction
      xvi. Impulsivity
      xvii. Activity level
      xviii. Play
      xix. Cognition
  **c.** Palpation
      **i.** Hepatosplenomegaly
      **ii.** Fontanelles and cranial sutures
      **iii.** Neurofibromas
  **d.** Cranial nerve testing
      **i.** Cranial nerve I (olfactory)
        (a) Not usually tested
        (b) If vials with distinctive fragrances are available, have child close eyes, pass a vial under child's nose, and ask child to identify it
      **ii.** Cranial nerve II (optic)
        (a) See Chapter 5 for details on eye examination techniques
        (b) Infants (Hobdell, 2001; Jarvis, 2003)
          (1) Optical blink reflex—shine light into eyes, watch for rapid closure
          (2) Regards face or close objects
          (3) Eyes follow moving object
        (c) Visual acuity
        (d) Visual fields by confrontation
        (e) Papillary reflex
          (1) Direct
          (2) Consensual (also tests third cranial nerve—oculomotor)
        (f) Funduscopic exam
          (1) Observe for papilledema
          (2) Optic atrophy
      **iii.** Cranial nerves III, IV, and VI (oculomotor, trochlear, and abducens)—eye movements
        (a) Oculomotor
          (1) Adduction—movement of the eye toward the nose
          (2) Upward and downward movements with outward gaze
          (3) Upward movements with inward gaze
          (4) Eye opening
        (b) Trochlear—downward movements with inward gaze
        (c) Abducens, abduction—movement of the eye away from the nose
        (d) Observe for:
          (1) Ptosis
          (2) Indicates an abnormality in CN III, which controls ability to open eyes
        (e) Asymmetric light reflex or abnormal cover/uncover test indicates an imbalance in extraocular muscles
        (f) Nystagmus
          (1) Involuntary eye movements, rapidly in one direction then slowly in opposite direction
          (2) Vertical or horizontal
          (3) One or two jerks at the extreme end of lateral gaze can be normal
        (g) Opsoclonus
          (1) Rapid chaotic movement of eyes in many directions

iv. Cranial nerve V (trigeminal)
 (a) Motor
   (1) Muscles used for chewing
   (2) Assess jaw movement
 (b) Sensory
   (1) Light touch
   (2) Pain and temperature in three distribution areas of the face:
     a) Ophthalmic
     b) Maxillary
     c) Mandibular
     d) Corneal reflex
 v. Cranial nerve VII (facial)
 (a) Motor—observe for asymmetry or weakness with facial movement
   (1) Frown
   (2) Raise eyebrows
   (3) Wrinkle the forehead (observe infants while crying or smiling)
   (4) Close the eyes
     a) Keep closed against resistance
     b) Ability to close eyes
   (5) Smile, show teeth, purse lips
   (6) Puff out cheeks against resistance
 (b) Sensory—taste
   (1) Sweet and salty on the tip of the tongue
   (2) Sour on the tip and on the borders of the tongue
   (3) Bitter on the back of the tongue and on the soft palate
 vi. Cranial nerve VIII (acoustic)
 (a) Cochlear division—hearing
   (1) Whisper test
   (2) Weber test—test of lateralization
     a) Place vibrating tuning fork on top of head or upper forehead
     b) Ask child if sound is heard equally in one or both ears
   (3) Rinne test—test of bone versus air conduction of sound
     a) Place vibrating tuning fork on mastoid process
     b) Ask child to say when no longer hears the hum or feels the vibration; note number of seconds
     c) Then place the tuning fork by the ear
     d) Ask child when can no longer hear the vibrations; note number of seconds
     e) Air conduction should be twice as long as bone conduction
 (b) Vestibular division tested if history of vertigo
   (1) Observe for nystagmus
   (2) Observe for unsteady gait
 vii. Cranial nerves IX and X (glossopharyngeal and vagus)
 (a) Swallowing
   (1) Ability to swallow
   (2) Uvula is midline
   (3) Soft palate and uvula should rise symmetrically when patient says "ah"
 (b) Gag reflex
   (1) Voice and taste on posterior third of tongue
   (2) Nasal quality may indicate an abnormality of vagus nerve
 viii. Cranial nerve XI (spinal accessory)

        (a) Sternomastoid and trapezius muscles controlling head and neck movement

        (b) Turn head against resistance

        (c) Shrug shoulders against resistance

    ix. Cranial nerve XII (hypoglossal)

        (a) Ability to stick out tongue and it remains midline

        (b) Infant—pinch nostrils; infant's mouth will open and tongue will rise to midline

**e.** Reflex testing

    i. Reflexes should be tested when child is relaxed and comfortable and extremities are positioned symmetrically

    ii. Deep tendon reflexes

    iii. Grade reflexes as follows:

        (a) 0 absent

        (b) 1+ present but diminished

        (c) 2+ normal

        (d) 3+ mildly increased but not pathologic

        (e) 4+ markedly increased, exaggerated jerk; clonus may be present

    iv. Specific reflexes:

        (a) Deep tendon reflexes—not usually tested in children younger than age 5; if tested, use fingers, not the reflex hammer (Jarvis, 2003)

            (1) Biceps (C6)

                a) Tap your index finger or thumb on the biceps tendon in the antecubital fossa

                b) Observe for contraction of the biceps muscle and flexion of the elbow

            (2) Brachioradialis (C6)

                a) Tap the brachioradialis tendon on the radial tuberosity (a few centimeters above the wrist on the thumb side)

                b) Observe for flexion and supination of the forearm

            (3) Triceps (C7)

                a) Tap the triceps tendon just above the elbow

                b) Observe for contraction of the triceps muscle and extension of the arm

            (4) Patellar (L3)

                a) Tap the patellar tendon just below the patella

                b) Observe for contraction of the quadriceps muscle and extension of the leg

            (5) Achilles (S1)

                a) Tap the Achilles tendon just above the heel

                b) Observe for plantar flexion of the foot

            (6) Clonus

                a) Test if the above reflexes are hyperreactive

                b) Flex knee at 45 degrees

                c) Briskly dorsiflex the ankle and maintain the foot in that position

                d) A rhythmic contraction of more than three beats is abnormal

        (b) Superficial reflexes

            (1) Babinski (L4, L5, S1, S2)

                a) Stroke the outer aspect of the foot from the heel across the ball of the foot

                b) Observe for extension of the great toe and fanning of the other toes

          c) A positive Babinski is normal in infants younger than 1 year of age but abnormal in children older than 1 year

      (2) Abdominal (T8-T12)

          a) Stroke the abdomen from lateral to medial above or below the umbilicus

          b) Observe for the normal response of deviation of the umbilicus toward the stimulus

      (3) Cremasteric (L1, L2)

          a) Stroke the inner aspect of the thigh downward

          b) Observe for the normal response of elevation of the testicle on the same side

  (c) Developmental reflexes

      (1) Rooting reflex

          a) Present at birth and disappears by 6 months

          b) Head moves toward side of mouth stroked with finger

      (2) Sucking reflex

          a) Present at birth and disappears by 10 months

          b) Sucking motion in response to stimulation of lips with finger

      (3) Palmar grasp reflex

          a) Present at birth and disappears by 4 months

          b) Infant grasps fingers placed in palm of hands

      (4) Moro (startle) reflex

          a) Present at birth and disappears by 4 to 6 months

          b) Flexion of arms and fingers in response to a loud noise or mimicking a falling motion

      (5) Tonic neck reflex

          a) Present at birth or appears at 1 to 2 months and disappears at 6 months

          b) Upper and lower extremities extend when head is turned toward that side, and the opposite arm and leg flex

      (6) Stepping reflex

          a) Present at birth and disappears by 3 months

          b) Stepping movements are made when infant's feet are pushed toward a flat surface when in a standing position

**v.** Abnormal involuntary movements

  (a) Fasciculations

      (1) Fine rippling movements that represent small muscle contractions

      (2) Observe for particularly in the tongue

  (b) Tics

      (1) Sudden stereotyped repetitive movements often involving the eyes, face, or mouth

      (2) Eye blinking

      (3) Mouth grimacing

      (4) Can also involve sudden rapid involuntary vocalizations

  (c) Chorea

      (1) Sudden and brief arrhythmic and asymmetric movements occurring most often in:

          a) Proximal extremities

          b) Neck

          c) Trunk

          d) Facial muscles

      (2) Disappears with sleep

        (d) Tremor

           (1) Rhythmic oscillation of a body part characterized by:

              a) The circumstances under which it occurs

                i) Rest

                ii) Posture

                iii) Action

              b) The frequency of the oscillations

                i) High

                ii) Low

      (e) Dystonia

           (1) Simultaneous and sustained contraction of both agonist and antagonist muscles

           (2) Resulting in a twisting movement or abnormal posture

      (f) Athetosis

           (1) Slow, twisting, writhing movements

      (g) Myoclonus

           (1) Sudden, brief, brisk muscle contractions

  **f.** Cerebellar function

    **i.** Coordination

      (a) Finger to nose testing—child should be able to smoothly and rapidly alternate touching finger to nose and touching his or her finger to your finger

      (b) Heel to knee to shin testing—child should be able to smoothly and rapidly slide the heel of one foot down the opposite leg from the knee to the shin

      (c) Rapid alternating movements

           (1) Child should be able to alternate patting the knees with the palms

           (2) Then with the backs of his hands and/or repeatedly touch the thumb to each finger on the same hand in rapid succession

      (d) In younger children assess coordination by asking them to draw or manipulate small toys

    **ii.** Balance

      (a) Romberg test

           (1) Ask child to stand erect, feet together and arms extended and the eyes open and then with eyes closed

           (2) Observe ability to maintain balance with eyes open and closed

           (3) Positive Romberg is abnormal and is present if patient becomes unsteady and tends to sway when eyes are closed

  **g.** Mental status—evaluation must be age appropriate

    **i.** Appearance

    **ii.** Level of consciousness

    **iii.** Thought processes

    **iv.** Mood and affect

    **v.** Communication

    **vi.** Level of attention

    **vii.** Judgment

    **viii.** Insight

    **ix.** Abstract reasoning

    **x.** Memory

  **h.** Assessment of muscles

    **i.** See Chapter 12 for details on testing muscle bulk, tone, strength, and Gower sign

      **ii.** Normal walking

      **iii.** Walking on toes and heels to identify muscle weakness

      **iv.** Tandem walking (heel to toe fashion)

      **v.** Running

   **i.** Sensation

      **i.** Light touch—use a wisp of cotton

      **ii.** Superficial pain—use a sharp object

      **iii.** Temperature—use a cold metal object such as a tuning fork

      **iv.** Vibration—use a tuning fork applied to bony prominences

      **v.** Position sense

        (a) Move joints up or down while patient's eyes are closed

        (b) Child should be able to correctly identify the direction of movement

      **vi.** Cortical sensation

        (a) Stereognosis

          (1) Ability to identify objects by manipulating and touching them

        (b) Graphesthesia

          (1) Ability to identify numbers, letter, or shapes drawn on the skin

        (c) Two-point discrimination

          (1) Ability to identify two points at 5 mm apart when touched with a sharp object

        (d) Infants and young children who cannot cooperate with testing may be evaluated by observing their response to different forms of sensory stimuli

---

# REFERENCES

Colyar, M. R. (2003). *Well-child assessment for primary care providers*. Philadelphia: F. A. Davis.

Goldbloom, R. B. (2003). *Pediatric clinical skills* (3rd ed.). Philadelphia: Saunders.

Fily, A., Truffert, P., Ego, A., et al. (2003). Neurological assessment at five years of age in infants born preterm. *Acta Paediatrica, 92*(12), 1433–1437.

Fuller, G. (2004). *Neurological examination made easy* (3rd ed.). Edinburgh: Churchill Livingstone.

Hobdell, E. (2001). Infant neurological assessment. *J Neurosci Nurs, 33*(4), 190–193.

Jarvis, C. (2003). *Physical examination and Health Assessment* (4th ed.). Amsterdam, Netherlands: Elsevier.

Larsen, W. J. (2001). *Human embryology*. New York: Churchill Livingstone.

Miyan, J. Embryology and neurulation. University of Manchester Institute of Science and Technology. Retrieved April 22, 2006, from www.bi.umist.ac.uk/users/mjfssjm4/OPT-NEU/Embryology.htm.

Moore, K. L., & Persaud, T V. N. (2003). *The developing human: Clinically oriented embryology*. Philadelphia: Saunders.

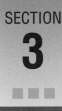

SECTION

**3**

# Special Topics in Health Promotion and Disease Prevention

# Core Concepts in Genetics

SUSAN M. HEIGHWAY, MS, APRN, BC-PNP, APNP

## HUMAN GENOME

1. Definition of human genome
   a. A person's total genetic complement, containing about 30,000 to 40,000 genes
   b. Consists of deoxyribonucleic acid (DNA) chemically bound to protein molecules
   c. Organized into distinct units called chromosomes
   d. Human Genome Project
      i. An international research effort to sequence and map all of the genes of *Homo sapiens*
      ii. Completed in April 2003
2. Role of DNA
   a. To store information (the genetic code)
   b. Transmit itself to subsequent generations
   c. Determine the precise nature of gene products, including protein structure
3. Chromosomes
   a. Distinct, physically separate microscopic structures in the nucleus of every cell
   b. Composed of chromatin that contains genetic information
   c. Visible only during cell division
   d. Each somatic cell contains *23 pairs* of chromosomes
      i. 22 autosomes and 2 sex chromosomes
      ii. Total of 46 chromosomes (called *diploid* number)
      iii. Autosomes
         (a) Chromosomes that resemble each other
         (b) Common to both sexes
         (c) Also called *homologous chromosomes*
         (d) Somatic cells divide by mitosis
            (1) All contents including chromosomes are duplicated
            (2) And distributed equally to the two identical daughter cells
            (3) Each daughter cell has exactly the same chromosomal content as the original cell

   **e.** A germ cell (i.e., gamete, mature egg or sperm) from each parent contributes
   - **i.** *One set* of 23 chromosomes (called *haploid* number)
   - **ii.** And one of two sex chromosomes: X or Y
     - **(a)** Combination of sex chromosomes determines the sex of the new infant
     - **(b)** Males 46, XY
     - **(c)** Females 46, XX
   - **iii.** Germ cells divide by meiosis
     - **(a)** Literally a reduction in size
     - **(b)** A two-step process
       - **(1)** Replication and segregation of each chromosome pair
       - **(2)** Formation of four gametes from the original cell
     - **(c)** Diploid chromosome number (46) reduces to the haploid number (23)
     - **(d)** Genetic exchange occurs between autosomes
     - **(e)** Results in chance distribution of genes

**4.** Gene
   - **a.** The basic unit of heredity
   - **b.** A segment of DNA
   - **c.** An ordered sequence of nucleotides
   - **d.** Arranged in a specific locus in a linear fashion along particular chromosomes
   - **e.** Structural genes encode cell components
   - **f.** Regulatory genes encode enzymes and hormones
   - **g.** Alternate forms of a gene at corresponding loci on homologous chromosome copies
     - **i.** Homozygous—when genes in a pair are identical
     - **ii.** Heterozygous—if one gene in a pair differs from the other
   - **h.** Activation of genes
     - **i.** The same genes are normally present in every somatic cell
     - **ii.** But are selectively expressed or "switched" on and off
     - **iii.** Very important for normal development

## HUMAN VARIATION

**1.** Genetic individuality
   - **a.** Pedigree—reflects a person's genetic inheritance pattern
     - **i.** A pictorial representation or diagram of the family history
     - **ii.** Determined by the chance distribution of genes
     - **iii.** Genetic and environmental factors can influence the inheritance pattern
   - **b.** Each individual is genetically and biochemically distinct from all other individuals (except for monozygous twins, triplets, etc.)
     - **i.** Karyotype
       - **(a)** Designation for a visual display of chromosome studies arranged in a standardized way
       - **(b)** The nomenclature includes
         - **(1)** The number of chromosomes
         - **(2)** The sex chromosomes contribution
         - **(3)** Any abnormalities found
     - **ii.** Genotype
       - **(a)** A specific pair of alleles (genes) at a single locus of homologous chromosomes
       - **(b)** Sometimes refers to a person's total genetic makeup or constitution

       iii. Phenotype—observable expression of a genetically determined trait
          (a) Visibly apparent (e.g., hair color)
          (b) Or biochemically detectable (e.g., blood type)
  **c.** Mutation
      **i.** A permanent change in genetic material
      **ii.** Occurs when an incorrect nucleotide base is inserted during DNA synthesis
      **iii.** Some produce a "gain of function" that may be advantageous or disadvantageous to the individual
      **iv.** Some produce a "loss of function," i.e., cannot produce a functional protein
  **d.** Dominant genes override characteristics of weaker (recessive) genes
  **e.** Dominant trait or characteristic
      **i.** Phenotype is apparent, or expressed when one copy of the gene is present at corresponding loci of homologous chromosomes
      **ii.** The dominant allele can be either in the homozygous or heterozygous state
  **f.** Recessive trait or characteristic
      **i.** Expressed only when two copies of the same gene are present at corresponding loci of homologous chromosomes
      **ii.** Each human is estimated to carry from five to seven recessive rare deleterious alleles in the heterozygous state
         (a) Usually remain undetected for generations
         (b) If he or she mates with another individual with same rare recessive allele, then they may have a child with a homozygous recessive disease
  **g.** A person's genetic constitution
      **i.** Determines the limits of range of response and potentials within which he or she can interact with environment
      **ii.** Maintains homeostasis, susceptibility, and resistance to disease
      **iii.** All people are not at equivalent risk for developing disease
      **iv.** No disease process is wholly genetic or wholly environmental

## CHROMOSOMAL AND GENETIC DISORDERS: GENERAL INFORMATION

**1.** Incidence and prevalence
  **a.** There are more than 4000 known genetic disorders
  **b.** Can affect anyone of any age, social, economic racial, ethnic, or religious background
  **c.** Expression of the disorder can be extremely variable from one person to another
  **d.** May be present in multiple family members or isolated to one family member
  **e.** These disorders affect all members of an individual's family along with the community and society as a whole
**2.** Etiology and pathophysiology
  **a.** Chromosomal abnormalities can be either:
      **i.** Numerical (aneuploidy)—extra or missing chromosomes
      **ii.** Structural
         (a) Deletions—portions missing
         (b) Duplications—portions added

      (c) Translocations—exchange of chromosome segments

      (d) Inversions—reversal of polarity within a chromosome

  **b.** Classic Mendelian inheritance patterns

    **i.** Autosomal recessive

      (a) Etiology

        (1) Occurs when the child has two copies of the specific mutated gene, one from each parent

        (2) Parents have 25% chance with each pregnancy of having an affected child

      (b) Pathophysiology

        (1) Often results in enzyme deficiency

        (2) Leads to biochemical abnormalities

          a) Insufficiency of a needed product

          b) Buildup of toxic materials

      (c) Presentations—Tay-Sachs, PKU, cystic fibrosis, sickle cell anemia

      (d) Incidence—usually affects males and females equally, but not always

      (e) Prevalence—history of disorder in previous generations rarely exists unless relatives have married (consanguinity)

    **ii.** Autosomal dominant

      (a) Etiology—disorder occurs when the individual has one or two abnormal genes

      (b) Pathophysiology—usually involves structural (physical) rather than enzymatic abnormalities

      (c) Presentation—achondroplasia, Huntington's disease, polydactyly

      (d) Incidence—usually affects males and females equally, but not always, such as in male pattern baldness

      (e) Prevalence

        (1) Disorder usually appears in every generation with little or no skipping

        (2) Transmitted by an affected person to half (50%) of his or her children on average

        (3) In individual families a 1:1 transmission ratio is not always seen

   **iii.** X-linked (sex-linked) disorders

      (a) Pathophysiology—involves abnormal genes located on an X, or female sex chromosome

      (b) Incidence

        (1) Females are carriers

          a) The abnormal gene on one X chromosome is compensated by the normal gene on the other X chromosome

        (2) Males are affected

          a) The abnormal gene on the X chromosome is invariably expressed

          b) The Y chromosome is small and mostly inactive

      (c) Presentations—muscular dystrophy, hemophilia, fragile X syndrome

  **c.** Nontraditional forms of inheritance

    **i.** Mitochondrial DNA mutations

      (a) Mitochondria are inherited solely through the mother via her egg

      (b) Genetic abnormalities in mitochondria of fathers is not passed on to their children

      (c) Examples: Leber optic atrophy and mitochondrial myopathy

    **ii.** Germ line mosaicism

      (a) Abnormal gene that is capable of causing a disease is present only in germ cells of an otherwise unaffected and healthy individual

(b) Examples: Duchenne muscular dystrophy and certain forms of osteogenesis imperfecta

   iii. Uniparental disomy

      (a) Inheritance of both chromosomes in a pair from same parent rather than inheriting one from each parent, as normally occurs

      (b) Recessive and abnormal genes are duplicated and expressed in the individual

      (c) Chances are greater for adverse outcomes such as birth defects, growth delay and mental retardation

      (d) Genomic imprinting

      (e) Variable phenotypic expression of an abnormal gene depending on whether the abnormal gene was inherited from father or mother

      (f) Gene expression is turned "on" in one case, and turned "off" in another

      (g) Example—chromosome 15 with a specific deleted gene results in Prader-Willi syndrome if it was inherited from father, or in Angelman syndrome if inherited from mother

   iv. Mutagenesis

      (a) Mutagens change DNA or chromosomes at any time during the life cycle

      (b) Examples—radiation, chemical and infectious agents

   v. Tetratogenesis

      (a) Teratogens are any substance that adversely affects fetal development, but does not alter the genetic material

      (b) Examples—drugs, alcohol, certain medications, maternal disease, or maternal infections

      (c) Consequences

         (1) No apparent effect

         (2) Prenatal or perinatal fetal death

         (3) Congenital anomalies

         (4) Altered fetal growth

         (5) Postnatal functional deficits and aberrations

         (6) Carcinogenesis

   vi. Multifactoral inheritance (hereditary-environmental interactions)

      (a) Several factors contribute to the total effect

      (b) No one factor is sufficient to produce the particular abnormalities

      (c) Probably occurs from the interaction of several genes with environmental factors

      (d) Examples—neural tube defects, cleft lip and palate, congenital hip dislocation

**3.** Presentation

  **a.** Diagnostic criteria

    **i.** No universal screening guidelines for detection of genetic disorders

    **ii.** Congenital anomaly—birth defect; abnormal variation in form or structure without inferring a specific cause

    **iii.** Minor anomaly

      (a) An external feature usually seen in the head, hands, feet, or face

      (b) Some may indicate presence of more serious problems (e.g., wide-set eyes, ear pits)

    **iv.** Major anomaly

      (a) Associated with significant disability

      (b) Serious functional problems

(c) And/or requires surgery or other medical treatment (spina bifida, congenital heart disease)

    v. Syndrome—a condition affecting two or more body systems and having one underlying cause

  **b.** Signs and symptoms

    **i.** Findings from the family history, medical history, developmental assessment, and physical examination indicate that further genetic evaluation is warranted for any child

    **ii.** Evidence of minor or major anomaly or syndrome

    **iii.** Ambiguous genitalia

    **iv.** Developmental delay or abnormal development, mental retardation

    **v.** Multiple family members with the same condition

    **vi.** Unusual growth patterns, such as short stature, especially when combined with more of the other factors.

    **vii.** Coma, vomiting, lethargy, unexplained metabolic acidosis, hyperammonemia, ketosis, seizures, hypoglycemia, or other combinations of metabolic signs and symptoms without an identifiable cause

    **viii.** Unusual dermatologic conditions (e.g., ichthyosis, unusual birthmarks, unusual scarring, skin tumors.)

    **ix.** Known chromosomal abnormality

    **x.** Any other suspicious signs or symptoms suggestive of genetic disorder that PNP believes need further evaluation

**4.** Diagnostic tests

  **a.** PNP usually does not order laboratory studies for genetic testing but should be familiar with them

  **b.** Biochemical testing—specific plasma and urine tests, skin or muscle biopsy with enzyme studies for questions about inborn errors of metabolism

  **c.** Chromosome analysis—when there are specific indicators, such as suspicion of a known syndrome, ambiguous genitalia, multiple anomalies, mental retardation, developmental delay, or low birth weight

  **d.** DNA analysis of blood—to look for abnormalities related to specific conditions (e.g., fragile X or Prader-Willi)

**5.** Indicators for referral for genetic evaluation or counseling

  **a.** Newborns/infants

    **i.** Newborns with prenatally suspected fetal abnormalities or growth retardation

    **ii.** Unusual facial features (dysmorphic features)—facial or skull asymmetry, premature closure of sutures, weakness or decreased facial expression, congenital cataracts, short palpebral fissures or epicanthal folds, wide-set eyes, low-set ears, ear pits, wide nasal bridge, unusual philtrum, cleft lip and palate)

    **iii.** Unusual growth pattern—small for gestational age, failure to thrive, large size, abnormalities in head growth (microcephaly or microcephaly), disproportionate growth

    **iv.** Skin—café-au-lait spots, ash leaf spots or loose, easily stretched skin that scars readily

    **v.** Physical abnormalities—congenital heart disease, clubfoot, neural tube defect, missing limbs, extra digits, ambiguous genitalia

    **vi.** Neurologic signs—unexplained hypotonia, seizure activity, absence of infantile automatisms or persistence beyond expected time of disappearance, asymmetry in movements

    **vii.** Identified through state newborn screening program as having an abnormal result for an inborn error of metabolism

   b. Childhood and adolescence
      i. Unusual head, neck, and face—coarse facies, abnormal dentition, persistent facial or cranial asymmetries
      ii. Sensory impairments
         (a) Hearing impairment not due to recurrent infection, meningitis, or trauma
         (b) Vision problems other than simple refractive errors or strabismus (e.g., unexplained optic atrophy, retinitis pigmentosa)
      iii. Unusual overall appearance, especially accompanied by short stature, failure to thrive, or slow psychomotor development
      iv. Unusual growth patterns
         (a) Tall, asymmetric, macrosomia and disproportionate
         (b) Short stature that is inconsistent with family height with or without an obvious bony dysplasia
      v. Known or suspected metabolic disorders
      vi. Neurodevelopmental
         (a) Mental retardation, developmental delays, and/or autism without an obvious etiology
         (b) Loss of developmental milestones or other evidence of a neurodegenerative disorder
      vii. Known chromosomal abnormality
      viii. Tumor or malignancy with a suspected genetic predisposition (e.g., retinoblastoma, Wilms' tumor)
   c. Indicators in the family history
      i. Multiple family members with the same condition
      ii. Known chromosomal abnormality
      iii. If parents'/child's problems have occurred in previous sibling
      iv. If parents are consanguineous (close blood relatives) or of similar ethnic origins, autosomal recessive pattern is possible
      v. If similar disorder has occurred in more than one generation
      vi. If more than one family member has same birth defect, but no regular pattern can be discerned, a multifactoral etiology can be suspected, e.g., neural tube defects, clefting malformations
      vii. Previous siblings who were miscarried or stillborn
6. PNP role in referral
   a. Components of the genetic evaluation
      i. Usually conducted by physician genetic specialist and genetic counselors through university medical centers, large medical facilities, or outreach clinics
      ii. Usually includes:
         (a) Review of the family history
         (b) Review of the individual's health and developmental history
         (c) Physical and neurologic examination
         (d) Laboratory tests as appropriate
         (e) Genetic counseling
   b. PNP role in genetic evaluation
      i. Consider the psychologic effect of a potential genetic disorder when discussing the referral with the family at risk because of history or at risk because of a child born with a genetic disorder
      ii. Exercise care not to make diagnoses or attempt to counsel
      iii. Facilitate the genetic evaluation process

    **iv.** Prepare the child/family for what to expect

    **v.** Communicate relevant information to the genetics team

    **vi.** Follow up with the family after genetics services have been provided

  **c.** PNP role in primary care after genetic counseling

    **i.** Once a specific etiology and disorder are identified, PNP can review etiology, prognosis and recurrence risk, medical management, and resources

    **ii.** Anticipate and discuss the emotional effect of the diagnosis on the individual and family

**7.** Influence on growth and development

  **a.** Physical and psychosocial outcomes can be improved through:

    **i.** Early detection

    **ii.** Appropriate medical treatment

    **iii.** Intervention programs

    **iv.** Supportive counseling

    **v.** Continued attention to primary care needs of the child

---

# REFERENCES

American Academy of Pediatrics Committee on Genetics, Section on Endocrinology, and Section on Urology. (2000). Evaluation of newborn with developmental anomalies of external genitalia. *Policy Statement, 106* (1), 138–142.

Behrman, R. E., Kliegman, R. M., & Jenson, H. B. (Eds.). (2004). *Nelson textbook of pediatrics* (17th ed.). Philadelphia: Saunders.

Centers for Disease Control and Prevention (CDC). An overview of the Human Genome Project. Retrieved March 13, 2006, from www.genome.gov/12011238.

National Coalition for Health Professional Education in Genetics (NCHPEG). (2000). *Core competencies in genetics essential for all health-care professionals.* Lutherville, MD: NCHPEG.

Genetics & Your Practice CD-ROM, Version 2.0. Designed for health care professionals working with patients from preconception/prenatal, infant/children to adolescent/adult. The curriculum provides practical information and resources to assist the busy professional in integrating genetics into their patient care. Can be obtained from the March of Dimes (call 1-800-367-6630, use order number 09-1177-99).

Jones, K. L. (1997). *Smith's recognizable patterns of human malformation* (5th ed.). Philadelphia: Saunders.

Williams, J. (2002). Education for genetics and nursing practice. *AACN Clin Issues, 13*(4), 492–500.

# WEB RESOURCES

National Human Genome Research Institute: www.genome.gov

National Organization on Rare Disorders: www.rarediseases.org

March of Dimes Birth Defects foundation: www.modimes.org

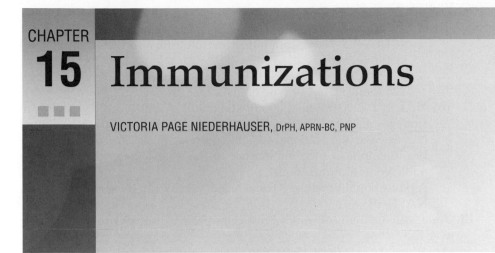

CHAPTER

**15** Immunizations

VICTORIA PAGE NIEDERHAUSER, DrPH, APRN-BC, PNP

1. General concepts
   a. Active immunizations
      i. A person's immunologic defenses are stimulated to prevent disease from future exposure
      ii. Immunizations that contain an infectious agent may be either live (attenuated) or killed (inactivated)
   b. Passive immunizations
      i. Human or animal antibody is given to an individual who has been exposed or is about to be exposed to a disease
      ii. Antibodies passed from mother to child during pregnancy can last for 6 months
      iii. Antibodies are passed from mother to child during breast-feeding
         (a) Encourage breast-feeding, especially in countries with lower levels of sanitation
   c. Herd immunity
      i. As more members of a community are vaccinated, the odds of the nonimmune person being exposed to a disease decrease
      ii. The community needs everyone to participate in immunization to help protect people who cannot protect themselves even through vaccination
      iii. No one can predict who will *not* become immune after vaccination
2. Immunizations and health disparities (Neiderhauser & Stark, 2005)
   a. Disparities in child and adolescent immunization rates occur among different ethnic/racial groups and socioeconomic groups
   b. Healthy People 2010 identified as a major priority to reduce the disparities in immunization rates
   c. Strategies are needed to improve access and compliance in these under- and unimmunized groups
3. Immunization compliance
   a. Resources for providers are available from several organizations
      i. Centers for Disease Control and Prevention Advisory Committee on immunization practices (CDC, 2006c)
      ii. NAPNAP
         (a) NAPNAP (2005) Position statement on immunization states that:
            (1) All children, adolescents and adults need to be immunized according to current Centers for Disease Control and Prevention

(CDC) Advisory Committee for Immunization Practices (ACIP) parameters

(2) All children need access to immunizations regardless of social and economic status, or type of insurance

(b) NAPNAP (2004) issued a joint statement in 2004 with the American College of Nurse Practitioners, the National Association of School Nurses, and the National Organization of Nurse Practitioner Faculties to emphasize the importance of focusing increased attention on adolescent immunizations

(c) A educational brochure "Teens Need Vaccines, too" is available from NAPNAP

   iii. American Academy of Family Physicians (2006) Clinical Care and Research website

   iv. American Academy of Pediatrics (2006) Immunization Initiatives website

   v. Immunization Action Coalition (2006)

   vi. National Network for Immunization Information (2005)

**b.** An educational brochure "Teens Need Vaccines, Too" is available from NAPNAP

**c.** Many issues affect immunization compliance in the pediatric population

   i. Vaccine refusal (Fredrickson, et al., 2004; Frenkel, 2004; Lieber, et al., 2003)

   ii. Complex immunization schedules

   iii. Provider apprehension and discomfort with multiple injections

   iv. Parental concerns and confusion

(a) Social issues

(1) School and daycare vaccination laws

a) By 1980 all 50 states had laws covering students first entering school and Head Start to grade 12 regarding immunization against:

   i) Diphtheria

   ii) Polio

   iii) Measles

   iv) Rubella

b) Some states have immunization requirements for college entrance

(2) "Exposure parties"—deliberately exposing children to a communicable disease, e.g., chickenpox

a) Reasons: to "get it over with," "to time the illness over summer vacation"

b) Puts children at needless risk of contracting serious illness with possible significant side effects

(b) Religious and cultural issues: www.immunizationinfo.org/immunization_policy-detail.

(1) Parens patriae—state asserts authority over child welfare

(2) No constitutional right exists for either a religious or philosophic exemption to school vaccination requirements, although some states allow it for:

a) Amish

b) Christian Scientists

(3) Exemptions

a) 50 states allow exemptions for medical reasons

         b)  48 states allow religious exemptions (not Mississippi and West Virginia)

         c)  20 states allow philosophic exemptions

   (c)  Popular press

       (1)  False belief that fetal tissue is still being used to produce vaccines (CDC, 2000a)

         a)  In fact, aborted fetal tissue obtained in the 1960s is the source of cell lines used today to produce vaccines

         b)  No new fetal tissue is needed now, or will be needed in the future

         c)  Vaccine manufacturers obtain human cell lines from the Food and Drug Administration (FDA)-certified cell banks

         d)  www.cdc.gov/nip/vacsafe/concerns/gen/humancell.htm

       (2)  Inflammatory bowel disease (IBD) (CDC, 2005e)

         a)  Measles-mumps-rubella (MMR) vaccine does not cause IBD

         b)  www.cdc.gov/nip/vacsafe/concerns/autism/ibd.htm

       (3)  Autism

         a)  Institute of Medicine (IOM) rejected a casual relationship between MMR vaccine and autism

         b)  IOM also rejected a causal relationship between thimerosal-containing vaccines and autism

         c)  www.immunizationinfo.org/iom_reports.cfm

       (4)  Rotavirus vaccine and intussusception

         a)  Rota Shield vaccine no longer recommended due to association between the two

         b)  In February 2006 a new Rotavirus vaccine was recommended by the Advisory Committee on Immunization Practices (ACIP) (CDC, 2006d)

           i)  RotaTeq (Merck & Co., Inc)

           ii)  Studies over 70,000 children and found no association of RotaTeq with intusseption

       (5)  Multiple sclerosis and the hepatitis B vaccine (CDC, 2005d)

         a)  The weight of the available scientific evidence does not support the suggestion that the two are causally related

         b)  www.cdc.gov/nip/vacsafe/concerns/ms/default.htm

       (6)  Sudden infant death syndrome (SIDS)

         a)  IOM evidence favors rejection of causal relationship of vaccines and SIDS

       (7)  Guillain-Barré syndrome (GBS) and influenza vaccines (CDC, 2005b)

         a)  More than 99% of patients with GBS have not received the influenza vaccine

         b)  Risk of developing GBS after influenza vaccine is rare

         c)  www.cdc.gov/nip/vacsafe/concerns/gbs/default.htm

       (8)  Febrile seizures and vaccines (CDC, 2001)

         a)  DPT (diphtheria, pertussis and tetanus) with whole cell pertussis, and MMR can temporarily increase the risk for fever-related seizures (febrile seizures)

         b)  A study showed that children did not have an increased risk for subsequent seizures or neurologic disabilities

         c)  However, DTP is no longer manufactured

         d)  The use of acellular pertussis (DTaP) has replaced DTP vaccine and has shown fewer side effects

         e)  www.cdc.gov/nip/issues/mmr-dtp/mmr-dtp.htm

(9) Oral polio vaccine and AIDS (CDC, 2004)
  a) 1990s *Rolling Stone* magazine featured an article that an experimental oral polio vaccine used in Africa in the late 1950s may have caused the AIDS epidemic
  b) Theory raised again in Edward Hooper's *The River*
  c) Investigations concluded that this is not true
  d) www.cdc.gov/nip/vacsafe/concerns/aids/poliovac-hiv-aids-qa.htm
v. Increasing number of vaccines and visits in the first few years of life, and parents reluctant to expose their infants to "so many shots"
vi. Implementation logistics and complexity
  (a) Vaccine ordering, storage, and handling issues
  (b) Inventory management
  (c) Vaccine expiration
  (d) Freezer/refrigerator temperature
  (e) Preparation time
  (f) Needlestick exposure
  (g) Record keeping/immunization tracking
vii. Missed opportunities for immunizations

d. Causes of missed opportunities
  i. Lack of simultaneous immunizations
    (a) When too many vaccines and injections are recommended over time, more missed opportunities will occur
  ii. Myths and misperceptions
    (a) Invalid precautions (runny nose, low-grade fever)
    (b) Invalid contraindications (allergy to nonvaccine substance)
    (c) Supposed adverse events from previous dose that were never documented
  iii. Reimbursement or cost issues
    (a) Vaccines are too costly for most practices and will not be stocked or offered
    (b) Children are referred to health department for vaccines, with no follow-up to ensure it was done
  iv. Lack of information or confusion about risk-benefit of new vaccines
    (a) Many forms to read, understand, and sign
    (b) Cultural and language barriers
  v. Lack of comprehensive immunization record keeping
    (a) Fragmented immunization records from multiple providers
    (b) Recommendations
      (1) Use of immunization registries for storing data from several sources
      (2) Recall/reminder systems for parents
      (3) Common immunization record card

e. Sites for vaccine administration
  i. Site depends on the age and size of the child and the type of vaccine administered
  ii. See Table 15-1 for the site and needle size for intramuscular and subcutaneous immunizations

f. Provider must document
  i. Name of vaccine
  ii. Date given
  iii. Vaccine information sheet date

■ **TABLE 15-1**
■ ■ **Sites for Immunization Administration**

| Type | Age | Site | Needle Size |
| --- | --- | --- | --- |
| Intramuscular | Birth-12 months | Vastus lateralis (muscle in the anterolateral aspect of the middle/upper thigh) | ⅞-1 inch<br>22-25 gauge |
| | 12–36 months | Vastus lateralis muscle or deltoid (if adequate muscle mass) | ⅝ inch for deltoid<br>1¼ inches<br>22-25 gauge |
| | >36 months | Dense portion of the deltoid, above the armpit, below the acromion process | ½ inch<br>22-25 gauge |
| Subcutaneous | Birth-12 months | Fatty area in anterolateral thigh | ⅝-¾ inch<br>23-25 gauge |
| | 12–36 months | Fatty area in anterolateral thigh or outer aspect of the upper arm | ⅝-¾ inch<br>23-25 gauge |
| | >36 months | Outer aspect of the upper arm | ⅝-¾ inch<br>23-25 gauge |

      iv. Manufacturer
      v. Lot number
      vi. Dose
      vii. Site
      viii. Signature and title of individual giving the immunization
   **g.** Handling and storage (CDC, 2006e)
      i. Standard household refrigerator/freezer is sufficient
        (a) Dormitory-style refrigerators are NOT recommended
        (b) Varicella especially must not be stored in a dormitory-style refrigerator
        (c) Maintain refrigerator compartment temperature between 35° to 46° F or 2° to 8° C
        (d) Never allow refrigerator temperature below 32° F
        (e) Maintain freezer compartment temperature at or below 5° F or −15° C
        (f) If freezer is not frost free then do not allow ice buildup greater than ¼ inch
      ii. Never store food or specimens in the same unit as vaccines
      iii. Never store vaccines in:
        (a) The doors
        (b) Airtight container
        (c) Crispers
      iv. Check temperature twice a day
      v. Establish a protection system that maintains the "cold chain"
      vi. Package vaccines properly for shipping and transportation
        (a) See CDC website at www.cdc.gov/nip, CDC National Immunization Information Hotline 800-232-2522 (English) 800-232-0233 (Spanish)
   **h.** Vaccines for Children (VFC) Act
      i. Immunization coverage is affected by availability and cost to families
      ii. No cost vaccines ordered by and obtained from the primary health care provider

        (a) Decreases referrals to public health centers

        (b) Improves continuity of care and promotes the medical home concept

    iii. Children who have health insurance that does not cover costs of immunizations may get free vaccines through VFC programs at:

        (a) Federally qualified health center (FQHC)

        (b) Rural health clinic (HC)

    iv. VFC programs provide immunizations for children who:

        (a) Are 18 years old or younger

        (b) Are eligible for Medicaid

        (c) Have no health insurance

        (d) Are Native American or Alaskan Native

    v. Vaccines not available through VFC

        (a) DT

        (b) Td

        (c) Meningococcal vaccine

    vi. Two other government vaccine programs are:

        (a) Vaccination Assistance Act Section 317

        (b) Funds that individual state legislatures provide to their health departments

i. Adverse events (CDC, 2005f)

    i. Must report adverse events requiring medical attention that occur within 30 days of immunization

    ii. Vaccine Adverse Event Reporting System (VAERS)

        (a) National vaccine safety surveillance program cosponsored by the CDC and the FDA

        (b) Collects and analyzes information from reports of adverse events following immunization administration

        (c) 85% of reports describe fever, local reactions, episodes of crying or mild irritability

        (d) 800-822-7967 or VAERS website www.vaers.org

        (e) Printable copies of report also from FDA: www.fda.gov/cber/vaers/vaers.htm and CDC, www.cdc.gov/nip

4. Immunization schedule (CDC, 2006a)

  a. Continuity of care and immunizations go hand in hand (Irigoyen, et al., 2004; Raucci, et al., 2004; Whitehill, et al., 2004)

  b. Routine immunization schedule

    i. The immunization schedule is revised at least yearly

    ii. PNP must monitor American Academy of Pediatrics (AAP) and CDC websites for periodic changes

    iii. Table 15-2 contains the routine vaccine schedule for children from birth to 18 years of age

  c. Delayed immunization schedule for children and adolescents who start late or who are more than 1 month behind (CDC, 2006b)

    i. Tables 15-3 and 15-4 give catch-up schedules and minimum intervals between doses for children who have delayed immunizations

        (a) There is no need to restart a vaccine series regardless of the time that has elapsed between doses

        (b) Use the chart appropriate for the child's age

    ii. DTaP: The fifth dose is not necessary if the fourth dose was given after the 4th birthday

    iii. IPV: For children who received an all-IPV or all-OPV series, a fourth dose is not necessary if third dose was given at age ≥4 years. If both oral polio

■ **TABLE 15-2**
■ ■ ■ **2006 Childhood and Adolescent Immunization Schedule**

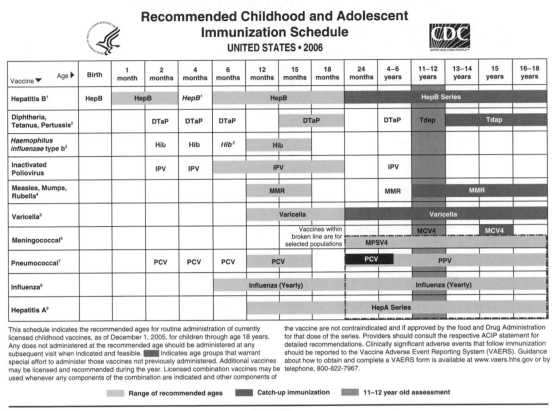

### Recommended Childhood and Adolescent Immunization Schedule
UNITED STATES • 2006

| Vaccine ▼    Age ▶ | Birth | 1 month | 2 months | 4 months | 6 months | 12 months | 15 months | 18 months | 24 months | 4–6 years | 11–12 years | 13–14 years | 15 years | 16–18 years |
|---|---|---|---|---|---|---|---|---|---|---|---|---|---|---|
| Hepatitis B[1] | HepB | HepB | | HepB[1] | | HepB | | | | | HepB Series | | | |
| Diphtheria, Tetanus, Pertussis[2] | | | DTaP | DTaP | DTaP | | DTaP | | | DTaP | Tdap | | Tdap | |
| Haemophilus influenzae type b[3] | | | Hib | Hib | Hib[3] | Hib | | | | | | | | |
| Inactivated Poliovirus | | | IPV | IPV | | IPV | | | | IPV | | | | |
| Measles, Mumps, Rubella[4] | | | | | | MMR | | | | MMR | | MMR | | |
| Varicella[5] | | | | | | Varicella | | | | | Varicella | | | |
| Meningococcal[6] | | | | | | | Vaccines within broken line are for selected populations | | MPSV4 | | MCV4 | | MCV4 | |
| Pneumococcal[7] | | | PCV | PCV | PCV | PCV | | | | PCV | PPV | | | |
| Influenza[8] | | | | | | Influenza (Yearly) | | | | | Influenza (Yearly) | | | |
| Hepatitis A[9] | | | | | | | | | | HepA Series | | | | |

This schedule indicates the recommended ages for routine administration of currently licensed childhood vaccines, as of December 1, 2005, for children through age 18 years. Any dose not administered at the recommended age should be administered at any subsequent visit when indicated and feasible. ▇ Indicates age groups that warrant special effort to administer those vaccines not previously administered. Additional vaccines may be licensed and recommended during the year. Licensed combination vaccines may be used whenever any components of the combination are indicated and other components of the vaccine are not contraindicated and if approved by the food and Drug Administration for that dose of the series. Providers should consult the respective ACIP statement for detailed recommendations. Clinically significant adverse events that follow immunization should be reported to the Vaccine Adverse Event Reporting System (VAERS). Guidance about how to obtain and complete a VAERS form is available at www.vaers.hhs.gov or by telephone, 800-822-7967.

▨ Range of recommended ages    ▇ Catch-up immunization    ▨ 11–12 year old assessment

---

**FOOTNOTES:**

Centers for Disease Control and Prevention: 2006 immunization schedule. Retrieved March 13, 2006, from http://www.cdc.gov/nip/recs/child-schedule-image1-ppt.jpg
For footnotes 1–9, see CDC website @ http://www.cdc.gov/nip/recs/child-schedule-imagen2-ppt.jpg

vaccine (OPV) and IPV were given as part of a series, a total of four doses should be given, regardless of the child's current age

iv. HepB: All children and adolescents who have not been immunized against hepatitis B should begin the hepatitis B vaccination series during any visit. Providers should make special efforts to immunize children who were born in, or whose parents were born in, areas of the world where hepatitis B virus infection is moderately or highly endemic

v. MMR: The second dose of measles-mumps-rubella (MMR) is recommended routinely at ages 4 to 6 years, but may be given earlier if desired

vi. Haemophilus influenzae type b (Hib): Vaccine is not generally recommended for children age ≥5 years

vii. Hib: If current age is less than 12 months and the first two doses were PRP-OMP (PedvaxHIB or ComVax), the third (and final) dose should be given at age 12 to 15 months and at least 8 weeks after the second dose

viii. PCV: Vaccine is not generally recommended for children age ≥5 years

ix. Td: A fourth dose is due at ages 15 to 18 months, but can be given as early as age 12 months if at least 6 months have elapsed since last dose. A final dose is given at age ≥ 4 years. For adolescents ages 11 to 12, Tdap is

■ **TABLE 15-3**
■ ■ **Catch-up Schedule for Childrens Age 4 Months Through 6 Years**

| Vaccine (Minimum Age for Dose 1) | Minimum Interval Between Doses | | | |
|---|---|---|---|---|
| | Dose One to Dose Two | Dose Two to Dose Three | Dose Three to Dose Four | Dose Four to Dose Five |
| **DTaP** (6 weeks) | 4 weeks | 4 weeks | 6 months | 6 months[1] |
| **IPV** (6 weeks) | 4 weeks | 4 weeks | 4 weeks[2] | |
| **HepB**[3] (birth) | 4 weeks | 8 weeks (and 16 weeks after first dose) | | |
| **MMR** (12 months) | 4 weeks[4] | | | |
| **Varicella** (12 months) | | | | |
| **Hib**[5] (6 weeks) | **4 weeks:** if first dose given at age <12 months<br>**8 weeks (as final dose):** if first dose given at age 12–14 months<br>**No further doses needed:** if first dose given at age ≥15 months | **4 weeks**[6]**:** if current age <12 months<br>**8 weeks (as final dose):** if current age ≥ 12 mo and second dose given at age <15 mo<br>**No further doses needed:** if previous dose given at age ≥15 mo | **8 weeks (as final dose):** only necessary for children age 12 months to 5 years who received 3 doses before age 12 months | |
| **PCV**[7] (6 wk) | **4 weeks:** if first dose given at age <12 months and current age <24 months<br>**8 weeks (as final dose):** if first dose given at age ≥12 months or current age 24–59 months<br>**No further doses needed:** for healthy children if first dose given at age ≥24 mo | **4 weeks:** if current age <12 mo<br>**8 weeks (as final dose):** if current age ≥ 12 mo<br>**No further doses needed:** for healthy children if previous dose given at age ≥24 mo | **8 weeks (as final dose):** this dose only necessary for children age 12 mo-5 yr who received 3 doses before age 12 mo | |

2006 Immunization Catch-up Schedule. Retrieved March 13, 2006, from Centers for Disease Control and Prevention website: http://www.cdc.gov/nip/recs/child-schedule-image3-ppt.jpg

1. DTaP: Fifth dose in not necessary if the fourth dose was administered after the fourth birthday.
2. IPV: For children who receive all-IPV or all-OPV series, a forth dose is not necessary if the third dose was administered at age 4 or older. If both IPV and OPV were given, a total of four doses should be given, regardless of the child's age.
3. HepB: Give the 3-dose series to all children and adolescents lass than 19 years of age if they were not previously vaccinated.
4. MMR: The second dose of MMR is recommended routinely at 4–6 years of age, but may be administered earlier if desired.
5. Hib: Vaccine not generally recommended for children five years and older.
6. Hib: If current age is less than 12 month and the first two doses were PRP-OMP (Pedvax-Hib or Comvax), the third and final dose should be given at 12 to 15 months and at least 8 weeks after the second dose.
7. PCV: Vaccine not generally recommended for children five years and older.

■ **TABLE 15-4**
■ ■ **Catch-up Immunization Schedule for Children Ages 4 Months Through 6 Years**

| Vaccine | Dose One to Dose Two | Dose Two to Dose Three | Dose Three to Dose Four |
|---|---|---|---|
| Td | 4 weeks | 6 months | [1]6 months if first dose given at age <12 months and current age <11 years; otherwise, 5 years |
| IPV[2] | 4 weeks | 4 weeks | IPV |
| HepB | 4 weeks | 8 weeks (and 16 weeks after first dose) | |
| MMR | 4 weeks | | |
| Varicella[3] | 4 weeks | | |

2006 Immunization Catch-up Schedule. Retrieved March 13, 2006, from Centers for Disease Control and Prevention website: http://www.cdc.gov/nip/recs/child-schedule-image4-ppt.jpg

1. Td: Adolescent Tdap may be substituted for any dose in a primary catch-up series or as a booster if age appropriate for Tdap. A five year interval from the last Td dose is encouraged when Tdap is used as a booster dose. See http://www.cdc.gov/nip for further information.
2. IPV: Vaccine not generally recommended for persons 18 years and older.
3. Varicella: Administered the two-dose series to all susceptible adolescents aged thirteen and older.

recommended; if missed, a single dose should be given between ages 13 to 18 years

   x. Tetanus, Diphtheria and acelluar Pertussis (Tdap): Licensed for use in 2005 due to the increase in pertussis cases in adolescents and young adults. This vaccine was added to the 2006 Recommended Childhood and Adolescent Immunization for children 11 to 12 years old who have completed the primary series of DTP/DTaP and have not received a Td Booster. In addition, 12 to 18 years old who have not received their Td booster should receive a booster dose of Dtap
   xi. IPV: Not generally recommended for people ages ≥18 years
   xii. Varicella: Give two-dose series to all susceptible adolescents age ≥13 years
 d. Vaccination of internationally adopted children
   i. Majority of vaccines used worldwide are produced with adequate quality control standards and are potent (CDC RR-2, 2004)
   ii. Only written documentation should be accepted as evidence of vaccination status
   iii. Repeating vaccinations is an acceptable option if status is unknown
5. Specific immunization information
 a. Diphtheria and tetanus toxoids and acellular pertussis vaccine (DTaP)
   i. Widespread use of the diphtheria and tetanus toxoids and acellular pertussis vaccine (DTaP) has reduced the incidence of pertussis in the United States by more than 95%
   ii. Currently most reported cases of pertussis occur in infants less than 12 months, 69% of who require hospitalization
   iii. Deaths due to diphtheria have also decreased dramatically from 14,000 cases in the 1920s to 2 cases in 2000
   iv. Likewise there were only 26 cases of tetanus reported in 2000 in the United States compared with hundreds of thousands of deaths worldwide prior to the vaccination

      **v.** The fourth dose of DTaP may be administered as early as age 12 months, provided 6 months have elapsed since the third dose and the child is unlikely to return at age 15 to 18 months

      **vi.** This immunization is given intramuscularly (IM)

      **vii.** Contraindications and precautions are found in Table 15-5 (CDC, 2005a)

  **b.** Diphtheria and tetanus (DT)

      **i.** This immunization is given to children younger than 7 years old in whom pertussis immunization is contraindicated

      **ii.** DT is given according to the DTaP schedule

      **iii.** This immunization is given IM

  **c.** Tetanus, diphtheria, and acellular pertussis (Tdap) & Tetanus diphtheria (Td)

      **i.** Tdap is recommended at age 11 to 12 years if at least 5 years have elapsed since the last dose of tetanus, diphtheria and pertussis–containing vaccine

      **ii.** There are currently 2 Tdap vaccines licensed for use in the United States

---

■ **TABLE 15-5**
■ ■ **Contraindications and Precautions for Immunizations**

| Vaccine | Contraindications/Precautions |
|---|---|
| **FOR ALL VACCINES** | |
| | **Contraindications:** Do not give if patient (1) has had an anaphylactic reaction to a prior dose or to any vaccine component or (2) severe latex allergy |
| | **Precautions:** Moderate or severe acute illness (minor illness is not a reason to postpone vaccination) |
| Diphtheria, tetanus acellular pertussis (DTaP) | **Contraindication for DTaP only:** previous encephalopathy within 7 days after DTP/DTaP<br>**Precautions for DTaP:** The following are precautions, not contraindications. When these conditions are present, the individual child's disease risk should be carefully assessed. In situations in which the benefit outweighs the risk (e.g., community pertussis outbreak), vaccination should be considered. |
| Diphtheria and tetanus (DT) | T ≥105° F (40.5° C) within 48 hr after previous dose<br>Continuous, inconsolable screaming or crying lasting ≥3 hr within 48 hr after previous dose<br>Previous seizure within 3 days after immunization |
| Tetanus and diphtheria toxoids (Td) | Pale or limp episode or collapse within 48 hr after previous dose<br>Unstable progressive neurologic problem (defer until stable)<br>Guillain-Barré syndrome (GBS) within 6 weeks after dose |
| Measles-mumps-rubella (MMR) | **Contraindications:**<br>Pregnancy or possibility of pregnancy within 4 wk (use contraception)<br>HIV is NOT a contraindication unless severely immunocompromised<br>Immunocompromised people (e.g., because of cancer, leukemia, lymphoma)<br>Anaphylactic reaction to neomycin or gelatin<br>**Precautions:**<br>If blood, plasma, and/or immune globulin were given in past 11 months, see ACIP statement *General Recommendations on Immunization* regarding time to wait before vaccinating (interval between IG and measles vaccine depends on the product)<br>Tuberculosis or positive tuberculin skin test (TST)<br>Note: MMR is not contraindicated if a TST test was recently applied. If TST and MMR weren't given on same day, delay TST for 4-6 wk after MMR (because MMR may temporarily suppress TST reactivity)<br>Thrombocytopenia or history of thrombocytopenic purpura<br>For patients on high-dose immunosuppressive therapy, consult ACIP recommendations regarding delay time. |

■ **TABLE 15-5**
■ ■ **Contraindications and Precautions for Immunizations—cont'd**

| Vaccine | Contraindications/Precautions |
|---------|-------------------------------|
| Inactivated polio vaccine | **Contraindication:**<br>Anaphylaxis to neomycin, streptomycin, or polymyxin B |
| Varicella | **Contraindications:**<br>Pregnancy or possibility of pregnancy within 4 wk<br>Anaphylactic reaction to neomycin or gelatin<br>HIV (can consider in children with asymptomatic or mild disease)<br>People immunocompromised due to high doses of systemic steroids, cancer, leukemia, lymphoma, or immunodeficiency. Note: For patients with humoral immunodeficiency, HIV infection, or leukemia, or for patients on high doses of systemic steroids, see ACIP recommendations<br>**Precautions:**<br>If blood, plasma, and/or immune globulin (IG or VZIG) were given in past 11 mo, see ACIP statement *General Recommendations on Immunization* regarding time to wait before vaccinating<br>For children taking salicylates, see ACIP recommendations |
| Influenza | **Contraindication:**<br>Severe anaphylactic reaction to chickens or egg protein can experience, on rare occasions, a similar type of reaction to killed influenza vaccines. Although influenza vaccine has been administered safely to such children after skin testing and even desensitization, these children generally should not receive influenza vaccine because of their risk of reactions, the likely need for yearly immunization, and the availability of chemoprophylaxis against influenza infection<br>**Precautions:**<br>GBS within 6 wk after dose |
| Meningococcal | Infrequent and mild adverse reactions occur, the most common of which is localized erythema for 1 to 2 days. Studies suggest that altering meningococcal immunization recommendations during pregnancy is unnecessary |
| Hepatitis B | **Contraindication:**<br>Anaphylactic reaction to baker's yeast |
| Hepatitis A | **Contraindication:**<br>Anaphylaxis to 2-phenoxyethanol or alum<br>**Precautions:**<br>Pregnancy |

Table adapted with permission from Summary for Rules for Childhood Immunization (September 8, 2005). Retrieved March 13, 2006, from http://www.immunize.org/nslt.d/n17/rules1.htm.
1. Td: Adolescent Tdap may be substituted for any dose in a primary catch-up series or as a booster if age appropriate for Tdap. A five year interval from the last Td dose is encouraged when Tdap is used as a booster dose. See http://www.cdc.gov/nip for further information.
2. IPV: Vaccine not generally recommended for persons 18 years and older.
3. Varicella: Administered the two-dose series to all susceptible adolescents aged thirteen and older.

    (a) ADACEL
        (1) Tetanus Toxoid, Reduced Diphtheria Toxoid and Acellular Pertussis Vaccine, Adsorbed (Tdap) (sanofi pasteur, Toronto, Ontario, Canada)
        (2) Licensed on June 10, 2005
        (3) For active booster immunization against tetanus, diphtheria, and pertussis as a single dose in persons aged 11–64 years

      (b) BOOSTRIX
        (1) Tetanus Toxoid, Reduced Diphtheria Toxoid and Acellular Pertussis Vaccine, Adsorbed (Tdap) (GlaxoSmithKline Biologicals [GSK], Rixensart, Belgium)
        (2) Licensed on May 3, 2005
        (3) For active booster immunization against tetanus, diphtheria, and pertussis as a single dose in persons aged 10–18 years
   iii. Subsequent routine Tetanus diphtheria (Td) boosters are recommended every 10 years
   iv. These immunizations are given IM

**d.** Polio
   i. The advent of poliovirus vaccination eliminated indigenous poliomyelitis in the Americas by 1994 largely due to the use of oral polio vaccines
   ii. Inactivated poliovirus vaccine (IPV) is currently the recommended polio vaccine in the U.S. due to the risk of vaccine associated paralytic poliomyelitis (VAPP) with administration of the oral form (OPV)
   iii. An all-IPV schedule is currently recommended in the United States although OPV is recommended by the World Health Organization for global eradication efforts
   iv. All children should receive four doses at ages 2 and 4 months, 6 to 18 months, and 4 to 6 years
   v. This immunization is given subcutaneously (subQ)

**e.** *Haemophilus influenzae* type B (Hib) conjugate vaccine (CDC, 2002)
   i. The introduction of widespread vaccination against Hib reduced the incidence of invasive Hib disease by 97% in the first 10 years of use
   ii. The vaccine is between 95% to 100% efficacious against typable, encapsulated Hib, the organism responsible for meningitis, epiglottitis, cellulitis, pneumonia, osteomyelitis, septic arthritis, bacteremia, and pericarditis
   iii. The vaccine does not protect against the unencapsulated, nontypable Hib strains responsible for otitis media, bronchitis, and sinusitis
   iv. Three Hib conjugate vaccines are licensed for infant use
      (a) HbOC (HibTiTER)
      (b) PRP-OMP (PedvaxHIB)
      (c) PRP-T (ActHIB & OmniHIB)
      (d) PRP-D (ProHIBIT) licensed for ages 12 to 60 months and not in primary series
      (e) If PRP-OMP (PedvaxHIB or ComVax [Merck & Co., Inc]) is administered at ages 2 and 4 months, a dose at age 6 months is not required
        (1) ComVax is Hib and HepB combined
   v. This immunization is given IM

**f.** Combination immunizations
   i. New sets always in development
   ii. ProQuad (Merck & Co., Inc & Co., Inc)
      (a) Combined live attenuated measles, mumps, rubella, and varicella (MMRV) vaccine
      (b) For use in children aged 12 months to 12 years
   iii. PRP-T combined with acellular pertussis
      (a) DTaP Tripedia called TriHIBIT
      (b) Used as fourth dose in series
   iv. DTP-HbOC
      (a) Tetramune
      (b) DTaP/Hib combinations should not be used at 2, 4, and 6 months but can be used as boosters

g. Measles-mumps-rubella (MMR)
 i. MMR have been virtually eliminated because of vaccinations against all three viruses
 ii. Occasional outbreaks have occurred generally among unimmunized individuals older than the age of 20, in prison, colleges, and the workplace
 iii. Two doses of the MMR vaccine result in 99% immunity
 iv. Adverse reactions to the three components of the vaccine include mild local reactions, delayed fever or rash, generalized lymphadenopathy and arthralgia, and transient orchitis
 v. The first MMR should be given beginning at age 12 months. The second dose of MMR is recommended routinely at age 4 to 6 years but may be administered during any visit, provided at least 4 weeks have elapsed since the first dose and that both doses are administered beginning at or after age 12 months. Those who have not previously received the second dose should complete the schedule by the 11- to 12-year-old visit.
 vi. This immunization is given subQ
h. Hepatitis B
 i. Hepatitis B virus (HBV) remains a significant cause of morbidity and mortality in the United States
 ii. Chronic disease from HBV, which can lead to cirrhosis and hepatocellular carcinoma, is more likely to occur if the virus is acquired early in life
 iii. Protection against HBV infection ranges from 80% to 95% for hepatitis B (HepB) vaccines licensed in the United States
 iv. Pain at the intramuscular injection site is the most common adverse side effect
 v. Infants born to HBsAg-negative mothers
  (a) First dose of HepB vaccine should be given as soon after birth as possible and before hospital discharge, but at least by age 2 months
  (b) If the infant receives the first dose at birth, it must be monovalent
  (c) The combination vaccine containing hepatitis B may be used as the first dose at 2 months of age and also to complete the series in infants receiving their first dose at birth
  (d) The second dose should be given at least 4 weeks after the first dose, except for combination vaccines, which cannot be administered before age 6 weeks
  (e) The third dose should be given at least 16 weeks after the first dose and at least 8 weeks after the second dose
  (f) The last dose in the vaccination series (third or fourth dose) should not be administered before age 6 months
 vi. Infants born to HBsAg-positive mothers
  (a) Should receive both the monovalent hepatitis B vaccine and 0.5 mL of hepatitis B immunoglobulin (HBIG) within 12 hours of birth
  (b) These immunizations should be given at separate sites
  (c) The second dose is recommended at age 1 to 2 months
  (d) The last dose in the vaccination series should not be administered before age 6 months
  (e) These infants should be tested for HBsAg and anti-HBs at 9 to 15 months of age
 vii. Infants born to mothers whose HBsAg status is unknown
  (a) Should receive the first dose of the HepB series within 12 hours of birth
  (b) Maternal blood should be drawn as soon as possible to determine the mother's HBsAg status; if the HBsAg test is positive, the infant should receive HBIG as soon as possible (no later than age 1 week)

        (c) Second dose is recommended at age 1 to 2 months
        (d) The last dose in the vaccination series should not be administered before age 6 months
  i. Pneumococcal (CDC, 2000b)
      i. *Streptococcus pneumoniae* causes about 17,000 cases of invasive disease including meningitis, bacteremia, and pneumonia in children younger than the age of 5
     ii. It is the most common bacterial cause of acute otitis media, sinusitis, and community-acquired pneumonia among all children and has replaced Hib as the leading cause of bacterial meningitis
    iii. Two pneumococcal vaccines
        (a) Pneumococcal conjugate vaccine (PCV7/Prevnar)
            (1) Seven valent vaccine for children younger than age 2 was released in the United States in 2000. It covers the most common serotypes involved in childhood illness
            (2) PCV7 is routinely recommended for all children 2 to 23 months and certain children 24 to 59 months
            (3) Vaccine efficacy is 97%. No serious adverse effects have been reported, only minor reactions including localized tenderness and redness at the injection site and fever
        (b) 23-valent pneumococcal polysaccharide (PPV/Pneumovax)
            (1) For use in children 24 months or older
            (2) Pneumococcal polysaccharide vaccine (PPV) is recommended in addition to PCV7 for certain high risk groups
                a) Sickle cell disease
                b) Functional or anatomic asplenia
                c) Nephrotic syndrome or chronic renal failure
                d) Immunosuppressive conditions
                e) HIV infections
                f) Cerebrospinal fluid leaks
        (c) These immunizations are given IM
  j. Varicella
      i. Varicella-zoster virus (VZV) causes a highly contagious, usually benign self-limited illness known as chickenpox
     ii. Complications include secondary bacterial infection, pneumonia, encephalomeningitis, glomerulonephritis, thrombocytopenia, purpura fulminans, cerebellar ataxia, arthritis and hepatitis, which can result in hospitalization and death
    iii. Routine vaccination has been shown to be cost effective and has reduced morbidity and mortality from VZV
     iv. Most common adverse reactions to the vaccine:
        (a) Local reaction
        (b) Local rash
        (c) Chickenpox-type lesions—few
        (d) Low-grade fever
      v. Varicella vaccine should be given to all children after the age of 12 months for whom there is no reliable history of chickenpox
     vi. Children 13 and older require two doses 4 weeks apart because of reduced seroconversion
    vii. This immunization is given subQ
   viii. Investigations are underway was to whether a two dose schedule for varicella should be required

  **ix.** A combined live attenuated measles, mumps, rubella and varicella vaccine was licensed in 2005 (CDC, 2005c)

**k.** Influenza

  **i.** Healthy children ages 6 to 23 months are recommended to receive influenza vaccine because children in this age-group are at substantially increased risk for influenza-related hospitalizations

  **ii.** Influenza vaccine is recommended annually for children age ≥6 months with certain risk factors (including but not limited to asthma, cardiac disease, sickle cell disease, HIV, diabetes, and household members of people in groups at high risk and can be administered to all others wishing to obtain immunity

  **iii.** Healthy children ages 6 to 23 months are encouraged to receive influenza vaccine if feasible because children in this age-group are at substantially increased risk for influenza-related hospitalizations

  **iv.** Children age ≤12 years should receive vaccine in a dosage appropriate for their age (0.25 mL if ages 6–35 months or 0.5 mL if ages ≥3 years)

  **v.** Children aged ≤8 years who are receiving influenza vaccine for the first time should receive two doses separated by at least 4 weeks

  **vi.** Contraindications: allergy to vaccine, vaccine components, chicken, eggs

  **vii.** This immunization is given IM

**l.** Hepatitis A

  **i.** This vaccine was added to the Recommended Childhood and Adolescent Immunization Schedule in 2006 for all children 12 months of age

  **ii.** In addition, recommended for children and adolescents in selected states and regions, and for certain high-risk groups; consult your local public health authority; also for children traveling to foreign countries where hepatitis A is endemic

  **iii.** Recommended for children and adolescents in selected states and regions, and for certain high-risk groups; consult your local public health authority; also for children traveling to foreign countries where hepatitis A is endemic

  **iv.** Children and adolescents in these states, regions, and high risk groups who have not been immunized against hepatitis A can begin the hepatitis A vaccination series during any visit

  **v.** The two doses in the series should be administered at least 6 months apart

  **vi.** This immunization is given IM

**m.** Meningococcal

  **i.** High risk group

   (a) College-bound, freshmen, living in dorm

  **ii.** Before 1999, only students entering two of the military academies routinely received vaccine. However, an increasing number of other military academies initiated vaccine programs

  **iii.** U.S. surveillance of meningococcal disease in college students began in 1998

  **iv.** Vaccines are effective against serogroup A, C, Y, and W-135 *Neisseria meningitidis*

  **v.** No vaccine is available for group B disease (B type causes one-third of meningococcal cases)

  **vi.** Providers should inform and educate students about the risks of meningococcal disease and discuss the availability of a safe and effective vaccine

  **vii.** Two vaccines are licensed for use in the United States

        (a) Meningococcal vaccine (MCV4, Menactra, Sanofi Pasteur)
            (1) Licensed in 2005 for people ages 11 to 55 years old
            (2) Recommended for all children 11 to 12 years old and unvaccinated high school entry students
            (3) All college freshman living in a dormitory should receive MCV4
        (b) Meningococcal polysaccharide vaccine (MPSV4)
            (1) Can be used as an alternative to MCV4 for college freshman living in dormitories
            (2) Recommended for children and adolescents ages 2 to 18 years
                a) Traveling to countries in which *N. meningitides* is hyper endemic or epidemic
                b) With terminal complement deficiencies and those with anatomic or functional asplenia
                c) who are infected with HIV
                d) Approved for use in children older than 2 years
            (3) Single dose of either vaccine is recommended

  **n.** Respiratory syncytial virus (RSV)
     **i.** Most common cause of bronchiolitis and pneumonia in infants and children younger than 12 months
    **ii.** Peak season from winter to early spring
   **iii.** Prevention of RSV is indicated for children with chronic lung disease and premature infants with or without chronic lung disease (<35 weeks of gestation)
    **iv.** Two types
        (a) RSV immune globulin intravenous (RSV-IGIV)
            (1) Given IV, one dose monthly
            (2) 15 mL/kg (750 mg/kg)
            (3) Begin before RSV season and continue until RSV season complete
            (4) MMR and varicella vaccines should be deferred for 9 months after the last dose
        (b) Anti-RSV humanized monoclonal antibody-palivizumab
            (1) Given IM, monthly during RSV season
            (2) 15 mg/kg
            (3) Does not interfere with response to vaccines

  **o.** Lyme disease vaccine
     **i.** Approved for children older than 15 years of age
    **ii.** Given on the basis of individual risk assessment
   **iii.** Recommended for people with known exposure to areas of moderate to high risk for tick-infested habitats
    **iv.** Given IM, three doses
        (a) Initial dose, second dose at 1 month after initial dose, third dose 12 months after initial dose

  **p.** Vaccine manufacturer numbers:

| | |
|---|---|
| **i.** Aventis-Pasteur | 800-822-2463 |
| **ii.** Bayer Corporation | 800-288-8371 |
| **iii.** GlaxoSmithKline | 800-825-5249 |
| **iv.** Merck & Co., Inc. | 800-672-6372 |
| **v.** Wyeth | 800-934-5556 |

**6.** Contraindications and precautions to immunizations (CDC, 2005a)
  **a.** Latex allergy
     **i.** Latex

         (a) Liquid sap from the commercial rubber tree

         (b) Latex is processed to form natural rubber latex and dry natural rubber

    ii. Dry natural rubber is used in syringe plungers and vial stoppers

    iii. Allergic reactions after vaccinations are rare

    iv. If severe anaphylaxis to latex is reported:

         (a) Vaccines supplied in vials or syringes that contain natural rubber should not be administered

         (b) Consider benefits of vaccination outweighing risk of allergic reaction

**b.** Contraindication is a condition in the infant, child, or adolescent that significantly increases the chance of a serious adverse event

**c.** Precaution is a condition in the infant, child or adolescent that may increase the likelihood of a serious adverse event or may interfere with the immunization's ability to produce immunity

**d.** Table 15–5 summarizes contraindications and precautions for immunizations

**e.** National Vaccine Injury Compensation Program

    i. Established by the National Childhood Vaccine Injury Act

    ii. No-fault system in which people thought to have incurred death or injury from the administration of a covered vaccine can seek compensation

    iii. Additional information available from www.hrsa.gov/osp/vicp or 800-338-2382

7. Tuberculosis (TB) screening

    **a.** Although TB screening is not an immunization, it is often included in immunization information and on immunization records

    **b.** The recommended tuberculosis skin test (TST) is Mantoux test containing 5 tuberculin units of purified protein derivative (PPD)

    **c.** This screening test is administered intradermally

    **d.** TST should be read at 48 to 72 hours after placement

    **e.** TST recommendations for high risk infants, children, and adolescents

        i. Immediate TST

           (a) Contact with known/suspected TB case

           (b) Clinical/radiographic findings suggestive of TB

           (c) Immigrants from endemic countries or contact with immigrants from endemic countries

        ii. Annual TST

           (a) HIV-positive children

           (b) Incarcerated youth

        iii. TST every 2 to 3 years

           (a) Children exposed to high risk people

        iv. TST at 4 to 6 years and 11 to 16 years

           (a) Children of parents who immigrated from high-prevalence areas

           (b) Frequent travel to endemic areas or contact with people who travel to these areas

    **f.** Interpretation of results

        i. Depends on epidemiologic and clinical factors

        ii. More than 15 mm induration

           (a) Considered positive in everyone

        iii. More than 10 mm induration

           (a) Considered positive in:

              (1) Children younger than 4 years old

              (2) People with other medical conditions

              (3) Parents or child born in high-prevalence area

(4) Frequent exposure to high risk adults

(5) Travel to high-prevalence areas of the world

   **iv.** ≥5 mm induration

      (a) Considered positive if:

         (1) Contact with known or suspected case of TB

         (2) Clinical findings suggestive of TB

         (3) Positive chest x-ray (active or previous active case)

## REFERENCES

American Academy of Family Physicians. (2006). Clinical care and research: Immunization resources. Retrieved on March 13, 2006, from www.aafp.org/x10615.xml.

American Academy of Pediatrics. (2006). Immunization initiatives. Retrieved on March 13, 2006, from www.cispimmunize.org.

Centers for Disease Control and Prevention (2000a). National immunization program use of human cell cultures in vaccine manufacturing. Retrieved March 13, 2006, from www.cdc.gov/nip/vacsafe/concerns/gen/humancell.htm.

Centers for Disease Control and Prevention. (2000b). Preventing pneumococcal disease among infants and young children. Recommendations of the Advisory Committee on Immunization Practices (ACIP), *49* (RR09), 1–38.

Centers for Disease Control and Prevention. (2001). Febrile seizures after MMR and DTP vaccinations. Retrieved March 13, 2006, from www.cdc.gov/nip/issues/mmr-dtp/mmr-dtp.htm.

Centers for Disease Control and Prevention. (2002). Prevention and control of influenza: Recommendations of the Advisory Committee on Immunization Practices (ACIP), *51* (RR03), 1-31.

Centers for Disease Control and Prevention (2004). Oral polio vaccine and HIV/AIDS: Questions and answers. Retrieved March 13, 2006, from www.cdc.gov/nip/vacsafe/concerns/aids/poliovac-hiv-aids-qa.htm.

Centers for Disease Control and Prevention. (2005a). Contraindications to vaccines chart. Retrieved March 13, 2006, from http://www.cdc.gov/nip/recs/contraindications_vacc.htm

Centers for Disease Control and Prevention. (2005b). Guillain-Barré syndrome (GBS) and influenza vaccine. Retrieved March 13, 2006, from www.cdc.gov/nip/vacsafe/concerns/gbs/default.htm.

Centers for Disease Control and Prevention (2005c). Licensure of a combined live attenuated measles, mumps, rubella, and varicella vaccine. Retrieved February 28, 2006 from http://www.cdc.gov/mmwr/preview/mmwrhtml/mm5447a4.htm

Centers for Disease Control and Prevention (2005d). Multiple sclerosis and the hepatitis B vaccine. Retrieved March 13, 2006, from www.cdc.gov/nip/vacsafe/concerns/ms/default.htm.

Centers for Disease Control and Prevention (2005e). National immunization program FAQs about measles vaccine and inflammatory bowel disease (IBD). Retrieved March 13, 2006 from www.cdc.gov/nip/vacsafe/concerns/autism/ibd.htm.

Centers for Disease Control and Prevention. (2005f).VAERS: Vaccine adverse effects reporting system. Retrieved March 13, 2006, from http://www.cdc.gov/nip/vacsafe/VAERS/CME-post-mktg-surv.htm

Centers for Disease Control and Prevention. (2006a). 2006 Childhood and Adolescent Immunization Schedule. Retrieved March 13, 2006, from http://www.cdc.gov/nip/recs/child-schedule.htm.

Centers for Disease Control and Prevention (2006b). *2006 immunization catch-up schedule.* Retrieved March 14, 2006, from http://www.cdc.gov/nip/recs/child-schedule.htm#catchup.

Centers for Disease Control and Prevention. (2006c). Advisory committee on immunization practices. Retrieved on March 13, 2006, from www.cdc.gov/nip/acip.

Centers for Disease Control and Prevention. (2006d). CDC's Advisory Committee recommends new vaccine to prevent rotavirus.

Retrieved on March 13, 2006 from http://www.cdc.gov/nip/pr/pr_rotavirus_feb2006.pdf

Centers for Disease Control and Prevention. (2006e). VACMAN: Vaccine management system. Retrieved March 13, 2006, from http://www.cdc.gov/nip/vacman/Default.htm

Fredrickson, D., Davis, T., Arnould C., et al. (2004). Child immunization refusal: Provider and parent perceptions. *Fam Med*, *36*(6), 431-439.

Frenkel, L. (Ed.) (2004). Immunization issues in the 21st century, part II. *Pediatr Ann*, *33*(9), 564-616.

Immunization Action Coalition. (2006). Home page. Retrieved on March 13, 2006 from http://www.immunize.org/index.htm

Irigoyen, M., Findley, S., Chen, S., et al. (2004). Early continuity of care and immunization coverage. *Ambu Pediatr*, *4*(3), 199-203.

Lieber, M., Colden, F., & Colon, A. (2003). Childhood immunizations: A parent education and incentive program. *J Pediatr Heath Care*, *17*(5), 240-244.

National Association of Pediatric Nurse Practitioners. (2004). Adolescent Immunizations: Nurses Can Make a Difference. Retrieved on March 13, 2006 from http://www.napnap.org/index.cfm?page=10&sec=54&ssec=465

National Association of Pediatric Nurse Practitioners. (2005). *Immunizations*. Retrieved March 13, 2006 from http://www.napnap.org/index.cfm?page=10&sec=54&ssec=66

National Network for Immunization Information (2005). IOM reports. Retrieved on February 28, 2006 from www.immunizationinfo.org/iom_reports.cfm

Niederhauser, V. & Stark, M. (2005). Narrowing the gap in childhood immunization disparities. *Pediatric Nursing*, 5, 380-386.

Raucci, J. Whitehill, J., & Sandritter, T. (2004). Childhood immunizations (part one). *J Pediatr Health Care*, *18*(2), 95-101.

Whitehill, J., Raucci, J. & Sandritter, T. (2004). Childhood immunizations (part two). *J Pediatr Health Care*, *18*(4), 192-199.

VICTORIA A. WEILL, MSN, RN, CPNP, APRN

## GENERAL NUTRITIONAL CONCERNS

1. Childhood overweight
   a. Definitions (CDC, 2006)
      i. The term *overweight* is preferred due to the negative connotation of the term *obesity*
      ii. Body mass index (BMI)
         (a) Weight in kilograms divided by height in meters squared ($kg/m^2$)
         (b) Standardized percentiles are available for age and sex
      iii. *At risk of overweight* for ages 2 to 20 years: BMI-for-age between the 85th and the 95th percentiles
      iv. *Overweight*: BMI-for-age at or above the 95th percentile
   b. Prevalence (CDC, 2006)
      i. Prevalence of overweight among young people has increased dramatically
      ii. Between 1980 and 1994, children and adolescents considered to be overweight increased by 100% in the United States
      iii. Between 1992 and 2002, 16% of children and adolescents ages 6 to 19 years were estimated to be overweight (National Center for Health Statistics, 2005)
   c. Etiology (Donohoue, 2004)
      i. Genetic factors control the set point for body weight
         (a) Energy expenditure has a positive relationship to body weight
         (b) Ethnic variability in resting energy expenditure is higher in African American than white prepubertal children
      ii. During childhood the body lays down all of the fat cells that will be in the body for life
         (a) However, fat cells do increase in size
         (b) If energy intake exceeds energy expenditure, excess fat intake is stored in the body
      iii. Maternal diabetes
      iv. Family overweight (AAP, 2004; Donohoue, 2004)
         (a) Risk is often expressed in terms of odds ratios, i.e., if the odds of an event are greater than one, e.g., 3.1, the event is *3.1 times more likely to happen than not*

(1) If one parent is overweight, the odds are 2.3 to 3.0 that the child will be obese in young adulthood

(2) If both parents of a 1- to 5-year-old child are overweight, the odds are 13.6 to 15.3 that the child will be obese in young adulthood

(3) In children younger than 5 years of age, parental obesity is a stronger predictor of obesity in adulthood than child's weight

(4) If child is overweight at ages 10 to 14, the odds are 22.3 that the child will be obese in young adulthood

  **v.** Environmental stimuli

    (a) Increased access to unhealthy foods

    (b) Decreased physical activity by children, including a decrease in required physical education by schools

      (1) Find ways to incorporate increased activity/exercise into a family activity

      (2) Visit Action for Healthy Kids website for community initiatives to improve nutrition & physical activity: www.actionforhealthykids.org

    (c) Increased popularity of TV, videos, video games, computers

      (1) Direct correlation between time spent watching television (inactivity) and excess consumption of calories (Crespo et al., 2001; Kennedy et al., 2002)

      (2) Greater than 4 hours of screen time per day is a risk factor

    (d) Advertising for sweets, soft drinks, cereals, fast foods focused on children

      (1) American companies spend $15 billion per year on marketing and advertising for children younger than age 12

      (2) Every year, the average child see 40,000 ads on television alone

      (3) See *Children and the Media Policy Brief* developed by the Children Now organization (www.childrennow.org)

  **vi.** Developmental processes

    (a) Increased independence and decision making by school-agers and adolescents

    (b) Susceptible to persuasion

**d.** Consequences for overweight children compared with other children

  **i.** More likely to be overweight as adults

  **ii.** Physiologic consequences (CDC, 2006)

    (a) More likely to have chronic illnesses later in life

    (b) More likely to have medical risks associated with cardiovascular disease

      (1) Nearly 60% of overweight children had at least one cardiovascular risk factor compared with 10% of those with a BMI $\leq$ 85th percentile

      (2) 25% of overweight children had two or more risk factors

    (c) Increased risk of the following health problems

      (1) Metabolic syndrome

        a) Triglycerides greater than 90 mg/dL

        b) High-density lipoprotein less than 40 mg/dL

        c) Waist circumference more than the 90th percentile for age and gender

        d) Glucose intolerance

         i) Diagnosis of diabetes, or

         ii) $HbA_{1C}$ greater than 6%

(2) Dyslipidemia

(3) Glucose intolerance

(4) Type 2 diabetes

(5) Hypertension

(6) Coronary heart disease

(7) Hepatic steatosis

(8) Cholelithiasis

(9) Early sexual maturation of females

(10) Some cancers (endometrial, breast, and colon)

(11) Osteoarthritis

(12) Infertility

(13) Obesity hypoventilation syndrome

(14) Sleep apnea

(15) Pseudotumor cerebri

iii. Psychosocial consequences

(a) These are significant

(b) Childwood overweight has been linked to:

(1) Social discrimination and bullying

(2) Negative self-image in adolescence that often persists into adulthood

(3) Parental neglect

(4) Behavioral and learning problems

(5) Depression

e. Prevention and treatment

i. Use the latest version of the U.S. Department of Agriculture and U. S. Food and Drug Association (2005) food pyramid as a guideline for selecting appropriate types of foods (available at www.nal.usda.gov/fnic/Fpyr/pyramid.html)

(a) The USDA has developed an individualized, interactive website to help children and adults develop a balanced diet, based on their age (2 and older), sex, and amount of daily activity. See www.mypyramid.gov.

(b) Goal is three meals plus two nutritious snacks per day

ii. Refer to new guidelines for energy and nutrient needs to plan and assess diets (See Appendix C in AAP, 2004)

(a) Dietary reference intake (DRI)—a new set of four nutrient-based reference values based on age and sex

(1) Estimated average requirement (EAR)—median usual intake value that should meet the requirements of half of all apparently healthy individuals

(2) Recommended daily allowance (RDA)—amount that is adequate for nearly all healthy individuals

(3) Adequate intake (AI)—reported when EAR or RDA have not been established

(4) Upper intake level (UL)—highest level of intake that should pose no risk of adverse health effects

iii. HEAT<sup>SM</sup>—NAPNAP's initiative for promoting *Healthy Eating and Activity Together* (NAPNAP, 2006) has resulted in evidence-based practice guidelines for children of all age-groups (Boxes 16-1 through 16-4)

(a) Early identification

(1) History, measurement, physical examination, and education

(b) Developmental issues and communication relevant to nutrition and activity

■ **BOX 16-1**
■ **"HEALTHY EATING AND ACTIVITY TOGETHER" INFANCY BRIEF GUIDE**

**EARLY IDENTIFICATION**
- Document family history relevant to risk of overweight *(gestational diabetes and diabetes mellitus highly significant for infants of Native American mothers)*
- Document gestational age and birth weight
- Perform length, weight, and head circumference and plot on CDC growth charts
- Educate parent about infant growth pattern, length for weight ratio, and rapid weight gain for infants under 6 months *(especially for Hispanic and African American infants)*

**DEVELOPMENT AND COMMUNICATION**
- Perform two-question screen for parent depression
- Document areas of strength and concern
- *Document personal attitudes, values, and beliefs; spiritual and cultural influences about nutrition, physical activity, and body shape and size; race; ethnicity; language and educational preferences*
- Educate parents about expected growth, physical, emotional, and developmental changes
- Educate parents about effective communication strategies
    - Infant engagement and disengagement cues, hunger and satiation cues
    - Infant self-calming; parents' response to crying
- *Counsel extended family members as well as parents about issues related to child's health*
- Refer family, as needed, to free or low-cost community nutritional and physical activity resources, including registered dieticians
- Counsel using Motivational Interviewing to address areas of concern:
    - Reinforce all positive health behaviors
    - Identify discrepancies between goals and behaviors
    - Develop a plan of action in partnership with the family

**NUTRITION AND FEEDING**
- Monitor nutritional intake
- Identify barriers to healthful infant nutrition
- Educate parents about nutritional intake:
    - **Breastfeed throughout the first year of life** *(strongly encouraged for Native American infants)*
    - Use only fully iron-fortified formulas if bottle feeding
    - **Delay introduction of solids until at least 4 months of age**
        - Fruits: gradual transition from 1 to 3 servin gs/day
        - Vegetables: 1 to 2 servings/day
        - Meat or other protein: 1 to 2 servings/day
    - Introduce variety in types and textures of foods
    - Portion size: 1–2 Tbsp =1 serving
    - Limit 100% fruit juice to 4–6 oz/day; avoid fruit drinks
    - **Avoid calorie-dense, nutrient-poor foods, e.g., French fries, soda**
- Educate parents regarding promising feeding practices
    - Gradually eliminate night feeding after 3 months of age; end at 6 months
    - No bottles in bed
    - **Recognize and respond to hunger and satiation cues**
    - Offer only healthful foods
    - Include older infant at family meals
- *Counsel with emphasis on positive health consequences of good nutrition, not infant weight*

**BOLD type indicates a strong evidence-based recommendation**
*Italic* type indicates a culturally appropriate recommendation

*Continued*

■ BOX 16-1
■ "HEALTHY EATING AND ACTIVITY TOGETHER" INFANCY BRIEF GUIDE—cont'd

**PHYSICAL ACTIVITY AND SEDENTARY BEHAVIOR**
■ Monitor physical activity and sedentary behavior
■ **Educate parents about age appropriate physical activity**
  ■ Tummy time
  ■ Floor time
  ■ Parent play with child
■ Educate parents about the value of parent modeling of being physically active and family activities
■ **Counsel parents to avoid TV and all forms of screen time for children <2 yrs**

**ADVOCACY**
■ Advocate for work and community environments that support breastfeeding mothers
■ Select daycare settings meeting standards for daily physical activity and no screen time

©2006 by the National Association of Pediatric Nurse Practitioners (NAPNAP). All rights reserved. (From pp. S22–S23 of *Journal of Pediatric Health Care, 20*(2), 2006)

■ BOX 16-2
■ "HEALTHY EATING AND ACTIVITY TOGETHER" EARLY CHILDHOOD BRIEF GUIDE

**EARLY IDENTIFICATION**
■ Document family history relevant to risk of overweight and update annually
■ Perform accurate length/height and weight at least annually; consider more frequent measurement if at risk of or overweight; document on the CDC growth charts
■ Perform assessment of risk of overweight and document on CDC growth chart; document on problem list if ≥ 85th percentile
  ■ Length for weight from 12-24 months
  ■ BMI for children >2 years of age
■ Examine growth chart for evidence of early adiposity rebound before age 5 years; document on problem list
■ Measure blood pressure at least annually from age 3 years; document BP > 90th% on problem list
■ Educate parents about the child's growth pattern, clearly identifying children at risk of overweight or overweight

**DEVELOPMENT AND COMMUNICATION**
■ Perform two-question screen for parent depression
■ Document areas of strength and concern
■ *Document personal attitudes, values, and beliefs; spiritual and cultural influences about nutrition, physical activity, and body shape and size; race; ethnicity; language and educational preferences*
■ Educate parents about expected growth, physical, emotional, and developmental changes and their impact on feeding and appetite
■ Educate parents about effective communication with the young child: foster toddler use of language to express needs and feelings, offer limited choices and simple directions
■ *Counsel extended family members as well as parents about issues related to child's health*
■ Refer family, as needed, to free or low-cost community nutritional and physical activity resources, including registered dieticians

**BOLD type indicates a strong evidence-based recommendation**
*Italic* type indicates a culturally appropriate recommendation

■ **BOX 16-2**
■ **"HEALTHY EATING AND ACTIVITY TOGETHER" EARLY CHILDHOOD BRIEF GUIDE—cont'd**

- ■ Counsel using motivational interviewing to address areas of concern
  - ■ Reinforce all positive health behaviors
  - ■ Identify discrepancies between goals and behaviors
  - ■ Develop a plan of action in partnership with the family

**NUTRITION AND FEEDING**
- ■ **Monitor nutritional intake for consistency with expert recommendations, and match with activity level at least annually**
- ■ Identify barriers to healthy eating
- ■ Educate parents regarding nutritional intake
  - ■ Consume 5 or more servings of fruits and vegetables/day
  - ■ At least half of grains consumed should be whole grain foods
  - ■ Provide foods with a variety of textures and flavors
  - ■ Milk, not more than 16 oz/day; low-or fat-free after 2 years of age
  - ■ Limit 100% fruit juice to 6 oz or less/day; avoid fruit drinks and soft drinks
  - ■ Limit fat intake; avoid foods high in saturated and trans fats; use soft margarine rather than lard, butter, or stick margarine
  - ■ Provide healthy snack foods
- ■ Educate parents regarding promising feeding practices
  - ■ **Parents are responsible for what, when, where; child is responsible for whether and how much**
  - ■ Balance energy intake in food with energy output in activity
  - ■ **Respect self-regulation of intake**
  - ■ Provide only healthy foods, and limited choices between 2 healthy alternatives
  - ■ Regular schedule of meals and snacks
  - ■ Eat family meals together regularly
  - ■ **Avoid restrictive and coercive food practices or use of food as a reward or for comfort**
  - ■ Limit fast food to no more than twice per week
- ■ *Counsel with emphasis on positive health consequences of good nutrition, not child's weight.*
- ■ *Counsel parents to offer traditional foods and not offer alternatives*

**PHYSICAL ACTIVITY AND SEDENTARY BEHAVIOR**
- ■ Monitor physical activity and sedentary behavior at least annually
- ■ Identify barriers to being physically active
- ■ Educate parents about age-appropriate physical activity
  - ■ At least 60 minutes of active, unstructured play and physical activity per day
- ■ Educate parents regarding physical activity as a family and parent as role model
- ■ *Counsel with emphasis on positive health consequences of increased physical activity, not weight (Hispanics, Native Americans)*
- ■ Educate parents about screen time practices and suseptibility of child to advertising:
  - ■ Avoid TV and other screen time for children < 2 years of age
  - ■ Limit TV and screen time to < 2 hours/day for children 2 years of age and older
  - ■ No TV in bedroom
  - ■ No TV during meals

**ADVOCACY**
- ■ Advocate for providing preschool age-children with childcare/preschool facilities that emphasize quality, daily physical activity (unstructured play and supervised active play) and avoid screen time
- ■ Advocate for optimal childcare/preschool menus, feeding, and eating routines

■ BOX 16-3
■ "HEALTHY EATING AND ACTIVITY TOGETHER" SCHOOL-AGE BRIEF GUIDE

**EARLY IDENTIFICATION**
- Document family history relevant to risk of overweight and update annually
- Measure height and weight at least annually; consider more frequent measurement if at risk of or overweight; document on the CDC growth charts
- Perform BMI calculation at least annually and document on CDC growth chart; document on problem list if ≥85th percentile
- Perform blood pressure at least annually; identify those with BP >90th percentile on problem list
- Perform and document Sexual Maturity Rating (Tanner Stage) annually
- Perform a fasting glucose level, total cholesterol, and/or lipid panel to assess for diabetes mellitus, hyperlipidemia, and metabolic syndrome if the child's BMI is ≥ 95th percentile
- Educate parent and child about growth pattern, clearly identifying status if at risk of or overweight

**DEVELOPMENT AND COMMUNICATION**
- Perform two-question screen for depression on parent and child
- Document areas of strength and concern
- Monitor child's social and emotional development
- *Document personal attitudes, values, and beliefs; spiritual and cultural influences about nutrition, physical activity, and body shape and size; race; ethnicity; language and educational preferences*
- Educate children and parents about expected growth, development, physical and emotional changes
- Educate parents and children about effective communication strategies
- Refer family, as needed, to free or low-cost community nutritional and physical activity resources, including registered dieticians
- *Educate families and children using the Pathways curriculum (Native Americans).*
- Counsel using Motivational Interviewing to address areas of concern
  - Reinforce all positive health behaviors
  - Identify discrepancies between goals and behaviors
  - Develop a plan of action in partnership with the family

**NUTRITION AND FEEDING**
- Monitor nutritional intake at least annually
- Identify barriers to healthy eating
- Educate children and parents regarding recommended nutritional intake:
  - Limit portion size
  - Consume 5 or more servings of fruits and vegetables per day
  - At least half of grains consumed should be whole grain foods
  - 3–4 dairy servings per day, fat-free for most; 800 mg calcium/day for ages 4–8 yrs 1200–1500 mg calcium/day for ages 8–12 yrs
  - Limit fast food to no more than twice per week
  - Consume healthful snacks
  - **Limit 100% fruit juice to 4–6 oz. or less/day; avoid fruit drinks and soda**
  - Limit fat intake; avoid foods high in saturated and trans fats; use soft margarine rather than lard, butter or stick margarine
- Educate children and parents regarding promising feeding practices:
  - Adapt food intake to match level of physical activity
  - Eat a healthy breakfast daily
  - Eat family meals together regularly
  - Prepare child to select and prepare healthful foods and drinks

**BOLD type indicates a strong evidence-based recommendation**
*Italic* type indicates a culturally appropriate recommendation

■ **BOX 16-3**
■ **"HEALTHY EATING AND ACTIVITY TOGETHER" SCHOOL-AGE BRIEF GUIDE—cont'd**

- Educate parents to avoid restrictive feeding practices or use of food for reward or comfort.
- *Counsel parents to offer traditional foods and not alternative foods*

**PHYSICAL ACTIVITY AND SEDENTARY BEHAVIOR**
- Monitor daily physical activity and sedentary behavior at least annually
- Identify barriers to being physically active
- **Educate children and parents about age appropriate physical activity**
  - **Engage in at least 60 minutes of intermittent moderate to vigorous physical activity per day**
- *Counsel with emphasis on positive health consequences of increased physical activity, rather than child's weight (Hispanics, African Americans)*
- Encourage parents to model healthy physical activity levels, and support child's activity participation
- Discuss media influence on health-related behavior, and educate children and parents regarding promising screen time practices
  - **Limit TV and screen time to ≤ 2 hours/day**
  - No TV in bedroom
  - No TV during meals
  - Parent monitoring of TV

**ADVOCACY**
- Advocate for retention of physical education in the schools
- Advocate for improved school lunches

■ **BOX 16-4**
■ **"HEALTHY EATING AND ACTIVITY TOGETHER" TEEN BRIEF GUIDE**

**EARLY IDENTIFICATION**
- Document family history relevant to risk of overweight and update annually
- Measure height and weight at least annually; consider more frequent measurement if at risk of or overweight; document on the CDC growth charts
- Perform BMI calculation at least annually and document on CDC growth chart; document on problem list if ≥ 85th percentile
- Perform blood pressure at least annually; document those with BP ≥ 90th percentile on problem list
- Perform and document Sexual Maturity Rating (Tanner Stage) annually
- Perform a fasting glucose level, total cholesterol and/or lipid panel to assess for diabetes mellitus, hyperlipidemia, and metabolic syndrome if the teen's BMI is ≥ the 95th percentile
- Educate parent and teen about growth pattern, clearly identifying status if at risk of or overweight

**DEVELOPMENT AND COMMUNICATION**
- Perform two-question screen for depression on parent and teen
- Document areas of strength and concern
- Monitor teen's social and emotional development

**BOLD type indicates a strong evidence-based recommendation**
*Italic* type indicates a culturally appropriate recommendation

*Continued*

- *Document personal attitudes, values, and beliefs; spiritual and cultural influences about nutrition, physical activity, and body shape and size; race; ethnicity; language and educational preferences*
- Educate teen and parents about expected growth, development, physical and emotional changes
- Educate parents about effective communication strategies with their teen
- *Counsel extended family members as well as parents about issues related to teen's health*
- Refer family, as needed, to free or low-cost community nutritional and physical activity resources, including registered dieticians
- Engage in Motivational Interviewing to address areas of concern
    - Reinforce all positive health behaviors
    - Identify discrepancies between goals and behaviors
    - Develop a plan of action in partnership with the family

## NUTRITION AND FEEDING
- Monitor nutritional intake at least annually
- Identify barriers to healthy eating
- Educate teen and parents regarding recommended nutritional intake
    - **Limit portion sizes**
    - **Consume 5 or more servings of fruits and vegetables per day**
    - At least half of grains consumed should be whole grain foods
    - 3–4 dairy servings per day, fat-free for most; 1200–1500 mg calcium/day
    - Limit fast food to no more than twice per week
    - Consume healthful snacks
    - **Limit 100% fruit juice to 4–6 oz. or less/day; avoid fruit drinks and soda**
    - Limit fat intake; avoid foods high in saturated and trans fats; use soft margarine rather than lard, butter, or stick margarine
- Educate teens and parents regarding promising feeding practices
    - Adapt food intake to match level of physical activity
    - Eat a healthy breakfast daily
    - Eat family meals together regularly
    - Prepare teen to select and prepare healthful foods and drinks
- Educate parents to avoid restrictive feeding practices, fad diets or use of food for reward or comfort
- *Counsel parents to offer traditional foods and not alternative foods*

## PHYSICAL ACTIVITY AND SEDENTARY BEHAVIOR
- Monitor daily physical activity and sedentary behavior at least annually
- Identify barriers to being physically active
- **Educate teens and parents about age appropriate physical activity**
    - **Engage in at least 60 minutes of intermittent moderate to vigorous physical activity per day**
- *Counsel with emphasis on positive health consequences of increased physical activity, rather than teen's weight (Hispanics, African Americans)*
- Encourage parents to model healthy physical activity levels and support teen activity participation.
- Discuss media influence on health-related behavior and educate teens and parents regarding promising screen time practices
    - **Limit TV and screen time to ≤2 hours/day**
    - No TV in bedroom
    - No TV during meals
    - Parent monitoring of TV

## ADVOCACY
- Advocate for partnerships among teens, schools, and the community to develop after-school programs that promote physical activity and improved nutrition

(1) Assessment, education
    (c) Nutrition essentials, optimal feeding, and eating behaviors
        (1) Assessment, education
    (d) Physical activity
        (1) Assessment, education, advocacy
2. Vegetarian diets (AAP, 2004; Moilanen, 2004)
    a. Infants and children on vegetarian diets need especially careful height and weight monitoring to ensure adequate growth
    b. In general, a vegetarian diet consists of plant foods
        i. Fruits
        ii. Vegetables
        iii. Nuts
        iv. Grains
        v. Legumes
    c. Vegans eat *no* animal products, including:
        i. Honey
        ii. Gelatin
        iii. Rennet—an enzyme that usually comes from animal sources
        iv. Animal fats
    d. Ovolactovegetarians will eat:
        i. Eggs
        ii. Dairy products
    e. Semivegetarians
        i. Avoid red meat
        ii. Usually include poultry
        iii. Fish
    f. Proteins
        i. Vegetarians need the same amount of protein as nonvegetarians
        ii. Lower amounts of protein in plant sources mean that a larger amount (weight or volume) of vegetable protein must be consumed
        iii. Food sources of plant protein
            (a) Fruits
            (b) Nuts and seeds
            (c) Legumes (lentils, peas, beans)
            (d) Cereals
            (e) Other vegetables
        iv. An understanding of the role of complementary vegetable proteins is essential
            (a) Meats contain all of the essential amino acids necessary to make *complete* proteins, which are necessary for growth
            (b) Plant protein is incomplete, i.e., one plant does not contain all of the essential amino acids
            (c) By combining different types of plant foods (beans with rice, for example) complete proteins can be constructed
    g. Advantages
        i. Properly planned ovolacto- or semivegetarian diet that is not overly restrictive can provide appropriate nutrients needed for growth for all age-groups
        ii. Decreases risk of some diseases or disorders
            (a) Overweight
            (b) Heart disease
            (c) Hypertension

        (d) Hypercholesterolemia

        (e) Gallstones

    h. Disadvantages

       i. Parent or adolescent must carefully plan diet

      ii. Lack of planning can lead to:

        (a) Nutritional deficiencies

        (b) Inadequate growth

     iii. Parents need to be especially vigilant for infants and toddlers

        (a) Few teeth

        (b) Immature digestive tract

        (c) Small stomachs

        (d) Must be fed frequently to obtain enough calories for energy and growth

     iv. Children younger than age 3 should not be fed nuts or seeds due to choking hazards

      v. Supplementation may be necessary to provide essential nutrients

        (a) Vitamin $B_{12}$

        (b) Folic acid

        (c) Iron

        (d) Zinc

        (e) Vitamin D

        (f) Occasionally calcium

3. Food allergy or food hypersensitivity (Anand & Routes, 2004)

    a. Pathophysiology

       i. Genetically predisposed individuals become sensitized to a specific allergen by exposure to it

      ii. Individuals prone to IgE-mediated allergic reactions are called atopic

     iii. Antigen-specific IgE antibodies bind to high-affinity receptors located on the surfaces of mast cells and basophils

     iv. Reexposure to the antigen causes release of chemical mediators

        (a) Histamine: causes contraction of smooth muscles of the airway and GI tract, increased vasopermeability and vasodilation, nasal mucus production, airway mucus production, pruritus, cutaneous vasodilation, and gastric acid secretion

        (b) Tryptase: a good marker of mast cell activation

        (c) Proteoglycans: include heparin and chondroitin sulfate

        (d) Chemotactic factors: release major basic protein; with neutrophils, can cause significant tissue damage in the later phases of allergic reactions

    b. Clinical manifestations

       i. GI tract

        (a) Severe diarrhea

        (b) Vomiting

      ii. Skin rash

        (a) Urticaria

        (b) Eczema (atopic dermatitis)

          (1) In 40% of infants with significant atopic dermatitis, food allergies are the cause (Heird, 2004b)

     iii. Respiratory tract

        (a) Throat swelling

    (b) Wheezing

    (c) Nasal congestion

   **iv.** Anaphylactic shock

    (a) Immediate—reaction occurs within minutes to 2 hours after ingestion

    (b) Delayed—reaction occurs within 2 hours to generally less than 48 hours

 **c.** Foods that may cause allergic reactions (APA, 2004; Heird, 2004b; Sampson & Leung, 2004)

   **i.** 90% of all food allergies caused by:

    (a) Milk

     (1) Cow's milk protein allergy most common food allergy in infants

     (2) All milk allergies will be evident by 12 months

     (3) Milk protein allergy is not the same as lactose intolerance, which is related to the type of sugar (lactose) in cow's milk

    (b) Peanuts—leading cause of fatal and near-fatal food allergy reactions in the United States

    (c) Eggs—evident by 18 months

    (d) Wheat

    (e) Soy

    (f) Nuts

    (g) Fish

   **ii.** Food allergens can carry through breast milk and cause allergic reactions in infants; therefore a breast-feeding mother should monitor her infant's symptoms with respect to her own food intake

   **iii.** Diagnosis

    (a) Sensitivity testing for IgE-mediated food allergy; use skin prick–puncture tests or radioallergosorbent tests

    (b) Food challenge can be done in the office with strict medical supervision

     (1) Patients avoid the suspected food(s) for at least 2 weeks

     (2) After intravenous access is obtained, graded doses of either a challenge food or a placebo food are administered (both are disguised or placed in capsules)

     (3) Ensure access to emergency medications (epinephrine, antihistamines, steroids, and inhaled β-agonists) and CPR equipment

     (4) Assess patient frequently for skin, GI, and respiratory changes

     (5) Terminate challenge when a reaction becomes apparent

     (6) Observe for delayed reactions

     (7) Confirm negative challenges with a meal-sized portion of the food

   **iv.** Treatment

    (a) Formula-fed infants

     (1) Change to protein hydrolysate formula

     (2) Should see improvement within 48 hours after food removed from diet

     (3) If necessary, work with allergist to identify troublesome food

    (b) Avoid suspected or confirmed foods

   **v.** Prognosis

    (a) About 85% of infants who are allergic to milk and eggs will develop a tolerance to them within the first 5 years of life

    (b) About 20% of infants who are allergic to peanuts will develop a tolerance to them

      vi. Prevention (Host & Halken, 2004)
        (a) Exclusive breast-feeding for 4 to 6 months offers some protection
        (b) Avoid introduction of high-allergen foods until later in life
          (1) Certainly until at least 4 months and maybe later
          (2) Especially peanuts

4. Breast-feeding
   a. Create a culture of breast-feeding (BF)
      i. Become knowledgeable about BF as a provider; a marketable skill for PNPs
      ii. Establish a BF-friendly office
        (a) Avoid distribution of formula samples
        (b) Avoid formula company–endorsed handouts
        (c) Surround mothers with people supportive of BF
      iii. NAPNAP released a Breastfeeding Position Statement in 2001 that will be updated in 2006
      iv. PNP should see BF infants at 3 to 5 days of life to prevent, identify, and correct BF problems (AAP, 2005)
   b. National goals for breast-feeding
      i. *Healthy People 2010* goals (U.S. Department of Health & Human Services, 2000)
        (a) 75% of new mothers will initiate BF
        (b) 50% still BF at 6 months
        (c) 25% breast-feed up to 1 year
      ii. NAPNAP (2001) Breastfeeding Position Statement "identifies breastfeeding as the natural and preferred method of infant feeding and human milk as superior to all substitute feeding options"
      iii. AAP (2005) recommends:
        (a) Exclusive BF for first 6 months
        (b) Support BF for as long as the mother desires
        (c) Teach mothers to examine their breasts for lumps during lactation
   c. Current rates in United States
      i. After decline in 1991, new resurgence in BF (Abluwalia, et al., 2003; AAP, 2005)
      ii. 18% increase in initiation of BF from 1993 to1998
      iii. 70% all women initiated BF in 2001
      iv. 33% some BF at 6 months
      v. More women from higher socioeconomic status BF, but new programs have increased the number of women from vulnerable groups who initiate BF
   d. Benefits of BF
      i. Human milk is specifically designed for human infants and cannot be duplicated
        (a) More than 100 different components in breast milk
      ii. Decreases illness in infant
        (a) Encourages mother-infant interaction
        (b) Newborns have immature immune systems
        (c) Human milk compensates for IgA not normally acquired until 4 months
          (1) IgA in breast milk blocks attachment of *Haemophilus influenzae* and streptococcus to respiratory epithelial cells
          (2) Mother can make antibodies against illnesses and pass them to infant through breast milk

(d) Decreases otitis media and upper respiratory tract infections
  (1) Otitis media is twice as common in non-BF infants compared with exclusive BF infants older than 4 months, independent of socio-economic status, gender, siblings, daycare, exposure to smoking
  (2) Infant with URI can better synchronize breathing with BF than with bottle-feeding
(e) Decreases gastrointestinal problems including gastroesophageal reflux
  (1) Protective against diarrheal illnesses
  (2) Breast milk is considered a clear fluid; therefore infant can continue BF through vomiting/diarrhea illness—not true of formula
  (3) Breast milk digested quicker than formula
(f) Decreases allergies—anti-inflammatory agents in breast milk help decrease atopy
(g) Breastfeeding infants during painful procedures provides analgesia (Gary, Miller, Phillip, & Blass, 2002)
(h) Breast-feeding decreases overweight—the longer infants breast-feed, lower incidence of infant overweight, independent of education and SES
(i) Economic reasons—formula costs approximately $1200 per year

**e.** Lactation
  **ii.** Supply and demand principle
    (a) Sucking causes pituitary to secrete oxytocin (hormone release)
    (b) Oxytocin causes alveoli to contract and cause an "outpouching" of the milk ducts (let-down)
    (c) Let-down is described as tingling, tightness, warmth, fullness in chest
    (d) Increased sucking due to let-down provides infant with hindmilk from alveoli
      (1) Fat content of hindmilk is 5%
      (2) Better for infant to suck longer on one breast
        a) Get higher fat hindmilk
        b) Start with second breast at next feeding
    (e) If no let-down, infant receives only foremilk
      (1) Fat content of foremilk is 2%
    (f) Milk supply
      (1) Increased sucking time at breast increases supply
      (2) Requires about 48 hours of increased sucking for infant to drive up supply
    (g) Amount of milk required
      (1) First 24 hours—only needs 37 mL breast milk for sufficient energy/fluids
      (2) Day 2—3 oz (90 mL)
      (3) Day 3—9 oz (270 mL)
      (4) Day 4—13 oz (390 mL)
  **iii.** Let-down reflex conditioning
    (a) Let-down can also be under emotional control
    (b) Oxytocin release enhanced by feelings of confidence but inhibited by pain and nicotine
    (c) Before BF, take warm shower or use warm compresses to soften breast
    (d) Find comfortable, quiet, safe place to nurse

   (e) Gently massage breast
      (1) Start where breast meets chest
      (2) Stroke toward nipple
      (3) Drink glass of fluid
   (f) Take 5 minutes to relax, think peaceful thoughts
   (g) Initially may take 3 to 4 minutes of vigorous sucking to elicit let-down
   (h) Once BF well established let-down will occur in seconds
 **f.** "Latching-on"
   **i.** Infant squashes nipple between tongue and roof of mouth
   **ii.** Improper position of infant's mouth on breast is number 1 cause of sore nipples
      (a) Teeth not an issue
   **iii.** To evaluate proper latching-on, mother should observe:
      (a) Infant with rhythmic suck and swallow
      (b) Gulping noise without clicking is expected
      (c) Infant's ears should wiggle
   **iv.** Poor latch
      (a) Key area of PNP intervention: follow BF families closely
      (b) Early hospital discharge means that some families go home with little practice and little opportunity for BF education
      (c) Help mother obtain a breast pump
         (1) Electric pump with double-headed tubing is preferable (faster than pumping by hand)
         (2) Use until latch better established
         (3) Pump 10 times every 24 hours
         (4) Mother can pump approximately 1 oz/hr
         (5) Feed infant expressed breast milk so infant has energy to learn new skill
            a) Use oral syringe
            b) Small cup
            c) Finger dipped in milk
 **g.** Scheduling BF: *on demand* is recommended rather than strict intervals
   **i.** BF when infant gives cues of being hungry
      (a) Sucking on the breast teaches infant to associate eating with hunger
      (b) Newborns are full of amniotic fluid so are usually not hungry
      (c) Mother needs to be more aggressive about offering breast to infant with passive temperament because often does not give hunger cues
   **ii.** Not necessary to BF "every 4 hours"
   **iii.** Suggested time intervals
      (a) In early days infant needs to nurse 8 to 12 times per day
         (1) Count from start of one feeding to start of next
         (2) Allow a maximum of 3 hours between feeds during the day
         (3) Wake after 4 hours during the day
         (4) Many infants *bunch feed* at night to fill up before a longer sleep period
         (5) Avoid nursing sooner than every 1½ to 2 hours; look for other reasons for crying
            a) Need for stimulation
            b) Diaper change
            c) Nap
            d) Cuddling
            e) Need to suck
      (b) Mother should not stop nursing unless she is too ill or dehydrated

**h.** How to determine adequate intake of breast milk
  **i.** Expect about 4 to 6 wet diapers/day (by age 5 to 7 days) (AAP, 2005)
    (a) New superabsorbent diapers may just feel heavier rather than wet
  **ii.** Infant satisfied for at least 2 hours
  **iii.** Weight loss >7% from birth weight indicates newborn needs VERY close surveillance; should not continue to lose weight after 10 days
  **iv.** Stools (normal)
    (a) Stools change from the black/green tarry meconium stools to seedy yellow-green within first few days
    (b) Is a concern if not yellow/green by 5 days
    (c) First 4 weeks infants should have at least 1–2 stools/day
    (d) After day 6 many infants will have a stool with each feeding
      (1) Pleasant odor
      (2) Mustard yellow to pale green
      (3) Soft
      (4) Curdy/seedy
      (5) Vigorous or explosive
    (e) After 1 month, if nursing well, 1 soft stool every 4 days or more can be normal (breast milk well absorbed)
**i.** BF premature infants is possible
  **i.** May need to pump and store milk initially
  **ii.** Many benefits from premature infant receiving pumped milk via nasogastric (NG) tube
**j.** Father involvement
  **i.** Discuss ways for father to be involved in feeding process
  **ii.** Consider pumping breast milk so father can bottle-feed
**k.** Physiologic jaundice—appears around third day of life (Hansen, 2005)
  **i.** Appears between the second and fifth days of life in both bottle- and breast-fed infants and clears by 2 weeks
  **ii.** Unconjugated serum bilirubin level greater than 30 mmol/L (1.8 mg/dL) during the first week of life
  **iii.** Appearance
    (a) Yellowish skin and sclera
    (b) Color change starts on the head and moves toward feet
    (c) True color of the skin can be observed by blanching (pressure on the skin with quick release)
  **iv.** Cause
    (a) Fetus has more red blood cells (RBCs) than newborn
    (b) RBCs normally break down and produce bilirubin
    (c) Bilirubin normally excreted via stool
    (d) But it takes up to 3 days for liver to handle load
    (e) Bilirubin is reabsorbed
    (f) Occurs with bottle- and breastfed infants, but BF may prolong it
  **v.** Diagnostic testing
    (a) Evaluate physiologic versus pathologic cause of jaundice
    (b) Bilirubin levels
  **vi.** Treatment
    (a) It usually causes no problems
    (b) Fluids will not help because bilirubin excreted via stool
    (c) Do not stop BF
    (d) Colostrum in breast milk is a natural laxative; increases defecation

      **vii.** Expected outcome
         (a) Usually will resolve in approximately 1 to 2 weeks in full-term infant
         (b) Requires 3 to 4 weeks in premature infants

  **l.** Thrush (*Candida albicans*) affects infant and mother
      **i.** Evidenced by white plaques on infant's buccal mucosa, tongue, gums
         (a) Plaques do not wipe off easily
         (b) May bleed or have erythematous base when removed
         (c) Satellite lesions and beefy, red rash in intertriginous folds of diaper area
      **ii.** Sharp, burning, consistent pain in breasts, not just while nursing
      **iii.** Refer mother to her primary care provider
      **iv.** Medications
         (a) Neonates
            (1) Nystatin suspension 100,000 units PO 4 times a day for at least 2 weeks
            (2) ½ dropper each side of mouth; rub in
         (b) Infants
            (1) Nystatin suspension 200,000 units PO 4 times a day for at least 2 weeks
            (2) 1 dropper each side of mouth; rub in
         (c) Diaper area
            (1) Nystatin cream 2 or 3 times a day with diaper change
      **v.** Boil all bottle nipples, pacifiers
         (a) Freezing will not kill fungus
      **vi.** Wash hands well before and after each contact with the infant or breasts

**m.** Breast engorgement
      **i.** Important area of anticipatory guidance and counseling
         (a) Mother's breast becomes too full and hard
         (b) Infant will be unable to latch well
         (c) Occurs at third to fifth day
         (d) Lasts 12 to 24 hours
      **ii.** Treatment
         (a) Continuous wearing of well-fitting bra for at least 24 to 48 hours
         (b) Prior to feeding:
            (1) Apply warm compresses to breast
            (2) Followed by gentle breast massage to increase milk flow and let-down
               a) Softens breast to improve ability to latch
               b) However, increases circulation to already congested breast
         (c) Frequent nursing
         (d) After feedings, treat swollen breast tissue with ice packs for 20 minutes
         (e) Pump breasts
            (1) Judicious pumping to extract a *small* amount of milk
               a) May decrease pain
               b) Make nipple grasp easier for infant
            (2) Too much pumping
               a) Will increase milk supply
               b) Worsen problem
            (3) Storage of pumped breast milk
               a) Glass or polypropylene plastic containers maintain IgA stability with freezing

b) Refrigeration as soon as possible is best
c) Freshly expressed milk
   i) Room temperature (<78° F) for 6 to 8 hours
   ii) Refrigerated 3 to 5 days (<39° F)
   iii) 2 weeks freezer inside refrigerator
   iv) 3 months freezer section of refrigerator with separate door
   v) 6 to 12 months (deep freeze at <0° F)

**n.** Sore nipples
   **i.** Observe BF for proper positioning of infant and proper latching-on
   **ii.** Wipe nipples with water after feeding to remove enzymes from infant's saliva
   **iii.** Rub nipples with small amount of expressed milk for healing
   **iv.** Dry breasts thoroughly
      (a) Avoid plastic-lined breast pads
      (b) Keep bra flaps down when possible

**o.** Blocked duct/mastitis
   **i.** Caused by an increase or decrease in milk demand or excessive pressure to one area
   **ii.** Symptoms
      (a) Fever
      (b) Flulike feeling
   **iii.** Signs associated with breast
      (a) Hard
      (b) Reddened
      (c) Tender areas
   **iv.** To relieve blockage
      (a) Continue to nurse; this is the best treatment
      (b) Use warm compresses
      (c) Massage
      (d) Change infant's position while feeding
      (e) Antibiotic treatment if necessary for fever or mastitis

**p.** Medications and BF
   **i.** Contraindicated medications
      (a) Radioactive compounds for diagnostic procedures
      (b) Drugs for early tuberculosis (TB)
      (c) Street drugs
      (d) Cancer chemotherapy
      (e) Lithium
      (i) Some antidepressants and antipsychotic agents
      (j) See AAP, 2001 for complete list
   **ii.** Alcoholic beverages are not recommended
      (a) Brain growth is greatest during first year of life
      (b) Will depress infant's CNS
   **iii.** Drugs that decrease milk supply
      (a) Decongestants/antihistamines
      (b) Some birth control pills (BCPs)
      (c) Progesterone-only BCPs are okay after milk supply is well established
      (d) Nicotine interferes with milk production
   **iv.** Little research exists on effect of herbs and "natural medicines" on BF infant
      (a) Not all herbs are innocuous
      (b) Dangers are unknown

     **v.** If temporary prescription drug is needed:

        (a) Try to pump and store milk before taking the medication

        (b) During treatment, pump and discard milk to maintain milk production

        (c) Ask if a route other than oral is possible, such as topical or inhaled

        (d) If can do once-per-day dosing

            (1) Take the dose before infant's longest sleep

            (2) Avoid nursing at time of peak serum level

**5.** Formula feeding issues

  **a.** Categories of formulas (all in general distribution fall into one of these categories)

     **i.** Normal newborn milk-based formula

     **ii.** Simple formula intolerance-soy based formula

     **iii.** Protein hydrolysate formula

  **b.** Evaluating formula (Morrow, 2004)

     **i.** All commercial formulas (even "generics") meet minimum nutritional standards set by Infant Formula Act

     **ii.** All formulas are evaluated in comparison with the composition of human milk as gold standard

     **iii.** Human breast milk: 20 cal/oz

        (a) Protein—mature breast milk protein is composed of:

            (1) 40% casein and 60% whey

            (2) Casein (curd) supplies amino acids for growth and development

            (3) Whey contains alpha-lactalbumin, lactoferrin, immunoglobulins, albumin, enzymes, growth factors, hormones

        (b) Fat—human milk fat is absorbed better than any other type of fat

        (c) Carbohydrate

     **iv.** Milk-based formula: 20 cal/oz; contains heated nonfat cow's milk

        (a) Protein

            (1) Cow's milk contains 80% casein and 20% whey

            (2) Formula casein and whey contents vary widely

        (b) Fat—vegetable oil may be added to formula to increase amount of linoleic acid and linolenic acid (essential fatty acids)

        (c) Added carbohydrate is lactose

     **v.** Soy-based formula—20 cal/oz

        (a) Contents

            (1) Protein—soy protein isolate

            (2) Fats—similar to cow's milk formula

            (3) Carbohydrate—sucrose and/or corn syrup

        (b) Nutritionally equivalent to cow's milk

        (c) Increasing theoretical concerns that phytoestrogens found in soy milk have impact on:

            (1) Growth and development

            (2) Reproduction

            (3) Thyroid disease

            (4) Immune system

        (d) No conclusive scientific evidence yet but soy formula should be used cautiously and only for specific indications listed below (Tuohy, 2003; Merritt & Jenks, 2004)

            (1) Galactosemia

               a) Hereditary lactose intolerance

               b) Extremely rare in infancy—fewer than 1/10,000

(2) Ovolactovegetarian families
   a) But most choose to breast-feed
(3) Temporary lactose deficiency
   a) Due to diarrheal illness
   b) If sibling has history of intolerance, start the next child on soy (Osborne & Sinn, 2004)
   c) Likely will not prevent allergy in next child
(4) Do not use with preterm infant weighing less than 1800 g
   a) Use preemie formula (see Section 5.e on p.198)
   b) Lactose important for calcium absorption
   c) Increased risk of rickets
   d) Bone demineralization
(5) Child with a documented cow's milk allergy (Host & Halken, 2004)
   a) 8% to 40% are also soy intolerant
(6) Colic—no evidence to support use of soy milk
(7) Increasing theoretical concerns that phytoestrogens found in soy milk have impact on:
   a) Growth and development
   b) Reproduction
   c) Thyroid disease
   d) Immune system
vi. Protein hydrolysate formula
   (a) Carbohydrate
      (1) No lactose
      (2) Various combinations of:
         a) Sucrose
         b) Corn syrup solids
         c) Cornstarch
         d) Tapioca starch
   (b) Fat
      (1) Medium chain triglyceride (MCT) oil
      (2) Vegetable oil for essential fatty acids
   (c) Protein
      (1) Hydrolyzed casein
         a) Predigested so cannot cause immune response
         b) Decreases fecal production due to decreased residue
   (d) Indications for use of protein hydrolysate formula
      (1) Severe allergy to cows milk protein
         a) Symptoms
            i) Blood in stool
            ii) Severe vomiting, diarrhea
            iii) Severe rash
            iv) Onset early in life
      (2) Significant malabsorption
         a) Hepatobiliary
         b) Gastrointestinal disease
   (e) Drawbacks—bad taste, expensive
c. Homemade formula
   i. Discourage use of homemade formulas from cow's milk or evaporated milk
   ii. Are nutritionally inadequate
   iii. High protein and sodium content may stress the kidneys

    **d.** Temporary illness formulas:
       **i.** Milk-based without lactose
         (a) Lactose intolerance very rare in infancy
         (b) Only used for temporary lactose deficiency caused by diarrheal illness
       **ii.** Soy based with added fiber
         (a) Shortens the duration of diarrheal illness
       **iii.** Milk-based with added rice
         (a) Used for infants with severe reflux
         (b) May or may not be helpful
    **e.** Preemie formulas—22 kcal/oz
       **i.** Higher calories, protein, calcium phosphorus
       **ii.** Better for catch-up growth than standard formula
       **iii.** Better bone mineralization
    **f.** Graduation formulas
       **i.** Iron fortified
       **ii.** Helpful for older infants not getting enough iron from complementary foods
       **iii.** Higher protein and minerals than regular formula
       **iv.** Clear advantage for infants or toddlers eating a variety of complementary foods
       **v.** Better than switching to cow's milk before age 12 months
       **vi.** May or may not be cheaper than formula (depends regionally)
    **g.** Formula switching
       **i.** Realize that new infants can be fussy but this is not always related to their formula
       **ii.** No evidence that switching formula categories (milk-based, soy-based, etc.) is effective
       **iii.** If switching is done, use the following guidelines:
         (a) If must switch formula have a clear rationale
         (b) Use formula 1 month before making a switch
         (c) Try a formula in the next category: milk based to soy based to protein hydrolysate
    **h.** Recommendations regarding of amount of formula intake
       **i.** Need *maximum* of 32 oz of formula per 24 hours
       **ii.** If infant takes more than 40 oz
         (a) Check nipple—opening may be too large
         (b) Increase water intake
           (1) Never give more than 4 oz of water per day to young infants
           (2) Causes electrolyte imbalance
         (c) Offer opportunities for nonnutritive sucking (hand, thumb, pacifier)
  **i.** Whole milk
       **i.** AAP (2004) recommends no whole cow's milk before age 12 months
         (a) Too low in iron, linoleic acid, and vitamin E
         (b) Too high in sodium, potassium, protein
       **ii.** No skim milk before age 2 years
         (a) Not enough calories
         (b) Infant will use own fat stores for energy
       **iii.** Goat milk
         (a) Deficient in folic acid
         (b) Deficient in vitamin $B_{12}$

6. Supplements
   a. Iron
      i. Breast-fed infants
         (a) No need for iron supplementation until at least 6 months of age if exclusively breast-fed
         (b) Iron in human milk has greater bioavailability
      ii. Formula-fed infants
         (a) In past 5 years amount of iron in low iron formula increased to 4 to 5 mg/L
      iii. Preterm infants definitely need additional iron by age 2 months
      iv. Full-term infants need additional iron by age 4 months
      v. According to AAP, there is no role for low iron formula, although it is available
         (a) All formula should have at least 10 to 12 mg/L
         (b) Iron in formulas does not cause GI disturbances despite beliefs by some parents and providers
   b. Fluoride (American Academy of Pediatric Dentistry, 2003)
      i. Identify sources and amounts of fluoride that children receive
         (a) Water (well or public sources)
         (b) Toothpaste, mouthwash
      ii. If water and/or total amount received is fluoride-deficient (<0.3 parts per million [ppm]) water, fluoride supplements should be:
         (a) Birth to 6 months: none
         (b) 6 months to 3 years: 0.25 mg/day
         (c) 3 to 6 years: 0.50 mg/day
         (d) 6 to 16 years: 1 mg/day
      iii. If water and/or total amount received is fluoride-deficient (0.3 to 0.6 ppm) water, fluoride supplements should be:
         (a) Birth to 6 months: none
         (b) 6 months to 3 years: none
         (c) 3 to 6 years: 0.25 mg/day
         (d) 6 to 16 years: 0.50 mg/day
      iv. See also Chapter 19 for more detail on fluorides and dental caries
   c. Vitamins (AAP, 2003)
      i. Breast-fed infants
         (a) Controversial; in general, supplementation with most vitamins is not necessary
         (b) Vitamin D (Gartner & Greer, 2003)
            (1) Synthesized by ultraviolet light on a cholesterol precursor in the skin; therefore exposure to sunlight is necessary to prevent rickets
            (2) With increased use of sunscreen and recommendations to decrease exposure to ultraviolet light the risk of Vitamin D deficiency has increased
            (3) Formula is supplemented, but breast milk is low in Vitamin D
            (4) Vitamin D supplement at 200 International Units beginning in the first 2 months of life and continuing through adolescence is necessary
         (c) Vitamin $B_{12}$
            (1) Strict vegetarian breast feeding mothers
               a) Infants are at risk for Vitamin $B_{12}$ deficiency and neurologic abnormalities

b) Monitor vitamin $B_{12}$ sufficiency with tests of infant's urinary methylmalonic acid

c) Parenteral or oral supplements for the infant may be necessary

ii. Formula fed infants—no vitamin supplements needed if:

(a) Younger than age 6 months and receiving formula with iron

(b) Older than age 6 months and getting adequate intake of complementary foods with iron

7. Failure to thrive (FTT) (Bauchner, 2004; Heird, 2004a)

a. Definition

i. Growth below the third or fifth percentile

ii. Growth rate that has decreased across two major growth percentiles

iii. Organic FTT—caused by an underlying medical condition

iv. Nonorganic FTT—no known medical cause; often called psychosocial FTT

b. Prevalence is unknown but could be 5% to 10% of low–birth weight children and children living in poverty

c. Etiology

i. Failure of a parent to offer sufficient calories

(a) Lack of knowledge of children's dietary needs

(b) Unusual dietary beliefs

(c) Lack of access to food

(d) Neglect

ii. Failure of child to take sufficient calories

(a) Difficulty swallowing

iii. Failure of child to retain sufficient calories

(a) Vomiting

(b) Diarrhea

(c) Malabsorption syndromes

d. Signs, symptoms, and differential diagnosis

i. Spitting, vomiting, food refusal, gastroesophageal reflux, chronic tonsillitis, food allergies

ii. Diarrhea, fatty stools, malabsorption syndromes, intestinal parasites, milk protein intolerance

iii. Snoring, mouth breathing, enlarged tonsils—adenoid hypertrophy, obstructive sleep apnea

iv. Recurrent wheezing, pulmonary infections—asthma, aspiration

v. Recurrent infections—HIV

vi. Travel to/from developing countries—parasitic or bacterial GI infections

e. Diagnosis

i. Organic FTT

(a) Conduct diagnostic tests to rule out organic cause as indicated by symptoms

ii. Nonorganic FTT

(a) Observation of parent-infant feeding sessions

(b) Treatment trial—weight gain in response to adequate caloric feedings

f. Treatment

i. Calm, comfortable feeding atmosphere for both infant or child and parent

ii. Organic FTT

(a) Treat the underlying organic cause

iii. Nonorganic FTT

(a) May need to be hospitalized for 5 to 10 days
    (1) Observe parent-infant/child interactions
    (2) Begin and sustain catch-up growth with adequate caloric feedings
    (3) Educate parents about appropriate foods and feeding styles
  **g.** Prognosis
    **i.** Negative effect on brain growth when FTT occurs during first year of life
    **ii.** Developmental delays
    **iii.** Social and emotional problems

# NUTRITION ISSUES RELEVANT TO CERTAIN AGE-GROUPS

**1.** Infant (birth to 4 months)
  **a.** Caloric need 110 kcal/kg body weight
  **b.** Breast-feeding (See Section 4 earlier)
    **i.** Number of times per day
    **ii.** Length
  **c.** Formula (see Section 5 earlier)
    **i.** Type of formula, e.g., Enfamil with Fe
      (a) Powdered—how is it prepared?
      (b) Concentrated—how is it prepared?
      (c) Ready to feed
    **ii.** Amount of formula
      (a) Number of ounces every number of hours, e.g., 4 oz every 4 hours
      (b) Rule of thumb: age in months + 3 oz every 4 hours (up to 5 months)
      (c) Total should not exceed 32 oz/day
  **d.** Juice and complementary foods (solids) are not recommended
  **e.** Infants less than 6 months should not be given free water (max 3–4 oz/day, if that) due to risk of electrolyte imbalance
  **f.** Pacifier or fingers can satisfy infant's desire or need to suck
  **g.** Indicators of adequacy of intake
    **i.** Gain of 30 g/day (1 oz/day) in first 3 months
    **ii.** Gain of 15 to 20 g/day in second 3 months
    **iii.** Six well-soaked diapers and yellowish stool daily
  **h.** Other growth parameters
    **i.** Lose up to 10% birth weight
      (a) Regain by 2 weeks if formula-fed
      (b) Regain by 3 to 4 weeks if BF
    **ii.** Length during first 6 months increases approximately 1 inch per month
    **iii.** Double birth weight by 5 to 6 months; triple by 1 year
  **i.** Breast-feeding infants nurse more during growth spurts to increase the milk supply needed to sustain their growth
    **i.** 10 days
    **ii.** 4 to 6 weeks
    **iii.** 3 months
**2.** Infant (4 months to 1 year)
  **a.** Caloric need 110 kcal/kg body weight
  **b.** Gains approximately 3 to 4 oz/week
  **c.** Starting complementary foods (solids)
    **i.** NAPNAP's *'Starting Solids; Nutrition Guide for Infants and Children 6 to 18 Months of Age* (2005) brochure provides information for parents about starting complementary foods in young infants

    **ii.** Breast milk and/or formula is sufficient until age 4 to 6 months

    **iii.** Formula-fed infants start closer to 4 months

    **iv.** Breast-fed infants start closer to 6 months

**d.** Signs of readiness for complementary foods

    **i.** Between 4 and 6 months of age

    **ii.** Can hold head up straight when sitting

    **iii.** Opens mouth when food approaches

    **iv.** Interested in food when others eat

**e.** Advantages of introducing complementary foods later

    **i.** Tongue thrust diminished (extrusion reflex)

    **ii.** Infant able to sit upright and refuse unwanted food

    **iii.** Rapid progression to table food

        (a) Bigger infants need texture variations

    **iv.** Avoid early sensitization to high-allergen foods such as eggs, peanuts, soy, wheat

    **v.** Lower risk for obesity

    **vi.** Mothers believe that infants sleep better through night, but this is not supported by research (sleeping through the night is related to reaching weight of about 11 lb)

**f.** Order of introducing new foods

    **i.** Typically has been regional/provider preference

    **ii.** Research indicates introduction of iron rich foods (fortified cereal/ meats) is an important reason to start these types of foods (Butte et al., 2004)

    **iii.** Sequence is less important than using single ingredient foods and waiting 2 to 4 days between each new food to monitor for reactions

    **iii.** Variety is important

**g.** In determining amounts to feed, teach parents to follow infant's cues of satiation

    **i.** Turning head away

    **ii.** Pushing spoon away

    **iii.** No longer opening mouth when spoon approaches

**h.** Foods to avoid or use with caution

    **i.** Allergy foods

        (a) To minimize the risk of developing of food allergies, avoid introducing foods that have a family history of food allergies until the following ages (AAP, 2000)

            (1) Wait until 6 months to start complementary foods

            (2) Dairy at 1 year

            (3) Eggs at 2 years

            (4) Peanuts/nuts/fish at 3 years

        (b) Introduce a new food only once every 2 to 4 days to clearly pinpoint any adverse reactions to a new food

    **ii.** Honey—avoid honey due to risk of botulism

    **iii.** Constipating foods

        (a) Many first foods tend to be constipating

        (b) Substitute with less constipating alternatives

            (1) Oatmeal instead of rice cereal

            (2) Plums instead of applesauce or bananas

**i.** Finger foods

    **i.** Any food can be considered a finger food if it:

        (a) Can be transferred by the child with the fingers from tray to mouth

        (b) Is soft enough to prevent choking

      **ii.** Finger foods can be started as soon as an infant has the fine motor control to move food from the high chair tray to his or her mouth

      **iii.** Safe to begin around 6 to 7 months

      **iv.** Allows infants to be independent in the eating process

  **j.** Choking foods

      **i.** Any food can cause choking

      **ii.** Foods that are round and slippery cause the most problems (hot dogs, bananas, grapes)

      **iii.** Foods that are sticky or hard are also problematic (candy, gum)

      **iv.** Young infants and toddlers are at greatest choking risk

        (a) Have small windpipes

        (b) Still mastering the feeding process

      **v.** Acquiring teeth does not guard against choking

      **vi.** Not until molars emerge (grinding teeth) should a child receive food that is not soft or pureed

      **vii.** For safety reasons, children should not be allowed to eat:

        (a) When walking or running

        (b) In the car seat

  **k.** Introduce juice in a cup

      **i.** Limit to 4 oz fortified 100% juice per day for vitamin C requirements

      **ii.** After controlling for maternal height, children who consume more than 12 oz/day of juice are shorter and more overweight than children who consume less

  **l.** At bed- or naptime give bottle containing only water to prevent dental caries

**3.** Toddler (1 to 3 years)

  **a.** Servings (see Table 16–1 for servings according to age- and food groups)

  **b.** Caloric need decreases to 100 kcal/kg (see Table 16–2)

  **c.** Goal: three meals plus two nutritious snacks per day

  **d.** Finger foods

      **i.** See Section 2.i. earlier

      **ii.** After age 1 finger foods should be the primary mode of feeding

      **iii.** Few toddlers are interested in eating from a spoon

  **e.** Choking foods—see Section 2.j. earlier

  **f.** Brazelton's recommendations for toddler period of intense negativity (Brazelton, 2002)

      **i.** Parents can relax knowing that the toddler will meet his or her nutritional needs if this minimum amount is eaten

        (a) 1 pint (16 oz) milk or milk product per day (includes milk, cheese, yogurt, ice cream)

        (b) 2 oz protein with iron (includes meat, egg, peanut butter)

        (c) 1 oz orange juice or an orange

        (d) Multivitamin

  **g.** Developmental reasons for not eating

      **i.** Physiologic anorexia

        (a) Not growing as fast as during infancy

        (b) Decreased caloric need

      **ii.** Increased physical activity

        (a) Too interested in other things

        (b) Difficulty sitting still

      **iii.** Exploring or playing with food is more fun than eating

      **iv.** Independent "no" stage

        (a) Don't battle with child over food

■ **TABLE 16-1**
■ ■ **Number of Servings and Serving Sizes for Age and Total Daily Calorie Intake**

| Food Groups | 1–3 years old*<br>Servings | 4–6 years old*<br>Servings | 6–21 years old 1600<br>Servings | 2000<br>Servings | 2600<br>Servings | 3100<br>Servings | Serving Size 1600-3100 Calorie Diets |
|---|---|---|---|---|---|---|---|
| Grains | 6<br>¼–½ slice bread<br>4 tbsp cooked cereal, rice, pasta<br>¼ cup dry cereal<br>1 or 2 crackers | 6 | 6 | 7–8 | 10–11 | 12–13 | 1 slice bread<br>1 cup of ready to eat cereal<br>½ cup rice, pasta, or cereal |
| Vegetables | 2–3<br>1 Tbsp/year age cooked vegetable | 3–5 | 3–4 | 4–5 | 5–6 | 6 | 1 cup raw leafy<br>½ cup cooked or raw other vegetables<br>¾ cup vegetable juice |
| Fruits | 2–3<br>½ piece fresh fruit<br>½ cup fruit canned, cooked<br>¼–½ cup juice | 2 | 4 | 4–5 | 5–6 | 6 | ¾ cup fruit juice<br>1 medium fruit<br>¼ cup dried fruit<br>½ cup fresh, frozen, canned fruit |
| Low-fat or fat-free dairy foods | 2<br>1–2 year olds should have whole milk<br>500 mg calcium/day | 2<br>800 mg calcium/d | 3<br>1,200–1500 mg calcium/d<br>9–18 years of age | 3 | 3 | 3–4 | 1 cup milk<br>1 cup yogurt<br>1½ oz cheese |
| Meat, poultry, fish, egg | 2 | 2 | 2 | 2 | 2 | 2–3 | 2–3 oz cooked meats, poultry, fish, 1 egg |
| Nuts, seeds, legumes | 2<br>a. 2 Tbsp cooked beans or peas<br>b. Only creamy peanut butter spread thinly on a cracker/ bread<br>c. Omit seeds and nuts | 2 | 3–4 | 4–5 | 1 | 1 | 1 Tbsp peanut butter<br>⅓ cup nuts<br>2 Tbsp seeds<br>½ cup cooked dry beans or peas |

*Because of the inconsistency in recommendations for calorie intake for young children among expert sources, the table focuses on the areas of agreement in terms of serving sizes and number of servings.

■ **TABLE 16-1**
■ ■ Number of Servings and Serving Sizes for Age and Total Daily Calorie Intake—cont'd

| Food Groups | 1–3 years old* Servings | 4–6 years old* Servings | 6–21 years old 1600 Servings | 2000 Servings | 2600 Servings | 3100 Servings | Serving Size 1600-3100 calorie diets |
|---|---|---|---|---|---|---|---|
| Fats, oils | Moderate use until 2 years of age (about 50% of total calories) | sparingly | 2 | 2–3 | 3 | 4 | 1 tsp soft margarine 1 Tbsp low-fat mayonnaise, salad dressing, vegetable oil |

American Academy of Pediatrics. (2004). *Pediatric nutrition handbook* (5th ed.). Elk Grove Village, IL: American Academy of Pediatrics.
Dietz, W.H., & Stern, L. (Eds.) (1999). *Guide to your child's nutrition.* New York: Villard.
U.S. Department of Health and Human Services and U.S. Department of Agriculture (HHS/USDA). (2005). *Dietary guidelines for Americans,* 2005. Retrieved October 20, 2005, from www.health.gov/dietaryguidelines/dga2005/document

■ **TABLE 16-2**
■ ■ Recommended Calories per Day Based on Gender, Age, and Level of Activity

| Gender | Age in years | Sedentary | Moderately Active | Active |
|---|---|---|---|---|
| Males | 2–3 | 1000 | 1000–1400 | 1000–1400 |
| | 4–8 | 1400 | 1400–1600 | 1600–2000 |
| | 9–13 | 1800 | 1800–2200 | 2000–2600 |
| | 14–18 | 2200 | 2400–2800 | 2800–3200 |
| | 19–30 | | 2600–2800 | 3000 |
| Females | 2–3 | 1000 | 1000–1400 | 1000–1400 |
| | 4–8 | 1200 | 1400–1600 | 1400–1800 |
| | 9–13 | 1600 | 1600–2000 | 1800–2200 |
| | 14–18 | 1800 | 2000 | 2400 |
| | 19–30 | 2000 | 2000–2200 | 2400 |

(b) Parents will not win because they cannot make toddlers eat
(c) Parents' job is to offer nutritious food choices
(d) Child must be in charge of determining his or her own intake
(e) Let child be involved in the cooking process—chopping, stirring, pouring—helps increase interest in food
v. Too much food on plate
(a) Overwhelms child
(b) Use small plates and utensils
vi. Too much fluid fills them up
(a) Offer maximum of 16 oz milk per day
(b) Offer maximum of 4 oz vitamin C fortified juice per day
vii. Consumes too many snack and/or "junk" foods in a day
h. Parental expectations about eating are too high (Garrow, 2004)

4. Preschoolers (ages 4 to 6 years) (AAP, 2004)
   a. Caloric needs—see Table 16–2 for caloric intake recommendations
   b. Servings—according to age and food groups (Table 16–1)
   c. Development
      i. Growth slowing down
      ii. More fully developed fine motor skills to handle utensils
      iii. Short attention span
      iv. Can sit at the table 15 to 20 minutes
      v. Psychosocial goal is development of individuation
   d. Unpredictable interest in eating
      i. Total daily energy intake usually fairly constant
      ii. Unable to choose a well-balanced diet; needs to be offered a variety of healthy foods
   e. Often resistant to new foods but should continue to be exposed to them
   f. May insist on eating only 4 or 5 favorite foods—this is a normal and temporary developmental issue for preschoolers
5. School-agers (ages 7 to 11 years) (AAP, 2004)
   a. Caloric needs—see Table 16–2 for caloric intake recommendations based on age and activity level
   b. Servings—see Table 16–1 for servings according to age, food groups, and caloric needs
   c. Development
      i. Cognitively able to understand nutrition concepts
      ii. Vary greatly in weight, height, growth velocity, body shape
      iii. Comparing themselves to peers
      iv. Begin to understand the concept of "dieting"
   d. Food choices
      i. Increased freedom over food choices
      ii. Parents should focus on helping school-agers to enjoy the *taste* of fruits and vegetables; school-agers perceive *healthfulness* and taste as opposites
      iii. Influenced by peers and others outside the family
      iv. Influenced by television
6. Adolescents (ages 12 to 21 years) (AAP, 2004)
   a. Caloric needs—see Table 16–1 for caloric intake recommendations based on age and activity level
   b. Servings—see Table 16–2 for servings according to age, food groups, and caloric needs
   c. Development
      i. Onset of puberty increases normal nutritional needs
      ii. Growth spurt increases normal nutritional needs
      iii. Levels of activity vary greatly, and alter caloric needs
      iv. Increased independence results in making most of own food choices
   d. National Health and Nutrition Examination Surveys between 1971 and 1991 showed that "of all age groups, adolescents had the highest prevalence of unsatisfactory nutritional status" (AAP, 2004, p. 151)
   e. Eating behaviors that increase during adolescence:
      i. Skip meals
      ii. Eat more meals outside home
      iii. Snack
      iv. Eat fast foods
      v. Fad diets

# REFERENCES

Ahluwalia,I.B.,Morrow,B.,Hsia,J.,Grummer-Strawn, L. M. (2003). Who is breast feeding? Recent trends from the pregnancy risk assessment and monitoring system. *J Pediatr, 142,* 486-491.

American Academy of Pediatric Dentistry. (2003). *Clinical guideline on fluoride therapy.* Chicago (IL): American Academy of Pediatric Dentistry.

American Academy of Pediatrics Committee on Drugs. (2001). The transfer of drugs and other chemicals into human milk. Policy statement. *Pediatrics, 108,* 776-789.

American Academy of Pediatrics Committee on Nutrition. (2000). Hypoallergenic infant formulas. Policy statement. *Pediatrics, 106,* 346-349.

American Academy of Pediatrics Committee on Nutrition. (2003). Prevention of pediatric overweight and obesity. Policy statement. *Pediatrics, 112,* 424-430.

American Academy of Pediatrics Committee on Nutrition. (2004). *Pediatric nutrition handbook* (5th ed.). Elk Grove Village, IL: American Academy of Pediatrics.

American Academy of Pediatrics Section on Breastfeeding. (2005). Breast feeding and the use of human milk. *Pediatrics, 115,* 496-506.

Anand, M. K., & Routes, J. M. (2004). Hypersensitivity reactions—immediate. Retrieved from eMedicine June 6, 2006, from www.emedicine.com/med/topic1101.htm.

Bauchner, H. (2004). Failure to thrive. In R. E. Behrman, R.M. Kliegman, & H.B. Jenson (Eds.), *Nelson textbook of pediatrics* (17th ed.) (pp. 133-134). Philadelphia: Saunders.

Brazelton, T.B. (2002). *Touch points. The essential reference.* Reading, MA: Addison-Wesley.

Butte, N., Cobb, K., Dwyer, J., Graney, L., Heird, W., & Rickard, K. (2004). The start healthy feeding guidelines for infants and toddlers *Journal of the American Dietetic Association, 104,* 442-54.

Centers for Disease Control and Prevention (2001). Recommendations for using fluoride to prevent and control dental caries in the US. *MMWR Recommendations and Reports, 50(RR-14),* 1-42.

Centers for Disease Control and Prevention. (2006). Overweight and obesity. Retrieved June 6, 2006, from www.cdc.gov/nccdphp/dnpa/obesity/index.htm.

Children Now. (2005). Brief: Interactive advertising and children: Issues and implications. Retrieved March 30, 2006, from http://www.childrennow.org/search.jsp?query=interactive+advertising.

Crespo, C. J., Smit, E., Troiano, et al. (2001). Television watching, energy intake, and obesity in U.S. children. *Arch Pediatr Adolesc Med, 155,* 360-365.

Dietz, W. H., & Stern, L. (Eds.). (1999). *Guide to your child's nutrition.* New York: Villard.

Donohoue, P. A. (2004). Obesity. In R. E. Behrman, R.M. Kliegman, & H.B. Jenson (Eds.), *Nelson textbook of pediatrics* (17th ed.). Philadelphia: Saunders, pp. 173-177.

Garrow, A. (2004). Coping patterns in mothers/caregivers of children with chronic feeding problems. *J Pediatr Health Care, 18*(3), 138-144.

Gartner, L.M., & Greer, F.R. (2003). Prevention of rickets and vitamin D deficiency: new guidelines for vitamin D intake. Clinical report. *Pediatrics, 111,* 908-910.

Gary, L., Miller, L.W., Phillip, B.L., Blass, E.M. (2002). Breastfeeding is analgesic in healthy newborns. *Pediatrics, 109,* 590-593.

Hansen, T. W. R. (2002). Jaundice, neonatal. Retrieved from eMedicine May 9, 2006, from www.emedicine.com/ped/topic1061.htm.

Heird, W. C. (2004a). Food insecurity, hunger and undernutrition In R. E. Behrman, R.M. Kliegman, & H.B. Jenson (Eds.), *Nelson textbook of pediatrics* (17th ed.). Philadelphia: Saunders, pp. 167-173.

Heird, W. C. (2004b). The feeding of infants and children. In R. E. Behrman, R.M. Kliegman, & H.B. Jenson (Eds.), *Nelson textbook of pediatrics* (17th ed.). Philadelphia: Saunders, pp. 157-167.

Host, A. & Halken, S. (2004). Hypoallergenic formulas—when, to whom and how long: after more than 15 years we know the right indication! *Allergy, 78,* 45-52.

Kennedy, C., Strzempko, F., Danford, C., & Kools, S. (2002). Children's perceptions of TV and health behavior. *J Nurs Schol, 34*(3), 297-302.

Merritt, R. J. & Jenks, B. H. (2004). Safety of soy based infant formulas containing isoflavens: the clinical evidence. *Journal of Nutrition, 134,* 1220S-1224S.

Moilanen, B. C. (2004). Vegan diets in infants, children, and adolescents. *Pediatrics in Review, 25,* 174-176.

Morrow, A. L. (2004). Choosing an infant or pediatric formula. *Journal of Pediatric Health Care.* 18, 49-52.

National Association of Pediatric Nurse Practitioners (NAPNAP). (2001). Position statement on breastfeeding. Retrieved on March 30, 2006 at http://www.napnap. org/index.cfm?page=10&sec=54&ssec=57

National Association of Pediatric Nurse Practitioners (NAPNAP). (2006). Identifying and preventing overweight in childhood: Clinical practice guideline. *Journal of Pediatric Health Care, 20*(2), S1-S63.

National Association of Pediatric Nurse Practitioners (NAPNAP). (2005). *Starting Solids: Nutrition guide for infants and children 6 to 18 months of age* (brochure). Cherry Hill, NJ: NAPNAP.

National Center for Health Statistics. (2005). Prevalence of overweight among children and adolescents: United States, 1999 - 2002. Retrieved on March 30, 2006 from http://www.cdc.gov/nchs/products/ pubs/pubd/hestats/overwght99.htm.

Osborn, D. A. & Sinn, J. (2004). Soy formula for prevention of allergy and food intolerance in infants. *Cochraine Database of Systematic Reviews: CD003741.*

Sampson, H. A., & Leung, D.Y.M. (2004). Adverse reactions to foods. In R. E. Behrman, R.M. Kliegman, & H. B. Jenson (Eds.), *Nelson textbook of pediatrics* (17th ed.) (pp. 789-792). Philadelphia: Saunders.

Tuohy, P. G. (2003). Soy infant formula and phytoestrogens. *Journal of Paediatric Child Health, 39,* 401-405.

U.S. Department Health & Human Services (HHS) Public Health Service, Office of Assistant Secretary for Health. (2000). *Healthy People 2010: Conference Edition.* Washington, D.C.: HHS.

U.S. Department of Health and Human Services and U.S. Department of Agriculture. (2005). *Dietary guidelines for Americans, 2005* (6th ed.). Washington, D. C.: U.S. Government Printing Office.

# Preconceptional and Prenatal Role of the PNP

MARY MARGARET GOTTESMAN, PhD, RN, CPNP, FAAN

## PRECONCEPTIONAL CARE

1. A teachable moment
   a. The preconceptional period lays the foundation for each child's health (Barash & Weinstein, 2002; Brundage, 2002; de Weerd, et al., 2002)
   b. Health encounters with adolescents and young adults are opportunities to ensure that their future children begin life with the best health possible (Hobbins, 2003; Moos, 2003; Muchowski & Paladine, 2003)
   c. Take this opportunity to identify and minimize risks
2. Identify and minimize risks
   a. Reproduction planning
      i. Encourage planned pregnancy
         (a) Consistent contraceptive use
         (b) Consistent condom use
         (c) Ideally, start prenatal vitamins before pregnancy
      ii. Assess relationship with sexual partner (McFarlane, et al., 2001; Saltzman, et al., 2003)
         (a) Coercion
         (b) Abuse
   b. Cardiovascular disease
      i. Anemia (Hindmarsh, et al., 2000)
         (a) Hemoglobin less than 11 mg/dL
         (b) Review diet, especially with vegans
         (c) Provide information on an iron-rich diet
         (d) Recommend additional iron and folate supplements, especially if on a daily multivitamin with iron already
      ii. Hypertension (Gabbe, et al., 2002; Korenbrot, et al., 2002)
         (a) Reinforce use of birth control and need to change medication prior to conception
         (b) At greater risk for preeclampsia, renal insufficiency, and fetal growth restriction
         (c) Methyldopa and calcium channel blockers are safer choices during pregnancy

        (d) Angiotensin-converting enzyme (ACE) inhibitors, angiotensin II receptor antagonists, and thiazide diuretics are associated with birth defects

    iii. Hyperlipidemia (Gabbe, et al., 2002)

        (a) Review low-fat, low-cholesterol diet recommendations

        (b) Evaluate safety of statins; reinforce use of birth control if Class D

**c.** Overweight (Lederman, et al., 2004; Watkins, et al., 2003)

    i. Evaluate overweight status; provide dietary counseling and advise increased physical activity for weight loss

    ii. BMI ≥30 kg/m$^2$ associated with increased risk for spina bifida, omphalocele, heart defects, and multiple anomalies

    iii. BMI 25 to 29.9 kg/m$^2$ associated with increased risk of heart defects and multiple anomalies

**d.** Metabolic, immune disorders (Sablock, et al., 2002)

    i. Diabetes mellitus (Gabbe, et al., 2002; Korenbrot, et al., 2002)

        (a) Advise to use birth control and plan pregnancy

        (b) Educate about self-monitoring, balance among diet, insulin/oral glycemics, and exercise

        (c) When desiring to become pregnant, advise of need to transition to insulin, if not already taking it, and the need for excellent glycemic control; advise insulin pump if not using currently

        (d) Advise of contraindications to pregnancy—blood urea nitrogen (BUN) greater than 30 mg/dL, creatinine clearance less than 30 mL/minute, coronary artery disease

        (e) Advise of risks to fetus from poorly controlled diabetes—congenital heart defects, congenital anomalies, fetal macrosomia

    ii. Thyroid disease (Gabbe et al., 2002)

        (a) Obtain thyroid-stimulating hormone (TSH) and T$_4$ levels, optimize thyroid replacement

        (b) Advise regarding dangers of both too little and too much thyroid hormone interfering with neuronal migration leading to abnormal function of the central nervous system

    iii. Phenylketonuria (Koch, et al., 2003; NIH, 2001; Widaman & Azen, 2003)

        (a) Lifelong metabolic control through dietary modifications benefits the individual in terms of cognitive performance and behavior

        (b) Advise regarding risks of uncontrolled phenylalanine levels to fetus including microcephaly, mental deficiency, and congenital heart defects

        (c) Encourage use of birth control and planned pregnancy

    iv. Kidney disease (Gabbe, et al., 2002)

        (a) Advise of complications with pregnancy for both the mother and fetus if BUN greater than 30 mg/dL, creatinine clearance less than 30 mL/minute, and/or serum creatinine greater than 1.5 mg/dL

        (b) Encourage use of birth control and planned pregnancy

        (c) If hypertensive, review medications for fetal teratogenicity and advise of need for change in therapy and excellent control prior to conception

    v. Asthma (Gabbe, et al., 2002)

        (a) Optimize control with comprehensive, written asthma care plan with stepped plan of care

        (b) The goal is to prevent maternal and fetal hypoxia through emphasis on preventive environmental and medical measures because many preventive medications are Class B, except for steroids, which are Class C

      (c) Potential problems during pregnancy for moderate and severe asthmatics include increased risk of preeclampsia, preterm delivery, and asthma exacerbations

      (d) Risks to the fetus include prematurity, low birth weight, hypoxia, hypoadrenalism, and increased risk of mortality

      (e) These effects are confounded by racial and lifestyle factors that are also associated with the risks listed above

  **vi.** Systemic lupus erythmatosus (SLE) (Gabbe, et al., 2002)

      (a) Encourage use of birth control and planned pregnancy after a 6-month remission period in symptoms

      (b) Review and advise patient regarding teratogenicity of medications, especially all NSAIDs, glucocorticoids, and methotrexate

      (c) Advise of potential dangers associated with pregnancy for the mother, especially renal failure, hypertension and eclampsia, and pulmonary hemorrhage or pneumonitis after delivery

      (d) Potential risks for the fetus include myocarditis, heart block, and congenital cardiac anomalies

  **vii.** Crohn's disease (Gabbe, et al., 2002)

      (a) Encourage use of birth control and planned pregnancy

      (b) Identify teratogenic medications and advise of need for change prior to pregnancy, especially mercaptopurine (Class D), and cyclosporine (Class C)

      (c) Optimize nutrition, 1 mg folate per day

  **viii.** Ulcerative colitis (Gabbe, et al., 2002)

      (a) Encourage use of birth control and planned pregnancy following a 6-month period of remission in symptoms

      (b) Identify teratogenic medications and advise of need for change prior to pregnancy

      (c) Optimize nutrition, 1 mg folate per day

**e.** Infectious disease (Brundage, 2002; Moos, 2003)

  **i.** Review all immunizations to ensure full immunity with particular attention to:

      (a) Rubella

      (b) Hepatitis B

      (c) Varicella

  **ii.** Screen sexually active males and females and treat for STIs (Brundage, 2002)

      (a) HIV/AIDS—if HIV positive, strongly recommend antiretroviral therapy during pregnancy to decrease the risk of transmission to the fetus (Peters, et al., 2003; AAP, 1999b; AAP, 2004a)

      (b) Syphilis—treat mother and all partners

      (c) Chlamydia—treat mother and all partners

  **iii.** Pneumococcal vaccine recommended before pregnancy for patients with functional and actual asplenia, e.g., sickle cell disease (Jackson & Vessey, 2004)

  **iv.** UTI (Brundage, 2002)

      (a) Emphasize need for preventive measures to avoid infection

      (b) Educate regarding need to complete treatment

**f.** Congenital disorders in the family history (AAP, 2004d)

  **i.** Refer for genetic counseling

**g.** Neurologic and mental disorders

  **i.** Seizure disorders (Korenbrot, et al., 2002)

(a) Optimize control with least teratogenic medications

(b) If at all possible, do not use multiple anticonvulsants and avoid use of carbamazepine, clonazepam, phenobarbital, phenytoin, primidone, and valproic acid

(c) Advise of increased risk for congenital anomalies, epilepsy in child

(d) Advise daily intake of 4 mg folate per day

   ii. Neural tube defect (Brent, et al, 2000; Chacko, et al., 2003)

(a) Advise of significantly increased risk of having a child with a neural tube defect

(b) Encourage use of birth control and planned pregnancy

(c) Recommend daily intake of 4 mg or more folate per day, ideally, before conception

   iii. Depression (Korenbrot, et al., 2002)

(a) Avoid use of benzodiazepines

(b) Maternal depression, anxiety, and emotional disorders associated with ADHD in children

**h.** Genetic disorders (AAP, 2004d)

   i. Referrals

(a) Refer to genetic counselor to ensure understanding of risks for fetus and potential treatments for the fetus and child

(b) Refer to perinatologist to review risks for mother and need for planned pregnancies and care as a high risk mother

   ii. Sickle cell—increased risk of hypertension, urinary tract and pulmonary infections with resulting trigger of crisis, pulmonary infarction (Gabbe, et al., 2002)

   iii. Thalassemias—increased risk of hypertension, urinary tract and pulmonary infections with resulting trigger of crisis, pulmonary infarction (Gabbe, et al., 2002)

   iv. Hemophilia

   v. Muscular dystrophy

   vi. Cystic fibrosis (CF)—in moderate and severe CF, increased risks to maternal health include respiratory decompensation, pulmonary hypertension, and preterm delivery (Gabbe, et al., 2002; Jackson & Vessey, 2004)

   vii. Tay-Sachs disease—carriers of Tay-Sachs defective gene may pass it on to a child; while most children with Tay-Sachs disease do not survive past age 6, a late onset Tay-Sachs disease has been observed in adults (National Human Genome Research Institute, 2006)

   viii. Down syndrome—increased risk of having a child with Down syndrome, advise contraceptive use and planned pregnancy, 4 to 6 mg folate per day; require more time and preparation for prenatal care experiences (AAP, 2001b)

   ix. Mental retardation—increased risk of having a child with mental retardation; advise contraceptive use and planned pregnancy, 4 to 6 mg folate per day; require more time and preparation for prenatal care experiences (Gabbe, et al., 2002)

   x. Marfan syndrome—autosomal dominant condition with high risk for perinatal aortic rupture; advise regarding adoption (AAP, 1996)

**i.** Medications contraindicated in pregnancy; advise of dangers to fetus and encourage use of birth control (Briggs, et al., 2002)

   i. Anticonvulsants

   ii. Isoretinoin (Accutane)

   iii. Herbal or macrobiotic supplements

   iv. ACE inhibitors
   v. Angiotensin II receptor antagonists
   vi. Thiazide diuretics
   vii. Benzodiazepines
   viii. Warfarin
j. Risk behaviors (AAP, 1998; AAP, 2001c; 2001e; Postlethwaite, 2003)
   i. Alcohol use (AAP, 2000b, 2001a; 2001e; Naimi et al., 2003; Rodier, 2004)
      (a) Address alcohol consumption during health visits; advise of legal consequences of underage drinking and dangers of drunk driving as well as riding with intoxicated drivers
      (b) Binge drinking is associated with increased risk of unplanned pregnancy
      (c) Advise all sexually active females of dangers to the fetus including mental retardation, growth retardation, malformations, and behavioral disorders; dose-related toxicity of alcohol for the fetus
      (d) Encourage use of birth control and planned pregnancy
      (e) Antabuse is a Class C medication
   ii. Illicit drug use (AAP, 1998; Rodier, 2004; Mone, et al., 2004)
      (a) Include discussion of illicit drug use in health visits
      (b) Advise sexually active females that cocaine and other illicit drugs are associated with increased risk for congenital anomalies
      (c) Recommend and refer to treatment programs to stop use
      (d) Encourage use of birth control and planned pregnancies
   iii. Tobacco chewing or smoking (AAP, 2001c; Maloni et al., 2003; NAPNAP, 2000; Yu et al., 2002)
      (a) Address tobacco use during health visits; advise of adverse effects and ease of becoming addicted
      (b) Advise of dangers to fetus and newborn—miscarriage, low birth weight, perinatal mortality, ADHD, and SIDS
      (c) Advise and support quitting smoking; nicotine patches, gum, and nicotine nasal sprays and inhalers are rated as Class D medications; bupropion is safe for use during pregnancy
3. Maximize healthy lifestyle behaviors
   a. Malnutrition is associated with increased risk for fetal loss, neonatal mortality, altered migration of neurons and inadequate myelination of the central nervous system, cardiovascular malformations, and predisposition to coronary disease (Mahajan, et al., 2004)
   b. Balanced diet emphasizing fruits, vegetables, and whole grains
      i. Daily intake of 1000 mg of calcium, generally three servings of calcium-rich foods per day
      ii. Folate intake of 400 mcg per day unless at increased risk for fetal defects; then increase to 4 mg per day
      iii. Adequate intake of iron-rich foods
      iv. Daily vitamin
      v. Identify pica habits and screen for toxin levels as indicated
      vi. Vegetarian/vegan diet—screen for deficiencies based on diet
      vii. Eating disorders
         (a) Refer for treatment
         (b) Optimize nutrition
      viii. Avoid excessive vitamin intake (Brundage, 2002)
         (a) Vitamin A no more than 3000 international units/day
         (b) Vitamin D no more than 4000 international units/day

    c. Dental health (AAP, 2003a; Champagne, et al., 2000; Jeffcoat, et al., 2001)
       i. Twice daily thorough brushing and flossing once per day
       ii. Use a toothpaste with fluoride approved by the ADA
       iii. Rinse mouth every night with an alcohol-free over-the-counter (OTC) mouth rinse with 0.05% sodium fluoride
       iv. Promptly treat dental caries
       v. Use chewing gums with xylitol rather than sugar
    d. Physically active lifestyle
       i. Advise 30 minutes of moderate daily exercise
       ii. Advise avoiding sedentary behavior or lifestyle
    e. Rest and sleep patterns
       i. Advise regular sleep habits and at least 8 hours of sleep nightly
       ii. Advise regarding teratogenicity if using hydroxyzine, benzodiazepines, flurazepam, and temazepam
       iii. Change to safer medications
       iv. When sleep problems persist, screen for mental health problems
       v. Refer to sleep medicine experts for persistent problems
    f. Psychosocial risks (AAP, 2003b; Gueorguieva, et al., 2003; Holzman, et al., 2001; Tiedje, 2003)
       i. Screen for extent of support network
       ii. Refer for counseling and support
       iii. Family violence
       iv. History of abuse, neglect—at risk to become an abusive or neglectful parent
       v. History of foster placement—at risk for poor parenting skills
       vi. Homelessness—at risk for abuse, survival sex, depression, substance abuse
    g. Minimize exposure to potentially hazardous environments and products that damage the central nervous and cardiovascular systems (Mone, et al., 2004; Rodier, 2004)
       i. Pets, especially cats—toxoplasmosis (Lopez, et al., 2000)
       ii. Radiation
       iii. Lead
       iv. Anesthetic gases
       v. Mercury
       vi. Pesticides, herbicides, fertilizers
       vii. Paint thinners and strippers, solvents
       viii. Polyvinyl chloride (PVC), polychlorinated biphenyl (PCB), polybrominated biphenyls (PBB)
       ix. Day care—cytomegalovirus (CMV), parvovirus B19
       x. Hot tubs

# PRENATAL CARE

1. Another teachable moment
    a. The prenatal period is a rich opportunity for parent support and education
    b. American Academy of Pediatrics supports the need for prenatal contact with expectant parents (AAP, 2001a)
2. Establish a professional relationship (AAP, 2003b)
    a. Include partner or other significant support people and encourage their attendance at health visits

    **b.** Provide an overview of office hours, telephone consultation, fees, hospital affiliations, emergency care; coverage on nights, weekends, and holidays

    **c.** Home visit for mothers on home bed rest for high risk conditions

**3.** Gather basic information (AAP, 2004c)

    **a.** Family medical history

        **i.** Quality of the parents' relationship

        **ii.** Concerns regarding the pregnancy, especially if unplanned or unwanted

        **iii.** Fears regarding inherited or transmitted disorders, including HIV

        **iv.** Attitudes toward tobacco, alcohol, and drug use

        **v.** Plans for labor, delivery, and rooming-in

        **vi.** Relationship between the parents and grandparents

        **vii.** Reaction of family members to the pregnancy

    **b.** Childhood recollections of how the parents were parented

        **i.** Experience in caring for children

        **ii.** Resources for caring for the child

        **iii.** Infant feeding choice (AAP, 1997; NAPNAP, 2001)

            **(a)** Encourage choice of breast-feeding and recommend a prenatal class to increase success

            **(b)** Discourage breast-feeding by HIV-positive women (AAP, 2004a; 2004b)

        **iv.** Safe water source; testing of well water, need for boiling before use

        **v.** Car seat and car safety

        **vi.** Postpartum adjustment and feelings

        **vii.** Lifestyle changes and expectations

        **viii.** Important cultural beliefs, values, and traditions about which the practitioner should be aware

        **ix.** Extent of support network

        **x.** Plans for employment, further education for parents, and child care

        **xi.** Sources of stress and instability—employment, housing, sibling relationships, discord between partners

    **c.** Parent education and support prior to delivery (NAPNAP, 2003)

        **i.** Describe newborn's appearance

        **ii.** Describe newborn's behavior immediately after birth and in the first 24 hours

        **iii.** Describe routine care provided directly after delivery and in the newborn nursery

        **iv.** Discuss the hospital visit by the pediatrician or PNP

        **v.** Advise regarding the timing of the first pediatric office visit after discharge

        **vi.** Address the advantages of breast-feeding; if appropriate, recommend a prenatal breast-feeding class

        **vii.** Describe the support available at the practice or the community for breast-feeding mothers (Li, et al., 2003)

        **viii.** Provide accurate and unbiased information about circumcision; address the performance of the procedure, benefits, and risks (AAP, 1999a)

        **ix.** Encourage participation in childbirth classes (Lu, et al., 2003)

    **d.** Parent skill building prior to delivery (NAPNAP, 2003)

        **i.** Discuss parents' plans and concerns regarding parenting

            **(a)** Discuss importance of the parent-child relationship

            **(b)** Identify important contributions of each partner to the child's development

        **ii.** Review home safety measures—burn and fall prevention, back-to-sleep, emergency numbers list by the phone (AAP, 2000a; Hauck, et al., 2003)

      iii. Review frequency and amount of infant feeding needs for breast-feeding or bottle-feeding as appropriate, hunger and satiation cues, burping

      iv. Review basic methods of coping with crying and reinforce that a prompt response cannot spoil the child; dangers of shaking babies

      v. Nighttime infant care and parent rest

      vi. Value of establishing daily care routines

      vii. Basic supplies and equipment

      viii. Conditions requiring a call to the pediatric office

   e. Identification and referral of parents with high risk circumstances

      i. Parents with a history of genetic or congenital abnormality (AAP, 2004d)

        (a) Refer to geneticist

        (b) Discuss abnormal results to assure parent understanding of potential risks and complications for the newborn

        (c) Assist with preparation for birth of a child with an abnormal condition

      ii. Single or teen parent (AAP, 2001a)

      iii. Relationship with own parents

        (a) Support from father of the baby

        (b) Experience of poor parenting

        (c) Plans for further education and care of child

        (d) Conflict with friends and family

        (e) Interest in parenting child

        (f) Knowledge of infant care and developmental needs

      iv. Parent history of substance abuse

      v. Parent history of abuse or neglect as a child

      vi. Current history of intimate partner violence

      vii. Parent history of mental retardation or mental illness

      viii. Inadequate basic resources

        (a) Refer to Women, Infants, and Children (WIC)—a special supplemental nutrition program

        (b) Temporary Assistance for Needy Families (TANF)

        (c) Shelters and housing assistance

        (d) Clothing resources

      ix. Lack of social support

        (a) Parent support group

        (b) Counseling

        (c) Assistance with developing network building skills

# REFERENCES

American Academy of Pediatrics (AAP). (1996). Health supervision for children with Marfan syndrome. *Pediatrics, 98*(5), 978-982.

American Academy of Pediatrics (AAP). (1997). Breastfeeding and the use of human milk. *Pediatrics, 100*(6), 1035-1039.

American Academy of Pediatrics (AAP). (1998). Tobacco, alcohol, and other drugs: The role of the pediatrician in prevention and management of substance abuse. *Pediatrics, 101*(1), 125-128.

American Academy of Pediatrics (AAP). (1999a). Circumcision policy statement. *Pediatrics, 103*(3), 686-693.

American Academy of Pediatrics (AAP). (1999b). Human immunodeficiency virus screening. *Pediatrics, 104*(5), 128.

American Academy of Pediatrics (AAP). (2000a). Changing concepts of sudden infant death syndrome: Implications for infant sleeping environment and sleep position. *Pediatrics, 105*(3), 358-361.

American Academy of Pediatrics (AAP). (2000b). Fetal alcohol syndrome. *Pediatrics, 106*(2), 358-361.

American Academy of Pediatrics (AAP). (2001a). Care of adolescent parents and their children. *Pediatrics, 10* (2), 429-434.

American Academy of Pediatrics (AAP). (2001b). Health supervision for children with Down syndrome. *Pediatrics, 107*(2), 442-449.

American Academy of Pediatrics (AAP). (2001c). Tobacco's toll: Implications for pediatricians. *Pediatrics, 10* (4), 794-798.

American Academy of Pediatrics (AAP). (2001d). The prenatal visit. *Pediatrics, 10* (6), 1456-1458.

American Academy of Pediatrics (AAP). (2001e). Alcohol use and abuse: A pediatric concern. *Pediatrics, 108* (1), 185-189.

American Academy of Pediatrics (AAP). (2003a). Oral health risk assessment timing and establishment of the dental home. *Pediatrics, 111* (3), 1113-1116.

American Academy of Pediatrics (AAP). (2003b). Family-centered care and the pediatrician's role. *Pediatrics, 112*(3), 691-696.

American Academy of Pediatrics (AAP). (2004a). Postexposure prophylaxis in children and adolescents for nonoccupational exposure to human immunodeficiency virus. *Pediatrics, 111*(6), 1475-1489.

American Academy of Pediatrics (AAP). (2004b). Human milk, breastfeeding, and transmission of human immunodeficiency virus type 1 in the United States. *Pediatrics, 112*(5), 1196-1205.

American Academy of Pediatrics (AAP). (2004c). Hospital stay for healthy term newborns. *Pediatrics, 113*(5), 1434-1436.

American Academy of Pediatrics (AAP). (2004d). Prenatal screening and diagnosis for pediatricians. *Pediatrics, 114*(3), 889-894.

Barash, J. H., & Weinstein, L. C. (2002). Preconception and prenatal care. *Primary Care, 29*(3), 519-542.

Brent, R., Oakley, G., & Mattis, D. (2000). The unnecessary epidemic of folic acid-preventable spina bifida and anencephaly. *Pediatrics, 106*(4), 825-827.

Briggs, G. G., Freeman, R. K., & Yaffee, S. J. (2002). *A reference guide to fetal and neonatal risk: Drugs in pregnancy and lactation* (6th ed.). Philadelphia: Lippincott Williams & Wilkins.

Brundage, S. C. (2002). Preconception health care. *Am Fam Phys, 65*, 2507-2514.

Chacko, M. R., Anding, R., Kozinetz, C. A., et al. (2003). Neural tube defects: Knowledge and preconceptional prevention practices in minority young women. *Pediatrics, 112*(3), 536-542.

Champagne, C. M., Madianos, P. N., Lieff, S., et al. (2000). Periodontal medicine: Emerging concepts in pregnancy outcomes. *J Intl Acad Periodontol, 2*, 9-11.

De Weerd, S., van der Bij, A. K., Cikot, R., et al. (2002). Preconception care: A screening tool for health assessment and risk detection. *Prevent Med, 34*, 505-511.

Gabbe, S.G., Niebyl, J. P., & Simpson, J. L. (Eds.). (2002). *Obstetrics: Normal and problem pregnancies.* (4th ed.) (Online). Philadelphia: Churchill Livingstone.

Gueorguieva, R. V., Sarkar, N. P., Carter, R. L., et al. (2003). A risk assessment screening test for very low birth weight. *Matern Child Nurs J , 7*(2), 127-136.

Hauck, F.R., Herman, S., Donovan, M., et al. (2003). Sleep environment and the risk of sudden infant death syndrome in an urban population: The Chicago infant mortality study. *Pediatrics, 111*(5), 1207-1214.

Hindmarsh, P. C., Geary, M. P., Rodeck, C. H., et al. (2000). Effects of early maternal iron stores on placental weight and structure. *Lancet, 356*(9231), 719-723.

Hobbins, D. (2003). Full circle: The evolution of preconception health promotion in America. *J Obstet Gynecol Neonatal Nurs, 32*(4), 516-522.

Holzman, C., Bullen, B., Fisher, R., et al. (2001). Pregnancy outcomes and community health: The POUCH study of preterm delivery. *Paediatr Perinatal Epidemiol, 15*(Suppl. 2), 136-158.

Jackson Allen, P. L., & Vessey, J. A. (5th ed.). *Primary care of the child with a chronic condition.* (5th ed.). St. Louis: Mosby.

Jeffcoat, M. K., Geurs, N. C., Reddy, M. S., et al. (2001). Periodontal infection and preterm birth: Results of a prospective study. *J Am Dental Assoc, 132*, 875-880.

Koch, R., Hanley, W., Levy, H., et al. (2003). The maternal phenylketonuria international study: 1984-2002. *Pediatrics, 112*(6), 1523-1135.

Korenbrot, C., Steinberg, A., Bender, C., & Newberry, S. (2002). Preconception care: A systematic review. *Matern Child Health J, 6*(2), 75-88.

Lederman, S.A., Akabas, S. R., Moore, B. J., et al. (2004). Summary of presentations at the conference on preventing childhood obesity, December 8, 2003. *Pediatrics, 14*(4), 1146-1173.

Li, R., Zhao, Z., Mokdad, A., Barker, L., & Grummer-Strawn, L. (2003). Prevalence of breastfeeding in the United States: The 2001 national immunization survey. *Pediatrics, 111*(5), 1198-1201.

Lopez, A., Dietz, V. J., Wilson, M., et al. (2000). Preventing congenital toxoplasmosis. *MMWR, 49,* 59-67.

Lu, M. C., Prentice, J., Yu, S. M., et al. (2003). Childbirth education classes: Sociodemographic disparities in attendance and the association of attendance with breastfeeding initiation. *Matern Child Health J, 7*(2), 87-93.

Mahajan, S. D., Singh, S., Shah, P., et al. (2004). Effect of maternal malnutrition and anemia on the endocrine regulation of fetal growth. *Endocr Res, 30*(2), 189-203.

Maloni, J. A., Albrecht, S. A., Kelly Thomas, K., et al. (2003). Implementing evidence-based practice: Reducing risk for low birth weight through pregnancy smoking cessation. *JOGNN, 32,* 676-682.

McFarlane, J., Parker, B., & Cross, B. (2001). *Abuse during pregnancy: A protocol for prevention and intervention.* (2nd ed.). White Plains, NY: March of Dimes Birth defects Foundation.

Mone, S. M., Gillman, M. W., Miller, T. L., et al. (2004). Effects of environmental exposures on the cardiovascular system: Prenatal period through adolescence. *Pediatrics, 113*(4), 1058-1069.

Moos, M. K. (2003). Preconceptional wellness as a routine objective for women's health care: An integrative strategy. *J Obstet Gynecol Neonatal Nurs, 32* (4), 550-556.

Muchowski, K., & Paladine, H. (2003). Importance of preconception counseling. *Am Fam Phys, 67*(4), 701-702.

Naimi, T. S., Lipscomb, L. E., Brewer, R. D., & Gilbert, B. C. (2003). Binge drinking in the preconception period and the risk of unintended pregnancies: Implications for women and their children. *Pediatrics, 111*(5), 1136-1141.

National Association of Pediatric Nurse Practitioners (NAPNAP). (2000). Position statement on prevention of tobacco use in the pediatric population. *J Pediatr Health Care, 14*(3), 29A-30A.

National Association of Pediatric Nurse Practitioners (NAPNAP). (2001). Position statement on breastfeeding. *J Pediatr Health Care, 15*(5), 22A.

National Association of Pediatric Nurse Practitioners (NAPNAP). (2003). Position statement on the PNP's role in supporting infant and family well-being during the first year of life. *J Pediatr Health Care, 17*(3), 19A-20A.

National Institutes of Health (NIH) (2001). National Institutes of Health consensus development conference statement: Phenylketonuria: Screening and management, October 16-18, 2000. *Pediatrics, 108* (4), 972-982.

National Human Genome Research Insititute. (2006). Learning about Tay-Sachs disease. Retrieved on May 9, 2006 at http://www.genome.gov/10001220.

Peters, V., Liu, K-L., Dominquez, K. et al. (2003). Missed opportunities for perinatal HIV prevention among HIV-exposed infants born 1996-2000, pediatric spectrum of HIV disease cohort. *Pediatrics, 111*(5), 1186-1191.

Postlethwaite, D. (2003). Preconception health counseling for women exposed to teratogens: The role of the nurse. *J Obstet Gynecol Neonatal Nurs, 32*(4), 523-532.

Rodier, P. M. (2004). Environmental causes of central nervous system maldevelopment. *Pediatrics, 113*(94), 1076-1083.

Sablock, U., Lindow, S. W., Arnott, P. I. E., & Masson, E. A. (2002). Prepregnancy counseling for women with medical disorders. *J Obstet Gynecol, 202*(6), 637-638.

Saltzman, L. E., Johnson, C. H., Gilbert, B.C., & Goodwin, M. M. (2003). Physical abuse around the time of pregnancy: An examination of prevalence and risk factors in 16 states. *Matern Child Health J, 7*(1), 31-42.

Tiedje, L. B. (2003). Psychosocial pathways to prematurity: Changing our thinking toward a lifecourse and community approach. *J Obstet Gynecol Neonatal Nurs, 32*(5), 650-658.

Watkins, M. L., Rasmussen, S. A., Honein, M. A., et al. (2003). Maternal obesity and risk for birth defects. *Pediatrics, 111*(5), 1152-1158.

Widaman, K. F., & Azen, C. (2003). Relation of prenatal phenylalanine exposure to infant and childhood cognitive outcomes: Results from international maternal PKU collaborative study. *Pediatrics, 112*(6), 1537-1543.

Yu, S. M., Park, C. H., & Schwalberg, R. H. (2002). Factors associated with smoking cessation among US pregnant women. *Matern Child Health J, 6,* 89-96.

**CHAPTER**

# 18

■ ■ ■

# Care of the Newborn Before Hospital Discharge

VALERIE MARBURGER, MS, RN, CPNP, NNP

Some PNPs specialize in newborn care. Within that role, they are present at deliveries to manage the newborn and conduct physical examinations immediately upon delivery, within the first few hours, and upon discharge. The PNP assures that appropriate preventive care and referrals are made and that the infant and mother are both ready to be discharged to home.

1. Assessment of the newborn immediately upon delivery (Tapero & Honeyfield, 2003; Thureen, et al., 2005)
   a. The Apgar score (AAP, 1996; Dubick, 2001)
      i. The Apgar was described by Dr. Virginia Apgar in 1952
      ii. A mnemonic for assessing the newborn at birth; includes five parameters as shown in Table 18-1
      iii. Each parameter is assigned a score of 0, 1, or 2
      iv. Total score can range from 0 to10
      v. All newborns are evaluated at 1 and 5 minutes
      vi. If score is less than 7 at 5 minutes, then reevaluate the Apgar at 10 and 15 minutes
      vii. By itself, a low Apgar score is *not* a good indicator of neurologic outcome
      viii. Concern for neurologic injury is indicated and close developmental follow-up warranted if all of following are present:
         (a) The Apgar score was 0 to 3 for more than 5 minutes
         (b) Profound metabolic acidosis
         (c) Neurologic dysfunction
         (d) Multisystem organ dysfunction
2. Resuscitation
   a. The Neonatal Resuscitation Program (NRP) was developed in 1987 as a collaborative effort of the American Academy of Pediatrics (AAP) and the American Heart Association (AHA) (AAP, 2005) to standardize delivery room stabilization of the newborn
   b. The NRP program is evidence based and recommends:
      i. At every delivery there should be a person who:
         (a) Has the primary responsibility for the infant
         (b) Is capable of initiating a resuscitation

■ **TABLE 18-1**
■ ■ **Components of the Apgar Score**

| | Sign | 0 Points | 1 Point | 2 Points |
|---|---|---|---|---|
| A | Activity (muscle tone) | Limp | Some flexion of extremities | Active motion |
| P | Pulse (heart rate) | Absent | <100 | >100 |
| G | Grimace (reflex irritability) | No response | Grimace | Sneeze, cough, pulls away |
| A | Appearance (skin color) | Blue, pale | Body pink, extremities blue | Completely pink |
| R | Respiration | Absent | Slow, irregular | Good, crying |

    ii. Either that person or someone else immediately available should have the skills required to:
      (a) Perform a complete resuscitation
      (b) Perform endotracheal intubation
      (c) Administer medications
   c. A PNP can obtain the additional NRP training to serve this function
3. Thermoregulation
   a. It is critical to monitor the newborn's temperature and the environmental temperature
   b. At birth infants can lose up to 1° F of body heat per minute
   c. This could predispose them to cold stress if precautions are not taken
   d. Cold stress signs
     i. Cold feet, followed by cold all over body
     ii. Decreased activity, poor suck, weak cry
     iii. Severe hypothermia
       (a) Face and extremities become bright red; slow, shallow breathing; slow heart rate
       (b) Hypoglycemia, metabolic acidosis, generalized internal bleeding, and respiratory distress
   e. The four principles of heat transference to and from the newborn's body and interventions to decrease heat loss are described in Table 18-2 (Blackburn, 2003)

■ **TABLE 18-2**
■ ■ **Principles of Heat Transference and Application to the Newborn**

| Principle | Definition | Prevention of Heat Loss |
|---|---|---|
| Conduction | Transfer of heat from the body to objects in contact with the body | Protect surfaces with warmed blankets |
| Convection | Heat is lost from the interior of the body to the surrounding air, and carried away by drafts | Warm inspired oxygen<br>Increase air temperature and decrease air currents<br>Swaddle and place cap on head |
| Evaporation | Moisture on the body surface vaporizes into surrounding air | Dry the infant immediately after birth<br>Use warmed, humidified air in Isolette |
| Radiation | Transfer of heat from the body surface to cooler surfaces *not* in contact with the infant | Keep infants away from exterior walls and windows |

    **f.** Gestational age (GA) plays an important role in heat production (Blackburn, 2003)

        **i.** Appropriate for GA and large for GA infants are born with brown fat stores

        **ii.** Brown fat able to dissipate as much as 100% of their stored energy for heat production

        **iii.** Small for GA and premature infants have not accumulated the brown fat stores and are at greater risk for hypothermia

        **iv.** Other infants at risk for hypothermia include:

            (a) Resuscitated newborns (hypoxic)

            (b) Hypoglycemic newborns

**4.** Brief physical examination in delivery room

    **a.** See Box 18-1 for "red flags" that signal need for intervention, assistance, and/or immediate referral to appropriate specialist

    **b.** Vital signs: normal ranges

        **i.** Heart rate 120 to 160 beats/minute

        **ii.** Respiratory rate 30 to 60 breaths/minute

        **iii.** Temperature 36.5° to 36.5° C (97.7° to 99.5° F)

        **iv.** Blood pressure not usually examined in the delivery room

    **c.** Inspect

        **i.** Respiratory effort

        **ii.** Color

        **iii.** Skin

        **iv.** Facial features

        **v.** Chest

        **vi.** Abdomen

        **vii.** Cord vessels—two arteries, one vein

        **viii.** Genitalia

        **ix.** Extremities

            (a) Tone and equality of movement

            (b) Count and spread of fingers and toes

        **x.** Spine—intact, no evidence of myelomeningocele

---

■ **BOX 18-1**
■ **RED FLAGS THAT SIGNAL NEED FOR REFERRAL TO SPECIALIST IMMEDIATELY AFTER DELIVERY**

- Respiratory distress
  - Grunting
  - Retractions
  - Flaring
  - Unequal breath sounds
- Cardiac
  - Pale or blue color
  - Capillary refill time >3 seconds
  - Greater than Grade II murmur
  - Shifted apical pulse
- Abdomen
  - Omphalocele
  - Scaphoid abdomen
  - Spine
  - Meningomyelocele
- More than three dysmorphic features

       **xi.** Void—many infants void as they are being delivered or soon after

       **xii.** Passage of meconium

  **d.** Auscultate

      **i.** Lungs

      **ii.** Heart

**5.** Vitamin K administration

  **a.** Vitamin K is given to all newborns to prevent hemorrhagic disease of the new-born (HDN), or more specifically, vitamin K deficiency bleeding (VKDB) (AAP, 2003; St. John, 2005)

  **b.** HDN occurs in 0.25% to 1.7% of infants, depending on prevalence of breast-feeding

  **c.** Etiology—vitamin K deficiency in breast milk (commercial formulas contain vitamin K; therefore, this is a disease almost exclusively of breast-fed infants)

  **d.** Classic HDN occurs 2 to 7 days after birth in breast-fed infants

      **i.** Generalized bleeding from:

         (a) Skin

         (b) Umbilicus

         (c) Circumcision site

         (d) Gastrointestinal tract

         (e) Other internal organs

      **ii.** Late-onset HDN

         (a) 2 to 12 weeks of age

         (b) Intracranial bleeding

  **e.** Risk factors for HDN

      **i.** Maternal anticonvulsant or anticoagulant therapy (occurs within first 24 hours)

      **ii.** Breast-feeding

      **iii.** Birth asphyxia

      **iv.** Prolonged labor

  **f.** Prevention of HDN

      **i.** Vitamin K injection (intramuscular) of 0.5 to 1 mg at birth

      **ii.** No evidence that the administration of vitamin K at birth increases the risk of childhood leukemia

**6.** Eye prophylaxis

  **a.** To prevent neonatal gonorrheal bacterial conjunctivitis and potential sequelae, newborns are routinely treated after birth with one of the following single-dose products:

      **i.** 1% silver nitrate drops

      **ii.** 0.5% erythromycin ointment

      **iii.** 1% tetracycline ointment

  **b.** Clinical trial (National Eye Institute, 1999)

      **i.** Showed that later development of eye infections was from external sources, not maternal, and that prophylaxis did not prevent them

      **ii.** Mothers who have tested negative for sexually transmitted diseases may choose to decline the administration of eye prophylaxis

**7.** Periods of reactivity shortly after birth

  **a.** Periods of awake and asleep are critical for the new infant's physical and social development

  **b.** First period

      **i.** Begins at birth to about 30 minutes after birth

      **ii.** Ideal time for mother and infant to get acquainted and for infant to begin to suckle at the breast

      **iii.** Characteristics of the infant

(a) Awake and alert

(b) Interested in feeding

(c) Respirations elevated 60 to 80 breaths per minute

(d) Heart rate elevated 160 to 180 beats per minute

c. Period of sleep lasts about 2 to 4 hours

   i. Deep sleep

   ii. Heart rate and respiratory rate within normal newborn range

   iii. Temperature may be slightly lower than normal

d. Second period of reactivity lasts about 4 to 6 hours

   i. Infant awake

   ii. Interested in feeding

   iii. May pass meconium stool

   iv. Heart rate and respiratory rate increase

   v. Increased secretions

   vi. May have periods of apnea

8. Glucose monitoring in the term or near-term well infant (Noerr, 2001)

  a. Glucose is vital for neonatal brain metabolism

    i. The nadir of blood glucose level is between 1 and 2 hours after birth

    ii. Normal glucose levels in the first 24 hours are between 30 and 50 mg/dL

    iii. Normal glucose levels after the first 24 hours are 45 to 60 mg/dL

    iv. Plasma glucose level of less than 30 mg/dL in the first 24 hours of life and less than 45 mg/dL thereafter constitutes hypoglycemia in the newborn (Cranmer & Shannon, 2005)

  b. Symptoms of hypoglycemia

    i. May be asymptomatic

    ii. Poor feeding, hypotonia, jitteriness, apneic spells, tachypnea, or seizures

    iii. These symptoms may also occur in newborns who have been asphyxiated, have sepsis or hypocalcemia, or are experiencing drug withdrawal

  c. Term infants most at risk for hypoglycemia are those with:

    i. Inadequate glucose production

      (a) Large for gestational age

      (b) Intrauterine growth restricted

      (c) Postmature

      (d) Cold stress

      (e) Perinatal stress (asphyxia, hypoxia)

      (f) Polycythemia

      (g) Inborn errors of metabolism

    ii. Increased glucose use

      (a) Infant of insulin-dependent diabetic mother

      (b) Maternal propranolol therapy

      (c) Rh incompatibility

    iii. Abnormal endocrine regulation of glucose metabolism

      (a) Adrenal insufficiency

      (b) Hypothyroidism

      (c) Panhypopituitarism

    iv. Idiopathic hypoglycemia

      (a) Delayed initial feeding

      (b) Local and regional maternal anesthesia

  d. Glucose thresholds are anywhere from 30 to 50 mg/dL

  e. Treatment

    i. Establish early regular breast-feeding (minimum of five feeds in the first 24 hours)

        ii. Offer glucose or sucrose with bottle or eyedropper if mother is unable to breast-feed

        iii. Any infant with a glucose level less than 25 mg/dL needs IV of 100 mg dextrose infusion/kg

        iv. Pancreatectomy if hypoglycemia cannot be controlled with medical therapy

9. Detailed physical assessment

    a. After the newborn is stabilized and has spent awake and alert time with mother, it is important for a thorough physical assessment to be done

    b. Inspect, auscultate, percuss, and/or palpate for symmetry, normal findings, normal variations, and congenital anomalies

        i. Lungs

           (a) Respiratory effort

           (b) Equal breath sounds

           (c) Equal chest movement

           (d) May auscultate coarse crackles for the first hour or two

        ii. Heart

           (a) Apical pulse easily auscultated with a regular rate and rhythm

           (b) Auscultate for murmurs

           (c) Note the point of maximum intensity (PMI)

        iii. Color

           (a) Know variations of normal and abnormal color within different racial groups

           (b) Acrocyanosis—blue-tinged hands and/or feet

           (c) Pallor

           (d) Jaundice

        iv. Skin

           (a) Hyperbilirubinemia practice guideline (AAP, 2004)

              (1) Promote and support successful breast-feeding

              (2) Measure the total serum bilirubin (TSB) or transcutaneous bilirubin (TcB) level in infants jaundiced in the first 24 hours

              (3) Recognize that visual estimation of the degree of jaundice can lead to errors, particularly in darkly pigmented infants

              (4) Interpret all bilirubin levels according to the infant's age in hours

              (5) Recognize that infants at less than 38 weeks of gestation, particularly those who are breast-fed, are at higher risk of developing hyperbilirubinemia and require closer surveillance and monitoring

              (6) Perform a systematic assessment on all infants before discharge for the risk of severe hyperbilirubinemia

              (7) Provide parents with written and verbal information about newborn jaundice

              (8) Provide appropriate follow-up based on the time of discharge and the risk assessment

              (9) Treat newborns, when indicated, with phototherapy or exchange transfusion

           (b) Erythema toxicum—benign, self-limited, asymptomatic skin condition that occurs only during the neonatal period in about 48% of newborns (Yan, 2002)

              (1) Small, sterile, erythematous papules, vesicles, and, occasionally, pustules

              (2) Surrounded by a distinctive diffuse, blotchy, erythematous halo

              (3) Transitory lesions—disappear in one area and appear elsewhere

(c) Milia—common, benign, tiny epidermoid cysts on facial skin of newborns (Cooper & Ratnavel, 2005)
(d) Mongolian spots—smooth, bluish gray, deep brown, or black macular patches
   (1) Primarily on back and buttocks of newborns of Asian, Indian, or African descent
   (2) Most fade by age 4 years, but may last into adulthood
**v.** Head and neck
 (a) Scalp
   (1) Abundance of hair
   (2) Hair whorls
   (3) Lesions
 (b) Caput succedaneum (Fuloria & Kreiter, 2002a)
   (1) Accumulation of blood or serum above the periosteum
   (2) Poorly demarcated soft tissue swelling that crosses suture lines
   (3) Pitting edema and overlying petechiae, ecchymoses, and purpura
   (4) No treatment required; usually resolves within days
 (c) Cephalhematoma (Fuloria & Kreiter, 2002a)
   (1) Rupture of blood vessels that traverse skull to periosteum
   (2) Well-demarcated swelling that does not cross suture lines
   (3) No skin discoloration
   (4) No treatment if uncomplicated
   (5) Potential complications: skull fracture, intracranial hemorrhage, hyperbilirubinemia
   (6) Usually reabsorb in 2 weeks to 3 months
 (d) Craniostosis—also called craniosynostosis; premature closure of the sutures of the skull
 (e) Fontanelles
   (1) Anterior—diamond shaped, top of head
   (2) Posterior—triangular, lower back of head; may be closed at birth
 (f) Neck
   (1) Range of motion
   (2) Cysts
   (3) Sinuses
**vi.** Eyes
 (a) Eyelids and orbits
 (b) External structures of the eyes
 (c) Motility
 (d) Eye muscle balance
 (e) Pupils—constrict and dilate appropriately
 (f) All infants should have an examination of the red reflex (AAP, 2002)
   (1) Darkened room
   (2) Infant's eyes open, best if opens naturally
   (3) Direct ophthalmoscopic exam 12 to 18 inches away from infant's eyes
   (4) Negative or normal when the reflections of the two eyes are symmetrical and red in color
 (g) If the following observations are made, refer infant to pediatric ophthalmologist
   (1) Dark spots in red reflex
   (2) Blunted red reflex on one side
   (3) No red reflex
   (4) Opacities or white spots (leukoma) within the area of the red reflex

    **vii.** Ears
        (a) Size
        (b) Shape
        (c) Position—normal: top of ears parallel with eyes
        (d) Inspect for:
            (1) Sinuses
            (2) Pits
            (3) Skin tags
            (4) Auditory canal
   **viii.** Nose—inspect for patency of nasal passages
    **ix.** Umbilical cord
        (a) At birth
            (1) Two arteries and one vein
            (2) If only one artery, test for renal anomalies and hearing defects
        (b) Outside the delivery room (Donlon & Furdon, 2002)
            (1) Evidence of drying begins at the cut edge
            (2) Odor may indicate infection
            (3) Inspect the base for erythema and warmth
            (4) Observe for drainage
                a) Clear fluid—could indicate a patent urachus (a canal connecting the fetal bladder with the allantois, a membranous sac that contributes to the formation of the umbilical cord)
                b) Purulent drainage—could indicate an infected urachal cyst or abscess
                c) Bilious or fecal drainage—could indicate a patent omphalomesenteric duct
        (c) Umbilical cord separation usually does not occur until 1 to 2 weeks of age
     **x.** Abdomen
        (a) Palpate for liver, spleen, kidneys
    **xi.** Genitalia
        (a) One of the first questions asked upon delivery is, "Is it a girl or boy?"
        (b) See Box 18-2 for characteristics of:
            (1) Apparent male
            (2) Apparent female
            (3) Indeterminate gender

---

■ **BOX 18-2**
■ **CRITERIA FOR DETERMINING SEX OF NEWBORN**

**APPARENT MALE**
- Bilateral nonpalpable testes in a full-term infant
- Hypospadias associated with separation of the scrotal sacs
- Undescended testis with hypospadias

**APPARENT FEMALE**
- Clitoral hypertrophy of any degree
- Foreshortened vulva with single opening
- Inguinal hernia containing a gonad

**INDETERMINATE**
- Ambiguous genitalia

(c) If gender is not readily apparent, immediate referral to a pediatrician or other specialist is essential to identify the genetic gender of the infant

(d) Ambiguous genitalia (AAP, 2000)

(1) "...a true social and medical emergency" (Hutcheson & Snyder, 2004, Section 2)

(2) Two primary causes

a) Congenital adrenal hyperplasia, which leads to salt-wasting nephropathy, hypotension, vascular collapse, and death

b) Mixed gonadal dysgenesis

(3) Each infant requires individual consideration based on physical examination, laboratory studies, and discussions with the parents

(4) Parents should be encouraged to not name the child or register the birth, if possible, until the sex is established and the parents have determined whether they want to rear the child as male or female

(e) Check for scrotal and inguinal masses (Benjamin, 2002)

xii. Anus

(a) Patent

(b) Fissure

(c) Skin tags

xiii. Trunk and spine

(a) Inspect for pilonidal sinus tracts, dimples, hair tufts, or areas suggestive of a meningocele

(b) Palpate spinal column

xiv. Hips (AAP, 2000)

(a) Developmental dysplasia of the hip (DDH) is the condition in which the femoral head has an abnormal relationship to the acetabulum

(b) Types of DDH include:

(1) Frank dislocation (luxation)

(2) Partial dislocation (subluxation)

(3) Instability

a) The femoral head comes in and out of the socket

b) Radiographic abnormalities of the acetabulum

(c) Hip examination (see Chapter 12)

(d) Risk factors for DDH

(1) Oligohydramnios

(2) Breech position (23%)

(3) First-degree family member with DDH

(4) Recommendations related to risk factors

a) Perform routine DDH physical exams

b) Positive family history of DDH: perform routine DDH physical exams

c) Breech presentation

i) Perform routine DDH physical exams

ii) Even with a negative physical exam obtain either:

*a)* An ultrasound examination at 6 weeks of age (a normal ultrasound does not eliminate the possibility of acetabular dysplasia)

*b)* Radiograph of the pelvis and hips at 4 to 6 months of age

(e) Early detection and treatment are essential

(1) All newborns need to be screened for DDH by physical examination

       (2) AAP recommendations for management of DDH (AAP, 2000)

          a) If a positive Ortolani or Barlow is found in the newborn or at the 2-week visit, the infant should be referred to an orthopedist

            i) Do not ultrasound

            ii) Do not obtain x-rays

            iii) Do not triple diaper

          b) If the results of the physical examination at birth are "equivocal" then repeat exam in 2 weeks

          c) If at the 2-week repeat exam the Ortolani and Barlow are negative but equivocal signs still exist:

            i) Refer to orthopedist

            ii) Obtain a real-time ultrasound at 3 to 4 weeks of age

  xv. Extremities

    (a) Muscle tone—holds limbs in anatomic position versus floppy

    (b) Syndactyly—fusion of digits

    (c) Polydactyly—extra digit

    (d) Amniotic band constricting blood flow into digit

    (e) Feet, toes (Gore & Spencer, 2004) (see Chapter 12)

       (1) Common newborn foot abnormalities include:

          a) Metatarsus adductus

          b) Clubfoot deformity

          c) Calcaneovalgus (flexible flatfoot)

          d) Congenital vertical talus (rigid flatfoot)

       (2) Most treatments are conservative, including observation, stretching, and splinting

       (3) Surgical correction should be referred to a specialist

       (4) Surgery not usually done for 6 to 9 months so that the child will better tolerate anesthesia

  xvi. Neurologic status

    (a) Note pitch of cry for abnormalities

    (b) Reflexes—absence of normal reflexes is a red flag for neurologic problems

       (1) Moro—startle reflex in response to loud noise, sensation of "falling"; hyperextends head, arms fly out, fingers spread, then arms move inward

       (2) Sucking—sucking occurs in response to examiner's finger touching roof of mouth

       (3) Rooting—stroking the cheek or corner of mouth causes infant to move head in same direction and open mouth

       (4) Palmar and plantar grasp—pressure on palm of infant's hand or area below toes of foot causes fingers to close or toes to curl inward

       (5) Tonic neck—when infant's head is turned to one side, the arm on that side stretches out and the opposite arm bends up at the elbow, like "fencing"

       (6) Stepping—infant lifts feet as if walking when held upright with feet on flat surface

       (7) Placing—when dorsal (back) side of the hand or foot is placed on the edge of a surface, such as a table, the infant will lift the extremity and place it on the flat surface

       (8) Babinski—when sole of foot is stroked, toes fan out

10. Newborn hearing screening
    a. American Academy of Pediatrics Joint Committee on Infant Hearing (2000) Position Statement recommends hearing screening for all newborns before discharge from hospital
    b. Objective physiologic measures must be used to detect unilateral or bilateral hearing loss of various severities, either:
       i. Otoacoustic emissions—either transient evoked or distortion product
       ii. Brainstem auditory–evoked response hearing test
11. Behavioral states (Young-Wardell & Fuchs, 2004)
    a. Parents should be informed about infant behavioral states and their relevance to caregiving as described below
    b. Quiet sleep
       i. Respirations regular
       ii. Lack of body activity
       iii. Lack of facial or eye movements
       iv. Relevance to caregiving
          (a) Poor feeding effort
          (b) Good time for trimming infant's nails
    c. Active sleep
       i. Irregular respirations
       ii. More body activity
       iii. Movement of face and eyes
       iv. Relevance to caregiving
          (a) Poor feeding effort
          (b) Parents think infant is awakening, but is not
    d. Drowsy
       i. Irregular respirations
       ii. Variable activity
       iii. Eyes glazed, open and close slowly
       iv. Relevance to caregiving
          (a) Easy to awaken
          (b) If left alone, may return to sleep state
    e. Quiet alert
       i. Regular respirations
       ii. Minimal body activity
       iii. Eyes wide and bright, very attentive
       iv. Extremely attentive to environment
       v. Relevance to caregiving
          (a) Feeding effort maximal
          (b) Best opportunity to socially interact with infant
    f. Active alert
       i. Irregular respirations
       ii. Much body activity
       iii. Eyes open, not attentive
       iv. Sensitive to environment
       v. Relevance to caregiving
          (a) Infant eats well
          (b) Infant not as socially interactive
    g. Crying
       i. Irregular respirations
       ii. Facial grimacing
       iii. Color changes

        iv. Variable sensitivity to environment
           (a) Relevance to caregiving
              (1) Infant needs attention immediately

12. Circumcision (AAP, 1999; Cantu, 2004)
   a. Circumcision—removal of the prepuce that normally covers the glans of the penis
   b. AAP currently stipulates that no medical evidence exists to recommend routine neonatal circumcision (Cantu, 2004)
      i. Potential benefits and risks both exist, but the procedure is not necessary to a child's well-being
      ii. Therefore, parents should determine, through informed choice, whether circumcision is in the best interest of their child
   c. The PNP's responsibility is to provide accurate, unbiased information
      i. Provide an opportunity to discuss and ask questions
      ii. Potential benefits of circumcision
         (a) Consistent with some religious beliefs and rituals
         (b) Child's genital appearance will be consistent with that of family or social peer group
         (c) Lower risk of urinary tract infection (but absolute risk is less than 1% if uncircumcised) (Cantu, 2004)
         (d) Lower risk of penile cancer (but absolute risk is extremely low if uncircumcised) (Cantu, 2004)
         (e) Lower risk of sexually transmitted infections, particularly HIV (but behavioral factors are more significant than circumcision status) (Cantu, 2004)
      iii. Potential risks of circumcision
         (a) Bleeding
         (b) Infection
      iv. If circumcision is elected:
         (a) It should only be performed on stable, healthy infants
         (b) The infant should be given procedural analgesia

13. Breast-feeding (See also Chapter 16)
   a. Human milk is preferred feeding for all infants
   b. It is the mother's decision whether to directly breast-feed, use expressed breast milk in a bottle, or to formula-feed with a bottle
   c. American Academy of Pediatrics' (2005) policy statement gives the primary care provider recommendations related to breast-feeding
      i. Breast feeding should begin as soon as possible after birth, preferably in the delivery room
      ii. Newborns should nurse 8 to 12 times per day about 10 to 15 minutes at each breast
      iii. Newborns should not spend more than 4 hours without feeding
      iv. When direct breast-feeding not available, then give expressed breast milk
   d. Formal evaluation of breast-feeding progress
      i. First 72 hours includes:
         (a) Time of each breast-feeding
         (b) Duration
         (c) Voids
         (d) Stools
      ii. No supplements unless a medical need arises
      iii. Avoid pacifier use until breast-feeding is well established

        iv. If discharged before 48 hours, need follow-up with primary care provider when the newborn is 2 to 4 days old

        v. Evaluate for need for iron, vitamin D, and fluoride supplementation

**14.** Planning for discharge

    **a.** The primary care provider decides when to send the infant home based on a complete evaluation of the mother-infant dyad

    **b.** If the infant is to be discharged before 48 hours the AAP (2004) has minimum criteria it recommends the dyad meet:

        i. The perinatal experience was uncomplicated and a vaginal delivery

        ii. The infant was a singleton between 38 and 42 weeks and size appropriate for gestational age

        iii. Vital signs within normal limits for the previous 12 hours

        iv. Respiratory rate less than 60

        v. Heart rate 100 to 160

        vi. Temperature within normal limits depending on method of measurement

        vii. The infant has voided and stooled

        viii. The infant has completed two feedings without difficulty

        ix. Normal physical exam

        x. If circumcised, no bleeding for at least 2 hours

        xi. No jaundice in first 24 hours

        xii. The mother is prepared to care for her infant at home and the following instruction is documented:

            (a) Breast- or bottle-feeding

            (b) Cord, skin, and genital care

            (c) Aware of signs indicating need to call primary care provider

            (d) Infant safety

        xiii. Laboratory data have been reviewed for abnormalities and action taken

            (a) Mother's prenatal labs including STIs, hepatitis B, blood type, and infant's blood type if indicated

            (b) Hepatitis B vaccine has been administered or appointment to administer has been scheduled

        xiv. Primary care provider for the infant has been identified and appointment scheduled within the next 48 hours after discharge

        xv. Family, environmental, and social risk factors have been assessed

        xvi. Discharge home should be delayed for further investigation and intervention if any of the following are identified:

            (a) Drug, alcohol use and abuse

            (b) History of child abuse or neglect

            (c) Mental illness in a parent

            (d) Lack of social support

            (e) No fixed income

            (f) History of untreated domestic violence

            (g) Teen mother

**15.** Transportation of the discharged infant

    **a.** "All newborns discharged from hospitals should be transported home in car safety seats that meet Federal Motor Vehicle Standard (FMVSS) 213 and that are selected to meet the specific transportation needs of healthy newborns, premature infants, or infants with special health care needs" (AAP, 1999, p. 986)

    **b.** See Chapter 19 for details on car seats

    **c.** Conduct a car seat test for preterm infants born less than 37 weeks of gestation and/or infants weighing less than 2500 g (AAP, 1996)

       i. Before discharge, infants should be placed in the car seat in which they will be traveling, and monitored by experienced personnel

         (a) For apnea, bradycardia, and oxygen desaturation

         (b) For a period of time longer than their expected duration of travel

       ii. If they demonstrate apnea, bradycardia, or oxygen desaturation then discharge must be delayed until the infant can pass the car seat test in the appropriate car safety seat or bed

**16.** Parent education

  **a.** Sleep

       i. Supine sleep position recommended to prevent SIDS, i.e., lying on back, face upward (AAP, 2000)

       ii. A secondary effect of SIDS prevention has been an increase in brachycephalic heads and other skull malformations due to supine position

         (a) To prevent these skull malformations, educate families regarding:

            (1) The importance of "tummy time" when the infant is awake

            (2) Alternate sleep positions from supine, to right side and left side

            (3) Assure the parents that although some developmental milestones may be delayed by the infant sleeping supine, there will be no difference by the time the infant is 18 months of age (Hunter & Malloy, 2002)

  **b.** Umbilical cord care (Donlon & Furdon, 2002)

       i. Wash hands

       i. Use soap and water to clean cord

       ii. Air dry

       iii. No alcohol necessary

       iv. Fold diaper down below the cord to avoid contaminating with urine and stool

       v. No tub baths until cord separates

       vi. "Red flags" for need to call PNP

         (a) Foul odor

         (b) Redness around base of cord

         (c) Drainage

         (d) If the cord has not separated by 3 weeks of age

  **c.** Care of the circumcised penis (AAP, 2001)

       i. Tip of the penis may appear raw or yellowish

       ii. If there is a bandage, change it with each diapering and use petroleum jelly to keep the bandage from sticking

       iii. If a plastic ring is attached, leave it on the penis; it will drop off within 5 to 8 days

       iv. The penis requires about 7 to 10 days to fully heal

  **d.** Care of uncircumcised penis

       i. Foreskin adheres to the penis and isn't retractable at birth

       ii. *Do not force* foreskin to retract; gently retract it

       iii. Gently wash and dry penis with each diaper change

       iv. Foreskin loosens as child grows

  **e.** See Box 18-3 for red flags that signal when parents should contact PNP

■ **BOX 18-3**
■ **RED FLAGS THAT SIGNAL WHEN PARENTS SHOULD CALL THE PEDIATRIC NURSE PRACTITIONER**

- Breathing abnormal
  - Too fast
  - Too hard
- Color pale or jaundice (yellow) on trunk and extremities
- Poor feeding
- Decreased general activity, lethargic
- Decreased urine output, no urine for 12 hours
- Watery stools
- Large, hard stools
- Temperature more than 100.6° or less than 98° F that does not quickly improve with clothing changes
- Persistent vomiting
- Projectile vomiting
- Extremely irritable, not consolable
- Looks and behaves "ill"

# REFERENCES

EDITOR'S NOTE: American Academy of Pediatrics Policies, Practice Guidelines and other recommendations are followed by PNPs. Many of these were written in the 1990s, but are still in effect as of July, 2005.

American Academy of Pediatrics. (2001). Circumcision: Frequently asked questions. Retrieved May 9, 2005, from www.medem.com/MedLB/article_detaillb.cfm?article_ID= ZZZ13FOPIUC&sub_cat=0.

American Academy of Pediatrics & American Heart Association. (2005). Neonatal Resuscitation Program. Retrieved on May 9, 2006 at http://www.aap.org/nrp/nrpmain.html

American Academy of Pediatrics Committee on Fetus and Newborn. (2004). Hospital stay for healthy term newborns (RE9539). *Pediatrics 113*(5), 1434-1436.

American Academy of Pediatrics Committee on Fetus and Newborn, American Academy of Pediatrics Committee on Obstetric Practice, American College of Obstetricians and Gynecologists. (1996). Use and abuse of the Apgar score. *Pediatrics 98*(1), 141-142.

American Academy of Pediatrics Committee on Genetics, Section on Endocrinology,

Section on Urology. (2000). Policy statement: Evaluation of the newborn with developmental anomalies of the external genitalia. *Pediatrics 106*(1), 138-142.

American Academy of Pediatrics Committee on Injury and Poison Prevention. (1999). Safe transportation of newborns at hospital discharge. *Pediatrics 104*(4), 987-987.

American Academy of Pediatrics Committee on Injury and Poison Prevention and Committee on Fetus and Newborn. (1996). Safe transportation of premature and low birth weight infants. *Pediatrics 97*(5), 758-760.

American Academy of Pediatrics Committee on Practice and Ambulatory Medicine, and Section on Ophthalmology. (2003). Policy statement: Eye examination in infants, children, and young adults by pediatricians. *Pediatrics, 111*(4), 902-907.

American Academy of Pediatrics. Committee on Quality Improvement, Subcommittee on Developmental Dysplasia of the Hip. (2000). Clinical practice guideline: Early detection of developmental dysplasia of the hip. *Pediatrics 105*(4), 896-905.

American Academy of Pediatrics. Joint Committee on Infant Hearing. (2000). Position statement: Principles and guidelines for early hearing detection and intervention programs. *Pediatrics, 106*(4), 798-817.

American Academy of Pediatrics. Provisional Committee for Quality Improvement and Subcommittee on Hyperbilirubinemia. (2004). Practice guideline: Management of hyperbilirubinemia in the newborn infant, 35 or more weeks gestation. *Pediatrics, 114*(1), 297-316.

American Academy of Pediatrics. Section on Breastfeeding. (2005). Policy statement: Breastfeeding and the use of human milk. *Pediatrics, 115*(2), 496-506.

American Academy of Pediatrics. Section on Ophthalmology. (2002). Policy statement, Red reflex examination of infants. *Pediatrics 109*(5), 980-981.

American Academy of Pediatrics. Task Force on Circumcision. (1999). Circumcision policy statement. *Pediatrics 103*(3), 686-693.

American Academy of Pediatrics. Vitamin K Ad Hoc Task Force. (2003). Controversies concerning vitamin K and the newborn. *Pediatrics 112*(1), 191-192.

Benjamin, K. (2002). Scrotal and inguinal masses in the newborn period. *Adv Neonatal Care, 2*(3), 140-148.

Blackburn, S.T. (2003). *Maternal, fetal, & neonatal physiology: A clinical perspective.* (2nd ed.). St. Louis: Saunders.

Cantu, S. (2004). Circumcision. Retrieved from eMedicine on July 6, 2005, at www.emedicine.com/ped/topic1791.htm.

Cooper, S., & Ratnavel, R. (2005). Milia. Retrieved from eMedicine on March 31, 2006, at www.emedicine.com/DERM/topic265.htm.

Cranmer, H., & Shannon, M. (2005). Pediatrics: Hypoglycemia. Retrieved from eMedicine on July 6, 2005, at http://master.emedicine.com/EMERG/topic384.htm

Donlon, C. & Furdon, S. (2002). Part 2: Assessment of the umbilical cord outside of the delivery room. *Adv Neonatal Care, 2*(4), 187-197.

Dubik, M. (2001). Apgar scores still useful. *AAP Grand Rounds, 5,* 50.

Fuloria, M., & Kreiter, S. (2002a). The newborn examination: Part I. Emergencies and common abnormalities involving the skin, head, neck, chest, and respiratory and cardiovascular systems. *Am Fam Phys, 65*(1), 61-68.

Fuloria, M., & Kreiter, S. (2002b). The newborn examination: Part II. Emergencies and common abnormalities involving the abdomen, pelvis, extremities, genitalia, and spine. *Am Fam Phys, 65*(1), 265-270.

Gore, A. I., & Spencer, J. P. (2004). The newborn foot. *Am Fam Phys, 69,* 865-872.

Hunter, J. & Malloy, M. (2002). Effects of sleep and play positions on infant development: Reconciling developmental concerns with SIDS prevention. *Newborn Infant Nurs Rev, 2*(1), 9-16.

Hutcheson, J., & Snyder, H. M. (2004). Ambiguous genitalia and intersexuality. Retrieved from eMedicine March 31, 2006, at www.emedicine.com/PED/topic1492.htm.

National Eye Institute. (1999). Clinical trial of eye prophylaxis in the newborn. www.nei.nih.gov/neitrials/viewStudyWeb.aspx?id=19.

Noerr, B. (2001). State of the science: Neonatal hypoglycemia. *Adv Neonatal Care, 1*(1), 4-21.

St. John, E. B. (2005). Hemorrhagic disease of the newborn. Retrieved from eMedicine July 6, 2005, at www.emedicine.com/ped/topic966.htm.

Tappero, E. & Honeyfield, M. E. (2003). *Physical assessment of the newborn* (2nd ed.). Santa Rosa, CA: NICU Ink Book.

Thureen, P., Deacon, J., Hernandez, J., & Hall, D. (2005). *Assessment and care of the well newborn* (2nd ed.). St. Louis: Elsevier Saunders.

Yan, A. C. (2006). Erythema toxicum. Retrieved from eMedicine March 31, 2006, at http://www.emedicine. com/PED/topic697.htm

Young-Wardell, C. D., & Fuchs, D. (2003). Biobehavioral assessment of the infant. *J Am Acad Child Adolesc Psychiatry, 42*(6), 746-747.

# Newborns and Infants

CYNTHIA A. DANFORD, PhD, RN, APRN, BC

1. Goals of the well child health care visit for newborns and infants (McCarthy, 2004; Muscari, 2000)
   a. Promote health and wellness in infants, ages birth to 12 months
   b. Provide continuity of care and avoid fragmentation of care (AAP, 2000)
   c. Help parents build confidence in caring for their infant
      i. Physically
      ii. Cognitively
      iii. Developmentally
   d. Encourage optimal family development
2. Recommended schedule for well baby examinations
   a. Guidelines from the Committee on Practice and Ambulatory Medicine of the American Academy of Pediatrics (AAP, 2000) assuming that the infant:
      i. Has adequate and competent parenting
      ii. Has no manifestations of important health problems
      iii. Is growing and developing satisfactorily
   b. Recommended schedule of visits based on infant's age
      i. 2 to 4 days
      ii. By 1 month
      iii. 2 months
      iv. 4 months
      v. 6 months
      vi. 9 months
      vii. 12 months
3. Overview of the process for a well baby examination (Green & Palfrey, 2002)
   a. Identify primary source of information and evaluate the adequacy of his or her information regarding the infant
      i. Parent
      ii. Grandparent
      iii. Significant other
   b. Chief complaint (if any)
   c. Family concerns
      i. Use of babysitters, daycare
      ii. Divorce and visitation
      iii. Sibling interaction

    **d.** Birth history
      **i.** Maternal history and pregnancy with this infant
        (a) Assess maternal age
        (b) Assess maternal past medical and social histories
        (c) Length of pregnancy with this infant
        (d) Planned or unplanned pregnancy
        (e) Amount of prenatal care
        (f) High risk prenatal behaviors
          (1) Drugs
          (2) Alcohol
          (3) Smoking
          (4) Caffeine
        (g) Perinatal infections and complications
        (h) Exposure to intimate partner violence
      **ii.** Infant birth history
        (a) Gestational age
        (b) Apgar scores
          (1) Score of less than 7 at 5 minutes indicates potential risk for dysfunction of central nervous system
        (c) Birth weight
        (d) Congenital anomalies or chronic conditions
    **e.** Family history
      **i.** Family composition
      **ii.** Other individuals in the home
      **iii.** Family illnesses or diseases
    **f.** Social history
      **i.** Exposure to smoke in or out of the home
      **ii.** Care providers
      **iii.** Daycare use
      **iv.** Violence exposure in or out of the home
      **v.** Exposure to pets
    **g.** Immunization history
      **i.** Past immunizations
      **ii.** Exposure to communicable diseases
    **h.** Review of newborn genetic screening (AAP, 2000) (Table 19-1)
    **i.** Nutritional assessment (see Chapter 16 for infant-specific information)
    **j.** Physical examination (see Section 4, following)
    **k.** Developmental screening and assessment (see Section 5, following)
    **l.** Observation/discussion of parent-infant interaction (see Section 6, following)
    **m.** Parent and/or provider concerns and anticipatory guidance (see Section 7, following)
      **i.** Crying
      **ii.** Colic
      **iii.** Sleeping
      **iv.** Sudden infant death syndrome (SIDS)
      **v.** Feeding
      **vi.** Pacifiers
      **vii.** Elimination
      **viii.** Teething
      **ix.** Oral health and dental caries
      **x.** Safety
      **xi.** Car seats

■ **TABLE 19-1**
■ ■ **Screening Recommendations for Each Scheduled Well Child Visit**

| | Screening Tests | | | | | | | | |
|---|---|---|---|---|---|---|---|---|---|
| Age | Development | Vision | Hearing | Genetic, Metabolic and Hemoglobinopathy | Oral Health Risk | Lead Risk | Lead Test | Anemia | TB Screening (PPD) |
| Newborn (hospital) | O | S | O | O (PKU + state required | | | | | |
| 2–4 days | O | S | O (if not done in hospital) | O (PKU + state required if not done in hospital) | | | | | |
| 1 mo | O | S | O (if not yet done) | | | O | | | |
| 2 mo | O | O | S | | | | | | |
| 4 mo | O | S | S | | | | | | |
| 6 mo | O | S | S | | OR | O | | OR (if WIC) | O |
| 9 mo | O | S | S | | | O (or 12 mo) | | O (or 12 mo) | |
| 12 mo | O | S | S | | O | O (if not 9 mo) | | O (if not 9 mo) | OR |

O, Objective, perform for all infants; OR, objective, perform for infants at risk; S, subjective, by history; PKU, phenylketonunia, WIC, Women, Infants, and Children.
Reproduced with permission from American Academy of Pediatrics. (2000). Recommendations for preventive pediatric health care. *Pediatrics, 105*(3), 645–646.

    **xii.** Infant walkers
    **xiii.** Water safety
    **xiv.** Poisons and toxic substances
  **n.** Administration of immunizations (see Chapter 15 for age-related immunization recommendations)
  **o.** Summary and preparation for the next visit
    **i.** Review developmental expectations and anticipated changes
    **ii.** Immunization expectations (see Chapter 15)
    **iii.** "Red flags" indicating need for follow-up with a health care provider (see Section 8, following)
**4.** Physical assessment
  **a.** Weight, length, head circumference
    **i.** See Chapter 4 for details
    **ii.** Graph measurements on age- and sex-appropriate growth charts
  **b.** Newborn reflexes (Table 19-2) (see also Chapter 18 for method of eliciting reflexes)
    **i.** Newborn should respond to sound, light, and noxious odors with a physical or physiologic response
    **ii.** All newborn reflexes should be assessed at all visits

■ **TABLE 19-2**
■ ■ **Newborn Reflexes**

| Reflex | Age Appears | Age Disappears | Comments |
|---|---|---|---|
| Rooting | Birth | 3–4 months | Sleeping infant may not respond to stimuli; absence indicates severe CNS disease or depressed infant |
| Sucking | Birth | 3–4 months | Sleeping or satisfied infant may not respond well; absence indicates CNS depression |
| Tonic Neck | Birth | 4–6 months | Persistence indicates CNS lesion; infant unable to get out of position is abnormal |
| Palmar grasp | Birth | 3–6 months | Should be strong and symmetric |
| Stepping | Birth | 6–8 weeks | Tests brainstem and spinal column; absence indicates paralysis or depressed infant |
| Moro | Birth | 4 months (sometimes as early as 1–3 months) | Asymmetry indicates paralysis or fractured clavicle; absence indicates brainstem problem; persistence is abnormal |
| Plantar grasp | Birth | 4 months | Tests spinal nerves S1–S2; suspect after 4 months |
| Babinski | Birth | Variable | Presence in young children and adults suspect for CNS lesion |

Adapted from Burns, C. E., Brady, M. A., Dunn, A.M., & Starr, N. B. (2004). *Pediatric primary care: A handbook for nurse practitioners* (3rd ed.). Philadelphia: Saunders; and Hill, N. H., & Sullivan, L. M. (2004). *Management guidelines for nurse practitioners working with children and adolescents* (2nd ed.). Philadelphia: F. A. Davis.

  iii. Present at birth and generally resolve by 6 months
  iv. Absence at birth indicates severe CNS disease
  v. Persistence beyond expected date of disappearance also indicates CNS alteration
  c. Review of systems according to Chapters 5 through 13
  d. Assessment of risk for dental caries formation: low, moderate, high risk
    i. Use the Caries Risk Assessment Tool (American Academy of Pediatric Dentistry, 2002)
5. Developmental screening and assessment
  a. Overview
    i. 12% to 16% of American children have developmental or behavioral disorders
    ii. The primary care setting is ideal for developmental and behavioral screening as it is where most children younger than 5 years are seen regularly
    iii. Denver II or a similar comprehensive developmental assessment should be performed at all visits (see Chapter 4)
    iv. See Table 19-3 for age-specific developmental milestones
    v. Note onset of significant milestones
    vi. All delays should be referred to the appropriate specialist
    vii. Coordinate care with community-based programs
      (a) Early Intervention Programs
        (1) Services are for children and sometimes for their families
        (2) Services include screening, diagnosis, treatment, rehabilitation, anticipatory guidance, and prevention of further delays when possible
      (b) Title V Block Grant Programs funded by the Maternal Child Health Bureau

| Age | Personal-Social | Language | Fine Motor | Gross Motor | Red Flags |
|---|---|---|---|---|---|
| Birth | Regards face | Alerts to bell | | Reflex head turn side to side | |
| 1 month | Spontaneous social smile by 6 weeks | | Tracks horizontally to midline<br>Hands tightly fisted | Lifts head when prone | |
| 2 months | Smiles and socializes when talked to | Cooing, searches with eyes for sound | Tracks past midline, tracks vertically<br>Hands unfisted half of time | Head bobs erect if held sitting | Rolling before 3 months may indicate hypertonia |
| 3 months | | Laughs, vocalizes when talked to | Reaches for bright objects; brings object to mouth<br>Holds rattle placed in hand<br>Hands unfisted most of time | Lifts shoulders up when prone | |
| 4 months | | Turns head to sound of voice or bell | "Rakes" at bright object, hands come together | Lifts up on elbows; head steady when upright | |
| 5 months | Plays with toes when supine | | Transfers object from one hand to the other | Lifts up on hands; rolls front to back; no head lag when pulled lying to sitting | Poor head control |
| 6 months | Discriminates social smile | Babbles, begins to imitate, chews | | Rolls back to front | |
| 7 months | Displays stranger anxiety; plays peek-a-boo (7–9 months) | | Radial-palmar grasp of cube<br>Rakes object into palm | Sits alone 30 seconds or more<br>Supports weight and bounces while standing<br>Feet to mouth | W-sitting may indicate adductor spasticity or hypotonia |
| 8 months | | Mama/dada nonspecific | Three-finger grasp<br>Holds one block in each hand | Crawls, sits well | |
| 9 months | | Understands the word "no" | Neat pincer grasp, uses thumb-finger apposition cubes<br>Bangs Cubes in midline | Pulls to stand | Persistence of primitive reflexes |
| 10 months | Waves good-bye, plays pat-a-cake, helps to dress | | | Creeps on hands and knees<br>Cruises<br>Walks with two hands held | |
| 12 months | Drinks from a cup | Mama/dada specific<br>Follows 1-word commands with gestures<br>3- to 5-word vocabulary | Gives object to mother<br>Marks with crayon<br>Attempts tower of two blocks | Beginning to walk alone<br>Walks with one hand held | Failure to develop protective reactions |

Adapted from Hill, N. H., & Sullivan, L. M. (2004). *Management guidelines for nurse practitioners working with children and adolescents* (2nd ed.). Philadelphia: F. A. Davis.

(1) Programs vary from state to state; see "State Snapshots of Maternal and Child Health" website at https://perfdata.hrsa.gov/mchb/mchreports/snapshots/snapShot.asp

(2) Examples include oral health services to improve access to dental care; "Help Me Grow" programs, newborn visitation, lead poisoning prevention

(c) Other community-based programs such as Head Start and Early Start

b. Comprehensive developmental assessment tools for infants

   i. See Chapter 4 for details on the following tests

   ii. Bayley Scales of Infant Development-II for mental, motor, and behavioral ratings (Bayley, 2005)

   iii. Ages and Stages Questionnaire—completed by parents when infant is ages 4, 6, 8, and 12 months to assess communication, gross motor movement, fine motor movement, problem solving, and personal-social behavior (Bricker & Squires, 1999)

   iv. Denver II—monitors language, fine motor, gross motor and personal-social behavior (Denver Developmental Materials, Inc., 2006)

c. Language and hearing screening

   i. CAT/CLAMS—Cognitive Adaptive Test/Clinical Linguistic and Auditory Milestone Scale (Kube, et al., 2000)

   ii. Typical skills (note that during the first years receptive skills are more advanced than expressive skills) (Berk, 2004; Blackwell & Baker, 2002)

    (a) 0 to 6 months

     (1) Various types of cries expressing hunger, hurt, wet diaper

     (2) Engages in social smiling and responds to adult facial expressions (2 to 3 months)

      a) Shows preference for mother's voice

      b) May turn and cease movement as mother speaks

     (3) Makes noises in response to voice satisfaction or displeasure, laugh (3 to 4 months)

     (4) Able to recognize and look for familiar sounds

     (5) Preference for highly intonated speech (4 to 6 months)

     (6) Enjoys many interactions

      a) Soft music

      b) Songs sung to them

      c) Individuals responding to their babbling, cooing, and gurgles

    (b) 2 to 12 months

     (1) Responds to own name

     (2) Coos, makes vowel sounds (2 months)

     (3) Understands names of familiar objects

     (4) Pays attention to conversation

     (5) Babbling includes consonant sounds (4 months)

     (6) Responds to words in usual situations: "No no."

     (7) Babbles expressively, begins preverbal gestures, begins word comprehension (8 to 12 months)

     (8) Understands some common words independent of context (11-13 months)

     (9) Says first recognizable word (12 months)

     (10) Interested in picture books

     (11) Teaching: encourage parents to:

      a) Address infant by name

      b) Use names of familiar objects

        c) Tell infant about the activities the parent is doing

        d) Show them picture books

        e) Sing songs

        f) Play peek-a-boo (4 months) and pat-a-cake (9 months)

  iii. Infants at risk for hearing loss should be screened (Cunningham, et al., 2003)

    (a) Risk factors for birth to 28 days

      (1) Family history of sensorineural hearing loss

      (2) In utero infection such as toxoplasmosis, rubella, cytomegalovirus, herpes, syphilis

      (3) Infants exposed to excessive noise in utero or as a newborn

      (4) Ear anomalies and other craniofacial anomalies

      (5) Hyperbilirubinemia requiring exchange transfusion

      (6) Birth weight less than 1500 g

      (7) Bacterial meningitis

      (8) Low Apgar scores: 0 to 3 at 5 minutes and to 6 at 10 minutes

      (9) Respiratory distress

      (10) Prolonged mechanical ventilation for more than 10 days

      (11) Ototoxic medications (gentamicin) administered for more than 5 days or used in combination with loop diuretics

      (12) Physical features associated with a syndrome (Down syndrome, Waardenburg syndrome)

    (b) Risk factors for 29 days to 4 months

      (1) Parental concern about hearing, speech, or language, and/or developmental delay

      (2) Any newborn risks as above

      (3) Recurrent or persistent otitis media with effusion for at least 3 months

      (4) Head trauma with fracture of temporal bone

      (5) Childhood infectious diseases (meningitis, mumps, measles)

      (6) Neurodegenerative disorders (Hunter syndrome)

      (7) Demyelinating diseases (Charcot-Marie-Tooth syndrome)

  iv. Refer infants if:

    (a) Lack or inconsistent response

    (b) Failure to achieve appropriate skills

    (c) Parental concern

**6.** Parent-infant interaction

  **a.** NAPNAP (2003) position statement on infant and family well-being in the first year of life

    **i.** "Infancy is a critical period that provides an important foundation for both physical and mental health throughout life"

    **ii.** The PNP has a critical role in assisting newborns to thrive within the family environment

  **b.** See Table 19-4 for age-specific observations of the parent-child interaction

    **i.** Observe how well parents are adjusting to their infant through each developmental stage

    **ii.** Evaluate the interaction and comfort level of both parents with infant

    **iii.** Assess emotional and behavioral response of parents to infant when infant is:

    (a) Smiling

    (b) Crying

    (c) Neutral

| Age | Supportive Parental Interactions | Positive Infant Responses |
|---|---|---|
| Newborn | Looking frequently at the infant<br>Having specific questions and observations about the individual characteristics of the infant<br>Touching, massaging, or gently rubbing the infant<br>Attempting to soothe the infant when the infant is upset | Looking content<br>Signaling needs<br>Feeding well<br>Responding to parent's attempts to soothe |
| 1 month | Talking to and smiling at the infant during the examination<br>Holding the infant during most of the visit<br>Comforting the infant effectively during stressful parts of the exam<br>Differentiating among different types of crying<br>Describing the infant's routine | Turning head toward parent's voice<br>Looking well cared for<br>Looking content<br>Responding to parent's attempts to soothe<br>Appearing well nourished<br>Searching for faces and actively regarding surroundings |
| 2 months | Describing feeling more confident with the infant<br>Describing the infant's routine<br>Talking to the infant and looking at the infant<br>Describing the infant's likes and dislikes | Gaining weight at an appropriate pace<br>Smiling |
| 4 months | Having fun with the infant<br>Thinking the infant is wonderful in one or more ways<br>Bringing toys and objects to amuse the infant<br>Naming specific games played with the infant<br>Describing funny or surprising behaviors that the infant does<br>Describing the infant's personality<br>Anticipating the infant's response to a particular event (e.g., undressing, a shot) | Recognizing parents<br>Having a well-shaped head as opposed to occipital flattening<br>Showing delight in social play with movement, smiles, giggles, and positive vocalizations<br>Looking well nourished |
| 6 months | Holding the infant for most of the exam<br>Comforting the infant after distress<br>Bringing and offering toys or appropriate objects<br>Responding to the infant's bids for attention<br>Allowing the infant to explore with his or her mouth<br>Tolerating the infant's exploration of the parent's face, hair, and so forth while setting limits in a positive way | Demonstrating awareness of the presence of strangers<br>Looking to the parent for comfort<br>Anticipating and adjusting to lifting and carrying<br>Babbling |
| 9 months | Allowing the infant to explore the environment safely<br>Being mindful of safety risks in the office (e.g., does not leave the infant unprotected on exam table)<br>Describing a good leave-taking ritual<br>Describing a comfortable bedtime routine and routine in case of night waking<br>Getting the infant to wave, play peek-a-boo, or play other games<br>Handling limit-setting comfortably | Demonstrating awareness of the presence of strangers<br>Looking to the parent for comfort<br>Reacting to separation from parent<br>Babbling syllables (e.g., ma-ma, da-da)<br>Smiling at own image in the mirror<br>Responding to his or her name<br>Pointing at objects |
| 1 year | Reading books to the child<br>Bringing age-appropriate toys<br>Reporting safety-proofing the house<br>Using appropriate limit-setting (e.g., moving the child away, distracting the child with an alternative activity)<br>Having appropriate behavioral expectations<br>Interpreting the child's behavior or utterances | Exploring the environment<br>Showing signs of using the parent as home base while exploring, checking back as necessary<br>Being able to self-soothe<br>Responding to his name<br>Sharing or using toys interactively with adults<br>Looking well cared for |

From Dion, S., & Stadtler, A. (2002). Age-specific observations of the parent-child interaction. In M. Jellinek, B. P. Patel, & M. C. Froehle (Eds.). *Bright futures in practice: Mental health,* Vol. II. Tool Kit. Arlington, VA: National Center for Education in Maternal and Child Health.

    c. Evaluate parent response to infant cues (sharing vocalizations, smiles, and facial expressions) (Gottesman, 1999)

        i. Some early infant behavior is innate and reflexive for the purpose of seeking food, security, warmth, and comfort, e.g., rooting, crying, Moro reflex, flailing of limbs

        ii. During the first year, infants begin to communicate purposively through verbalizations and nonverbal behavior

    d. Evaluate extent of reciprocal responses between infant and parents

    e. Relationship between infant; and parent-infant interactions (Carey, 1988; Chess & Thomas, 1986; Kochanska, et al., 2005 )

        i. Refers to behavioral style or the way an individual experiences and responds to the internal and external environment

        ii. Origin

            (a) Approximately half of one's behavioral style is genetically determined

            (b) Remaining sources include psychosocial environment, nonhuman environment, and the infant's physical condition

        iii. Stability—low in the early days and weeks of life, increasing by 2 to 3 years of age

        iv. Affects how the parents feel about themselves and how they function as parents

            (a) Agreeable, flexible infants tend to make their parents feel happy, competent, and successful

            (b) Irritable, inflexible infants tend to adversely influence their parents' self-esteem, satisfaction as parents, marital relationship, mood, and decision to return to work

            (c) Poor fit between the infant's temperament and the caregivers is a common source of parent-child interaction distress and behavior problems in the child

        v. Anticipatory guidance

            (a) Introduce parents to the process of "reading" their infant's behavioral cues or how the infant functions and then responds to stimuli

            (b) Note: Research indicates that newborn behavior has little correlation with later infant behavior so parents need to be reminded to be flexible in their interpretation

            (c) Temperament behaviors that most likely need to be accommodated rather than changed by the parents include less soothable crying and irritability and irregular eating and sleeping patterns

            (d) Temperament should not be misconstrued as something abnormal

                (1) Behavioral disturbance may involve the infant's temperament and may help to determine realistic goals for intervention

                (2) An improved fit between the environment and the infant may result in decreased and disappearing adverse behavior

    f. Address parenting concerns as infant changes and develops

        i. Stranger anxiety/fear arises at approximately 6 to 8 months

            (a) Less pronounced in the infant who attends daycare

        ii. Object permanence—at 8 months infants realize that an object is permanent and will look for it when out of the line of vision

            (a) Separation anxiety arises at approximately 8 to 9 months

            (b) Indicates clear attachment to a familiar caregiver

    g. Play activities appropriate for infants from newborn to 1 year (Glassy, et al., 2003):

        i. Newborns

            (a) Learn through imitation

(b) Cuddle infant, sing and vocalize with infant to increase parent-infant bond

(c) Mobiles to stimulate vision (follows objects by 2 months)

ii. Young infant

(a) Talk, sing, read to infant

(1) Songs with movement by 4 months

(2) Clapping songs

(b) Peek-a-boo by 4 months

(c) Brightly colored picture books, board books (can distinguish colors by 5 months)

(d) Stuffed animal or favorite blanket for comfort

(e) Crib gym

iii. Older infant

(a) Talk, sing, read to infant

(b) Games, music:

(1) Waves goodbye by 7 months

(2) Pat-a-cake by 7 months

(3) Puts objects in container by 7 to 10 months; dumping toys; stacking toys

(4) Balls, toys that roll by 9 months

(5) Scribbles with a crayon by 12 months

(6) Push-pull toys by 12 months

(7) Chasing games by 12 months

(c) Set simple rules, limits

h. Infant exercise programs are *not* supported by the AAP as being beneficial for infant development

i. Other anticipatory guidance

i. Remind parents to rest when the infant rests

ii. Breast-feeding mothers need proper nutrition to be able to provide for the infant

iii. Assist development of parenting role

(a) Use *Bright Futures* as a guide for age-appropriate teaching

(b) Parenting support groups are useful for some parents

iv. Organized plans help parents connect with the infant's developmental needs

7. Parent and/or provider concerns and anticipatory guidance

a. Crying (Soltis, 2004)

i. Physiology of crying (Ludington-Hoe, et al., 2002)

(a) A series of four movements that resembles a Valsalva maneuver

(b) Accompanied by physiologic changes

(1) Increased heart rate and blood pressure

(2) Reduced oxygen level

(3) Elevated cerebral blood pressure

(4) Initiation of the stress response

(5) Depleted energy reserves and oxygen

(6) Interrupted mother-infant interaction

(7) Potential brain injury and cardiac dysfunction

(c) All normal infants cry

ii. Typical pattern of crying in young infants (Soltis, 2004)

(a) An increase in crying duration until about 6 weeks of age

(b) A gradual decrease in duration of crying until 4 months of age

(c) During the day, crying is most prevalent during late afternoon and evening

      (d) Various types of cries believed to express hunger, hurt, wet diaper, need for attention, or simply an expression of vigor

   **iii.** Crying interventions

      (a) Answer infant cries swiftly, consistently, and comprehensively

      (b) Hold the infant skin-to-skin (i.e., kangaroo care)

      (c) Swaddling

      (d) Pacifier

      (e) Sugar water or a sweet-tasting nonsucrose solution

      (f) Heartbeat sounds

      (g) Distraction by lullabies or mother's voice

      (h) Rhythmic movement

      (i) Reduction of external stimuli

   **iv.** Anticipatory guidance

      (a) Review normal crying patterns of infants to avoid unreasonable parental expectations

      (b) A crying or upset infant should never be shaken as a disciplinary measure

         (1) Reinforce importance of not shaking infants to avoid shaken baby syndrome

         (2) Ensure that all caregivers of the infant are also aware of this issue

      (c) Remind parents to never leave their child with an individual with a history of abuse

      (d) Inconsolable infants should be evaluated by a PNP (Ateah, et al., 2003)

      (e) Infants are unable to learn social behavior, thus parents must learn to interpret infant behaviors

      (f) Infants are unable to be patient and accept delayed gratification—this develops during next several years

      (g) Meeting the infant's needs takes priority over discipline

**b.** Colic (Leung & Lemay, 2004)

   **i.** Definition

      (a) Episodes of uncontrollable crying or fussing

      (b) Otherwise, a healthy and well-fed infant less than 3 months old

      (c) Episodes last more than 3 hours per day, and more than 3 days per week for at least 3 weeks

      (d) May be accompanied by excessive bloating, flatulence, abdominal pain

      (e) Typically resolves by 3 to 4 months of age

   **ii.** Etiology unknown

   **iii.** Interventions

      (a) Supportive counseling of parents is necessary because this is very stressful to family

      (b) Reassurance that the child is not "sick" and that the symptoms will subside

      (c) Interventions similar to those in Section 7.a.iii. earlier

      (d) Survey research of PNPs and pediatricians (Lobo, et al., 2004)

         (1) PNPs more likely to recommend behavioral and environmental approaches

         (2) Pediatricians more likely to prescribe medications and recommend parental interventions

         (3) Formula changes were rarely recommended by either PNPs (6.7%) or pediatricians (5.7%)

**c.** Normal sleep, sleeping problems, co-sleeping, and SIDS prevention

   **i.** Normal sleep (Davis, et al., 2004a; 2004b)

(a) Essential for normal growth and development, emotional health, and immune function
(b) A period of rest, but also of intense higher cortical brain activity
(c) Normally is irregular and inconsistent in infants
(d) Regulated by:
    (1) Circadian rhythm based on a light/dark cycle
    (2) Homeostatic process of sleep debt accumulated during waking hours and relief of this debt by sleep

ii. Normal sleep requirements (Davis, et al., 2004a)
    (a) 1 month of age—8 hours during night, 7.75 hours during day; longest sleep period is about 2 to 4 hours
    (b) 6 months of age—10 hours during night, 4.25 hours during day; longest sleep period is about 6 hours; should fall asleep on their own
    (c) 12 months of age—10.25 hours during night, 3.5 hours during day

iii. Sleep problem is a sleep pattern that (Davis, et al., 2004b)
    (a) Interferes with the refreshing nature of sleep for the infant
    (b) Significantly disrupts the sleep of others

iv. SIDS (sudden infant death syndrome)
    (a) A rare occurrence during the first month of life with peak incidence between 2 and 4 months of age
    (b) Risk factors include:
        (1) Prone sleeping position
        (2) Sleeping on a soft surface
        (3) Overheating
        (4) Maternal smoking
        (5) Prematurity
        (6) Low birth weight
        (7) Young maternal age
        (8) Late or no prenatal care
        (9) Male sex

v. Focused history
    (a) Where infant sleeps and with whom the infant shares a room
    (b) Position for sleeping, e.g., back, prone, side
    (c) Ability to fall asleep and stay asleep in own crib
    (d) Sleep times, awake times, nap times
    (e) Self-soothing behaviours
    (f) Use of sleep aids: blanket, stuffed animal, sleeping with a bottle
    (g) Parent participation in helping infant fall asleep (rocking, holding)
    (h) Parental response to crying during night
    (i) Co-sleeping (Poppell, 2002)
        (1) Believed to strengthen the parent-child bond
        (2) Cultural variations
            a) Japanese children lie next to their mothers during infancy and early childhood
            b) Black children fall asleep with a parent and stay with them throughout part or all of the night more than white children
            c) Appalachian children from eastern Kentucky often sleep with their parents for the first 2 years of life

vi. Anticipatory guidance
    (a) Sleep problem interventions (Davis, et al., 2004b; Pohl & Renwick, 2002)

(1) Develop consistent bedtime routines
(2) "Graduated extinction" method to help infants fall asleep and stay asleep in own crib—infant learns self-soothing methods and associates crib environment with waking up
   a) Place infant in crib when partially asleep
   b) Make scheduled checks on infant
   c) During crying episodes, do not rock, feed, or hold infant
   d) Gradually decrease intervals between checks
(b) AAP (2005) does not recommend co-sleeping of infant with parents in same bed
   (1) Risk of overlying the infant, which can lead to suffocation
   (2) Infant experiences less slow-wave sleep and more frequent night-time arousals
(c) Review crib safety
   (1) Slats should be no greater than 2⅜ inches (60 mm) apart
   (2) Keep crib sides raised
   (3) Mattress should be firm and fit snugly in crib
(d) Review SIDS prevention techniques (AAP, 2004; Moon, 2001)
   (1) Infant should sleep in parents' room, but in a separate bed
   (2) Sleep position should be wholly on the back for every sleep
   (3) Avoid use of soft bedding such as pillows, quilts, comforters, sheepskins, and porous mattresses
   (4) Avoid use of soft toys or toys with loops or string cords
   (5) Avoid overheating the infant
      a) Keep room temperature comfortable
      b) Caution against use of excessive clothing or blankets on an infant; use infant sleep sacks rather than blankets
   (6) Offer a pacifier at naptime and bedtime (delay until age 1 month if breastfeeding)
   (7) Protect infant from second-hand smoke
   (8) Avoid SIDS monitors and other similar devices for SIDS prevention

**d.** Feeding and feeding problems
  **i.** For details, see Chapter 16, Nutrition
  **ii.** See NAPNAP (2001) position statement on the PNP's role in support of breast-feeding as the ideal form of nutrition for infants

**e.** Pacifiers
  **i.** Studies suggest that pacifiers stent the upper airway and thus may prevent SIDS
  **ii.** Some studies link pacifier use with increased susceptibility to otitis media, increased dental malocclusion, and shortened duration of breast-feeding

**f.** Elimination and elimination problems
  **i.** Normal urination
    (a) Infants on formula or breast-fed should urinate six to eight wet diapers per day
    (b) Urine output equals approximately 50 to 300 mL/day
  **ii.** Normal bowel patterns
    (a) Breast-fed infants
      (1) First few weeks of age, stools are frequent throughout the day
      (2) As infants grow, stools are less frequent, ranging from once a day to once every several days
      (3) Stools are soft, sticky, or watery, curdlike in texture, and light yellow
      (4) Odor is not unpleasant and may have a sour smell

        (b) Formula-fed infants
- (1) During first month, two to four stools per day is common
- (2) As infants grow, stools become less frequent ranging from one to three per day
- (3) Stools are firmer, darker, and more odorous than stools in breast-fed infants
- (4) Stool color ranges from brown, greenish, to dark yellow depending on formula type
- (5) Soft and semiformed

        (c) Iron supplements darken stools in both breast- and formula-fed infants

        (d) Stools change in consistency and color as solid foods are introduced, becoming firmer and darker

        (e) Infants have involuntary bowel and bladder control

        (f) By 9 to 12 months infants may establish their own unique regular pattern of stooling and urinating

  iii. Constipation or diarrhea—see Chapter 30 for illnesses of the gastrointestinal tract

**g.** Teething
- **i.** Primary tooth eruption begins approximately 6 months of age
  - (a) First to erupt are the lower central and lateral incisors
  - (b) Followed by the upper center and lateral incisors at about 8 months of age
- **ii.** Infant may present with a fever, drooling, irritability, or mouthing of objects
- **iii.** Cold teething rings may ease discomfort or restlessness
- **iv.** Fluids should be encouraged
- **v.** Acetaminophen can help ease the discomfort

**h.** Oral health and dental caries (see also Chapter 16, Section 6.b)
- **i.** General (Fluoride Recommendations Work Group, 2001)
  - (a) In children, dental caries are reported to be five times more common than asthma and seven times more common than hay fever
  - (b) The Centers for Disease Control and Prevention suggest that dental caries is likely the most prevalent of infectious diseases
  - (c) During 1999–2002, the prevalence of dental caries increased with age (Beltrán-Aguilar, et al., 2005)
    - (1) 41% of children aged 2 to 11 years
    - (2) 42% of children and adolescents aged 6 to 19 years
    - (3) Approximately 90% of adults
- **ii.** Groups at risk for dental caries designated by the American Academy of Pediatrics
  - (a) Children with mothers with a high caries rate
  - (b) Children who sleep with a bottle or breast-feed throughout the night
  - (c) Children in families of low socioeconomic status
  - (d) Children with special health care needs
  - (e) Children with demonstrable caries, plaque, demineralization, and/or staining
  - (f) Later-order offspring
- **iii.** Dental history of the mother has a direct correlation with the infant; therefore assessing mother's dentition and oral hygiene habits is appropriate:
  - (a) Oral hygiene practices
  - (b) Fluoride exposure
  - (c) Sugar intake
  - (d) Dietary practices

(e) Use of dental services

(f) Number and location of dental caries

iv. All infants should receive an oral health risk assessment by 6 months of age by a qualified pediatric health care professional (AAP, 2003)

(a) Early referral to a pediatric dentist if in one of the at-risk groups

(b) Refer as early as 6 months and no later than 6 months after the first tooth erupts or 12 months, whichever comes first

v. Mechanism of development of dental caries (Fluoride Recommendations Work Group, 2001)

(a) Bacteria that cause dental caries reside in dental plaque

(b) Plaque is a sticky organic matrix of bacteria, food debris, dead mucosal cells, and salivary components that adheres to tooth enamel

(c) Bacterial by-products (i.e., acids) dissolve the hard surfaces of teeth

(d) Unchecked, the bacteria can penetrate the dissolved surface, attack the underlying dentin, and reach the soft pulp tissue

(e) Dental caries can result in loss of tooth structure, pain, and tooth loss and can progress to acute systemic infection

vi. Mechanism of prevention of dental caries (Fluoride Recommendations Work Group, 2001)

(a) Fluoride inhibits or even reverses the process by which cariogenic bacteria metabolize carbohydrates to produce acid and affects bacterial production of adhesive polysaccharides

(b) Saliva is a major carrier of topical fluoride

(c) Fluoride, when present in the mouth, is also retained and concentrated in plaque

vii. Recommendations and anticipatory guidance

(a) Breast-feeding or bottle-feeding formula or juice during sleep may cause dental caries

(b) Infants of any age should not be put to bed with a bottle

(c) Infant gums and primary teeth can be cleaned with a soft damp cloth or soft toothbrush

(1) Begin to brush child's teeth twice daily as soon as the first teeth erupt

(2) Floss between teeth once a day as soon as teeth contact one another

(3) Good family oral hygiene contributes to good infant oral hygiene

(d) Dietary considerations

(1) After the eruption of the first teeth provide fruit juices only during meals

(2) Carbonated beverages should be excluded from the infant's diet

(3) Ideally, infants should have their mouth cleaned with a damp cloth after feedings

viii. Fluoride (Fluoride Recommendations Work Group, 2001)

(a) Everyone should receive frequent exposure to small amounts of fluoride

(b) Primary care providers (and parents) should know the fluoride concentration in their primary source of drinking water

(1) Optimal level is 2 ppm

(2) This information is the basis for all individual and professional decisions regarding use of other fluoride modalities (e.g., mouth rinse or supplements)

(c) Fluoride toothpaste should not be used in children younger than 2 years if drinking water is above optimal

    (d) If fluoride toothpaste is used, place no more than a pea-sized amount (0.25 g) of toothpaste on the toothbrush and remove excess toothpaste after brushing

    (e) Begin fluoride use at 6 months as indicated

    (f) In areas where the natural fluoride concentration is below optimal, children should use alternative sources of drinking water

**i.** General safety issues

  **i.** A study of data from more than 23,000 injuries and 636 deaths the leading cause of injury changes approximately every 3 months from birth to 12 months of age (Agran, et al., 2003)

    (a) Infants' developmental capabilities are directly related to the common types of injuries that they receive

      (1) Medication poisoning was the single highest cause of injury for any age group

      (2) Infants age 3 to 5 months are most likely to be battered

      (3) Falls from furniture were most common between age 6- to 8-months

  **ii.** Anticipatory guidance for age-related safety issues must occur at each well child visit

**j.** Car seat safety (AAP, 2006) (see also Chapter 22, Section 4.c.viii)

  **i.** Infant-only seats

    (a) Car seats should be placed in the backseat only

    (b) Seats are only rear facing

    (c) For babies up to 20 to 22 pounds

    (d) Come with a three- or five-point harness

    (e) Small, portable, and fit newborns best

    (f) Features

      (1) Detachable base should fit snugly in the car

      (2) Higher weight and height limits for those infants exceeding weight/height before 1 year

      (3) Harness slots should be at or below the infant's shoulders and give room for growth

      (4) Handles should be down during travel; check instructions for variations

  **ii.** Convertible seats

    (a) Bigger and heavier than infant-only seats and may be used for larger children

    (b) May be too large to fit the newborn properly; newborn should be able to recline comfortably

    (c) Use rear facing until the infant is 1 year and at least 20 pounds or more

    (d) For a small infant the best choice is a five-point harness for safety

    (e) A car seat with an overhead shield can hit the baby's face in a crash

  **iii.** Car seat caution

    (a) Shopping carts

      (1) Avoid placing an infant and car seat in the fold-down seat of a shopping cart

      (2) Avoid using built-in infant seats in shopping carts

      (3) The high position of the car seat and the weight of the infant causes the cart to be top-heavy and increase the chance of the cart tipping over

      (4) Shop with infants using a stroller or a backpack or frontpack

(b) Unsafe car seats
  (1) Older than 10 years is too old. Some manufacturers recommend use for only 5 to 6 years. See manufacturer's recommendations.
  (2) Do not use if car seat has been in a crash
  (3) Do not use if there is no label with the manufacture date, seat name, or model number; this information is important to check on recalls
  (4) Do not use if the car seat does not come with instructions
  (5) Do not use if the car seat has any cracks in the frame
  (6) Do not use if there are any missing parts
(c) To check on recalls contact the Auto Safety Hot Line 888-327-4236 or the National Highway Traffic Safety Administration at www.nhtsa.dot.gov/people/injury/childps/recall/canister.htm

iv. Special considerations
  (a) Premature infants
    (1) Use car seats without a shield
    (2) Newborn should be observed in a car seat before hospital discharge to ensure semireclining position does not cause bradycardia or breathing difficulties
    (3) A crash-tested car bed should be used for the infant who needs to travel flat
    (4) An adult should ride in the backseat with the infant
  (b) Special-needs infants
    (1) Easter Seals offers programs for children with special health needs: 800-221-6827
    (2) Automotive Safety for Children Program 317-274-2977
    (3) AAP brochure: "Safe Transportation of Children with Special Needs: A Guide for Families"

**k.** Infant walkers
  i. Parents perceive that infant walkers keep their child safe and help them learn to walk
  ii. There is no research that supports these parental perceptions
  iii. American Academy of Pediatrics (2001) has called for a ban on production and use of baby walkers due the risk of major and minor injury
    (a) In the U. S., nearly 200,000 infants were seen in emergency rooms for injuries from baby walkers between 1990 and 2001 (Shields & Smith, 2006)
      (1) Three-fourths of the infants fell down the stairs while in the walker
      (2) Head injuries were most common; some were fatal
    (b) Research indicates that walkers do not help infants learn to walk but may delay normal motor and mental development (Shields & Smith, 2006)
    (c) Parents who insist on using a walker need to select one that meets the ASTM F977-96 performance standards to prevent falls downstairs
      (1) Adult supervision is necessary during walker use, but does not completely prevent injury due to the high rate of speed an infant can move (approx 3 feet/second)
      (2) Barriers such as stair gates should be used for added safety
      (3) Stationary infant walker-like devices that do not roll are a safer alternative
        a) Allows the infant to bounce, swivel, and tip
        b) Eliminates stair-related injuries

l. Water safety (See also, Chapter 22, Section 4.c.ii. for further information)
   i. Research data indicate that children less than 1 year of age most frequently drown in bathtubs and buckets (AAP, 2004)
   ii. Constant supervision of infants in or near water is essential
     (a) Parents should be alerted to the dangers of standing water
     (b) All water should be removed from buckets immediately after use
     (c) Infants should never be left alone in bathtubs or near open standing water of any type, including toilet bowls
     (d) Effectiveness of swimming instruction for infants has not been determined and should not be a means to ensure water safety
   iii. All pools should be enclosed with a four-sided fence, 4 feet high and climb-proof, with openings of no more than 4 inches below the fence and between the posts
     (a) Pool covers are not a safe alternative to fences
     (b) Gates should be self-latching and self-closing
     (c) Parents should learn CPR and keep U.S. Coast Guard equipment such as life jackets and a shepherd's crook at the poolside

m. Home safety
   i. Playpens should have small openings less than $\frac{1}{4}$ inch (6 mm)
   ii. Infant should not be left in playpen or crib with drop side down
   iii. Hot water heater thermostat should be lower than 120° F
     (a) Water should be tested for warmth before bathing to avoid burns
     (b) Never leave infants unattended in the bathtub or pool
   iv. Maintain a smoke-free environment
   v. Avoid direct sunlight
     (a) Put a hat on the infant when outside
     (b) Keep skin covered with lightweight, light-colored clothing
     (c) Apply sunscreen (fragrance free with a minimum sun protection factor of 15) whenever infant is exposed to sun
   vi. Infants and young children should never be left alone with other children or pets
   vii. Infants should not be held while caregiver is drinking hot liquids or smoking
   viii. Remove all guns from the home
   ix. If a gun is in the home make sure it is locked up, unloaded, with ammunition safely stored in a separate place and the key kept with the parent
   x. Keep toys with small parts out of reach
   xi. Keep sharp objects out of reach
   xii. Use safety locks on cabinets and drawers
   xiii. Cover electrical outlets
   xiv. Keep plastic bags and latex balloons out of the infant's reach
   xv. Lower the infant mattress at 6 months
   xvi. Install gates at the top and bottom of stairways
   xvii. Remove dangling cords from infant's reach
     (a) Telephone
     (b) Electrical
     (c) Window blinds
   xviii. Avoid leaving heavy or hot objects on tablecloths that could be pulled down
   xix. Prevent infection
     (a) Wash toys with soap and water regularly
     (b) Avoid large crowds, especially with a newborn

    (c) Discourage visits from friends and family members with colds or illness

  **xx.** Pets

    (a) Keep pet food and pet food dishes away from child

    (b) Keep infant away when pets are eating

**n.** Poisons and toxic substances

  **i.** General rules

    (a) Keep local poison control number near the telephone

    (b) Keep all poisonous substances locked safely out of the infant's reach, including:

      (1) Medications

      (2) Alcohol

      (3) Poisons

      (4) Cleaning aids

      (5) Paint

      (6) Health and beauty aids

    (c) Never store poisons in containers that contained other substances

    (d) Be aware of poisonous plants that may be in the home or outside environment

  **ii.** Phthalates (Shea, 2003)

    (a) Phthalates are used in the production of plastics to make them durable and flexible

    (b) Research results about the safety of phthalates are inconclusive

    (c) AAP reports that further research is needed on the exposure of infants and young children to phthalates

    (d) Two components of phthalates affect children more than adults:

      (1) Diethylhexyl phthalate (DEHP) is found in toys and in medical equipment such as intravenous fluid bags

      (2) Diisononyl phthalate (DINP) is used in making toys

    (e) Neonates are at risk if medical equipment is used that is high in phthalates

    (f) Infants and young children are at risk due to mouthing soft toys

    (g) Manufacturers in the United States and Canada have removed these compounds from infant bottles and nipples, teethers, and toys intended for mouthing

    (h) The less-toxic DINP has been substituted for DEHP in some toys

  **iii.** Lead (Kemper, et al., 2005) (see also Chapter 22, Section 4.i)

    (a) An environmental health problem for young children

    (b) At age 12 months, all infants should be tested for elevated blood lead levels

    (c) All children 6 to 72 months of age in HUSKY Part A Medicaid must be assessed for lead exposure risk, and at a minimum, screened at 12 months

    (d) Lead levels greater than 10 mcg/dL are considered elevated and require follow-up

      (1) A study of 3682 children covered by Medicaid in Michigan (Kemper, et al., 2005)

      (2) All had elevated blood lead levels but only 53.9% received follow-up

      (3) Follow-up testing was lower for Hispanic or non-white versus white children, urban versus rural children, and for children living in high- versus low-risk lead areas

      (4) See Chapter 22 (Toddlers, Preschoolers, and School-agers) for more information about lead poisoning prevention

8. "Red flags" indicating need for follow-up with a health care provider
   a. Fever of 100.4° F (38° C) or higher rectally
   b. Seizure
   c. Skin rash or ecchymotic spots
   d. Change in activity or behavior that raises a parent's concern
   e. Excessive irritability or lethargy
   f. Failure to eat
   g. Vomiting
   h. Diarrhea
   i. Dehydration
   j. Jaundice in newborn
   k. Cough

## REFERENCES

Agran, P. F., Anderson, C., Winn, D., Trent, R., et al. (2003). Rates of pediatric injuries by 3-month intervals for children 0 to 3 years of age. *Pediatrics, 111,* e683-e692.

American Academy of Pediatric Dentistry. (2002). Policy on the use of a caries-risk assessment tool (CAT) for infants, children and adolescents. Retrieved March 31, 2006, from www.aapd.org/members/referencemanual/pdfs/02-03/Caries%20Risk%20Assess.pdf.

American Academy of Pediatrics Section on Pediatric Dentistry. (2003). Oral health risk assessment timing and establishment of the dental home. *Pediatrics, 111*(5), 1113-1116.

American Academy of Pediatrics. (2005). Car safety seats: A guide for families - 2006. Retrieved April 2, 2006 from www.aap.org/family/carseatguide.htm.

American Academy of Pediatrics Clinical Report (2003). Hearing assessment in infants and children: Recommendations beyond neonatal screening. *Pediatrics, 111*(3), 436-440.

American Academy of Pediatrics Committee on Children with Disabilities. (2001). Developmental surveillance and screening of infants and young children. *Pediatrics, 108*(1), 192-196.

American Academy of Pediatrics Committee on Injury, Violence and Poison Prevention. (2001). Injuries associated with infant walkers. *Pediatrics, 108*(3), 790-792.

American Academy of Pediatrics Committee on Injury, Violence and Poison Prevention. (2004). Prevention of drowning in infants, children and adolescents. *Pediatrics, 112*(2), 437-439.

American Academy of Pediatrics Task Force on Sudden Infant Death Syndrome. (2005). The changing concept of Sudden Infant Death Syndrome: Diagnostic coding shifts, controversies regarding the sleeping environment, and new variables to consider in reducing risk. *Pediatrics, 116*(5), 1245-1255.

Ateah, C. A., Secco, L. & Woodgate, R. L. (2003). The risks and alternatives to physical punishment use with children. *J Pediatr Health Care, 17*(3), 126-132.

Bayley, N. (2005). Bayley scales of infant development-II. Available through Psychological Assessment Resources, Inc. at www3.parinc.com/products/product.aspO?Productid=BSID-II.

Beltrán-Aguilar, E. D., Barker, L. K., Canto, M. T., et al. (2005). Surveillance for Dental Caries, Dental Sealants, Tooth Retention, Edentulism, and Enamel Fluorosis, United States, 1988-1994 and 1999-2002. *MMWR, 54*(03), 1-44.

Berk, L. E. (2004). *Development through the lifespan* (3rd ed.). Boston: Allyn & Bacon.

Blackwell, P. B., & Baker, B. M. (2002). Estimating communication competence of infants and toddlers. *J Pediatr Health Care, 16*(1), 29-35.

Bricker, D., & Squires, J. (1999). *Ages & stages questionnaires: A parent-completed, child-monitoring system* (2nd ed.). Baltimore: Paul H. Brookes.

Burns, C. E., Brady, M. A., Dunn, A. M., & Starr, N. B. (2004). *Pediatric primary care: A handbook for nurse practitioners* (3rd ed.). Philadelphia: Saunders.

Carey, W. B. (1998). Teaching parents about infant temperament. *Pediatrics, 102*(5), 1311-1316.

Chess, S., & Thomas, A. (1986). *Temperament in clinical practice.* New York: Guilford Press.

Cunningham, M., Cox, E. O., the Committee on Practice and Ambulatory Medicine, & the Section on Otolaryngology and Bronchoesophagology. (2003). Hearing assessment in infants and children: Recommendations beyond neonatal screening. *Pediatrics, 111*(3), 436-440.

Davis, K. F., Parker, K. P., & Montgomery, G. L. (2004a). Sleep in infants and young children: Part One: Normal sleep. *J Pediatr Health Care, 18*(2), 65-71.

Davis, K. F., Parker, K. P., & Montgomery, G. L. (2004b). Sleep in infants and young children: Part Two: Common sleep problems. *J Pediatr Health Care, 18*(3), 130-137.

Denver Developmental Materials, Inc. (2006). Denver-II. Retrieved May 11, 2006, from www.denverii.com/DenverII.html.

Dion, S., & Stadtler, A. (2002). Age-specific observations of the parent-child interaction. In M. Jellinek, B. P. Patel, & M. C. Froehle (Eds.). *Bright futures in practice: Mental health,* Vol. II. Tool Kit. Arlington, VA: National Center for Education in Maternal and Child Health.

Fluoride Recommendations Workgroup. (2001). Recommendations for using fluoride to prevent and control dental caries in the United States. *MMWR, 50*(RR14), 1-42.

Glassy, D., Romano, J., & the American Academy of Pediatrics Committee on Early Childhood, Adoption, and Dependent Care. (2003). Selecting appropriate toys for young children: The pediatrician's role. *Pediatrics, 111*(4), 911-913.

Gottesman, M. M. (1999). Enabling parents to "read" their baby. *J Pediatr Health Care, 13*(3), 148-151.

Green, M., & Palfrey, J. S. (Eds.). (2002). *Bright futures: Guidelines for health supervision of infants, children, and adolescents* (2nd ed., rev.). Arlington, VA: National Center for Education in Maternal and Child Health.

Hill, N. H., & Sullivan, L. M. (2004). *Management guidelines for nurse practitioners working with children and adolescents* (2nd ed.). Philadelphia: F. A. Davis.

Kemper, A. R., Cohn, L. M., Fant, K. E., et al. (2005). Follow-up testing among children with elevated screening blood lead levels. *JAMA, 293,* 2232-2237.

Kochanska, G., Friesenborg, A. E., Lange, L. A., et al. (2004). Parents' personality and infants' temperament as contributors to their emerging relationship. *J Personal Social Psychol, 86* (5), 744-59.

Kube, D. A., Wilson, W. M., Petersen, M. C., & Palmer, F. B. (2000). CAT/CLAMS: Its use in detecting early childhood cognitive impairment. *Pediatric Neurol, 23*(3), 208-215.

Leung, A. K. C., & Lemay, J. F. (2004). Infantile colic: A review. *J Royal Soc Health, 124*(4), 162-266.

Lobo, M. L., Kotzer, A. M., Keefe, M. R., et al. (2004). Current beliefs and management strategies for treating infant colic. *J Pediatr Health Care, 18*(3), 115-122.

Ludington-Hoe, S. M., Cong, O, & Hashemi, F. (2002). Infant crying: Nature, physiologic consequences, and select interventions. *Neonatal Network, 21*(2), 29-36.

McCarthy, P. L. (2004). The well child. In R. E. Behrman, R. M. Kliegman, & H. B. Jenson (Eds.). *Nelson textbook of pediatrics* (17th ed.). Philadelphia: Saunders, pp. 20-22.

Moon, R. Y. (2001). Are you talking to patents about SIDS? *Contemp Pediatr, 18*(3), 122-129.

Muscari, M. E. (2000). *Advanced pediatric clinical assessment: Skills and procedures.* Philadelphia: Lippincott Williams & Wilkins.

National Association of Pediatric Nurse Practitioners. (2001). *Breastfeeding.* Retrieved January 8, 2006 from http://www.napnap.org/index.cfm?page=10&sec=54&ssec=57

National Association of Pediatric Nurse Practitioners. (2003). *The PNPs role in supporting infant and family well-being during the first year of life.* Retrieved January 8, 2006 from http://www.napnap.org/index.cfm?page=10&sec=54&ssec=70

Pohl, C. A., & Renwick, A. (2002). Putting sleep disturbances to rest. *Contemp Pediatr, 19*(11), 74-94.

Poppell, S. L. (2002). Bed-sharing with infants. *MCN, Am J Matern Child Nurs, 27*(3):193.

Shea, K. M. (2003). Pediatric exposure and potential toxicity of phthalate plasticizers. *Pediatrics, 111*(6), 1467-1474.

Shields, B. J., & Smith, G. A. (2006). Success in the prevention of infant walker-related injuries: an analysis of national data, 1990-2001. *Pediatrics, 117*, e452-e459.

Soltis, J. (2004). The signal functions of early infant crying. *Behavioral and Brain Sciences, 27*(4), 443-458.

# Preterm Infant Follow-up Care

MARY ENZMAN HAGEDORN, PhD, RN, HNC, CNS, CPNP

1. Prematurity (March of Dimes PeriStats, 2006)
   a. About 12.3% of all births were premature in 2003, i.e., fewer than 37 completed weeks of gestation
   b. Classifications of prematurity based on gestation (Table 20-1)
      i. Preterm
      ii. Very preterm
   c. Classifications of prematurity based on birth weight (see Table 20-1)
      i. Low birth weight (LBW)
      ii. Very low birth weight (VLBW)
      iii. Extremely low birth weight (ELBW)
   d. Prematurity rate increased by 13% between 1992 and 2002
   e. Rates are highest for Blacks (17.6%) compared with Native Americans (12.9%), Hispanics (11.4%), whites (10.7%), Asians (10.2%)
   f. 49% to 95% of preterm infants survive after premature birth depending on their weight at birth
   g. Advances in neonatal intensive care have dramatically improved the survival rates of preterm infants but they are likely to have special needs in one or more body systems (DeLoian, 2002; Hagedorn, et al., 2002)
2. Common medical problems of preterm infants after discharge
   a. Chronic lung disease (CLD)/bronchopulmonary dysplasia (BPD)
      i. 17% to 54% of premature graduates of the NICU suffer from CLD or BPD (Hagedorn, et al., 2002)
      ii. A disorder of premature infants that is characterized by respiratory distress and impaired gas exchange
      iii. An iatrogenic disease caused by oxygen toxicity and barotraumas resulting from pressure ventilation
      iv. Signs and symptoms: excessive bronchial secretions, narrowed airways, and ineffective oxygen and carbon dioxide exchange
      v. Severe forms result in a dependence on supplemental oxygen, decreased exercise tolerance, increased work of breathing, and a vulnerability to infections
      vi. Alters the infant's energy use with implications for feeding, nutrition, growth, cardiovascular function, behavior, and neurodevelopmental issues

■ **TABLE 20-1**
■ ■ **Glossary Related to Preterm Infants**

| Term | Definition | Incidence and Prevalence |
|---|---|---|
| Preterm infant | Less than 37 completed weeks of gestation | 9246 born per week 12.1% of all births |
| Very preterm infant | Less than 32 completed weeks of gestation | 1497 born per week |
| Low birth weight | Birth weight <2500g | 6040 born per week 50% of all NICU admissions |
| Very low birth weight | Birth weight <1500g | 1126 born per week 25% of all NICU admissions |
| Extremely low birth weight | Birth weight <1000g | 1% of all NICU admissions |
| Chronological or birth age | Time since birth | |
| Gestational age | Estimated time since conception; postconceptual age | |
| Corrected age | Age corrected for prematurity | |

Deloian, B (2002). The premature infant. In J. Fox (Ed.). *Primary health care of infants, children, & adolescents.*
St. Louis: Mosby; and March of Dimes PeriStats available at www.marchofdimes.com/peristats/pdflib/195/99.pdf.

vii. Most infants with BPD/CLD slowly grow out of their worst symptoms of chronic lung disease through a regimented comprehensive treatment plan aimed at maintaining adequate nutrition, minimizing cardiac demands, and preventing respiratory infections

viii. Pharmacologic therapy for respiratory problems in preterm infants (Table 20-2)

ix. In a small number of infants, the respiratory insufficiency is so severe that cardiac function is compromised and a steady downhill progression occurs

b. Acute respiratory infections

i. Preterm infants are more susceptible to pneumonias (Atkuri & Ferguson, 2006)

ii. Can result in severe and sometimes catastrophic outcomes in the presence of CLD

iii. VLBW infants are highly susceptible to RSV and bronchitis in the first year of life

c. Apnea of prematurity

i. About 23% of premature infants have apnea

ii. Most cases of apnea in premature infants are idiopathic (40% of apnea episodes are central; 50% are mixed; and 10% are obstructive)

iii. Identifiable causes include gastroesophageal reflux, anemia, sepsis, meningitis, upper airway obstruction, hypoxia, and bronchospasm (Hagedorn, et al., 2002)

iv. Despite apnea monitoring being controversial and an unproven method of preventing SIDS, many premature infants with documented apnea are discharged with provisions of at-home monitoring

v. Newer apnea monitors are capable of recording respiratory and heart rates, and oximetry

vi. Infants with apnea often respond to caffeine (loading dose of 20-40mg/kg is given and a maintenance dose of 5–8 mg/kg/day is administered 24 hours after loading dose) (Hagedorn, et al., 2002)

vii. Parents should be competent in management of apnea monitors and in age-appropriate CPR

**■ TABLE 20-2**
**■ ■ Respiratory Medications Commonly Used for Premature Infants**

| Drug | Dosage | Comments |
|---|---|---|
| **Apnea** | | |
| Caffeine citrate | 5–8 mg/kg/day | Administer in the morning because sleep pattern may be disturbed<br>Can cause tachycardia, hyperglycemia, jitteriness, seizures |
| **Bronchodilator** | | |
| Albuterol (Proventil, Ventolin) | 0.1 mg/kg up to 5 mg in 2 ml of NS q 4–6 hr | Drug of choice for bronchospasm<br>Can cause hyperactivity and tachcardia |
| **Histamine Inhibitor** | | |
| Cromolyn 20 mg/2ml | 10–20 mg/tid | Prevents release of inflammatory mediators and reduces airway hypersensitivity<br>Can cause uticaria, rash, throat irritation |
| **Diuretics** | | |
| Furosemide | 2–4 mg/kg/dose PO bid | Treatment for CHF symptoms, fluid overload in BPD/CLD<br>Can cause metabolic alkalosis, hypokalemia, hypocalcemia, hypochloremia, hyponatremia, renal calcifications, ototoxicity |
| **Thiazides** | | |
| Chlorothiazide | 5–20 mg/kg/dose PO bid | Less potent than furosemide, promotes potassium and bicarbonate excretion with sodium and chloride, spares calcium<br>Can cause electrolyte imbalance, hypercalcemia, hyperglycemia, decreased magnesium level, hypersensitivity, GI upset, glycosuria |
| Hydrochlorothiazide | 1–2 mg/kg/dose PO bid | Can cause electrolyte imbalance, hypercalcemia, hyperglycemia, metabolic alkalosis, increased urinary losses of sodium, potassium, magnesium, chloride, phosphorus, and bicarbonate; spares calcium |
| Spironolactone | 1–5 mg/kg/ dose PO bid | Weak diuretic; causes increased sodium chloride and water loss; spares potassium<br>Can cause irritability, lethargy, vomiting, diarrhea, rash |
| Bumetanide | 0.015 to 0.1 mg/kg/day PO | 40 times the potency of furosemide; used in neonates and infants who are refractory to furosemide therapy<br>Same side effects as furosemide |

   **d.** Patent ductus arteriosus (PDA) (see Chapter 42)
      **i.** The transitional process between intrauterine and extrauterine life requires the closure of the PDA that in utero connected the aorta and the pulmonary artery
      **ii.** The PDA may not close in the premature infant
      **iii.** Closure may be accomplished through medication or a surgical ligation
   **e.** Chronic cardiac insufficiency, cor pulmonale, or congestive heart failure
      **i.** Cor pulmonale: heart becomes enlarged, pumps less efficiently, and causes total body fluid overload, which further compromises pulmonary function (Hagedorn, et al., 2002)
      **ii.** In infants with chronic cardiac insufficiency, recovery of normal cardiac function parallels recovery of pulmonary function

    **f.** Necrotizing enterocolitis (NEC)

        **i.** A destructive infection of the small bowel, with associated signs of severe illness, excessive bleeding, cardiovascular collapse, or respiratory decompensation

        **ii.** VLBW and ELBW infants are susceptible due to immaturity of the digestive system, and increased vulnerability to tissue injury

        **iii.** NEC occurs in 1 in 1000 live births; in VLBW infants it is 5 in 100 live births

        **iv.** The ileocecal region is most commonly involved (50%), followed by the large and small intestines (25%)

        **v.** Up to 15% of infants with NEC will have necrosis of the bowel and significant risk of death or short bowel syndrome (Bensard, et al., 2002)

        **vi.** More than half the infants will respond to medical treatment, but of those, 30% develop strictures that require surgical management

        **vii.** Survival rates of VLBW infants have improved from 50% to 80% over the past two decades

        **viii.** ELBW infants still have a mortality rate of 50% (Bensard, et al., 2002)

    **g.** Gastroesophageal reflux (GER)

        **i.** Reflux often presents as regurgitation but can also manifest as apnea, aspiration pneumonia, or worsening BPD/CLD

        **ii.** Common in preterm infants

        **iii.** Giving the infant smaller, more frequent feedings may be useful, along with 30-degree angle positioning for up to an hour after feedings

        **iv.** Pharmacologic therapy for GER (see Table 20-3)

        **v.** Surgery may be required in severe cases of reflux when weight gain cannot be established

    **h.** Retinopathy of prematurity (ROP)

        **i.** ROP is a disease of prematurity in which the incidence is inversely proportional to the gestational age (Hagedorn, et al., 2002)

        **ii.** Occurs in 9% to 24% of premature infants born at 32 weeks of gestation or less and leads to blindness in 1% to 4%

        **iii.** Highest incidence in infants younger than 28 weeks of gestation and in VLBW and ELBW infants

        **iv.** ROP is classified by location of disease in the retina (zone), by degree (stage) of vascular abnormality, and the extent of developing vasculature (clock hour) (National Eye Institute, 2005)

            **(a)** Stage I—mildly abnormal blood vessel growth

            **(b)** Stage II—moderately abnormal blood vessel growth

---

■ **TABLE 20-3**
■ ■ **Medications for Gastrointestinal Reflux**

| Drug | Dosage | Comments |
|---|---|---|
| Metoclopramide | 0.1 mg/kg divided q 8hr | GI smooth muscle stimulant |
| Omeprazole | 0.3–3 mg/kg divided q 12hr PO | Gastric acid pump inhibitor Recommended starting dose 0.7 mg/kg PO in morning |
| Ranitidine | 3–4 mg/kg divided q 8hr PO | $H_2$ agonist |

From Bensard, D, Calkins, C, Partrick, D, Price, F (2002). Neonatal Surgery. In G. Merenstein & S. Gardner (Eds.), *Handbook of neonatal intensive care* (5th Ed.) (p. 707). St. Louis: Mosby Yearbook.

          (c) Stage III—severely abnormal blood vessel growth; the abnormal blood vessels grow toward the center of the eye instead of following their normal growth pattern along the surface of the retina

          (d) Stage IV—partially detached retina; traction from the scar produced by bleeding, abnormal vessels pull the retina away from the wall of the eye

          (e) Stage V—completely detached retina and the end stage of the disease; if not treated, the infant can have severe visual impairment and even blindness

      v. Treatment with laser/cryotherapy is associated with a 50% decrease in retinal detachment; however long-term visual consequences of laser surgery are unknown (Hagedorn, et al., 2002)

      vi. Screening examinations of preterm infants for ROP is essential

      vii. A pediatric ophthalmologist is essential for ongoing management of ROP

  i. Strabismus and amblyopia

      i. Both are more common in premature infants

      ii. Because strabismus can be a sign of intraocular pathology, ophthalmologic consultation is indicated

      iii. In VLBW infants, strabismus at 6 weeks of age typically resolves by 9 months of age

      iv. Strabismus present at 9 months of age will probably persist

  j. Intraventricular hemorrhage (IVH)

      i. IVH arises from fragile immature blood vessels whose integrity was disturbed by a disorder of prematurity that might include hypoxia; low blood pressure, or infection

      ii. The incidence of IVH in VLBW ranges from 30% to 50%

      iii. Less than 10% of VLBW infants with mild IVH result in hydrocephalus

      iv. With grade IV bleeds, 50% to 60% of preterm infants die, and 65% to 100% of survivors will develop hydrocephalus

      v. Premature ELBW infants experience higher rates of neurologic and neurosensory impairments

      vi. Neurologic sequelae include seizures, hydrocephalus, cerebral palsy, periventricular leukomalacia, and mental retardation

          (a) 17% to 23% of VLBW infants have sequelae

          (b) 20% to 41% in ELBW infants have sequelae

  k. Hernias

      i. Inguinal

          (a) More common in male infants with a history of prematurity and ventilatory assistance

          (b) The incidence is 30% in VLBW and ELBW infants

          (c) Approximately 10% to 50% of inguinal hernias are bilateral

          (d) Premature infants have very small internal rings and the risk of incarceration is high; therefore these infants should be referred for surgical intervention

      ii. Umbilical hernias

          (a) Rarely incarcerate; therefore can be managed with observation

          (b) Usually reduce spontaneously by the time the child reaches 3 to 5 years of age

  l. Undescended testicles

      i. Premature birth slows the descent of the testicles and only 26% of testes are intrascrotal by the time the premature male reaches term age

       **ii.** By 1 year, 94% of testes are intrascrotal

       **iii.** Surgical consultation should be considered if testicles have not descended by age 1

  **m.** Anemia

       **i.** Factors that lead to anemia include lower iron stores due to prematurity; lower erythropoietin production compared with term infants; and frequent blood sampling during the NICU stay

       **ii.** During primary care and preterm follow-up visits, tachycardia, poor feeding, poor weight gain, and apnea with bradycardia may indicate the presence of anemia

       **iii.** A blood count should be checked if these symptoms are identified

       **iv.** Iron supplementation reduces the level and duration of anemia

          **(a)** Recommended dosage is 2 to 4 mg/kg/day for 12 to 15 months

          **(b)** Many preterm infants continue to be more vulnerable to respiratory and gastrointestinal infections throughout infancy that may require rehospitalization for treatment

  **n.** Many preterm infants require multiple medications and/or durable medical equipment (e.g., apnea monitors, nebulizers, feeding pumps, and suction) in their homes after discharge and over the first year of life

  **o.** Some conditions may not manifest until infancy or childhood (e.g., cerebral palsy, sensorimotor disabilities, developmental disabilities, attention deficit disorder, asthma)

**3.** Premature infant follow-up programs

  **a.** Emerged to provide focused, holistic comprehensive care in conjunction with the infant's primary care provider such as a pediatric nurse practitioner

  **b.** The primary goal for families and premature infants is normalization (Deloian, 2002)

  **c.** Preterm infants with growth and weight concerns should have more frequent health maintenance visits compared to full-term newborns

  **d.** Coordination of health care and timely intervention and follow-up is an important role for the PNP

  **e.** Abnormalities found during initial screening frequently require consultation with other specialists and follow-up programs designed for integrated management of the complex needs of the preterm infant

  **f.** The PNP must be sensitive to the issues of parental support and family dynamics

  **g.** Inquiries about potential social problems should be part of every visit to detect clues of family strain, neglect, or abuse

**4.** First preterm infant follow-up visit

  **a.** Guidelines for a typical newborn or infant well-child visit (Chapter 19) should be followed

  **b.** Concerns unique to preterm infants will be listed below

  **c.** Maternal birth history related to this birth

       **i.** Alcohol or drug exposure

       **ii.** Therapeutic medications (e.g., corticosteroids)

       **iii.** Complications of pregnancy

       **iv.** Pregnancy-induced hypertension

       **v.** Preterm labor

       **vi.** Placenta previa, or placental abruption

       **vii.** Smoking

       **viii.** Poor maternal weight gain

       **ix.** Violence or trauma affecting mother

    **x.** TORCH (toxoplasmosis, rubella, cytomegalovirus, herpes simplex, and others, such as syphilis) infections

    **xi.** Complications of delivery (hemorrhage)

  **d.** Infant birth history

    **i.** Complications during labor and delivery (e.g., asphyxia, low Apgar scores, traumatic or prolonged delivery)

    **ii.** Determine the age of the child (see Table 20-1)

      (a) Chronologic age

      (b) Gestational age

      (c) Age-corrected for prematurity (Box 20-1)

  **e.** Infant's history since discharge from NICU

    **i.** Illnesses

    **ii.** Emergency department visits, operations and hospitalizations

    **iii.** Accidents—precipitating factors and sequelae

  **f.** Developmental screening and assessment (see Chapter 19, Section 5 for details)

    **i.** Use developmental screening tools that have been standardized for preterm infants (e.g., Bayley, First Step)

    **ii.** In the study, Perception of Child Vulnerability Among Mothers of Former Premature Infants (Allen, et al., 2004):

      (a) Preterms were more likely to have worse developmental outcomes at age 1 if their mothers perceived them as being medically vulnerable

      (b) Mothers who were most anxious when their babies were discharged from the hospital also were most likely to perceive them as medically vulnerable a year later

      (c) Efforts to reduce parental perception of child vulnerability should be targeted toward more anxious parents

      (d) Interventions may prevent unnecessary health care and result in improved developmental outcomes in premature infants

    **iii.** A study showed that at age 7, children who were born at less than 29 weeks of gestation were more likely to be bullied by their peers than those born full term (Nadeau, et al., 2004)

  **g.** Immunizations—request history of immunizations given in the NICU

  **h.** Allergies to medications, food, and environmental factors

  **i.** Current habits

    **i.** Nutrition: formula or breast-feeding (calculate calories/kg/day), vitamin and/or iron supplements, solid foods

    **ii.** Feeding: parental satisfaction, feeding routines, self-feeding, feeding problems (e.g., gagging, bottle or food refusal, oral aversion, swallowing or chewing problems, vomiting, gastroesophageal reflux, colic, delayed self-feeding)

■ **BOX 20-1**
■ **EXAMPLE OF A FORMULA FOR ADJUSTING AGE FOR PREMATURITY**

---

34-week-gestation infant = 40–34 = 6 weeks, or 1 month and 2 weeks early
Chronologic age: 6 months 3 weeks
          Less: *1 month 2 weeks*
          Corrected age: 5 months 1 week

---

Adapted from Deloian, B (2002). The premature infant. In J. Fox (Ed.). *Primary health care of infants, children, & adolescents.* St. Louis: Mosby

      iii. Sleep-wake cycle: pattern, habituation, nighttime rituals, problems in sleep pattern or duration

      iv. Elimination: patterns, problems with constipation, retention, diarrhea

      v. Muscle tone: hypotonia, hypertonia, spasticity, tremors, lack of muscle coordination (tripping, falling)

      vi. Behavior

        (a) State of transitions and control, problems with transition in activities

        (b) Irritability, touch aversion, environmental aversion

        (c) Inattentiveness, lack of concentration, alertness, responsiveness to caregiver

**j.** Growth problems or delays

**k.** Continuing medical conditions

**l.** Medications

    **i.** Review dosages, effectiveness, and side effects of current medications

    **ii.** Revise dosages relative to child's growth

    **iii.** Educate parents on medication purposes, dosages, side effects, etc.

**m.** Physical examination

    **i.** See Chapters 5 to 13 for details on systems review

    **ii.** Aspects of physical examination unique to the preterm infant are described below

      (a) Graph height, weight, head circumference, and weight-length ratio using *corrected* age until 2 to 3 years of age

      (b) Growth charts (Centers for Disease Control and Prevention, 2006)

        (1) The CDC's revised growth charts can be used with LBW infants, but were not standardized for VLBW infants (available at www.cdc.gov/growthcharts)

        (2) There are charts for VLBW infants (Ehrenkranz, 1999) but they only extend to about 120 days uncorrected postnatal age or up to body weight of 2000 g

        (3) The Infant Health and Development Program (IHDP) growth charts may be used for VLBW infants from an age corrected for gestation of 40 weeks to 36 months, but norms are based on data collected in 1985, which was before current medical and nutritional care practices were being used

        (4) If CDC charts are used for VLBW infants after that point, recognize that their patterns of growth will be similar, but measurements may fall in the lower percentiles

      (c) Throat—evaluate suck-swallow rhythm, tongue thrust, oral aversion, uvula movement, hyperactive or hypoactive gag reflex

      (d) Respiratory tract

        (1) Observe for symmetry of chest movement, respiratory distress, retractions, stridor

        (2) Monitor closely for RSV—wheezing, rhinorrhea, pharyngitis, cough, sneezing, and low-grade fever

      (e) Neck and shoulders—delayed or poor head control, tight scarf sign, decreased shoulder tone (distress in being placed prone), difficulty bringing hand to midline

      (f) Trunk—arching, decreased range of motion, hypotonia (decreased strength, delayed sitting)

      (g) Extremities—hypertonia, hypotonia, passive tone, hand-mouth coordination, eye-hand coordination, gait, hyperreflexia, clonus

    (h) Reflexes
      (1) Delayed integration of primitive reflexes: Moro reflex, asymmetric tonic neck, palmar or plantar grasp, placing, step
      (2) Delayed emergence of protective reflexes (Dzinkowski, 2000):
        a) Landau reflex—if infant is held in a horizontal prone position, the infant will lift head and extend the neck and trunk. When the neck is passively flexed, the entire body will flex. This reflex is present by 6 months and hypotonicity (low tone) indicates motor system deficits
        b) Parachute reflex—infant is held around the waist in a horizontal prone position and then lowered slowly, head first to the surface. By age 6 to 8 months the infant should respond by extending the arms and hands to break the "fall." If this response is asymmetric, it indicates an unilateral motor abnormality
        c) Propping reflexes—anterior propping: when sitting up, infant will extend the arms forward to catch himself and prevent falling forward; followed by lateral propping: infant extends the arm laterally to catch himself; develops at 5 to 7 months of age
    (i) Sensory systems
      (1) Touch—observe for aversive behaviors to touch, especially around mouth, difficulty being held, poor sensory integration
      (2) Hearing assessment (AAP, 2000)
        a) Premature infants require more extensive hearing evaluations
        b) 5% of premature infants born before 32 weeks of gestation have hearing loss by 5 years of age
        c) Brainstem auditory-evoked response hearing test should be repeated at 3 to 4 months of age
        d) Tympanometry and acoustic reflex should be tested at each visit
        e) Premature infants are more prone to ear infections, which may contribute to the hearing loss
      (3) Visual assessment—refer to ophthalmologist if:
        a) Abnormal findings
        b) Infant less than 32 week of gestation and received oxygen
        c) Infants less than 28 weeks of gestation
        d) Repeat exam again at 3 to 6 months of age

**n.** Laboratory tests
    **i.** A complete blood cell (CBC) and reticulocyte count should be checked between 2 and 4 months or sooner if Epogen was used
    **ii.** Hemoglobin and hematocrit should be checked according to chronologic age
    **iii.** Oxygen saturation levels should be monitored if the infant has chronic lung disease

**o.** Immunizations—the following vaccines should be given in full doses according to chronologic age and schedule (Kirmani, et al., 2002):
    **i.** Diphtheria, tetanus, and acellular pertussis (DTaP)
    **ii.** Hepatitis B
    **iii.** *Haemophilus influenzae* type B (Hib)
    **iv.** Inactivated polio vaccine (IPV)
    **v.** Prevnar to prevent pneumococcal meningitis and pneumonia
    **vi.** Influenza vaccine for infants older than 6 months of age with bronchopulmonary disease (BPD) or chronic lung disease (CLD) or other chronic illnesses

vii. RSV vaccine—see AAP policy statement (AAP, 2003; Meissner, et al., 2003)

    (a) Palivizumab is preferred for children with a history of preterm birth *and* two or more risk factors for RSV

    (b) Monthly administration of palivizumab during the RSV season results in a 45% to 55% decrease in the rate of hospitalization attributable to RSV

**5.** Nutritional needs of preterm infants

  **a.** Breast-feeding is the first choice for premature infants

    **i.** Breast milk protects against infection

    **ii.** Breast-fed infants have better developmental scores at 18 months of age than formula-fed infants

    **iii.** The infant should be encouraged to nurse every 2 to 3 hours

    **iv.** Most mothers of premature infants need reassurance and support with breast-feeding

  **b.** Vitamin, mineral, and iron requirements are same as normal infants (see Chapter 16 for details)

  **c.** Caloric requirements

    **i.** Preterm infants need 110 to 150 kcal/kg/day to achieve adequate growth

    **ii.** Infants with BPD/CLD, GER, cerebral palsy, cardiac problems, formula intolerance, or other chronic illnesses may require 200 kcal/kg/day

    **iii.** Breast milk and standard formulas contain 20 kcal/oz

    **iv.** Human milk fortifier may be added to breast milk

    **v.** Similac Neosure (24 cal/oz) or Enfamil 22 is most often used for the first year of life

    **vi.** Formula companies provide dilution instructions for use with preterm infants

    **vii.** The calorie content of formulas can be increased by adding polycose, vegetable oils, or medium chain triglyceride oils

    **viii.** Most preterm infants do not tolerate formulas containing more than 30 kcal/oz

  **d.** Hyperosmolality of the higher calorie formulas can predispose the preterm infant to a higher risk for hyperosmolar dehydration

  **e.** In the infant with CLD or short gut, vomiting and diarrhea may result in the rapid development of severe dehydration; therefore close monitoring is required

  **f.** ELBW infants may require nasogastric or gastrostomy feeding during the night to promote weight gain (Daley & Kennedy, 2000)

  **g.** Feeding difficulties

    **i.** Feeding is the most common problem for the VLBW infant at home due to easy fatigability and poor state regulation (Daley & Kennedy, 2000; Deloian, 2002)

    **ii.** The length and frequency of feedings must be increased

  **h.** Introduction of solids should occur at 6 months after due date

  **i.** Cow's milk can be started at 12 months after the due date

  **j.** Preterm infants require more catch-up time and require formula beyond 12 months of age

**6.** Role of PNP in primary care of premature infants

  **a.** On discharge from the NICU, primary care settings should be the medical home of preterm infants and manage referrals to specialists and community agencies

  **b.** PNP role (Ritchie, 2002)

      **i.** PNP can assume the role of primary care provider for many preterm infants

      **ii.** Collaboration and communication are important ingredients in the goal of providing comprehensive, family-focused care

      **iii.** For each patient, maintain a list of active diagnoses, health needs, and referrals made

         (a) Some referrals may need to be reactivated periodically

         (b) Physical therapy and occupational therapy are priorities

      **iv.** Encourage parents to keep a notebook with similar information, including the NICU discharge summary, immunizations, referral names and contact information, etc.

      **v.** Assist parents to serve as advocates for their child

      **vi.** Uncover parent concerns and help them recognize the need for referrals and resources

      **vii.** Help parents navigate health care service systems

   **c.** Resources that are often needed by the family of a premature include:

      **i.** Parent support groups and parents of premature infants

      **ii.** Community health or home health nursing

      **iii.** Occupation and physical therapists

      **iv.** Speech and language therapists

      **v.** Vision and hearing interventions

      **vi.** Regional centers or community centers focusing on developmental disabilities

      **vii.** Early Intervention Program for Infants and Toddlers with Disabilities—government supported program designed to provide preventive and treatment services to children and families (see www.nectac.org/&sim;pdfs/idea/303pp.pdf)

      **viii.** Literature and resources

      **ix.** Family/individual counseling (stress management, family dynamics, grief)

         (a) Preterm infants are at risk for child abuse

         (b) Teach parents about normal infant crying and the dangers of shaken baby syndrome (see Chapter 19, Section 7 for more details on this topic)

**7.** Long-term implications/prognosis:

   **a.** ELBW and VLBW infants often have myriad medical and developmental conditions with conflicting reports on the outcomes

   **b.** Most research literature concludes that 50% to 70% of ELBW infants will have multiple medical conditions and neurologic sequelae that require a variety of services and interventions (Kilbride, et al., 2004)

   **c.** More than 50% of VLBW and ELBW infants from a large cohort evaluated at 30 months corrected age had disabilities in mental and psychomotor development, neurofunctioning, sensory (visual and hearing loss), and speech delays (Wood, et al., 2000)

   **d.** Other studies have described higher numbers of ELBW infants with behavioral, fine motor, and educational difficulties

   **e.** Newer studies have also found similar issues with the neurologic and developmental disabilities in the ELBW infant

   **f.** 44% to 56% of a population of VLBW infants manifested CP, mental retardation, blindness and deafness; 37% of VLBW infants in a research cohort had undergone at least one surgical procedure, 8% had undergone two, and 6% had undergone three procedures during the first year of life. These surgeries include strabismus correction, ear tube placement, tonsillectomy and adenoidectomy, hernia repair, circumcision, and surgery for undescended testicles

g. Overall outcomes improve for the LBW infant when compared with VLBW and ELBW infants; the statistics improve dramatically for LBW infants

## REFERENCES

Allen, E. C., Manuel, J. C., Legault, C., et al. (2004). Perception of child vulnerability among mothers of former premature infants. *Pediatrics, 113*(2), 267-273.

Ambalabanan, N., Nelson, K.G., Alexander, G., et al. (2000). Prediction of neurologic morbidity in extremely low birth weight infants. *J Perinatol, 20*(8), 496-503.

American Academy of Pediatrics Committee on Infectious Diseases and Committee on Fetus and Newborn. (2003). Revised indications for the use of palivizumab and respiratory syncytial virus immune globulin intravenous for the prevention of respiratory syncytial virus infections. *Pediatrics, 112*(6), 1442-1446.

American Academy of Pediatrics. Joint Committee on Infant Hearing. (2000). Position statement: Principles and guidelines for early hearing detection and intervention programs. *Pediatrics, 106*(4), 798-817.

Atkuri, L. V., & Ferguson, L. E. (2006). Pediatrics, pneumonia. Retrived from Medicine on April 1, 2006 at http://www.emedicine.com/emerg/topic396.htm

Bensard, D., Calkins, C., Partrick, D., & Price, F. (2002). Neonatal surgery. In G. Merenstein & S. Gardner (Eds.). *Handbook of neonatal intensive care* (5th ed.). St. Louis: Mosby Yearbook, pp. 702-724.

Centers for Disease Control and Prevention. (2006). 2000 growth charts: United States. Retrieved April 1, 2006, from www.cdc.gov/growthcharts.

Daley, H., & Kennedy, C. (2000). Meta-analysis: Effects of interventions in premature infant feeding. *J Perinatal Neonatal Nurs, 14*(3), 62-70.

Deloian, B. (2002). The premature infant. In J. Fox (Ed.). *Primary health care of infants, children, & adolescents.* St. Louis: Mosby.

Dzinkowkski, R. C. (2000). Symptoms and signs of cerebral palsy if present in infants and toddlers. Retrieved June 6, 2006, from www.geocities.com/aneecp/symptoms.htm. Originally published as: Dzinkowkski, R. C., Smith, K. K., Dillow, K. A., & Yucha,

C. B. (1996). Cerebral palsy: A comprehensive review. *Nurse Pract, 21*(2), 45-59.

Ehrenkranz, R.A., Younes, N., Lemons, J.A., et al. (1999). Longitudinal growth of hospitalized very low birth weight infants. *Pediatrics, 104,* 280-289.

Hagedorn, M., Gardner, S., & Abman, S. (2002). Respiratory diseases. In G. Merenstein & S. Gardner (Eds.). *Handbook of neonatal intensive care* (5th ed.). St. Louis: Mosby, pp. 485-575.

Kilbride, H. W., Thorstad, K., & Daily, D. K. (2004). Preschool outcome of less than 801-gram preterm infants compared with full-term siblings. *Pediatrics, 113*(4), 742-747.

Kirmani, K. I., Lofthus, G., Pichichero, M. E., Voloshen, T., & D'Angio, C. T. (2002). Seven-year follow-up of vaccine response in extremely premature infants. *Pediatrics, 109*(3), 498-504.

March of Dimes PeriStats. (2006). Retrieved April 1, 2006, from www.marchofdimes.com/peristats/pdflib/195/99.pdf.

Meissner, H. C., Long, S. S., & American Academy of Pediatrics Committee on Infectious Diseases and Committee on Fetus and Newborn. (2003). Revised indications for the use of palivizumab and respiratory syncytial virus immune globulin intravenous for the prevention of respiratory syncytial virus infections. *Pediatrics, 112*(6), 1447-1452.

Nadeau, L., Tessier, R., Lefebvre, F., & Robaey, P. (2004). Victimization: a newly recognized outcome of prematurity. *Devel Med Child Neurol, 46*(8), 508-513.

National Eye Institute. (2005). Retinopathy of prematurity. Retrieved April 1, 2006, from www.nei.nih.gov/health/rop/index.asp#5.

Ritchie, S. K. (2002). Primary care of the premature infant discharged from the neonatal intensive care unit. *MCN, Am J Matern Child Nurs, 27*(2), 76-85.

Wood, N. S., Marlow, N., Costeloe, K., et al. (2000). Neurologic and developmental disability after extreme preterm birth. EPIcure Study Group. *N Engl J Med, 343*(6), 378-384.

# Child Abuse and Neglect

SANDRA L. ELVIK, MS, RN, CPNP

1. Definitions of child abuse and neglect
   a. The Federal Child Abuse Prevention and Treatment Act [CAPTA]) defines child abuse and neglect as causing a child to suffer past or recent harm due to acts of omission or commission on the part of a parent or caretaker that results in death, serious physical or emotional harm, sexual abuse, or exploitation (Hornor, 2005)
   b. Child abuse and neglect is more commonly called child maltreatment and has several subgroups
      i. Physical abuse—the infliction of physical injury
         (a) Physical punishment
         (b) Over-discipline
         (c) Other methods that harm a child
         (d) Examples:
             (1) Punching, kicking, beating
             (2) Biting
             (3) Burning
             (4) Shaking (shaken baby syndrome)
      ii. Neglect (Dubowitz, et al., 2000)
         (a) Noncompliance with health care recommendations
         (b) Delay or failure in getting health care
         (c) Inadequate food
         (d) Drug-exposed newborns and older children
         (e) Inadequate protection from environmental hazards
         (f) Inadequate supervision
         (g) Abandonment
         (h) Inadequate hygiene
         (i) Inadequate clothing
         (j) Educational needs not being met
     iii. Sexual abuse and exploitation - engaging children in sexual activity, including pornography (Leder, et al., 2001a; McColgan & Giardino, 2005):
         (a) That they cannot comprehend
         (b) For which they are developmentally unprepared
         (c) For which they cannot give informed consent
         (d) That violates societal taboos

iv. Emotional and psychologic abuse
  (a) Inadequate affection, nurturance, love
  (b) Includes bizarre forms of punishment, such as locking a child in a closet
  (c) Adult caretaker who yells at or belittles a child (Elvik, 1998)
  (d) Effects of chronic lack of parental nurturing may not be identified until years later, even into adulthood
v. Munchausen by proxy
  (a) Falsifying symptoms in child for psychologic benefit of parent

c. Discipline versus abuse
  i. Corporal punishment is often used as a disciplinary method by parents and other care providers
  ii. Corporal punishment is "the use of physical force with the intention of causing a child to experience pain, but not injury, for the purpose of correction or control of the child's behavior" (Straus, 1994)
  iii. NAPNAPs (2001) position statement on corporal punishment strongly opposes its use, based on the physical and psychological risk to children and on research that shows a relationship with long-term effects of impulsive and antisocial behavior
  iv. PNPs should assess families' disciplinary practices, "counsel parents to avoid those that are harmful, ineffective, or abusive and to educate parents on effective, age-appropriate alternative strategies" (NAPNAP, 2001b)

d. Incidence of child abuse (Rubin, et al., 2003)
  i. United States Department of Health and Human Services reports that among 906,000 children confirmed by child protective service agencies as being maltreated in 2003:
    (a) 61% were neglected; 19% were physically abused; 10% were sexually abused; and 5% were emotionally or psychologically abused
  ii. Of an estimated 1,500 children confirmed to have died from maltreatment:
    (a) 36% of these deaths were from neglect, 28% from physical abuse, and 29% from multiple maltreatment types
  iii. Males and females have similar rates of victimization

2. Historical perspective
  a. Maltreatment of children has been recorded since ancient times (Feldman, 1977)
    i. Infanticide was used to prevent depletion of family resources or to eliminate sickly children
    ii. Children through history have been sent to the streets as prostitutes or used in other ways as "marketable commodities" for the parents' benefit
    iii. Children were used for cheap labor as portrayed in Victorian literature, most notably by Charles Dickens
  b. The landmark case of Mary Ellen McCormick in 1874 (Kempe, et al., 1962)
    i. A young child was being severely beaten by her stepmother
    ii. No help from outside agencies because beatings could not be proven
    iii. Intervention was finally given by the New York Society for the Prevention of Cruelty to Animals on the basis that Mary Ellen could be considered an animal
      (a) The abusive mother's custodial rights were eventually terminated and Mary Ellen was adopted by a Methodist minister

        (b) The case was the basis for the formation of the New York Society for the Prevention of Cruelty to Children

        (c) Later it became the American Humane Society

  **c.** Child abuse as a problem recognized by health care professionals as "Battered Child Syndrome" came to the forefront in 1961 (Kempe, et al., 1962)

    **i.** "The Battered Child" was published in *JAMA*

    **ii.** Directed physicians to be responsible for evaluating children with suspicious injuries, to write the diagnosis of "battered child," and to report those injuries

    **iii.** Mandatory reporting laws were enacted in all 50 states between 1963 and 1968

    **iv.** Reporting laws targeted physicians and other health care providers

    **v.** Federal Child Abuse Prevention and Treatment Act initiated in 1974 and last amended in 2003

  **d.** New sources of risk to children stems from electronic media (McColgan & Giardino, 2005)

    **i.** Children ages 2 to 18 spend 38 hours per week (5 hours/day) using electronic media

    **ii.** Computers are in 71% of U.S. households with children ages 8 to 17

    **iii.** 67% of households have access to the Internet

    **iv.** Dramatically increases risks of exposure to:

        (a) Material that is inappropriate or encourages dangerous or illegal activities

        (b) Exposure to harassment through email, chat rooms

        (c) Engaging in activity that has legal ramifications

        (d) Exposure to predators who may lure children into meeting them in person

    **v.** Parents have a responsibility to monitor their children's access to and use of electronic media

**3.** Etiology of child abuse

  **a.** Child abuse crosses all social, economic, educational levels

  **b.** Certain characteristics are associated with increased risk for child maltreatment:

    **i.** Perpetrators of abuse

        (a) Young or inexperienced parent

        (b) Substance abuse

        (c) Intimate partner violence

        (d) Abused as children themselves

        (e) Stress

        (f) Depression

    **ii.** Abused children

        (a) Premature

        (b) Developmental delay

        (c) Congenital physical anomalies

        (d) Unusual temperament

        (e) Illegitimate or unwanted pregnancy

        (f) Attention-deficit, hyperactivity

        (g) Resemblance to someone the caretaker does not like

        (h) Bonding failure

        (i) Problem pregnancy

        (j) Difficult delivery

        (k) Placement in foster care

    iii. Caretaker factors
        (a) Little understanding of normal development of children
        (b) Expectations of their children are too high
        (c) Experienced severe punishment as a child
        (d) Poor impulse control
        (e) Free expression of violence
        (f) Social isolation
        (g) Poor social-emotional support system
        (h) Low self-esteem
        (i) Lack of educational achievement
        (j) History of psychiatric illness
        (k) Substance abuse
        (l) Lack of prenatal care
        (m) Single-parent home with mother head of household
        (n) Previous involvement with child protection services
        (o) Parent-child relationship role reversal
    iv. Environmental factors
        (a) Chronic stress
        (b) Unemployment
        (c) Divorce
        (d) Poverty
4. Clinical evaluation: general
    a. History (Hornor, 2005)
        i. PNP must be willing to admit that "good parents" can abuse their children
           (Elvik, 1998)
        ii. Complete history from parent or caretaker
            (a) Interview methods
                (1) Best if child and adult can be interviewed separately
                (2) Allow parent to lead the interview
                (3) If possible interview the child alone
                (4) Using open-ended nonleading questions
            (b) Timeline of injury
                (1) Note any delay in obtaining medical care
                (2) Who was present when injury occurred
                (3) Witnesses
            (c) History of present illness
            (d) Review of symptoms
            (e) Medical history
            (f) Family history
            (g) History of injury-related disorders
            (h) Suspicious information:
                (1) The child reports inflicted physical injury or sexual contact
                (2) A caretaker reports an incident that is incompatible with the
                    injury
                (3) The history of a physical injury is not consistent with child's level
                    of development
                (4) The account of how injury occurred changes over time
        iii. Family tree
            (a) Current living situation
            (b) Number of siblings with same or different fathers
            (c) Number of parental partners
        iv. Screen for emotional abuse or neglect

   **b.** General assessment
      **i.** Thorough physical examination
         (a) Body diagrams to illustrate site of injuries
         (b) Color photography
      **ii.** Note personal hygiene
      **iii.** Note child's behavior
         (a) Normal growth and developmental milestones
         (b) Appropriateness for child's age
   **c.** Behavioral manifestations
      **i.** Not specific to abuse, may be caused by other stressors
      **ii.** Suspicious behaviors:
         (a) Change in the child's normal pattern of eating, sleeping, toileting, interaction with others
         (b) School problems, runaway, suicide attempts
         (c) Excessive masturbation or sexualized activities (to the exclusion of most other solitary activities); inappropriate play for age
         (d) Anger, rage
         (e) Substance abuse
         (f) Withdrawal from family or peers
         (g) Genital and/or anal symptoms
         (h) Dressing inappropriately for the weather to cover up bruises
   **d.** Physical manifestations—variable depending on the type of child maltreatment
**5.** Clinical evaluation of the child with a fracture
   **a.** Accidental fractures increase as the child becomes more mobile
      **i.** Fractures in infants are suspect until proven otherwise
   **b.** Presentation:
      **i.** Immobility of limb
      **ii.** Swelling
      **iii.** Pain or crying with movement
   **c.** Diagnostic studies
      **i.** Skeletal x-rays
      **ii.** May be used in conjunction with:
         (a) Bone scan
         (b) CT scan of head
         (c) Serum calcium level
         (d) Alkaline phosphate
   **d.** Radiologic manifestations (Care, 2002; Thompson, 2005)
      **i.** Incompatibility between observed injury and reported history
      **ii.** Findings highly specific to abuse
         (a) Metaphyseal-epiphyseal lesions
         (b) Rib fractures
         (c) Sternal fractures
         (d) Scapula fractures
         (e) Medial or lateral clavicle fractures
         (f) Spinous process fractures
      **iii.** Findings moderately specific to abuse
         (a) Bilateral fractures
         (b) Multiple fractures
         (c) Vertebral body fractures
         (d) Hand or foot fractures
         (e) Fractures of varying ages
         (f) Complex skull fractures

iv. Differential diagnoses
   (a) Accidental injury
   (b) Physiologic periosteal new bone formation in infancy
   (c) Osteogenesis imperfecta
   (d) Menke's kinky hair syndrome
   (e) Copper deficiency
   (f) Rickets
   (g) Scurvy
   (h) Renal osteodystrophy
   (i) Congenital syphilis
   (j) Osteomyelitis
   (k) Leukemia
   (l) Bony metastases
   (m) Congenital insensitivity to pain
   e. Refer to orthopedics or emergency department
6. Clinical evaluation of bruises
   a. Compare the injury with historical information and child's developmental level—is the bruise likely to have been caused by the mechanism given?
      i. Accidental bruises are usually over bony prominences, like elbows and knees
      ii. Toddlers commonly have accidental bruises on anterior tibias or foreheads from falling
   b. Nonaccidental or inflicted bruises are in more "hidden" body surfaces like buttocks, inner thighs, behind the ears (Thompson, 2005)
   c. Mouth, dental, oral injuries are often overlooked and include:
      i. Bruises or petechiae of the inner lips and gums, or frontal dental ridge
      ii. Puncture lesions of the inner lips from teeth
      iii. Tears to the frenulum, fractured or avulsed teeth
   d. Suspicious bruises (Thompson, 2005)
      i. Patterned rather than irregular round lesions with amorphous borders
      ii. Bilateral or symmetric bruises are more consistent with abusive injuries
      iii. Numerous factors make specific timing or dating of a bruise difficult
   e. Differential diagnosis for suspicion of child abuse (Thompson, 2005)
      i. Hereditary collagen problems
      ii. Accidental injury
      iii. Osteogenesis imperfecta
      iv. Ehlers-Danlos—connective tissue disorder, articular hypermobility, skin extensibility, and tissue fragility
      v. Hematologic disorders
         (a) Anemia
         (b) Thrombocytopenia
         (c) Bleeding disorders, e.g., hemophilia
      vi. Infections (meningococcemia)
      vii. Phytophotodermatitis—rash from sun exposure to skin following contact with plants or their juices, e.g., lemons, limes, celery
      viii. Cultural practices
         (a) Cao Gaio—coining
      ix. Mongolian spots
   f. Diagnostic tests include:
      i. Complete blood count (CBC) with differential
      ii. Platelet count
      iii. PT/PTT (prothrombin time/partial thromboplastin time)
   g. Refer to appropriate specialist

7. Clinical evaluation of bite marks
   a. Physical assessment
      i. Small, linear lesions within a complete or partial arc
      ii. Size of arc may assist with determining who or what bit the child
      iii. Consultation with a forensic dentist (odontologist) is usually required
   b. Differential diagnosis
      i. Human bite
      ii. Animal or rodent bites (Van As, et al., 2006)
         (a) The configurations of bite patterns are different in animals as they bite and tear, using canine teeth
         (b) More trauma to the wound site
      iii. Diagnostic tests
         (a) Fresh or unwashed bites can be swabbed for possible DNA evidence
   c. Treatment (Tablitz, 2004)
      i. Detailed history of the injury and photograph
      ii. Gram stain and culture
      iii. Copious irrigation and debridement
      iv. Consider wound closure or refer to subspecialty, e.g., plastic surgery
      v. Elevate and immobilize wound
      vi. Antibiotic treatment specific to common pathogens of source
      vii. Consider rabies and tetanus prophylaxis
   d. Follow-up in 24 to 48 hours
8. Clinical evaluation of burn injury (Daria, 2004; Hettiaratchy & Dziewulski, 2004).
   a. Etiology (Elvik, 1998; Thompson, 2005)
      i. About one-quarter of burns are abusive in origin (Thompson, 2005)
      ii. Abusive burns occur as "discipline"
      iii. A peak time for abusive burns is during toilet training
   b. Intentional (abusive) burn compared to accidental burns
      i. Deeper and more symmetric than accidental burns
      ii. Patterned or circumferential around a digit or extremity
      iii. Occur in protected areas (genitals, thighs) less likely to be accidental
      iv. Immersion burns have precise margins and areas of spared skin due to the defensive position of the body when placed into the hot liquid
      v. Due to the configuration of immersion burns, they are referred to as "glove," "stocking," or "doughnut" burns
      vi. Forced contact with a hot surface can result in a patterned burn such as a cigarette burn or stove top burner
   c. Differential diagnosis
      i. Accidental burn
         (a) Accidental burns occur in young children because of their inquisitive nature
         (b) Commonly, burns from accidental contact are on fingertips and palms
         (c) Children younger than 4 years old are disproportionately represented
            (1) Reach up to a table or stove and spill hot liquids on them
            (2) Large burn area from the initial contact with the skin
            (3) Path of the liquid narrows as it cools, causes an "arrow-down" pattern
      ii. Staphylococcal scalded skin syndrome
      iii. Impetigo

        **iv.** Cultural practices, e.g., Chinese practice of moxibustion

           (a) Small cone-shaped amount of moxa herb is placed on top of an acupuncture point and burned

           (b) May lead to localized scarring, blisters, and scarring after healing

  **d.** Diagnostic tests

     **i.** Skin cultures for suspected infection

  **e.** Treatment—see Chapter 32

  **f.** Refer to burn specialists if indicated

**9.** Clinical evaluation of head injury

  **a.** Head trauma is the leading cause of death in child abuse cases (Rubin, et al., 2003)

  **b.** Visible bruising of the scalp is rare, seen in only about 10% to 15% of patients

  **c.** Accidental falls usually cause minor injury (Reece & Sege, 2000)

     **i.** When skull fractures occur, they are linear

     **ii.** Do not include intracranial/retinal hemorrhages

  **d.** Shaken baby syndrome (SBS) (Sinal, et al., 2000)

     **i.** Definition

        (a) Closed head injuries in children ages birth to 4 years that result from vigorous shaking of an infant

        (b) Life-threatening condition that involves admission to the hospital, often to the intensive care unit

        (c) Constellation of injuries

           (1) Subdural or epidural hemorrhages

           (2) Retinal hemorrhages

           (3) Fractures (especially to ribs)

     **ii.** Etiology

        (a) Males are most likely the perpetrators

        (b) Infant typically lives with biologic mother and biologic father or mother's boyfriend

     **iii.** Presentation

        (a) Usually mimics infectious process in infant

           (1) Lethargy

           (2) Decreased interest in or ability to feed

           (3) Full or bulging anterior fontanelle

           (4) Seizures

           (5) Loss of muscle tone

     **iv.** Differential diagnosis for head injury due to child abuse

        (a) Accidental head injury

        (b) Sepsis

        (c) Hematologic problems (vitamin K deficiency)

        (d) Other inborn errors

     **v.** Diagnostic tests

        (a) Skull and skeletal radiographs

        (b) CT of the head

        (c) Review newborn screening results and administration of vitamin K at delivery

        (d) Ophthalmology consultation

     **vi.** Prognosis

        (a) Approximately 60% of infants with head injuries due to abuse die from the injuries or have lifelong sequelae

           (1) Mental retardation

(2) Blindness

(3) Developmental delays

    **vii.** Refer to appropriate specialist

      (a) Neurologist

      (b) Neurosurgeon

**10.** Clinical evaluation of Munchausen syndrome by proxy (MBP) (Schreier, 2005)

    **a.** Falsifying symptoms in child when there is nothing medically wrong with the child

    **b.** Consequently, health care providers become the agent of harm to the child due to unnecessary treatment, diagnostic tests, medication, surgery, etc.

    **c.** Rare, but reported in pediatric psychiatry literature

    **d.** First described in 1977 in England by Roy Meadow

    **e.** Medical diagnosis terms for the child victim

      **i.** Pediatric condition falsification (PCF)

      **ii.** "Masquerade syndrome"

      **iii.** Amplification or falsification of an illness by a parent

      **iv.** Fastidious disorder by proxy (FDP)

    **f.** Assumptions about the in caregiver who harms her or his child through PCF

      **i.** Done for self-serving psychologic needs

      **ii.** To get help for caregiver's self due to being overwhelmed

      **iii.** To get help for the child who caregiver thinks is not being treated adequately

      **iv.** Caregiver has delusional belief that the child is ill

      **v.** Caregiver has a compulsive need to be considered by providers as an ideal parent

      **vi.** Primary motivation may be an intense need for attention

    **g.** Munchausen syndrome in teens

      **i.** Newly recognized condition that may be a continuation by the teen who was a child victim of MBP

      **ii.** Self-harming behavior has many etiologies (suicide attempts, attention seeking, peer rituals, Munchausen)

**11.** Clinical evaluation of the neglected child

    **a.** Child neglect is a continuum of behaviors, from failing to provide a child's basic needs to willfully placing a child in danger of physical harm (Dubowitz, et al., 1999)

      **i.** "Basic needs" usually refers to food, clothing, shelter, medical care/immunizations, and education

      **ii.** Other areas are sometimes included

        (a) Lack of nurturing

        (b) Failure to provide developmentally appropriate stimulation or play

        (c) Inadequate supervision of the child

        (d) Child abandonment

        (e) Refusal or delay in seeking health care

    **b.** The most common entity associated with neglect is failure-to-thrive (FTT)

      **i.** FTT is defined as the child's height and/or weight below the fifth percentile on a standardized growth chart

      **ii.** Organic FTT is not due to neglect, but suggests such causes as:

        (a) Cardiac lesions

        (b) Neurologic deficits

        (c) Fetal alcohol syndrome (FAS)

        **iii.** Nonorganic or environmental FTT
           (a) No organic cause
           (b) Usually stems from psychosocial issues in the family
           (c) Infant "shuts down" mentally and physically from lack of nurturing and stimulation
           (d) Maternal depression is often the root cause of FTT

  **c.** Differential diagnosis
      **i.** Malnutrition
      **ii.** Prenatal substance use
      **iii.** Cardiac
      **iv.** Neurologic
      **v.** Genetic factors

**12.** Clinical evaluation of the sexually abused child
  **a.** Types of sexual abuse
      **i.** Involvement in child pornography
      **ii.** Exposure to voyeurism, exhibitionism
      **iii.** Fondling, fingering
      **iv.** Sexual intercourse
         (a) Extragenital—genital to genital contact without penetration
         (b) Vaginal penetration
         (c) Anal penetration
         (d) Oral penetration

  **b.** Presentation of alleged sexual abuse occurs in several ways
      **i.** Children may disclose their molestation to a third party, such as a teacher or school nurse
         (a) Disclosures should always be taken seriously
         (b) Interview should be done by specially trained individuals (forensic training)
      **ii.** Nonspecific physical symptom may be the impetus for a visit to the health care provider
         (a) Recurrent abdominal pain
         (b) Enuresis
         (c) Encopresis
         (d) Eating disorders
         (e) Vaginal itching or rash
      **iii.** Nonspecific behavioral symptoms may be the impetus for a visit to primary care provider
         (a) Sexualized play
         (b) Excessive masturbation
         (c) Self-mutilation
         (d) Insertion of foreign objects in vagina, urethra, or anus (differentiate from age-appropriate curiosity about body openings)
         (e) Poor school performance
         (f) Depression, anger, suicide attempt, overdose
      **iv.** During a well child visit, the PNP may note a physical finding that suggests sexual abuse

  **c.** Physical assessment
      **i.** Examine entire body
      **ii.** Special focus on external genitalia and anal areas
         (a) Should be done routinely at every health care visit
         (b) Knowledge of the child's baseline physical findings will alert the PNP for possible abuse or other problems

(c) Proper assessment of the female external genitalia is done by gently separating the labia majora
(d) Digital internal examination is never indicated in a prepubertal child
(e) All females are born with hymens, the majority of which develop an opening just before birth
(f) Normal hymenal shapes (Figure 21-1)
   (1) Redundant—thick due to maternal estrogen, pale, folded on itself (Adams, 2004)
   (2) Crescentic
   (3) Annular
   (4) Septate
(g) Note that the hymen is often normal in appearance even when sexual abuse has occurred
(h) Occasionally, a hymen can be imperforate
   (1) No opening to the vagina
   (2) Considered a congenital anomaly and should be evaluated (Elvik, 1998)
iii. Maturation and development:
   (a) Hymens are redundant at birth
   (b) By about 2 years of age, the configuration changes to crescentic or annular
   (c) At puberty, the hymen returns to its redundant appearance due to estrogen
      (1) The redundant hymen is very elastic
      (2) Penetration can occur without signs of trauma
iv. Unusual genital and/or anal findings are most often nonspecific for sexual abuse
   (a) Genital erythema is associated with poor hygiene which can be especially problematic with overweight females

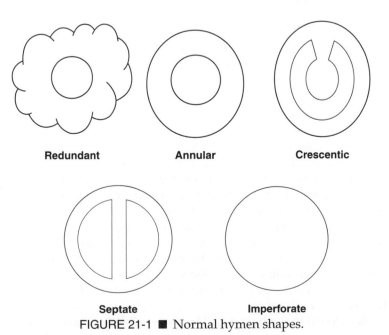

Redundant    Annular    Crescentic

Septate    Imperforate
FIGURE 21-1 ■ Normal hymen shapes.

      (b) Vaginal discharge can be caused by autoinoculation of organisms from other areas, such as the respiratory tract

      (c) Anal fissures are commonly seen with constipation

   v. A lack of unusual physical findings is typical in many sexually abused children (Kellogg, et. al., 2005)

      (a) Due to the various acts of molestation

      (b) Due to anatomic variations in children

      (c) Does not rule out child abuse, but is a finding in a given case at the time of the physical examination (Giardino & Finkel, 2005)

  vi. Genital and/or anal trauma

      (a) More likely when assaulted by a stranger

      (b) Findings include (Christian, et al., 2000):

         (1) Bruising

         (2) Genital tears

         (3) Bleeding

  vii. Differential diagnosis for sexual abuse

      (a) Self-inflicted trauma

      (b) Accidental trauma

      (c) Vaginitis from harsh soaps

      (d) Laundry detergents

      (e) Prolonged contact with sand or chlorine

      (f) Frequent use of bubble bath

      (g) Pruritus of vaginal or anal areas due to:

         (1) Infestation by pinworms

         (2) Constipation or diarrhea causing anal fissures

         (3) Infection

            a) Organisms specific to sexually transmitted diseases

            b) Normal flora, such as *Escherichia coli*

 viii. Diagnostic tests—should be done by specialist in child sexual abuse

      (a) Vaginal culture

      (b) Chlamydial immunofluorescence

      (c) Pregnancy test

      (d) Rectal culture

      (e) Blood test for syphilis, HIV, and hepatitis

13. Role of the pediatric nurse practitioner in child abuse

  a. All 50 states have mandated reporting laws for child abuse and neglect

  b. Licensed health care providers are mandated to report "suspicious" cases

  c. Suspicious defined as—based on the provider's training and experience, one would likely be suspicious or concerned about the possibility of abuse or neglect

    i. When history, behavioral manifestations, and/or physical findings are suspicious, the case must be reported

    ii. Other agencies such as law enforcement and child protective services will investigate and determine if the suspicions are substantiated

    iii. Individuals who report are not held liable whether or not abuse or neglect is substantiated, unless the report was made with malice intended

    iv. 8% to 30% of physicians said that they failed to report suspected child abuse at some time during their career (Flaherty & Sege, 2005)

  d. Barriers to recognition of abuse (Flaherty & Sege, 2005)

    i. Lack of knowledge and training in recognition of abuse

    ii. Psychologic barriers

      (a) Denial that parent could be responsible for abuse

(b) Familiarity with the family
(c) Stirs up ambivalent feelings about own family and/or children
(d) Anxiety caused by countertransference of fear, guilt, shame, and sympathy
iii. Family racial and socioeconomic factors
(a) Racial bias—several studies showed that physicians were more likely to miss abusive head trauma in children whose families were white and intact
e. Barriers to reporting of abuse (Flaherty & Sege, 2005)
i. Physical abuse and sexual abuse reported more often than physical neglect, emotional abuse, or medical neglect
ii. Threshold effect on what is considered acceptable parenting (discipline) practices
iii. Specialty—pediatricians less likely to report failure to thrive than are family practice or emergency department physicians
iv. Race and socioeconomic status—overall, Black and/or poor children are not overrepresented
v. Lack of knowledge and training about reporting rules
vi. Reluctance to hurt the family by reporting abuse
vii. Worry that the child will be hurt further by reporting abuse
viii. Worry that child will not return to the practice for essential care
ix. Negative previous experiences with Child Protective Services (CPS)
x. Misunderstanding of CPS role
xi. Requires extra office time and interrupts patient flow
xii. Some health care plans do not pay for needed diagnostic tests to validate suspicions
xiii. Time required to testify in court is costly
f. Documentation in cases of child maltreatment is critical to all parties involved
g. Expertise in forensic examination and evidence collection is essential
i. Defer examination and refer immediately to an emergency department or sexual abuse center
ii. Registered nurses can obtain advanced education and clinical preparation in forensic examination of sexual assault victims through sexual assault nurse examiner (SANE) programs
h. Genital examination
i. Lesions should be described completely in terms of:
(a) Size
(b) Shape
(c) Color
(d) Location on the body
ii. If the provider is familiar with hymen configuration, description of the hymen shape and color should be done along with the presence or absence of:
(a) Discharge
(b) Bruising
(c) Lesions
(d) It is never acceptable to indicate "hymen intact" or "hymen not intact" because this gives no real information about the genital area
i. Documentation should be legible and clearly written because the information contained in the medical record will be read by a number of nonmedical professionals, including attorneys and judges

    **j.** Immediate needs of the patient should be addressed including:
        **i.** Life-threatening injuries
        **ii.** Need for consultation with other specialists such as orthopedics or gynecology
    **k.** General management (Leder, et al., 2001a)
        **i.** Emotional support for the child and family
            (a) Crisis counseling at the time of the incident or disclosure
            (b) Referral to child abuse specialist
        **ii.** Treat the medical needs
        **xiii.** Prevent STDs
        **iv.** Emergency contraception
    **l.** Advocacy for all concerned is important (Care, 2002; Dubowitz, 2002)
        **i.** Individual child
        **ii.** Parent
        **iii.** Family
        **iv.** Community
        **v.** Society
    **m.** Preventive teaching
        **i.** Discipline at home—avoid corporal punishment, verbal abuse
        **ii.** "Good" and "bad" touch
    **n.** Research has shown that the team approach to child maltreatment has several benefits
        **i.** Use of experts decreases perpetrator's possible defense strategies
        **ii.** Working in teams helps prevent early "burnout" of the individual professional in these highly emotional and sensitive cases
        **iii.** More coordinated efforts on the part of the various agencies involved decreases anxiety for the child and his/her family

**14.** Long-term sequelae
    **a.** Childhood abuse or neglect is a risk factor for behavioral and emotional problems in later life
    **b.** Requires multidisciplinary treatment (Scheid, 2003)
    **c.** Common sequelae
        **i.** Personality disorders
        **ii.** Mood disorders (Conway, et al., 2004)
            (a) Depression
            (b) Posttraumatic stress disorder (PTSD)
                (1) Intrusive recall of the event
                    a) Nightmares
                    b) Flashbacks
                (2) Changes in emotions
                    a) Irritability
                    b) Feeling numb
                (3) Aggressive behavior
                (4) Inappropriate sexual behavior
                (5) Changes in arousal
                    a) Feeling on edge
                    b) Insomnia
                    c) More likely to startle
                    d) Inattentiveness
                    e) Hyperactivity
                (6) Decrease in self-care
                    a) Poor hygiene

        b) Enuresis
        c) Encopresis
      (7) Future aspirations lost
   **iii.** Reactive attachment disorder (RAD)
      (a) Abnormalities in relationships
        (1) Indifferent to caregivers
        (2) Too friendly to strangers
      (b) Failure to thrive
   **iv.** Mood disturbances
      (a) Mood instability
      (b) Anxiety symptoms
        (1) Separation anxiety
        (2) Social phobia
        (3) Panic attacks
   **v.** Substance abuse in older children and teens

# REFERENCES

Care, M. (2002). Imaging in suspected child abuse: What to expect and what to order. *Pediatr Ann, 31,* 651-659.

Christian, C. W., Lavelle, J. M., De Jong, A. R., et al. (2000). Forensic evidence findings in prepubertal victims of sexual assault. *Pediatrics, 106*(6, No. 1, Pt 1), 100-104.

Conway, M., Mendelson, M., Giannopoulos, C., et al. (2004). Childhood and adult sexual abuse, rumination on sadness, and dysphoria. *Child Abuse Negl, 28,* 393-410.

Daria, S., Sugar, N., Feldman, K., et al. (2004). Into hot water head first: Distribution of intentional and unintentional immersion burns. *Pediatr Emerg Care, 20,* 302-310.

Department of Health and Human Services (DHHS) (US), Administration on Children, Youth, and Families (ACF). Child maltreatment 2003 [online]. Washington (DC): Government Printing Office; 2005. [cited 2005 April 5]. Available from: URL: www.acf.hhs.gov/programs/cb/pubs/cm03/index.htm.

Dubowitz, H. (Ed.) (1999). *Neglected children.* Thousand Oaks, CA: Sage Publications. (One of the best works on neglect)

Dubowitz, H. (2002). Preventing child neglect and physical abuse: A role for pediatricians. *Pediatr Rev, 23,* 191-195.

Dubowitz, H., Giardino, A., & Gustavson, E. (2000). Child neglect: Guidance for pediatricians. *Pediatr Rev, 21,* 111-116.

Elvik, S. L. (1998). Child maltreatment. In T. E. Soud & J. S. Rogers (Eds.). *Manual of pediatric emergency nursing.* St. Louis: Mosby.

Feldman, K. W. (1997). Evaluation of physical abuse. In M. E. Helfer, et al. (Eds.). *The battered child* (5th ed.). Chicago: University of Chicago Press. (A classic source)

Flaherty, E. G., & Sege, R. (2005). Barriers to physician identification and reporting of child abuse. *Pediatr Ann, 34*(5), 349-356.

Giardino, A. P., & Finkel, M. A. (2005). Evaluating child sexual abuse. *Pediatr Ann, 34*(5), 382-394.

Hettiaratchy, S., & Dziewulski, P. (2004). Pathophysiology and types of burns. *BMJ, 328,* 1427-1429.

Hornor, G. (2004). Sexual behavior in children: Normal or not? *J Pediatr Health Care, 18,* 57-64.

Hornor, G. (2005). Physical abuse: Recognition and reporting. *J Pediatr Health Care, 19,* 4-11.

Jackson, S. (2004). A USA national survey of program services provided by child advocacy centers. *Child Abuse Negl, 28,* 411-421.

Kellogg, N. & the AAP Committee on Child Abuse and Neglect. (2005). The evaluation of sexual abuse in children. *Pediatrics, 116*(2), 506-512.

Kempe, C. H., Silverman, F. N., Steele, B. F., et al. (1962). Landmark article July 7, 1962: The battered-child syndrome. *JAMA, 251*(4), 3288-3294. (A classic article)

Leder, M., Knight, J., & Emans, S. (2001a). Sexual abuse: Management strategies and legal issues. *Contemp Pediatr, 18,* 77-92.

Leder, M., Knight, J., & Emans, S. (2001b). Sexual abuse: When to suspect it, how to assess for it. *Contemp Pediatr, 18,* 59-76.

Maguire, S., Mann, M., & Kemp, A. (2005). Are there patterns of bruising in childhood which are diagnostic or suggestive of abuse? A systematic review. *Arch Dis Child, 90,* 182-186.

McColgan, M. D., & Giardino, A. P. (2005). Internet poses multiple risks to children and adolescents. *Pediatr Ann, 34*(5), 406-414.

Mudd, S., & Findlay, J. (2004). The cutaneous manifestations and common mimickers of physical child abuse. *J Pediatr Health Care, 18,* 123-129.

Nelms, B. (2003). Keeping children safe: Protecting from sexual abuse. *J Pediatr Health Care, 17,* 275-276.

Oaksford, K., & Frude, N. (2003). The process of coping following child abuse: A qualitative study. *J Child Sex Abus, 12,* 41-72.

Reece, R. M., & Sege, R. (2000). Childhood head injury: accidental or inflicted? *Arch Pediatr Adoles Med, 154,* 11-15.

Rubin, D.M., Christian, C.W., Bilaniuk, L. T., et al. (2003). Occult head injury in high-risk abused children. *Pediatrics,* 111(6, Pt.1), 1382-1386

Scheid, J. (2003). Recognizing and managing long-term sequelae of childhood maltreatment. *Pediatr Ann, 32,* 391-401.

Schreier, H. (2002). Munchausen by proxy defined. *Pediatrics, 110,* 985-988.

Shanel-Hogan, K. (2004). What is this red mark? *J Cal Dent Assoc, 32,* 304-305.

Sinal, S., Petree, A., Harman-Giddens, M., et al. (2000). Is race or ethnicity a predictive factor in Shaken Baby Syndrome? *Child Abuse Negl, 9,* 1241-1246.

Spataro, J., Mullen, P., Burgess, P., et al. (2004). Impact of child sexual abuse on mental health: Prospective study in males and females. *Brit J Psychiatry: J Ment Sci, 184,* 416-421.

Straus, M.A. (1994). Beating the devil out of them: corporal punishment in American families. San Francisco, Jossey-Bass Publisher.

Thompson, S. (2005). Accidental or inflicted? *Pediatr Ann, 34*(5), 372-381.

Trenchs, V., Curcoy, A., Pou, J., et al. (2005). Retinal haemorrhages as proof of abusive head injury. *J Pediatr, 146,* 437-438.

Turner, J., & Reid, S. (2002). Munchausen's syndrome. *Lancet, 359,* 346-349.

Tyler, K., Whitebeck, L., Hoyt, D., & Cauce, A. (2004). Risk factors for sexual victimization among male and female homeless and runaway youth. *J Interpers Violence, 19,* 503-520.

U.S. Department of Health & Human Services (HHS) (2003). Child maltreatment 2001: Reports from the states to the national child abuse and neglect data system. Washington, DC: U.S. Government Printing Office.

van As, A.B., Kalebka, R.R., vader Heyde (2006). Animal attacks: a red herring of child abuse? *S Afr Med J, 96*(3), 184-186.

Walker, J., Carey, P., Mohr, N., et al. (2004). Gender differences in the prevalence of childhood sexual abuse and in the development of pediatric PTSD. *Arch Women Ment Health, 7,* 111-121.

Westcott, H., & Jones, D. (1999). The abuse of disabled children. *J Child Psychol Psychiatry, 40,* 497-506.

# Toddlers, Preschoolers, and School-agers

JUDY PITTS, MSN, RN, CPNP

1. Goals of the well child health care visit for toddlers, preschoolers, and school-agers
   a. Health promotion
      i. NAPNAP's recently released evidence-based clinical practice guideline provides detailed information about nutrition and exercise in four age groups, infants, preschool children, school age children, and adolescents (NAPNAP, 2006)
   b. Health maintenance (Table 22-1) (Green & Palfrey, 2002)
      i. Assessment of growth parameters (see Chapter 4 for guidelines)
      ii. Immunizations (see Chapter 15 for age-specific details)
      iii. Health screening (Table 22-1) (Glascoe & Macias, 2003)
   c. Developmental assessment (see Chapter 4 for recommendations)
   d. Discussion of parental concerns
   e. Thorough history and physical exam
      i. Talk to the child as well as the parents; interviewing techniques should be developmentally appropriate for the child's age (Instone, 2002)
      ii. See Chapters 5 through 13 for assessment of each body system
   f. Anticipatory guidance
2. Recommended schedule for well child examinations
   a. Guidelines from the Committee on Practice and Ambulatory Medicine of the American Academy of Pediatrics (AAP, 2000) assuming that the child:
      i. Has adequate and competent parenting
      ii. No manifestations of important health problems
      iii. Is growing and developing satisfactorily
   b. Recommended schedule of visits based on child's age
      i. 15 months
      ii. 18 months
      iii. 24 months
      iv. 3 years
      v. 4 years
      vi. 5 years
      vii. 6, 8, and 10 years

■ **TABLE 22-1**
■ ■ **Recommended Health Maintenance and Screening During Toddler and Preschool Years**

| Age | Health Maintenance | Recommended Screenings |
|---|---|---|
| 15 months | Height, weight, head circumference<br>Immunizations if not up-to-date | Lead screening if high risk and if not done in the past 6 months<br>Vision, hearing (subjective & by history)<br>Developmental assessment |
| 18 months | Height, weight, head circumference<br>Immunizations if not up-to-date | Hb/Hct<br>Vision, hearing (subjective & by history)<br>Developmental assessment |
| 24 months | Height, weight, BMI, head<br>circumference<br>Immunizations if not up-to-date | Lead screening<br>Hb/Hct<br>Cholesterol if high risk<br>Vision, hearing (subjective & by history)<br>Developmental assessment |
| 3 years | Height, weight, BMI, BP | Dental exam<br>Lead screening if high risk<br>Vision, hearing tests<br>Hb/Hct<br>Cholesterol if high risk<br>Developmental assessment |
| 4 years | Height, weight, BMI, BP | Lead screening if high risk<br>Vision, hearing tests<br>Hb/Hct<br>Cholesterol if high risk<br>Developmental assessment |
| 5 years | Height, weight, BMI, BP<br>Immunizations (DtaP #5,<br>IPV #4, MMR #2) | Lead screening if high risk<br>Vision, hearing tests<br>TB screening if high risk<br>Hb/Hct<br>Urinalysis<br>Cholesterol if high risk<br>Developmental assessment |
| 6, 8,<br>10 years | Height, weight, BMI, BP | Vision, hearing tests<br>Hb/Hct for high risk children<br>Cholesterol if high risk<br>Developmental assessment |

Reprinted with permission from: American Academy of Pediatrics Committee on Practice and Ambulatory Medicine. (2000). Recommendations for preventive pediatric health care. *Pediatrics, 105*(3), 645–646. Also available at http://aappolicy.aappublications. org/cgi/content/full/ pediatrics;105/3/645.

3. Developmental assessment
   a. A strong knowledge base of developmental principles and developmental characteristics of children throughout childhood is critical for:
      i. Developmental assessment (see Chapter 4 for assessment tools)
         (a) Gross motor development (Box 22-1)
         (b) Fine motor development (Box 22-2)
            (1) Moves from unrefined movement to more specific and purposeful movements
            (2) Become more adept in using their hands and fingers to help control their environment
         (c) Speech and language development (Box 22-3)
         (d) Personal and social development (Box 22-4)

■ **BOX 22-1**
■ **GROSS MOTOR DEVELOPMENTAL MILESTONES OF TODDLERS AND PRESCHOOLERS**

| Age | Developmental milestones |
|---|---|
| 12 months | Walking alone |
| 15 months | Walks backward |
| 18 months | Runs |
| 21 months | Walks up stairs with help |
| 24 months | Walks up and down steps without help |
| 30 months | Jumps with both feet off ground |
| 3 years | Pedals a tricycle |
| 4 years | Hops, skips |
| 5 years | Jumps over low obstacles |

■ **BOX 22-2**
■ **FINE MOTOR DEVELOPMENTAL MILESTONES OF TODDLERS AND PRESCHOOLERS**

| Age | Developmental Milestone |
|---|---|
| 12 months | Mature pincer grasp |
| 15 months | Scribbles imitation |
| 18 months | Scribbles spontaneously |
| 21 months | Tower, five blocks |
| 24 months | Imitates stroke with pencil |
| 30 months | Unbuttons |
| 3 years | Copies circle |
| 4 years | Buttons clothing |
| 5 years | Ties shoes |

■ **BOX 22-3**
■ **SPEECH AND LANGUAGE DEVELOPMENTAL MILESTONES OF TODDLERS AND PRESCHOOLERS**

| Age | Developmental Milestone |
|---|---|
| 12 months | Uses two words other than "mama," "dada" |
| 15 months | Uses 4 to 6 words |
| 18 months | Puts 2 words together |
| | Knows 8 body parts |
| | 20 words by 20 months |
| 21 months | 50-word vocabulary |
| 24 months | Follows two-step commands |
| 30 months | Uses pronouns appropriately |
| 3 years | 250-word vocabulary |
| 4 years | Sings song from memory |
| 5 years | Prints first name |

      ii. Observation of strong and subtle cues of developmental delays
     iii. Anticipatory guidance
  **b.** Toddler
      i. Starts as the child begins toddling around at approximately 1 year and continues through the second year

■ **BOX 22-4**
■ **PERSONAL AND SOCIAL DEVELOPMENTAL MILESTONES OF TODDLERS AND PRESCHOOLERS**

| Age | Developmental Milestone |
|-----|------------------------|
| 12 months | Comes when called |
| 15 months | Uses spoon, cup independently |
| 18 months | Imitates parent chores |
| 21 months | Asks for food |
| 24 months | Parallel play |
| 30 months | Gives first and last names |
| 3 years | Group play, shares |
| 4 years | Tells tall tales |
| 5 years | Abides by rules |

    ii. A very fascinating time when the child:
      (a) Has a drive to achieve goals beyond current skills, e.g., walk, talk, climb
      (b) Begins to assert his or her own will
   iii. Toddlers are learning to:
      (a) Talk
      (b) Coordinate and refine and gross motor skills
      (c) Control elimination
      (d) Control their own behavior
      (e) Right from wrong
      (f) Explore the fantasy world
      (g) Explore their own environment
      (h) Master their environment while maintaining self-esteem
   iv. Challenging age-group for parents and health care providers
      (a) When a toddler embraces his or her feelings, everyone is aware
      (b) Usually cannot reason with a toddler who can only see the situation from his own perspective
      (c) Parents can often get caught up in their dilemma
      (d) Parents need to recognize these difficult times as a part of normal development
    v. Play is a major tool for learning—usually parallel play
   vi. Growth slows down, as does the appetite
      (a) Growth is at a steady rate of about 3 to 5 pounds and 2 to 3 inches per year
      (b) Growth occurs in peaks and valleys
      (c) Appetite will have peaks and valleys
      (d) Plot growth yearly on a standardized growth chart to observe the growth velocity
      (e) Often will slow down in their growth velocity during toddler stage
      (f) Watch growth velocity to be sure that it does not fall more than two standard deviations below the previous growth curve or below the third percentile
      (g) Toddlers often look chubby with a potbelly
      (h) Occipital frontal head circumference usually follows a similar percentile as height

    **vii.** Speech, language, and cognitive development are intertwined

        (a) At about age 2, the toddler moves from Piaget's sensorimotor stage to the preoperational stage

        (b) Learn by exploring through their senses and increasing motor abilities

        (c) Sensorimotor activities underlay language, imitation of factions observed earlier, and make-believe play

        (d) Learn through symbols or mental representations in their environment

        (e) Learn through imitation and by exploring their environment

        (f) Active imagination

        (g) Egocentric, animistic and magical thinking

        (h) Language is the most flexible means of mental representation

        (i) Playing, reading and talking are essential for speech development

        (j) Refer for speech and hearing evaluation if there is no speech by 18 months

  **viii.** Personal and social

        (a) Erikson's stage of autonomy versus shame and doubt

        (b) Behavior is often difficult for parents to handle

        (c) Expect resistance as the toddler is learning self-control and self-confidence

        (d) A parent who is too controlling or lenient can hinder the toddler's passage through this stage

        (e) Emerging competencies are in speech and toilet training

    **ix.** Nutrition issues (Gottesman, 2002)

        (a) The appetite slump common to toddlers is a significant issue

        (b) No more than 4 to 6 ounces of juice should be given because it will decrease the appetite

        (c) Toddlers need approximately 1000 calories a day

        (d) It is best to offer small frequent meals with three meals and two snacks each day

        (e) Mealtime can be a challenge but should not be a battle

        (f) It is the parent's responsibility to offer well-balanced meals and the toddler's responsibility to eat or not eat

        (g) Does not like new foods (neophobic)

        (h) It may take several attempts before trying something new

        (i) Portion size should be about one-quarter the adult portion

        (j) Needs only 1 to 2 ounces of meat daily

        (k) Cut food into bite-size pieces; finger foods

        (l) By 12 to 15 months most children should be off the bottle

        (m) Milk intake dramatically decreases; solids increase

        (n) Calcium (Carakushansky, 2003)

            (1) Retention is lower but increases until puberty

            (2) By 12 months, needs about 800 mg/day

            (3) Can get it in two to three servings of milk products each day

**c.** Preschooler

    **i.** Chronologic age is 3 to 5 years

    **ii.** Vocabulary, coordination, intellectual thinking, and social skills are being developed

    **iii.** Excited about learning and discovering

    **iv.** By age 5 years:

        (a) Know their full name, address, and phone numbers

        (b) Can tell stories

        (c) Beginning to draw figures that represent people, animals, and objects

        (d) Understand that pictures, numbers, words, and letters are symbols of real things and ideas

        (e) Begin "reading" on their own

     **v.** May recognize a few words such as their name or words on signs

   **vi.** Parents need to provide an environment to help develop the confidence that preschoolers need to:

        (a) Make their own decisions

        (b) Make new friends

        (c) Develop talents

        (d) Build self-esteem

  **vii.** Physical development

        (a) Grow at a steady rate of about 3 to 5 pounds and 2 to 3 inches per year

        (b) Grow in peaks and valleys

        (c) Appetite is variable but eat better than as a toddler

        (d) Starts to lose the potbellied appearance

 **viii.** Gross and fine motor skills become more refined

        (a) Can draw pictures of people, animals, and objects

        (b) Can use scissors to cut

   **ix.** Speech, language, and cognitive development

        (a) Piaget's preoperational stage

        (b) Thinking still not logical

        (c) Asks many questions

        (d) Intelligible speech

        (e) Talkative and animated

        (f) Sings songs

        (g) Tells stories

        (h) Still has active imagination

    **x.** Personal social development

        (a) Becomes more social and starts to play competitively

        (b) Erikson's initiative versus guilt stage

        (c) Begins to initiate instead of imitate

        (d) Developing a conscience and a sexual identity

        (e) Can tell a story and sing a song from memory

        (f) Likes to help with household chores

   **xi.** Nutritional issues

        (a) Appetite usually improves and mealtime is not such a challenge

        (b) Watch for excessive weight gain

        (c) Bad habits in the preschool years can continue into the school-age years

        (d) Still need two to three glasses of low-fat milk a day and should avoid soda pop, especially with caffeine

        (e) No more than 1 hour of television a day

        (f) A research study showed a significant correlation between more than 8 hours per week of television watching and overweight in 3-year-olds (Reilly, et al., 2005)

  **d.** School-ager

    **i.** Children ages 6 to 11 or 12 (prepubertal)

        (a) Main task is to learn basic skills of reading, writing, arithmetic

        (b) If children do not do well academically, they need to develop other skills that make them feel competent like dancing, art, music, and sports

        (c) Important years for the development of self-esteem

  **ii.** Physical development

        (a) Growth is at a steady rate of about 3 to 5 pounds and 2 to 3 inches per year

        (b) Growth is normally slow but steady until they approach adolescence

        (c) Overweight is often a problem—usually starts in this age-group

  **iii.** Gross motor development

        (a) Gross motor skills become more refined

        (b) Strength improves

        (c) Coordination improves

        (d) Participates in sports

  **iv.** Fine motor development

        (a) Fine motor skills become more refined

        (b) Learn to print, then write cursive

        (c) Develop more coordination in upper extremities

        (d) Become more adept in using their hands and fingers to help control their environment

  **v.** Speech, language, and cognitive development

        (a) Piaget's concrete operational stage—understands concrete better than abstract phenomena

        (b) Language is the most flexible means of mental representation

        (c) Playing, reading, and talking continue to be important for learning and speech development

        (d) Learning skills needed for adulthood

        (e) Speech therapy is recommended if dysfluency, stuttering

        (f) Starts thinking logically

  **vi.** Personal and social development

        (a) Erikson's stage of industry versus inferiority

        (b) Trying to develop a sense of self worth by developing new skills

        (c) Need to find something that the child can do well

        (d) Ability to play in groups—competition

        (e) Development of friendships

        (f) Understands right from wrong

        (g) Learns to follow the rules

        (h) Learns responsibility

  **vii.** Nutrition issues

        (a) Needs two to three glasses of low-fat milk each day

        (b) Needs three meals and at least one snack per day

        (c) Portion sizes should be half of the adult portion

        (d) Vitamins not needed if eats well

        (e) Calcium—needs 800 to 1200 mg each day

        (f) Encourage activity

        (g) Watch for obesity

        (h) 1 to 2 hours of TV or computer games each day

**4.** Common health concerns

  **a.** Oral health

    **i.** The first dental visit recommended at 3 years and then every 6 months

    **ii.** Children with malocclusion, dental caries, or dental injuries should see a dentist earlier than 3 years

      iii. As soon as teeth come in, parents need to start brushing them

      iv. Normally the first teeth come in between 6 and 15 months

      v. Children should brush and floss their teeth after each meal and after eating concentrated sugars

      vi. If the child's water source is fluoridated, a fluoride supplement is not necessary

      vii. Fluoride toothpaste should not be used until the toddler learns to expectorate the toothpaste instead of swallowing (see Chapter 19, Section 7.h. for more detail on fluorides and dental caries)

**b.** Pacifiers and bottles

      i. After 6 months, pacifiers should be limited to bedtime and discontinued as soon as possible

      ii. Offering a transitional object often helps while weaning off a bottle or pacifier

      iii. To avoid dental decay, children should be weaned off the bottle by 12 months

**c.** Safety issues (AAP, 2003)

      i. Poisons (see also Chapter 19, Section 7.n. i–ii)

        (a) Each year, unintentional poisonings from medicines and household chemicals kill about 30 children and prompt more than 1 million calls to the nation's poison control centers

        (b) Discuss at every health supervision exam for the toddler and preschooler

        (c) Children 18 to 35 months are at greatest risk for accidental ingestion of medications and poisonous products

        (d) Toddlers are at high risk because they are learning through investigating their environment and they do not have the judgment or the skill to handle it safely

        (e) Parents should be advised on how to child-proof and poison-proof their home, yard, garage, and automobile

        (f) Give parents the number of the local poison control center

        (g) Most deadly poisons

          (1) Medications

          (2) Antifreeze

          (3) Windshield washer solution

          (4) Alcohol-containing products and beverages

          (5) Petroleum products such as gasoline, lamp oil, kerosene, turpentine, lighter fluid

      ii. Water and sun safety (See also Chapter 19, Section 7.l. for more information on water safety)

        (a) More children drown in the tub than anywhere else

        (b) Even a bucket with water in it can be a danger for a top-heavy toddler

        (c) Never leave a toddler or a preschooler unattended around water or while in tub

        (d) Water heaters should be turned down to 120° F (49° C)

        (e) Children 12 to 17 months are at greatest risk for hot liquid and vapor injuries

        (f) Temperature of water and time it takes to burn an infant's or child's skin

          (1) 150° F (66° C) 2 seconds

          (2) 140° F (60° C) 6 seconds

          (3) 125° F (52° C) 2 minutes
          (4) 120° F (49° C) 10 minutes
    (g) Most parents are aware of the importance of watching children around swimming pools or around any water or boats
          (1) All children younger than the age of 12 should wear an approved lifejacket while boating
    (h) Water and sun go hand in hand
    (i) Children older than the age of 6 months should wear sunscreen (SPF 15 or higher) and protective clothing such as a hat and t-shirt to avoid sunburn
    (j) Sunscreen should be reapplied every several hours while in the sun
    (k) Avoid the sun if possible during peak hours (11 AM-2 PM)

iii. Choking
    (a) Many infants and children die each year from choking
    (b) Deaths are preventable if parents watch their children more closely and keep dangerous toys, foods, and household items out of their reach
    (c) Many toys intended for use by children can be extremely hazardous if improperly used or used without supervision
    (d) Test the size of toys for children younger than 2 years by placing the toy inside a toilet paper roll
          (1) If the toy fits inside the roll it is too small
          (2) If the toy does not slide through the roll then it is normally too big for the child to swallow

iv. Shopping carts—small children must be strapped into grocery carts at all times; use an adult's belt if cart has no safety strap

v. Beds
    (a) Cribs should have tight-fitting mattresses and the spaces between the slats should not be wider than 2⅜ inches
    (b) Children should not play or sleep in a bunk bed until they are school age

vi. Bike helmets
    (a) Wearing bike helmets as soon as a child starts riding is a good habit to start
    (b) Parents should be encouraged to set a good example by wearing helmets and practicing safe behaviors in front of their children

vii. Trampoline
    (a) AAP (1999) policy states that a trampoline should not be used at home, inside or outside
    (b) During anticipatory guidance, advise parents never to purchase a home trampoline or allow children to use home trampolines

viii. Car seats (see also Chapter 19, Section 7.j. for other details)
    (a) More children are killed as passengers in car crashes than from any other type of accident
    (b) Every child needs to be in the right restraint for age and weight
    (c) Children younger than the age of 1 year and less than 20 pounds should be in a rear-facing infant seat or a convertible seat
    (d) Many new cars and vans are equipped with built-in forward-facing car seats—designed for infants older than 12 months or those who weigh more than 20 pounds
    (e) Once the child is 12 months old and 20 pounds he or she can be in a forward-facing car seat

    (f) A forward-facing seat, a combination seat, or a belt-positioned booster seat should be used once the child outgrows the convertible seat

    (g) A booster seat is recommended until seat belts fit well, which is until the child weighs approximately 80 pounds

    (h) Children have outgrown their car seats when the tops of their ears are above the top of the car seat or their shoulders are above the strap slots

    (i) The car seat needs to be installed correctly, according to vehicle's owner's manual

    (j) Parents should always test the harness and the seat belt for snug fit after it is installed

    (k) The car seat should not move more than several inches any way once it is installed

    (l) The bottom of the car seat attaches to anchors on the right and left backseat and a tether at the top of the car seat holds the top of the car seat in place

  (m) LATCH (lower anchors and tethers for children)

      (1) LATCH is a new system that simplifies installation of car seats without the use of seat belts

      (2) All automobiles and safety seats manufactured after September 1, 2002, are required to have LATCH

      (3) Older car seats or car seats not made for LATCH will not work with this system and the seat belt should then be used

    (n) The car seat is very stable when installed properly

    (o) If the center seat doesn't have anchors, a child safety seat may be installed using a seat belt

    (p) Position of safety seat in the vehicle

      (1) Never place a toddler in the front seat in a car with passenger-side airbags

      (2) A child less than 80 pounds should not be in the front seat with passenger-side airbags

      (3) The safest place for a child less than 12 years or 80 pounds is in center of the backseat

      (4) If there is no backseat, deactivation of the passenger-side airbag is advised

      (5) If the vehicle is equipped with side airbag, a child will be safest in the back, center seat

      (6) The safety of children traveling in automobiles with side-releasing airbags has not been established

**ix.** Safety while traveling by air

    (a) Every child should be placed in an FAA-approved safety seat when flying

    (b) Whereas many airlines provide free tickets to children younger than age 2, these tickets do not include a seat

    (c) For safety during takeoff, landings, and possible turbulence, it is important to purchase a seat so the child can be ensured a place to sit

    (d) Some airlines have their own safety seats and others require that you bring your own

    (e) Parents should check with the airline before departure

    (f) Bringing child's own car seat ensures that the child will have a car seat available once the destination is reached

**x.** Safety on the streets—children 36 to 47 months are at greater risk for pedestrian injuries

**d.** Toilet training

    **i.** The key to toilet training is readiness

    **ii.** Most toddlers have the muscle control to regulate their bladders between the ages of 18 and 36 months

    **iii.** The following are signs of readiness, and the more signs of readiness displayed by the toddler, the easier it will be to toilet train

        (a) Child shows interest and knows what it means to go to the bathroom

        (b) Able to understand and follow simple directions

        (c) Able to communicate needs

        (d) Able to sit for short periods

        (e) Wants to please parents

        (f) Has bowel movements at regular times every day

        (g) Able to remain dry through naps or for about 2 hours

        (h) Knows when he or she urinates or defecates

    **iv.** Once the child is showing signs of readiness the parent should start pre-toilet training activities

        (a) The parents should purchase a potty chair and place it in the bathroom

        (b) The toddler should be allowed to sit on the potty chair with clothes at first

        (c) Purchasing a child's book or video about going to the toilet is helpful in teaching names for elimination and to encourage to child to use the toilet

    **v.** After keeping track of the toddler's toileting habits, place the toddler on the toilet without a diaper at a time he or she is likely to eliminate

    **vi.** If the child eliminates in the toilet, a great deal of praise should be given

    **vii.** If the child is ready, this is a very easy process

**e.** Sleep problems

    **i.** The main sleep problems during the toddler and preschool period are:

        (a) Difficulties going to sleep

        (b) Waking after they are asleep

        (c) Nightmares

        (d) Night terrors

        (e) Sleepwalking

    **ii.** There is no perfect time to put a toddler in a big bed

    **iii.** If the child is climbing out of bed or does not fit in the crib, it is time to move to big bed

    **iv.** Most children go to a big bed sometime between 2 and 3 years

    **v.** Having a routine for bedtime often helps with going to sleep

    **vi.** Need to be consistent with the bedtime routine and always put the child to bed while awake

    **vii.** All children have sleep cycles that cause them to be in deep and wakeful periods all night

    **viii.** If the child cries or tries to get out of bed the parent must put him or her back to bed with no rewards like additional stories or parent getting into bed with the child

    **ix.** They will eventually learn how to get to sleep

    **x.** Children who have self-soothing techniques have fewer problems with getting themselves back to sleep

    **xi.** Toddlers have overactive imaginations, so they are prone to have nightmares

xii. Nightmares usually happen toward the end of the night, and toddlers may need to be comforted but they usually can fall right back to sleep

xiii. Nightmares can be remembered

xiv. Night terrors happen more often in the preschooler or older child

    (a) Night terrors happen early in the night, and the child will wake up in a panic

    (b) The child may shake, scream, cry and not recognize the parent

    (c) The child will not remember the night terror the next day

    (d) Sometimes the child is so out of control that the parent mistakes it for a seizure

    (e) Nightmares are more frightening for the child, and night terrors are more frightening for the parent

**f. Discipline**

i. When the child becomes frustrated in attempts to achieve behaviors or milestones, temper tantrums or misbehaviors often occur

ii. Need to provide guidance, avoid frustrating situations, and provide reasonable choices to control temper tantrums (Green, et al., 2001)

iii. Discipline is begun during the toddler years

iv. One of the greatest gifts that parents can give their children is teaching them how to behave

v. Discipline is teaching and should not be punitive but done with love

vi. While the toddler is young, diversion is the best form of discipline

vii. After the toddler is 24 months, time-out may be used

viii. Most 24-month-olds will not sit alone so the parent must stay with them for the allotted time (1 minute for each year of age)

ix. As the child gets older taking away privileges is an appropriate form of discipline

x. Spanking teaches a child that it is okay to hit

**g. Developmental disorders**

i. By the age of toddlerhood many developmental disorders will display themselves

ii. Mental retardation will present with delays in speech and personal social development

iii. Cerebral palsy is a disorder of movement and posture

iv. Cerebral palsy usually presents with delays in gross and fine motor development

v. Communication disorders are seen with mental retardation, autism, and pervasive developmental disorders

vi. If developmental delays are diagnosed and treatment is begun early, often the child can reach a full potential

**h. Learning problems**

i. The main task of the school-ager is to learn basic skills such as reading, writing, and math

ii. These skills will help the child prepare for adulthood

iii. Not all children find it easy to learn

iv. When a child has difficulty in school, all efforts should be taken to help the child succeed

v. Attention deficit hyperactivity disorder (ADHD) is one of the more common problems interfering with learning (see Chapter 49 for more information on ADHD)

**i. Lead poisoning** (see also Chapter 19, section 7, h.iii)

i. Epidemiology (Marcus, 2004)

        (a) Lead poisoning is the most common environmental illness in children in the United States

        (b) Prevalence greatest in Black, non-Hispanic, followed by Mexican American, then white non-Hispanic

  **ii.** Risk factors (from KeepKidsHealthy.com Lead Poisoning Screening Quiz)

        (a) Lives in or often visits a house that was built before 1950

        (b) Lives in or often visits a house that was built before 1978 and is being remodeled

        (c) Has playmates or friends that have high lead levels

        (d) Lives in a zip code where more than 27% of the housing was built before 1950

        (e) Is a member of a high risk group, including living in poverty, receiving aid from Medicaid and/or WIC

        (f) Eats or chews on nonfood things (pica), such as paint chips or dirt

        (g) Has family members that work at a place or has a hobby that involves pottery, stained glass, foundry, soldering, welding, lead ammunition, fishing weights or toy soldiers, auto repair, etc.

        (h) Lives or plays near an area with any of the following:

            (1) Smelter

            (2) Hazardous waste site

            (3) Lead industry

            (4) Place where batteries are manufactured or repaired

            (5) House construction site

            (6) Heavily traveled major highway

            (7) Place where cars are abandoned or repaired

       (i) Consumes any of the following products:

            (1) Medicines (especially home remedies) imported from another country, including:

                a) Pay-loo-ah (fever and rash treatment)

                b) Azarcon (a Mexican treatment for intestinal blockage that is 90% lead)

                c) Asian folk remedies, including ghasard (a brown powder used to aid digestion), bali goli (a round, flat black bean that is dissolved in water) and kandu (a red powder used to treat stomachaches)

                d) Middle Eastern folk remedies, including farouk (teething) and bint al zahab (colic)

                e) Cosmetics like surma or kohl

       (j) Eats foods that are cooked or stored in imported or glazed pottery

       (k) Eats foods or candy that are canned or produced outside the United States

       (l) Frequently chews on keys (which often contain small amounts of lead)

       (m) Lives in a home in which the plumbing has lead pipes, lead solder, or lead-containing holding tanks

 **iii.** Signs and symptoms

        (a) Often occurs with iron deficiency anemia

        (b) Hemoglobin is rarely less than 9 g/dL

        (c) Anemia is normochromic or normocytic or may be microcytic and hypochromic

        (d) Mean corpuscular hemoglobin (MCH) decreased slightly

(e) Anemia usually seen when lead levels are 50 to 80 mcg/dl

(f) Symptoms

    (1) Often there are no symptoms

    (2) Listlessness

    (3) Loss of appetite

    (4) Irritability

    (5) Problems with coordination, balance

    (6) Behavioral changes

    (7) Developmental delays

    (8) Growth delays

**iv.** Blood lead level (CDC, 2005; Marcus, 2005)

(a) Preferably done by venipuncture

    (1) Less than 10 mcg/dl is normal

    (2) More than 10 mcg/dl, rescreen, intervention, search for source

    (3) From 15 to 19 mcg/dl, rescreen, educational and nutritional intervention; reportable to local health department

    (4) See Chapter 19, Section 7 for information about follow-up on lead screening results

    (5) The following levels require referral to emergency medicine or other appropriate specialist

        a) 20 to 44 mcg/dl, evidence of increased exposure to lead; remedy environment; consider chelation

        b) 45 to 69 mcg/dl, chelation therapy; environmental intervention

        c) Greater than 70 mcg/dl, emergency treatment should begin

**v.** Treatment (Marcus, 2004)

(a) Primary treatment is removal from the lead exposure

(b) Initiated with levels greater than 45 mcg/dl

(c) Succimer (2,3 dimercaptosuccinic acid) administered orally 10 mg/kg PO q8h, days 1 to 5; 10 mg/kg PO q12h days 6 to 14

(d) Blood levels of Hb increase when treatment discontinued

(e) Dimercaprol and calcium edetate are no longer preferred method

(f) Environmental intervention: remove paint chips, peeling paint, mop and dust with high-phosphate cleaner (>5%) obtained at hardware store (some automatic dishwasher soaps have >5% phosphates)

(g) Diet high in calcium and iron

(h) Multivitamin with Fe

(i) Discontinue use of pacifier

(j) Keep child's hands clean

(k) Test other children in the home

(l) Flush water pipes daily before using water for drinking or cooking

(m) Use cold tap water for cooking

---

## REFERENCES

American Academy of Pediatrics. (2003). Rates of pediatric injuries by 3 month intervals for children 0–3 years of age. *Pediatrics, 111* (6), e683-e692. Also available at http://pediatrics.aappublications. org/cgi/content/abstract/111/6/e683.

American Academy of Pediatrics, Committee on Nutrition. (1999). Calcium requirements of infants, children and adolescents. *Pediatrics, 104*(5), 1152-1157. Also available at http://aappolicy.aappublications. org/cgi/content/ full/pediatrics;104/5/1152.

American Academy of Pediatrics Committee on Practice and Ambulatory Medicine. (2000). Recommendations for preventive pediatric health care. *Pediatrics, 105*(3), 645-646. Also available at http://aappolicy.aappublications. org/cgi/content/full/pediatrics;105/3/645.

Carakushansky, M., O'Brien, K. O., & Levine, M. A. (2003). Vitamin D and calcium: Strong bones for life through better nutrition. *Contemp Pediatr, 20* (3), 37-53.

Centers for Disease Control and Prevention. (2005). CDC Childhood Lead Poisoning Prevention Program. Retrieved July 1, 2005, from www.cdc.gov/nceh/lead/lead.htm.

Glascoe, F. P., & Macias, M. M. (2003). How you can implement the AAP's new policy on developmental and behavioral screening. *Contemp Pediatr, 20* (4), 85-66.

Gottesman, M. M. (2002). Helping toddlers eat well. *J Pediatr Health Care, 16,* 92-96.

Green, M., & Palfrey, J. S. (Eds.). (2002). *Bright futures: Guidelines for health supervision of infants, children and adolescents* (2nd ed., rev.). Arlington VA: National Center for Education in Maternal and Child Health.

Green, M., Sullivan, P. D., & Eichberg, C. G. (2001). What to do with the angry toddler. *Contemp Pediatr, 18* (8), 65-84.

Instone, S. L. (2002). Developmental strategies for interviewing children. *J Pediatr Health Care, 16,* 304-305.

Marcus, S. (2005). Toxicity: Lead. Retrieved June 6, from www.emedicine.com/EMERG/topic293.htm.

National Association of Pediatric Nurse Practitioners (NAPNAP). (2006). Healthy Eating and Activity Together (HEAT^sm) Clinical Practice Guideline: Identifying and Preventing Overweight in Childhood. Cherry Hill, NJ: NAPNAP.

Reilly, J. J., Armstrong, J., Dorosty, A. R., et al. (2005). Early life risk factors for obesity in childhood: Cohort study. *BMJ, 330* (7504), 1357.

Satter, E. (2000). *Child of mine: Feeding with love and good sense* (rev.ed.). Palo Alto, California: Bull Publishing.

# Mental Health Promotion and Mental Health Screening for Children and Adolescents

BERNADETTE MAZUREK MELNYK, PhD, RN, CPNP/NPP, FAAN, FNAP AND
ZENDI MOLDENHAUER, PhD, RN-CS, PNP/NPP

1. Mental health disorders and psychosocial morbidities in children and teens
   a. Definition of mental health (Satcher, 2003; Shives & Issacs, 2002)
      i. The successful performance of mental function, resulting in:
         (a) Productive activities
         (b) Fulfilling relationships with others
         (c) Self-direction
         (d) Problem-solving ability
      ii. The ability to adapt to change and to cope successfully with adversity
2. Incidence and background of mental health disorders
   a. Approximately 1 out of 4 children (i.e., 13 million) in the United States are affected by mental health or psychosocial morbidities that impair functioning at home and school (U.S. Office of the Surgeon General, 1999)
      i. Depression (see Chapter 41)
      ii. Anxiety disorders (see Chapter 41)
      iii. Effects of divorce
      iv. ADHD (see Chapter 49)
      v. Substance abuse
      vi. Eating disorders (see Chapter 45)
      vii. Sexual and physical abuse (see Chapter 21)
      viii. Risk-taking behaviors
      ix. Suicide is the third leading cause of death (Centers for Disease Control and Prevention [CDC], 2001) (see Chapter 41)
         (a) After motor vehicle accidents and homicides
         (b) In youth ages 15 to 19 years
         (c) Males more than females; 12.9 versus 2.7 per 100,000
   b. Virtually every U.S. classroom has one or two children, ages 9 to 17 years, with serious emotional problems (President's New Freedom Commission on Mental Health, 2002)

    **c.** Mental health problems or psychosocial morbidities are beginning to surpass physical health problems in children and youth (Melnyk, et al., 2003)

    **d.** Incidence is underestimated due to inadequate screening, intervention, and referral by primary care providers (U.S. Department of Health and Human Services [HHS], 1999)

    **e.** Approximately 70% of youth in need of treatment do not receive mental health services (Melnyk, et al., 2002)

    **f.** Insufficient numbers of child mental health care providers (Weitzman, 2003)
        **i.** Only 6300 psychiatrists in the United States
        **ii.** More than 30,000 are needed

    **g.** More than 12,700 children were placed into the child welfare or juvenile justice systems in 2002 so that they could receive mental health services (U.S. GAO Report to Congressional Requesters, 2003)

    **h.** Race or ethnicity and mental health disorders (Satcher, 2003)
        **i.** More common in Blacks than whites
        **ii.** Blacks are less likely to seek treatment

    **i.** Cost associated with mental health illnesses (U.S. Office of the Surgeon General, 1999).
        **i.** Estimated to be $69 billion per year
        **ii.** An additional $12.6 million is allocated to substance abuse treatment

    **j.** Despite ongoing prevention and intervention efforts:
        **i.** Numbers of children with mental health problems are increasing
        **ii.** Costs of screening, treatment, and prevention are climbing

    **k.** Case finding (Kelleher, et al., 2000; Melnyk et al., 2003; HHS, 2003)
        **i.** Children are most likely to receive assessment and treatment of these problems in primary care practices and schools
        **ii.** Emphasizes the urgent need for providers in these sites
        **iii.** Need providers competent in screening and implementing successful evidence-based early interventions

**3.** Risk and protective factors for child and adolescent mental health disorders

    **a.** Risk factors
        **i.** Poor self-esteem
        **ii.** Lack of other developmental assets
            (a) Resiliency
            (b) Connectedness to a parent
            (c) Positive coping skills
        **iii.** Altered parenting
            (a) Overprotective
            (b) Controlling
            (c) Rigid
            (d) Permissive
            (e) Lack of supervision
            (f) Limit setting
        **iv.** Parental conflict, separation, divorce
        **v.** Parents who have mental health problems, including use of substances
        **vi.** Chronic illness or child or family member with handicap
        **vii.** Hospitalization or life-threatening medical procedures
        **viii.** Learning disabilities
        **ix.** Deteriorating grades
        **x.** The presence of multiple stressors or recent stressful life events
            (a) Recent move
            (b) Death or illness of a family member or close friend

■ **TABLE 23-1**
■ ■ **Mental Health Screening Instruments for Primary Care—cont'd**

| Instrument and Author | Format | Logistics | Meaning of Scores | Reliability and Validity Evidence |
|---|---|---|---|---|
| Keep Your Children/ Yourself Safe and Secure questionnaire (KySS)(Melnyk, et al., 2002) Completed by parents or children | For ages 10–20 60 items on mental health knowledge and attitudes scored as strongly disagree = 1 to strongly agree = 5 13 items on worry about common mental health problems scored as not at all =1 to always = 5 | Taps mental health knowledge, attitudes, worries, communication, and needs items Fifth-grade reading level May be obtained through application from NAPNAP at www.napnap.org | Completing the KySS itself is an intervention in that it raises awareness of these problems and prompts children and parents to ask providers about them (Melnyk, et al., 2002) | Well-established face and content validity Reliability of worry items: alpha coefficient = 0.87 for children; 0.90 for parents |

     **v.** Other screening tools for specific mental health disorders available from U.S. Office of the Surgeon General (2006)
        (a) Depression
        (b) Anxiety disorders
        (c) Suicide
  **5.** Mental health interviewing in primary care
    **a.** When conducting an interview with a child or teen, it is critical to:
      **i.** Inform the child that your conversation is confidential
        (a) Unless he or she tells you that someone has hurt him or her
        (b) And/or that he or she wants to hurt him- or herself or someone else
      **ii.** If this information is revealed, you must tell the child that you will need to talk to another professional about it
    **b.** HEADSS is a short interview screen for teens
      **i.** Home
        (a) Where the child or teen is living
        (b) Who lives in the home
        (c) How is the child or teen getting along with people in the home
        (d) Is the environment supportive of the child
        (e) Has the teen ever run away or been incarcerated?
      **ii.** Education
        (a) How the teen is functioning in school in terms of grades
        (b) Teacher and peer relations
        (c) Suspensions
        (d) Missed school days, etc.
     **iii.** Activities
        (a) Extracurricular and sports activities that the teen is involved in
        (b) What the teen does with his friends, etc.
        (c) Amount of physical activity and screen time in which child/teen is involved
      **iv.** Drugs
        (a) What substances are used by the teen, family, and friends including:
          (1) Street, over-the-counter, and prescription drugs

        (2) Alcohol

        (3) Cigarettes

        (4) Caffeine

        (5) Inhalants

  v. Sexuality

    (a) Has the teen had sex; if yes, when was the first time?

    (b) Sexual preference

    (c) Use of contraceptives

    (d) Number of partners

    (e) Ever forced to have sex

    (f) History of sexually transmitted diseases

    (g) Use of condoms

    (h) History of pregnancy and abortion

    (i) History of sexual or physical abuse

  vi. Suicide

    (a) Any suicidal ideations or history of suicidal attempts?

    (b) If suicidal ideations, does the teen have a plan and is there access to a gun?

c. Critical mental health screening questions for parents (or age-appropriate adaptations)

  i. Do you have any concerns or worry:

    (a) About your child's mental or emotional health or his or her behaviors?

    (b) Has there been a change in how he or she usually is at home or at school?

    (c) If yes, proceed to the following questions.

  ii. What is the history and background to the parent's concern(s)?

    (a) What? What specifically occurs? What precipitated it? What are the associated symptoms (e.g., headaches, stomachaches)?

    (b) Where? At home, school, daycare?

    (c) When? Time of day? During a transition?

    (d) Is this an ongoing concern or an event that happened recently that is worrisome

    (e) Who? Who is with the child when it occurs? Who is involved?

    (f) How? How does the parent (and others) react?

    (g) Why? What are the parents' and child's ideas about why this is occurring?

  iii. Name three words that describe your child

  iv. What do you see as your child's strengths (e.g., self-esteem, coping skills)?

  v. What factors may place him or her at risk for emotional or behavior problems?

  vi. Have there been any recent life events or changes that have caused stress in your child and family?

    (a) Separation

    (b) Birth of a sibling

    (c) Illness or death of a family member or the child's friend

    (d) Hospitalization

    (e) Motor vehicle accident

  vii. How is your child's attention span (rule of thumb: 1 minute per each year of age)?

  viii. Does your child have any behaviors that worry you?

  ix. How would you describe your child's personality and temperament?

    (a) Optimistic versus pessimistic

    (b) Difficult versus easy-going

      ii. Educational testing to evaluate aptitude and ability

     iii. Neuropsychologic tests with trained specialists as indicated from the screening questionnaires or interview

6. Medical screening

  a. A suspected mental health disorder requires ruling out medical health conditions as an etiologic factor:

       i. Vision or hearing problems

      ii. Anemia

     iii. Hypothyroidism

     iv. Mononucleosis and chronic fatigue syndrome

      v. Eating disorders

     vi. Substance abuse

    vii. Premenstrual syndrome

   viii. Diabetes mellitus

     ix. Head trauma

      x. CNS lesions

     xi. Seizures

    xii. Cushing's syndrome

   xiii. HIV and AIDS

   xiv. Mitral valve prolapse

    xv. Systemic lupus erythematosus

   xvi. Chronic conditions

  xvii. Developmental delays

 xviii. Failure to thrive

  b. Obtain a general health history, including:

       i. A thorough review of all systems, e.g., has your child ever had or does he or she now have problems with his or her:

        (a) Head (e.g., headaches, head injuries)

        (b) Eyes (e.g., difficulty seeing, blurry vision)

        (c) Ears (e.g., ear infections), etc.

      ii. Has your child ever been hospitalized or had any surgeries?

     iii. Does your child have any type of chronic illness?

     iv. What medications does your child take?

       (a) At what dosage?

       (b) Does he or she experience any side effects from the medications?

      v. Assess prenatal, natal, and developmental history, including whether the child attained developmental milestones on time

  c. Conduct a thorough physical examination, including laboratory tests as indicated

7. Conducting a mental status exam

  a. Appearance (e.g., how is the child dressed and groomed?)

  b. Attitude and interaction (e.g., is the child cooperative, guarded, or avoidant?)

  c. Activity level or behavior

       i. Calm

      ii. Active

     iii. Restless

     iv. Presence of psychomotor activity

      v. Abnormal movements

     vi. Tics

  d. Speech

       i. Loud or quiet, flat in tone or full of intonation, slow or rushed

      ii. How are words formed?

      **iii.** Does the child understand what is being said?

      **iv.** Does the child express himself or herself appropriately?

  **e.** Thought processes

      **i.** Coherent

      **ii.** Disorganized

      **iii.** Flight of ideas (rapid skipping from topic to topic)

      **iv.** Blocking (inability to fill memory gaps)

      **v.** Loosening associations (the shifting of topics quickly even though unrelated)

      **vi.** Echolalia (mocking repetition of another person's words)

      **vii.** Perseveration (repetition of verbal or motor response)

  **f.** Thought content including:

      **i.** Delusions (false, irrational beliefs, such as "I am Superman")

      **ii.** Obsessions (persistent thoughts or impulses)

      **iii.** Perceptual disorders (including hallucinations [altered sensory perceptions], such as hearing voices inside or outside his or her head that others do not)

      **iv.** Phobias (irrational fears)

      **v.** Hypochondriasis (excessive worry about personal health without an actual reason)

  **g.** Impulse control: ability to control impulses

      **i.** Aggressive

      **ii.** Hostile

      **iii.** Sexual impulses

  **h.** Mood or affect

      **i.** Depressed

      **ii.** Anxious

      **iii.** Flat

      **iv.** Ambivalent

      **v.** Fearful

      **vi.** Irritable

      **vii.** Elated

      **viii.** Euphoric

      **ix.** Inappropriate

  **i.** Suicidal and or homicidal behavior or ideation

  **j.** Cognitive functioning

      **i.** Orientation to surroundings

      **ii.** Attention span or concentration

      **iii.** Memory (recent and remote)

      **iv.** Ability to abstract

      **v.** Insight or judgment

  **k.** Make astute observations of parent-child interaction

      **i.** Warm

      **ii.** Nurturing

      **iii.** Conflict

      **iv.** Rejecting

      **v.** Appropriate use of limit setting

      **vi.** In tune with child's feelings and needs

      **vii.** Affectionate

      **viii.** Eye contact and other body language.

  **l.** If further testing is warranted from the history and physical exam, refer to a mental health specialist

8. General approach to management of mental health disorders in primary care
   a. Primary prevention
      i. Parenting
      ii. School
      iii. Environment
      iv. Primary care
   b. Secondary prevention, essential components
      i. Early detection
      ii. Intervention
   c. Tertiary prevention: intervention once major loss or trauma or abuse is sustained
   d. Support and therapeutic communication with child and family
   e. Appropriate referral to mental health specialists or other services
   f. Psychoeducation (informing parents about what to expect with the condition)
   g. Psychotherapy
   h. Psychopharmacology
   i. Follow-up is very important
   j. Follow evidence-based guidelines to manage children with mental health problems
      i. National Guideline Clearinghouse for evidence-based clinical practice guidelines
      ii. Sponsored by Agency for Health Care Research and Quality and the AMA
      iii. Available at www.guideline.gov
9. Prevention of psychologic disorders in children and adolescents
   a. Prevention should:
      i. Occur at the primary, secondary, and tertiary levels
      ii. Intervene at the family, school, community, and primary care levels
   b. Primary prevention
      i. Should start during pregnancy or at birth with parenting education and support
         (a) Anticipatory guidance about infant temperament
         (b) Normal developmental milestones and characteristics
         (c) Positive parenting strategies to facilitate self-esteem and close relationships
      ii. It is easier to prevent behaviors that have never started and it is never too early to begin parent effectiveness training
   c. Specific preventive strategies
      i. Use *Bright Futures in Practice: Mental Health*
         (a) Guidelines for the mental health of children in a developmental context
         (b) By the Health Resources and Services Administration (HRSA)/ Maternal-Child Health Bureau (MCHB)
         (c) Available at www.brightfutures.org/mentalhealth
         (d) Information on early recognition and intervention for specific mental health problems and mental disorders
         (e) Tool kit for health professionals and families for use in screening, care management, and health education
      ii. Use the Keep Your Children/Yourself Safe and Secure (*KySS*) *Guide for Mental Health Screening, Early Intervention, and Health Promotion* (Melnyk, 2004)

        (a) Obtained from the National Association of Pediatric Nurse Practitioners (NAPNAP) at www.napnap.org

        (b) User-friendly guide

            (1) Key information

            (2) Screening tools

            (3) Early evidence-based intervention strategies or resources

            (4) Educational handouts that can be duplicated for parents and school-aged children and teens, and families

            (5) Tips on reimbursement for the prevention and treatment of mental health problems

            (6) Important information on prescribing medication for common child and adolescent mental health problems

iii. Screen for mental health or psychosocial morbidities at every visit

iv. Raise awareness of these problems

        (a) Posters in practice settings

        (b) Handouts

        (c) Parenting classes

v. Assist children, parents, and communities to build developmental assets in children

        (a) Teach children effective communication strategies

        (b) Problem-solving skills

        (c) Refusal skills

        (d) Coping strategies

        (e) Provide children and teens with opportunities for involvement in community activities

vi. Use the *Guide to Positive Youth Development* (ACT for Youth, 2003)

        (a) From the ACT for Youth Upstate Center of Excellence

        (b) Available at www.actforyouth.net

vii. Implement prevention strategies for children at highest risk for psychopathology and for those who experience traumatic events, including:

        (a) MVAs

        (b) Hospitalization

        (c) Rape

        (d) Family and neighborhood violence

viii. Encourage parents to be actively involved in their children's lives

        (a) Monitor their activities (who, what, when, and where)

        (b) Monitor the things that they are reading, watching, and listening

        (c) Mentor and model healthy behaviors

        (d) Require a 48-hour advance notice for sleeping over at a friend's house, because most drug and alcohol parties come together at the last minute

ix. Facilitate mentors for children and teens

        (a) Those who have mentors are less likely to use illegal drugs and alcohol

        (b) Are less likely to skip school

x. Encourage parents to:

        (a) Set developmentally appropriate limits and enforce them consistently

        (b) Become informed and to define their position on at-risk behaviors (e.g., zero tolerance)

        (c) Avoid double standards (e.g., do as I say, not as I do)

        (d) Avoid making excuses for their children (if they think there is a problem with their child, there usually is)

(e) Frequently communicate their expectations to their children regarding their behaviors and school performance

(f) Become acquainted with their children's friends and the parents of their children's friends (hold meetings to determine group rules)

(g) Do not allow their children and teens to watch R-rated movies, especially children younger than 13 years of age

xi. Help parents to assist their children in dealing with the current stressful events in their lives and in our society

xii. Emphasize importance of daily physical activity and exercise in releasing stress and anxiety

xiii. Encourage family activities and outings

xiv. Encourage service to others, belonging to sport, club, hobby group, and religious involvement

xv. Provide opportunities for children to be successful

(a) Encourage mastery skill development

(b) Teach coping and problem-solving strategies as well as refusal skills

(c) Build relationships with youth

xvi. Encourage journaling and creative expression with school-aged children and teens

xvii. Detect abuse and neglect early

(a) Address poverty; refer to social workers for assistance

(b) Build strong families with supports and resources

xviii. Participate in NAPNAP's KySS campaign

(a) Available at www.napnap.org

(b) See Melnyk et al., 2003

xix. Use quality resources to promote access to mental health in your state

xx. Become familiar with the Children's Defense Fund

(a) Children's Mental Health Resource Kit: Promoting Children's Mental Health Screens and Assessments

(b) Helps providers increase access and availability of mental health screens for children through Medicaid and the Children's Health Insurance Program (CHIP)

(c) See www.cdfhealth@childrensdefense.org or call 202-662-3575.

xxi. Familiarize parents with quality parenting resources:

(a) *Adventures in Parenting*

(1) By the National Institute of Child Health and Human Development (NICHD)

(2) Booklet that incorporates 30 years of research evidence on effective parenting techniques to stimulate healthy development

(3) Can be downloaded for free at www.healthfinder.gov/docs/doc06425.htm

(4) Or call the NICHD Information Resource Center at 800-370-2943

(b) *Common Sense Parenting* by Raymond Burke and Ron Herron (2000)

(c) *Bright Futures Handouts for Families* available at www.brightfutures.org

(d) *Parent Soup*

(1) An on-line resource with excellent parenting information

(2) What to expect at every stage of development

(3) See www.parentsoup.com

(e) *Creating Opportunities for Parent Empowerment (COPE)*
 (1) Evidence-based programs for parents with children experiencing stressors
  a) Parental separation and divorce
  b) Hospitalization
  c) Critical illness
 (2) Also for parents experiencing the birth of a low–birth weight premature infant
 (3) Copies can be obtained from Dr. Bernadette Melnyk at Arizona State University http://nursing.asu.edu

## REFERENCES

ACT for Youth Downstate Center for Excellence, ACT for Youth Upstate Center of Excellence (2003). *A guide to positive youth development.* New York: Mount Sinai Adolescent Health Center.

American Medical Association (1994). *Guidelines for adolescent preventive services (GAPS).* Retrieved April 6, 2006 from www.ama-assn.org/ama/pub/category/1980.html.

Burke, R., & Herron, R. (2000). *Common sense parenting,* 2nd ed. Boys Town, NE: Boys Town.

Centers for Disease Control and Prevention. (1999). Suicide deaths and rates per 100,000. Retrieved October 15, 2004, from www.cdc.gov/nchs/data/hus/tables/2003.

Department of Health and Human Services (1999). *Mental Health: A Report of the Surgeon General.* Rockville, MD: Department of Health and Human Services, Substance Abuse and Mental Health Services Administration, Center for Mental Health Services, National Institute of Mental Health. Available at: www.surgeongeneral.gov/library/mentalhealth/toc.html#chapter3.

Glascoe, F. P. (2001). *Parents Evaluation of Developmental Status.* Nashville: Ellsworth & Vandemeer Press.

Jellinek, M. (2002). Pediatric Symptom Checklist. In M. Jellinek, Ed. *Bright futures in practice: Mental health.* Georgetown University: The National Center for Education in Maternal & Child Health. Retrieved on April 6, 2006 from http://www.brightfutures.org/mentalhealth/pdf/professionals/ped_sympton_chklst.pdf

Kelleher, K. J., McInerny, T. K., Gardner, W. P., et al. (2000). Increasing identification of psychosocial problems: 1979–1997. *Pediatrics, 105,* 1313-1321.

Melnyk, B. M., Brown, H., Jones, D., et al. (2003). Improving the mental/psychosocial health of U.S. children and adolescents: Outcomes and implementation strategies from the National KySS Summit. *J Pediatr Health Care (Suppl), 17*(6), S1-S24.

Melnyk, B. M., Feinstein, N. F., Tuttle, J., et al. (2002). Mental health worries, communication, and needs of children, teens, and parents during the year of the nation's terrorist attack: Findings from the national KySS survey. *J Pediatr Health Care, 16*(5), 222-234.

Navon, M., Nelson, D., Pagano, M., & Murphy, M. (2001). Use of the pediatric symptom checklist in strategies to improve preventive behavioral health care. *Pediatric Serv, 52*(6) 800-804.

Pollack, C. L., & Kaye, D. L. (2002). Management and assessment of child mental health problems in the pediatric office. In D. L. Kaye, M. E. Montgomery, & S. W. Munson (Eds.). *Child and adolescent mental health.* Philadelphia: Lippincott Williams & Wilkins.

President's New Freedom Commission on Mental Health. *Interim report: Fragmentation and gaps in care for children.* Retrieved on April 6, 2006 from http://www.mentalhealth.samhsa.gov/publications/allpubs/NMH02-0144/gaps.asp

Ryan-Wenger, N. A. (2001). Use of children's drawings for measurement of developmental level and emotional status. *J Child Fam Nurs, 4*(2), 139-149.

Satcher, D. (2003). *Mental health. A lifespan approach.* Keynote presentation. Rochester,

New York: KySS Invitational Summit, March 29, 2003.

Shives, L. R., & Issacs, A. (2002). *Psychiatric and mental health nursing*. Philadelphia: Lippincott.

United States General Accounting Office (GAO) (2003). *Report to congressional requesters: Child welfare and juvenile justice*. Retrieved April 6, 2006, from http://www.gao.gov/new.items/d03397.pdf

U.S. Department of Health and Human Services (2003). *Compendium of AHRQ Research Related to Mental Health* (AHRQ Pub. No. 03-0001).

U.S. Department of Health and Human Services (HHS). (2000). *Healthy People 2010*. Available online at www.healthypeople.gov.

U.S. Department of Health and Human Services. (1999). *Mental Health: A Report of the Surgeon General—Executive Summary*. Rockville, MD: U.S. Department of Health and Human Services, Substance Abuse and Mental Health Services Administration, Center for Mental Health Services, National Institutes of Health, National Institute of Mental Health.

U.S. Department of Health and Human Services. (2006). Office of the Surgeon General. Retrieved on April 6, 2006 from http://www.surgeongeneral.gov/library/reports.htm

Weitzman, M. (2003). Who is and who isn't providing mental health services to our nation's children. Invited presentation. Rochester, New York: National KySS Summit, March 28.

# Sports Participation: Evaluation and Monitoring

JULIE NOVAK, DNSc, RN, MA, CPNP, FAANP

1. Scope of sports participation
   a. More than 30 million children and teens younger than age 18 participate in some form of organized sports, and the number is rising
   b. The fastest rise in participants has occurred in high school girls and children younger than age 10 (Metzl, 2002; Noonan, 2003)
   c. Age of beginning involvement
      i. T-ball begins at age 4 or 5
      ii. American Youth Soccer Organization begins at age 5
      iii. Pop Warner football and ice hockey leagues begin at age 7 or 8
   d. Increasing numbers of child athletes are:
      i. Engaging in intense training for a single sport on a year-round basis
      ii. Participating in multiple sports in a single season
   e. Most important aspects of sports participation
      i. Developmental and psychosocial benefits
      ii. Optimal sports participation can enhance a child's sense of community
   f. Sports participation should:
      i. Be a value-added activity contributing to healthy physical and emotional development
      ii. Promote a stable self-concept and feelings of self-worth
2. Motivations for sports participation
   a. Intrinsic factors
      i. Competence motivation
      ii. Test abilities against others
      iii. Participate for the excitement of the game
      iv. To have fun
      v. Girls are more goal oriented
      vi. Boys are more motivated to win
      vii. Personal benefits include: (Metzl, 2002)
         (a) Valuing preparation
         (b) Building resilience
         (c) Attitude control
         (d) Leadership opportunities
         (e) Understanding teamwork and camaraderie

      (f) Long-term thinking (sacrificing immediate gratification for long-term gain)

      (g) Valuing diversity

      (h) Stress relief

      (i) Improve skills, sometimes leading to mastery

      (j) Fitness and healthy habits

  **b.** Extrinsic factors

     **i.** Approval of significant adults

     **ii.** Peer approval; multiple peer groups including:

      (a) School

      (b) Sports

      (c) Church or synagogue

     **iii.** Ribbons and trophies

     **iv.** Spend time with old friends and make new friends, leading to sense of identity and balance (Metzl, 2002; Sullivan & Anderson, 2000)

**3.** Readiness to participate in sports

  **a.** Requires an individual assessment of the child's physical, cognitive, social, and motor development (AAP, 2001b; Sullivan & Anderson, 2000)

  **b.** Physical readiness

     **i.** See Chapter 12 for assessment of the musculoskeletal system

     **ii.** Many children acquire the motor skills necessary for sports participation by age 6

  **c.** Cognitive readiness

     **i.** By age 5, concepts of comparison and competition are developed

     **ii.** At age 6

      (a) Most children understand rules

      (b) If an activity has no rules, they often create them

  **d.** Social readiness

     **i.** Children younger than 7 generally lack the social and cognitive skills for:

      (a) Competition

      (b) Teamwork

      (c) Rapid decision making

     **ii.** Children as young as 7 and 8

      (a) Can participate on "select, elite teams"

      (b) Play high-level competitive sports year-round

     **iii.** Children often naturally select and modify activities so they can participate successfully and have fun (Metzl, 2002)

  **e.** Competition

     **i.** Must be designed for children rather than adults

     **ii.** Most children younger than the age of 10 appreciate competition less than adolescents

     **iii.** Controlled competition; Special Olympics is an excellent example

     **iv.** By age 15 years, 75% of children who have been involved in organized sports drop out, often reporting too much pressure to excel and win (Metzl, 2002)

**4.** Adult involvement

  **a.** Sports can have a positive influence on children if adults:

     **i.** Teach fundamental skills

     **ii.** Role-model a positive, respectful, courteous attitude based on positive reinforcement and consistency

     **iii.** Foster the child's sense of accomplishment

      iv. Prevent injury by ensuring that child has adequate:
- (a) Conditioning
- (b) Hydration
- (c) Supervision
- (d) Stringent control of games by officials or referees
- (e) Trainers on-site

      v. Balance sports with noncompetitive activities (and avoid making these activities competitive) such as:
- (a) Art
- (b) Music
- (c) Theater

5. Influence of the media
   a. Pressure to play may lead to injuries
   b. Pressure to perform may lead to injuries
   c. Unrealistic expectations may lead to injuries
   d. Effect on body image and self-concept
   e. Worldwide effect on developing children
   f. Hero worship
   g. The "just win" mentality has trickled down from professional and college levels with an emphasis on winning

6. Benefits of sports participation (AAP, 2001b)
   a. Sports participation is correlated with:
      i. Increased academic performance
      ii. Decreased school dropout and teen pregnancy rates
      iii. Decreased involvement in risk behaviors
      - (a) Smoking
      - (b) Substance use
   b. Greater total energy expenditure than those who do not participate, which correlates with: (Ara, et al., 2004; Metzl, 2002)
      i. Less body fat
      ii. Lower body weight
      iii. Lower incidence of overweight and obesity throughout life
      iv. Lower incidence of depression throughout life
   c. Strength and resistance training
      i. Among children as young as 8 years is a safe and effective method of increasing strength and improving athletic performance (Bernhardt, et al., 2001)
      ii. Baseline strength can be increased by 30% to 40% (Faigenbaum, et al., 2001)
      iii. Properly prescribed and supervised strength and resistance training can: (Story, Holt, and Sofka, 2002)
      - (a) Improve body composition
      - (b) Increase muscular strength and endurance
      - (c) Reduce risk of injury
      - (d) Enhance overall fitness and performance in sports and recreational activities
      iv. Recommendation for healthy participants of all ages: A minimum of 1 set of 8 to 10 exercises (multijoint and single joint) that involve the major muscle groups should be performed two or three times per week (Hass, et al., 2001)
      v. Beneficial if the program focuses on sports-specific tasks
      vi. If poorly supervised, strength training programs often lead to injury

    **c.** Unique aspects of female athletes

        **i.** 1972 adoption of Title IX of the Educational Amendment Act

        **ii.** Title IX requires colleges and universities to provide equal access of all races and both genders to all aspects of higher education including sports team participation and associated scholarship support

      **iii.** Women's sports participation increased by 700% in the 1970s and 1980s

      **iv.** In 1972 there were approximately 25,000 female high school athletes; in 2000 there were more than 3 million

       **v.** Sport is a great way for girls and women to build strong, healthy bodies, self-esteem and a lifelong love of physical activity

      **vi.** Optimal diet for female athletes

        **(a)** A balanced diet of 3000 kcal/day is required to obtain the RDA benefits of 15 mg iron and 750 mg calcium per day (Story, Holt, & Sofka, 2002)

        **(b)** Foods rich in iron include:

          **(1)** Lean meat, shrimp, fish, chicken breast, turkey, eggs, dried fruit and peas, kidney beans, cream of wheat, and fortified cereal

          **(2)** Sources of vitamin C, including citrus, fortified fruit juices, strawberries, cantaloupe, green peppers, broccoli, and cabbage, taken with meals increase the absorption of nonmeat sources of iron

          **(3)** Liver is no longer recommended due to its high cholesterol content and potentially high level of environmental toxins

        **(c)** Foods rich in calcium include dairy products, calcium-fortified soy milk and orange juice, tofu processed with calcium, blackstrap molasses, sesame seeds and sesame butter, almonds and almond butter, and some vegetables including broccoli, okra, collard and mustard greens, kale, and rutabaga

**9.** PNP role in sports health promotion

  **a.** Advocate

    **i.** Sports health policy development and implementation for optimal participation

    **ii.** Increased participation in and funding for youth sports should be a high priority particularly in light of the well-documented national epidemic of childhood obesity

  **b.** Researcher

    **i.** There is a lack of data on the full scope of the effect of sports participation by children, particularly for young females

    **ii.** A need to explore creative funding mechanisms to support projects, provide health and injury data to state and national tracking systems, and to suggest ways of improving quality assurance systems and program evaluation

  **c.** Educator

    **i.** Inform children, teens, parents, coaches, schools, legislators, and the community about the importance of sports health protection for all children

    **ii.** Encourage parents to ask questions (National Athletic Training Association, 2005; National Youth Sports Safety Foundation, 2005)

      **(a)** What is the level of the coach's preparation?

      **(b)** Does the coach's training include first aid and CPR?

      **(c)** How does the coach handle injuries?

      **(d)** What is the protocol for returning to sports following injury?

      **(e)** Is there an on-site health care provider?

      **(f)** Are there emergency medications on hand for asthma and allergy sufferers?

(g) What are the inclement weather guidelines especially for lightning storms and extreme heat?

(h) Who takes care of the field to make sure it is hazard-free for playing?

(i) Is the athletic equipment safe, properly fitted, and in good repair?

(j) Are there supervised preseason and in-season conditioning programs?

d. Collaborator

    i. A multidisciplinary approach to childhood sports health, including physicians, nurses, psychologists, nutritionists, coaches, athletic directors, athletic trainers, and physical therapists, is critical

    ii. A collaborative model, focusing on the best interests and short- and long-term health goals of the athlete while educating parents and coaches, is critical

e. Consultant

    i. Serve as a consultant to schools, parent groups, community leaders, legislators

    ii. Many of these groups have no health care providers among their numbers

    iii. The PNP can provide important insight into needs, safety and health of children

f. Advisor (Novak, 2001)

    i. PNPs can become members of school boards, athletic boards, and local, state, and national policymaking boards and committees

    ii. Remind all involved adults that sports lead to broader longer-term opportunities for success far beyond winning including:

        (a) Developing a sense of being the best that one can be

        (b) Fulfilling potential

        (c) Improving skills

        (d) Developing camaraderie and teamwork

        (e) Doing something that one is passionate about

        (f) Building character, persistence, and perseverance

    iii. Recommend a curriculum for coaches that includes (Thompson, 1995)

        (a) Communication and teaching

        (b) Physical and psychologic child development principles

        (c) Fitness

        (d) Sportsmanship

        (e) Cooperation

        (f) Nonviolent conflict resolution

        (g) Basic first aid is optimal

g. Care provider (Thompson, 1995)

    i. Conduct preparticipation sports exams

    ii. Provide acute care on the field

    iii. Provide long-term care for a chronic condition as a result of sports participation

    iv. Injury assessment in the primary care setting

    v. Refer children as necessary to orthopedics, neurology, cardiology, emergency department, hospital, rehabilitation

h. Role model

    i. PNPs who include regular physical activity in their own schedules:

        (a) Provide more physical activity counseling

        (b) Provide more relevant counseling

(3) Concussion symptoms or mental status abnormalities (including amnesia) on examination last more than 15 minutes

   (c) Grade III

      (1) Any loss of consciousness

         a) Brief (seconds)

         b) Prolonged (minutes)

  ii. Management of concussion

    (a) Grade I concussion

      (1) Remove from contest

      (2) Examine immediately and at 5-minute intervals for the development of mental status abnormalities or postconcussive symptoms at rest and with exertion

      (3) May return to contest if mental status abnormalities or postconcussive symptoms clear within 15 minutes (controversial)

    (b) Grade II concussion

      (1) Remove from contest and disallow return that day

      (2) Examine on-site frequently for signs of evolving intracranial pathology

      (3) A trained person should reexamine the athlete the following day

      (4) A health care provider should perform a neurologic examination to clear the athlete for return to play after 1 full asymptomatic week at rest and with exertion

    (c) Grade III concussion

      (1) Transport the athlete from the field to the nearest emergency department by ambulance if still unconscious or if worrisome signs are detected (with cervical spine immobilization, if indicated)

      (2) A thorough neurologic evaluation should be performed emergently, including appropriate neurologic imaging procedures when indicated

      (3) Hospital admission is indicated if any signs of pathology are detected, or if the mental status of the athlete remains abnormal (American Academy of Neurology, 1997)

    (d) When evaluating concussion, symptoms of headache more than 3 hours, difficulty concentrating more than 3 hours, retrograde amnesia, loss of consciousness (Asplund, et al., 2004)

      (1) May indicate a more severe injury or prolonged recovery

      (2) Use great caution before returning these athletes to the contest

    (e) The often-fatal second-impact syndrome occurs when a second, seemingly insignificant, head injury takes place before total resolution of symptoms of a previous head injury

 c. Mononucleosis

  i. See Chapter 33 for symptoms, diagnosis, and treatment of mononucleosis

  ii. Assessment criteria for return to play includes assessment of: (AAP, 2001; Halstead & Bernhardt, 2002)

    (a) Energy level

    (b) Splenomegaly

    (c) Type of sport (contact vs. noncontact)

  iii. A patient with an acutely enlarged spleen should avoid all sports due to potential risk of rupture

  iv. A patient with chronically enlarged spleen needs individual assessment before playing collision, contact, or limited contact sports

d. Atlantoaxial instability in Down syndrome
  i. Trisomy 21 (Down syndrome) is strongly associated with instability of the upper cervical spine
  ii. Incidence of atlantoaxial instability ranges from 10% to 25% (Thompson, 2004)
  iii. The Special Olympics maintains a requirement that all athletes with Down syndrome receive x-rays of the cervical spine to identify atlanto-axial instability
e. Tobacco use
  i. Less prevalent in student athletes than the general student and adolescent population
  ii. Smokeless tobacco (snuff, quid, and chaw) use is prevalent among youth engaged in particular sports (e.g., baseball)
  iii. Educational programs must target students in the primary grades, e.g., Tar Wars sponsored by the American Academy of Family Practice
  iv. Cessation programs using the Internet, instant messaging, CD-ROM, and telephone counseling are more often requested by youth as opposed to weekly classes (Novak, 2002)
  v. Interventions (Novak, 2002)
    (a) Must be focused, with ongoing support during the first 2 to 4 weeks of the quit attempt
    (b) Add pharmacologic interventions for teens who are addicted to tobacco
    (c) NAPNAP (2004) Position Statement on the Prevention of Tobacco Use in the Pediatric Population calls for PNPs to take an active role in anti-tobacco activities
f. Performance-enhancing substances
  i. Definition: stimulants or ergogenic aids designed to give athletes a chemically induced advantage in competition (Armsey & Hosey, 2004; Metzl, 2002)
  ii. Caffeine
    (a) Diuretic properties cause dehydration
    (b) Leads to reduced strength and stamina and hyperthermia
  iii. Nicotine
    (a) Addictive
    (b) Far greater health risk than performance benefits
  iv. Ephedrine
    (a) Herbal teas
    (b) Cold medications
    (c) Nutritional supplements such as ginseng and ginkgo biloba
    (d) Recently banned in many products
    (e) It is linked to:
      (1) Seizures
      (2) Heat exhaustion
      (3) Stroke
  v. Amphetamines
    (a) Most potent
    (b) Banned
  vi. Creatine
    (a) Remains the most popular nutritional supplement among young athletes, with sales of more than $400 million annually

(b) A study of 1103 children and adolescents (grades 6–12) found that 5.6% were using creatine

(c) Improving sports performance was the cited goal in 75% of cases

(d) Users were found at all grade levels (Metzl, et al., 2001)

vii. Anabolic steroids

(a) Anabolic steroids contribute to increased muscle size and strength

(b) Although older teens are the heaviest users, more than 500,000 students in grades 8 to 10 used them in 2000, the National Institute on Drug Abuse reported in its educational initiative (NIDA, 2000)

(c) Adverse effects have been reported in virtually every organ system and some are irreversible (Novak, 2003)

(d) Major effects of anabolic steroid use include: (Metzl, 2002)

(1) Increased muscle mass

(2) Hirsutism

(3) Deepened voice

(4) Acne

(5) Aggression

(6) Psychologic lability (hormone rage)

(7) Decreased sex drive

(8) Depression with cessation of use

(9) Increased risk of hepatic cancer and cardiovascular disease

(e) Side effects include:

(1) Increased blood pressure and cholesterol

(2) Decreased high-density lipoproteins

(3) Gastrointestinal distress

(4) Water retention that overloads kidneys

(5) Cardiac damage

(6) Increased sports and stress injuries because muscle development exceeds tendon strength

(f) There may be little effect on overall athletic performance unless *strength* is the primary factor in determining success

viii. $\beta_2$-agonists

(a) May cause anabolic effect

(b) Stimulant effects

ix. $\beta$-blockers

(a) Can enhance fine motor control

(b) They are banned substances in higher levels of competition

x. Adrenocorticotropic hormone (ACTH) and human chorionic gonadotropic hormone (HCG)

(a) Increase height

(b) Increase muscle mass

(c) Increase body weight

xi. Diuretics

(a) Induce rapid weight loss and reduce fluid retention secondary to anabolic-androgenic steroid use

(b) Most commonly used in wrestling

(c) Hallmarks of diuretic abuse include: (Metzl, 2002)

(1) Excessive urination

(2) Rapid weight loss in a short period

(3) Syncope due to orthostatic hypotension

xii. Epogen—synthetic erythropoietin

(a) Increases RBC mass and oxygen-carrying capacity

       (b) 18 cardiovascular deaths in cyclists attributed to epogen since 1987

       (c) Use is difficult to detect

**g.** Sudden cardiac death in young competitive athletes (Berger, et al., 2004)

  **i.** Etiology

       (a) Cardiomyopathy

       (b) Coronary artery anomalies

       (c) Cardiac mass

       (d) Ruptured aorta

       (e) Aortic stenosis

       (f) Myocarditis

       (g) Mitral valve prolapse

  **ii.** Cardiovascular history—inquire about and seek parental verification (Lyznicki, et al., 2000)

       (a) Family history of premature death (sudden or otherwise)

       (b) Family history of heart disease in surviving relatives

       (c) Significant disability from cardiovascular disease in close relatives younger than age 50 years

       (d) Specific knowledge of the occurrence of conditions in family (i.e., hypertrophic cardiomyopathy, long QT syndrome, Marfan's syndrome, or clinically important arrhythmias)

       (e) Personal history of heart murmur

       (f) Personal history of systemic hypertension

       (g) Personal history of excessive fatigability

       (h) Personal history of syncope, excessive or progressive shortness of breath (dyspnea), or chest pain or discomfort, particularly if present with exertion

 **iii.** 18% of athletes with sudden cardiac death had cardiovascular symptoms within the preceding 36 months including:

       (a) Chest pain

       (b) Exertion dyspnea

       (c) Syncope (9% had 1–10 syncopal or near-syncopal episodes)

       (d) Dizziness

  **iv.** Cardiovascular screening

       (a) Have you ever passed out during exercise?

       (b) Have you ever been dizzy during exercise?

       (c) Have you ever had chest pain during exercise?

       (d) Do you tire more quickly than your friends?

       (e) Have you ever had racing of your heart or skipped beats?

# REFERENCES

AAP: American Academy of Pediatrics, Committee on Sports Medicine and Fitness (2001a). Medical conditions affecting sports participation. *Pediatrics, 107*, 1205-1209.

AAP: American Academy of Pediatrics. Committee on Sports Medicine and Fitness and Committee on School Health. (2001b). Organized sports for children and preadolescents. *Pediatrics, 107*(6), 1459-1452.

American Academy of Neurology. (1997). Guidelines for the management of concussion in sports: American Academy of Neurology Practice Parameter. *Neurology, 48*, 581-585.

American Academy of Orthopedic Surgeons. (2005). Patient education library. Retrieved July 21, 2005, from http://orthoinfo.aaos. org.

Ara, I., Vincente-Rodriquez, G., Jimenez-Ramirez, J., et al. (2004). Regular participation in sports is associated with enhanced physical fitness and lower fat mass in prepubertal boys. *Int J Obes Relat Metabol Disord, 28*(12), 1585-1593.

Armsey, T. D., & Hosey, R. G. (2004). Medical aspects of sports: epidemiology of injuries, preparticipation physical examination, and drugs in sports. *Clin Sports Med, 223*(2), 255-279, vii.

Asplund, C. A., McKeag, D. A., & Olson, C. H. (2004). Sport-related concussion: Factors associated with prolonged return to play. *Clin J Sport Med, 14*(6), 339-343.

Berger, S., Kugler, J. D., Thomas, J. A., & Friedberg, D. Z. (2004). Sudden cardiac death in children and adolescents: Introduction and overview. *Pediatr Clin North Am, 51*(5), 1201-1209.

Bernhardt, D. L. (2004). *Concussion.* Retrieved from eMedicine on April 17, 2006 at http://www.emedicine.com/sports/topic27-Clinical.htm

Birch, K. (2005). Female athlete triad. *BMJ, 330*(7485), 244-246.

Centers for Disease Control and Prevention (2005). National Center for Injury Prevention and Control Activity Report: 2001. Retrieved June 6, 2006, from www.cdc.gov/ncipc/pub-res/unintentional-activity/07-state-programs.htm.

Faigenbaum, A. D., Zaichowsky, L. D., Wescott, W. L., et al. (2001). The effects of a twice-a-week strength-training program on children and adolescents. *Pediatrics, 107*, 1470-1472.

Gittes, E. B. (2004). The female athlete triad. *J Pediatr Adolesc Gynecol, 17*(5), 363-365.

Halstead, M. E., & Bernhardt, D. T. (2002). Common infections in the young athlete. *Pediatr Ann, 31*(1), 42-48.

Harmon, K. G. (1999). Assessment and management of concussion in sports. *Am Fam Phys, 60*(3), 887-894.

Hass, C. J., Feigenbaum, M. S., & Franklin, B. A. (2001). Prescription of resistance training for healthy populations. *Sports Med, 31*(14), 953-964.

Lyznicki, J. M., Neilson, N. H., & Schneider, J. F. (2000). Cardiovascular screening of student athletes. *Am Fam Phys, 62*(4), 765-772.

Metzl, J. D. (2002). *The young athlete.* Boston: Little, Brown and Company.

Metzl, J. D., Small, E., Levine, S. R., & Gershel, J. C. (2001). Creatine use among young athletes. *Pediatrics, 108*(2), 421-425.

National Association of Pediatric Nurse Practitioners (NAPNAP) (2004). *Position statement on the prevention of tobacco use in the pediatric population.* Retrieved on June 6, 2006, at http://www.napnap.org/Docs/pos-tobacco.pdf

National Athletic Training Association. (2005). *Safety checklist for high school sports.* Retrieved July 21, 2005, from www.nata.org/publicinformation/files/safetychecklist.pdf.

National Institute on Drug Abuse (NIDA) (2000). *Steroid abuse and addiction,* www.nida.gov/research reports/Steroids/AnabolicSteroids.html.

National Youth Sports Safety Foundation. (2005). *A primer for safety on youth sports.* Available for $2 from www.nyssf.org/wframeset.html.

Noonan, D. (September 22, 2003). When safety is the name of the game. *Newsweek,* 64-66.

Novak, J. (2003). Cited by Wendy L. Bonifazi in "Quest for big muscles yields big problems." *Nurs Spect.* Retrieved June 6, 2006, from http://community. nursing-spectrum.com/MagazineArticles/article.cfm?AID=12642.

Novak, J. C. (2001). PNPs: activists in the local, national, and global arenas. *J Pediatr Health Care, 15*(5), 17A-18A.

Novak, J. C. (2002). The tobacco user's cessation helpline (TOUCH): A pilot study to developing effective interventions. *Purdue Nurse.* West Lafayette: Purdue University.

Peer, K. S. (2004). Bone health in athletes. Factors and future considerations. *Orthop Nurs, 23*(3), 174-181.

Sherman, R. T., & Thompson, R. A. (2004). The female athlete triad. *J School Nurs, 20*(4), 197-202.

Stollo, N. K. (2003). When competition is queen: Health issues in women athletes. *Adv Nurse Pract, 11*(7), 32-36, 39.

Story, M., Holt, K., & Sofka, D. (Eds.). (2002). *Bright futures in practice: Nutrition* (2nd ed.). Arlington, VA: National Center for Education in Maternal and Child Health.

Sullivan, J. A., & Anderson, S. J. (2000). *Care of the young athlete.* American Academy of Orthopedic Surgeons and the American

Academy of Pediatrics. Elk Grove Village, IL: AAP Publishing.

Thompson, G. H. (2004). The neck. In R. E. Behrman, R. M. Kliegman, & H. B. Jenson (Eds.). *Nelson textbook of pediatrics* (17th ed., p. 2289). Philadelphia: Saunders.

Thompson, J. (1995). *Positive coaching: Building character and self-esteem through sports, the Stanford experience*. Portola Valley, CA: Warde Publishers.

Vitulano, L. A. (2003). Psychosocial issues for children and adolescents with chronic illness: self-esteem, school functioning and sports participation. *Child Adolesc Clin North Am, 12*(3), 585-592.

Wind, W. M., Schwend, R. M., & Larson, J. (2004). Sports for the physically challenged child. *J Am Acad Orthop Surg, 12*(2), 126-132.

# CHAPTER 25

# Early Adolescents, Late Adolescents, and College-age Young Adults

NAOMI A. SCHAPIRO, RN, MS, CPNP

1. Rationale for emphasis on adolescent health promotion
   a. Period of significant growth and change, physically, emotionally, cognitively, and socially
   b. Incidence of serious medical problems low
   c. Lifelong health habits established during adolescence influence chronic disease in future (Rosen & Neinstein, 2002)
   d. Dramatic cognitive, social, physical, and pubertal changes introduce new goals, needs, and opportunities
   e. Preventable "new morbidities" are taking over as leading causes of death during adolescence (Anderson, 2002) (Table 25-1)
      i. Accidents
      ii. Homicides
      iii. Suicides
   f. New morbidities are primarily psychosocial in origin and are related to risky behaviors and factors that increase risk
   g. *Healthy People 2010* (U. S. Department of Health and Human Services, 2000) critical youth objectives
      i. Decrease the proportion of youth who:
         (a) Engage in binge drinking of alcohol
         (b) Use illicit drugs
         (c) Use tobacco
      ii. Decrease deaths from:
         (a) Homicides
         (b) Motor vehicle accidents
         (c) Suicide
      iii. Decrease the proportion of youth who are "at risk for overweight" and "overweight" according to CDC criteria (See Chapter 16, Section 1) (Neumark-Sztainer, et al., 2002)
      iv. Increase the proportion of youth who engage in vigorous activity three times per week for 20 minutes or more

■ **TABLE 25-1**
■ ■ **Leading Causes of Death in Adolescents and Related Risky Behaviors**

| Causes of Death | Ages 10–14 | Ages 15–19 | Ages 20–24 | Related Risky Behaviors |
|---|---|---|---|---|
| Accidents | 38.2% (1)* | 49.8% (1) | 41.5 % (1) | 30.7% rode in car with drunk driver in past 30 days<br>13.3% drove after drinking in past 30 days<br>17.2% of male students 9.5% of female students and 13% of all students rarely or never wear seat belts |
| Murders | 5.6% (4) | 14.1% (2)<br>Black males<br>44% (1) | 17% (2)<br>Black males<br>48.9% (1) | 17.4% of students had carried a weapon in past 30 days<br>29.3% of male students 6.2% of female students and 6.4% of all students carried a weapon to school in past 30 days |
| Suicides | 7.2% (3) | 14.1% (3) | 13.4% (3) | 19% of high school students seriously considered suicide in past 12 months |
|  | Second leading cause of death for white male and all Native American youth, ages 15–24<br>Suicide and sexual orientation: ↑ rate of youth victimization associated with ↑substance use and ↑suicidal behavior among gay and bisexual youths | | | 8.8% of high school students attempted suicide in past 12 months<br>58% of all suicides in US in 1997 committed with a firearm<br>Young women more likely to attempt, but 5 times more young men ages 15-19 succeed |

*(1) denotes ranking within age group.

    **v.** Increase the proportion of youth who:
        (a) Abstain from sex
        (b) Use condoms
**2.** Periodicity of examinations
    **a.** Guidelines for Adolescent Preventive Services (GAPS)
        **i.** Developed and promoted by the American Medical Association's Department of Adolescent Health (1997)
        **ii.** American Academy of Pediatrics (AAP), Bright Futures, American Association of Family Physicians (AAFP), American Medical Association (AMA) are in general agreement
        **iii.** A list of 24 recommendations intended to organize, restructure, and redefine health care delivery for 11- to 21-year-old patients
        **iv.** Provides preventive service recommendations and a flow sheet that is useful for implementing and documenting these services during office visits
        **v.** Enables identification of at-risk adolescent patients and provides them with information about changing unhealthy behaviors

      vi. Health questionnaires are available in English and Spanish for younger adolescents, middle and older adolescents, and parents and guardians

     vii. Yearly well child visits are recommended

       (a) Screen yearly for:

         (1) Height

         (2) Weight

         (3) Body mass index (BMI)

         (4) Blood pressure

         (5) Hearing

         (6) Vision

         (7) Urinalysis (recommended only by AAP)

         (8) Hematocrit or hemoglobin

           a) Once between 11 and 21 years

           b) Consider yearly in menstruating females (Wu, et al., 2002)

         (9) Tuberculosis

       (b) Tests for youth at particular risk

         (1) Cholesterol

         (2) Sexually transmitted infections (STIs)

           a) Urine screening now available for some STIs, e.g. *Chlamydia trachomatis* and *Neisseria gonorrhoeae*

           b) For sexually active teens consider the following STIs depending on local prevalence (Burstein & Murray, 2003):

             i) Chlamydia

             ii) Gonorrhea

             iii) Syphilis

             iv) Human papillomavirus (HPV)—relationship between HPV and low-grade dysplasia in young women (Saslow et al, 2002; Shafer, 2000)

             v) HIV

           c) Papanicolau (Pap) test—recommended 3 years after beginning sexual activity or at age 21 (Saslow, et al., 2002)

           d) Indications for pelvic exam without Pap test include dyspareunia, pain, vaginal discharge

       (c) Psychosocial assessments every year

         (1) Tobacco use

         (2) Alcohol use

         (3) Drug use

         (4) Sexual activity

         (5) School performance

         (6) Eating disorders

         (7) Depression

         (8) Physical, sexual, or emotional abuse

         (9) Suicidal ideation

       (d) Immunizations (see Chapter 15 for details on routine immunizations)

       (e) Complete physical examination three times during adolescence

    viii. An understanding of adolescent physical, psychosocial, and cognitive development guides assessment, health promotion, and disease prevention interventions

**3.** History taking with adolescents and college-age young adults

  **a.** Reasons for encouraging confidential portions of the interview (without parents or guardians) (Klein & Wilson, 2002)

    **i.** Perceived lack of confidentiality is a barrier to care

      ii. Adolescents most want to discuss drugs, smoking, healthy dietary habits with provider only

     iii. 63% of teens who engage in risky behaviors have not spoken to provider about them

**b.** Legal and ethical background for adolescent privacy, consent, and assent (Dickey & Deatrick, 2000; English, 2000)

       i. Common law traditionally has given mature minors (14 years and up) some rights to make decisions about health care

      ii. Constitutional right to privacy applies to adolescents as well as adults in some instances

     iii. Ethical principle of autonomy supports adolescent's right to make decisions consistent with developmental abilities

     iv. Utilitarian ethical principle supports confidential interview to facilitate disclosure of sensitive but important information

      v. Emancipated minor

        (a) Legally married

        (b) Member of the Armed Forces

        (c) Legal emancipation

           (1) Living apart from parent or guardian

           (2) Legally self-supporting

      vi. Mature minor

        (a) Living apart from parents, with or without permission

        (b) Managing own affairs

        (c) Income from any source

     vii. All 50 states give adolescents some rights to privacy/consent for confidential issues (English, 2000, Maradiegue, 2003)

        (a) Many states have laws mandating reporting of consensual sexual activity depending on: (American Academy of Family Physicians, et al., 2004)

           (1) Age of minor

           (2) Sexual partner, i.e. adult, family member

        (b) Federal policy gives parents control over all medical records (Dailard, 2003)

           (1) Including confidential information

           (2) Individual states may override this

        (c) Health Insurance Portability and Accountability Act (HIPAA)

           (1) Confidentiality/privacy rules affect most providers, protect release of information

           (2) Protects school employees in limited situations (HIPAA-related billing)

        (d) Family Educational Rights and Privacy Act (FERPA)

           (1) Applies to PNPs employed by schools

           (2) May apply to school-based health centers

           (3) Parents have access to school records

           (4) Records may be shared without student/parental permission within school, to law enforcement, depending on state law

        (e) Exceptions to confidentiality

           (1) Patient expresses suicidal ideation or intent to harm self

           (2) Patient expresses intent to harm someone else

           (3) Patient suffered:

              a) Physical abuse

              b) Emotional abuse

              c) Sexual abuse

              d) Reportable neglect

    **c.** Principles for the order of interview questions
        **i.** Rapport building with teen, using areas of interest
        **ii.** Start with chief complaint or most pressing concern
        **iii.** In general, move from less sensitive to more sensitive questions
    **d.** Tailor the interview to the youth's developmental stage (Goldenring & Rosen, 2004)
        **i.** See Box 25-1 for key issues at four developmental stages
        **ii.** Use more concrete language for early adolescents
        **iii.** Be sensitive to varying exposures to risky behaviors
            **(a)** For younger teens, start with, "Do you know anyone who…?"
            **(b)** For older teens or with history of risky behaviors, use a more direct approach
    **e.** Questioning techniques
        **i.** Use a combination of open-ended and closed questions
        **ii.** Gender neutral, avoid assumptions about family structure and sexual orientation of teen
        **iii.** Try to use teen's terminology, without trying to sound like an adolescent
    **f.** Warn of exceptions to confidentiality before raising sensitive issues
    **g.** Avoid too much distance
        **i.** Write as little as possible during the interview
        **ii.** Watch own body language, eye contact, and that of teen
    **h.** Many mnemonics are available to avoid missing important information, e.g., HEADS, PACES, SAFETEENS (Box 25-2), CAGE, CRAFFT (Box 25-3)

---

■ **BOX 25-1**
■ **KEY TOPICS FOR DISCUSSION DURING PRIMARY CARE VISIT BASED ON AGE-GROUP**

**EARLY ADOLESCENT**
Anticipatory guidance about puberty, body changes
Encourage critical thinking about messages in media
Exercise, group physical activities
Encourage healthy food choices
   Discourage skipping meals
   Avoid excessive restrictions
Encourage delay of experimentation with drugs, alcohol, smoking, sex
Inform of availability of confidential support services
Condom demonstration if indicated
Appropriate safety messages
   Seat belts
   Helmets

**MIDDLE ADOLESCENT**
Encourage planning
   Educational goals
   Career, job goals
Think through short-term consequences of actions
More receptive to discussions about healthy food choices
Exercise
Injury prevention in sports
Encourage safer choices
Sexual activity
Avoid substance use connected to sexual activity or motor vehicles
Job safety
Volunteer opportunities

■ **BOX 25-1**
■ **KEY TOPICS FOR DISCUSSION DURING PRIMARY CARE VISIT BASED ON AGE-GROUP—cont'd**

**LATE ADOLESCENT, YOUNG ADULT, COLLEGE BOUND**
Pre-college immunizations, screening tests
Binge drinking, drug issues on campus
   "Freshman 15" – typical weight gain of about 15 pounds in first year of college attributed to dorm life and poor diet
Transitioning relationships with parents, new responsibilities at age 18
Wanted, unwanted sexual activity
Availability of confidential support services
Transition to adult care

**LATE ADOLESCENT, YOUNG ADULT, NOT COLLEGE BOUND**
Post–high school plans, or plans to get diploma, GED
Non-college career options
Work, peer group
Wanted, unwanted sexual activity
Availability of confidential support services
Substance use issues
Housing if living in foster care or temporary situation
Transitional plans for health insurance
Transition to adult care

■ **BOX 25-2**
■ **MNEMONICS USEFUL IN THE COMPREHENSIVE EVALUATION OF ADOLESCENT AND YOUNG ADULT**

**HEADS**
**H** = Home, habits
**E** = Education, employment, exercise
**A** = Accidents, ambition, activities, abuse
**D** = Drugs (tobacco, alcohol, others), diet, depression
**S** = Sex, suicide, safety

**PACES**
**P** = Parents, peers
**A** = Accidents, alcohol/drugs
**C** = Cigarettes
**E** = Emotional issues
**S** = School, sexuality

**SAFE TEENS**
**S** = Sexuality
**A** = Accident, abuse
**F** = Firearms/homicide
**E** = Emotions (suicide/depression)
**T** = Toxins (tobacco/alcohol, others)
**E** = Environment (school, home, friends)
**E** = Exercise
**N** = Nutrition
**S** = Shots (immunization status and school performance

■ **BOX 25-3**
■ **CAGE AND CRAFFT MNEMONICS FOR ALCOHOL OR DRUG USE ASSESSMENT**

**CAGE**
■ Have you felt a need to **Cut** down on drinking?
■ Have you been **Annoyed** by criticism of your drinking?
■ Have you felt **Guilty** about drinking?
■ Have you felt the need for a morning **Eye-opener?**

**CRAFFT**
■ Have you ridden in a **Car** with someone high?
■ Do you drink or use drugs to **Relax** or fit in?
■ Do you drink or use drugs while **Alone?**
■ Do you **Forget** things you did while on alcohol or drugs?
■ Do **Family** or **Friends** tell you to cut down?
■ Have you been in **Trouble** from drinking or drugs?

4. Adolescent physical development
   a. Girls
      i. Onset of puberty varies widely, between ages 8 and 13 years
      ii. Growth spurt between Sexual Maturity Rating (SMR) (formerly Tanner stages) 3 and 4 (see Chapter 9, Figure 9-4 and Chapter 26, Figure 26-1)
      iii. Norms for height, weight, and BMI are available on charts from CDC; www.cdc.gov/growthcharts
      iv. Norms for blood pressure are available from Muntner and colleagues (2004)
      v. See Chapter 29, Section 3 for details on hyperlipidemia
      vi. Menarche—beginning of menstrual periods
         (a) Average age is 12 years
         (b) Range from 9 to 16 years
         (c) Occurs between SMR stages 3 and 4
      vii. Reach 85% of adult height at menarche
         (a) Closing of epiphyses about 2 years later
      viii. Continue to develop
         (a) Hips and breasts continue to develop throughout puberty
         (b) Body fat increases
   b. Boys
      i. Onset of puberty varies widely, between ages 9 and 13 years
      ii. Growth spurt between SMR stages 4 and 5 (See Chapter 9, Figure 9-2)
      iii. Norms for height, weight, and BMI are available on charts from CDC; www.cdc.gov/growthcharts
      iv. Norms for blood pressure are available from Munter and colleagues (2004)
      v. See Chapter 29, Section 3 for details on hyperlipidemia
      vi. Spermarche—involuntary ejaculation ("wet dream")
         (a) Average age is 13 years
         (b) Range from 11 to 15 years
         (c) Occurs between SMR stages 2 and 3
      vii. May not reach full skeletal maturity until age 18 to 20 years
      viii. Adds muscle mass mostly after completion of skeletal growth

5. Adolescent cognitive and psychosocial development (Radzik, et al., 2002)
   a. Early adolescence (ages 10 to 13 years)
      i. Shift from dependence on parents to desire for independent behavior
         (a) Increase in frequency of conflicts with parents
      ii. Increased importance of peer group, primarily same-sex relationships
      iii. Major body image concerns due to varying rates of pubertal changes in this age group
      iv. Increased
         (a) Need for privacy
         (b) Daydreaming
         (c) Mood swings
         (d) Sexual feelings
      v. Developing ability to reason abstractly versus concrete thinking
      vi. Poor impulse control
      vii. Little future orientation
   b. Middle adolescence (ages 14 to 16 years)
      i. Conflicts with parents
         (a) Decrease in frequency
         (b) Increase in intensity
      ii. More comfort with body, but continuing self-image preoccupation
      iii. Intense peer group involvement
         (a) Mixed gender
         (b) Clubs
         (c) Sports and other group activities
         (d) Gangs
      iv. Increased dating
      v. Sexual experimentation
      vi. Continued intellectual development, beginnings of individuality
      vii. Feelings of omnipotence and immortality, increased risk taking
   c. Late adolescence (ages 16 to 23 years)
      i. Increased integration of dependence or independence, appreciation of family
      ii. Largely finished with pubertal growth and development
      iii. Peer group values less important, individual values more developed
      iv. Adult cognitive abilities, more future orientation
      v. More realistic educational and vocational goals
      vi. Beginning financial independence
      vii. Vulnerable time for teens without clear educational and vocational goals
         (a) High school graduation nears
         (b) Loss of childhood "safety nets"
6. Risky behavior and risk factors
   a. Biomedical and epidemiologic models are useful to understand the links among risky behaviors, risk factors, and health outcomes
   b. Role of risky behaviors in adolescence
      i. To gain peer acceptance and respect
      ii. To establish autonomy from parents
      iii. To repudiate norms and values of conventional authority
      iv. Coping
         (a) Anxiety relief
         (b) Frustration
      v. To mark transition out of childhood to more adult status

    c. Awareness of behavior as a risk factor increases with age, but may not change behavior

    d. Negative outcomes of risky behaviors

        i. Physical (disease, disability)

        ii. Social (school expulsion, limited job opportunities)

        iii. Legal record

    e. Positive outcomes of risky behaviors

        i. Increased self-esteem

        ii. Learn self-control

        iii. Evaluate cost versus benefit of behaviors

    f. Surveys completed by adolescents about risky behavior; see Table 25-2 for details on the following sources:

        i. National or State Youth Risk Behavior Surveillance System

        ii. Monitoring the Future Survey

        iii. National Longitudinal Study of Adolescent Health

        iv. Kaiser Family Foundation studies

7. Health risks related to adolescent developmental levels

    a. Physical development

        i. Interest in risk-taking behavior is related to stage of pubertal development

          (a) Early developers at higher risk due to less cognitive ability to control impulses

■ **TABLE 25-2**
■ ■ **Sources of Data About Adolescent Health Risk Behavior**

| Study | Population | Frequency, Methodology | Focus of Study | Access Information and Sponsor of Study |
|---|---|---|---|---|
| Youth Risk Behavior Surveillance System (YRBSS) | High school students | Every 2 years, anonymous self-report questionnaire in school | Includes, sex, alcohol, drug, safety, diet, and exercise | www.cdc.gov/nccdphp/dash/yrbs (Centers for Disease Control & Prevention) |
| Monitoring the Future | 50,000 8th, 10th, 12th graders, follow-up to college, young adults | Yearly in-school survey, follow-up mailed survey to selected sample of senior class | Primarily drug and alcohol use and related attitudes | http://monitoringthe future.org (University of Michigan, sponsored by National Institute on Drug Abuse) |
| National Longitudinal Study of Adolescent Health | 7th to 12th graders surveyed in 1994–95 with longitudinal follow-up Wave III 2001–02 | Combination of in-school and at-home surveys, interviewed teens and parents, collect some objective data | Forces that influence health-related behaviors | www.cpc.unc.edu/projects/addhealth (University of North Carolina, sponsored by National Institute of Child Health and Human Development) |
| Kaiser Family Foundation/ | Adolescents, ages 15–17 sample small (500) | Part of monthly omnibus adolescent phone surveys nationwide | Attitudes about sexuality, cover sexual behaviors not found on other surveys | www.kff.org or www.seventeen.com/sexsmarts |

        (b) Late developers may be at lower risk due greater ability to control impulses

    ii. Girls who develop early

        (a) Treated as older, even by parents

        (b) Less popular with age mates

        (c) Increased risk for sexual activity with older males

    iii. Boys who develop early

        (a) More popular in middle school

        (b) May have social difficulties in high school as other boys "catch up"

    iv. Boys who develop late

        (a) Increased risk for being the victim of social bullying

        (b) Risk for social isolation

**b.** Disconnection from school or post–high school education often a precursor to risky behaviors (Bonny, et al., 2000)

**c.** Clustering of behaviors, such as substance use and sexual activity

    i. 89% of youth ages 15 to 24 years say peers mix substance use and sexual activity (Kaiser Family Foundation, 2002)

    ii. Youth say peers are less likely to use condoms if they engage in sexual activity while "high"

**d.** Exposure to dating violence associated with:

    i. Higher rates of substance abuse

    ii. Eating disorders (Silverman, et al., 2001)

**e.** Lesbian, gay, bisexual, transgender youth who report victimization by peers report higher rates of:

    i. Alcohol use

    ii. Drug use

    iii. Suicidal behavior (Bontempo & D'Augelli, 2002)

**f.** Negative childhood events

    i. Young men have an increased risk of fathering a child in adolescence who have suffered adverse childhood events, including: (Anda, et al., 2002)

        (a) Abuse

        (b) Parental separation

        (c) Death in family or close friend

        (d) Drug use

**g.** Need to fit in, meet internal or external standards about appearance (Anstine & Grinenko, 2000); PNPs should ask about:

    i. Satisfaction with appearance

    ii. Satisfaction with weight

    iii. Relationship between appearance, weight, and self-esteem

    iv. How much does thinking about weight affect teen's self-esteem

    v. Overeating (Neumark-Sztainer, et al., 2002)

        (a) Eating in secret

        (b) Binge-purge cycle

    vi. Protein and vitamin supplements

    vii. Weight-reducing efforts (Neumark-Sztainer, et al., 2003)

        (a) Laxatives and diuretics

        (b) History of excessive exercise

    viii. Diet history (see Chapter 45 for information on eating disorders)

        (a) Belief that he or she should be dieting

        (b) Number of diets in past year

        (c) Types of diets

8. Home, school, job, and leisure time issues relevant to adolescents and young adults
   a. Home
      i. Immigrant teens may be living with adult siblings or extended family
      ii. Changes in family of origin
         (a) Divorce
         (b) Custody
         (c) Death of parent
      iii. Teens living with boyfriend or girlfriend and family
      iv. Separation or reunification with parents due to:
         (a) Immigration
         (b) Incarceration
         (c) Illness
      v. Exposures
         (a) Intimate partner violence
         (b) Drug
         (c) Alcohol use
      vi. Changes in youth's level of independence
         (a) Driving safety, driving rules set by parents
         (b) If married or in college, may want to move to family practice or adult health care
   b. School
      i. Home school, public, parochial, vocational, college, trade school
      ii. Sports or other extracurricular activities
         (a) A measure of connection to school
         (b) Extra motivation for attendance and grades
      iii. Issues that may affect educational success
         (a) Special education
         (b) 504 plan of the Rehabilitation Act of 1973 states that the curriculum must be the same for all students at each grade, but that individualized instructional and environmental accommodations must be made for children with disabilities
         (c) English as a second language
      iv. Grade point average (GPA)
         (a) If low
            (1) Attendance problems
            (2) Work too difficult
            (3) Not doing work
            (4) Involved in outside employment
         (b) Any recent increase or decrease in GPA
      v. Patterns of school failure
         (a) Teen has always done poorly
            (1) Dyslexia or other major neurologic or learning disability
            (2) Major behavioral or psychologic issues
            (3) Long term trauma (e.g., abuse)
            (4) Frequent moves
            (5) Migrant family
            (6) Illegal immigrant family
            (7) Homeless
         (b) Gradual decline (through middle school, high school)
            (1) ADD without hyperactivity
            (2) Other organizational or executive function issues
            (3) Minor learning disabilities

(4) These may surface because schoolwork is more complex and requires more organizational skills
  (c) Sudden decline
    (1) Depression or other behavioral or psychologic issue
    (2) Acute trauma
    (3) Sexual assault
    (4) Death
    (5) Divorce in family
    (6) Drug, alcohol use
**c.** Jobs
  **i.** More than 20 hours per week not recommended if in school
  **ii.** Schedule, location, other hazards
  **iii.** Realism of plans after high school graduation
    (a) Taking right courses and activities
    (b) Taking SATs or college applications on time (Muscari & Berkstresser, 2001)
    (c) Vocational training
  **iv.** Unrealistic or no plans
    (a) Loss of health insurance at high school graduation or 18 if not in school
    (b) Possible loss of parental support, housing
    (c) Transitions for youth in foster care
**d.** Leisure time
  **i.** Balance between work, school, leisure activities
  **ii.** How does teen spend free time?
    (a) Hobbies, talents
    (b) School, church, or community activities
      (1) Measure of connection to school
      (2) Connections to community, supports
      (3) Adult role models outside of family
  **iii.** Friends—name friends, best friend
  **iv.** Exercise (Timperio, et al., 2004)
    (a) 30 to 60 minutes of moderate to intense daily exercise?
    (b) Exercise other than physical education (PE) during school
    (c) Access to safe, affordable facilities?
    (d) Intensity of exercise (may be a form of purging)
9. Current trends in alcohol, tobacco, and other drug use (Grunbaum, et al., 2004)
  **a.** Alcohol
    **i.** 74.9% of high school students report having drunk alcohol
    **ii.** Pattern of alcohol or drug abuse often different from adult patterns
      (a) Late adolescents and young adults often focus on binge drinking (Nelson, et al., 2005)
      (b) A significant portion of high school students report binge drinking in past 30 days
        (1) Male (29%)
        (2) Female (27.5%)
      (c) Not very concrete about timing, e.g., "long time ago" can be 2 weeks to 3 years
    **iii.** Assess alcohol risk behavior (see Box 25-3: CAGE, CRAFFT mnemonics)
  **b.** Tobacco
    **i.** More than a third of high school students have used some form of tobacco

      ii. Secondary gains for tobacco use
        (a) Rebel image for nonconformist youth
        (b) Weight control issues for girls
        (c) Seen as stress reliever
        (d) Camouflage for social insecurity

  c. Marijuana
    i. Use rose during the '90s, but now may be declining or leveling off (40.2% of high schools students have used marijuana, 22.4% in the past 30 days)
    ii. Negative effects on memory, motivation
    iii. Prolonged withdrawal period (>6 weeks)
    iv. Can be detected in urine up to 2 to 3 weeks after use
    v. Some teens, parents, providers do not recognize marijuana as significant drug of abuse (Dennis, et al., 2002)

  d. "Club drugs" (Grunbaum et al., 2004; Strote, et al., 2002; Tellier, 2002)
    i. Rising in popularity, especially for college-age students
      (a) Ecstasy (MDMA)—11.1% of high school students have used this
      (b) Ketamine
      (c) GHB—Gamma hydroxy butyrate
      (d) Methamphetamines
      (e) Mixtures, including heroin and sildenafil (Viagra)
      (f) Nationwide, cocaine, heroine are less prevalent in teens, but regional use varies

  e. Inhalants, e.g., glue, paint, propellants, are used by 12.1% of students
  f. Associated drug and alcohol issues
    i. Motor vehicle accidents
    ii. Fights
    iii. Arrests
    iv. Suspensions
  g. Many teens reluctant to embrace abstinence programs
  h. Issues of dual diagnosis for teens with substance abuse, e.g., learning disorders, depression

10. Current trends in adolescent sexual behavior
  a. 32.8% of ninth graders and 61.6% of high school seniors have had intercourse at least once (Grunbaum et al., 2004)
  b. Among 15- to 19-year-olds, 4.5% of men, 10.6% of women have had some same sex contact (Mosher, et al., 2005)
  c. Average age for first sexual activity is 16.32 years (Lonczak, et al., 2002)
  d. Of 15 to 17 year-olds who have not had intercourse, 20.7% of boys, 18% of girls have had oral sex experience (Mosher, et al., 2005)
  e. One fourth of teens say that oral sex is part of a casual or serious relationship (Kaiser Family Foundation, 2002)
  f. 34% report having done "something sexual" in a casual encounter
  g. Approximately 900,000 U.S. teenagers become pregnant each year in the U.S. (Lonczak, et al., 2002)
  h. Adolescents and young adults account for two thirds of all reported STIs (Lonczak, et al., 2002)
  i. Condom use (DeVisser & Smith, 2000)
    i. 63% of students having sex used a condom at last intercourse
    ii. 38% of college students reported "late" condom use on at least one occasion, i.e. applied after initial penetration
    iii. 13% of all condom use was "late"

        iv. Between 10 and 11% of heterosexual 15- to 19-year-olds engage in anal intercourse (Mosher, et al., 2005)

           (a) Associated with less frequent condom use

           (b) Correlated with an increased number of sexual partners

  **j.** Screening and intervention issues

    **i.** Consensual sexual activity

       (a) Broaden sexuality questions, may uncover *intention* to have sex for those who have not had sex yet

          (1) Through-the-clothes non-intercourse behaviors

          (2) Under-clothes or clothes-off non-intercourse behaviors

          (3) "Have you ever had sex or *come close* to having sex?"

          (4) Oral sex

          (5) Vaginal sex

          (6) Anal sex

       (b) Same-gender or cross-gender sexual contact

       (c) Focus on behaviors (number, gender of partners) rather than labels (straight, gay, bisexual) (Garofalo & Harper, 2003)

       (d) Recent studies show teens in "long-term relationships" (>3 weeks) are less likely to use condoms

    **ii.** Sexual abuse, nonconsensual sexual activity

       (a) May refuse or be reluctant to undress for general physical examination

       (b) Clinician will generally need to report past abuse if teen younger than 18 and not previously reported (warn teen before asking)

       (c) Implications for teen's current ability to negotiate appropriate partners, safer sex

       (d) Implications for comfort level or ability to have healthy sexual relationships

       (e) May not be able to tolerate pelvic or genital exam

**11.** Current trends in youth safety (Grunbaum, et al., 2004)

  **a.** Bullying (Nansel, et al., 2001)

    **i.** Being teased is a precursor to being bullied

    **ii.** Being bullied is associated with social isolation, and poor social and emotional adjustment

    **iii.** Health Behavior of School-aged Children survey of a representative sample of 15,686 U.S. children in grades 6 through 10 (Nansel, et al., 2001)

       (a) Estimated that 10.6% of the nation's 20 million children in that age-group bully others "sometimes" and 8.8% bully others once a week or more

       (b) Boys were more involved in bullying behavior and being bullied than girls

       (c) Boys tend to be bullied by physical contact (slaps, being pushed)

       (d) Girls are bullied verbally (rumors, sexual comments)

       (e) Black children are less likely to be bullied than other groups

       (f) Hispanic males are more likely to be the bullies

       (g) No rural, urban, or suburban differences were found

  **b.** Students who had missed school in past 30 days because they felt unsafe

    **i.** 10.2% of Latinos

    **ii.** 9.8% of Blacks

  **c.** 33.2% had been in a physical fight in past 12 months

    **i.** 40.5% of male students

    **ii.** 25.1% of female students (increased from 2001)

    **d.** 41.7% of self-identified lesbian, gay, bisexual, or transgender youth do not feel safe at their school (Sexuality Information and Education Council of the United States, 2001)
        **i.** 45.9% report daily verbal harassment
        **ii.** 13.7% report experiencing physical assault
    **e.** Dating violence
        **i.** Seven separate studies showed that the incidence of being a victim of dating violence varies depending on the sample and research method (Hickman, et al., 2004)
           (a) Physical violence: 5% to 28%
           (b) Sexual violence: 2% to 12%
        **ii.** Gender differences vary widely
        **iii.** More research is needed on this topic
    **f.** Screening and intervention issues regarding safety
        **i.** Guns in home
           (a) Increased risk for suicide
        **ii.** Physical fighting in home between:
           (a) Siblings
           (b) Parents
           (c) Parent-child
        **iii.** Alcohol and drug use
           (a) Parents
           (b) Siblings
           (c) Other family members
        **iv.** Housing issues
           (a) Safety of building
           (b) Smoke and carbon monoxide detectors
           (c) Peeling paint
           (d) Mold
        **v.** Neighborhood issues
           (a) Gang violence
           (b) Drug dealing
        **vi.** Teen involved in physical fights
           (a) Home
           (b) Neighborhood
           (c) School
    **g.** Screening and intervention issues regarding gang involvement
        **i.** Teen may be very reluctant to disclose involvement
        **ii.** Teen, peers, siblings, or cousins involved in gangs
           (a) Prevalence in neighborhood, school
           (b) Local boundaries
           (c) Providers may need update from police and/or youth agencies
        **iii.** Configuration of gang
           (a) Neighborhood versus regional or international gang
           (b) Trends to more violence between factions of larger gangs
           (c) Single ethnic versus multiethnic gang
        **iv.** Teen wearing gang insignia
           (a) Dress
           (b) Tattoos
           (c) Writing or drawings
           (d) "Claiming a color" or close identification without actual membership

      v. Initiation rites, rituals for joining or leaving gang (may cause harm to self, property, or others)

12. Current trends in adolescent and young adult depression and suicide
    a. See Chapter 41 for details on epidemiology, screening, and diagnosis of depression and suicide ideations
    b. Review of treatment interventions for suicide prevention can be found in Gould, et al., 2003

13. Harm reduction theory and principles to decrease risky behavior and promote safety
    a. Harm reduction theory
        i. Approach from grassroots work with injection drug users during HIV epidemic
        ii. Nonmedical use of psychoactive drugs inevitable
        iii. Nonmedical use of drugs will produce societal harm
        iv. Pragmatic drug policies based on consequences, not their "message"
        v. Drug users part of larger community, protect health of community by protecting health of drug users
        vi. Wide range of interventions needed to address harms of drug use
    b. Harm reduction principles (Marlatt, 1996)
        i. Public health alternative to moral and criminal and disease models of drug use and addiction
            (a) Abstinence as ideal outcome, but accepts alternatives that reduce harm
            (b) "Bottom-up" approach based on advocacy, rather than "top-down" policy
            (c) Promotes low threshold access to services to decrease barriers to access
        ii. Decrease stigma
            (a) Drug use
            (b) Addiction
            (c) High risk sexual practices
        iii. Consolidate approach to a variety of high risk behaviors and their consequences
    c. Harm reduction in practice
        i. Safer sex (condoms and barrier methods) and contraception
        ii. Avoidance of combining substance use and driving or sex
        iii. Decreased drug and alcohol use
        iv. Needle exchange for injection drug use

14. Strategies for helping adolescents and young adults to make positive changes
    a. Brief motivational interventions (Boekeloo, et al., 2004)
        i. Adaptation of "Stages of Change" approach (Pender, et al., 2002)
            (a) Teens view health care providers as credible sources of information
            (b) Teens often in the exploratory or initiating phases of risky behaviors
            (c) Teachable moments in health care
            (d) Patient-centered interventions increase teen's sense of autonomy and control
    b. Motivational interview (Sindelar, et al., 2004)
        i. Establish rapport
        ii. Opening statement (teen's permission to discuss subject)
        iii. Assess current behavior and progress (e.g., third pregnancy test in 4 months)
        iv. Give feedback (e.g., prolonged URI secondary to smoking)

  **v.** Assess readiness to change (scale of 1 to 10, ruler scale, etc.)

  **vi.** Tailor intervention approach

   (a) Not ready—raise awareness, inform, and encourage

   (b) Unsure—explore ambivalence, look into future, next step

   (c) Ready—identify change options, help develop action plan

  **vii.** Close the encounter

 **c.** Point out positive strengths and resources

  **i.** Use information from history and physical examination

   (a) Positive family relationships

   (b) Positive connections in community

   (c) Religious organizations

   (d) Positive achievements, supports at school

   (e) Positive peer connections

  **ii.** Look for hidden strengths, protective decisions, even for troubled youths

  **iii.** Encourage support of adult role models outside as well as inside of family (Zimmerman, et al., 2002)

  **iv.** Discuss the risks and identify ways to capitalize on the strengths to find solutions and decrease risk

**15.** Working with parents to increase positive outcomes

 **a.** Parents of preadolescents (<10 years)

  **i.** Encourage parental discussions regarding puberty, body changes

  **ii.** Encourage parents to transmit values on sexual and drug behavior

  **iii.** Encourage parental monitoring of and discussion about media with child

  **iv.** Encourage child's development of hobbies, sports and skills, especially in groups

 **b.** Parents of early adolescents (10 to 13 years)

  **i.** Supervision more difficult, as organized child care ends, but crucial during after-school hours

  **ii.** Encourage after-school activities

  **iii.** Involvement of other adult role models

   (a) Church

   (b) Mentors

   (c) Coaches

   (d) Extended family (Zimmerman, et al., 2002)

 **c.** Parents of middle to late adolescents

  **i.** Parent moves from "disciplinarian" to "consultant"

  **ii.** Loss of control over teen's activities, decisions, less legal control after age 18

  **iii.** Cultural clashes with expectations of mainstream U.S. culture and expectations or traditions of immigrant families

  **iv.** Empathize with parental frustrations, challenges

  **v.** Often more enjoyment of the relationship as teen matures

---

## REFERENCES

American Academy of Family Physicians, American Academy of Pediatrics, American College of Obstetricians and Gynecologists, & Society of Adolescent Medicine. (2004). Position Paper: Protecting adolescents: Ensuring access to care and reporting sexual activity and abuse. *J Adol Health*, *35*, 420-423.

American Medical Association (AMA) Department of Adolescent Health. (1997). *Guidelines for adolescent preventive services (GAPS) recommendations monograph.* Chicago: AMA. Also available www.ama-assn.org/ama/upload/mm/39/gapsmono.pdf.

Anda, R. F., Chapman, D. P., Felitti, V. J., et al. (2002). Adverse childhood experiences and risk of paternity in teen pregnancy. *Obstet Gynecol, 100,* 37-45.

Anderson, R. N. (2002). Deaths: Leading causes for 2000. *Natl Vital Stat Rep, 50.*

Anstine, D., & Grinenko, D. (2000). Rapid screening for disordered eating in college-aged females in the primary care setting. *J Adolesc Health, 26,* 338-342.

Boekeloo, B. O., Bradley, O., Jerry, J., et al. (2004). Randomized trial of brief office-based interventions to reduce adolescent alcohol use. *Arch Pediatr Adolesc Med, 158*(7), 635-642.

Bonny, A. E., Britto, M. T., Klostermann, B. K., et al. (2000). School disconnectedness: Identifying adolescents at risk. *Pediatrics, 106,* 1017-1021.

Bontempo, D. E., & D'Augelli, A. R. (2002). Effects of at-school victimization and sexual orientation on lesbian, gay, or bisexual youth's health risk behavior. *J Adolesc Health, 30,* 364-374.

Burstein, J. R., & Murray, P. J. (2003). Sexually transmitted disease pathogens among adolescents. *Pediatr Rev, 24,* 75-82.

Dailard, C. (2003). New medical records privacy rule: The interface with teen access to confidential care. *The Guttmacher Report on Public Policy, March,* 6-7.

Dennis, M., Babor, T. F., Roebuck, M. C., & Donaldson, J. (2002). Changing the focus: The case for recognizing and treating cannabis use disorders. *Addiction, 97* (Suppl 1), 4-15.

DeVisser, R. O., & Smith, A. M. A. (2000). When always isn't enough: Implications of the late application of condoms for the validity and reliability of self-reported condom use. *AIDS Care, 12,* 221-224.

Dickey, S. B., & Deatrick, J. (2000). Autonomy and decision making for health promotion in adolescence. *Pediatr Nurs, 26,* 461-467.

English, A. (2000). Reproductive health services for adolescents: Critical legal issues. *Obstet Gynecol Clin North Am, 27,* 195-211.

Garofalo, R., & Harper, G. W. (2003). Not all adolescents are the same: Addressing the unique needs of gay and bisexual male youth. *Adolesc Med, 14*(3), 595-611.

Goldenring, J. M. & Rosen, D. S. (2004). Getting into adolescent heads: An essential update. *Contemporary Pediatrics, 21*(1) 64-80.

Gould, M. S., Greenberg, T., Velting, D. M., & Shaffer, D. (2003). Youth suicide risk and preventive interventions: A review of the past 10 years. *J Am Acad Child Adolesc Psychiatry, 42,* 386-405.

Grunbaum, J. A., Kann, L., Kinchen, S. A., et al. (2004). *Youth Risk Behavior Surveillance - United States, 2003* (53 (SS-2): Morbidity and Mortality Weekly Report Center for Disease Control Surveillance Summaries.

Hickman, L. J., Jaycox, L. H., & Aronoff, J. (2004). Dating violence among adolescents: Prevalence, gender distribution, and prevention program effectiveness. *Trauma Violence Abuse, 5*(2), 123-142.

Kaiser Family Foundation. (2002). Millions of young people mix sex with alcohol or drugs: With dangerous consequences. Presented on February 7, 2002 at the conference titled, Dangerous liaisons: Substance abuse and sexual behavior. Sponsored by the National Center on Addiction and Substance Abuse at Columbia University, New York and the Kaiser Family Foundation. Press release retrieved on April 18, 2006 at http://www.outproud.org/pdf/CASANewsRelease.pdf

Klein, J. D., & Wilson, K. M. (2002). Delivering quality care: Adolescents' discussion of health risks with their providers. *J Adolesc Health, 30,* 190-195.

Lonczak, H. S., Abbott, R. D., Hawkins, J. D., et al. (2002). Effects of the Seattle Social Development Project on sexual behavior, pregnancy, birth and sexually transmitted disease outcomes by age 21 years. *Arch Pediatr Adolesc Med, 156,* 438-447.

Maradiegue, A.N. (2003) Minor's rights versus parental rights: Review of legal issues in adolescent health care. *J Midwifery and Women's Health, 48,* 170-177.

Marlatt, G. A. (1996). Harm reduction: Come as you are. *Addictive Behaviors, 21,* 779-788.

Mosher, W. D., Chandra, A., & Jones, J. (2005). Sexual behavior and selected health measures: Men and women 15-44 years of age, United States, 2002. Advance data from vital and health statistics; no 362. Hyattsville, MD: National Center for Health Statistics.

Muntner, P., He, J., Cutler, J. A., et al. (2004). Trends in blood pressure among children and adolescents. *JAMA, 291*(17), 2107-2113.

Muscari, M. E., & Berkstresser, M. (2001). The precollege examination: Fostering a healthy transition. *J Pediatr Health Care, 15,* 63-70.

Nansel, T. R., Overpeck, M., Pilla, R. S., et al. (2001). Bullying behaviors among US youth: prevalence and association with psychosocial adjustment. *JAMA, 285* (16), 2094-3000.

Nelson, T. F., Naimi, T. S., Brewer, R. D., & Wechsler, H. (2005). The state sets the rate: The relationship of college binge drinking to state binge drinking rates and selected state alcohol control policies. *Am J Public Health, 95*(3), 441-446.

Neumark-Sztainer, D., Story, M., Hannan, P. J., & Croll, J. (2002). Overweight status and eating patterns among adolescents: Where do youths stand in comparison with Healthy People 2010 objectives? *Am J Public Health, 92,* 844-851.

Neumark-Sztainer, D., Wall, M. M., Story, M., & Perry, C. L. (2003). Correlates of unhealthy weight-control behaviors among adolescents: Implications for prevention programs. *Health Psychol, 22,* 88-98.

Pender, N. J., Murdaugh, C. L., & Parsons, M. A. (2002). *Health promotion in nursing practice* (4th ed.). Upper Saddle River, N.J.: Prentice-Hall.

Radzik, M., Sherer, S., & Neinstein, L. S. (2002). Psychosocial development in normal adolescents. In L. S. Neinstein (Ed.). *Adolescent health care: A practical guide* (4th ed.). Philadelphia: Lippincott Williams & Wilkins, pp. 53-58.

Rosen, D. S., & Neinstein, L. S. (2002). Preventive health care for adolescents. In L. S. Neinstein (Ed.). *Adolescent health care: A practical guide* (4th ed.). Philadelphia: Lippincott Williams & Wilkins, pp. 79-125.

Saslow, D., Runowicz, C. D., Solomon, D., et al. (2002).American Cancer Society guideline for the early detection of cervical neoplasia and cancer. *CA: A Cancer Journal for Clinicians, 52,* 342-362.

Sexuality Information and Education Council of the United States (SIECUS). (2001). *Lesbian, gay, bisexual and transgender youth issues.* SIECUS Report, Volume 29, Number 4. Retrieved April 18, 2006, from www.siecus.org/pubs/fact/fact0013.html

Shafer, M. A. (2000). With urine based screening, do sexually active adolescent girls still need annual pelvic examinations? No: recommending annual exams is not evidence based. *West J Med, 173,* 293.

Silverman, J.G., Raj, A., Mucci, L.A., & Hathaway, J.E. (2001). Dating violence against adolescent girls and associated substance use, unhealthy weight control, sexual risk behavior, pregnancy, and suicidality. *JAMA, 286,* 572-579.

Sindelar, H. A., Abrantes, A. M., Hart, C., et al. (2004). Motivational interviewing in pediatric practice. *Curr Probl Pediatr Adolesc Health Care, 34*(9), 322-339.

Strote, J., Lee, J. E., & Wechsler, H. (2002). Increasing MDMA use among college students: Results of a national survey. *J Adolesc Health, 30,* 64-72.

Tellier, P-P. (2002). Club drugs: Is it all ecstasy? *Pediatr Ann, 31,* 550-556.

Timperio, A., Salmon, J., & Ball, K. (2004). Evidence-based strategies to promote physical activity among children, adolescents and young adults: Review and update. *J Sci Med Sport, 7*(1), Suppl., 20-29.

U.S. Department Health & Human Services Public Health Service, Office of Assistant Secretary for Health. (2000). *Healthy People 2010: Conference Edition.* Washington, DC: HHS.

Wu, A. C., Lesperance, L., & Bernstein, H. (2002). Screening for iron deficiency. *Pediatr Rev, 23,* 171-177.

Zimmerman, M. A., Bingenheimer, J. B., & Notaro, P. C. (2002). Natural mentors and adolescent resiliency: A study with urban youth. *Am J Community Psychol, 30,* 221-243.

# Sexuality and Birth Control

JEAN B. IVEY, DSN, CRNP

## SEXUALITY AND SEXUAL HEALTH

1. Most sources agree that sexuality includes knowledge, beliefs, attitudes, values, and behaviors related to sexual identity and sexual expression
   a. Deals with anatomy, physiology, and the biochemistry of the sexual response system
   b. Roles, identity, personality, individual thoughts and feelings, behaviors and relationships, and communication patterns also contribute
2. Sexual health encompasses the absence of sexually transmitted diseases and reproductive disorders, control of fertility, avoidance of unwanted pregnancies, and sexual expression without exploitation, oppression, or abuse (Nusbaum & Hamilton, 2002)
3. Physical sexual development in children and adolescence
   a. Embryology of sexual organ development (see Chapter 9)
   b. Hormonal changes in both sexes (Plant, 2002; Rogol, et al., 2002)
      i. Gonadotropin-releasing hormone produced by the hypothalamus
      ii. Stimulates anterior pituitary to produce and secrete
         (a) TSH—thyrotropin-stimulating hormone
         (b) FSH—follicle-stimulating hormone
         (c) LH—luteinizing hormone
         (d) At puberty, thyrotropin-releasing hormone (TRH) stimulates release of TSH and prolactin, which triggers sexual development
   c. Males
      i. Hormones
         (a) LH stimulates the Leydig cells of the testicles to cause maturation of the testicles and production of testosterone
         (b) FSH stimulates sperm production
         (c) Estrogen, progesterone, testosterone, and other androgens from the gonads stimulate development of secondary sex characteristics
            (1) Muscle growth
            (2) Bone growth
            (3) Larynx enlargement and vocal cord thickening
            (4) Skin thickening and oil secretion
            (5) Axillary and facial hair growth

    ii. Spermatogenesis occurs after an increase in pituitary FSH and androgen is produced by the Leydig cells.

      (a) Testosterone is needed for the Sertoli cells to function

      (b) Increased pituitary FSH causes the Sertoli cells in testicles to increase germ cell proliferation and maturation

      (c) Leydig cells produce androgen

      (d) Androgen receptors in the seminiferous tubules cause an increase in the number and maturity of the sperm

      (e) Sertoli cells in prepubertal testicles also produce inhibin B

        (1) Inhibin B controls FSH production by a negative feedback mechanism

        (2) Serum inhibin B levels have a strong positive correlation with testicular volume and sperm counts

  iii. Assessing testicular function

      (a) Physiology

        (1) Testicular function begins at about 7 to 8 weeks of gestation with the production of testosterone by the testicles

        (2) Testosterone levels increase, then levels fall at birth

        (3) Pituitary gonadotropin causes another rise in testosterone until about 3 months of age, and then gradually decreases

        (4) Testosterone levels rise again at the onset of puberty until reaching adult level

      (b) History

        (1) Timing and extent of sexual maturity and onset of puberty should be documented regularly

        (2) Adolescents' reports of libido, sexual function, strength, and energy are also significant

        (3) Comparison with mean onset of puberty in adolescents of similar cultural, racial, and socioeconomic status may be useful

        (4) A history of hypospadias, epispadias and cryptorchidism or microphallus may indicate problems with Leydig cell function

  iv. Assessing sexual development in the male: sexual maturity ratings (SMR) (Tanner stages) (see Chapter 9, Figure 9-2)

      (a) Stage 1: Prepubertal

      (b) Stage 2: Testicular and scrotal enlargement is first sign of puberty

        (1) PNP may use an orchiometer to record approximate volume of testicles

        (2) Sparse straight pubic hair, slightly pigmented at the base of the penis

      (c) Stage 3: Lengthening of the penis

        (1) Scrotal enlargement

        (2) Pubic hair darker and coarser, curlier, over entire pubis

      (d) Stage 4: Increased diameter of the penis

        (1) Glans larger and wider

        (2) Scrotum darker

        (3) Pubic hair curlier but limited to pubis

      (e) Stage 5: Penis, testicles, and scrotum adult sized

        (1) Pubic hair spread to inner thighs, toward the umbilicus

        (2) Adult quality and amount of pubic hair

      (f) Tanner/SMR should be instituted in school-age males along with a discussion of pubertal changes as a part of anticipatory guidance for the patients and their parents

(g) Onset of puberty can begin as early as 8 years or as late as 16 or 17 years

(h) Adolescent males have a slower, steadier rate of skeletal growth than females, which peaks at Tanner/SMR stage 5

(i) Concerns about late timing of sexual maturation and growth

    (1) Genetic and familial patterns are also influential

    (2) Inquire about parental age of maturation

    (3) Measure serum alkaline phosphatase, bone age, and growth patterns

        a) May contribute to the evaluation of growth potential in an adolescent

    (4) Measure plasma testosterone levels and plasma LH and compare with norms

    (5) Gonadotropin stimulation can be used to determine Leydig cell capacity

    (6) Obvious delays in sexual maturation should be referred to a pediatric/adolescent endocrinologist

**d.** Females

    **i.** Hormones

        (a) Anterior pituitary stimulation and production of TSH, adrenocorticotropic hormone (ACTH), and the gonadotropic hormones cause:

            (1) Cyclical maturation of ovarian follicles

            (2) Production of progesterone and estrogen

        (b) Androgens and thyroxin cause the adolescent growth spurt and development of secondary sexual characteristics

        (c) Female development includes

            (1) Broadening of the shoulders, hips, and thighs

            (2) Skeletal growth spurt in females peaks between Tanner/SMR stages 2 and 3

            (3) Lean body mass decreases from approximately 80% to approximately 75% by the end of puberty

            (4) Continual increase in body fat

            (5) Body fat levels are related to the onset of menses and regular ovulatory cycles

            (6) Adolescents with a low amount of body fat frequently experience pubertal delays and irregular ovulatory cycles

    **ii.** Female sexual development

        (a) Begins with the differentiation of ovaries from testicles during the seventh week of gestation

        (b) Thelarche: development of breast buds

            (1) Usually occurs between the ages of 9 and 11 years

            (2) Tanner/SMR stages (Figure 26-1)

                a) Stage 1: Prepubertal, no breast tissue

                b) Stage 2: Breast buds

                c) Stage 3: Enlargement of the breast and areola with no separation of their contours

                d) Stage 4: Projection of the areola, with the papilla forming a secondary mound above the level of the breast

                e) Stage 5: Breast adult-like in appearance with the areola recessed to the general contour of the breast, breast enlarged

                f) Breasts frequently grow unevenly and girls need to be reassured that generally, they will equalize

                g) Timing of the onset of breast development has no relationship to the eventual size of the mature breast

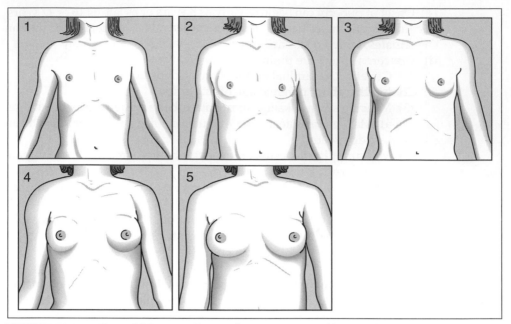

FIGURE 26-1 ■ Sexual Maturity Rating/Tanner stages of breast development. (From Berkowitz C. (2000). *Pediatrics: A primary care approach*, (ed 2.) St. Louis: Saunders).

      (c)  Adrenarche or pubarche: appearance of pubic hair
- (1) Usually occurs about 6 months after the breast buds appear
- (2) Tanner/SMR stages (see Chapter 9, Figure 9-4))
  - a) Stage 1: No pubic hair is visible
  - b) Stage 2: Sparse, long, slightly pigmented, downy, straight or slightly curly hair along the labia
  - c) Stage 3: Hair is coarser, curlier, and darker and spreads over most of the pubic bone
  - d) Stage 4: Hair is adult-like in appearance but does not extend onto the thighs
  - e) Stage 5: Hair is adult-like in appearance and extends over the thighs

      (d)  Thelarche and adrenarche stages are compared to arrive at a single Tanner/SMR stage for the female

      (e)  The *earlier* stage is reported when the two are not equal

**4.** Sexuality and typical psychosocial development in children (Blythe & Rosenthal, 2000; Ryan, 2000)

  **a.** Infancy (birth to ages 1 to 1½)
- **i.** Freud
  - (a) Oral stage of psychosexual development
  - (b) Sexual pleasure derived primarily from sucking, gumming, biting
- **ii.** Piaget
  - (a) Sensorimotor stage of cognitive development
  - (b) Learn through physical interaction and experience
  - (c) Trial-and-error behaviors lead to repetition of *successful* behaviors
  - (d) Successful behaviors are those that meet the infant's own needs, or those that are reinforced by adults
  - (e) Develop concept of object permanence, i.e., that objects exist even when out of sight

          **iii.** By 6 to 9 months infants "discover" their genitals

          **iv.** Derive pleasure from rubbing or stroking them

          **v.** Parents should avoid sending negative messages about genitals

             (a) Demonstrating an aversion to looking at them

             (b) Negative expressions

             (c) Complaints about odor

             (d) Communicate that these body parts are unacceptable or shameful

  **b.** Toddler (ages 1½ to 3 years)

        **i.** Freud

           (a) Anal stage of psychosexual development

           (b) Derive sexual pleasure primarily from releasing or withholding bowel movements

        **ii.** Piaget

           (a) Preoperational stage

           (b) Beginning use of symbols and language to communicate

           (c) Egocentric—cannot comprehend other points of view than one's own

           (d) Memory and imagination developing

        **iii.** Gaining control over urination and defecation are major developmental tasks

        **iv.** Curious about their bodies

        **v.** Name their body parts

        **vi.** Learn proper names or slang names for genitals

        **vii.** Masturbation a common, normal, self-soothing activity

        **viii.** Begin to learn social norms for behavior in public

           (a) Not to expose their own or others' genitals

           (b) Not to touch their own or others' genitals

        **ix.** Age 2

           (a) A child's sex role identity is established

           (b) Begin to learn behaviors associated with that sex in their culture

  **c.** Preschool (ages 3-5 years)

        **i.** Freud

           (a) Phallic stage of psychosexual development

           (b) Derive sexual pleasure from manipulation of the genitals

        **ii.** Piaget

           (a) Preoperational stage of cognitive development continues

        **iii.** Sexual identity and sex role behaviors part of preschool socialization

        **iv.** Play imitates adult roles and relationships

        **v.** Curious about the opposite sex

        **vi.** Giggle over "bathroom words" such as "pee-pee" or "poop"

        **vii.** Modest; dislike or refuse to get undressed in front of strangers

        **viii.** Mimic adult sexual behaviors, such as kissing and stroking

        **ix.** Playing "doctor" among peers

           (a) Normal behavior

           (b) Motivation is curiosity

           (c) Parents should not overreact, but simply redirect children's play

        **x.** Masturbation is very common

           (a) Parents should not forbid masturbating or shame the child

           (b) Tell child when and where he or she may engage in that behavior

        **xi.** PNP teaching issues

           (a) Children imitate the behavior they see

           (b) Parents should model healthy sexual behavior

(c) Healthy sexual development requires seeing others treated with respect and love

(d) Preschool or daycare exposes to other children and their families, teachers, and workers

    (1) Children may imitate other role models

    (2) Parents should explain why some of these behaviors are unacceptable

(e) Children's awareness of inappropriate behavior toward their bodies

    (1) Teach children to recognize when it is inappropriate for others to touch or look at their bodies

    (2) Teach them ways to be assertive, set limits, and exit from an uncomfortable situation

(f) Children need reasonable and consistent consequences for their negative behavior

(g) Positive experiences with relationships, feeling valued and respected decreases the likelihood of victimization and sexual acting out in the teen years

  **d.** School-aged child (ages 5 to puberty)

    **i.** Freud

      (a) Latency stage of psychosexual development

      (b) Need for sexual pleasure is suppressed

      (c) Energy is used for social development and learning

      (d) Most child development experts disagree with the notion that sexual pleasure is suppressed

    **ii.** Piaget

      (a) Concrete operational stage of cognitive development

      (b) Learning to think logically about concrete phenomena

      (c) Manipulates symbols of concrete phenomena

      (d) Understands principles of cause and effect related to concrete phenomena

    **iii.** Puberty in girls usually begins between 9 and 13 years, and in boys, between 10 and 15 years

    **iv.** Begin to establish more intimate relationships with peers, first as same sex "best friends" and later with "boyfriends" or "girlfriends"

    **v.** Learn new values, communication patterns, ways of relating to others

      (a) Experiment with acceptable and undesirable behaviors

      (b) Motivation for experimentation may be to reach personal or group goals

  **e.** Early, middle, and late adolescence

    **i.** Stages of adolescence

      (a) Early: ages 10 to 14 years

      (b) Middle: ages 15 to 17

      (c) Late: ages 18 to early 20s

    **ii.** Most sexuality issues and concerns are the same for all stages of adolescence

    **iii.** A systematic review of research suggests that changes in the social and sexual behavior of adolescents is, in part, due to neurophysiologic changes (Nelson, et al., 2005)

      (a) The increase in gonadal steroids influences changes in the limbic system

      (b) Emotions and interpretation of social situations originate in the limbic system

        (c) Maturation of the prefrontal cortex allows for more complex responses to social information

    iv. Freud

        (a) Genital stage of psychosexual development

        (b) Renewed sexual interest and desire

    v. Piaget

        (a) Formal operations stage of cognitive development

        (b) Able to appreciate more abstract situations

        (c) Understands cause and effect with concrete and abstract phenomena

        (d) Can predict future consequences of current behavior

**f.** Early adolescence

    i. Frequently frightened by the changes in their body, their feelings, and mood swings that accompany hormonal surges

    ii. Increased modesty, embarrassment, and fear that they are abnormal are common

    iii. Need factual information about their bodies

    iv. Boys may be embarrassed about physical changes, erections, and night-time emissions

        (a) PNP should initiate discussion about these

        (b) Reassure that these are normal and indicate beginning of puberty

    v. Girls may be embarrassed about physical changes and beginning of menses

    vi. Or girls may be concerned about when menses will occur, such as in school

        (a) PNP should initiate discussion about these potential concerns

        (b) Provide tips on how to use and discreetly carry menstrual products

    vii. Need to know how to deal with erections, "wet dreams," menses, other physical changes, and peer comments and behaviors

**g.** Middle adolescence

    i. Frequently involved in dating

    ii. May experiment with various levels of sexual activity

    iii. PNP should include discussion about the dating scene, decision making, risk taking, safety and assertiveness

    iv. PNP should offer to help the adolescent discuss sexual activity with parents

    v. Delayed puberty becomes an issue in this age-group

    vi. Involvement in activities where they must undress or shower together is often a source of angst

**h.** Late adolescence

    i. Period when intimate and serious relationships are frequently formed

    ii. Sexual activity is often the norm

**i.** All adolescents

    i. Sexual identity: it is important for the PNP to recognize that gender and sexual identity are not the same thing

    ii. Identity development

        (a) Experimentation and moratorium

        (b) Process of establishing a self-concept and sense of identity includes establishing a sexual identity

        (c) Experimentation with behaviors and roles is normal

    iii. Relationships with same-sex peers are strong

    iv. Dating and steady, but often short-term relationships with opposite sex are "practice" for future long-term commitment to a partner

    **v.** These relationships are a common source of emotional upheaval

    **vi.** Sexual debut

        (a) Abstinence—PNP should promote abstinence as a defense against:

            (1) STI

            (2) Unwanted pregnancy

            (3) Risky behaviors

        (b) Masturbation

            (1) Many teens told masturbation is wrong and may have disabling consequences

            (2) PNP should explain that masturbation is normal and safe

        (c) Mutual masturbation

            (1) Adolescents choose as an alternative to intercourse

            (2) PNP should be able to discuss this option with adolescents

        (d) Oral sex

            (1) Adolescents often do not consider oral sex to be sexual activity

            (2) Fail to realize STIs can be transmitted through oral sex

            (3) May not take preventive measures

        (e) Pornography

            (1) Pornography is readily available in print and electronically

            (2) Most adolescents have an opportunity to view it

            (3) PNP should discuss pornography and its negative effect on attitudes and beliefs toward others

            (4) Adolescents need information about legal ramifications of accessing pornographic sites or materials

    **vii.** In case adolescents cannot be abstinent, discuss alternative methods of contraception and preventing STI

    **viii.** Clearly explain and/or demonstrate how to use these methods

    **ix.** Provide, or tell adolescents how to access contraceptives

    **x.** Provide, or tell adolescents how to access and use, pregnancy tests

    **xi.** Provide pregnant adolescents with information about alternatives

    **xii.** PNPs must be advocates for adolescents faced with difficult decisions and conflicting values

**j.** Sexual risk-taking behavior

    **i.** Adolescents are believed to have the following cognitive characteristics that predispose them to risk taking behavior, although there is much debate about the validity of these theories (Vartanian, 2000)

        (a) Personal fable—none of life's troubles will affect the adolescent because he/she feels special and unique

        (b) Imaginary audience—belief that others are always watching and evaluating their behavior

        (c) Egocentric

        (d) Not all are at formal operations stage of cognitive development and have difficulty understanding cause-and-effect relationships among abstract concepts

        (e) Omnipotence fantasies

        (f) Need for acceptance

        (g) Fluctuations in self-efficacy, depending on the task (Faryna & Morales, 2000)

    **ii.** Prevalence and incidence

        (a) Adolescents and young adults account for two thirds of all reported STIs (Nusbaum & Hamilton, 2002)

        (b) Youth Risk Behavior Surveillance—U.S., 2001 (Grunbaum, et al., 2002)

        (1) Grades 9 through 12, CDC school-based survey

        (2) 45.6% had sexual intercourse, 48.5% male, 42.9% female

        (3) 14.2% had sexual intercourse with four or more partners

        (4) 33% had sexual intercourse in the past 3 months

        (5) 57.9% had used a condom during last sexual intercourse

        (6) Black students were more likely than white or Hispanic students to report condom use

        (7) 18.2% of sexually active students or their partners used birth control pills

        (8) 25.6% had used alcohol or drugs at last sexual intercourse

        (9) 4.7% reported that they had been pregnant or had gotten someone else pregnant

       (10) Prevalence of pregnancy varied from 2.2% to 7.4% with state of residence

     (c) FACCT 2001 Robert Wood Johnson Foundation National Strategic Indicators (Bethell, et al., 2000)

        (1) Project surveyed 2000 adolescents, ages 1 to 17 years

        (2) 33.6% reported risky health behaviors that included early sexual activity and pregnancy

        (3) 49.9% had sexual intercourse at some time

        (4) 36.3% were currently sexually active

        (5) 58% reported using a condom at last intercourse

     (d) The National Adolescent Health Information Center's 2003 monograph (Ozer, et al., 2003)

        (1) 60.5% of adolescents have had sexual intercourse at least once

        (2) 47.9% were currently sexually active

        (3) 21.6% of seniors report having had four or more sexual partners in their lifetime

        (4) Non-Hispanic Blacks were sexually active at earlier ages and at higher rates than whites

        (5) 57.9% reported condom use

  **k.** Tips on taking a sexual health history (Box 26-1)

  **l.** Other implications for practice

     **i.** Adolescents are frequently sexually active

    **ii.** Anticipatory guidance and reinforcement about healthy choices and preventive measures are needed

   **iii.** Availability of information and access to contraceptives is important

   **iv.** Discussing the influence of drugs and alcohol on risk taking is important

    **v.** Adolescents' cultural and religious norms may conflict with PNP's desire to follow recommendations from primary care clinical guidelines

   **vi.** Adolescents need to trust the PNP before they will frankly discuss these issues

  **vii.** PNP must be clear about the extent to which confidentiality can be maintained

 **viii.** PNP may need to advocate for adolescents' privacy during well child and episodic visits

**5.** External influences on sexuality and sexual development

  **a.** Family influences (Jaccard & Dittus, 2000; O'Sullivan, et al., 2001)

     **i.** Children learn what it means to be male or female from their parents and extended family members first

    **ii.** Families behave in different ways that give children messages about sexuality from birth

■ **BOX 26-1**
■ **TIPS ON TAKING A SEXUAL HEALTH HISTORY**

- A proactive and preventive approach is required in primary care settings
- Ask questions about sexual activity
  - Gender of partner(s)
  - Number of partner(s)
  - Change in desire or frequency
  - Pain with intercourse
  - Oral or anal sex
  - Ever forced to have sex
- Use of devices or substances to enhance sexual pleasure
  - Difficulty achieving erection and/or orgasm
  - Any questions or concerns about your sexual functioning
- Ask questions about risk for STI
  - Risk factors for HIV
  - Ever tested for HIV
  - Like to be tested for HIV
  - Had any STIs
  - How do you protect yourself from HIV and other STIs

Adapted from Nusbaum, M. R. H., & Hamilton, C. D. (2002). The proactive sexual health history. *Am Fam Phys, 66,* p. 1706.

    iii. "Good" versus "bad" labels applied to behavior, dress, feelings, relationships with self and others influence children's identity of self

    iv. Family mores may be supported by or in conflict with cultural and social mores

    v. When adults become aware of children's sexual behaviors, they should be able to evaluate the behaviors in order to (Ryan, 2000):

        (a) Differentiate between developmentally appropriate versus problematic sexual behaviors

        (b) Respond consistently to what they see or hear

        (c) Validate or correct the sexual learning that children are demonstrating

    vi. Parents can be taught how to communicate with their children about sexuality in age-appropriate ways (Green & Documet, 2005)

**b.** Peer influences

    i. Children compare themselves to other children beginning in the toddler period and increasingly as they grow older

    ii. When they visit others' homes and see others' parents and siblings they compare their behavior to their families' and draw conclusions about the validity of what they have been told previously

    iii. Preschoolers enjoy bathroom word jokes and respect privacy and modesty

    iv. By the school-age period they openly question deviations from what they expect

    v. They experiment with sexually explicit words and tell sexually oriented jokes

    vi. Adolescents vary widely in levels of sexual maturation

    vii. Peers may tease or bully those who are dissimilar to themselves or their own group of friends

    **viii.** Adolescents adopt the views of their peers and experiment with their sexuality in dress, conversation, and physical contact, which may progress to sexual intercourse

**c.** Social influences

    **i.** The social milieu of children and adolescents affects what they view as normal and acceptable appearance and behavior

    **ii.** Social constraints on behavior and rules about dress and relationships are powerful and carry powerful sanctions for nonconformity

    **iii.** The media have been credited with desensitizing children and adolescents to nudity, violence, and blatant sexual activity in public venues

    **iv.** Research is needed to validate the relationship between media exposure and sexual risk-taking behavior (Escobar-Chavez, et al., 2004)

    **v.** Internet and late-night television offer soft and hard pornography

    **vi.** Sports figures and teen idols publicize sexual exploits, illegitimate children, and frequent mate changes

    **vii.** Conservative religious groups forbid seemingly innocent activities such as going to movies or dancing

    **viii.** The gamut of attitudes and behaviors is wide ranging and confusing to children

**d.** Cultural influences

    **i.** Individual and familial behaviors are affected by the dominant culture and the culture of their immediate and extended families

    **ii.** It is important to assess the cultural beliefs about sexuality, sexual activity during adolescence, and contraception as a part of the history

    **iii.** Racial and ethnic groups vary widely in their acceptance of sexuality and attitudes toward adolescent pregnancy and fatherhood

    **iv.** It is inappropriate to assume that individuals hold beliefs based on their racial background or ethnicity

        **(a)** Important to interview parents and adolescents separately

        **(b)** Inquire about:

            **(1)** Their individual beliefs

            **(2)** Family beliefs

            **(3)** Their perception of each other's beliefs

        **(c)** This information will guide the PNP in approaching sensitive topics

        **(d)** May be helpful with assisting family members to resolve conflicts about topics related to sexuality

**e.** Sex education

    **i.** Use a Positive Youth Development framework in anticipatory guidance

        **(a)** Clarify the questions children have

        **(b)** Answer questions honestly

        **(c)** Do not overwhelm them with too much detail if not ready for it

        **(d)** Clarify misconceptions

        **(e)** Build on the strengths and abilities of adolescents to promote effective decision making and resistance to negative influences

        **(f)** Enumerate the adolescent's strengths and compare them with identified risk factors

        **(g)** Help the adolescent find resources and support in areas of risk behaviors

    **ii.** The internet as a resource for sexual information (Gilbert, et al., 2005)

        **(a)** Users of the www.iwannaknow.org website over a three month period completed an online survey

        **(b)** The 1,242 respondents between ages 13 and 17 years accessed information on the following topics (in decreasing order of frequency): Sexual expression, teen sexuality, virginity, relationships, contraception, STD information

iii. Parental guidance related to children's sexuality and sexual development

(a) It may be necessary to prompt parents to discuss sexual development and sexuality at routine visits

(b) Teach parents the identifying markers of pubertal development

(c) Provide materials or discuss how to approach adolescents about this topic

(d) Print and electronic resources are readily available and usually free or very low cost

(e) It may be necessary to offer to discuss these topics with adolescents whose parents do not feel able to do so

iv. School-based sex education

(a) Curricula should provide more than basic biologic information

(b) Should help with decision making, options, assertiveness, and locating resources

(c) Availability of individual counseling and discussion groups is important

(d) Parents, school boards, and state departments of education often dictate the extent to which children are given information about sexuality and sexual decision making in their textbooks and health classes

v. Community-based sex education

(a) Youth service organizations that sponsor recreational and sports activities may provide sex education information or classes

(b) Faith based: churches and synagogues

(1) May offer their own versions of sex education to the children

(2) May welcome health professionals who will provide classes within their moral or values framework

(3) Abstinence-only educational programs (Santelli, et al., 2006)

a) For moral and/or religious reasons, some programs teach only about abstinence as a prevention against pregnancy and STIs

b) Exclusion of information about other methods is construed by some as withholding essential information

(c) Adolescents living in residential settings, such as juvenile custody

(1) May be able to access health care providers for basic care and information

(2) Individual counseling is important

(3) Group classes may be provided

6. Atypical sexuality and psychosocial development in children

a. Early maturing school-aged children

i. Have social, emotional, and physical differences from their normal or late-maturing peers

ii. Dress and behave differently

iii. May be teased or bullied by less well-developed peers

iv. May attract attention of older students

v. Deal with hormonal fluctuations that may affect their emotions

vi. Parents and teachers may fear early maturation will lead to sexual activity or affect peers' behavior toward them

vii. Parents need help discussing puberty calmly with these children

viii. Adults begin treating children who are physically mature as if they were much older and often have unrealistic expectations for their behavior

  ix. PNP role
    (a) Explain puberty and human reproduction to school-age children during well child checkups
    (b) Alert parents at well child checkups of the need to prepare their school-agers for pubertal changes

**b.** Failure or delay of physical development
  i. When physical development is apparently delayed, explore common causes first
  ii. May be compounded by primary or secondary amenorrhea in the female
  iii. A common cause is malnutrition
    (a) An inadequate amount of body fat and inadequate intake of nutrients can delay the onset and continuation of pubertal development
    (b) A diet diary and nutritional consultation may identify this problem
    (c) Adolescents with eating disorders are particularly prone to delayed puberty
  iv. A common cause is excessive exercise
    (a) Athletes with a low percentage of body fat also may experience delayed puberty
    (b) The diet may be balanced but inadequate calories are consumed to compensate for energy expended
    (c) A record of dietary intake, exercise, and periodic weights may identify this problem
  v. Refer to an endocrinologist or geneticist for further evaluation

**c.** Gynecomastia
  i. Benign breast enlargement is seen in 75% to 85% of adolescent males
  ii. An increase in glandular and adipose tissue results in an increase in serum estrogen
  iii. Serum estrogen causes breast enlargement
  iv. Estrogen levels are higher in overweight males
  v. PNP should assess the extent to which this potentially embarrassing condition interferes with the adolescent's normal social and emotional development
  vi. PNP can empathize, suggest ways to decrease weight, and camouflage the breast enlargement
  vii. Reassure the adolescent that the condition generally lasts about a year and resolves spontaneously

**d.** Precocious puberty (Kaplowitz, 2003)
  i. Manifested by appearance of pubic and axillary hair as early as age 7 or 8 in girls and age 9 for boys
  ii. Accelerates growth
  iii. Referral to a pediatric endocrinologist is essential
  iv. Anticipatory guidance to assist the child and family with planning for physical and psychosocial ramifications of these events is important

**e.** Physically or mentally challenged adolescents
  i. Modifications of anticipatory guidance
    (a) Explanations of physical changes should be on a developmentally appropriate level
    (b) Adolescents require preparation, education, and support to negotiate puberty
    (c) Their vulnerability to molestation or sexual abuse should be addressed
    (d) Discuss ways adolescents can avoid or exit themselves from uncomfortable situations

        (e) An interdisciplinary approach that involves the PNP, educators, specialists, parents, and the adolescents is optimal

    ii. Education for parents

        (a) Parents need to know what to expect with their adolescent

        (b) Discuss how they can address their adolescent's needs, problems, and vulnerabilities

        (c) Discuss decision points likely to arise, e.g., need for birth control

        (d) Discuss resources available to parents

**f.** Ambiguous genitalia

    i. Ambiguous genitalia may be diagnosed at birth

    ii. Genetic testing usually done to determine sex

    iii. Parents need emotional support and guidance while they make decisions about whether to raise child as a girl or boy

    iv. If not diagnosed at birth, the problem may become apparent when secondary sex characteristics fail to develop or take on the appearance of the opposite sex

    v. Refer to an endocrinologist when the condition is recognized

    vi. Parents and child will need emotional support and guidance while they make decisions about how to define the child's sexual identity

**g.** Sexual orientation

    i. Experimentation

        (a) Some adolescents engage in same-sex sexual behavior

            (1) As an exploration of "forbidden" behavior

            (2) As a short-lived peer group activity

        (b) Experimentation by the unsure adolescent

            (1) Adolescents who have close relationships with same sex individuals often report feeling attracted to individuals of their same sex

            (2) May be ashamed or frightened by these feelings and afraid that they are deviant or unacceptable to others

            (3) It is important for the PNP to acknowledge that these feelings are common

            (4) One experience does not predict future sexual behavior

            (5) PNPs should help adolescents discuss these feelings and experiences in a nonjudgmental manner

    ii. Self-identification as homosexual or bisexual

        (a) Youth recognize, self-label and accept their homosexuality or bisexuality earlier than did youth of previous generations (Savin-Williams & Cohen, 2004)

        (b) PNPs should make it clear that they accept and welcome clients who are homosexual or bisexual

        (c) Key issues include decision making about relationships, who to tell, STI prevention, self-esteem

## BIRTH CONTROL

**1.** Decision making about birth control

    **a.** PNP responsibilities

        i. Provide factual information to allow intelligent choices and minimize side effects

        ii. Ask adolescent which method he or she prefers (Hacker, et al., 2000)

        iii. Assess adolescent's ability to:
           (a) Make decisions
           (b) Follow directions
       iv. Consent about birth control and information about sexuality and birth control vary from state to state (Gold & Sonfield, 2001)
        v. Discussions
           (a) Separately with adolescent and then parents
           (b) Followed by a joint discussion
  **b.** Parental influences
        i. Parents may demand that adolescents who are not sexually active use birth control in anticipation of such activity
       ii. Others are convinced their child would never be sexually active
           (a) PNP must help some parents face the reality of their child's behavior
           (b) Parents should be informed of research findings that suggest children of parents who expect abstinence are less likely to become sexually active (Karofsky, et al., 2000)
       iii. Parents may have preconceived ideas
           (a) About birth control methods
           (b) Side effects that are no longer valid
  **c.** Peer influences
        i. Adolescents often request the same type of birth control that a friend or relative is using
       ii. Often have partial information or misinformation about the method
       iii. Need a summary of options, risks, benefits, side effects
  **d.** Media promotions may lead to request for specific products
  **e.** Marketing
        i. Internet marketing may influence decisions
           (a) Conservative pleas for abstinence
           (b) Mail out or call in prescription methods with no written prescription
           (c) Physician "consultants" write the prescriptions
           (d) Cost is usually higher than prescriptions available locally
       ii. Others offer discounts for mail orders from written prescriptions
           (a) Most volume discounts are minimal

**2.** Birth control methods
  **a.** Free information
        i. Ensure that the source is reputable
       ii. Planned Parenthood at www.plannedparenthood.org
           (a) Birth control options, effectiveness, advantages, possible problems
           (b) Sections on choices, guidelines for sex partners, and abstinence
       iii. Birth control options at www.birthcontrol.com
       iv. Women's Health Center at Mayo Clinic at www.mayoclinic.com
        v. Printed materials, including charts comparing methods free or inexpensive
           (a) Drug companies
           (b) Feminine products
           (c) Contraceptive manufacturers
       vi. See Table 26-1 for birth control options (Greydanus, et al., 2001; Kollar, 2002)
  **b.** Barrier methods
        i. Male condoms
           (a) Readily available in many stores
           (b) Adolescents use condoms frequently, more or less effectively
           (c) Condom use regardless of birth control method should be consistently recommended

■ **TABLE 26-1**
■ ■ **Birth Control Options for Adolescents**

| Method & Trade Names | Active Ingredient | Side Effects | Effectiveness | Return to Fertility | Cost |
|---|---|---|---|---|---|
| Condoms (Male: Trojan, Life-styles) (Female: Reality) (Male or female: Panty) | Latex Latex-free: silicone or polyurethane Synthetic resin AT-10, up to 10 times thinner than most regular latex condoms, anti-allergenic | Latex allergy | Male condom: 86%–98% (with spermicide use) Female: 75%–95% (with spermicide use) | Immediate | Male condom: 12/$7 ~$484/yr Female condom: 3/$14 ~$974/yr Panty: $10 ($4.95 refills) $4-$8 for spermicide |
| Hormonal implants (Norplant, Implanon) | Implanon: etonogestrel 69 mcg good for 3 years, 3 rods instead of 5 | Irregular bleeding, headaches, depression, weight gain or loss, visibility or scarring at insertion site | 99.95% | | $500-$750 exam & insertion, $100-$200 for removal (lasts 5 yr) $170/yr |
| Hormonal: injections (Depo-Provera) | Progestin | Irregular/absent periods, weight gain, depression, headaches | 99.7% effective for 12 weeks (Depo-Provera) | 2- to 3-month delay | $50 per injection $258/yr |
| Hormonal injections (Lunelle) temporarily off the market | Medroxyprogesterone acetate/estradiol cypionate | Irregular/absent periods, weight gain or loss, nausea, breast tenderness, mood changes | >99% | 2- to 3-month delay | $30-$35 per injection $420/yr |
| Hormonal: combination pills (Alesse, Loestrin, Triphasil, Nordette, Ortho Tricyclin, Ovral, Demulen, many others) | Estrogen-progestin 28-day pill packs preferred for adolescents | Irregular/absent periods, weight gain or loss, nausea, breast tenderness, mood changes | 95%-99% | Immediate | $15-$25/mo $300 |
| Hormonal: mini pill (Micronor, Ovrette) | Progestin | | 99.5% | Immediate | $15-$25/mo $300 |
| Intravaginal (Nuva Ring) | Ethinyl estrodiol etonogestrel | Spotting, breakthrough bleeding; weight gain | 93% | 2–3 months | $65 $780 |
| Transdermal: patch (Ortho Evra) | Norelgestromin/ ethinyl estradiol | Should be similar to OCP but not known | Should be similar to OCP | Immediate expected | $21 each $756 |
| Diaphragm | | Can't use when infection is present, risk of bladder infection | 80%–94% | Immediate | $733 |
| Cervical cap | | | 80%–90% nulliparous 60–80% others | | $1146/yr |

■ **TABLE 26-1**
■ ■ **Birth Control Options for Adolescents—cont'd**

| Method & Trade Names | Active Ingredient | Side Effects | Effectiveness | Return to Fertility | Cost |
|---|---|---|---|---|---|
| Lea's shield | Silicone barrier | Best for nulliparous | 9%–94% (with spermicide) | Immediate | $58, last 1 year |
| IUD (Mirena, Paragard, Progestasert) | Copper (good for 10 yr) or levonorgestrel (good for 5 yr) | Not recommended for nulliparous women; slight weight gain; lighter/absent periods, some spotting at first | 99.7% good for 5 years | Immediate | Copper $54/yr Progesterone $408/yr |
| Emergency contraception (Preven) | Ethinyl estradiol/ levonorgestrel or etonogestrel or misoprostol | | | | $50 |

Adapted from Kollar, L. M. (2002). *New contraceptive options for adolescents.* Paper presented at the meeting of the National Association of Pediatric Nurse Practitioners Annual Nursing Conference, Orlando, FL, with updates from current literature.

(d) Teaching
    (1) How to negotiate with a partner to use a condom
    (2) How to put it on
    (3) What to do if a condom breaks
    (4) Changing condoms for repeated intercourse
    (5) Use of lubricants and spermicides
    (6) Protection that condoms do and do not provide
    (7) Latex-free (silicone) male condoms are available
  **ii.** Female condoms
    (a) Less readily available in stores
    (b) Provide more control over pregnancy risks and susceptibility to STI
    (c) More difficult to apply and remove safely
    (d) Probably not the best contraceptive for adolescents
    (e) May be the answer to male refusal to use a condom
    (f) Latex-free (polyurethane) female condoms are more susceptible to breakage
  **iii.** Diaphragms and cervical caps
    (a) Requires fitting, practice, and appropriate application and removal
    (b) Effectiveness ranges from 80% to 94% in nulliparous women
    (c) Adolescents may have difficulty
      (1) Complying with application of spermicides
      (2) With proper insertion
      (3) With removal timing and technique
  **iv.** Contraceptive sponge
    (a) Soft, disposable polyurethane foam
    (b) Contains the widely used spermicide nonoxynol-9
    (c) Moistened with water and inserted into the vagina
    (d) Protects against pregnancy for the next 24 hours without the need to add spermicide cream or jelly
    (e) Continued effectiveness with repeated acts of intercourse

   **c.** Hormonal methods
- **i.** Transdermal patches
  - (a) Ortho Evra patch (norelgestromin/ethinyl estradiol)
  - (b) May have difficulty keeping them attached to skin
  - (c) Have higher levels of estrogen than most birth control pills (van den Heuvel, et al., 2005)
  - (d) Recent reports of thromboembolism and thrombophlebitis associated with this product
- **ii.** Intradermal implants (progestin)
  - (a) Requires physician or specially trained NP for insertion and removal
  - (b) Effective for long-term contraception (Norplant, 5 years)
  - (c) Side effects have been a problem for many women, and early removal is common
  - (d) Adolescents may not accept these side effects
  - (e) May be good for adolescents who fear needles but can't reliably use other methods
- **iii.** Injection
  - (a) Depo-Provera injection is required every 12 weeks
  - (b) Injections required each month
  - (c) One-time dosing very effective with adolescents
  - (d) Fear of needles may make it less attractive
  - (e) Depletes calcium stores
  - (f) Average weight gain is 8 pounds
- **iv.** Intravaginal ring (Dieben, et al., 2002)
  - (a) NuvaRing (ethinyl estradiol/etonogestrel)
  - (b) Inserted monthly, removed after 3 weeks
  - (c) Must remember to remove after 3 weeks and reinsert after fourth week
  - (d) Some adolescents do not like to touch themselves, so are hesitant to use these
- **v.** Emergency contraception
  - (a) IUD insertion within 7 days of intercourse (rarely used in adolescents)
  - (b) Levonorgestrel
  - (c) Preven (ethinyl estradiol/levonorgestrel)
    - (1) Two different regimens have been recommended
      - a) Take a double dose of the medication as soon as possible after intercourse (within 120 hours)
      - b) Take a single dose and repeat it in 12 hours
      - c) No difference in efficacy has been reported
      - d) Regimen number 1 may be more appropriate for adolescents who may not remember the second dose
      - e) Fewer side effects are seen with progestin-only pills
- **vi.** Oral contraceptive pills
  - (a) Mini pills (progestin only)
  - (b) Combination pills (estrogen/progestin)
    - (1) Yasmin (drospirenone/ethinyl estradiol )
      - a) Note: recent reports of increased thrombophlebitis with this product
      - b) Initial weight loss of 5 pounds is common due to diuretic effect but regained after 6 months
    - (2) Requires consistent use
    - (3) Complaints of weight gain with some combination pills
    - (4) Acne clears and periods become regular
    - (5) Not for all adolescents, particularly smokers

        (c) Every-3-month option
- (1) Seasonale
- (2) Cycle: 91-day oral contraceptive regimen
- (3) Tablets containing a progestin (levonorgestrel) and an estrogen (ethinyl estradiol) for 12 weeks (84 days), followed by 1 week (7 days) of placebo (inactive) tablets
- (4) Menstrual period about every 3 months
- (5) May have more unplanned bleeding and spotting between periods than with monthly regimen

        (d) Intrauterine device (IUD)
- (1) Mirena (levonorgestrel)
- (2) Paragard (copper)
- (3) Progestasert (progesterone)
- (4) Note: not usually recommended for nulliparous women because the uterus may be too small for the device

**3.** Birth control failure

  **a.** Pregnancy

    **i.** Approximately 900,000 U.S. adolescents become pregnant each year (Lonczak, et al., 2002)

    **ii.** PNP must be aware of:
- (a) Sensitivity and specificity of pregnancy tests
- (b) Optimal length of time required for accuracy of pregnancy tests
- (c) Laws about disclosing results
- (d) Rights of adolescents and parents
- (e) Adolescent's ability or reluctance to share this information with parents
  - (1) Offer support and presence during this process
  - (2) Or encourage to share information with another trusted adult
- (f) Laws about age of pregnant adolescent versus father of the child
  - (1) Local Children's Protective Agency may need to be informed if child sexual abuse or rape is suspected

    **iii.** Evaluate adequacy of adolescent and family's resources (personal, financial, educational, nutritional, medical, etc.)

    **iv.** Refer to social worker if necessary

    **v.** Refer for prenatal care

    **vi.** Continue to see adolescent for primary care
- (a) Evaluate adolescent's acceptance of pregnancy
- (b) Evaluate adolescent's ability to care for infant

  **b.** Adoption

    **i.** PNP must be aware of:
- (a) Local and area resources
- (b) Rights of adolescent parents
- (c) Vulnerability of adolescent to coercion to release or not to release infant for adoption

  **c.** Abortion

    **i.** Availability and regulations vary by state

    **ii.** PNP must be aware of:
- (a) Local and area resources
- (b) Parental notification laws
- (c) When counseling before an abortion procedure is required
- (d) Vulnerability of adolescent to coercion to have an abortion

# REFERENCES

Bethell, C., Lansky, D., Hendryx, M. (2000). *RWJF priority and program area performance indicators summary report.* Retrieved April 19, 2006, from http://www.markle.org/resources/facct/index.php.

Blythe, M. J. & Rosenthal, S. L. (2000). Female adolescent sexuality. *Adolesc Gynecol 27* (1), 125-139.

Dieben, T. O., Roumen, F. J., & Apter, D. (2002). Efficacy, cycle control and user acceptability of a novel combined contraceptive vaginal ring. *Obstet Gynecol, 100*(3) 585-593.

Escobar-Chavez, S. L., Torolero, S., Markham, C., & Low, B. (2004). Impact of the media on adolescent sexual attitudes and behaviors. Report submitted to the Centers for Disease Control and Prevention. Available at www.medinstitute.org/media/MediaExecSum.htm.

Faryna, E. L., & Morales, E. (2000). Self-efficacy and HIV-related risk behaviors among multiethnic adolescents. *Cultur Divers Ethnic Minor Psychol, 6*(1), 42-56.

Gilbert, L. K., Temby, J. R. E., Rogers, S. E. (2005). Evaluating a teen STD prevention Web site. *J Adolesc Health, 37*(3), 236-242.

Gold, R. B., & Sonfield, A. (2001). Reproductive health services for adolescents under the State Children's Health Insurance Program. *Fam Plan Perspect, 33*(2), 81-87.

Green, H. H., & Documet, P. I. (2005). Parent peer education: Lessons learned from a community-based initiative for teen pregnancy prevention. *J Adolesc Health, 37* (3 Suppl), S100-107.

Greydanus, D. E., Patel, D. R., & Rimsza, M. E. (2001). Contraception in the adolescent: an update. *Pediatrics, 107* (3), 562-573.

Grunbaum, J. A., Kann, L., Kinchen, S. A., et al. (2002). *Youth risk behavior surveillance—United States,* 2001. Retrieved June 6, 2002, from www.cdc.gov/mmwr/preview/mmwrhtml/ss5104a1.htm.

Hacker, K. A., Mare, Y, Strunk, N., & Horst, L. (2000). Listening to youth: Teen perspectives on pregnancy prevention. *J Adolesc Health, 26*(4), 279-288.

Jaccard, J., & Dittus, P. J. (2000). Adolescent perceptions of maternal approval of birth control and sexual risk behavior. *Am J Pub Health, 90*(9), 1426-1430.

Kaplowitz, P. B. (2003). Precocious puberty. Retrieved on June 6, 2006, from www.emedicine.com/ped/topic1882.htm.

Karofsky, P. S., Zeng, L., & Kosorok, M. R. (2000). Relationship between adolescent-parental communication and initiation of first intercourse by adolescents. *J Adolesc Health, 28*(1), 41-45.

Kollar, L. M. (2002). *New contraceptive options for adolescents.* Paper presented at the meeting of the National Association of Pediatric Nurse Practitioners Annual Nursing Conference, Orlando, FL.

Lonczak, H. S., Abbott, R. D., Hawkins, J. D., et al. (2002). Effects of the Seattle Social Development Project on sexual behavior, pregnancy, birth, and sexually transmitted disease outcomes by age 21 years. *Arch Pediatr Adolesc Med, 156,* 438-447.

Nelson, E. E., Leibenluft, E., McClure, E. B., & Pine, D. S. (2005). The social re-orientation of adolescence: A neuroscience perspective on the process and its relation to psychopathology, *Psychol Med, 35*(2), 163-174.

Nusbaum, M. R. H., & Hamilton, C. D. (2002). The proactive sexual health history. *Am Fam Phys, 66,* 1705-1712.

O'Sullivan, L. F., Meyer-Bahlburg, H. F. L., & Watkins, B. X. (2001). Mother-daughter communication about sex among urban African American and Latino families. *J Adolesc Res, 16*(3), 269-292.

Ozer, E. M., Park, M. J., Paul, T., et al. (2003) *America's adolescents: Are they healthy?* San Francisco: University of California, San Francisco, National Adolescent Health Information Center.

Plant, T. M. (2002). Neurophysiology of puberty. *J Adolesc Health, 31*(6S), 185-191.

Rogol, A. D., Roemmich, J. N., & Clark, P.A. (2002). Growth at puberty. *J Adolesc Health 31*(6S), 192-200.

Ryan, G. (2000). Childhood sexuality: A decade of study. Part I—Research and curriculum development. *Child Abuse Negl, 24*(1), 33-48.

Ryan, G. (2000). Childhood sexuality: A decade of study. Part II—Dissemination and future directions. *Child Abuse Negl, 24*(1), 49-61.

Santelli, J., Ott, M. A., Lyon, M., et al. (2006). Abstinence and abstinence-only education: A review of U. S. policies and programs. *J Adolesc Health, 38*(1), 72-81.

Savin-Williams, R. C., Cohen, K. M. (2004). Homoerotic development during childhood and adolescence. *Child & Adolesc*

*Psychiatric Clinics of North America, 13*(3), 529-549, vii.

Vartanian, L. R. (2000). Revisiting the imaginary audience and personal fable constructs of adolescent egocentrism: a conceptual review. *Adolescence, 35*(140), 639-661.

# Diagnosis and Management of Common Illness in Children and Adolescents

# Common Illness of the Head, Eyes, Ears, Nose, and Throat

JO ELLEN LEE, MSN, RN, CPNP

## DISORDERS OF THE EYE

1. Signs and symptoms: red eye, "pinkeye," discharge from eye, swollen eye, with or without pain
   a. Related signs and symptoms—erythema of the ocular adnexa, conjunctiva, sclera, cornea, or inflammation of deeper structures, exudates
   b. Focused history and physical examination—see Chapter 5 with special attention to:
      i. History
         (a) Onset and progression
         (b) Age
         (c) Environment
            (1) Season
            (2) Daycare
            (3) Exposures—family, friends with similar signs and symptoms
         (d) Signs and symptoms
            (1) Nature of redness
            (2) Presence of eye pain
            (3) Vision changes
            (4) Itching
            (5) Discharge
            (6) Foreign body sensation
            (7) Photophobia
            (8) Fever
            (9) Ear pain
            (10) Rhinorrhea
            (11) Nasal congestion
         (e) Juvenile rheumatoid arthritis
         (f) Neonate—parent history of STD and/or vaginal discharge
      ii. Physical examination (Figure 27-1)
         (a) Temperature, pulse, respiratory rate
         (b) Site of redness

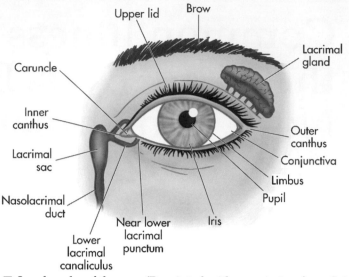

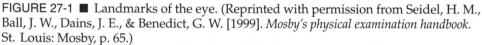

FIGURE 27-1 ■ Landmarks of the eye. (Reprinted with permission from Seidel, H. M., Ball, J. W., Dains, J. E., & Benedict, G. W. [1999]. *Mosby's physical examination handbook.* St. Louis: Mosby, p. 65.)

   (c) Conjunctival injection
    (1) Cloudy
    (2) Redness
    (3) Blanched
   (d) Unilateral or bilateral
   (e) Nature of discharge
    (1) Clear
    (2) Watery
    (3) Mucoid
   (f) Purulent otitis media often associated with conjunctivitis (Cook & Walsh, 2005)
   (g) Head and neck—check for lymphadenopathy
   (h) Rhinorrhea
   (i) Congestion
  **c.** Differential diagnoses for red eye (Box 27-1)
   **i.** Conjunctivitis (Silverman & Bessman, 2005)
    (a) Definition—inflammation of the conjunctiva (mucous membranes of the eye)
    (b) Signs and symptoms—redness and swelling of the conjunctiva and discharge, typically bilateral
    (c) Pathophysiology—exposure to an agent activates the inflammatory response that causes dilation and exudation from conjunctival blood vessels
    (d) Etiology and characteristics
     (1) Chemical conjunctivitis
      a) Due to silver nitrate drops used for chemoprophylaxis of newborn's eyes for prevention of ophthalmia neonatorum
      b) Noninfectious, mild, self-limited
     (2) Bacterial conjunctivitis
      a) Bilateral or unilateral

■ **BOX 27-1**
■ **DIFFERENTIAL DIAGNOSIS OF RED EYE**

| Disorder/Cause | Ocular Adenexa | Conjunctiva | Cornea | Uveal Tract/ Pupil |
|---|---|---|---|---|
| Infections/ inflammation | Hordeolum chalazion<br>Chalazion<br>Blepharitis<br>Phthiriasis<br>Sinusitis (frontal)<br>Periorbital cellutitis<br>Preseptal cellulitis<br>Dental abscess<br>Contact dermatitis<br>Seborrhea | Conjunctivitis | Keratitis<br>Syphilis | Iridocyclitis<br>Reiter's syndrome |
| Trauma | Frequent eye-rubbing<br><br>Blunt trauma | Blunt trauma<br>or laceration | Contact lenses<br>Corneal ulcer<br>Corneal abrasion<br>Chemical irritant | Hyphema (pupil) |
| Tumors | Neuroblastoma<br>Leukemia<br>Neurofibroma | Orbital tumors | | |
| Miscellaneous | Cavernous sinus<br>thrombosis<br>Prolonged<br>crying | Subconjunctival<br>hemorrhage<br>(due to severe<br>cough, blood<br>dyscrasias,<br>vomiting) | | |
| Toxic/environment/drugs | | Scopolamine,<br>atropine,<br>smog,<br>cosmetics,<br>smoke,<br>chemicals<br>Contact lenses | | |
| Allergic/inflammatory | | Allergic<br>conjunctivitis,<br>keratocon-<br>junctivitis<br>sica and<br>other dry<br>eye disorders<br>Nasal inflammation,<br>Sjögren's<br>syndrome<br>Other collagen<br>vascular<br>disorders<br>Kawasaki disease<br>Juvenile rheumatoid<br>arthritis<br>Stevens-Johnson<br>syndrome<br>Inflammatory<br>bowel disease | | |

b) Discharge and matting of eyelids
c) Very contagious
d) Usually self-limiting—lasts 8 to 10 days
e) Serious complications are rare
f) Organisms
   i) Staphylococcus
   ii) Streptococcus
   iii) *Haemophilus influenzae*
(3) Ophthalmia neonatorum
  a) Newborn inclusion conjunctivitis
   i) *Chlamydia trachomatis* infection from the mother
   ii) Develops between 5 and 14 days of age
   iii) Lid swelling, chemosis, mucous discharge
  b) *Neisseria gonorrhoeae* infection from mother
   i) Infants less than 4 weeks of age
   ii) Hyperpurulent discharge
   iii) Remains a significant cause of blindness worldwide
(4) Viral conjunctivitis
  a) Extremely common and highly contagious
  b) Starts unilaterally
  c) Typically no discharge or matting of eyelids
  d) May have a mucous discharge
  e) Associated with an upper respiratory infection (URI)
  f) May have an enlarged preauricular lymph node
  g) Outbreaks occur in families, schools, daycare
  h) Adenovirus the most common cause
  i) Herpes simplex virus
  j) Lasts about 14 days with or without treatment
(5) Allergic or toxic conjunctivitis
  a) Bilateral
  b) Cardinal symptom is itching
  c) Epiphora, foreign-body sensation, mucous discharge
  d) Vernal keratoconjunctivitis
   i) Inflamed cornea and conjunctiva
   ii) Cobblestone papillae in conjunctiva
   iii) Bumps in the limbal area
   iv) Intense itching, pain, photophobia, corneal ulcers
   v) Associated with seasonal allergies
  e) Often unidentified sources
  f) Associated with atopic dermatitis
  g) Contact lens solution
(6) Preseptal cellulitis
  a) Early eyelid edema and erythema
  b) Looks like conjunctivitis, especially in young children, who are difficult to examine

**d.** Diagnostic tests
  **i.** It is critical to rule out gonococcal infections because of the destructive nature of this eye disease and associated systemic infections
  **ii.** Gram stain of discharge from eye
   (a) Always done for ophthalmia neonatorum
   (b) Diagnosis is gonococcus if gram-negative intracellular diplococci are observed

     (c) Diagnosis is likely chemical (if neonatal) or viral if polymorphonu-clear leukocytes without bacteria are observed

     (d) Diagnosis is chlamydia if intracytoplasmic paranuclear inclusion bodies are observed

   iii. Culture and sensitivity of discharge from eye

     (a) Thayer-Martin medium—gonococcus

     (b) Viral cultures for herpesvirus and adenovirus not clinically useful

     (c) Chlamydia culture technique not widely available

   iv. Immunofluorescence staining—chlamydia

   v. Scraping or smears of the conjunctiva reveal numerous eosinophils and may isolate an offending allergen

**e.** Treatment (see Chapter 54, Table 54-10 for topical eye medications)

   i. Principles

     (a) To decrease problem of bacterial resistance, avoid chronic use of empiric broad-spectrum antibiotics for conjunctivitis that is typically self-limiting (chemical, adenovirus, allergic)

     (b) Avoid steroids; steroids activate or accelerate unrecognized herpes simplex virus infections; chronic use may raise intraocular pressure or cause cataracts

     (c) Refer to ophthalmology for tonometry (intraocular pressure) if symp-toms include epiphora, photophobia, eye pain, excessive blinking or squeezing eyelids, headaches

     (d) Chemical conjunctivitis—self-limiting; no treatment required

     (e) Bacterial conjunctivitis

       (1) Erythromycin 0.5% ophthalmic ointment, tetracycline 1%, poly-myxin B ophthalmic solution or ointment

       (2) Gonococcal—IV penicillin G or ceftriaxone

       (3) Chlamydia—oral erythromycin, or erythromycin or tetracycline ophthalmic ointment; if recurrent, treat with trimethoprim-sulfamethoxazole

     (f) Viral conjunctivitis

       (1) Mild cases—treat with saline solution, artificial tears; refrigerate the eye drops to be more soothing; cool compresses

       (2) Moderate and severe cases

         a) Decongestants and antihistamines given topically or systemi-cally, Naphcon, Naphcon-A, Vascon, Vascon-A

          i) To avoid rebound congestion, these products should not be used for more than 3 days

         b) Topical mast cell stabilizers useful for maintenance therapy or vernal conjunctivitis

         c) Cromolyn sodium for prevention of symptoms

         d) Nonsteroidal antiinflammatory drugs (NSAIDs) can be used for late-phase treatment of itching and burning

         e) Topical steroids are sometimes used in severe cases of allergy but they must be used with caution because of possible side effects; at maximum they should be used for 1 week

       (3) Adenovirus—no specific treatment recommended

       (4) Herpes simplex—refer to ophthalmologist

   ii. Prognosis

     (a) Complications are extremely rare from common bacterial, viral, or allergic conjunctivitis

  (b) Ophthalmia neonatorum (gonococcal conjunctivitis)
   (1) Benign if recognized early and treated
   (2) Devastating if misdiagnosed or treatment delayed
   (3) Failure to diagnose gonococcal conjunctivitis may lead to corneal perforation, and blindness
  (c) Chronic chlamydial conjunctivitis
   (1) Leads to scarring and corneal opacity
   (2) Chlamydia pneumonia develops in 20% of these patients up to 6 months later
  (d) Viral conjunctivitis may rarely lead to conjunctival scarring
  (e) Maintain a high threshold of suspicion for herpes-induced blepharitis or keratitis
  (f) Herpes simplex viral conjunctivitis
   (1) May lead to significant visual loss from recurrence
   (2) Corneal scarring even with proper therapy
  (g) Allergic conjunctivitis—refer to an allergist or ophthalmologist if:
   (1) Treatment is unresponsive
   (2) Worsening symptoms
   (3) Corneal abrasions
   (4) Impaired vision
   (5) Need for corticosteroids
   (6) Severe keratoconjunctivitis (dryness of conjunctiva and cornea, corneal ulcers)
   (7) Atypical manifestations
   (8) If already receiving steroids and additional therapy is required
 **iii.** Follow-up
  (a) No routine follow-up recommended for most common causes of conjunctivitis
  (b) Daily follow-up is necessary if due to gonococcal, chlamydia, and herpes simplex
  (c) Epidemic viral conjunctivitis—frequency of follow-up is dictated by severity of symptoms (daily to weekly)
  (d) Follow atypical conjunctivitis closely until more serious disease can be excluded
**f.** Lacrimal duct obstruction
 **i.** Signs and symptoms
  (a) Epiphora—excessive tearing when not crying
  (b) Purulent drainage in corner of eye or crusted eyelids and eyelashes
  (c) Dacryocystitis—infection of lacrimal sac; redness at inner canthus, swelling at side of nose
  (d) Dacryocystocele—blue swelling next to inner canthus; seen most often at birth
 **ii.** Pathophysiology—blockage of the portion of the tear drainage system extending from the lacrimal sac to the nose
 **iii.** Etiology
  (a) Failure of complete canalization of the nasolacrimal duct (congenital dacryostenosis)
  (b) Mechanical blockage of a too narrow duct; affects approximately 5% of newborns
 **iv.** Diagnostic tests
  (a) Dye disappearance test (DDT)—fluorescein stain is applied to the conjunctival cul-de-sac and the patient is observed for 5 minutes

(1) Negative test (normal): the tear meniscus will remain relatively unstained

(2) Positive test: the height of the stained tear meniscus will either increase or fail to increase but remains stained

(b) Culture any unexplained discharge or drainage

  v. Treatment

(a) Initially

(1) Lacrimal sac massage—wash hands; place index finger on the side of child's nose and firmly massage down toward the corner of the nose

(2) Warm compresses

(3) Either ophthalmic antibiotic drops or ointment is appropriate when ocular discharge increases

(b) If still symptomatic at about 12 months of age, refer to pediatric ophthalmologist

(1) Probing and irrigation are performed

(2) If above fails, then Silastic tube may be inserted

(3) If these fail, dacryocystorhinostomy is performed to prevent recurrent infections, dacryocystitis and maceration of the lids from excessive tearing

  vi. Follow-up

(a) Infants should be reevaluated at each well child visit and at least by 12 months of age so that referral for surgery can be made if necessary

  vii. Prognosis

(a) Spontaneous resolution in approximately 95% of patients by 12 months of age

(b) Surgery is successful for 85% to 95% if done by about 13 months of age

**g.** Periorbital cellulitis, orbital cellulitis (Givner, 2002)

  i. Definition, signs and symptoms:

(a) Periorbital (preseptal) cellulitis

(1) Acute infection and inflammation involving the eyelid and the surrounding tissue anterior to the orbital septum without involvement of the eye or orbital contents

(2) Periorbital induration, erythema, warmth, tenderness

(b) Orbital cellulitis

(1) Acute inflammation of the orbital contents posterior to orbital septum

(2) Periorbital induration, erythema, warmth, tenderness

(3) Proptosis (bulging eye), swollen conjunctiva, weakness of eye muscles, decreased visual acuity

  ii. Etiology

(a) Periorbital cellulitis

(1) Hematogenous spread, such as bacteremia

(2) Spread of focal infection secondary to:

   a) Trauma

   b) Insect bite

(b) Orbital cellulitis

(1) Extension from paranasal or ethmoid sinus infection

(c) A pathogen is isolated in only about 30% of cases, and only two thirds of those will have a positive blood culture

(d) Most common bacterial pathogens are:

       (1) *Streptococcus pyogenes* (group A)

       (2) *Staphylococcus aureus* (staph A)

          a) Staph A and group A strep should be strongly considered when there is a focal skin infection

       (3) *Streptococcus pneumoniae*—most common cause of periorbital cellulitis

       (4) *H. influenzae* type B (Hib)

          a) Less likely—the incidence of Hib disease has dramatically decreased since the start of routine Hib-conjugate vaccination of infants in 1990

          b) *S. pneumoniae* and Hib are more likely in cases of hematogenous spread

    (e) Fungi should be considered if the patient is immunocompromised

iii. Prevalence

    (a) Periorbital cellulitis is more common than orbital cellulitis

    (b) Periorbital cellulitis occurs most often in young children, average age is 21 months

    (c) Orbital cellulitis occurs most often in older children; average age is 12 years

iv. Diagnostic tests

    (a) Special attention to visual examination and eye movements

    (b) Culture purulent eye material

    (c) Not useful to culture local wound infection

    (d) Complete blood count

       (1) Usually have a WBC count between $10,000/mm^3$ and $15,000/mm^3$

       (2) WBC greater than $15,000/mm^3$ is suggestive of associated bacteremia

    (e) Blood culture

    (f) Refer to pediatrician if the following are indicated:

       (1) Lumbar puncture indicated when meningitis cannot be ruled out clinically and the patient is febrile and irritable and appears toxic

       (2) CT scan to help differentiate between periorbital and orbital cellulitis

       (3) CT scan will also reveal presence of sinusitis, proptosis, orbital or subperiosteal abscess, or foreign body

       (4) Orbital sonography to determine orbit involvement

v. Treatment

    (a) Outpatient management should be considered if:

       (1) No signs of orbital infection or toxicity

       (2) Close follow-up can be ensured within 12 to 24 hours

       (3) Antibiotics (see Chapter 54, Table 54-3)

          a) Antibiotics should be β-lactamase–resistant and should cover *Streptococcus, Staphylococcus,* and *H. influenzae*

          b) Give an IM or IV dose of a third-generation cephalosporin (e.g. ceftriaxone) immediately

          c) 10-day course of oral antibiotics may be considered at follow-up, e.g., amoxicillin-clavulanate or erythromycin-sulfamethoxazole

    (b) Refer for admission to hospital for IV antibiotics if child appears toxic or has evidence of disseminated disease, if there is a purulent wound near the involved eyelid, or if close follow-up cannot be assured

      vi. Follow-up
        (a) Ordinarily, improvement is evident within 24 to 48 hours
        (b) Patients should be seen daily until:
          (1) Clear signs of clinical resolution
          (2) Blood cultures have been negative for 48 hours if previously positive culture
     vii. Prognosis
        (a) Excellent prognosis in patients with an uncomplicated course
        (b) Complications include:
          (1) Development of orbital cellulitis from periorbital cellulitis
          (2) Disseminated bacterial infection (e.g., sepsis or meningitis)
          (3) Loss of vision
          (4) Subperiosteal or orbital abscess
          (5) Epidural and subdural abscess
          (6) Thrombosis in the retina or sinus
  **h.** Blepharitis
     **i.** Definition, signs and symptoms
        (a) Inflammation or infection of the eyelid margins
        (b) Erythema, crusting, and scaling at the lid margins, irritation, burning, and itching of the eye
     **ii.** Pathophysiology and etiology
        (a) Thirty meibomian glands are located in each tarsal plate of the eye; pilosebaceous glands of Zeis and apocrine glands of Moll are located within the distal eyelid margin
        (b) These glands produce the lipid component of tears
        (c) Occlusion of these glands will cause an accumulation of secretions
        (d) Simple squamous blepharitis (seborrheic blepharitis)
          (1) Occurs mostly in older children with other signs and symptoms of seborrhea
          (2) Associated with eczema
        (e) Ulcerative blepharitis
          (1) Most common cause of chronic conjunctivitis in children
          (2) Usually due to a secondary infection by *S. aureus* or *Staphylococcus epidermidis*
          (3) Children who rub their eyes frequently are at risk for developing blepharitis
          (4) Purulent inflammation of the glands of the lid margin results in ulcerations
          (5) Also associated with contact lens and cosmetic use
          (6) Associated with Down syndrome
        (f) Observe for other irritants of the lid margin
          (1) Lice
          (2) Seborrhea
          (3) Contact dermatitis
    **iii.** Diagnostic tests
        (a) Gram stain of conjunctival scrapings for bacteria
        (b) Giemsa stain of conjunctival scrapings to evaluate leukocytic response and presence of neutrophils
        (c) Bacterial and viral cultures of the lid margin
     **iv.** Treatment
        (a) A combination of antimicrobials and lid hygiene is recommended for several weeks until blepharitis is completely resolved

       (b) Topical antistaphylococcal antibiotic, two or three times a day (see Chapter 54, Table 54-10)

          (1) Ophthalmic ointment is more soothing than solution

          (2) Ointment will cause blurred vision (mechanical blurring, not pathologic)

          (3) Oral antibiotics may be required in severe cases

       (c) Lid hygiene

          (1) Removal of scales and crust with a moist cotton swab

          (2) Soap, or dilute baby shampoo provides the best results

          (3) Most patients prefer a commercial preparation of lid scrub for the convenience and ease of daily use

          (4) Warm (not hot) compresses for 15 minutes, twice a day

          (5) Tarsal massage—gentle massage of skin of lower lid

       (d) Treat underlying seborrhea of the scalp and eyebrows with selenium sulfide shampoo

       (e) Use hypoallergenic makeup

    **v.** Follow-up

       (a) Needed to ensure compliance with prescribed regimen

       (b) Improvement may be seen as soon as a few days

    **vi.** Prognosis

       (a) Benign, but frequently recurrent or chronic

       (b) Prevention by handwashing, avoidance of eye rubbing, and eye hygiene

**i** Chalazion

  **i.** Pathophysiology, signs and symptoms

       (a) Obstruction of meibomian glands of upper or lower lids

       (b) Inflammation causes secretion of contents of meibomian glands to form a subcutaneous nodule (lipogranuloma)

       (c) May start as tender and erythematous, then become painless nodules

  **ii.** Treatment

       (a) Small chalazia may resolve without treatment

       (b) Warm (not hot) compresses two or three times a day for 20 minutes for 2 to 3 days

       (c) Lid hygiene as is done with blepharitis

  **iii.** Follow-up

       (a) Needed only if condition not responding to treatment or complications occur

       (b) Refer to ophthalmologist for surgical excision or corticosteroid injections

  **iv.** Prognosis

       (a) Usually benign

       (b) Fragile, vascular granulation tissue called pyogenic granuloma that enlarges and bleeds rapidly can occur if a chalazion breaks through the conjunctival surface

**j.** Hordeolum (stye)

  **i.** Pathophysiology, signs and symptoms

       (a) An acute localized inflammation of one or more sebaceous glands (meibomian or zeisian) of eyelids or eyelashes

       (b) Acute, erythematous, tender lump that forms a furuncle

  **ii.** Etiology

       (a) Most common infectious pathogen is staphylococcus

       (b) Highest incidence is in children and adolescents

      **iii.** Diagnostic tests

        (a) Culture not necessary

      **iv.** Treatment

        (a) Furuncle often ruptures spontaneously when it becomes large and a point develops

        (b) Removal of an eyelash near the furuncle frequently promotes rupture

        (c) Antimicrobials (Johns Hopkins ABX Guide, 2006)

          (1) Usually not necessary unless accompanied by cellulitis

          (2) Topical antibiotics for external hordeolum or mild internal hordeolum include erythromycin ophthalmic ointment or sulfacetamide 10% ophthalmic ointment

          (3) Systemic antibiotics for moderate or severe internal hordeolum include dicloxacillin or cephalexin

        (d) Warm moist compresses for 15 minutes three or four times a day

        (e) Eye hygiene—cleanse eyelids with baby shampoo once a day (as done with blepharitis)

        (f) Discourage use of eye makeup until hordeolum is resolved

        (g) Dispose of old eye makeup

        (h) Handwashing, discourage eye-rubbing

     **v.** Follow-up

        (a) Not needed unless condition does not resolve or becomes recurrent

        (b) Refer for incision and drainage if it does not rupture after forming a point

      **vi.** Prognosis—usually benign, but can become a recurrent condition

  **k.** Eye trauma (Moeller & Rifat, 2003)

     **i.** Prevalence

        (a) Most eye injuries occur in the anterior globe and are nonperforating

        (b) Corneal abrasions make up about 83% of all nonperforating anterior globe injuries

        (c) 30% of blindness in children younger than age 10 is due to trauma

        (d) Sports and activities in which ocular trauma is common include:

          (1) BB guns

          (2) Archery

          (3) Darts

          (4) Motorcycling

          (5) Bicycling

          (6) Racquet sports

          (7) Boxing

          (8) Basketball

          (9) Baseball

        (e) Diagnostic tests

          (1) Topical anesthetic used for examination only—never use for pain control

          (2) Fluorescein stain with Wood's lamp to visualize epithelial injury of cornea, such as abrasions, ulcers

          (3) If cause is herpes simplex virus-1 (HSV-1), staining shows a dendritic ulcer

          (4) Possible radiographs to visualize foreign body

          (5) Visual acuity—to determine any deviation from normal

          (6) Ophthalmic examination—determine other orbital or ocular injuries

      (f) Treatment – refer to ophthalmologist

      (g) Prognosis

         (1) Children are at high risk for ocular complications, including:

           a) Rebleeding

           b) Glaucoma

           c) Corneal blood staining with resultant amblyopia

**ii.** Corneal abrasion (Howell, 2005)

    (a) Pathophysiology, signs and symptoms

       (1) Loss of epithelial lining from corneal surface of eye

       (2) Significant pain, tearing, light sensitivity (photophobia), foreign body sensation, decreased visual acuity

       (3) Conjunctival injection (redness), iritis , eyelid swelling

    (b) Etiology—commonly caused by paper, toys, fingernails, brushes, contact lenses, ultraviolet light (tanning)

    (c) Treatment

       (1) Topical antimicrobials are commonly used but their necessity is controversial

       (2) Research shows that patching the eye is not necessary

       (3) Refer to ophthalmologist if signs and symptoms not resolved within 24 hours

**iii.** Keratitis

    (a) Pathophysiology, signs and symptoms

       (1) Inflammation and ulceration of the cornea

       (2) Begins as a well-defined infiltration at the center or edge of the cornea

       (3) Subsequently suppurates and forms an ulcer that may penetrate deep into the corneal tissue

       (4) May spread to involve the width of the cornea

       (5) Signs and symptoms same as corneal abrasion

    (b) Etiology

       (1) Most common cause is HSV-1

       (2) Other viruses, bacteria, and fungi also can cause keratitis

       (3) Most common risk factor is trauma

       (4) Other common causes

         a) Allergic reaction

         b) Conjunctivitis

         c) Systemic infection

         d) Use of corticosteroids

    (c) Can cause a dramatic alteration in visual acuity and can progress to corneal ulceration and blindness

    (d) Treatment

       (1) Immediate referral to ophthalmologist for appropriate treatment

       (2) Delay in referral can lead to corneal opacification, scarring, loss of vision

       (3) Never place a patch over keratitis or a corneal ulcer

       (4) Steroids should never be used

**iv.** Foreign body in eye

    (a) Pathophysiology

       (1) Surface foreign body (FB)

         a) FB is nonadherent or loosely adherent to cornea or conjunctival epithelium

         b) Most likely sources include dirt, sand, grass

  (2) Penetrating—FB cuts into but not through cornea or sclera
  (3) Perforating—FB cuts through cornea or sclera and into globe
(b) Treatment
  (1) Surface FB
      a) Remove foreign body via irrigation with normal saline
      b) Place eye shield for 24 to 48 hours for protection until reevaluation
  (2) Penetrating or perforating FB
      a) Refer to ophthalmology immediately
      b) Place eye shield on injured eye

v. Hyphema
  (a) Pathophysiology and etiology
      (1) Rupture of iris or ciliary body blood vessels, causing accumulation of blood in the anterior chamber of eye
      (2) Often caused by balls, fists, sticks, towels
      (3) May also occur with bleeding disorders and sickle cell disease
  (b) Treatment
      (1) Refer to ophthalmologist
      (2) May resolve itself within 5 to 6 days
      (3) Surgery may be necessary to remove blood that has collected
      (4) Hospitalization often necessary

vi. Black eye (ecchymoses)
  (a) Pathophysiology—bruising of periorbital region from trauma
  (b) Treatment of uncomplicated ecchymosis
      (1) Cold compresses for 24 to 48 hours
      (2) Then warm (not hot) compresses until swelling resolves
      (3) Elevate head
      (4) Inform parents or patient that ecchymosis and edema may spread, usually downward due to gravity

vii. Chemical irritation
  (a) Pathophysiology—burns of the eyelids, conjunctiva and/or cornea
  (b) Symptoms—burning, tearing, photophobia
  (c) Etiology
      (1) Caused by steam, intense heat, common household agents
      (2) Amount of damage directly related to duration of exposure
  (d) Treatment
      (1) An acute ocular emergency
      (2) Topical anesthetic may reduce pain from injury and irrigation
      (3) Copious irrigation with normal saline for 20 to 30 minutes
      (4) Patch and refer to ophthalmologist immediately
      (5) Severe chemical injury to eye requires hospitalization
  (e) Complications
      (1) After chemical burn, *Pseudomonas* contamination is common and may lead to corneal ulcerations; usually prevented with topical antibiotics (see Chapter 54, Table 54-10)

viii. Tumor (retinoblastoma) (Aventura, Roque, & Aaberg, 2006)
  (a) Pathophysiology
      (1) Most common primary ocular malignancy of childhood
      (2) Congenital growth that arises from a multipotential precursor cell (mutation in the long arm of chromosome 13 band 13q14)
      (3) Exhibits a variety of growth patterns within the eye

(b) Signs—dysmorphic appearance, white reflex (leukocoria), strabismus, poor vision, nystagmus, unilateral mydriasis, white spots on iris, anorexia, failure to thrive

(c) Incidence
  (1) 250 to 500 new cases per year
  (2) If bilateral, diagnosed at an average age of 13 months
  (3) If unilateral, diagnosed at an average age of 24 months
  (4) 90% diagnosed before age 5 years

(d) Treatment—immediate referral to pediatric ophthalmologist

2. Symptoms: poor vision, changes in vision
   a. Focused history and physical examination—see Chapter 5 with special attention to:
      i. Symptom assessment
         (a) When, where, and at what age was vision loss or change first noticed?
         (b) How has this changed?
         (c) Other ocular abnormalities recognized and treated
         (d) One or both eyes
         (e) Number of waking hours symptoms are present
      ii. Recent trauma
      iii. Current medications
      iv. Sensitivity to light (photophobia)
      v. Excessive tearing or lid squeezing
   b. Focused physical assessment
      i. Visual acuity screening
         (a) Accurate monocular and binocular visual acuities are the most sensitive indicators of amblyopia
         (b) If results of vision screening by medical assistant suggests abnormality, retest by PNP is warranted
      ii. Detailed eye examination (see Chapter 5)
      iii. Refer to ophthalmology or optometry for more extensive examination, diagnosis, and treatment
   c. Strabismus
      i. Definition—ocular misalignment
         (a) Exotropia—eyes deviate outward
         (b) Esotropia—eyes deviate inward
         (c) Hypotropia—eyes deviate inward
         (d) Hyperopia—eyes deviate upward
         (e) Pseudostrabismus—eyes appear to be crossed due to exaggerated epicanthal folds on either side of bridge of nose; no ocular deviation, e.g., Asians
      ii. Pathophysiology
         (a) Normal for intermittent and alternating esotropia or exotropia to be present in first 4 to 6 months of life
         (b) A supranuclear (visual cortex) inability to use the eyes together usually results in comitant strabismus (i.e., degree of ocular misalignment does not vary with the direction of gaze)
         (c) An infranuclear disorder of the extraocular muscles or their respective cranial nerves results in noncomitant strabismus (i.e., degree of misalignment varies depending on direction of gaze or which eye is fixating on the target)
         (d) Interruption of visual development in an eye (e.g., retinoblastoma tumor)

iii. Prevalence
  (a) 4% of the population has some form of more than 100 types of strabismus
  (b) Approximately 30% of children with strabismus have family members with strabismus
  (c) Inheritance is multifactorial, with a strabismic parent having a 12% to 17% chance of having a child with strabismus (versus 4% in the general population)
  (d) Most forms of strabismus are comitant and begin in either infancy or early childhood
  (e) Suppression of vision in one eye is an adaptation to diplopia; without correction, permanent loss of vision is probable
  (f) Acquired strabismus after age 6 months is usually from cataracts, retinoblastoma, anisometropia, or high refractive errors
iv. Diagnostic tests
  (a) Cover/uncover test and corneal light reflex (see Chapter 5)
  (b) Refer to ophthalmology for further testing
v. Treatment
  (a) Prompt diagnosis and treatment offers the best results, although no therapy will "cure" most forms of childhood strabismus because the synaptic problem affecting binocular function in the visual cortex cannot be reversed
  (b) Goal: improve vision
    (1) Medical
      a) Can correct significant refractive errors as early as 4 to 6 months of age
      b) "Penalization" of the preferred eye with patching or cycloplegic drops improves amblyopia
    (2) Surgical
      a) Correction of conditions that interfere with vision (cataracts, vitreous hemorrhage)
      b) Correction of conditions that degrade images (retinal detachment, upper lid ptosis, hemangioma)
    (3) Goal: correct the misalignment
      a) Medical
        i) Spectacles with or without bifocal or optical prism
        ii) Topical miotic drops can manipulate accommodation and improve ocular alignment in some forms of esotropia
        iii) Visual training exercises have some, but limited usefulness
      b) Surgical
        i) Extraocular muscle surgery to mechanically move the eyes into a more advantageous position for the brain to process images
        ii) Successful with one operation in 75% to 80% of patients
        iii) 20% to 25% require two operations
vi. Primary care concerns
  (a) Chronic strabismus is disfiguring and results in decreased self-esteem, poor self-image, and aberrant social interaction
  (b) Common *misinformation* about strabismus
    (1) Children will "grow out of it"—they won't; treatment is essential

(2) Strabismus is just "lazy eye" (amblyopia)—it isn't the same thing (see following)

(3) Strabismus is due to serious underlying problems—that is not likely

(c) Contact with social services for blind and visually impaired individuals must be made for children, even if they are only *suspected* of being visually impaired

(1) Encourage families to make the contact even when the child may be too young to provide objective data of the extent of disability

d. Amblyopia

i. Definition—amblyopia occurs when the retina transmits only a blurred image to the brain; a neuropathologic process unique to infancy and childhood resulting in decreased vision in one or both eyes

ii. Pathophysiology

(a) Visual system cell growth and synaptogenesis (cortical vision) is initiated at birth and is finished by 9 years of age

(b) Normal and equal visual input is necessary for proper cell growth and synaptogenesis of the visual pathways in the brain

(c) If, during this period, one eye (or both) is not capable of normal and equal visual input, synaptogenesis and cell growth is disturbed, resulting in deficient vision

(d) The younger the cortical vision system, the more sensitive it is to abnormal input

(e) The period of cortical visual development between birth and 17 weeks of life is the "sensitive or critical period"

(f) Amblyopia will develop after only 1 week of abnormal visual input in an infant less than 1 year old

(g) The clinical rule is that a week of abnormal visual input per year of life is amblyogenic

(h) If a congenital or neonatal amblyogenic stimulus is not treated before the end of the sensitive period, it is impossible to recover full and normal vision

iii. Prevalence

(a) Present in 2% of the population and is the leading cause of preventable visual loss in children

(b) Strabismic amblyopia is the most common

(1) 50% of people with strabismus also have amblyopia

(2) Occurs in infants and children (up to 9 years) with strabismus

(c) There is no hereditary predisposition to primary amblyopia

(d) This is an acquired disease

(e) An increased prevalence in family members of similar amblyogenic conditions is associated with strabismus in the child

iv. Prognosis

(a) Untreated amblyopia results in irreversible visual loss with an increased risk of complete visual disability if the good eye is traumatized or affected by disease

(b) Final visual acuity is dependent on the combination of:

(1) Amblyogenic factor

(2) Age at presentation

(3) Compliance with amblyopia treatment

(4) In general the earlier the diagnosis and treatment the better the prognosis

**e.** Cataracts
    **i.** Definition, signs and symptoms
        (a) Opacity of the clear, crystalline lens of the eye
        (b) Some are small and nonprogressive and do not cause visual symptoms
        (c) Central opacity of 3 mm or more is clinically significant and decreases visual acuity
    **ii.** Pathophysiology
        (a) Opacity represents a derangement of the normal developmental growth of the crystalline fibers of the central lens nucleus or peripheral cortex
        (b) Frequently classified according to their morphology or etiology
        (c) Age at which cataract began may be detected by its location within the lens
    **iii.** Etiology, prevalence
        (a) About one third are congenital
            (1) Primary inherited congenital cataracts are usually autosomal dominant
            (2) Some are autosomal and rarely, X-linked recessive varieties
        (b) One third are associated with systemic genetic metabolic, or maternal infectious disorders
        (c) About one third are idiopathic
            (1) A small number occur along with other primary ocular abnormalities and some metabolic disorders
        (d) Others are secondary to steroids, radiation, and localized trauma
    **iv.** Refer to ophthalmology for further testing, diagnosis, and treatment
    **v.** Prognosis
        (a) With newborn cataracts, visual restoration becomes progressively more difficult to impossible after 8 to 12 weeks because of irreversible deprivation amblyopia
        (b) Deprivation amblyopia is a concern with any other type of cataract if not removed and/or treated quickly
        (c) Can achieve corrected visual acuities of 20/40 or better for bilateral cataracts and 20/40 to 20/200 for monocular cataracts
        (d) In all cases, the onset or presence of nystagmus before the cataract is removed is an ominous sign of a poor outcome
        (e) Cataract surgery involves removal of the lens and its posterior capsule, or removal of both lens and capsule
            (1) If capsule remains, a replacement lens can be implanted
            (2) Capsule itself may develop a secondary cataract
            (3) An eye with no lens is prone to glaucoma and retinal detachment, either of which can cause permanent visual loss
        (f) Parental and educational support services may be needed for those with residual visual handicap
        (g) Special local, state, and federal services for the visually handicapped and/or blind may be required because not all children who have successful surgical results will have good vision
**f.** Congenital glaucoma
    **i.** Definition—elevated intraocular pressure
    **ii.** Signs—epiphora (excessive tearing), photophobia, blinking spasms
    **iii.** Pathophysiology and etiology
        (a) Aqueous humor, a clear fluid produced by the ciliary body at the posterior base of the iris, passes through the pupil and exits through

the trabecular meshwork and Schlemm's canal located at the anterior junction of the cornea and the iris

(b) Improper drainage of aqueous humor leads to elevated intraocular pressure, enlargement of the eye, and damage to optic nerve fibers

(c) Primary congenital glaucoma caused by structural abnormalities of trabecular network, iris, or cornea

(d) Glaucoma is associated with systemic abnormalities such as:
   (1) Aniridia
   (2) Rubella
   (3) Sturge-Weber syndrome—a neurologic disorder indicated at birth by seizures accompanied by a large port-wine stain birthmark on the forehead and upper eyelid of one side of the face

(e) Glaucoma may be acquired secondary to ocular abnormality such as cataract

iv. Prevalence
   (a) 1 : 10,000 live births
   (b) 1 : 2 female to male ratio
   (c) 70% are bilateral
   (d) Primary congenital glaucoma accounts for about half of all cases of glaucoma

v. Refer immediately to ophthalmology for further testing, diagnosis, and medical or surgical treatment

vi. Prognosis
   (a) Guarded; even if pressure is well controlled, the child must be carefully followed for amblyopia, abnormal refractive errors, and recurrence of glaucoma
   (b) Complications
      (1) Unrecognized and untreated amblyopia (the most serious threat to child's vision)
      (2) High degrees of myopia
      (3) Anisometropia (difference in refractive error between both eyes)
      (4) Buphthalmos (enlargement of the fibrous coats of the eye, and corneal scarring)
      (5) Continued, long-term surveillance is essential
      (6) Ensure that potential systemic medicines do not raise intraocular pressure
   (c) Contact with social services for blind and visually handicapped individuals must be made for children even if they are only *suspected* of being visually impaired

g. Nystagmus (Curtis & Wheeler, 2005)
   i. Definition, signs and symptoms—involuntary, horizontal, vertical, rotary, or mixed rhythmic movement of eyes noted on eye examination
   ii. Pathophysiology
      (a) Oscillation is a common, normal finding in the newborn, but persistence beyond the neonatal period indicates pathology
      (b) Classified according to direction of movement
         (1) Horizontal—abnormality of the peripheral labyrinth, or a lesion of the vestibular system in the brainstem or cerebellum, or a serious side effect of drugs, particularly phenytoin
         (2) Vertical—indicative of brainstem dysfunction
      (c) May be familial
      (d) Associated with:

(1) Albinism

(2) Refractive errors

(3) Central nervous system (CNS) abnormalities

(4) Various diseases of inner ear and retina

  **iii.** Refer immediately to ophthalmologist and/or neurologist

  **iv.** Prognosis

   (a) Nystagmus intensity (frequency × amplitude) often improves spontaneously with increasing age but depends on etiology

   (b) Nystagmus that presents after age 6 months is considered late infantile or childhood nystagmus and has a graver prognosis

**h.** Refractive errors

 **i.** Noted with visual acuity screening test

  (a) Hyperopia (farsightedness)

   (1) Visual image is focused behind the retina

   (2) Able to see objects clearly at a distance, but not at close range

  (b) Myopia (nearsightedness)

   (1) Visual image is focused in front of the retina

   (2) Able to see objects clearly up close, but not at a distance

  (c) Astigmatism

   (1) Due to an irregular curvature of the cornea or lens

   (2) Causes light rays to bend in different directions

 **ii.** Etiology

  (a) Hyperopia

   (1) Axial length of eye too short

   (2) Insufficient convexity of the refracting surface of the cornea

   (3) Familial pattern common

   (4) Mild hyperopia commonly found in children; spontaneous resolution usually by 6 years of age

  (b) Myopia

   (1) Axial length of eye too long

   (2) Increased curvature of the refracting surface of the cornea

   (3) Familial pattern common

   (4) Frequently associated with prematurity

   (5) May be present at birth; usually appears around 8 to 10 years of age

  (c) Astigmatism

   (1) Familial developmental variations in the curvature of the cornea

   (2) Retina cannot focus

   (3) Rare, but may be caused by soft tissue masses of upper lid, e.g., chalazion, hemangioma

 **iii.** Refer to ophthalmologist or optometrist for further testing, diagnosis, and correction

 **iv.** Prognosis

  (a) Detection of visual problems in children at an early age is essential to prevent the development of otherwise avoidable permanent visual loss

  (b) Support and reassurance according to the child's developmental level are needed during the period of adjustment to contact lenses or eyeglasses

  (c) Once vision is stabilized, then yearly optometric eye exams are recommended

**i.** Blindness (amaurosis)

      **i.** Definition and symptoms

        (a) Varies from inability to distinguish light from darkness, partial or no vision

          (1) Noted in newborn examination (no response to moving object)

          (2) Noted in vision screening tests when visual acuity appears to worsen over time

        (b) Legal blindness is distant acuity 20/200 in better eye or visual field that includes an angle of no greater than 20 degrees

        (c) Primary blindness—present at birth

     **ii.** Etiology and prevalence

        (a) One third of blindness in children is from trauma

        (b) Variety of pathologic causes: cataracts, glaucoma, retinopathy of prematurity, retinoblastoma, detached retina, cranial nerve II damage, infection, hydrocephalus, genetic abnormality

    **iii.** Refer immediately to ophthalmologist

    **iv.** Prognosis—early identification and treatment, if possible, is the key to a good prognosis

## DISORDERS OF THE EAR

**1.** Symptoms: earache, draining ear, hearing loss

  **a.** Symptom assessment

    **i.** Location—one ear, both ears, inside the ear, outer ear

    **ii.** Duration—acute onset suggests recent trauma or infection, number of prior infection, and time of last infection

    **iii.** Severity of pain (evaluated by parent or child) on a scale of 1 to 10

    **iv.** Drainage—characteristics

    **v.** Hearing loss

    **vi.** Associated symptoms—fever, pain in other sites, URI, sore throat, hoarseness, dizziness, itching, drooling

    **vii.** Exposure at home or at school to others with infection

    **viii.** Aggravating or alleviating factors

    **ix.** Changes in behavior

  **b.** Focused physical assessment (Figure 27-2)

    **i.** Temperature

    **ii.** External ear—swelling, redness, drainage, position of pinna, lesions on pinna, pain with movement of pinna (palpation or traction)

    **iii.** Ear canal—swelling, drainage, erythema, areas of trauma

    **iv.** Tympanic membrane (TM)—color, mobility with pneumatic otoscopy, landmarks, bulging, foreign body, lesions behind the tympanic membrane (Jones & Kaleida, 2003)

  **c.** Differential diagnoses for earache: acute otitis media, otitis externa, mastoiditis

  **d.** Acute otitis media (AOM) (Auinger, et al., 2003)

    **i.** Pathophysiology

      (a) Eustachian tube dysfunction results in fluid accumulation in the middle ear

      (b) Proliferation of microorganisms results in infection, inflammation of the mucoperiosteum, and pain

    **ii.** Incidence and etiology

      (a) More than 5 million AOM cases occur annually in U.S. children

        (1) Results in more than 10 million antibiotic prescriptions

        (2) About 30 million office visits

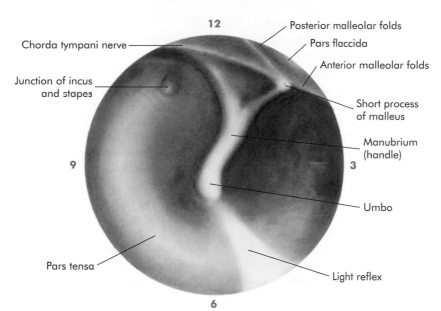

**12**

Chorda tympani nerve

Posterior malleolar folds

Pars flaccida

Anterior malleolar folds

Junction of incus and stapes

Short process of malleus

Manubrium (handle)

**9**

**3**

Umbo

Pars tensa

Light reflex

**6**

FIGURE 27-2 ■ Landmarks of the ear. (Reprinted with permission from Seidel, H. M., Ball, J. W., Dains, J. E., & Benedict, G. W. [1999]. *Mosby's physical examination handbook.* St. Louis: Mosby, p. 77.)

    (b) Bacterial
        (1) *S. pneumoniae* (30%)
        (2) *H. influenzae* (20%)
        (3) *Moraxella catarrhalis* (7%)
        (4) Group A streptococcus (2%)
        (5) Enteric gram-negative (1%)
        (6) *S. aureus* (1%)
    (c) Viral
        (1) Respiratory syncytial virus (RSV)
        (2) Influenza
        (3) *Mycoplasma pneumoniae*
        (4) Fungal (rare)
    (d) Risk factors not amenable to change
        (1) Genetic predisposition, e.g., Down Syndrome
        (2) Cleft palate
        (3) Premature birth
        (4) Incidence in males greater than in females
        (5) Native American or Inuit ethnicity
        (6) Siblings in the household
        (7) Low socioeconomic status
        (8) Family history of AOM
        (9) Ages 6 months to 3 years of age because of the normally horizontal position of the eustachian tube
      (10) Incidence during winter months greater than in other seasons
    (e) Risk factors amenable to change
        (1) Supine bottle-feeding (breast-feeding for first 6 months is recommended)

(2) Bottle propping

(3) Pacifier use after age 6 months

(4) Environmental tobacco smoke

(5) Daycare

iii. Assessment

(a) History and physical exam will usually be enough to make a diagnosis of AOM

(b) American Academy of Family Practice and AAP (2004) have approved criteria for *diagnosis* of AOM that requires three characteristics:

(1) History of acute onset

(2) Signs of middle ear effusion (at least one of four):

a) Bulging TM

b) Air and fluid level visible behind TM

c) Otorrhea

d) Limited mobility of TM – difficult to test if ear canal is narrow, poor seal of otoscope, presence of cerumen

(3) Sign of middle ear inflammation (at least one of two):

a) Erythema of TM

b) Distinct otalgia that interferes with sleep or activity

(c) An evaluation of pain level is essential

iv. Diagnostic tests

(a) Confirm AOM with testing

(1) Audiometry—hearing loss

(2) Tympanometry—measures middle ear pressure and TM compliance

(b) Lateral neck x-ray to rule out suspected retropharyngeal mass or abscess if suspected

(c) Note: blood tests are not routinely useful

(d) Refer to pediatrician or EENT specialist for:

(1) Tympanocentesis for bacterial culture and sensitivity (C&S)

(2) Imaging of head if intracranial pathology is suspected

v. Treatment

(a) Refer to otolaryngologist if:

(1) Child is seriously ill or appears toxic

(2) Persistent failure of antimicrobial therapy

(3) Child is at risk for unusual organisms

a) Neonates

b) Immunocompromised

(b) Goals related to antibiotic treatment are to minimize unnecessary use of antibiotics and prevent development of resistant microorganisms

(c) American Academy of Family Practice and AAP (2004) have approved evidence-based guidelines for *treatment* of uncomplicated AOM for children ages 2 months to 2 years

(1) Pain management is important (see Chapter 55 for details on analgesics)

a) Acetaminophen or ibuprofen

b) Benzocaine otic drops for children older than age 5 years

(2) Observation option—"watchful waiting" for 48 to 72 hours

a) Criteria

i) Children are otherwise healthy

ii) Children ages 6 months to 2 years with nonsevere illness at presentation and an uncertain diagnosis

iii) Children 2 years of age or older without severe symptoms at presentation or with an uncertain diagnosis

  b) 80% of children whose AOM is not treated immediately with antibiotics get better on their own and have no increased risk of a serious infection
  c) Parents expect a prescription, but one study found that they accept a watchful waiting recommendation if they are given a "clear explanation of the problem and a plan of action" (McCormick, et al., 2005)
 (3) First line of antibiotic therapy is high-dose amoxicillin (80-90 mg/kg/day)
  a) Generally effective against susceptible and intermediate resistant pneumococci
  b) Safe, inexpensive, has an acceptable taste, and narrow microbiologic spectrum
  c) If child is allergic to amoxicillin and the allergic reaction is not a type I hypersensitivity reaction, prescribe cefdinir, cefpodoxime, or cefuroxime
  d) Optimal duration of therapy for patients with AOM is uncertain
  e) Symptoms should stabilize within the first 24 hours of therapy and begin to improve during the second 24 hours
 (4) Second line of therapy
  a) If no improvement by 48 to 72 hours, there is another disease present or the chosen therapy was not adequate
  b) Choice of antibiotic should be based on the likely pathogen(s) present or the provider's clinical experience
  c) Antibiotics for 10 to 14 days
 (5) No recommendations for complementary or alternative medicines due to insufficient evidence
 (d) Minimize risk factors that are amenable to change
 (e) Observe for signs and symptoms of complications
  (1) Perforation
  (2) Hearing loss
  (3) Mastoiditis
  (4) Epidural abscess
  (5) Cholesteatoma
  (6) Meningitis
  (7) Facial nerve paralysis
  (8) Language delay
  (9) Labrynthitis
  (10) Lateral sinus thrombosis
**e.** Otitis media with effusion (OME)
 **i.** Definition, signs and symptoms
  (a) Presence of fluid in the middle ear
  (b) *Without* other signs or symptoms of AOM
  (c) Usually no pain or fever
  (d) Feeling of ear fullness, pressure, or popping
 **ii.** Pathophysiology
  (a) Eustachian tube dysfunction changes the middle ear mucosa
   (1) Mucosa becomes secretory with increased mucus production
   (2) Mucus becomes viscous as the mucosa absorbs water
   (3) Negative pressure in the middle ear results in fluid accumulation by effusion
   (4) Fluids become stuck behind the tympanic membrane

   (b) Mild to moderate hearing loss with concomitant language delays may occur with OME, contributing to behavioral difficulties, poor attention, and poor school performance
   (c) Fluid is usually sterile
iii. Etiology, prevalence
   (a) OME accounts for 25% to35% of all cases of otitis media
   (b) OME is the natural consequence of both treated and untreated acute otitis media
   (c) 3% to 40% have OME associated with allergic rhinitis
iv. Focused physical examination
   (a) American Academy of Pediatrics (AAP), the American Academy of Family Physicians (AAFP), and the American Academy of Otolaryngology—Head and Neck Surgery (AAO-HNS) have developed evidence-based clinical practice guidelines on the diagnosis and treatment of OME (2004)
      (1) Use pneumatic otoscopy as the primary diagnostic method for OME
      (2) TM is often cloudy with distinctly impaired mobility
      (3) An air fluid level or bubble may be visible in the middle ear
   (b) If diagnosis is still unclear, tympanometry may be helpful
      (1) After age 4 months, tympanometry with a standard 226-Hz probe tone is reliable
      (2) Younger than age 4 months, specialized equipment with a higher probe tone frequency is required
   (c) Tympanogram is flat or shows negative pressure
   (d) Audiogram may show hearing loss of 15 to 30 decibels
   (e) At each assessment, document the laterality (unilateral or bilateral), duration of effusion, and presence and severity of associated symptoms
v. Treatment
   (a) AAP, AAFP, AAO-HNS Practice Guidelines (2004)
   (b) Identify children at increased risk for developmental delay or disorder because of physical, sensory, cognitive, or behavioral factors that are not caused by OME but can make the child less tolerant of hearing loss or vestibular problems secondary to middle-ear effusion
   (c) Management of children with OME who are at increased risk for developmental delays should include:
      (1) Speech and language therapy concurrent with managing OME
      (2) Hearing aids or other amplification device for hearing loss independent of OME
      (3) Insertion of tympanostomy tubes
      (4) Hearing testing after resolution of OME to document improvement
   (d) Management of children with OME who are *not* at risk for developmental delay
      (1) Watchful waiting for 3 months from the date of effusion onset or diagnosis
         a) Any intervention for OME (medical or surgical) other than observation has the potential for harm
         b) About 75% to 90% of residual OME after an episode of AOM resolves spontaneously within 3 months
      (2) Antihistamines and decongestants are ineffective for OME and are not recommended for treatment
      (3) Antimicrobials and corticosteroids do not have long-term efficacy and are not recommended for routine management

(4) No recommendations for complementary or alternative medicines due to insufficient evidence

(5) Reexamine at 3- to 6-month intervals until:

    a) Effusion is no longer present

    b) Significant hearing loss is identified (refer to otolaryngologist)

    c) Structural abnormalities of the eardrum or middle ear are suspected (refer to otolaryngologist)

(e) Encourage parents to:

    (1) Decrease background noises

    (2) Speak louder than usual (if needed)

    (3) Focus on the child's face when speaking

(f) Recommend the child be given preferential seating in school and be spoken to face to face

**f.** Otorrhea (draining ear) (Schroeder & Darrow, 2004)

  **i.** Etiology

    (a) Otitis externa (see section g. below)

      (1) Severe pain

      (2) Sense of fullness in ear

    (b) Cholesteatoma (see section h. below)

      (1) Mild drainage

      (2) White "pearl" observed under upper left side TM

    (c) Foreign body in ear

    (d) Perforated TM (see section i. below)

    (e) Tympanostomy tube in TM (see section j. below)

      (1) Occurs in 75% of children with tubes placed in TM

      (2) Reduced by use of antibiotic drops at time of placement

      (3) Increases with acute URI

      (4) Usually painless

      (5) Resolves spontaneously in most cases

    (f) Chronic suppurative otitis media (CSOM)

      (1) Diagnosis used after 6 weeks of otorrhea through a perforated TM

      (2) Treat with 10- to 14-day course of systemic antibiotics

    (g) Granular myringitis

      (1) Clear or purulent otorrhea

      (2) Flat granulation of surface of a thickened but intact TM

      (3) Treat with debridement of ear; treat granulations with caustic or antiseptic agents (silver nitrate, trichloroacetic acid, gentian violet, steroids)

    (h) Cerebrospinal fluid otorrhea and perilymphatic fistula

      (1) Clear discharge from ear that reappears quickly after it is removed

      (2) Sensation of fullness in ear

      (3) May have dizziness, hearing loss, or recurrent meningitis

  **ii.** Treatment

    (a) Most critical step in diagnosis and management of otorrhea is debridement of ear canal—use swabs, suction, irrigation

    (b) Topical antibiotics are usually indicated (concentrations of antibiotics are 100 to 1000 times greater than with systemic therapy)

    (c) Expandable methylcellulose otowick or sponge maximizes exposure of the ear canal to medication and decreases drainage

(d) See specific diagnoses for other treatment and follow-up recommendations

**g.** Otitis externa

  **i.** Pathophysiology, signs and symptoms

    (a) Disruption of the squamous epithelium of the auditory canal

    (b) Alteration in the canal pH increases susceptibility to microbial invasion, which results in inflammation and pain

  **ii.** Etiology

    (a) Excess moisture

      (1) Swimming

      (2) Immersion during bathing, hairwashing

    (b) Foreign body

    (c) Cerumen

      (1) A protective substance in the ear canal

      (2) Provides an acidic environment and lysozymes that prevent microbial invasion

      (3) Removal of cerumen and cleaning with soapy water disrupts the canal's acidic pH and removes antimicrobial enzymes

      (4) Excessive cleaning disrupts the surface epithelium

    (d) Bacterial

      (1) *Pseudomonas aeruginosa*

      (2) *S. aureus*

      (3) Gram-negative enterics

      (4) Group A streptococci

    (e) Viral

      (1) HSV

      (2) Varicella

      (3) Herpes zoster

    (f) Fungal

      (1) *Candida albicans*

      (2) *Aspergillus niger*

    (g) Foreign bodies and aggravating factors increase risk factors

  **iii.** Diagnostic tests

    (a) Usually not necessary

    (b) Bacterial culture and sensitivity and Gram stain in cases that do not respond to conventional therapy

    (c) Culture immunocompromised patients

    (d) Fungal, viral culture in selected, refractory cases that do not respond to conventional therapy

  **iv.** Treatment

    (a) Remove purulent debris

    (b) Antibiotic otic drops (see Chapter 54, Table 54-11 for details)

    (c) If canal is swollen it may prohibit entry of antibiotic drops

      (1) Use antibiotic corticosteroid drops, especially if canal is swollen

      (2) Place a cotton wick in canal to facilitate entry of drops into the canal

      (3) Change wick every 48 hours

    (d) Fungal infections

      (1) Acetic acid drops are good for preventing and treating fungal infections

      (2) Antifungal drops (e.g., clotrimazole 1% solution)

(e) Oral antibiotics that cover strep and staph are indicated only if there is associated:
  (1) Cellulitis
  (2) Adenitis
  (3) Acute otitis media
(f) Refer to otolaryngology for IV antibiotics if there are severe complications or malignant otitis externa
v. Follow-up
  (a) Expect improvement of symptoms in 24 to 48 hours after initiation of antibiotics
  (b) Watch for:
    (1) Fever
    (2) Severe or local inflammation especially if child is:
      a) Immunocompromised
      b) Chronically ill
    (3) Cellulitis of surrounding tissues
    (4) Adenitis
    (5) Malignant otitis externa
    (6) Stenosis of auditory canal (with recurrent infections)
    (7) Transient hearing loss
  (c) Prevention
    (1) Use water-impermeable earplugs when:
      a) Swimming
      b) Water sports
    (3) 2% acetic acid drops (or 70% ethyl alcohol) after swimming or immersion of ears helps to restore acidic pH
h. Cholesteatoma (Roland, 2006)
  i. Signs and symptoms
    (a) Hallmark symptom is either unremitting or recurrent, painless, otorrhea
    (b) Conductive hearing loss is a common symptom
    (c) Dizziness is not common but indicates serious erosion into ossicles
    (d) Otorrhea that is unresponsive to antibiotics
    (e) TM perforation occurs in more than 90% of patients
  ii. Pathophysiology (Box 27-2)
  iii. Etiology—not clear, but various theories regarding its formation
    (a) Congenital
    (b) Acquired
      (1) Inflammatory process
      (2) Perforation
      (3) Failure of normally desquamated tissue to drain from middle ear
  iv. Refer immediately to otolaryngologist for surgical excision
  v. Prognosis
    (a) Prompt diagnosis and treatment are essential to prevent multiple complications
    (b) Cholesteatoma could invade and destroy the temporal bone and other structures
    (c) Could spread to intracranial cavity and cause infection
    (d) May lead to facial nerve paralysis
i. TM perforation (Howard, 2006; Schroeder & Darrow, 2004)
  i. Normal physiology of the TM—the TM has two zones that could become perforated

■ **BOX 27-2**
■ **DIFFERENTIAL DIAGNOSES AND PATHOPHYSIOLOGY FOR HEARING LOSS**

| Differential Diagnoses | Pathophysiology |
|---|---|
| Congenital (Dhooge, 2003; Kenna, 2004) | 1. Genetic: cause of >50% of all incidents of congenital hearing loss in children<br> a. Autosomal dominant<br> b. Autosomal recessive<br> c. X-linked<br> d. Mitochondrial<br>2. Intrauterine infections (e.g., rubella, herpes simplex, CMV, toxemia)<br>3. Rh incompatibilities<br>4. Prematurity<br>5. Maternal diabetes<br>6. Anoxia |
| Infection | 1. Acute otitis media (OM) may cause ischemia in the tympanic membrane (TM) and fluid in the middle ear, thus transmission of sound waves is diminished<br>2. Chronic suppurative OM (CSOM)<br>3. TM may perforate from the fluid pressure (preceded by severe pain) (Howard, 2005)<br>4. Bacterial infection (e.g., meningitis, encephalitis)<br>5. Viral infections of the child (e.g., measles, mumps, varicella, influenza) |
| Toxins | Aminoglycoside antimicrobials, cisplatin |
| Cholesteatoma (Roland, 2006) | 1. A destructive lesion of the skull base that can erode and destroy structures within the temporal bone, mostly in middle ear and mastoid area<br>2. Cystlike mass with lining of stratified squamous epithelium, filled with desquamated debris<br>3. As mass enlarges, pressure on bony structures can damage them<br>4. Enzyme activity at margin of cholesteatoma causes bone erosion<br>5. Infection increases enzyme activity<br>6. Erosion into brain is a serious risk |
| Traumatic perforation of TM (Howard, 2006) | 1. Blows to the ear that cause sudden increased pressure on the TM (e.g., being struck with the flat of the hand; head hitting the water surface, ear down)<br>2. Severe water pressure (e.g., scuba divers)<br>3. Exposure to severe atmospheric overpressure from an explosion can tear the TM<br>4. Cerumen removal methods (e.g., cerumen pick, cotton swabs, irrigation) |
| Tympanostomy tubes | Deliberate incision in the TM to place pressure-equalizing tubes |
| Continuous noise (Roland, 2004) | 1. Most prone to noise injury is the portion the cochlea sensitive to frequencies of about 4000 Hz<br>2. Outer hair cells are more susceptible to noise exposure than inner hair cells<br>3. Stereocilia of outer hair cells become "disarrayed and floppy" and respond poorly to noise (metabolic exhaustion)<br>4. High-frequency noise is more damaging than low-frequency noise<br>5. Hearing loss can be *temporary* if source of noise is removed |
| Acoustic trauma (Roland, 2004) | 1. One-time brief exposure to >140 dB for <0.2 second followed by immediate bilateral, *permanent* hearing loss<br>2. Impulse noise—blast effect, explosion<br>3. Impact noise—collision of metals<br>4. Causes tearing of TM and damage to ossicles and cell walls, and mixing of perilymph and endolymph that may destroy hair cells |

      (a) Pars tensa is a tough and resilient fibrous layer with an almost transparent mucosal layer inside and squamous epithelium outside

      (b) Pars flaccida is a smaller zone with no fibrous layer that lies above the suspensory ligaments of the malleus

  **ii.** Symptoms

      (a) Audible whistling sounds during sneezing and nose blowing

      (b) Decreased hearing ability

      (c) Frequent ear infection with colds and when water enters the ear canal

      (d) Copious purulent drainage that may also be sanguineous

      (e) Uncomplicated perforations are never painful

      (f) Pain indicates a concurrent disease process

  **iii.** Differential diagnosis and pathophysiology (see Box 27-2)

  **iv.** Diagnostic tests

      (a) Culture discharge—most common organisms are:

        (1) *P. aeruginosa*

        (2) *S. aureus*

      (b) Purified protein derivative (PPD) skin test to rule out TB

      (c) CT scan of mastoid to rule out mastoiditis

  **v.** Treatment

      (a) Patients with central nervous system sequelae, refer immediately

      (b) Hospitalization may be necessary

      (c) Oral antibiotics and antibiotic ear drops may be required

      (d) Uncomplicated perforated TM tends to heal itself and requires no treatment (Howard, 2006)

      (e) Surgical repair may be done

      (f) Prevention of infection while TM is healing

        (1) Cotton plugs with petroleum jelly when bathing and hairwashing (soap decreases surface tension of water and allows it to enter middle ear)

        (2) Discourage swimming (use fitted earplugs if unavoidable)

        (3) Diving, jumping into water, and underwater swimming forbidden

        (4) Ear irrigations are prohibited with current or history of perforated TM

      (g) If not responsive, suspect mastoiditis or cholesteatoma

  **vi.** Follow-up

      (a) Follow-up every week for 3 months; most heal within 2 weeks

      (b) Refer to otolaryngologist

        (1) Unresolved perforation after 1 year

        (2) Surgical repair delayed until 9 to 12 years of age

  **vii.** Prognosis (Howard, 2006)

      (a) Some perforated TMs do not heal, but with preventive efforts against infection, need not be a problem

      (b) Surgically repaired TMs perforate again in as many as 10% of patients

      (c) Site of perforation and associated risk of cholesteatoma

        (1) Central—relatively safe from cholesteatoma formation

        (2) Peripheral, especially in pars flaccida—increased risk

**j.** Tympanostomy tubes

  **i.** See Box 27-2 for description

      (a) One million tubes inserted annually

      (b) Short term—intended to remain in eardrum 8 to 15 months

      (c) Long term—intended for more than 15 months

      **ii.** Indications

        (a) Failed antibiotic prophylaxis of 4 months or longer

        (b) Allergy to penicillin or sulfonamides

        (c) Associated hearing loss of 20 dB

        (d) Other complications

        (e) With increasing numbers of resistant bacteria, possibility of more frequent use of tubes

      **iii.** Treatment

        (a) Fitted earplugs for swimming to prevent infection

        (b) If drainage occurs from tubes, treat with antibiotic otic suspension and hydrocortisone

        (c) Most tubes remain in place for specified period

        (d) If chronic otorrhea occurs, tubes may need to be removed

**k.** Mastoiditis

    **i.** Pathophysiology

      (a) Infection of the mastoid air cells that can range from an asymptomatic illness to a severe life-threatening disease

      (b) Develops when the accumulation of purulent exudate in the middle ear does not drain through the eustachian tube or through a perforated TM, but spreads to the mastoid bone

      (c) Can progress to a coalescent phase when the air cells are destroyed

      (d) May then progress to subperiosteal abscess or to a chronic mastoiditis

    **ii.** Etiology, prevalence

      (a) Rare—occurs in 0.2% to 0.4% of children

      (b) Unusual in very young due to incomplete pneumatization of the mastoid air cells

      (c) Caused by an extension of the inflammation of AOM into mastoid air cells

      (d) Common organisms:

        (1) Group A β-hemolytic streptococcus

        (2) *S. pneumoniae*

        (3) *S. aureus*

        (4) Anaerobic bacteria

        (5) Enteric bacteria

      (e) Cholesteatomas may contribute to the development of mastoiditis by impeding mastoid drainage of pus or erosion of underlying bone

      (f) Tuberculosis

    **iii.** Diagnostic tests

      (a) CBC—leukocytosis with neutrophil predominance

      (b) Erythrocyte sedimentation rate (ESR)—increased with acute inflammation

      (c) X-ray of mastoid can indicate damage but fairly unreliable

      (d) PPD—if tuberculosis suspected

      (e) Refer to otolaryngology for:

        (1) Middle-ear aspirate Gram stain and culture

        (2) Bone scan

        (3) Lumbar puncture—to rule out diagnosis of meningitis in a toxic-looking child

    **iv.** Treatment

      (a) Refer to otolaryngology

        (1) Essential to accomplish middle-ear drainage (with or without tube placement early in the process)

(2) Parenteral antibiotics to treat most likely organism

(b) Audiograms should be done routinely to check for hearing loss

v. Prognosis

(a) Appropriate and early treatment of otitis media with timely follow-up to identity treatment failure decreases the chance of mastoiditis

(b) Complications of chronic mastoiditis

(1) Subperiosteal abscess

(2) Coalescence of infection

(3) Facial nerve palsy

(4) Meningitis

(5) Intracranial abscess

(6) Venous thrombosis

(7) Irreversible hearing loss

l. Hearing loss

  i. Normal physiology of hearing (Howard, 2006)

(a) TM is a stiff, but flexible, translucent diaphragm that moves synchronously with sound waves, which manifest as variations in air pressures

(b) TM vibrations are transmitted through the attached malleus and other ossicle bones to the cochlea

(c) In the cochlear hair cells, vibratory mechanical energy changes to electrochemical energy that travels via the eighth cranial nerve to the brain

  ii. Classification of hearing loss

(a) Conductive loss—normal bone conduction, but transmission of sound waves through the canal, middle ear, and inner ear is obstructed; usual range is 15 to 40 dB loss

(b) Sensorineural loss—cochlea hair cells and/or auditory nerve damage; may range from mild to profound loss

(c) Mixed—components of conductive and sensorineural hearing loss are present

  iii. Etiology (see Box 27-2)

  iv. Focused assessment—see Chapter 5 with special attention to the following:

(a) Focused history

(1) Suddenness of onset (Roland, 2004)

(2) Age of onset

(3) Hearing status of parents

(4) Maternal infections during pregnancy

(5) Neonatal or child's history of infections

(6) Noise on jobsite (OSHA requires hearing protection if noise in the workplace exceeds 85 dB)

(7) Use of portable radios and cassette, CD, or MP3 players can play at levels greater than 85 dB, but even adolescents rarely set them that high, and exposure times are short (Roland, 2004b)

(8) Speech and social development

(9) Signs of hearing loss

a) Substitution of words with gestures, especially after age 15 months

b) Does not respond to questions

c) Inattention

(b) Focused physical assessment

(1) External examination of ear

    a) Congenital malformations
      i) Structural abnormalities of external ear
      ii) External canal abnormalities
      iii) Craniofacial malformations
  (2) Internal examination of ear
  (3) Throat—secondary infection
  (4) Audiometric testing to measure amount of loss (Jacobson & Jacobson, 2004)
    a) Normal (no hearing loss [HL]): 0 to 15 dB
    b) Minimal HL: 16 to 25 dB
    c) Mild HL: 26 to 30 dB
    d) Moderate HL: 31 to 50 dB
    e) Moderate to severe HL: 51 to 70 dB
    f) Severe HL: 71 to 90 dB
    g) Profound HL: more than 91 dB

v. Differential diagnoses and pathophysiology for hearing loss (see Box 27-2)

vi. Referrals
  (a) Sudden hearing loss is an otologic emergency and should be immediately referred to an otolaryngologist (Carr, 2004)
  (b) Refer others to appropriate specialist, depending on the diagnosis

vii. Prognosis
  (a) Spontaneous recovery rates for sudden sensorineural hearing loss range from 47% to 63% (Carr, 2004)
  (b) Negative prognostic factors include:
    (1) Age younger than 15 years or older than 65 years
    (2) Elevated ESR (>25)
    (3) Vertigo or vestibular changes
    (4) Hearing loss in the opposite ear
    (5) Severe hearing loss

viii. Prevention—"The most effective ear protection is the ear protection the person will wear" (Roland, 2004)

# DISORDERS OF THE NOSE

1. Signs and symptoms: runny nose, itching nose, sneezing, snoring
  a. Focused assessment—see Chapter 5 with special attention to:
    i. Focused history
      (a) Duration of symptoms
      (b) Amount, color, thickness, and odor of nasal drainage
      (c) Unilateral or bilateral drainage
      (d) Exacerbating and relieving factors
      (e) Snoring with sleep
      (f) Nose or mouth breathing
      (g) Halitosis
      (h) Changes in sense of taste or smell
      (i) Fever
      (j) Medication use
        (1) Antihistamine
        (2) Nasal decongestant
    ii. Focused physical examination
      (a) Quantity, viscosity, and color of drainage

(b) Swelling of turbinates

(c) Color of nasal mucosa

(d) Allergic crease on nose

(e) Allergic salute

(f) Excoriation of nares

(g) Postnasal drip

(h) Color, exudates in posterior pharynx

(i) Tonsillar enlargement

(j) Erythema of conjunctiva, drainage

(k) Dennie lines

(l) Allergic shiners

(m) Breath sounds—wheeze

(n) Temperature

**b.** Differential diagnoses for rhinitis

   **i.** Viral infection

   **ii.** Allergic rhinitis

   **iii.** Vasomotor rhinitis

   **iv.** Infectious sinusitis

   **v.** Foreign body in nose

   **vi.** Nasal polyps or tumor

   **vii.** Deviated nasal septum

   **viii.** Medications

      (a) Rhinitis medicamentosa—rebound nasal congestion

      (b) Oral contraceptives

      (c) Antihypertensives

      (d) NSAIDs

**c.** Allergic rhinitis (AR) (Zagaria & Buonanno, 2005)

   **i.** Pathophysiology, signs and symptoms

      (a) Immunoglobulin E (IgE)–mediated response to inhaled allergens or irritants

      (b) T cells differentiate into $T_H2$ cells and interleukins 4, 5, and 9

      (c) Early phase occurs within minutes of exposure

         (1) IgE-sensitized mast cells degranulate and release cysteinyl leukotrienes, prostaglandins, cytokines, and histamine

         (2) Histamine is primarily responsible for sneezing; rhinorrhea; itching eyes, nose, and palate; some congestion

      (d) Late phase—congestion

         (1) Nasal mucosa becomes infiltrated with inflammatory cells (basophils, eosinophils, neutrophils, mast cells, mononuclear cells)

         (2) Histamine's action on receptors $H_1$ to $H_4$ causes increased proinflammatory cytokines that maintain the congestion

         (3) Nasal epithelium becomes hypertrophied from mast cells and eosinophils

   **ii.** Etiology, prevalence, incidence

      (a) 50% of cases are due to allergens

         (1) Occurs in 50% of children and 20% of adults

         (2) Incidence peaks at ages 12 to 15

         (3) About $6.3 to $7.9 billion per year is spent directly and indirectly on AR

        (4) Seasonal—"hay fever," predicted seasonal pattern of symptoms

          a) Trees in spring, grass in summer, ragweed in fall

          b) More common after age 6

        (5) Perennial—symptoms last 9 months or longer

          a) House dust mites, cockroaches, molds, animal dander

          b) May occur in children younger than age 6

    (b) Genetic predisposition—family history of atopic dermatitis, asthma and allergic rhinitis (29% chance if present in one parent; 47% chance if present in two parents vs. 13% chance if no family history)

  **iii.** Diagnostic tests

    (a) Primarily a clinical diagnosis

    (b) CBC with differential

      (1) Elevated eosinophils

      (2) Elevated total IgE

    (c) Nasal smear for eosinophils—10% considered confirmatory

    (d) Refer to allergist for skin prick testing, intradermal testing, and in vitro antigen-specific antibody assays *only if the results would change the practitioner's treatment plan*

  **iv.** Treatment

    (a) First-line therapy—environmental control to minimize exposure to allergens

      (1) Remove carpets, drapes, stuffed animals

      (2) Plastic covers on mattresses and pillows

      (3) Decrease humidity with air conditioner, air purifiers, avoidance of tobacco smoke

    (b) Medications (see Chapter 54, Table 54-4 for details)

      (1) See Allergic Rhinitis and Its Impact on Asthma (ARIA) guidelines (2001) issued by the World Health Organization

      (2) Intranasal glucocorticosteroids are the most effective agent for AR

        a) Inhibit release of mediators from basophils and inhibit influx of other inflammatory cells to reduce nasal inflammation and nasal hypersecretions

        b) Prevent early-and late-phase reactions

        c) Once-daily doses are available

        d) Can be used with antihistamines

        e) Examples: betamethasone, budesonide, triamcinolone

      (3) Systemic glucocorticosteroids are *not* recommended

      (4) $H_1$ antihistamines—bind to $H_1$ receptors to prevent histamine binding and release; decrease hypersecretions

        a) Systemic first- and second-generation, intranasal, ophthalmic forms

        b) First-generation antihistamines have a sedative effect, e.g. diphenhydramine, hydroxyzine, chlorpheniramine

        c) Second-generation antihistamines are preferred because they are peripheral histamine blockers with little or no CNS or sedative effects, e.g., fexofenadine, loratadine

      (5) Decongestants

        a) Systemic or intranasal forms have vasoconstriction effects that shrink swollen mucosa and improve breathing

        b) Rhinitis medicamentosa—rebound congestion that occurs with prolonged use of intranasal decongestants (>3 to 5 days)

        c) Pseudoephedrine is the safest variety

(6) Mast cell stabilizers, e.g., cromolyn sodium nasal spray
    a) Use for severe and chronic AR if other medications are unsuccessful
    b) Used for prevention, not treatment of symptoms—prevents antigen-triggered mast cell degranulation and release of allergic mediators
    c) Takes 2 to 3 weeks to take effect
(7) Leukotriene inhibitors, e.g., montelukast, zafirlukast
    a) Use as an alternative to, or in combination with, intranasal glucocorticosteroid
    b) Antagonist to leukotrienes at the receptor sites to cause vasoconstriction and decrease mucosal swelling
(c) Refer to allergist for allergen-specific immunotherapy—hyposensitization to the allergen, especially dust mites, animal dander, pollens, molds, insect stings
(d) Prognosis
    (1) "…early, aggressive treatment of allergic rhinitis may prevent or slow asthma development and improve quality of life…" (Elder, et al., 2002, p. 3)
    (2) Chronic problem with exacerbations is common
    (3) Continual medical therapy helps to alleviate or diminish symptoms

**d.** Nonallergic rhinitis (Woodall & Meyers, 2005)
  **i.** Prevalence and pathophysiology
    (a) Occurs in 5% to 10% of the population; symptoms similar to allergic rhinitis, but no IgE mediation, as documented by allergen skin testing
    (b) Seven subclassifications, including infectious rhinitis, nonallergic rhinitis with eosinophilia syndrome (NARES), occupational rhinitis, hormonal rhinitis, drug-induced rhinitis, gustatory rhinitis, and vasomotor rhinitis
    (c) Vasomotor rhinitis may be due to dominance of the parasympathetic system causing vasodilation and nasal mucosa swelling
  **ii.** Treatment
    (a) No single recommended treatment
    (b) Treatment should be based on patients' specific symptoms
    (c) Autonomic self-regulation may be effective
      (1) Nasal airway resistance can be reduced up to 50% through isotonic exercise, which is mediated by increases in sympathetic tone, e.g., changes from erect to supine position; lying on right side results in lower pressure in the left nostril
      (2) Nasal compliance is decreased with cold air and increased with hot air
      (3) Nasal blood flow is not affected by hot air, but decreases in the presence of cold air

**e.** Foreign body in the nose
  **i.** Common in toddlers and preschoolers
  **ii.** Typical items include food, crayons, small toy parts, erasers, paper wads, beads, beans, pebbles, alkaline button batteries (e.g., watch batteries)
  **iii.** Unilateral foul discharge from naris may be first clue of a nasal foreign body
  **iv.** Button batteries can cause tissue damage and should be removed immediately

    **v.** Removal techniques
       (a) Head mirror or light will provide visualization of object
       (b) May need nasal decongestant initially to decrease swelling
       (c) Removal by forceps, nasal suction, or magnet
    **vi.** If unable to remove, refer to otolaryngologist

## DISORDERS OF THE THROAT

**1.** Symptoms: sore throat, neck pain, stiff neck
    **a.** Focused assessment—see Chapters 12 and 13, with special attention to:
       **i.** Focused history
         (a) Location, onset, duration, progression of neck pain, stiffness and/or swelling
         (b) Limitation of neck movement
         (c) Associated signs and symptoms
            (1) Fever
            (2) Dysphagia
            (3) Ear pain
            (4) Rash
            (5) Difficulty breathing
            (6) Cough
            (7) Fatigue
            (8) Drooling
            (9) Stridor
            (10) Facial edema
            (11) Trauma
         (d) Exposures at home, school, daycare, work
       **ii.** Focused physical examination
         (a) Temperature
         (b) Systemically toxic appearance
         (c) Range of motion of neck
         (d) Pain on palpation
         (e) Palpation of the neck, head, clavicle, and axillary lymph nodes for pain, redness, size, fluctuance
         (f) Neck or head hyperextension
         (g) Pharynx
            (1) Difficulty swallowing
            (2) Tonsillar size
            (3) Erythema of posterior and anterior pharynx
            (4) Exudates
            (5) Petechiae in or on pharynx and/or tonsils
            (6) Swelling in pharynx area
            (7) Uvula—swelling, deviation
            (8) Teeth—caries, abscessed gums
         (h) Lungs
    **b.** Differential diagnoses
       **i.** Muscle pull or strain, torticollis (see Chapter 34, Section 4)
       **ii.** Acute pharyngeal infection (epiglottitis, pharyngitis, tonsillitis, peritonsillar or retropharyngeal abscess, cervical lymphadenitis, parotitis, mononucleosis) (see also, Chapter 33, Section 3)
       **iii.** Congenital brachial cleft, thyroglossal duct cyst

        iv. Hemangiomas, cystic hygroma

        v. Meningitis, encephalitis

c. Epiglottitis

    i. Pathophysiology

        (a) Is an acute life-threatening bacterial infection

        (b) Results in narrowing of the glottic opening due to cellulitis and edema of the aryepiglottic folds, arytenoids, and hypopharynx

    ii. Etiology, incidence, and prevalence

        (a) Etiologic agents include:

            (1) *H. influenzae* type b

            (2) *S. aureus*

            (3) *S. pneumoniae*

            (4) *S. pyogenes* (group A β-hemolytic streptococcus [GABHS])

            (5) Group C β-hemolytic streptococcus

        (b) *C. albicans* may be etiologic agent in immunocompromised patients

        (c) *Pasteurella multocida* after exposure to nasopharyngeal secretions from a cat

        (d) Incidence reduced by 98% since the implementation of *H. influenzae* vaccine

        (e) Year-round occurrence

        (f) Disease due to *S. pyogenes* occurs most often in early school-age children during the winter and early spring

        (g) Affects boys and girls equally in all geographic areas

        (h) Rare in Alaskan Natives, Native Americans

        (i) Occasional secondary cases in households or daycare centers

        (j) May be more frequent in children with sickle cell anemia, asplenia, immunoglobulin defects, leukemia

    iii. Diagnostic tests

        (a) NOTE: Do not attempt throat culture if epiglottitis is suspected

        (b) Lateral neck radiograph shows characteristic "thumb sign" of edematous epiglottis with narrowing of the posterior airway and ballooning of the hypopharynx

        (c) CBC shows increased white blood cell count with left shift

        (d) Blood cultures positive 90% of time for the causative organism

    iv. Treatment

        (a) Immediate transport to emergency department; personnel experienced in airway management should accompany the child at all times

        (b) Airway management—maintain child upright; never supine; oxygen therapy

        (c) Perform emergent cricothyrotomy if obstruction occurs before controlled airway management

    v. Prognosis and follow-up

        (a) Mortality is estimated at 8%, but should approach zero with appropriate airway management

        (b) Universal immunization with *H. influenzae* type B vaccine

        (c) Antibiotic prophylaxis for:

            (1) Index cases

            (2) Intimate contacts

            (3) Susceptible children in household or childcare setting

d. Pharyngitis, tonsillitis (Bisno, et al., 2002)

    i. Pathophysiology—inflammation of the mucous membranes and underlying structures of the pharynx and tonsils

    **ii.** Etiology

      (a) Viral infection—adenovirus, enterovirus, herpangina, herpesvirus, influenza, Epstein-Barr

      (b) Bacterial infection—group A β-hemolytic streptococcus (GABHS), *N. gonorrhoeae* or *N. meningitidis*, mycoplasma, chlamydia, *C. diphtheriae*, *H. influenzae*—nontypable)

      (c) Secondary to chronic rhinitis (allergic, nonallergic), sinusitis, tumor

    **iii.** Diagnostic tests

      (a) Throat culture or quick strep test

        (1) NOTE: Do not attempt a throat swab if child is drooling or having difficulty breathing

        (2) If rapid strep test is negative, back-up culture should be done due to risk of false negative

        (3) Carrier state—identify low colony count on culture or streptozyme test for streptococcal antibodies

        (4) Infants may need culture of nasal secretions instead of the pharynx due to higher carrier rates in the nasopharynx

        (5) Cultures of asymptomatic contacts of patients with GABHS are not indicated except:

          a) An outbreak in a school or daycare

          b) Contacts with a history of nonsuppurative complications

      (b) CBC—use only if child appears toxic, otherwise not useful

      (c) Epstein-Barr virus (EBV) testing is most effective if patient has had symptoms for more than 7 days

      (d) Influenza testing

    **iv.** Treatment

      (a) Fever management

        (1) Tylenol 10 to 15 mg/kg/dose every 4 hours

        (2) Ibuprofen 10 mg/kg/dose every 6 hours

      (b) Pain management

        (1) Analgesics as per fever management

        (2) Saltwater gargle

        (3) Anesthetic sprays or lozenges

      (c) Treatment of specific etiology

        (1) Viral—symptomatic treatment only

        (2) GABHS, i.e., *Streptococcus pyogenes* α (see Chapter 54, Table 54-3 under the heading of "Microorganism sensitivity)

          a) Penicillin V for 10 days PO

            i) Children 250 mg bid or tid

            ii) Adolescents and adults 250 mg tid or qid, or 500 mg bid

          b) Allergic to penicillin (PCN)—give erythromycin; dose varies with formulation

          c) Others: clarithromycin, cephalosporins—first generation, azithromycin, IM benzathine penicillin G, mixtures of benzathine and procaine penicillin G

          d) Secretions are infectious until after 24 hours of antibiotics

      (d) Fluid and nutrition therapy as needed

    **v.** Follow-up

      (a) Patients with GABHS

        (1) Clinical improvement usually rapid after start of antibiotics

        (2) Cure rate is excellent

          a) Except in noncompliant patients

        b) Rare coinfection with pathogens that elaborate β-lactamase or in cases of a new infection acquired from family or classroom contact (rare)

    (3) No need to perform posttreatment cultures in asymptomatic patients in areas where acute rheumatic fever is low

    (4) Watch for suppurative complications
        a) Cervical adenitis
        b) Mastoiditis
        c) Peritonsillar abscess

    (5) Morbidity associated with:
        a) Acute rheumatic fever (ARF)
        b) Acute poststreptococcal glomerulonephritis

    (6) Long-term penicillin prophylaxis is required for patients with a history of rheumatic fever

    (7) Child can return to school after 24 hours of antibiotic therapy

**e.** Peritonsillar abscess
    **i.** Pathophysiology, signs and symptoms
        (a) Infectious complication of pharyngitis or tonsillitis due to accumulation of purulence in the tonsillar fossa, causing a cellulitis that leads to abscess
        (b) Sore throat with bulging posterior soft palate, deviation of uvula to contralateral side with fluctuance
        (c) Can become an airway emergency
    **ii.** Etiology, prevalence
        (a) Bacteria—GABHS, staphylococcus, anaerobic bacteria
        (b) More common in adolescents, but may occur in younger ages
    **iii.** Diagnostic tests
        (a) WBC count usually elevated with a left shift
        (b) Rapid strep test
        (c) Refer to otolaryngologist for further diagnosis and treatment:
            (1) Gram stain and culture of aspirate
            (2) CT scan or ultrasound to differentiate between cellulitis and abscess
    **iv.** Treatment
        (a) Needle aspiration and/or drainage
        (b) IV therapy with penicillin, nafcillin, oxacillin, specific for organism
        (c) Tonsillectomy if not responding to IV antibiotics in 24 to 48 hours
        (d) Analgesia
        (e) Hydration
    **v.** Prognosis
        (a) Swift and complete recovery can be expected
        (b) Recurrence not uncommon

**f.** Retropharyngeal abscess
    **i.** Pathophysiology
        (a) Inflammation of the posterior aspect of the pharynx and suppurative retropharyngeal lymph nodes
        (b) Can become an airway emergency
    **ii.** Etiology and prevalence
        (a) Relatively rare infection
            (1) Most common in children younger than 4 years of age
            (2) Secondary to untreated pyogenic adenitis
        (b) Causative pathogens
            (1) GABHS

            (2) Anaerobic organisms

            (3) *S. aureus*

        (c) In older children, usually a superinfection from penetrating injury to posterior wall of the oropharynx

        (d) Possible complication of bacterial pharyngitis

    **iii.** Diagnostic tests

        (a) CBC with differential shows elevated WBC

        (b) Lateral neck radiography shows that the retropharyngeal space is wider than C4 vertebral body

        (c) Computed tomography (CT) scan to visualize abscess

    **iv.** Treatment

        (a) Emergency referral to otolaryngologist

        (b) Emergency hospital admission

        (c) IV antibiotics with surgical incision and drainage if needed

        (d) Analgesics for pain

    **v.** Prognosis and expected course

        (a) Complete recovery if treated early

        (b) Can recur in younger ages

  **g.** Cervical lymphadenitis

    **i.** Pathophysiology—inflammation and swelling of one or more cervical lymph nodes

    **ii.** Etiology and prevalence

        (a) Prevalent among preschool children

        (b) Pathogens

            (1) *S. pyogenes* and *S. aureus*—80% of cases

            (2) *Mycobacterium tuberculosis*

            (3) Other organisms: viral, fungal, parasitic

        (c) Secondary to local infections of ear, nose, throat (see Chapter 33, Section 3)

    **iii.** Diagnostic tests

        (a) CBC with differential shows moderate to marked elevation in WBCs

        (b) Mantoux test to rule out tuberculosis

        (c) Mono spot to rule out mononucleosis

        (d) Throat culture or quick strep test to rule out GABHS if other symptoms are consistent

        (e) Serology tests if infection is not resolving

            (1) EBV

            (2) Toxoplasmosis

            (3) Cytomegalovirus (CMV)

            (4) Histoplasmosis

        (f) Aspiration of node if fluctuant

        (g) Aerobic and/or anaerobic culture

    **iv.** Treatment

        (a) If no evidence of systemic infection, treat empirically with oral antibiotics (dicloxacillin, amoxicillin clavulanate, cephalexin for a minimum of 10 days and for no less than 5 days after resolution of symptoms)

        (b) Analgesics for fever and pain

        (c) Application of cold compresses

        (d) Surgical aspiration may be necessary

    **v.** Follow-up

        (a) Measure and follow node size

        (b) Most resolve over time without any complications

        (c) Refer to otolaryngologist for biopsy if not improving

# REFERENCES

Allergic Rhinitis and its Impact on Asthma (ARIA) Independent Expert Panel. (2001). Allergic rhinitis and its impact on asthma. *J Allergy Clin Immunol, 108*(5), S147-S334.

American Academy of Pediatrics (AAP) and the American Academy of Family Physicians (AAFP), Subcommittee on Management of Acute Otitis Media. (2004). Practice guideline on diagnosis and management of acute otitis media. *Am Fam Phys, 69*(11), 2713-2715.

American Academy of Pediatrics (AAP), American Academy of Family Physicians (AAFP), and American Academy of Otolaryngology—Head and Neck Surgery (AAO-HNS) Subcommittee on Otitis Media with Effusion. (2004). Practice guideline on diagnosis and management of otitis media with effusion. *Am Fam Phys, 69*(12), 2929-2931.

Auinger, P., Lanphear, B. P., Kalkwarf, H. J., & Mansour, M. E. (2003). Trends in otitis media among children in the United States. *Pediatrics, 112* (3), 514-520.

Aventura, M. L., Roque, M. R., & Aaberg, T. M. (2006). *Retinoblastoma*. Retrieved Juve 6, 2006, from www.emedicine.com/oph/topic346.htm.

Bisno, A. L., Gerber, M. A., Gwaltney, J. M., et al. (2002). Practice guidelines for the diagnosis and management of group A streptococcal pharyngitis (IDSA Guidelines). *Clin Infect Dis, 35*(2), 113-125.

Carr, M. M. (2004). *Inner ear, sudden hearing loss*. Retrieved April 21, 2006, from www.emedicine.com/ent/topic227.htm.

Cook, K. A., & Walsh, M. (2005). *Otitis media*. Retrieved from eMedicine on April 19, 2006, at http://www.emedicine.com/emerg/topic351.htm.

Curtis, T., & Wheeler, D. T. (2005). *Nystagmus, congenital*. Retrieved April 21, 2006, from www.emedicine.com/oph/topic688.htm.

Dhooge, I. J. (2003). Risk factors for the development of otitis media. *Curr Allergy Asthma Rep, 3*, 321-325.

Elder, M. A., Mellon, M. H., & Spector, S. L. (2002). The link between rhinitis and asthma. *Patient care for the nurse practitioner, November special edition*, 1-15. Montvale, NJ: Thomson Medical Economics.

Givner, L. B. (2002). Periorbital versus orbital cellulitis. *Pediatr Infect Dis J, 21*, 1157-1158.

Howard, M. L. (2006). Middle ear, tympanic membrane, perforations. Retrieved from eMedicine on June 6, 2006, at http://www.emedicine.com/ent/topic206.htm.

Howell, R. M. (2005). *Corneal abrasion*. Retrieved June 6, from www.emedicine.com/EMERG/topic828.htm.

Jacobson, J., & Jacobson, C. (2004). Evaluation of hearing loss in infants and young children. *Pediatr Ann, 33*(12), 811-821.

Jones, W. S., & Kaleida, P. H. (2003). How helpful is pneumatic otoscopy in improving diagnostic accuracy? *Pediatrics, 112*(3), 510-513.

Kenna, M. A. (2004). Medical management of childhood hearing loss. *Pediatr Ann, 33*(12), 822-832.

McCormick, D. P., Chonmaitree, T., Pittman, C., et al. (2005). Nonsevere acute otitis media: A clinical trial comparing outcomes of watchful waiting versus immediate antibiotic therapy. *Pediatrics, 115*(6), 1455-1465.

Moeller, J. L., & Rifat, S. F. (2003). Identifying and treating uncomplicated corneal abrasions. *Physician Sports Med, 31*(8), 15-17.

Pelton, S. I. (2002). Acute otitis media in an era of increasing antimicrobial resistance and universal administration of pneumococcal conjugate vaccine. *Pediatr Infect Dis J, 21*(6), 599-604, 613-614.

Roland, P. S. (2006). *Cholesteatoma*. Retrieved June 6, 2006, from www.emedicine.com/ped/topic384.htm.

Roland, P. S. (2004). Inner ear, noise-induced hearing loss. Retrieved September 27, 2005, from www.emedicine.com/ent/topic723.htm.

Schroeder, A., & Darrow, D. H. (2004). Management of the draining ear in children. *Pediatr Ann, 33*(12), 843-853.

Silverman, M. A., & Bessman, E. (2005). *Conjunctivitis*. Retrieved from eMedicine on April 19, 2006, at http://www.emedicine.com/emerg/topic110.htm.

Woodall, B. S., & Meyers, A. D. (2005). *Nonallergic rhinitis*. Retrieved April 21, 2006, from www.emedicine.com/ent/topic402.htm.

Zagaria, M. A. E., & Buonanno, A. P. (2005). A patient-oriented approach to the management of allergic rhinitis. *Clin Rev, 15*(9), 58-70.

# Common Illness of the Pulmonary System

JO ELLEN LEE, MSN, RN, CPNP

1. Symptom and sign: cough, wheezing
   a. Focused assessment (see Chapter 6 for history and physical examination of the pulmonary system) (Schwartz, et al., 2005)
   b. Symptom assessment
      i. Characteristics
         (a) How long has the cough or wheeze been present?
         (b) Color change during a coughing or wheezing episode
         (c) Timing—day, night, intermittent, persistent, seasonal
         (d) Place—inside, outside, home, school
         (e) Triggers—allergens, infections, cold air, exercise, emotional factors, pets
         (f) Cough (Spiro, 2003)
            (1) Quality—harsh, dry, productive, paroxysmal
            (2) Expectorant—color, consistency, amount, hemoptysis
         (g) Medication used—type, dosage, effectiveness
         (h) Immunization status
      ii. Associated signs and symptoms—presence and duration of:
         (a) Rhinorrhea (color) and nasal congestion
         (b) Earache with or without drainage
         (c) Sore throat with or without difficulty swallowing and/or hoarseness
         (d) Shortness of breath
         (e) Chest tightness
         (f) Fever
         (g) Headache
         (h) Muscle aches with or without malaise
         (i) Vomiting and diarrhea
         (j) Abnormal stools
   c. Family and child history
      i. Asthma, reactive airway disease, allergies, atopy
      ii. Bronchopulmonary dysplasia (BPD)
      iii. Tuberculosis
      iv. Smoking habits
      v. Cystic fibrosis

      **vi.** Chronic pulmonary diseases
     **vii.** Environmental concerns
        (a) Passive smoke
        (b) Chemical inhalation
 **d.** Focused physical assessment
       **i.** Color and perfusion
      **ii.** Temperature, blood pressure
     **iii.** Growth status, pubertal status
     **iv.** Respiratory rate, pattern, effort
      **v.** Adventitious breath sounds
      **vi.** Quality of voice
     **vii.** Rash, including eczema
    **viii.** Allergic shiners, Dennie lines, nasal crease
      **ix.** Lymphadenopathy
       **x.** Evaluation of adventitious sounds—rales, wheeze, rhonchi, altered breath sounds, symmetry
      **xi.** Evidence of respiratory compromise and adequacy of airway and ventilation
     **xii.** Rhinorrhea—cloudy or clear
    **xiii.** Boggy nasal mucosa
    **xiv.** Liver and spleen may be pushed down by hyperinflated lungs
 **e.** See Table 28-1 for differential diagnoses, age-related frequency of diagnosis, pulmonary characteristics, and other signs and symptoms
 **f.** Upper respiratory infection (URI)
      **i.** Acute viral infection of upper respiratory tract
     **ii.** Signs and symptoms (see Table 28-1)
    **iii.** Etiology
        (a) Causative pathogens
          (1) More than 100 infectious pathogens, with rhinovirus the most common
          (2) Parainfluenza
          (3) Respiratory syncytial virus (RSV)
          (4) Coronaviruses
          (5) Adenoviruses
          (6) Enteroviruses
          (7) Influenza
          (8) *Mycoplasma pneumoniae*
          (9) Reovirus
        (b) Transmission: pathogen shed in large amounts through nasal secretions and easily spread through self-inoculation and to others from fingers and hands to objects
        (c) Universal susceptibility: children average five to eight infections per year, with a peak incidence during the first 2 years
        (d) Increased susceptibility associated with active and passive smoke exposure
        (e) More frequent in crowded situations
        (f) Seasonal—peaks in early fall, late January and early April
     **iv.** Diagnostic tests
        (a) Viral cultures expensive, generally unnecessary
        (b) If suspicious of non-viral etiology, consider:
          (1) Throat and nose culture
          (2) Drug screen (rhinorrhea, cough associated with drug withdrawal)

■ **TABLE 28-1**
■ ■ **Differential Diagnoses for Cough and Wheezing, Age-Related Frequency, and Characteristic Signs and Symptoms**

| Diagnosis | Most Typical Age-Group | Pulmonary Characteristics | Other Signs and Symptoms |
|---|---|---|---|
| Upper respiratory infection | All ages | **Cough,** nonproductive, worsens at night due to postnasal drip<br>Sore throat<br>Congestion | Acute onset<br>Pharyngitis<br>Rhinorrhea<br>Conjunctivitis<br>Fever |
| Pertussis | Infants | Catarrhal stage progresses to paroxysmal stage with severe **coughing** episodes and inspiratory "whoops" that may persist for weeks<br>Cyanosis | Catarrhal stage: mild URI symptoms with cough for about 2 weeks; low-grade fever<br>Vomiting when sucking or crying precipitates coughing episodes<br>Poor feeding<br>Conjunctival hemorrhages<br>Facial petechiae |
| Allergy | All ages | **Cough,** worsens at night | Itching<br>Conjunctivitis<br>Nasal congestion<br>Rhinorrhea |
| Asthma | All ages | Dry, nonproductive **cough** may be the only symptom<br>**Wheezing**<br>Tachypnea<br>Cyanosis | Activity worsens symptoms |
| Sinusitis | School-agers | Acute sinusitis:<br>**Cough** during day; may be worse at night<br>Chronic sinusitis:<br>**Cough** during day and night<br>Associated with intractable **wheezing** | Acute sinusitis:<br>Fever<br>Clear or mucopurulent rhinorrhea or postnasal drip<br>Facial pain, headache<br>Sore throat, halitosis<br>Chronic sinusitis:<br>Malaise, fatigue, anorexia<br>May have low grade fever<br>Sore throat<br>Swelling of middle turbinates<br>Nasal discharge varies day to day |
| Influenza | All ages | Dry **cough** with clear lungs or nonproductive, dry cough | Sudden onset of fever; lasts about 5 days<br>Chills<br>Malaise<br>Headache<br>Myalgia<br>Rhinorrhea<br>Pharyngitis<br>Conjunctivitis |
| Bronchiolitis | Infants up to age 2 | Nonproductive **cough**<br>**Wheezing**<br>Tachypnea | Rhinitis<br>Otitis<br>Conjunctivitis and/or |

■ **TABLE 28-1**
■ ■ **Differential Diagnoses for Cough and Wheezing, Age-Related Frequency, and Characteristic Signs and Symptoms—cont'd**

| Diagnosis | Most Typical Age-Group | Pulmonary Characteristics | Other Signs and Symptoms |
|---|---|---|---|
| | | Retractions<br>Nasal flaring<br>Prolonged expiratory phase<br>Variable cyanosis<br>Apnea<br>Crackles | Pharyngitis |
| Croup | Infants<br>Toddlers | Mild cases:<br>    Barking **cough**<br>    Hoarseness<br>    No dyspnea<br>    Hypoxia<br>More severe cases:<br>    Barking **cough**<br>    Inspiratory stridor<br>    Dyspnea<br>    Hypoxemia | Abrupt onset<br>Symptoms worsen at night<br>    and with anxiety<br>Rhinorrhea<br>Hoarse voice<br>Poor appetite<br>Low grade fever (usually)<br>Dehydration in mild and more<br>    severe cases |
| Pneumonia | All ages | **Cough**, productive, hemoptysis<br>Persistent cough if chlamydia<br>**Wheezing**<br>Tachypnea<br>Retractions<br>Grunting<br>Nasal flaring<br>Crackles<br>And/or diffuse or localized<br>    decrease in breath sounds | May also have concurrent URI<br>Purulent sputum if bacterial<br>    cause<br>Fever<br>Pleuritic pain |
| Bronchitis | All ages<br>Common <5 years of age | Brassy, nonproductive **cough** that<br>    worsens and becomes<br>    productive<br>**Wheezing**<br>Coarse, bronchial breath sounds<br>    in periphery of lungs<br>Dyspnea | Initial phase may include<br>    URI symptoms<br>Rhinorrhea or nasal<br>    congestion<br>Fever<br>Malaise<br>Sore throat<br>Chest pain<br>Myalgias or arthralgias |
| Foreign body aspiration | Toddlers, adolescents | If bronchial:<br>Nonproductive **cough**<br>Unilateral **wheezing**<br>Decreased breath sounds<br>If tracheal:<br>Partial or total obstruction of<br>    breathing | |
| Gastroesophageal reflux disease | Infants <1 year of age | Chronic cough | Regurgitation<br>Abdominal pain<br>Heartburn<br>Dysphagia<br>Hoarseness<br>Pharyngitis<br>Halitosis<br>Dental erosion<br>Otitis media |

*Continued*

■ **TABLE 28-1**
■ ■ **Differential Diagnoses for Cough and Wheezing, Age-Related Frequency, and Characteristic Signs and Symptoms—cont'd**

| Diagnosis | Most Typical Age-Group | Pulmonary Characteristics | Other Signs and Symptoms |
|---|---|---|---|
| Measles | School-agers, young adolescents | Hacking **cough** | Irritability<br>Coryza<br>High fever<br>Conjunctivitis<br>Photophobia<br>Koplik's spots in the mouth<br>Toxic appearance<br>Generalized morbilliform rash |
| Psychogenic cough | Adolescents | Chronic dry, hacking **cough**<br>Cough disappears when sleeping | Increases with stress |
| Tracheoeso-phageal fistula | Infants | Episodes of **coughing**<br>Rattling respiration<br>Choking<br>Cyanosis | Symptoms worsen during feeding |
| Tuberculosis | All ages | Productive **cough** | Daily fevers<br>Night sweats<br>Weight loss |
| Cystic fibrosis | All ages | All:<br>  Frequent respiratory infections<br>Infants <1 year:<br>  **Coughing**<br>  **Wheezing**<br>Childhood, adulthood:<br>  Chronic, productive **cough**<br><br>  **Wheeze**<br>  Dyspnea on exertion | All:<br>  Salty sweat<br>Neonatal:<br>  Meconium ileus<br>  Viscid meconium<br>Early infancy:<br>  Steatorrhea, foul smelling stools<br>  Failure to thrive<br>Childhood, adulthood:<br>  Steatorrhea, foul smelling stools<br>  Weight loss in spite of high calorie intake<br>  Excessive flatus<br>  Abdominal pain and/or distention<br>  Delayed puberty<br>  Infertility |

    **v.** Treatment—primarily supportive
        (a) Analgesics for sore throat, muscle aches, and fever greater than 101° F (38.3° C)
        (b) Relief of nasal congestion
            (1) Saline nose drops with gentle nasal aspiration
            (2) Cool-mist humidification
        (c) Maintain hydration; also helps to liquefy secretions
        (d) Antibiotics not recommended because cause is almost always viral, and because of cost, side effects, and antibacterial resistance (Spurling, et al., 2004)

(e) Antihistamines and decongestants are not recommended for infant or young child; may provide symptomatic relief for older children and adolescents

(f) If symptoms persist beyond 7 to 10 days, consider secondary infection

(g) Prevention
(1) Handwashing
(2) Good hygiene and cleaning of clothes, toys, and play areas
(3) Limited exposure to crowded situations

(h) Prognosis—usually self-limiting

g. Pertussis (Bocka, 2005)
i. Highly contagious bacterial infection characterized by paroxysmal coughing episodes ending in an inspiratory "whoop"
ii. Signs and symptoms (see Table 28-1)
iii. Etiology
(a) Caused by *Bordetella pertussis*
(b) Transmission: person-to-person contact via aerosolized droplets
(c) Incubation: 6 to 20 days, usually 7 to 10 days
(d) Most contagious during the catarrhal stage
(e) 35% of cases are younger than 6 months of age
(f) Highest mortality occurs in infants less than 6 months of age
iv. Diagnostic tests
(a) Chest x-ray—thickened bronchi and evidence of atelectasis and bronchopneumonia
(b) White blood cell (WBC) count with marked leukocytosis
(1) Usually in the paroxysmal period
(2) Persists for 3 to 4 weeks
(c) Nasopharyngeal culture of direct fluorescent antibody (DFA) stain—positive in initial stage of illness
v. Treatment
(a) Antibiotic therapy—erythromycin (or Septra if allergic); or other macrolides
(b) Prophylaxis of household and daycare contacts
(c) Isolate, and no return to school or daycare until 5 days of antibiotic treatment are complete, whether child is treated at hospital or at home
(d) Supportive therapy to include:
(1) Fluids and nutrition
(2) Oxygen supplementation
(3) Ventilatory support
(e) Household and other close contacts should receive prophylactic treatment of erythromycin regardless of immunization status
(f) Report all cases to state health department
(g) Immunization: if not up to date on DTaP, give a booster dose
vi. Follow-up
(a) The paroxysmal stage can last up to 4 weeks and the convalescent stage up to several months
(b) Complications
(1) Pneumonia
(2) Hypoxic encephalopathy
(3) Otitis media
(4) Tuberculosis activation

(5) Epistaxis, hemoptysis

(6) Hernia

(7) Reinduction of paroxysmal coughing with upper respiratory infections

(8) Seizures

(9) Cerebral hemorrhage

(10) Coma and death

(c) The complications of pertussis are more likely to occur in the younger infant and therefore tend to have a more serious, protracted course

h. Allergy (see Chapter 27)

i. Asthma (see Chapter 36)

j. Sinusitis (Goodhue & Brady, 2004; Ramadan, 2005)

  i. Pathophysiology

  (a) Part of the natural history of a cold or allergic rhinitis

  (b) Inflammation and edema of the mucous membranes lining the paranasal, maxillary, or ethmoid sinuses

  (c) Obstructs normal drainage

  (d) Bacterial overgrowth in sinuses

  (e) Maxillary and ethmoid sinuses most frequently involved

  ii. Signs and symptoms (see Table 28-1)

  iii. Types

  (a) Acute sinusitis: symptoms last more than 10 but less than 30 days

  (b) Chronic sinusitis: symptoms last more than 30 days

  iv. Etiology, prevalence

  (a) Common pathogens—similar to those found in otitis media

    (1) Acute infection

      a) *Streptococcus pneumoniae*

      b) *Haemophilus influenzae*

      c) *Moraxella catarrhalis*

    (2) Chronic—anaerobes due to low oxygen content and low pH of fluid

      a) Group A β-hemolytic streptococci

      b) *Staphylococcus aureus*

  (b) 5% to 10 % of URIs in children develop into sinusitis

  (c) May be secondary to:

    (1) Allergies

    (2) Adenoidal hypertrophy

    (3) Anatomic abnormalities

    (4) Dental abscess

    (5) Diving

    (6) Swimming

  (d) Higher incidence in boys

  v. Diagnostic tests

  (a) X-rays not useful except for maxillary sinusitis

  (b) CT scan necessary only for complicated sinusitis

  vi. Treatment

  (a) Uncomplicated acute sinusitis—antibiotic therapy for 14 days—amoxicillin or erythromycin

  (b) Should have noticeable improvement in 3 to 4 days

  (c) If unresponsive, chronic sinusitis, or in area of high prevalence of β-lactamase–producing *H. influenzae*, use amoxicillin-clavulanate, cefuroxime axetil, or a newer macrolide

(d) Decongestants, antihistamines
    (1) Not useful in acute sinusitis
    (2) May be useful in chronic sinusitis
(e) Treat pain with acetaminophen or ibuprofen
(f) Humidifier at night to decrease drying of mucosa
(g) Increase oral fluid intake

  **vii.** Prognosis
    (a) Refer to otolaryngologist if condition becomes recurrent or chronic
    (b) Complications may include orbital cellulitis, intracranial symptoms

**k.** Influenza (Fleming, et al., 2005)
  **i.** Highly contagious, viral illness
  **ii.** Signs and symptoms (see Table 28-1)
  **iii.** Etiology
    (a) Epidemic influenza caused by influenza types A and B
    (b) Seasonal: mid-October through mid-February
    (c) Transmission by direct person-to-person contact via airborne droplet or by articles contaminated with nasopharyngeal secretions
    (d) School-age children most likely to be infected during an outbreak
    (e) Incubation period 1 to 3 days
    (f) Infectious 24 hours before onset of symptoms and while symptoms are most severe

  **iv.** Diagnostic tests
    (a) Nasopharyngeal cultures obtained within first 72 hours of illness may reveal influenza
    (b) Diagnosis is usually based on clinical signs and available prevalence data

  **v.** Treatment
    (a) Supportive therapy
      (1) Bed rest
      (2) Fluids
      (3) Fever management with acetaminophen or ibuprofen
    (b) Amantadine, rimantadine, and zanamivir are antiviral prophylactic drugs that diminish the severity of influenza A, but are not effective for influenza B (U. S. Federal Food and Drug Administration, 2006)
      (1) Not approved for infants less than 12 months of age
      (2) Dosages 5 mg/kg/day (<40 kg); 200 mg/day (≥40 kg)
    (c) Immunization—people in high risk groups should be vaccinated yearly, as should household contacts

  **vi.** Follow-up
    (a) Influenza A infections last longer than influenza B and C
    (b) Observe for signs and symptoms of complications
      (1) Pneumonia
      (2) Otitis media
      (3) Sinusitis
      (4) Myositis
      (5) Reye's syndrome
      (6) Convulsions with fever
      (7) Secondary bacterial infection
      (8) Drug toxicity
    (c) Persistence of the fever does not necessarily mean a secondary bacterial infection has occurred
    (d) Cough may last up to 2 weeks
    (e) Lethargy and malaise may persist up to 2 weeks

l. Bronchiolitis (Fleming, et al., 2005; Steiner, 2004)
  i. An acute viral infection of the lower airways
  ii. Signs and symptoms (see Table 28-1)
  iii. Etiology
    (a) Primarily caused by RSV
    (b) Other causes
      (1) Parainfluenza
      (2) Adenovirus
      (3) Rhinovirus
      (4) Influenza
    (c) Seasonal—most commonly occurs in midwinter to early spring
    (d) Almost all children have had one episode of bronchiolitis before the age of 3 years
    (e) Hospitalization more common for infants less than 6 months of age and those with cardiorespiratory disease
  iv. Diagnostic tests
    (a) Based on history and clinical observations
    (b) Chest x-ray shows peribronchial thickening, air trapping, segmental atelectasis
    (c) Pulse oximetry shows decreases in oxygen saturation as disease process worsens
    (d) WBC may or may not be increased
    (e) Viral culture with rapid diagnostic technique may be positive for:
      (1) RSV
      (2) Influenza
  v. Treatment
    (a) Primarily supportive
      (1) Oxygen
      (2) Keep airways clear; suction nares
      (3) Fluid and nutritional support
      (4) Bronchodilators, depending on the response
      (5) Corticosteroids are commonly used, but a systematic review of the evidence showed that they are of no benefit for infants and children with acute viral bronchiolitis (Patel, et al., 2004)
    (b) Hospitalization is recommended for infants if (Steiner, 2004):
      (1) Age less than 3 months
      (2) Gestational age less than 34 weeks
      (3) Cardiopulmonary disease, immunodeficiencies
      (4) Respiratory rate >70 breaths per minute
      (5) Wheezing and respiratory distress associated with oxygen saturation < 92% on room air
      (6) Hypercarbia
      (7) Atelectasis or consolidation on chest radiography
      (8) Lethargic appearance
    (c) Ribavirin may be given if hospitalized with severe disease
    (d) Only infants at high risk for contracting RSV are eligible for *preventive* treatment with palivizumab (Synagis) (Steiner, 2004)
      (1) Less than 2 years of age with chronic lung disease treated within 6 months of RSV season
      (2) Infants born at 28 weeks gestation or earlier may benefit if palivizumab is given during their first RSV season whenever it occurs during first year of life

   (3) Infants born at 29 to 32 weeks gestation may benefit if palivizumab is given during their first RSV season whenever it occurs during first 6 months of life

   (4) Infants born at 32 to 35 weeks gestation may be treated if two of the following risk factors are present: day care; school-aged siblings, exposure to environmental pollution, abnormal airways, severe neuromuscular problems

 **vi.** Prognosis and expected course

  (a) Most infants improve within 3 to 5 days

  (b) Complications to watch for

   (1) Impending respiratory failure (may be sudden)

   (2) Sudden deterioration suggesting atelectasis due to mucous plugging

   (3) Fatigue may occur in infants who have prolonged and extensive disease

   (4) Worsening hypoxemia

   (5) Apnea

  (c) Those who need mechanical ventilation may have difficulties with extubation due to excessive secretions and atelectasis

  (d) Those with severe disease requiring hospitalization are predisposed for further lower respiratory tract problems

**m.** Croup

 **i.** Acute upper airway obstruction typically caused by a viral infection of the larynx

 **ii.** Signs and symptoms (see Table 28-1)

 **iii.** Etiology

  (a) Parainfluenza type 1 most common organism

  (b) Less common

   (1) Parainfluenza types 2 and 3

   (2) RSV

   (3) Adenovirus

   (4) Influenza A and B

   (5) Measles

  (c) Rare: *M. pneumoniae, S. aureus, H. influenzae*

 **iv.** Diagnostic tests

  (a) WBC count may be normal or elevated

  (b) Pulse oximetry shows hypoxia with severe disease

  (c) Radiographic image of airway shows classic narrowing of the trachea to a sharp point—"steeple sign"

  (d) Viral cultures or rapid test of nasopharyngeal secretions

 **v.** Treatment

  (a) Mild case—outpatient care

   (1) Adequate oral hydration

   (2) Antipyretics

   (3) Humidity

   (4) Family education regarding worsening respiratory distress

  (b) Moderate to severe disease—hospitalize for supportive care:

   (1) Oxygen supplementation; 1% to 5% require intubation

   (2) Intravenous fluids

  (c) Medication

   (1) Nebulized racemic epinephrine or budesonide

        a) A rebound phenomenon with worsening of stridor and respiratory distress after initial relief may occur up to 2 hours post-treatment in some patients

        b) Several studies have shown that children can be safely discharged home 3 to 4 hours after racemic epinephrine treatment

    (2) Corticosteroids—a systematic review of research evidence shows that dexamethasone and budesonide are effective in relieving symptoms of mild and moderate croup as early as 6 hours, decrease number of return office visits or hospitalization, decrease length of time spent in hospital (Russell, et al., 2003)

    (3) Antibiotics are not indicated unless a bacterial infection is present

  (d) Handwashing and avoid touching face to prevent spread

  **vi.** Prognosis and expected course

    (a) In most cases the illness is self-limited, lasting 3 to 5 days

    (b) Recurrence rate highest if hospitalized, and if intubated

    (c) Recurrent croup suggests an underlying anatomic problem

**n.** Pneumonia

  **i.** Signs and symptoms (see Table 28-1)

  **ii.** Aspiration pneumonia

    (a) Common causative agents

      (1) Food

      (2) Saliva

      (3) Gastric contents

      (4) Other substances into the air passages

    (b) Associated circumstances or settings

      (1) Most frequently in children with upper airway abnormalities or neurologic deficits

      (2) Severe gastroesophageal reflux (GER)

      (3) Other esophageal problems

      (4) May also occur subsequent to the inhalation of smoke or hydrocarbons

      (5) Near-drowning episodes

      (6) Alcohol ingestion by adolescents

    (c) Incidence

      (1) 4% preschool children

      (2) 1% to 2 % of school-age years

  **iii.** Infectious pneumonia—infection usually involves small airways in children but may also infect the larger airways and/or the alveoli

    (a) Etiology

      (1) Common viral agents

        a) RSV

        b) Parainfluenza types 1, 2, and 3

        c) Influenza A and B

        d) Adenovirus types 1, 2, 5, and 6

      (2) Bacterial agents

        a) Newborns

          i) Group B streptococci

          ii) Gram-negative enteric bacilli

          iii) Chlamydia trachomatis

          iv) Ureaplasma

          v) Rarely syphilis

      b) Infants and young children ≤6 years of age:
         i) *S. pneumoniae* (primary cause)
         ii) *H. influenzae* (incidence of type B disease has dramatically decreased since introduction of vaccine)
     c) Preschool through young adulthood
         i) Mycoplasma
         ii) Chlamydia
     d) Older children and adolescents
         i) *S. pneumoniae* most likely
         ii) More rarely *S. aureus*
         iii) Anaerobes
     e) Immunocompromised or malnourished children—opportunistic organisms should be considered, such as:
         i) *Pneumocystis jiroveci*
         ii) Yeast
         iii) Dimorphic soil fungi

(b) Diagnostic tests

    (1) Chest x-ray shows that atelectasis, opacification, and intrathoracic structures will shift toward the atelectic area
      a) Aspiration
         i) Pneumonia develops in portion of lung that is dependent at time of aspiration
         ii) Otherwise will show diffuse or localized mottled infiltrates with or without atelectasis
      b) Viral
         i) Begins with scattered perihilar and peribronchial infiltrations
         ii) In later stages, more localized infiltrations
      c) Bacterial
         i) Characterized by patchy infiltrates in infants
         ii) Lobar consolidation with *S. pneumoniae* or *H. influenzae*
         iii) Hilar adenopathy with *H. influenzae* or staph
         iv) Pleural effusion may be present
    (2) WBC count may or may not be elevated, with increased neutrophils and lymphocytes
    (3) Viral cultures of nasopharyngeal secretions
      a) Rapid identification with immunofluorescence
      b) Enzyme immunoassay less sensitive for RSV or influenza
    (4) Blood cultures
      a) If bacterial pneumonia is suspected
      b) Positive in only 10% to 15% of cases
    (5) Sputum culture
      a) Warranted if cough is productive
      b) Rarely beneficial in younger children
      c) Perform a Gram stain and culture
      d) Acid-fast bacillus (AFB) for tuberculosis
    (6) Positive cold agglutinin screen or titer
      a) Greater than 1:32 suggestive of *M. pneumoniae*
    (7) Pulse oximetry shows decreased oxygen saturation with severe disease

(c) Treatment

    (1) Refer to pulmonologist if child is immunocompromised or appears toxic

        (2) Antimicrobial treatment based on etiology
- a) Penicillin (*S. pneumoniae*)
- b) Macrolides or azalides (*M.* or *Chlamydia pneumoniae*)
- c) Amoxicillin or cephalosporin (*H. influenzae*)
- d) IV antibiotics if staph, or very severe case

        (3) Currently no antiviral medication for treatment of pneumonia

        (4) Bronchodilators and chest physiotherapy may improve airway clearance

        (5) Other supportive therapy may include additional fluids, oxygen

(d) Prognosis

        (1) Most children resolve pneumonia without any complications

        (2) X-rays may be abnormal for up to 6 weeks (serial x-rays not recommended)

        (3) Complicated pneumonias may be associated with restrictive or obstructive lung diseases

        (4) Pulmonary function tests should be done on a case-by-case basis

        (5) Pneumococcal vaccine should be given to immunocompromised patients and those with chronic illness, especially sickle cell disease

        (6) Children with sickle cell disease should take prophylactic penicillin for protection against encapsulated organisms, including pneumococcus

**o.** Bronchitis
- **i.** Acute—transient inflammation of the larger lower airways
- **ii.** Chronic—persists for more than 2 weeks; rarely an isolated entity in children, but rather a symptom of some other condition
- **iii.** Signs and symptoms (see Table 28-1)
- **iv.** Etiology
  - (a) Most commonly viral
    - (1) Adenovirus
    - (2) Influenza A and B
    - (3) Parainfluenza type 3
    - (4) RSV
    - (5) Rhinovirus
  - (b) Bacterial agents
    - (1) *M. pneumoniae*
    - (2) *B. pertussis*
    - (3) *C. pneumoniae*
    - (4) *Corynebacterium diphtheriae*
  - (c) Acute bronchitis occurs most frequently in the winter and early spring
  - (d) Rates are higher among males
- **v.** Diagnostic tests
  - (a) Diagnosis primarily based on history and physical
  - (b) Chest x-ray may be normal or show some peribronchial thickening
  - (c) Pulmonary function tests (PFTs) may be normal or may indicate an obstructive pattern; PFT may or may not improve after bronchodilators
- **vi.** Treatment
  - (a) Avoidance of respiratory irritants
  - (b) Increase fluid intake
    - (1) Expectorants usually not helpful
    - (2) Antihistamines should not be used because they dry secretions

        (c) Bronchodilators—a systematic review of research evidence showed that $\beta_2$-agonists are not useful for children with bronchitis unless there is evidence of airflow obstruction (Smucny, et al., 2004)

        (d) Inhaled steroids may be indicated for chronic bronchitis

        (e) Antibiotics are not usually helpful for viral illnesses

        (f) Antibiotics (with efficacy against *Mycoplasma* and *Chlamydia* spp.) are useful if bacterial etiology is suspected

        (g) Increased humidity (vaporizer)

    **vii.** Prognosis

        (a) Most patients recover uneventfully without any treatment

        (b) Small infants may require frequent position changes to facilitate pulmonary drainage

        (c) Children with repeated cases of bronchitis should be evaluated for respiratory tract anomalies and other conditions of the upper and lower respiratory tracts and trachea

**p.** Foreign body aspiration (FBA)

    **i.** Inhalation of a foreign body that lodges in the upper trachea or lower airways, resulting in total or partial airway obstruction, local injury, and inflammation

    **ii.** Signs and symptoms (see Table 28-1)

    **iii.** Etiology and prevalence

        (a) Food or object with pliable, slick, or cylindrical surface

            (1) Latex balloons are most common

            (2) Peanuts

            (3) Other nuts

            (4) Hot dogs

            (5) Candy

            (6) Grapes

        (b) 80% of cases are less than 3 years of age

        (c) 66% of cases are male

    **iv.** Diagnostic tests

        (a) Pulse oximetry shows decreased oxygen saturation with significant obstruction

        (b) Chest x-ray

            (1) Only 10% of aspirated objects are radiopaque

            (2) Unilateral changes in aeration from obstruction

        (c) Expiratory chest, decubitus, or fluoroscopy (imaging throughout the complete respiratory cycle)

            (1) Obstructive emphysema (failure to deflate)

            (2) Atelectasis is typical

    **v.** Treatment

        (a) Institute cardiopulmonary resuscitation if needed

        (b) Immediate transport to hospital for evaluation and removal

        (c) Or refer for rigid bronchoscopy, evaluation, and removal if there is convincing history of foreign body aspiration, regardless of radiographic findings

        (d) After removal, the following may be useful:

            (1) Antiinflammatory medication

            (2) Humidification

            (3) Bronchodilators

            (4) Antibiotics if evidence of pneumonia or bronchitis

(e) Be aware of complications that can occur secondary to FBA
  (1) Pneumonia
  (2) Atelectasis
vi. Follow-up
  (a) Chest x-ray in 6 to 8 weeks
    (1) Evaluate resolution of previous findings
    (2) Sooner if child is not improving
vii. Prevention
  (a) Remove small items from environment of small child
  (b) Child must sit while eating
  (c) Adult supervision while child is eating
  (d) Cut food in small pieces for young children
  (e) Avoid commonly aspirated foods and objects (no latex balloons, etc.) in children less than 3 years of age
q. GER disease (see Chapter 30)
r. Measles (rubeola)
  i. An acute, highly contagious viral disease
  ii. Signs and symptoms (see Table 28-1)
  iii. Etiology, incidence
    (a) Caused by *Morbillivirus*
    (b) Transmission: direct contact with infected secretions or via airborne droplets
    (c) Infected individuals are contagious 3 to 5 days before appearance of rash, to 4 days after appearance of rash
    (d) Increased incidence during winter and spring
  iv. Diagnostic tests
    (a) Presence of measles-specific IgM antibody suggests recent infection
    (b) Usually diagnosed by presence of symptoms and characteristic rash
  v. Treatment
    (a) Refer to pediatrician
    (b) No specific antiviral therapy available
    (c) Management of uncomplicated measles is primarily supportive
      (1) Bed rest
      (2) Adequate hydration
      (3) Acetaminophen or ibuprofen for fever and body aches
      (4) Antitussive therapy
    (d) Reportable to state health department
  vi. Prognosis and follow-up
    (a) In uncomplicated measles, the patient begins feeling better with a fading of rash on the third and fourth days
    (b) Otitis media is most common complication
    (c) Educate caretakers regarding complications
      (1) Otitis media
      (2) Encephalitis
      (3) Pneumonia
    (d) Prevention—measles immunization
s. Psychogenic cough (Holmes & Fadden, 2004)
  i. Symptoms
    (a) Honking or barking cough
    (b) Most patients with this condition do not cough during sleep, are not awakened by cough, and generally do not cough during enjoyable distractions

  **ii.** Prevalence

   (a) Psychogenic cough occurs less frequently in adults than in children

   (b) Lower rates of resolution in adults

 **iii.** Diagnosis—important to rule out organic causes before assuming it is psychogenic

 **iv.** Treatment

   (a) Evaluate sources of stress and effectiveness of coping strategies

   (b) Behavior modification

**t.** Tracheosophageal fistula (TEF)

 **i.** Failure of complete separation of the primitive foregut into trachea and esophagus at 4 to 8 weeks gestation, resulting in an opening between the trachea and esophagus

 **ii.** Signs and symptoms (see Table 28-1)

 **iii.** Etiology and incidence

   (a) Major types include:

    (1) Esophageal atresia (EA) and distal TEF (87%)

    (2) Pure EA without TEF (8%)

    (3) EA with proximal TEF with or without distal TEF (2%)

   (b) Incidence 1:3000 to 1:4000

   (c) Slight male predominance

   (d) No inheritance pattern established, but the most likely gene belongs to the *HOX D* group

   (e) 50% associated with other anomalies, mostly cardiac and gastrointestinal

   (f) 10% have VATER or VACTERYL syndrome, which involves anomalies of the vertebrae, anus, cardiac system, trachea and esophagus, renal system, and limbs

   (g) Also associated with:

    (1) Trisomy 13, 18, and 21

    (2) CHARGE syndrome (coloboma of eye, heart defects, atresia of the choanae, retardation of growth and development, ear abnormalities and deafness)

    (3) Schisis syndrome

    (4) Potter syndrome

 **iv.** Diagnostic tests

   (a) Plain chest x-rays are all that are usually needed to make a diagnosis

    (1) May show tracheal compression and deviation

    (2) Absence of a gastric bubble

    (3) Aspiration pneumonia in the posterior segments of the upper lobes

   (b) Do not order contrast studies—they carry the risk of aspiration pneumonitis and pulmonary injury

 **v.** Treatment—immediate referral to pediatric surgery

 **vi.** Prognosis

   (a) Some cases need staged surgery

   (b) Mortality and morbidity greater with prematurity, severe lung disease, and presence of life-threatening and major associated anomalies

   (c) More predisposed to croup and stridor—treat aggressively

   (d) Long-term morbidity

    (1) Chronic cough (may be barky or croupy)

    (2) Chronic intermittent stridor secondary to tracheomalacia

    (3) Dysphagia and reflux in almost 50% as adults

    (4) Increased airway resistance and rapid gastric emptying in those with gastric transposition

   **u.** Tuberculosis (TB)

      **i.** A chronic, granulomatous infection that may cause pulmonary, extrapulmonary, or disseminated disease

         (a) Primary infection—positive TB skin test without clinical, radiographic, or laboratory evidence of disease

         (b) Tuberculosis disease

            (1) Pulmonary—hilar adenopathy with or without parenchymal lesion

            (2) Extrapulmonary (miliary TB) may involve any organ of the body

      **ii.** Signs and symptoms (see Table 28-1)

      **iii.** Etiology and prevalence

         (a) Caused by *Mycobacterium tuberculosis*

         (b) Transmission: inhalation of aerosol droplets through person to person contact

         (c) All pediatric TB cases are acquired through contact with an infected adult

         (d) TB rates for all ages in the United States are highest in urban, low-income areas

         (e) Increased TB risk associated with

            (1) Minority ethnic groups in the United States and immigrants from high risk countries

            (2) Homeless and prison populations

            (3) Infants and adolescents

            (4) Human immunodeficiency virus (HIV) or immunosuppression

            (5) IV drug use

            (6) Many chronic illnesses

      **iv.** Diagnostic tests

         (a) Tuberculin skin test by Mantoux

         (b) Testing recommended annually for at-risk groups, or exposure to at-risk groups

         (c) Depending on risk factors, positive tests of 5 mm, 10 mm, and 15 mm are indicators of infection

         (d) Chest x-ray may show lobar or segmental parenchymal lesion, lymphadenopathy, pleural effusion, or miliary disease (snowflake appearance)

         (e) Positive acid-fast bacillus culture of sputum or early morning gastric aspirate

      **v.** Treatment

         (a) Referral to an infectious disease specialist for treatment plan

         (b) All cases reported to health department

         (c) For asymptomatic infection, 6 months treatment with isoniazid (INH) or rifampin for INH-resistant TB

      **vi.** Prognosis and follow-up

         (a) When the regimen is followed, a complete cure is achieved in 97% to 98% of patients

         (b) Yearly screening chest x-ray

         (c) Bacille Calmette-Guérin (BCG) vaccine is a live vaccine from attenuated strains of *Mycobacterium bovis* recommended only for:

            (1) Infants and children who are purified protein derivative (PPD) negative, but are continually and intimately exposed to contagious adults or to adults with INH and rifampin-resistant TB

            (2) Those who cannot take long-term preventive medication

  **v.** Cystic fibrosis (see Chapter 43)

2. Sign: dyspnea
   a. Focused assessment—see Chapter 6 for details on pulmonary assessment (Schwartz, et al., 2005)
   b. Differential diagnoses for dyspnea
      i. Asthma (see Chapter 36)
      ii. Bronchiolitis (see section 1.l. above)
      iii. Croup (see section 1.m. above)
      iv. Pneumonia (see section 1.n. above)
      v. Bronchitis (see section 1.o. above)
      vi. Foreign body aspiration (see section 1.p. above)
      vii. Cystic fibrosis (Chapter 43)
      viii. Diaphragmatic hernia
      ix. Congestive heart failure
      x. Pneumothorax
      xi. Pleural effusion
   c. Diaphragmatic hernia (Steinhorn, 2004)
      i. Herniation of the abdominal contents into the thoracic cavity through an opening in the diaphragm
      ii. Pathophysiology
         (a) Diaphragm forms between 7 and 10 weeks of gestation
         (b) Diaphragm is composed of pleuroperitoneal folds and the septum transversum
         (c) Bochdalek hernia develops when midgut returns to the abdominal cavity prematurely or diaphragmatic development is delayed
            (1) Bowel is trapped in the thoracic cavity, preventing the pleuroperitoneal folds from connecting with the thoracic wall
            (2) Allows a communication between the thoracic and abdominal cavities
            (3) Results in bowel in the thoracic cavity (usually on left side) and bilateral lung hypoplasia
         (d) Morgagni hernia is result of a defect in the septum transversum
            (1) Liver, bowel, and omentum in the thoracic cavity (usually on right side)
            (2) Less lung hypoplasia seen than with Bochdalek hernias
      iii. Signs and symptoms
         (a) Cyanosis and respiratory distress usually in first minute of life
         (b) Scaphoid abdomen
      iv. Etiology and incidence
         (a) Bochdalek hernias
            (1) Most common—90% of all cases of congenital diaphragmatic hernia
            (2) Incidence 1 per 2000 to 4000 live births
            (3) 80% to 90% of cases on the left side
            (4) Slightly more common in males
            (5) 40% of cases are associated with congenital malformation
            (6) 5% to 16% associated with chromosomal abnormality
            (7) 18% associated with a congenital heart disease
         (b) Morgagni hernias
            (1) Accounts for 2% of all diaphragmatic hernias
            (2) More common in females
         (c) Estimated 2% recurrence rate in first-degree relatives

      **v.** Diagnostic tests

        (a) Chest x-ray reveals a mass (bowel) in thoracic cavity

        (b) Arterial blood gas

          (1) $Po_2$ shows evidence of severe hypoxia

          (2) $Pco_2$ elevated

          (3) pH reveals significant acidosis (both respiratory and metabolic)

    **vi.** Treatment—refer immediately to pediatric surgery

   **vii.** Prognosis

        (a) Improvement depends on the extent of pulmonary hypoplasia and pulmonary hypertension

        (b) Bochdalek hernias—33% to 65% survival

        (c) Morgagni hernias—excellent prognosis

**d.** Congestive heart failure (CHF)

    **i.** Clinical syndrome that reflects the inability of the heart to meet metabolic requirements of the body

    **ii.** Etiology

        (a) Congenital heart defects with volume or pressure overload (most common)

        (b) Acquired heart disease (less common cause)

        (c) Others

          (1) Tachyarrhythmias, complete heart block in infancy

          (2) Severe anemia, hydrops fetalis

          (3) Acute hypertension

          (4) Bronchopulmonary dysplasia

          (5) Acute cor pulmonale

          (6) Arteriovenous malformations

   **iii.** Diagnostic tests

        (a) Chest x-ray

          (1) Cardiomegaly almost always present

          (2) Pulmonary vascular congestion dependent on etiology

        (b) Echocardiogram

          (1) Assess ventricular function

          (2) Chamber enlargement

          (3) Anatomy

        (c) Electrocardiogram

          (1) Not diagnostic

          (2) May help assess etiology

    **iv.** Treatment—refer to cardiologist or pulmonologist for further diagnostics and treatment

**e.** Pneumothorax (Chang & Barton, 2005)

    **i.** Pathophysiology

        (a) Air enters the pleural space via ruptured alveoli or via the chest wall from trauma

        (b) Usually collapse of the lung on the affected side seals the leak

        (c) If a "ball-valve" mechanism ensues, however, air can accumulate in the thoracic cavity, causing a tension pneumothorax

    **ii.** Etiology

        (a) Spontaneous

          (1) Secondary to rupture of apical blebs, i.e., accumulation of air between layers of visceral pleura that are not confined by connective tissue

          (2) Occurs with cystic fibrosis

      (b) Mechanical trauma
         (1) Penetrating injury
         (2) Blunt trauma
      (c) Barotrauma (mechanical ventilation)
      (d) Iatrogenic
         (1) Central venous catheter placement
         (2) Bronchoscopy with biopsy
      (e) Infection
         (1) *S. aureus*
         (2) *S. pneumoniae*
         (3) *M. tuberculosis*
         (4) *B. pertussis*
         (5) *P. jiroveci*
      (f) Airway occlusion
         (1) Mucous plugging
         (2) Foreign body
         (3) Meconium aspiration
      (g) Malignancy
   iii. Incidence
      (a) Spontaneous pneumothorax occurs in 5 to 10/100,000; male greater than female 6:1
      (b) Peak incidence at 16 to 24 years of age
      (c) Cystic fibrosis—occurs in 20% of patients older than 18 years of age
   iv. Diagnostic tests
      (a) Chest x-ray
         (1) Radiolucency of the affected lung
         (2) Lack of lung markings in the periphery of the affected lung
         (3) Collapsed lung on the affected side
         (4) Possible pneumomediastinum with subcutaneous emphysema
      (b) Arterial blood gases
         (1) $Po_2$ is frequently decreased
         (2) $Pco_2$ elevated with respiratory compromise, decreased from hyperventilation
      (c) Pulse oximetry shows low oxygenation
      (d) Electrocardiogram (ECG)
         (1) Diminished amplitude of the QRS voltage
         (2) Rightward shift of the QRS axis (if left sided)
         (3) Chest CT
   v. Treatment
      (a) Stabilize the patient and refer immediately to emergency department or pulmonologist
      (b) Oxygen
         (1) Until saturations are higher than 95%
         (2) Breathing 100% oxygen can speed reabsorption of intrapleural air into the bloodstream
   vi. Prognosis
      (a) If simple, spontaneous pneumothorax, recovery is excellent
      (b) Other causes; prognosis is related to the underlying cause
f. Pleural effusion
   i. Pathophysiology
      (a) There is normally 1 to 15 mL of fluid in the pleural space

    (b) Alteration in the flow and/or absorption of this fluid leads to fluid accumulation in the pleural cavity

    (c) Two types

       (1) Transudate—mechanical forces of hydrostatic and oncotic pressures are altered, favoring liquid filtration

       (2) Exudate—damage to the pleural surface occurs that alters its ability to filter pleural fluid; lymphatic drainage is diminished

          a) Exudative stage—simple parapneumonic effusion; pleural fluid glucose and pH normal

          b) Fibropurulent stage—increase in fibrin, polymorphonuclear neutrophils (PMNs; leukocytes), bacterial invasion of pleural cavity; fluid glucose and pH falls, lactate dehydrogenase (LDH) increases

          c) Organizing stage—fibroblasts grow; pleural peal

  **ii.** Etiology and prevalence

    (a) Most common cause is pneumonia, followed by:

       (1) Congenital heart disease

       (2) Malignancy

    (b) For empyema, most common organisms include:

       (1) *S. aureus* (28%)

       (2) *S. pneumoniae* (20%)

       (3) *H. influenzae* (13%)

  **iii.** Diagnostic tests

    (a) Imaging—chest radiograph, ultrasound, CT scan

    (b) Refer to pulmonology for thoracentesis, pleural biopsy and pleural fluid analysis

  **iv.** Treatment

    (a) Refer to pulmonology for hospitalization and treatment

    (b) Diet—if the diagnosis is chylothorax (leakage of lymphatic fluid from the thoracic duct into the pleural space), the diet needs to be supplemented for 4 to 5 weeks with medium chain triglycerides

  **v.** Prognosis

    (a) Expect improvement usually within 1 to 2 weeks

    (b) May have fever spikes up to 2 to 3 weeks

    (c) Properly treated infectious etiology; excellent prognosis

    (d) Others—depend on underlying disease process

**3.** Sign: apnea

  **a.** Pathophysiology

    **i.** Breathing disorder characterized by cessation of airflow lasting more than 20 seconds

      (a) Central apnea

        (1) Lack of airflow secondary to cessation of breathing

        (2) Absence of drive to breathe from the CNS

      (b) Obstructive apnea

        (1) Lack of airflow secondary to airway obstruction

        (2) Paradoxical chest-wall motion frequently seen

        (3) Respiratory drive present

    **ii.** Mixed apnea—central and obstructive events occurring together

  **b.** Focused assessment—see Chapter 6 for details on pulmonary assessment (Schwartz, et al., 2005)

    **i.** Child's history

        (a) Age of infant or child
        (b) Gestational age
        (c) Evidence of infection
            (1) Fever
            (2) URI
            (3) GI symptoms
        (d) Prior history of GER or seizures
        (e) Presence of snoring
        (f) Headaches or daytime sleepiness
        (g) Change in school performance
    ii. Symptom assessment
        (a) Length of apnea—estimated or timed?
        (b) Movement of the chest with or without airflow
        (c) Paradoxical movement of the chest
        (d) Color change
        (e) Awake or asleep when the event occurred
        (f) Change in the patient's muscle tone (floppy vs. stiff)
        (g) Episode related to:
            (1) Feeding
            (2) Choking
            (3) Gagging
            (4) Coughing
            (5) Vomiting
            (6) Crying
        (h) Change in the patient's mental status during or after the event
        (i) Urinary or stool incontinence during the event
    iii. Focused physical assessment
        (a) See Chapter 6 for pulmonary assessment
        (b) Craniofacial abnormalities
            (1) Micrognathia
            (2) Macroglossia
        (c) Choanal atresia or stenosis
        (d) Evidence of nasal or pharyngeal obstruction
            (1) Congestion
            (2) Rhinorrhea
            (3) Foreign body
            (4) Enlarged tonsils and adenoid tissue in toddlers and older children

**c.** Diagnostic tests
    i. Arterial blood gases reveal the significance of the event
    ii. CBC with differential to identify anemia, polycythemia, infection
    iii. Electrolytes—bicarbonate, glucose
    iv. Oxygen saturation
    v. End-tidal $CO_2$ tension
    vi. pH probe (if GER suspected)
    vii. X-rays of chest, lateral neck reveal infection, aspiration, obstruction, tonsillar and adenoid hypertrophy, patency of nasopharyngeal airway
    viii. Refer to pulmonologist for polysomnography, imaging

**d.** Treatment
    i. Refer to appropriate specialist depending on the suspected underlying cause
    ii. Home apnea monitors

(a) Monitoring technology now allows for the storing of information on a microchip, which can be downloaded for the provider to review
(b) Use is controversial
(c) Indications
    (1) Any infant perceived to be at high risk for sudden infant death syndrome (SIDS) or severe apparent life-threatening event (ALTE)
    (2) One or more siblings who died of SIDS
    (3) Symptomatic premature infants
    (4) Central hypoventilation syndrome
    (5) Infants and young children who have tracheotomies
(d) When to discontinue—controversial
    (1) Dependent on the underlying cause of apnea
    (2) Possible conflicts with other treatments
e. Etiology—see following and Box 28-1

■ **BOX 28-1**
■ **ETIOLOGY OF APNEA**

Prematurity
Breath-holding spells
Gastroesophageal reflux
Foreign body aspiration
Laryngomalacia
Tracheomalacia
Apparent life-threatening event
Sudden infant death syndrome
Infection
　Meningitis
　Viral meningoencephalitis
　Respiratory syncytial virus (RSV)
　Pertussis
CNS
　Malformations
　Seizure
　Cerebral or intraventricular hemorrhage
　Masses
　Congenital central hypoventilation
　Werdnig-Hoffman
　Familial dysautonomia
　Laryngeal chemoreflex
Asphyxia—accidental, abuse
Pharmacologic
　Accidental drug ingestion
　Ethanol
　Sedatives
　Narcotics
　Toxins
Metabolic
　Hypoglycemia
　Hypoxia
　Hypocarbia
　Overheating
Anemia
Genetic and familial disorders

**f.** Apnea of prematurity
  **i.** Pathophysiology—due to immaturity of CNS and pulmonary systems
    (a) Central apnea in which the lack of airflow is secondary to cessation of breathing
    (b) Or may be due to the absence of drive to breathe from the CNS
  **ii.** Prevalence—more than 50% of premature infants will develop apnea
  **iii.** Treatment
    (a) Stimulants—caffeine, theophylline
    (b) Supplemental oxygen is helpful for both obstructive and central apnea, especially if oxygen desaturation occurs
    (c) Apnea monitor
  **iv.** Prognosis
    (a) Some infants may exhibit apnea of more than 20 seconds without apparent adverse effects
    (b) Most infants outgrow apnea of prematurity and immaturity at term or within 1 or 2 months of age
**g.** Breath-holding spells (BHS)
  **i.** Pathophysiology
    (a) Simple BHS are involuntary (reflexive) events in which the child becomes apneic and often bradycardic at end of expiration
    (b) BHS are classified as severe when they are prolonged and associated with loss of consciousness, seizure activity
    (c) Often divided into cyanotic spells or pallid spells, based on child's appearance during the episodes
      (1) Cyanotic spells thought to be related to an autonomic dysregulation leading to prolonged expiratory apnea
      (2) Pallid spells thought to be related to an overactive vagal response resulting in bradycardia or asystole
    (d) Anemia has been reported to worsen the severity and frequency of BHS
  **ii.** Etiology and prevalence
    (a) Usually initiated by anger, frustration, fear, or minor injury
    (b) Lifetime prevalence of up to 25% during childhood
    (c) Severe BHS occur in less than 1% of the population
    (d) Onset is typically between 6 months and 2 years of age; rare after age 6 years
    (e) Cyanotic spells more common than pallid spells
  **iii.** Diagnostic tests
    (a) CBC (anemia and iron deficiency)
    (b) EEG (seizures)
    (c) ECG (cardiac pathology–long-QT syndrome)
  **iv.** Treatment
    (a) Lower child to the floor to prevent falling
    (b) Clear the mouth of food or foreign bodies during episode to prevent aspiration
    (c) Evaluate need for CPR if loss of consciousness is longer than 1 minute
    (d) Reassure parents
      (1) These spells will not harm the child
      (2) Normal breathing resumes after loss of consciousness
    (e) Referral to a mental health professional if parents unable to discipline child for fear of inducing BHS

      (f) Medications
        (1) Iron for treatment of anemia
        (2) Atropine for use in severe pallid BHS
    **v.** Prognosis
      (a) No clear evidence of long-term sequelae
      (b) Some reports of neurodevelopmental abnormalities and rarely death in children with severe BHS do exist, but the association of these outcomes with the BHS is very controversial

**h.** GER—see Chapter 30

**i.** Foreign body aspiration—see section 1.p on p. 427

**j.** Laryngomalacia and tracheomalacia
    **i.** Pathophysiology and etiology
      (a) Laryngomalacia
        (1) Variable extrathoracic airway obstruction that may lead to apnea
        (2) Long flaccid omega-shaped epiglottis that prolapses posteriorly and curves to the lumen on inspiration
        (3) Most common congenital anomaly of the larynx
        (4) Most common noninfectious cause of stridor in infants
      (b) Tracheomalacia
        (1) Variable intrathoracic airway obstruction
        (2) During exhalation, the tracheal wall experiences a positive pressure that results in an external dynamic compression of the lumen
        (3) Result of prolonged artificial ventilation, especially in a premature infant
    **ii.** Diagnostic tests
      (a) Chest x-ray
        (1) Usually normal in both laryngomalacia and tracheomalacia
        (2) Useful to rule out other abnormalities that can create external airway compression
      (b) Refer to pulmonologist for other diagnostic tests, e.g., laryngoscopy, bronchoscopy, airway fluoroscopy, barium swallow, MRI
    **iii.** Treatment
      (a) Observation and reassurance are frequently the only intervention indicated in the majority of cases
      (b) Patients who require tracheotomy might benefit from continuous positive airway pressure (CPAP)
      (c) Humidification of secretions may help some patients
    **iv.** Prognosis and follow-up
      (a) Usually excellent in cases of isolated laryngomalacia and/or tracheo-malacia
      (b) Patients with tracheoesophageal fistula often persist with tracheal dysfunction beyond corrective surgery (Sharma & Duerkson, 2006)
      (c) Assist with solving feeding difficulties and monitor weight gain

**k.** ALTE
    **i.** Apneic events that to the child's caretaker appear life-threatening
    **ii.** *Incorrectly* referred to as "near-miss" SIDS or "aborted SIDS" events
    **iii.** In a study of 14 children who experienced an ALTE and 12 controls, the long-term outcome by midpuberty showed neurologic deficits in the ALTE group, particularly in gross motor movements (Milioti & Einspieler, 2005)

l. SIDS
- **i.** Sudden and unexpected death of an infant (<1 year) that remains unexplained after a complete postmortem investigation, including autopsy, death scene evaluation, and review of the case history
  - (a) May see punctate petechial hemorrhages
- **ii.** Etiology
  - (a) Unknown
  - (b) Multiple theories, including:
    - (1) Central apnea
    - (2) Upper airway obstruction and cardiac arrhythmias
    - (3) Metabolic diseases
    - (4) Environmental factors
      - a) Hyperthermia
      - b) Unsafe bedding
      - c) Prone sleeping position
- **iii.** Incidence
  - (a) 5000 deaths per year in the United States
  - (b) 1.4 cases per 1000 live births
  - (c) 90% of cases occur before 6 months of age
  - (d) Peak incidence: 2 to 4 months of age
- **iv.** Treatment
  - (a) Resuscitation is almost always initiated before receiving the infant at the hospital
  - (b) If rigor mortis or lividity is present, resuscitation efforts should not be initiated
  - (c) The medical examiner must be notified of all suspected SIDS deaths
  - (d) The family will need emotional support—refer to a local SIDS group if available
- **v.** Prevention
  - (a) Avoid a prone sleeping position for young, healthy infants
  - (b) Provide a safe sleeping environment, i.e., no pillows
  - (c) Apnea monitors for infants who have experienced an ALTE have *not* been shown to decrease mortality related to SIDS

# REFERENCES

Bocka, J. (2005). *Pediatrics, pertussis*. Retrieved June 19, 2006, from www.emedicine.com/emerg/topic394.htm.

Chang, A. K., & Barton, E. D. (2005). *Pneumothorax, iatrogenic, spontaneous and pneumomediastinum*. Retreived from eMedicine on April 24, 2006 from http://www.emedicine. com/emerg/topic469.htm.

Fleming, D. M., Pannell, R. S., Elliot, A. J., & Cross, K.W. (2005). Respiratory illness associated with influenza and respiratory syncytial virus infection. *Arch Dis Child, 90*(7), 741-746.

Goodhue, C. J., & Brady, M. A. (2004). Respiratory disorders. In C. E. Burns, A. M. Dunn, M. A. Brady, et al. (Eds.). *Pediatric primary care: A handbook for nurse practitio-ners* (3rd ed.). Philadelphia: Saunders, pp. 811-838.

Holmes, R. L., & Fadden, C. T. (2004). Evaluation of the patient with chronic cough. *Am Fam Phys, 69*(9), 2159–2168.

Milioti, S., & Einspieler, C. (2005). The long-term outcome of infantile apparent life-threatening event (ALTE): A follow-up study until midpuberty. *Neuropediatrics, 36*(1), 1–5.

Patel, H., Platt, R., Lozano, J. M., & Wang, E. E. (2004). Glucocorticoids for acute viral bronchiolitis in infants and young children. *Cochrane Database Syst Rev, 3*, CD004878.

Ramadan, H. H. (2005). Pediatric sinusitis: Update. *J Otolaryngol, 34*(Suppl 1), S14-S17.

Russell, K., Wiebe, N., Saenz, A., et al. (2003). Glucocorticoids for croup. *Cochrane Database Syst Rev, 14*, CD001955.

Schwartz, M. W., Bell, L. M., Bingham, P. M., et al. (2005). *The 5 minute pediatric consult* (4th ed.). Philadelphia: Lippincott Williams & Wilkins.

Sharma, S., & Duerkson, D. (2006). Tracheoesophageal fistula. Retrieved June 19, 2006, from www.emedicine.com/med/topic3416.htm.

Smucny, J., Flynn, C., Becker, L., & Glazier, R. (2003). Beta2-agonists for acute bronchitis. *Cochrane Database Syst Rev, 1*, CD001726.

Spiro, C. E. (2003). Evaluating chronic cough: A systematic approach. *Clin Rev, 13*(10), 52-57.

Spurling, G. K., Del Mar, C. B., Dooley, L., & Foxlee, R. (2004). Delayed antibiotics for symptoms and complication of respiratory infections. *Cochrane Database Syst Rev, 4*, CD004417.

Steiner, R. W. P. (2004). Treating acute bronchiolitis associated with RSV. *American Family Physician, 69*(2), 325-332.

Steinhorn, R. H. (2004). *Congenital diaphragmatic hernia*. Retrieved June 19, 2006, from www.emedicine.com/ped/topic2603.htm.

U. S. Food and Drug Administration. (2006). Influenza (flu) antiviral drugs and related information. Retrieved on April 21, 2006, at http://www.fda.gov/cder/drug/antivirals/influenza/

# Common Illness of the Cardiovascular System

ANNETTE BAKER, MSN, RN, PNP AND JULI-ANNE K. EVANGELISTA, MS, APRN, BC, PNP

1. Symptoms: syncope (fainting), dizziness, visual disturbances
   a. Focused history
      i. Child's history
         (a) Previous experiences with dizziness, syncope
         (b) Systemic disease
         (c) Connective tissue disorders such as Marfan syndrome
         (d) Eating disorders
      ii. Family history
         (a) History of sudden unexpected death under age 40
         (b) Congenital deafness
         (c) Cardiomyopathy
         (d) Common history of recurrent toddler or adolescent syncope that was "outgrown"
   b. Symptom assessment
      i. Environment
         (a) Time
         (b) Place
         (c) Temperature—typically a hot environment
         (d) Activity
            (1) Standing for long periods
            (2) Physically active
      ii. Presyncopal signs and symptoms can serve as:
         (a) Clues to the pathophysiology
         (b) Target for preventive therapy efforts
         (c) An assessment of the severity of symptoms
      iii. Syncope episode (falls to ground, "passes out")
         (a) Definition—transient and abrupt loss of consciousness caused by a decrease in cerebral blood flow, resulting in collapse and relatively prompt recovery over a period of seconds
         (b) Length of loss of consciousness
         (c) Injury
      iv. Postsyncopal signs and symptoms
   c. Focused physical assessment
      i. Orthostatic vital signs
         (a) Measure heart rate and blood pressure in supine position

   (b) Then ask the patient to move directly to standing position
   (c) Repeat the heart rate and blood pressure at 1 and 3 minutes
ii. Brief neurologic examination is appropriate
iii. Detailed cardiac examination with patient in several positions, i.e., standing, sitting or lying on left side
   (a) Examine for transient murmurs from dynamic subaortic stenosis and mitral valve prolapse
iv. Common diagnostic tests used by cardiology
   (a) Electrocardiogram (ECG)
   (b) Echocardiography
   (c) Treadmill exercise testing
   (d) Head-up tilt test
   (e) Cardiac catheterization
d. Prevalence (Soteriades, et al., 2002)
   i. Syncope represents a common cause of referral for children seen in the cardiology outpatient setting; for example, at Children's Hospital in Boston
      (a) 3,820 clinic visits by 1,923 children over 13 years were for syncope
      (b) Syncope accounts for 5% of all new patients
   ii. 20% to 50% of all adults state that they have had at least one syncopal episode (Miller & Kruse, 2005)
e. Pathophysiology
   i. The core physiology of any true syncopal event is abruptly ineffective cerebral blood flow resulting from:
      (a) Ineffective cardiac output (cardiac syncope)
      (b) Ineffective cardiovascular control (neurally mediated syncope)
      (c) See Table 29-1 for likelihood of specific symptoms associated with these two causal mechanisms
      (d) The specific cause is unknown in 13% to 31% of patients even after thorough investigation (Miller & Kruse, 2005)

■ **TABLE 29-1**
■ ■ **Signs and Symptoms Characteristic of the Two Major Causes of Syncope**

|  | Neurally Mediated Syncope | Cardiac Syncope |
| --- | :---: | :---: |
| **Premonitory Signs and Symptoms** | +++ | ± |
| Light-headedness | +++ | +/± |
| Palpitations | + | ++ |
| Occurs while upright | +++ | + |
| Occurs while sitting | +/± | + |
| Emotional trigger | ++ | ++ |
| Exercise trigger | + | ++ |
| **Residual Findings** |  |  |
| Pallor | +++ | +/± |
| Incontinence | − | + |
| Disorientation | − | + |
| Fatigue | ++ | ± |
| Diaphoresis | ++ | ± |
| Injury | + | ++ |

    **ii.** Cardiac syncope (Miller & Cruse, 2005)
- (a) Symptoms
  - (1) Characterized by an abrupt onset of collapse
  - (2) Few premonitory symptoms
- (b) Typical history
  - (1) Acute collapse
  - (2) Often with activity or exercise
  - (3) With nearly immediate recovery
  - (4) Palpitations are sometimes noted
  - (5) Not diagnostic in any clear fashion
  - (6) For transient events, recovery is similarly rapid
- (c) Prevalence—overall, 10% to 30% of syncope is categorized as cardiac (Miller & Kruse, 2005)
- (d) Pathophysiology
  - (1) Transpires secondary to combinations of:
    - a) Obstruction to left ventricular filling (pulmonary hypertension, tachycardia)
    - b) Left ventricular ejection (aortic stenosis or hypertrophic cardiomyopathy)
    - c) Ineffective contraction (profound bradycardia, dilated cardiomyopathy, pathologic tachyarrhythmia) with an underlying substrate that is either:
      - i) Structural
      - ii) Functional, or
      - iii) Electrical conduction system-related
  - (2) Responses to arrhythmias, and other transient impairments in cardiac output, are in part determined by the effectiveness of baroreflex controls
  - (3) Classified as aborted sudden cardiac death if:
    - a) Significant residual of confusion
    - b) Disorientation
    - c) Need for CPR
    - d) Palpitations (all four of these symptoms increase suspicion of a serious arrhythmia; none are diagnostic)
    - e) Occurrence with exercise, injury, urinary incontinence
    - f) Onset while sitting or supine
    - g) Most critical distinction is whether there is historical or examination evidence of heart disease
- (e) Treatment—therapy is directed at the underlying disorder

   **iii.** Neurally mediated syncope (also called reflex-mediated syncope)—common fainting, neurocardiogenic syncope (Hamer & Bray, 2005; Kapoor, 2003; Miller & Kruse, 2005)
- (a) Term used for this type emphasizes the dominant disordered cardiac and vascular regulation that results in symptoms, of, e.g.:
  - (1) Vasovagal syncope
  - (2) Cardioinhibitory syncope
  - (3) Pallid breath-holding spells (or reflex anoxic seizures)
  - (4) Vasodepressor syncope
  - (5) Postural orthostatic tachycardia syndrome (POTS)
- (b) Prevalence—about 36% to 62% of syncope is categorized as reflex-mediated (Miller & Kruse, 2005)

(c) Vasodepressor or vasovagal syncope (Connolly, et al., 2003; Flevari, et al., 2002)
  (1) Pathophysiology
    a) Initiated by blood pooling in the extremities, typically when standing
    b) Results in decreased right ventricular filling, then decreased left ventricular filling
    c) Triggers left ventricular sensory activation to the brainstem, carotid body, and carotid sinus activation
    d) Initially results in decreased vagal or parasympathetic activation and increased sympathetic or catecholamine activation to raise heart rate, increase venous and arteriolar tone, and enhance left ventricular contractility
    e) Homeostatic response causes a modest increase in heart rate and narrowing of pulse pressure with patient recovery and ability to stand upright
    f) If unsuccessful, homeostatic mechanisms increase, but a paradoxical parasympathetic (vagal) stimulation may result:
      i) Slows heart rate with or without sympathetic withdrawal
      ii) Decreased vascular tone and lowered blood pressure
  (2) Etiology
    a) Most classic form of syncope
    b) Exacerbated by anxiety and hyperventilation
    c) Active use of the skeletal muscle pump (jogging, isometrics) can enhance venous return and raise systemic blood pressure, blunting the initial responses
    d) Medications or concomitant medical disorders can also exacerbate or blunt the cyclic swings in cardiac and vascular control
(d) Convulsive syncope
  (1) Pathophysiology
    a) Mechanisms are complex
    b) Some patients have both sinus tachycardia and profound atrioventricular (AV) block
    c) Symptom and rhythm correlation (Connolly, et al., 2003, Kapoor, 2003)
      i) Variable rhythm
      ii) Combined with the failure of pacemakers to completely eliminate symptoms in syncope
  (2) Etiology—acute pain, anxiety, fear
(e) POTS and recurrent symptoms
  (1) Characteristics
    a) Greater than 30 to 40 beat per minute heart rate increase with a 6-minute stand test
    b) Many patients experience minimal syncope, but have recurrent presyncopal symptoms, e.g., palpitations or exercise intolerance
  (2) Prevalence
    a) Adolescent female dominance
(f) Exercise-induced and exercise-associated syncope
  (1) Pathophysiology

a) Normal cardiovascular response to exercise is:
  i) Vasodilation
  ii) Increased sympathetic output
  iii) Blood flow shifts to the legs
    *a)* Skeletal muscle pump action enhances venous return, increases cardiac output
    *b)* Postexercise, pump function immediately decreases and can result in venous pooling
(2) Incidence of death during exercise in young people (Maron, 2003)
  a) Incidence is unknown, but rare
  b) Media attention to rare deaths has increased awareness of this potential health problem
(g) Psychogenic syncope and situational syncope
  (1) Pathophysiology
    a) Acute anxiety may result in prolonged cardiac pauses, bradycardia
    b) Over time, acceleration and embellishment of symptoms make it appear that syncope results from panic or anxiety
    c) Physical examination, lab testing, and monitoring are neither consistent nor diagnostic of clear pathology
  (2) Prevalence, etiology
    a) In young adults, measures of anxiety are a better predictor of future faints than syncope during head-up tilt test (Kouakam, et al., 2002)
    b) Emotional trigger, e.g., the sight of blood
(h) Toddler syncope (DiMario, 2001b; Kelly, et al., 2001)
  (1) Also called "pallid breath-holding spells," "white syncope," "reflex anoxic seizures,"
  (2) Characterized by
    a) Well-recognized stereotypic syndrome of paroxysmal collapse
    b) A trivial physical or emotional trauma triggers an aborted cry, pallor, and opisthotonoid posture (head and lower limbs bend backward and trunk arches forward)
    c) Resolves after about 1 minute
    d) Often followed by sleep
    e) Rarely accompanied by true seizures
    f) Contrasts and overlaps with classic breath-holding spells in which there is ongoing crying with cyanosis, breath holding, and then syncope
  (3) Prevalence (DiMario, 2001b)
    a) Prevalence may be up to 5% of toddlers
    b) Onset is typically between age 6 months and 3 years
    c) Boys and girls are equally affected
    d) Ends by age 5 years for more than 65%, and for the majority by age 8 years
    e) After 8 years generally classified as convulsive syncope
  (4) Treatment
    a) Explanation and parental reassurance by the primary care provider when episode is typical and isolated
    b) If recurrent, evaluate for anemia, arrhythmia, and epilepsy
    c) Iron therapy may be useful if iron deficiency is also present

(5) Prognosis
  a) Although the level of bradycardia can be quite impressive, most toddlers have infrequent episodes that resolve without specific therapy
  b) Nearly 20% of toddlers with breath-holding spells will have some syncope as adolescents
(6) Follow-up
  a) Family therapy may be needed if home environment or parenting style appears to be a precipitating factor
  b) If repeated spells, refer to cardiologists or neurologists for further evaluation

iv. General treatment recommendations for neurally-mediated syncope
  (a) Few double-blind, placebo-controlled studies are available for children due to the episodic, self-resolving nature of the disorder
  (b) Therapy recommendations are based on limited trials and on the underlying pathophysiology
  (c) Some strategies may be used by primary care providers; others are best managed by specialists
    (1) Nonpharmacologic, nondevice therapy
      a) Cornerstone of therapy is education
        i) Nature of syncopal events
        ii) Ways to either prevent or abort spells (depends upon the cause)
      b) The vast majority of patients will have significant relief with a combination of:
        i) Overhydration, including:
          a) Increased fluid
          b) Decreased caffeine
          c) Increased sodium intake
        ii) Antigravity maneuvers—NOTE: symptoms caused by arrhythmia are not usually affected by these maneuvers
          a) Isometric leg or arm contractions
          b) Staged shifts from supine to upright
          c) Squatting or lying down with onset of presyncopal symptoms
          d) Compression stockings
          e) "Tilt training" with supervised upright time leaning against a wall can be beneficial (Numata, et al., 2000)
          f) Upright, weight-bearing aerobic exercise
          g) Cognitive-behavioral therapy through psychiatry or psychology—critical for situational, psychogenic syncope
    (2) Medical approach
      a) Pacemaker, e.g., rare, but may be used for severe toddler syncope (DiMario, 2001a)
    (3) Pharmacologic therapy (Massin, 2003)
      a) Volume enhancement, e.g., fludrocortisone
      b) Limit excessive catecholamine drive with β-blockers, e.g., atenolol, pindolol
      c) Blood pressure augmentation, e.g., midodrine hydrochloride
      d) Rarely anticholinergic therapy
      e) Therapy is typically continued for approximately 1 year, followed by trials of decreasing therapy

2. Symptom: chest pain (Evangelista, et al., 2000; Morel & Bye, 2000)
   a. Prevalence
      i. Chest pain is a common complaint in the pediatric age-group
      ii. Primary complaint in 650,000 pediatric encounters yearly
      iii. Accounts for 5% to 15% of children referred to a pediatric cardiology clinic (Yildirim, et al., 2004)
      iv. Relationship to pubertal status and sex (Rhee, 2005)
         (a) Children with advanced puberty report more symptoms than children who are early or on time
         (b) Boys report more musculoskeletal pain (including chest pain) than girls
         (c) Girls report more headaches
      v. Only about 1% of emergency department visits by children are for chest pain
      vi. Physically and emotionally distressing symptom
         (a) Rarely indicates serious cardiac problems
         (b) Perceived as "heart pain" to most children and their families
         (c) Presents a diagnostic challenge to the health care provider
      vii. Public awareness of sudden cardiac death in young healthy children may contribute to a family's anxiety about childhood chest pain
         (a) By the time a patient reaches the primary care or cardiology office, the anxiety level of the family is high
         (b) Appropriate care for this group of patients must address not only the etiology but also reassurance about the nature of what is often a self-limited condition
   b. Focused history
      i. Accurate history is the most important component of the clinical assessment to identify the cause of chest pain
      ii. If possible, history should be obtained from the patient rather than the parents, who may be prone to interpret their child's symptoms in light of their own experiences or anxiety
      iii. Child's history
         (a) Recent fever or illness
         (b) Chest wall trauma
         (c) Recent stressful life event
         (d) Previous cardiac surgery
         (e) Previous inflammatory process of the coronary arteries (i.e., Kawasaki disease)
      iv. Family history
         (a) Known cardiac history, e.g., cardiomyopathy
         (b) Syncope or abnormal heartbeats
         (c) Sudden or early death
         (d) Genetic or connective tissue disorders, i.e., Marfan syndrome
   c. Symptom analysis (Box 29-1)
      i. Note—in most circumstances, chest pain is present for many months if not years before parents seek input, supporting a noncardiac cause
      ii. Manner of onset may suggest an etiology
         (a) Acute – typical of a cardiac cause
         (b) Chronic
         (c) Gradual or sudden

■ **BOX 29-1**
■ **SYMPTOM ANALYSIS FOR CHEST PAIN**

1. When was the onset of pain?
2. When does it occur?
3. What might have precipitated the pain?
   - Injury or strain (musculoskeletal)
   - Response to rest or analgesics (musculoskeletal)
   - Emotional circumstances, e.g., family disruption
   - School difficulties
   - Illness of a friend or relative
   - Depression (psychogenic)
   - Eating, drinking
4. How often does it happen?
   - Continuous
   - Constant
   - Intermittent
   - Recurrent
5. Describe the type of pain
   - Burning
   - Stabbing
   - Sharp
   - Squeezing
   - Dull
   - Cramping
   - Ache
6. Describe the intensity of the pain
   - Use scale of 1 to 10
   - Ask for reference points for pain at levels 1 and 10
7. Where is the pain located, i.e., midsternal, left anterior, etc.?
8. Where does it hurt the worst?
9. Can you point to it with one finger?
10. Is the pain localized or diffuse?
11. Does the pain radiate anywhere?
12. How long does the pain last, i.e., seconds, minutes, hours?
13. Is the pain made worse by deep breathing, exercise, or activity?
14. Any associated symptoms?
    - Palpitations
    - Dizziness
    - Syncope
    - Epigastric pain
    - Nausea
    - Vomiting
    - Fatigue
    - Fever
    - Cough
    - Coryza
    - Shortness of breath
    - Orthopnea or dyspnea on exertion
    - Rapid heartbeat, dizziness, syncope on exertion

      iii. Radiating pain
- (a) Cardiac chest pain is generally midprecordial and can radiate to the left arm
- (b) Severe crushing pain radiating to the back is experienced with aortic tears
- (c) Subcostal pain is generally chest wall related

      iv. It is often helpful to ask parents if they are worried about the pain and if so, why; this line of questioning may disclose emotional factors that influence the symptoms

**d.** Focused physical examination

      **i.** Inspection
- (a) Appearance of the patient may suggest a connective tissue disorder, e.g., tall individual with:
  - (1) Dolicocephaly—elongated head
  - (2) Pectus excavatum
  - (3) Carinatum
- (b) Inspect the chest wall for trauma or asymmetry

      **ii.** Palpation
- (a) Chest wall for tenderness, i.e., costochondral borders
- (b) A palpable thrill supports left ventricular outflow tract obstruction
  - (1) Left sternal border or
  - (2) Base bilaterally or
  - (3) Suprasternal notch

      **iii.** Auscultation
- (a) Heart arrhythmias, murmurs, rubs, or gallops may suggest underlying heart disease by their hyperdynamic quality and displacement of the point of maximal intensity in patients with volume-overloaded lesions
  - (1) Ventricular hypertrophy
    - a) Apical heave—right ventricle
    - b) Parasternal heave—left ventricle
  - (2) Underlying cardiac disease
    - a) Loud $S_2$ associated with pulmonary hypertension
    - b) Muffled heart sounds are found in with moderate to large pericardial effusions
  - (3) Systolic clicks
    - a) Bicuspid aortic valve prolapse
    - b) Mitral valve prolapse
  - (4) Harsh systolic ejection murmur
    - a) Valvular or subvalvular aortic stenosis
    - b) Heard along the left sternal border
    - c) Radiation to the base and neck
  - (5) Mitral regurgitation
    - a) Heard at the apex
    - b) Radiation to the left axilla
    - c) Murmurs associated with posterior mitral leaflet abnormalities
      - i) Heard at the left mid- to upper sternal border
      - ii) Related to a more anterior- and superior-directed regurgitant jet
  - (6) Aortic regurgitation
    - a) Mild to moderate degree regurgitant murmur
    - b) Murmur radiates from the right base, down the left lower sternal border toward the apex

        (7) $S_3$ gallops
          a) Moderate mitral regurgitation
          b) Dilated cardiomyopathy
        (8) $S_4$ gallops
          a) Less common
          b) Noted in hypertrophic cardiomyopathy
          c) Severe aortic stenosis
        (9) Friction rub associated with acute pericarditis
     (b) Auscultate lungs for rales, wheezes, decreased breath sounds, pneumonia, and other evidence of congestive heart failure (CHF)
   **iv.** Palpation
     (a) Abdomen for referred pain or discomfort to the chest
     (b) Costochondral junctions to elicit tenderness
 **e.** Diagnostic tests
   **i.** Ordered by PNP
     (a) Electrocardiogram
     (b) Chest x-ray
   **ii.** Ordered by referred specialty providers
     (a) Echocardiograph
     (b) Exercise testing
 **f.** Differential diagnoses (see Table 29-2 for cardiac and noncardiac causes)
 **g.** Treatment and management
   **i.** Vast majority of childhood chest pain is not cardiac in origin
     (a) Management primarily includes:

■ **TABLE 29-2**
■ ■ **Differential Diagnosis of Pediatric Chest Pain**

| Cardiac Causes | Observations |
| --- | --- |
| 1. Cardiomyopathy | |
|   a. Hypertrophic | Marked increase in myocardial oxygen demand exceeds coronary flow during exercise, resulting in angina |
| | Exacerbated by midcavitary obstruction |
| | Leads to increased myocardial work |
| | Increased myocardial oxygen consumption |
| | Coronary artery compression produced by myocardial bridging may cause myocardial ischemia and angina |
|   b. Dilated | Decreased cardiac muscle mass |
| | Capacity of the heart to deliver adequate coronary blood flow is impaired by diminished stroke volume |
| 2. Acute myocarditis | Generally of viral origin, usually the result of concomitant pericarditis |
| | Pain due to imbalance between myocardial demand and cardiac output |
|   a. Valvular | Severe aortic valve or subaortic obstruction |
| | Limitation of cardiac output during exercise in the setting of left ventricular hypertrophy |
| | Severe mitral regurgitation |
|   b. Pericardial | Acute inflammation of the pericardium |
| | Cause could be viral, bacterial, autoimmune, surgical insult |
| | Pain due to opposition of the inflamed parietal and visceral pericardial surfaces |
| | Effusion separates the surfaces, so pain is diminished or absent |

■ **TABLE 29-2**
■ ■ **Differential Diagnosis of Pediatric Chest Pain—cont'd**

| Cardiac Causes | Observations |
|---|---|
| c. Coronary | |
| i. Kawasaki disease | Results in the formation of coronary abnormalities |
| | Occurs in 2%-4% of those receiving IV gamma globulin within 10 days of fever onset |
| | Occurs in 20%–25% of those not treated within 10 days of fever onset |
| ii. Giant aneurysm | >8 mm diameter |
| | At risk for late progressive stenosis at the distal or proximal ends of the aneurysm |
| | Exercise will produce chest pain in those with critical narrowing |
| 3. Congenital coronary artery abnormalities | Uncommon (Basso, et al., 2000) |
| | Chest pain during exercise related to: |
| | • Compression of an artery between the aortic and pulmonic roots |
| | • Insufficient flow through a kinked acute angle takeoff of the artery |
| | • Spasm of the artery |
| | Rarely, left coronary artery may arise from the pulmonary artery |
| | Presents in infancy with heart failure following LV infarction |
| | Can remain silent until later in childhood when symptoms of pain with exercise begin |
| a. Aortic abnormalities | Acute severe chest pain that may radiate to the back, due to: |
| | Dissection of the aorta in Marfan's syndrome |
| | Other connective tissue disorders |
| | Turner's syndrome |
| | Familial aneurysmal diseases |
| | A sinus of Valsalva aneurysm can rupture unexpectedly into the right atrium or ventricle |
| b. Rhythm abnormalities | Children may complain of chest pain during acute events of supraventricular tachycardia |
| | Pain or discomfort from coronary ischemia may be related to: |
| | • Diminished ventricular diastolic filling |
| | • Low cardiac output |
| | • Other causes: |
| |   • Ventricular tachycardia most common after repair or palliation of congenital lesions |
| |   • Cardiomyopathy |
| |   • Long QT syndrome |
| |   • Severe electrolyte disturbances |

| Noncardiac Causes | |
|---|---|
| 1. Chest wall origin | Most common explanation for chest pain in 31% of children (Pantell & Goodman, 2004) |
| | May involve connective tissue, bone, muscle |
| | Traumatic or atraumatic |
| a. Costochondritis | Inflammation at the costochondral junction |
| | Common in adolescent athletes |
| | Lifting heavy objects (Morel & Bye, 2000) |
| b. Precordial catch syndrome | Sharp pain of short duration |
| | Sometimes exercise induced |
| | May be relieved with deep inspiration |
| c. Slipping rib syndrome | Caused by trauma or tension on the fibrous connections to the 8th, 9th, or 10th rib; not attached to the sternum but to each other |
| | With unrestrained motion of a rib, pain is due to irritation of the intercostal nerves |

*Continued*

■ **TABLE 29-2**
■ ■ **Differential Diagnosis of Pediatric Chest Pain—cont'd**

| Cardiac Causes | Observations |
|---|---|
| d. Hypersensitive xiphoid | Uncommon, but xiphoid or sternum may be hypersensitive |
| | Usually improves spontaneously |
| e. Pectus deformities | Occasional pain accentuated by exercise (Mansour, et al., 2003) |
| f. Sickle cell disease | Acute chest syndrome |
| | Frequent cause of hospital admissions and death |
| | An important cause of death in this group of children |
| g. Breast conditions | More common in females, but occurs in males |
| | Causes: infection, pubertal growth, menstrual changes, pregnancy |
| h. Traumatic chest pain | Very common in adolescents |
| | Causes include muscle strains, tears or spasm, rib fractures |
| 2. Pulmonary | |
| a. Reactive airway disease | Pain related to persistent cough, dyspnea, pneumothorax, exercise-induced bronchospasm |
| b. Other pulmonary causes | Pulmonary embolus |
| | Hypercoagulability |
| | Pleural disease |
| | Pleural effusion |
| | Pleural irritation |
| | Pneumothorax |
| 3. Gastrointestinal | |
| a. Gastroesophageal reflux with esophagitis | Produces a burning sensation in the retrosternal area |
| | Sometimes exacerbated by supine positioning |
| b. Peptic ulcer disease | Most frequently associated with *Helicobacter pylori* infection |
| | Important source of pain localized to epigastric region, lower chest |
| c. Esophageal spasm | Can produce marked chest pain |
| 4. Psychogenic | Among pediatric patients in a cardiology clinic with chest pain, many are psychogenic in origin (Pantell & Goodman, 2004) |
| | Often related to a significant life event |
| | This diagnosis not always well accepted |
| | Family and child often very anxious about cause |
| | Some noninvasive testing may be necessary to show no underlying disease as cause for pain |
| | Requires building of trust and rapport with child and family |
| 5. Hyperventilation syndrome | Chest pain may be a presenting symptom |

        (1) Explanation of the diagnosis and reassurance to the child and family
        (2) Reassurance that chest pain is common in this age-group
      (b) Alleviates much of the stress and anxiety around this issue
      (c) Decreases the frequency and severity of symptoms
      (d) Prognosis is generally excellent
    **ii.** Costochondritis—treatment with a short course of a nonsteroidal antiinflammatory (NSAID) may be helpful (see Table 55-5 for dosing guidelines for NSAIDs)
  **h.** Refer to appropriate specialty if indicated by history and physical examination
**3.** Sign: hyperlipidemia noted on screening test
  **a.** Childhood lipid screening
    **i.** Health problem—atherosclerotic heart disease is the leading cause of morbidity and mortality in the adult population in America

    **ii.** Abnormalities in the lipid profile are an important indicator of the development of atherosclerotic disease

        **(a)** Atherosclerosis begins as a silent process and patients are asymptomatic until advanced stages of the disease

        **(b)** Autopsy studies have shown that fatty streaks begin to appear in the aorta and coronary arteries during childhood and adolescence

   **iii.** Cholesterol levels, especially high and low end of the spectrum, follow similar percentiles from childhood into adulthood if not identified and treated early (Nicklas, et al., 2002)

        **(a)** Aim of cholesterol screening and lipid-lowering treatment in pediatrics

            **(1)** To detect children at the highest risk for developing cardiovascular disease

            **(2)** To minimize their individual risk factors (Box 29-2)

        **(b)** Lipid screening remains a highly controversial area in pediatrics

        **(c)** Institute for Clinical Systems Improvement (2004) consensus statement recommends:

            **(1)** No universal screening of lipid values

            **(2)** Selective screening for all children older than the age of 2 years

            **(3)** Target patients at the highest risk

                **a)** Family history of early heart disease (<55 years old in a first- or second-degree relative) or elevated cholesterol (Hopkins, 2003; Marais, et al., 2004)

                **b)** Genetic family history is unknown (i.e., adopted)

                **c)** Individual risk factors (see Box 29-2)

        **(d)** Initial screen for total cholesterol and high-density lipoprotein cholesterol

---

■ **BOX 29-2**
■ **RISK FACTORS FOR CORONARY HEART DISEASE**

Family history in a first- or second-degree relative
   Elevated cholesterol
   Diabetes
   Heart disease
   Hypertension
   Premature atherosclerotic disease
Individual risk factors:
   Elevated LDL cholesterol (>110 mg/dL)
   Low HDL cholesterol (<35 mg.dL)
   Elevated Lp(a)
   At risk for overweight (BMI <85%) or overweight (BMI >85%)
   Smoking
   Lack of physical exercise
   Male gender
   Elevated blood pressure
   Diabetes type 1 or type 2
   Renal disease
   Hypertension
   History of Kawasaki disease

(1) Obtaining both values gives the practitioner a better idea of individual risk

(2) Accurate in the nonfasting state

**b.** Focused history

   **i.** Family history (first- or second-degree relative) (Wiegman, et al., 2003)

      (a) Elevated cholesterol, heart disease, hypertension, or diabetes

      (b) Premature atherosclerotic disease, younger than 55 years

**c.** Focused physical examination

   **i.** Physical examination is typically normal

   **ii.** Special attention to:

      (a) Examination of the tendons and knuckles for xanthomas

      (b) Inspection of the eyes for arcus corneae, a grey opaque line around the margin of the cornea, separated by an area of clear cornea; related to lipid degeneration

      (c) Inspect for acanthosis nigricans on neck and under the arms of overweight children—a sign of insulin resistance

**d.** Pathophysiology

   **i.** Cholesterol profile

      (a) Cholesterol is a fatlike substance that is transported in the serum by lipoproteins i.e., molecules containing both fats and proteins

      (b) Lipids play a role in cell membranes and formation of bile salts and steroid hormones

      (c) The major types of lipoproteins in the serum include: LDL, HDL, VLDL, chylomicrons (triglycerides), which make up TC (total cholesterol)

         (1) Low-density lipoprotein (LDL) cholesterol

            a) Major cholesterol-carrying lipoprotein in the plasma

            b) Elevated LDL levels are atherogenic and directly associated with increased risk of coronary disease

            c) LDL cholesterol is therefore the primary target of lipid-lowering therapy

            d) Easy to remember as L = "lousy" cholesterol

            e) Can be measured directly, but usually calculated using a formula:

            f) TC − (VLDL + HDL)

         (2) High-density lipoprotein (HDL) cholesterol

            a) Serves a protective function

               i) HDL cholesterol acts as a scavenger

               ii) Transports cholesterol from vessels to liver for secretion in the bile

            b) Inverse relationship between HDL levels and heart disease; therefore considered a negative risk factor

            c) Lower in males than females

            d) Drop in males during puberty

            e) Easy to remember as H = "healthy or happy" cholesterol

         (3) Very-low-density lipoprotein (VLDL) cholesterol

            a) Synthesized in the liver

            b) Responsible for transport of majority of plasma triglycerides when fasting

            c) Precursors of LDL

            d) VLDL remnants are atherogenic

            e) When fasting blood drawn, one can divide the triglyceride value by 5 (providing triglycerides are <400 mg/dL) to obtain the VLDL cholesterol

(4) Chylomicrons
  a) Largest and highest in density
  b) Rich in triglycerides and are formed in the intestine from dietary fat
  c) Triglycerides are increased by:
    i) Increased sugar intake
    ii) Increased carbohydrate intake
    iii) Increased body weight
    iv) Some medications
    v) Recent illness
(5) Lipoprotein (a)
  a) Density is between HDL and LDL
  b) Carries a protein that reduces body's ability to dissolve blood clots
  c) May be a marker or cause of heart disease—still under investigation
(6) Total cholesterol
  a) Standard formula is: Total cholesterol = LDL + HDL + VLDL

(d) American Heart Association guidelines for acceptable, borderline and high total and LDL cholesterol levels for children ages 2 through 19 (Table 29-3)
(e) Risk ratios are helpful in determining treatment because they take into account HDL values:
  (1) Total cholesterol/HDL cholesterol—ideal for children is about 1.5 to 1
  (2) LDL cholesterol/HDL cholesterol—ideal for children is 3.5 to 1

e. Etiology
  i. Dyslipidemia, hyperlipidemia, and early cardiovascular disease tend to aggregate in families as a result of common genetic and environmental factors
  ii. Genetic factors
    (a) Majority of lipid abnormalities in children are inherited in a dominant fashion, affecting 50% of offspring
    (b) Several types of genetic dyslipidemias
      (1) Familial hypercholesterolemia (FH) is an autosomal dominant disease
        a) Heterozygous FH
          i) Occurs in 1 per 500 people, leading to defective LDL receptor function in the liver and increased levels of LDL

■ **TABLE 29-3**
■ ■ **American Heart Association Guidelines for Cholesterol Levels for Children Ages 2 to 19 Years**

|  | Total Cholesterol (mg/dL) | LDL Cholesterol (mg/dL) |
|---|---|---|
| Acceptable | <170 | <110 |
| Borderline | 170–199 | 110–129 |
| High | ≥200 | ≥130 |

From Cardiovascular Health in Childhood: A statement for health professionals from the Committee on Atherosclerosis, Hypertension, and Obesity in the Young (AHOY) of the Council on Cardiovascular Disease in the Young, 2002, American Heart Association. Reproduced with permission.

ii) Some families with FH have the additional risk factor of a low HDL

iii) Without treatment, as many as 50% of FH patients will have early heart disease as adults

b) Homozygous FH

i) Extremely rare and serious

ii) Occurs in 1 per 1 million people

iii) Results in cholesterol levels greater than 600 mg/dL

iv) Tendon and cutaneous xanthomas are apparent by school age

v) Can develop symptoms of coronary artery disease in childhood

vi) No cure; usually undergo regular plasmapheresis (every 2 to 3 weeks)

vii) Sometimes combined with lipid-lowering medication

(2) Familial combined hyperlipidemia

a) Dominant disorder

b) High LDL cholesterol and/or

c) High triglycerides

(3) Familial hypertriglyceridemia

a) Elevated triglycerides

b) Often also have low levels of HDL cholesterol

(4) Familial hypoalphalipoproteinemia

a) Low HDL cholesterol (an independent risk factor)

(5) Metabolic syndrome (de Ferranti, et al., 2004)

a) More prevalent in the pediatric population in recent years

b) Characterized by a group of risk factors:

i) High triglycerides

ii) Low HDL cholesterol

iii) Abdominal obesity

iv) Insulin resistance

v) Glucose intolerance

vi) Hypertension

vii) Sedentary lifestyle

viii) Increase in inflammatory markers

iii. Secondary causes of dyslipidemia in children older than 2 years old

(a) Endocrine disorders, especially:

(1) Hypothyroidism

(2) Renal disease

(3) Diabetes mellitus

(4) Obstructive liver disease

(5) Systemic infections

(6) Certain medications

f. Diagnostic tests

i. Serum cholesterol panel

(a) Lipid values should not be obtained within 3 weeks of febrile illnesses because acute illnesses can affect the lipid profile by lowering total cholesterol and raising triglycerides

(b) Ideally, the patient should be seated for at least 5 minutes before blood drawing

(c) Total cholesterol and HDL cholesterol can be obtained at any time of day and are not affected by eating

(d) In order to obtain triglyceride values and calculated LDL levels, the patient should fast (except for water) for 9 to 12 hours before blood drawing

(e) When triglycerides are greater than 400 mg/dL, the calculation of LDL is not accurate and a direct LDL-cholesterol measurement or a lipoprotein electrophoresis should be done to ascertain LDL values

ii. Other tests to rule out secondary causes

(a) Screening TSH

(b) Liver function tests

(c) Renal functions tests

(d) Urinalysis

iii. Measuring cholesterol

(a) Accurate measurement of cholesterol is critical in determining those patients who require further intervention

g. Treatment and management (Belay, et al., 2004)

i. Nonpharmacologic

(a) Children with LDL-cholesterol values greater than 130 mg/dL or LDL greater than 100 in a child with diabetes should receive individualized treatment from a lipid specialist

(b) Lifestyle modification remains the mainstay of therapy for children and adolescents with elevated cholesterol

(c) Children and families should have individualized nutritional counseling regarding the recommendations for a "heart-healthy" diet

(1) Emphasis should be placed on choosing foods that provide "right fat" such as olive and canola oil because monounsaturated fats have a beneficial effect on HDL cholesterol levels

(2) Saturated fat should be limited to less than 7% of dietary intake

(3) Dietary cholesterol intake should not exceed 200 mg per day

(4) The optimal diet should be rich in whole grains, fruits, and vegetables

(5) Skim milk is recommended for children older than 2 years to ensure adequate calcium and vitamin D intake

(6) Foods high in concentrated sugars such as juice, soda, sugary cereals, cookies, and cakes should be discouraged, especially for children with elevated triglyceride values

(d) Regular aerobic exercise is recommended (at least 30 minutes a day, 5 days a week)

(e) Education regarding the importance of avoidance of smoking should begin at a young age

(f) See Chapter 16, section 1, for detailed information on prevention and management of overweight, and NAPNAP's HEAT Campaign practice guidelines

ii. Lipid-lowering medication (McCrindle, et al., 2003)

(a) Lipid-lowering medications are recommended for children:

(1) More than 10 years old

(2) Whose LDL cholesterol remains greater than 160 mg/dL with a positive family history of early heart disease

(3) Or LDL greater than190 mg/dL without a family history of early heart disease

(4) Despite 6 to 12 months of lifestyle modification

(b) Isolated high triglycerides

(1) Treated with diet

(2) Medications are reserved for those with an increased risk of pancreatitis (TG >400 mg/dL)

(c) Bile acid resins, ezetimibe, and statins are the most commonly used lipid lowering medications for childhood and adolescence

(d) Niacin is not used anymore in the pediatric population because of the high incidence of liver inflammation as well as the disturbing side effect of flushing

(e) Fibric acid derivatives also are not used in children because of elevations in liver function tests

4. Sign: high systolic or diastolic blood pressure noted on screening

  a. Hypertension in children and adolescents (Chobanian, et al., 2003; Morgenstern, 2002; Varda & Gregoric, 2005)

    i. Normative data for systolic and diastolic blood pressure (BP) readings for age and gender are now available in Muntner, et al., 2005

    ii. Definitions (assumes a pattern with repeated measurements)

      (a) Normal—BP less than the 90th percentile

      (b) Prehypertension—BP between 90th and 95th percentiles (about 5% of cases)

      (c) Stage I hypertension—BP ≥95th percentile to 5 mm Hg greater than the 99th percentile (about 5% of cases)

      (d) Stage II hypertension—BP more than 5 mm Hg higher than the 99th percentile

    iii. Hypertension is a significant risk factor for cardiovascular disease in adulthood

    iv. Hypertensive children are more likely to become hypertensive adults

    v. Hypertension is also part of the "metabolic syndrome," a constellation of symptoms that also includes overweight, larger than normal waist circumference, insulin resistance and dyslipidemia

  b. Etiology of hypertension

    i. "White coat" hypertension

      (a) Includes patients whose BP is greater than the 95th percentile in the office, but less than the 90th percentile normally

    ii. Primary or essential hypertension (Flynn, 2002)

      (a) Prevalence is about 1% to 2% of children in the United States

      (b) Elevated BP—more than the 95th percentile

      (c) No identifiable cause

      (d) Diagnosis of the majority of older children and adolescents with hypertension

      (e) Tends to be more prevalent in children with other risk factors, such as overweight

    iii. Secondary hypertension (Flynn, 2002)

      (a) Has an identifiable cause

      (b) Requires prompt evaluation and institution of therapy

      (c) More prevalent in infants, and young children younger than 6 years old, and older children and adolescents who have significantly elevated readings

      (d) Coarctation of the aorta accounts for one third of infant cases

      (e) Even after coarctation repair, many children require pharmacologic therapy to manage residual hypertension

      (f) Most common cause in young children overall is renal disease

  c. Focused history

    i. Family history

          (a) Incidence and age of onset of first- or second-degree family members with:
- (1) Hypertension
- (2) Diabetes
- (3) Coronary artery disease or stroke
- (4) Overweight
- (5) Sleep apnea
- (6) Endocrine disorders

  **ii.** Child's medical history
- (a) Previous hospitalizations
- (b) Umbilical artery catheterization in the neonatal period
- (c) Frequent urinary tract infections
- (d) Frequent headaches
- (e) Visual changes
- (f) Current medications
- (g) Overweight
- (h) Use of nutritional supplements
- (i) History of episodic flushing
- (j) Sleep disorders, frequent snoring
- (k) Smoking
- (l) Presence of other individual hypertension risk factors
  - (1) Prematurity
  - (2) Congenital heart disease
  - (3) Renal disease
  - (4) Increased intracranial pressure
  - (5) Systemic illness that may affect blood pressure (BP)

**d.** Focused physical assessment

  **i.** Measurement of BP (Park, et al., 2001)
- (a) Monitor BP yearly in all children more than 3 years of age
- (b) Monitor BP in younger children if they have any individual risk factors for hypertension
- (c) Norms for child and adolescent BP are available from Muntner, et al., 2005)
- (d) BP standards are based on auscultatory readings (See Chapter 11 for details on BP measurement)
- (e) Systolic BP is the first sound or "tapping" heard during cuff deflation
  - (1) Korotkoff 1 (K1)
  - (2) Occurs at the moment of ventricular systole
- (f) Diastolic BP is the disappearance of Korotkoff sounds (K5)
  - (1) Occurs at the end of ventricular diastole
- (g) Obtain baseline blood pressure measurements in both arms and one leg (note: leg pressures are generally 10 to 20 mm Hg higher)
- (h) Determine BP percentile based on age, gender, and height
- (i) If blood pressure is elevated
  - (1) Repeat on two additional separate occasions
  - (2) If elevation is severe or patient is symptomatic, an immediate workup is indicated

  **ii.** Ambulatory BP monitoring (Saarel, et al., 2004) (See Chapter 11 for details)

  **iii.** Plot height and weight on growth charts

  **iv.** Calculate body mass index (BMI) and plot on BMI charts for children ≥2 years

    **v.** Inspection

      (a) Assess for truncal obesity and acanthosis nigricans (sign of insulin resistance), which are components of metabolic syndrome

      (b) Assess for edema, café-au-lait spots, bruising (related to underlying renal disease or systemic disease)

      (c) Examine optic fundi for tortuosity, narrowing, hemorrhages, papilledema

    **vi.** Palpation

      (a) Thyroid gland for enlargement, masses

      (b) Abdomen for masses, bruits, enlarged kidneys

      (c) Assess presence or strength of femoral pulses

    **vii.** Auscultation

      (a) Thorough cardiac exam to include heart rate, rhythm, murmurs, or clicks

      (b) Carotid bruits

**e.** Diagnostic tests

    **i.** Laboratory

      (a) Blood urea nitrogen (BUN), creatinine, electrolytes, urinalysis to asses renal function

      (b) Urine culture to assess infection

      (c) CBC to assess anemia

      (d) Thyroid stimulating hormone TSH to assess thyroid function

      (e) Drug screen in patients with suspected substance abuse (i.e., cocaine or stimulants)

      (f) Plasma and urine catecholamines or plasma and urine steroid levels to rule out secondary causes in young children or in children with significant hypertension

      (g) Serum aldosterone (high), cortisol (normal), and renin (low) to diagnose primary hypertension

      (h) Fasting lipid profile to assess for dyslipidemia (additional risk factor)

    **ii.** X-rays, scans, etc.

      (a) Renal ultrasound to rule out congenital anomaly, hydronephrosis, or unequal renal size

      (b) Dynamic signal analyzer (DSA) scan, and/or scintigraphy (with or without angiotensin-converting enzyme [ACE] inhibition)

      (c) Renal magnetic resonance angiography (MRA) (best for abnormalities of main renal artery and its primary branches)

      (d) Newer computed tomography (CT) scan methods (3-D or spiral CT with contrast)

      (e) Angiography remains the "gold standard"

      (f) Polysomnography may be indicated in patients with a history of a sleep disorder

      (g) Echocardiogram to assess left ventricular hypertrophy

      (h) Retinal exam to look for end organ effects

      (i) Enhanced MRI (magnetic resonance imaging) or MIBG (Metaiodobenzylguanidine) scanning if pheochromocytoma is suspected

    **iii.** Recommendations for management and testing are based on the degree of BP elevation (National High Blood Pressure Education Program Working Group, 2004)

      (a) Prehypertension (90th to 95th percentile)

        (1) Lifestyle counseling (diet, exercise, no smoking)

        (2) Recheck BP in 6 months

        (3) Labs: fasting lipids and glucose only if overweight

        (4) In patients with known diabetes or kidney disease:

           a) Echocardiogram for LV hypertrophy

           b) Retinal exam

    (b) Stage 1 hypertension (95th to 5 mm Hg higher than the 99th percentile)

        (1) Recheck BP on two more visits with 1 to 2 weeks

        (2) Lifestyle counseling (diet and exercise)

        (3) Labs: BUN, creatinine, electrolytes, CBC, fasting lipid profile, glucose, urinalysis, urine culture

        (4) Referral to an expert within 1 month during which repeat measurements and diagnostic tests can be performed

           a) Renal ultrasound

           b) Echocardiogram for LV mass

           c) Retinal examination

           d) Additional lab or testing in young children with higher suspicion of secondary causes:

               i) Plasma and urine catecholamines and steroids

               ii) Additional renovascular imaging

  (c) Stage 2 hypertension (>5 mm Hg higher than the 99th percentile value)

        (1) Recheck BP within a week or immediately if symptomatic

        (2) Lifestyle counseling (diet and exercise)

        (3) All labs and tests from stage 1 evaluation are indicated

        (4) Prompt referral to an expert for evaluation and initiation of antihypertensive therapy (within 1 week)

**f.** Treatment

    **i.** No long-term studies available in children with treated versus untreated hypertension

    **ii.** Only a few medication trials in the pediatric population, and most provide only short-term data

    **iii.** Treatment guidelines and use of medications are mainly extrapolated from adult data

    **iv.** Initial management

      (a) Assess risk factors

      (b) Determine secondary cause of hypertension if present

      (c) Detect end organ effects such as increased LV mass

      (d) Counsel regarding lifestyle modification

      (e) DASH diet (Dietary Approach to Stop Hypertension) at www.DashForHealth.com

      (f) Heart-healthy diet

      (g) Reduced dietary sodium

      (h) Avoid or stop smoking

      (i) Encourage regular aerobic exercise

      (j) Indications for pharmacologic intervention

        (1) Evidence of end organ effects (i.e., increased LV mass)

        (2) Symptomatic hypertension

        (3) Secondary hypertension

        (4) Persistent hypertension despite lifestyle modifications

        (5) Presence of additional risk factors (i.e., diabetes)

      (k) Goal of therapy

        (1) To decrease blood pressure to less than the 95th percentile in healthy patients

(2) To decrease blood pressure to more than the 90th percentile in patients with evidence of end organ effects or those with additional risk factors such as diabetes or renal disease

(l) Classes of pharmacologic agents (Table 29-4)

(1) Thiazide diuretics

(2) ACE inhibitors—teratogenic

(3) ARBs (angiotensin receptor blockers)—teratogenic

(4) β-blockers

(5) Calcium channel blockers

(m) Initiation of therapy

(1) Start with the lowest recommended dose

(2) Current information on pediatric doses are summarized in the Fourth Report on the Diagnosis, Evaluation and Treatment of High Blood Pressure in Children and Adolescents, Table 9, http://pediatrics.aappublications. org/cgi/content/full/114/2/ S2/555

(3) Monitor response to therapy by BP monitoring and assessing "target organ" effects (i.e., LV mass)

(4) Lab values should be monitored as indicated for the particular pharmacologic agent

5. Signs and symptoms: prolonged fever, rash, red eyes, changes in the mucous membranes, changes in the extremities, lymphadenopathy

a. A high index of suspicion is required to diagnose Kawasaki disease in a timely manner to prevent coronary artery aneurysms (Newburger & Fulton, 2004)

i. Kawasaki disease is an inflammation of the blood vessels

■ **TABLE 29-4**
■ ■ **Common Agents for Treatment of Hypertension in Children in the Primary Care Setting**

| Drug Class | Drug Name | Notes | Relative Cost |
|---|---|---|---|
| Thiazide-type diuretics | Hydrochlorothiazide (HCTZ) (daily) | Monitor electrolytes periodically | $ |
| Angiotensin-converting enzyme (ACE) inhibitors | Captopril (tid) Enalopril (daily-bid) Lisinopril (daily) | Contraindicated in pregnancy First choice for children with ventricular dysfunction/heart failure Monitor potassium, creatinine | $$ |
| Angiotensin-receptor blockers | Losartan (daily) Irbesartan (daily) | Contraindicated in pregnancy Monitor potassium, creatinine | $$$ |
| Calcium channel blockers | Amlodipine (daily) Extended-release nifedipine (daily-bid) | May cause tachycardia | $$$ |
| β-blockers | Propranolol (daily) Atenolol (daily-bid) | May cause lethargy Decreases heart rate Should not be used with type 1 diabetes Noncardioselective β-blockers (propranolol) are contraindicated in asthma | $ |

      **ii.** It is a multisystem, acute, self-limiting disease

  **b.** Signs and symptoms

      **i.** Acute phase—fever begins and diagnostic criteria become evident; classic criteria include the following:

          (a) Bilateral conjunctivitis

             (1) Nonexudative

             (2) May have evidence of anterior uveitis by slit-lamp exam

          (b) Changes in mucous membranes

             (1) Lips may be cracked and erythematous

             (2) Erythema of the oropharynz

             (3) Generally no blisters in the mouth

             (4) "Strawberry tongue"

                a) Sloughing of thc filiform papillae

                b) Prominent fungiform papillae

          (c) Changes in the extremities

             (1) Hands and feet are swollen and beefy red

             (2) Periungual (fingertips and toes) desquamation occurs in week 2 or 3

          (d) Rash

             (1) Often accentuated in the groin with local desquamation

             (2) Never vesicular or bullous

          (e) Cervical lymphadenopathy

             (1) At least one lymph node >1.5 cm

             (2) Nonsuppurative

      **ii.** Associated signs and symptoms

          (a) Elevated sedimentation rate (resolves gradually over 6–8 weeks)

          (b) Elevated C-reactive protein

          (c) Anemia (can persist until the resolution of inflammation)

          (d) Elevated liver function tests

          (e) Thrombocytosis (peaks 2 to 3 weeks after onset of fever)

          (f) Elevated white blood cell count with a left shift, increased neutrophils

          (g) Low albumin

          (h) Urethritis with sterile pyuria: microscopic examination reveals mononuclear cells

          (i) Irritability (can persist for up to 8 weeks)

          (j) Aseptic meningitis

          (k) Joint pain

          (l) Arthritis (temporary)

          (m) Desquamation (approximately 2 to 3 weeks after onset of fever)

             (1) Periungual

             (2) Groin area

          (n) Vomiting

          (o) Abdominal pain

          (p) Diarrhea

          (q) Hydrops of the gallbladder

          (r) Sensorineural hearing loss (rare)

  **c.** Pathophysiology

      **i.** Inflammation of the blood vessels (vasculitis)

          (a) Acute, diffuse vasculitis of the small arteriolds, venules and medium-sized arteries throughout the body, with a predilection for the coronary arteries

(b) Bloodwork reflects increased inflammatory marker

(c) Symptoms reflect inflammation (liver, gall bladder, mucous membranes, skin)

ii. Inflammation of joints

(a) Small joint arthritis (30% of cases)

(b) Sometimes progresses to the large weight-bearing joints (temporary)

iii. Cardiac Complications

(a) Damage to the medium-sized arteries—with a predilection for the coronary arteries

(b) Coronary artery aneurysms occur in 20 to 25% of untreated children as a result of damage to the vessel wall

(c) In affected vessels, dilation occurs gradually and coronary artery dimensions reach their largest size approximately 4 weeks after illness onset

(d) Myocarditis is involved in most cases to some degree (usually subclinical; decreased left ventricular function on echocardiogram)

(e) Other cardiac issues may include valvular regurgitation (usually transient), pericarditis, effusions and ECG changes

iv. Thrombocytosis is common in the second and third week of illness, when platelet counts can climb to over 1 million

(a) Elevated platelet counts combined with a dilated, aneurysmal vessel

(b) Predisposes these children to coronary thrombosis and myocardial ischemia

(c) Symptoms of MI may be subtle, especially in young children, e.g., pallor, diaphoresis, vomiting, chest pain and/or pressure

d. Epidemiology of Kawasaki disease (Lane, et al., 2005)

i. Etiology

(a) Unknown

(b) No evidence of spread from person to person

(c) Some experts believe that Kawasaki disease may represent a final "common pathway" in response to a common illness in a genetically susceptible host

(d) A large family-based genotyping study of Kawasaki disease (Burns, et al., 2005)

(1) Included triads of a child with Kawasaki disease and both parents

(2) Suggested a genetic susceptibility related to the *IL-4* gene or regions linked to *IL-4*

ii. Prevalence and incidence

(a) In the United States, the incidence of Kawasaki disease is estimated from hospital discharge data because there is no required reporting of the illness

(b) An estimated 4248 hospitalizations associated with Kawasaki disease occurred in the year 2000 (Holman, et al., 2003)

(c) Kawasaki disease occurs in children of all racial groups, but it is markedly more prevalent in Japan and in children of Japanese ancestry

(d) Approximately 75% of children who develop Kawasaki disease are younger than age 5, with a median age of 2 years

(e) More common during the winter and early spring months

(f) Incidence of boys to girls is 1.5 to 1.7 : 1

(g) Siblings and twins have a higher risk of Kawasaki disease, suggesting that genetic factors may play a role in susceptibility (Newburger, et al. 2004)

(h) Associated with recent carpet cleaning, living near a stagnant body of water, higher socioeconomic background; no cause and effect has been established

iii. Morbidity

(a) Kawasaki disease now surpasses acute rheumatic fever as the leading cause of acquired heart disease in children in the United States and Japan

(b) Incidence of coronary artery aneurysms is highest in infants; however, recent data have also shown a higher incidence of coronary artery aneurysms in children older than 6 years (possibly related to late diagnosis)

(c) In Japan the recurrence rate is approximately 3% and approximately 1% in United States

iv. Mortality

(a) Overall mortality is 0.3% and is almost always related to cardiac effects of the illness

e. Focused history

i. Date that fever began

ii. Timing of appearance of signs and symptoms

f. Focused physical examination

i. Multisystem, with special attention to:

(a) HEENT

(b) Lymph nodes

(c) Skin

(d) Extremities

g. Diagnostic tests

i. Erythrocyte sedimentation rate (ESR)

ii. C-reactive protein (CRP)

iii. Complete blood count (CBC)

iv. Albumin

v. Blood culture

vi. Throat culture to rule out strep pharyngitis if suspected

vii. Liver function tests

viii. Ophthalmology examination (optional) to document the presence of anterior uveitis (may aid in the diagnosis of difficult cases)

ix. Echocardiogram to measure coronary artery dimensions, left ventricular function, valvular function, and the presence of pericardial effusion

(a) At the time of diagnosis

(b) 1 to 2 weeks later

(c) 4 to 6 weeks after illness onset

(d) More frequently as indicated

h. Diagnostic criteria (Box 29-3)

i. NOTE: Many patients with aneurysms never meet the diagnostic criteria

ii. Consider the diagnosis of Kawasaki Disease in any child with prolonged fever.

iii. Expected clinical features may not all be present at a single point in time

iv. American Heart Association (AHA) has published an algorithm to help guide testing and diagnosis of incomplete cases (Newberger, et al., 2004)

v. Watchful waiting is sometimes necessary before a diagnosis can be made

i. Differential diagnoses

i. Scarlet fever

ii. Toxic shock syndrome

■ **BOX 29-3**
■ **CLASSIC CLINICAL CRITERIA FOR DIAGNOSIS OF KAWASAKI DISEASE[1]**

- Fever persisting at least 4 to 5 days
- Presence of at least four of the following principal features[2]:
  - Changes in extremities
    - Acute: erythema of palms and soles, edema of hands and feet
    - Subacute: periungual peeling of fingers and toes in second and third week
  - Polymorphous exanthem
  - Bilateral bulbar conjunctival injection without exudate
  - Changes in the lips and oral cavity: erythema and cracking of lips, strawberry tongue, diffuse injection of oral and pharyngeal mucosa
  - Cervical lymphadenopathy (>1.5 cm in diameter), usually unilateral

[1] These criteria should be used as a guideline. Not all of the features need to be present at once. Atypical or incomplete Kawasaki disease should be considered in children with fewer than four features of criteria, prolonged fever, and no alternative diagnosis

[2] Children with fever for at least 5 days and fewer than four principal features can be diagnosed as having Kawasaki disease when coronary artery abnormalities are detected by two-dimensional echocardiography or angiography
Source: Newburger, J. W., Takahashi, M., Gerber, M. A., et al. (2004). Diagnosis, treatment, and long-term management of Kawasaki disease: A statement for health professionals. From the Committee on Rheumatic Fever, Endocarditis, and Kawasaki Disease, Council on Cardiovascular Disease in the Young, American Heart Association, Pediatrics, 2004, *114*(6), 1708–1733.

    **iii.** Staphylococcal scalded skin syndrome
    **iv.** Viral illnesses including adenovirus, measles, enterovirus, mononucleosis
    **v.** Bacterial adenitis
    **vi.** Juvenile rheumatoid arthritis
    **vii.** Rocky Mountain spotted fever
        (a) If the coronary artery measurements are normal at the 6-week echocardiogram, aspirin is discontinued and patients are seen at infrequent intervals (1 year and every 5 years)
**j.** Treatment and management
    **i.** See American Heart Association recommendations for the diagnosis, treatment and long-term management of Kawasaki disease (Newburger, et al., 2004)
    **ii.** Initial therapy goals
        (a) Decrease systemic inflammation
            (1) Fever duration is a strong predictor of coronary outcome; longer fever duration is associated with increased risk of aneurysm formation
        (b) Reduce the risk of aneurysm formation during the acute illness
    **iii.** Intravenous immunoglobulin (IVIG) therapy
        (a) Administer IVIG, 2 g/kg over 8 to 12 hours
        (b) Within the first 10 days of illness (counting the first day of fever as day 1)
        (c) IVIG shortens the duration of fever and decreases the risk of coronary artery aneurysms three- to fivefold
        (d) IVIG should still be administered after the tenth day of illness if the patient is still febrile, has signs or symptoms of inflammation and/or has coronary changes
        (e) Effectiveness (Fong, et al., 2004)
            (1) Very effective in the majority of cases

    (2) Approximately 10% of children have continual or recrudescent fever

   (f) Retreatment with same dose of IVIG is recommended if:

    (1) Fever is still present or patient has recrudescent (recurrent) fever 36 hours after treatment is completed

    (2) Coronary abnormalities develop

 iv. Aspirin therapy

  (a) Aspirin has been used historically in Kawasaki disease

  (b) In acute phase of illness, high doses of aspirin (80-100 mg/kg/day divided q6h) are used for its anti-inflammatory effect

   (1) Continue until afebrile for 48 hours

   (2) Use of aspirin does not lower the incidence of coronary abnormalities

  (c) Low dose aspirin (3-5 mg/kg/day) is used for its antiplatelet effect

   (1) Initiated after a 48-hour afebrile period

   (2) Discontinue 6 to 8 weeks after illness onset in patients without coronary abnormalities

 v. Antithrombotic therapy

  (a) Indicated in children with coronary artery aneurysms

  (b) Long-term antithrombotic therapy is required because of the risk of thrombosis in dilated vessels

  (c) Risk of thrombosis increases with the size of the aneurysm

  (d) Low-dose aspirin (3-5 mg/kg/day) remains the most common treatment

   (1) Additional medications may be added to aspirin, depending on the size of the coronary aneurysm(s)

   (2) Clopidogrel (Plavix) and dipyridamole (Persantine) have been used in conjunction with aspirin in patients with moderate-sized aneurysms

  (e) Children with giant aneurysms (>8 mm) are at the greatest risk of thrombosis

   (1) Usually started on heparin therapy

   (2) Long-term, these children are maintained on Coumadin and aspirin with an International Normalized Ratio (INR) goal of 2 to 2.5

  (f) Risks and benefits of each particular anticoagulation regimen are weighed on an individual basis

 vi. Additional therapies for children who do not respond to IVIG after two doses, and continue to have fever and/or enlarging coronary arteries

  (a) Because the numbers of children in this category are small, there are few studies to guide therapy

  (b) An expert to guide therapy should be consulted

 vii. Immunizations

  (a) For children on aspirin therapy

   (1) Require yearly influenza vaccine

   (2) Aspirin should be temporarily discontinued and substituted with another regimen for 6 weeks if the varicella vaccine is to be given

  (b) After high-dose IVIG therapy, live viral vaccines (MMR, varicella) should be deferred for 11 months

 viii. Long-term management issues (Baker, et al., 2003)

  (a) Parents of children with coronary aneurysms should be taught cardiopulmonary resuscitation (CPR)

  (b) Over years, damaged vessel walls may try to heal

(1) Healing occurs by myointimal proliferation, making the vessel walls thicker and less reactive than a normal vessel

(2) Stenoses can develop, especially at the distal ends of the aneurysm, increasing risk for MI

(3) These children may be at risk for premature atherosclerosis (Cheung, et al., 2004)

(c) Other conditions include valvular regurgitation (usually transient), pericarditis or effusions and ECG changes

(d) A heart-healthy lifestyle is recommended for all children to minimize their additional risk factors for coronary disease

(1) No smoking

(2) Screen cholesterol profile one year after illness

(3) Regular exercise for most children

(4) Heart healthy diet

ix. Prognosis

(a) Children are divided into five risk levels, depending on their coronary artery outcome to guide the frequency and type of follow-up:

(1) Level 1 includes children who never had any coronary abnormalities

a) Excellent prognosis

(2) Level 2 has transient dilation with normalization of measurements by the 6- to 8-week echocardiogram

(3) Level 3 has a small to medium aneurysm with no more than one aneurysm per coronary artery

(4) Level 4 has one or more giant or complex aneurysms in the same vessel, without obstruction

(5) Level 5 includes those children who have had coronary artery obstruction

(b) See AHA guidelines (Newburger, et al., 2004) for follow-up recommendations, some of which are managed by specialty physicians

6. Symptom and signs: sensation of rapid heart rate; heart rate too fast to count; in infants: poor feeding, pallor, diaphoresis

a. Supraventricular tachycardia (SVT) is the likely diagnosis (Kantoch, 2005)

i. Young and older children can report a sensation of unusually rapid heart rate

ii. However, the PNP must have a high index of suspicion to diagnose SVT in infants

b. Definition of SVT—ventricular rate in excess of the age-related normal ranges

c. Focused history, signs, and symptoms

i. Young and older children

(a) Tachycardia

(1) Occurs with a sudden onset and resolution

(2) Heart rate that is "too fast too count"

(3) Tends to occur at rest

(4) Not related to exercise

(5) Has no particular pattern

(b) Often older children complain of palpitations after completion of exercise

(c) Chest pain

(d) Presyncope

(e) Dizziness

(f) Light-headedness

        (g) Diaphoresis

        (h) Nausea

        (i) Possible orthostatic hypotension

        (j) Rarely have signs of congestive heart failure

    **ii.** Infant signs of SVT

        (a) Poor feeding

        (b) Pallor

        (c) Diaphoresis (due to a heightened catecholamine state)

        (d) Symptoms of congestive heart failure

           (1) Lethargy

           (2) Irritability

**d.** Focused physical assessment

    **i.** Physical examination results may be normal

    **ii.** Inspection—large jugular venous pulsations

    **iii.** Auscultate heart rate for full minute

        (a) Upper limits of normal are approximately:

           (1) Neonates to 1 year—180 beats per minute (BPM)

           (2) 1 to 3 years—150 BPM

           (3) 4 to 6 years—130 BPM

           (4) 7 to 10 years—110 BPM

           (5) ≥11 years—100 BPM

        (b) Tachycardia may be the only finding in children who are otherwise healthy and have significant hemodynamic reserve

        (c) Children who have limited hemodynamic reserve may be tachypneic and hypotensive

        (d) An $S_3$ may be present

    **iv.** Auscultate the lungs—crackles may be heard secondary to heart failure

    **v.** Attend to ruling out other disease processes that can explain an adaptive arrhythmia, such as:

        (a) Sinus tachycardia

        (b) Infection and/or fever:

           (1) Infants can manifest sinus rhythm rates as high as 230 to 240 BPM

           (2) Young children up to 200 BPM

           (3) Teenagers up to 180 BPM

           (4) Heart rates above these parameters during infection or fever generally indicate a rhythm abnormality

        (c) Anemia

        (d) Endocrine problems

**e.** Differential diagnosis

    **i.** Primary care PNPs may diagnose an SVT, but further diagnosis and treatment should be referred to a pediatric cardiac specialist

    **ii.** See Box 29-4 for potential diagnoses

**f.** Treatment

    **i.** Managed by the emergency department or cardiac specialists

    **ii.** Acute episodes

        (a) Vagal maneuvers

        (b) Adenosine

        (c) Verapamil

        (d) Propranolol

        (e) Cardioversion

    **iii.** Chronic SVT management

■ **BOX 29-4**
■ **MECHANISMS OF THE DEVELOPMENT OF SUPRAVENTRICULAR TACHYCARDIA (SVT)**

| | |
|---|---|
| Wolff-Parkinson-White syndrome | Sinus node reentry |
| Concealed Wolff-Parkinson-White syndrome | Intra-atrial reentry |
| | Typical AV node reentry |
| Mahaim fibers tachycardia (nodoventricular) | Atypical AV node reentry |
| | Atrial flutter |
| Permanent junctional reciprocating tachycardia | Atrial fibrillation |
| | Atrial ectopic |
| Antidromic tachycardia | Chaotic atrial |
| Atriohisian pathway | Junctional ectopic |

      (a) Antiarrhythmic agents
      (b) Radiofrequency catheter ablation
  **g.** Prognosis (Ganz & Gugneja, 2005)
      **i.** Prognosis depends on the underlying structural heart disease
      **ii.** Children with symptomatic Wolff-Parkinson-White (WPW) syndrome have a small, but real, risk of sudden death
      **iii.** Children with episodic SVT, but a structurally normal heart, have an excellent prognosis
**7.** Signs and symptoms: fever, painful joints, rash, swollen lymph nodes, muscle weakness
  **a.** Any combination of these signs and symptoms calls for investigation of the diagnosis of acute rheumatic fever (ARF) (Blosser & Freitas-Nichols, 2004; Goodhue & Brady, 2004)
  **b.** Definition—systemic connective tissue disease
      **i.** Prodromal stage—group A β-hemolytic streptococci (GABHS) infection
      **ii.** Acute stage—inflammation of heart, joints, CNS, skin and subcutaneous tissues
      **iii.** Sequelae—rheumatic heart disease, damage and scarring of the mitral valve, CHF
      **iv.** Recurrent—may recur after a subsequent GABHS infection
  **c.** Prevalence and etiology
      **i.** ARF occurs mostly in children ages 5 to 15 years
      **ii.** Develops in 0.2 to 2 per 100,000 children who had a GABHS infection
      **iii.** Develops in 0.2 % to 0.3% of children who were not treated for GABHS infection
      **iv.** Chances of recurrent ARF with a subsequent GABHS infection are 50%
      **v.** ARF is a complication of a GABHS infection of the pharynx or tonsils
         (a) Untreated or partially treated
         (b) Latent period of 10 to 20 days after the infection
         (c) Evidence of progressive symptoms appears about 3 to 5 weeks after the infection
      **vi.** Evidence of genetic susceptibility
  **d.** Symptoms and signs (Box 29-5)
      **i.** Incidence of some manifestations:
         (a) Arthritis of large joints—65%
         (b) Carditis—50%
         (c) Chorea—15% to 30%
         (d) Cutaneous nodules—5%
         (e) Subcutaneous nodules—less than 7%

      ii. Erythema marginatum
         (a) Evanescent, macular lesions
         (b) Appear in a snakelike pattern on trunk and proximal aspects of the extremities
         (c) Change to clear in center and red on the margins
         (d) Develop, then disappear in minutes or hours
  **e.** Focused history
      **i.** History of sore throat, tonsillitis
      **ii.** Treated or untreated with antibiotics
      **iii.** Previous history of ARF
  **f.** Focused physical examination
      **i.** Inspection
         (a) Skin, especially trunk and extremities
         (b) Motor behavior
      **ii.** Auscultate
         (a) Heart
         (b) Lungs

■ **BOX 29-5**
■ **JONES CRITERIA FOR RHEUMATIC FEVER**

**EVIDENCE OF PRECEDING GABHA INFECTION**
Positive throat culture or rapid streptococcal antigen test result; elevated or rising streptococcal antibody titer

**MINOR MANIFESTATIONS**
Arthralgia; fever; elevated acute-phase reactants; elevated erythrocyte sedimentation rate; elevated C-reactive protein

**MAJOR MANIFESTATIONS**
CARDITIS
Tachycardia out of proportion to degree of fever; cardiomegaly; new murmurs or change in preexisting murmurs; muffled heart sounds; precordial friction rub; precordial pain; changes in electrocardiogram (esp. prolonged PR interval)

POLYARTHRITIS
Swollen, hot, red, painful joints; after 1-2 days, affects different joints (migratory); favors large joints (knees, elbows, hips, shoulders, wrists)

ERYTHEMA MARGINATUM
Erythematous macules with clear center and wavy, well-demarcated border; transitory; nonpruritic; primarily affects trunk and extremities (inner surfaces)

CHOREA
Sudden, aimless, irregular movements of extremities; involuntary facial grimaces; speech disturbances or emotional lability; muscle weakness (can be profound); muscle movements exaggerated by anxiety and attempt at fine motor activity; relieved by rest

SUBCUTANEOUS NODES
Nontender swelling; located over bony prominence; may persist for some time and then gradually resolve

From Dajani AS et al: Guidelines for the diagnosis of rheumatic fever: Jones criteria, updated 1992, Circulation 87:302-307, 1993.
*The presence of two major or one major and two or more minor criteria with evidence of preceding group A β-hemolytic streptococcal (GABHS) infection indicates a high probability of rheumatic fever.

      **iii.** Palpate

         (a) Joints

         (b) Skin

         (c) Muscle strength

         (d) Bony prominences

  **g.** Diagnostic tests

      **i.** Rapid strep test during acute phase—positive

      **ii.** Throat culture—two thirds may be negative during

      **iii.** Antistreptolysin (ASO) test—elevated

      **iv.** Acute phase reactants

         (a) Erthyrocyte sedimentation rate (ESR)—elevated

         (b) CRP—elevated

      **v.** Chest x-ray

      **vi.** Echocardiogram

  **h.** Diagnosis

      **i.** Differential diagnosis

         (a) ARF

         (b) Juvenile arthritis

         (c) Systemic lupus erythematosus

         (d) Infective endocarditis

         (e) Lyme disease

      **ii.** Diagnosis of ARF is based on Jones criteria (see Box 29-5)

         (a) Evidence of preceding GABHS infection is required, plus:

         (b) Two major criteria met, or

         (c) One major and two minor criteria met

  **i.** Treatment (see Chapter 54, Table 54-3 for details on medications)

      **i.** Antibiotic therapy

         (a) Benzathine penicillin G intramuscular is antibiotic of choice

         (b) Erythromycin if child is allergic to penicillin

      **ii.** Antiinflammatory therapy

         (a) Aspirin for arthritis

         (b) Corticosteroids for severe carditis

      **iii.** Refer to cardiac specialist for CHF symptoms

      **iv.** Bed rest for severe carditis and CHF, or if severe chorea develops

  **j.** Prevention of ARF

      **i.** Initial ARF: treat GABHS pharyngitis with penicillin V or erythromycin

      **ii.** Recurrent ARF

         (a) Treat children with history of ARF and new GABHS infection with benzathine penicillin G intramuscular every 2 to 28 days

         (b) Prophylactic antibiotic for 3 to 5 years if transient cardiac involvement; lifelong if persistent cardiac involvement

         (c) Additional prophylactic antibiotic before de ntal or surgical procedures to prevent bacterial endocarditis

---

# REFERENCES

Baker, A. L., Gauvreau, K., Newburger, J. W., et al. (2003). Physical and psychosocial health in children who have had Kawasaki disease. *Pediatrics, 111*(3), 579-583.

Basso, C., Maron, B.J., Corrado, D., & Thiene, G. (2000). Clinical profile of congenital coronary artery anomalies with origin from the wrong aortic sinus leading to sudden death in young competitive athletes. *J Am Coll Cardiol, 35* (6), 1493-1501.

Belay, B., Belamarich, P., & Racine, A. D. (2004). Pediatric precursors of adult atherosclerosis. *Pediatr Rev, 25*, 4-16.

Blosser, C. G., & Freitas-Nichols, J. (2004). Cardiovascular disorders. In C. E. Burns, A. M. Dunn, M. A. Brady, et al. (Eds.). *Pediatric primary care: A handbook for nurse practitioners* (3rd ed.).Philadelphia: Saunders, pp. 769-810.

Burns, J. C., Shimizu, C., Shike, H., et al. (2005). Family-based association analysis implicates IL-4 in susceptibility to Kawasaki disease. *Genes Immun, 6*(5), 438-444.

Cheung, Y. F., Yung, T. C., Tam, S. C., et al. (2004). Novel and traditional cardiovascular risk factors in children after Kawasaki disease: Implications for premature atherosclerosis. *J Am Coll Cardiol, 43*(1), 120-124.

Chobanian, A. V., Bakris, G. L., Black, H. R., et al. (2003). Seventh report of the Joint National Committee on Prevention, Detection, Evaluation, and Treatment of High Blood Pressure. *Hypertension, 42*, 1206-1252.

Connolly, S. J., Sheldon, R., Thorpe, K. E., et al. (2003). Pacemaker therapy for prevention of syncope in patients with recurrent severe vasovagal syncope: Second Vasovagal Pacemaker Study (VPS II): A randomized trial. *JAMA, 289*(17), 2224-2229.

de Ferranti, S. D., Gauvreau, K., Ludwig, D. S., et al. (2004). Prevalence of the metabolic syndrome in American adolescents: Findings from the Third National Health and Nutrition Examination Survey. *Circulation, 110*, 2494-2497.

DiMario, F. J., Jr. (2001a). Breath-holding spells and pacemaker implantation. *Pediatrics, 108*(3), 765-766.

DiMario F. J., Jr. (2001b). Prospective study of children with cyanotic and pallid breath-holding spells. *Pediatrics, 107*(2), 265-269.

Evangelista, J. A., Parsons. M., & Renneburg, A. K. (2000). Chest pain in children: Diagnosis through history and physical examination. *J Pediatr Health Care, 14*(1), 3-8.

Flevari, P. P., Livanis, E. G., Theodorakis, G. N., et al. (2002). Baroreflexes in vasovagal syncope: two types of abnormal response. *Pacing Clin Electrophysiol, 25*(9), 1315-1323.

Flynn, J. T. (2002). Differentiation between primary and secondary hypertension in children using ambulatory blood pressure monitoring. *Pediatrics, 110*(1), 89-93.

Fong, N. C., Hui, Y. W., Li, C. K., & Chiu, M. C. (2004). Evaluation of the efficacy of treatment of Kawasaki disease before day 5 of illness. *Pediatr Cardiol, 25*(1), 31-34.

Ganz, L., & Gugneja, M. (2005). *Paroxysmal supraventricular tachycardia.* Retrieved August 31, 2005, from www.emedicine.com/med/topic1762.htm#section~follow-up.

Goodhue, C. J., & Brady, M. A. (2004). Atopic disorders and rheumatic diseases. In C. E. Burns, A. M. Dunn, M. A. Brady, et al. (Eds.). *Pediatric primary care: A handbook for nurse practitioners* (3rd ed.). Philadelphia: Saunders, pp. 587-621.

Hamer, A. W., & Bray, J. E. (2005). Clinical recognition of neurally mediated syncope. *Intern Med J, 35*(4), 2160-221.

Holman, R. C., Curns, A. T., Belay, E. D., et al. (2003). Kawasaki syndrome hospitalizations in the United States, 1997 and 2000. *Pediatrics, 112*(3), 495-501.

Hopkins, P.N. (2003). Familial hypercholesterolemia—Improving treatment and meeting guidelines. *Int J Cardiol, 89*, 13-23.

Inglefinger, J. R. (2004). Pediatric antecedents of adult cardiovascular disease—Awareness and intervention. *N Engl J Med, 350*(21), 2123-2126.

Institute for Clinical Systems Improvement (ICSI). (2004). *Lipid screening in children and adolescents.* Bloomington, MN: ICSI.

Kantoch, M. J. (2005). Supraventricular tachycardia in children. *Indian J Pediatr, 72*(7), 609-619.

Kapoor, W. N. (2003). Is there an effective treatment for neurally-mediated syncope? *JAMA, 289*(17), 2272-2275.

Kelly, A. M., Porter, C. J., McGoon, M. D., et al. (2001) Breath-holding spells associated with significant bradycardia: Successful treatment with permanent pacemaker implantation. *Pediatrics, 108*(3), 698-702.

Kouakam, C., Vaksmann, G., Pachy, E., et al. (2000). Long-term follow-up of children and adolescents with syncope; predictor of syncope recurrence. *European Heart Journal, 22*(17), 1618-1625.

Lane, S. E., Watts, R., & Scott, D. G. (2005). Epidemiology of systemic vasculitis. *Curr Rheumatol Rep, 7*(4), 270-275.

Lurbe, E., & Redon, J. (2002). Reproducibility and validity of ambulatory blood pressure monitoring in children. *American Journal of Hypertension, 15* (2 Pt 2), 69S-73S.

Lutwick, L. I., & Ravishankar, J. (2005). *Rheumatic fever.* Retrieved September 1, 2005, from www.emedicine.com/med/topic3435.htm.

Mansour, K.A., Thourani, V.H., Odessey, F.A. et al. (2003). Pectus deformities of the anterior chest wall. *Ped Resp* Red, 4(3), 237.

Maron, B.J. (2003). Sudden death in young athletes. *N Engl J Med 349*, 1064-1075.

Marais, A. D., Firth, J. C., & Blom, D. J. (2004). Homozygous familial hypercholesterolemia and its management. *Semin Vasc Med, 4*(1), 35-42.

Massin, M. (2003). Neurocardiogenic syncope in children: "Current concepts in diagnosis and management. *Paediatr Drug, 5*(5), 327-334.

McCrindle, B. W., Ose, L., & Marais, A. D. (2003). Efficacy and safety of atorvastatin in children and adolescents with familial hypercholesterolemia or severe hyperlipidemia: A multicenter, randomized, placebo-controlled trial. *J Pediatr 143*, 74-80.

Miller, T. H., & Kruse, J. E. (2005). Evaluation of syncope. *Am Fam Phys, 72*(8), 1492-1502.

Morel, K., & Bye, M. R. (2000). Solving the puzzle of pediatric chest pain. *J Resp Dis Pediatr, 2*, 66-75.

Morgenstern, B. (2002). Blood pressure, hypertension, and ambulatory blood pressure monitoring in children and adolescents. *Am J Hypertens, 15* (2 Pt 2),:64S-66S.

Muntner, P., He, J., & Cutler, J. A. (2005). Trends in blood pressure among children and adolescents. *JAMA, 291*(17), 2107-2113.

National High Blood Pressure Education Program Working Group on High Blood Pressure in Children and Adolescents: The Fourth Report on the Diagnosis, Evaluation, and Treatment of High Blood Pressure in Children and Adolescents. *Pediatrics, 114*, 555-576.

Newburger, J. W., & Fulton, D. R. (2004). Kawasaki disease. *Curr Opin Pediatr, 16*(5), 508-514.

Newburger, J. W., Takahashi, M., Gerber, M. A., et al. (2004). Diagnosis, treatment, and long-term management of Kawasaki disease: A statement for health professionals. From the Council of Cardiovascular Disease in the Young, Committee on Rheumatic Fever, Endocarditis and Kawasaki Disease. *Circulation, 110*, 2747-2771. Also published in *Pediatrics*, 2004, *114*(6),1708-1733.

Nicklas, T. A., von Duvillard, S. P., & Berenson, G. S. (2002). Tracking of serum lipids and lipoproteins from childhood to dyslipidemia in adults: The Bogalusa Heart Study. *Int J Sports Med, 23*(Suppl 1), S39-S43.

Pantell, R. H., & Goodman, B. W. (2004). Adolescent chest pain: A prospective study. *Pediatrics, 71*, 881887.

Park, M. K., Menard, S. W., & Yuan, C. (2001). Comparison of auscultatory and oscillometric blood pressures. *Arch Pediatr Adolesc Med, 155*, 50-53.

Rhee, H. (2005). Relationships between physical symptoms and pubertal development. *J Pediatr Health Care, 19*(2), 95-103.

Saarel, E. V., Stefanelli, C. B., Fischbach, P. S., et al. (2004) Transtelephonic electrocardiographic monitors for evaluation of children and adolescents with suspected arrhythmias. *Pediatrics, 113*(2), 248-251.

Shulman, S. T. (2003). Is there a role for corticosteroids in Kawasaki disease? *J Pediatr, 142*(6), 601-603.

Soteriades, E. S., Evans, J. C., Larson, M. G., et al. (2002). Incidence and prognosis of syncope. *N Engl J Med, 347*(12), 878-885.

Varda, N. M., & Gregoric, A. (2005). A diagnostic approach for the child with hypertension. *Pediatr Nephrol, 20*(4), 499-506.

Wiegman, A., Rodenburg, J., de Jongh, S., et al. (2003). Family history and cardiovascular risk in familial hypercholesterolemia: Data in more than 1000 children. *Circulation 107*, 1473-1478.

Williams, C. L., Hayman, L. L., Daniels, S. R., et al. (2002). Cardiovascular health in childhood: A statement for health professionals from the Committee on Atherosclerosis, Hypertension, and Obesity in the Young (AHOY) of the Council on Cardiovascular Disease in the Young, American Heart Association. *Circulation, 106*, 143-160.

Yildirim, A., Karakurt, C., Karademir, S., et al. (2004). Chest pain in children. *Int. Pediatr., 19*(3), 175-179.

# Common Illness of the Gastrointestinal System

LEIGH SMALL, PhD, RN, CPNP

1. Sign: poor weight gain
   a. Failure to thrive (FTT)
      i. Definition: malnutrition and inadequate physical growth (Krugman & Dubowitz, 2003)
      ii. A decline on weight-for-age growth chart across two centiles or below the second centile for at least 3 months (Ammaniti, et al., 2004)
      iii. Other criteria are also used: less than fifth percentile, less than third percentile
      iv. Two general types used historically, but in fact most cases are a combination of both
         (a) Organic FTT—due to physiologic pathology
         (b) Nonorganic (NOFTT)—no physiologic pathology is found
      v. Pathophysiology and differential diagnoses (Krugman & Dubowitz, 2003)
         (a) Inadequate caloric intake—negligence, poverty, incorrect preparation of formula, behavior problems, disturbed parent-child relationship (see Chapter 21 related to child neglect)
         (b) Inadequate absorption, e.g., cystic fibrosis (CF), celiac disease, cow's milk protein allergy, vitamin or mineral deficiencies, biliary atresia
         (c) Excess metabolic demand—hyperthyroidism, chronic infection, renal disease, hypoxemia from congenital heart disease (CHD), or chronic lung disease
         (d) Defective utilization—genetic abnormalities, congenital infections, metabolic disorders
      vi. Etiology is multifactorial; theories include:
         (a) Dysfunctional mother-child feeding interactions (Ammaniti, et al., 2004)
            (1) Theory—feeding is a fundamental factor in development of the mother-infant relationship and stabilization of the infant's biologic rhythms
            (2) In a controlled study of 333 mother-child pairs, feeding interactions were videotaped and analyzed for affective state of mother,

interactional conflict, child's food refusal behaviors, and affective state of the dyad

(3) Compared with control mothers:

a) Mothers of NOFTT children showed significantly more negative affect, lower ability to interpret infant cues

b) The NOFTT dyad communications were significantly more conflictual, noncollaborative, and nonempathic

c) NOFTT children showed more food refusal behaviors, poorer nutritional intake, and difficulty with state regulation during meals

(b) Extremes of parental attention, i.e., negligence or hypervigilance (Krugman & Dubowitz, 2003)

(c) Maternal depression (O'Brien, et al., 2004)

(1) Theory—depression affects quality of maternal-child interaction, which has a negative effect on infant feeding

(2) In a controlled study of 763 children, mothers of NOFTT children were significantly more depressed (21.4% vs. 11.1%) than mothers of control children

**vii.** Focused history and physical as shown in Chapter 8, with special attention to potential pathophysiologic mechanisms and associated differential diagnoses listed previously

(a) Other focus areas (Krugman & Dubowitz, 2003)

(1) Calculate degree of malnutrition; compare current weight with expected weight at the 50th percentile; Gomez criteria:

a) Less than 60% of expected—severe FTT

b) 61% to 75%—moderate FTT

c) 76% to 90%—mild FTT

(2) Assess diet and feeding patterns in detail

(3) Arrange to observe a feeding interaction between mother and infant suspected of having NOFTT

(4) Developmental assessment—delays are common

**viii.** Treatment

(a) For catch-up growth, increase caloric intake to 150% of normal requirement

(b) Referral to a multidisciplinary team may be needed to work successfully with child and parents

**ix.** Prognosis

(a) Infants with NOFTT are at risk for short stature, behavior problems, developmental delay

2. Signs: infant irritability, inconsolable crying

   **a.** Differential diagnoses (Box 30-1)

   **b.** Focused history and physical as shown in Chapter 8, with special attention to differential diagnoses (Boynton, et al., 2003; Fox, 2003; Mulligan, et al., 2003; Schwartz, 2003)

   **c.** Infantile colic (Petersen-Smith, 2004) (See Chapter 19)

   **i.** Presentation

   (a) Definition—an apparently healthy infant less than 3 months of age who experiences episodes of paroxysmal severe crying lasting greater than 3 hours, three or more times a week

   (b) Other signs and symptoms include demanding frequent feedings, fussy while feeding, excessive gas, inconsolable, tense

   **ii.** See Chapter 19 for other details about colic

■ **BOX 30-1**
■ **DIFFERENTIAL DIAGNOSES FOR INFANT IRRITABILITY AND INCONSOLABLE CRYING**

Normal crying
Infantile colic
GI tract disturbances/intestinal obstruction
- Gastroesophageal reflux disease (GERD)
- Formula intolerance, sensitivity, or allergy
- Breast-feeding mother's intake of substances and foods
- Gastroenteritis
- Constipation
- Flatus
- Overfeeding/underfeeding
- Hirschsprung's disease
- Malrotation/volvulus
- Intussusception
- Pyloric stenosis
- Meckel's diverticulum
- Incarcerated hernia

Testicular torsion
Infectious diseases
- Otitis media
- Sepsis
- Meningitis
- Increased intracranial pressure
- Peritoneal infection
- URI or other infection
- Pyelonephritis/UTI

Trauma
- Corneal abrasion
- Child abuse
- Unobserved injury
- Head injury
- Lead toxicity
- Drug reaction (i.e., immunizations)

    iii. Treatment

        (a) Tell parents that you recognize that the stress of having an infant with colic is often severe

            (1) Acknowledge that they are likely to feel angry, hostile, and guilty

            (2) Tell them that the risk of abuse is increased with colicky infants

            (3) Introduce them to the National Center for Shaken Baby Syndrome website (2006) and the Period of PURPLE Crying document for advice

                a) Based on years of research of normal, healthy infants

                b) P = peak, U = unpredictability, R = resistance to soothing, P = painlike expression, L = long crying bouts, E = evening

        (b) Offer parent support by frequent phone calls until resolved—emphasize that:

            (1) Infant is healthy

            (2) It is a fairly common problem

            (3) Infant is not rejecting the parent

            (4) Symptoms *will* go away

(5) It is normal for parent to feel varied emotions, including fear, sadness, anger, helplessness

(c) Consistency in care provision and routines

(d) Establish sleep routines

(e) Comforting and soothing techniques

(1) Some infants with colic are soothed by repetitive sounds or motion

(f) Reduce stimulation

(g) Trial of different formulas—this is controversial because research shows effectiveness in only about 5% of infants with colic

(h) Change in feeding techniques

(1) Feed slowly

(2) Burp frequently

(3) Recognize infant cues of satiety

(4) Avoid overfeeding

(i) Medications have not been shown to be effective

(j) A study of PNP and pediatrician beliefs and management strategies for colic showed that PNPs were more likely to use behavioral and environmental approaches than pediatricians (Lobo, et al., 2004)

iv. Prognosis—typically resolves abruptly or gradually to 6 months of age

3. Symptoms: nausea, vomiting and/or diarrhea (Boynton, et al., 2003; Fox, 2003; Mulligan, et al., 2003; Schwartz, 2003)

a. Vomiting accounts for more than 3 million ambulatory pediatric visits each year

b. Nausea is an unpleasant psychic sensation that one might vomit

c. Reflux is passage of gastric contents into the esophagus

d. Regurgitation is passage of refluxed gastric contents into the oropharynx

e. Vomiting is the forceful ejection of gastric contents out of the mouth

i. Physical, psychic, and environmental circumstances stimulate the bilateral chemoreceptor trigger zones in the brainstem, which signal the bilateral vomition centers in the reticular formation of the medulla

ii. These mechanisms then result in vomiting

iii. Differential diagnoses for vomiting (Box 30-2)

iv. Focused history and physical as shown in Chapter 8, with special attention to differential diagnoses

v. Treatment

(a) Identify and eliminate the cause of vomiting

(b) Correction of dehydration and electrolyte imbalance are of primary concern with infants and children with vomiting (see section 3.g. below)

f. Diarrhea (Berman, 2003; Petersen-Smith, 2004; Sears, 2005)

i. Definition—increase in frequency, volume and/or liquidity of stool

ii. Presentation

(a) Acute

(1) Loss of stool more than 10g/kg/day in infants, more than 200 g/day in children

(2) An episode lasting less than 2 weeks

(3) Accounts for 20% of acute care office visits in children younger than 2 years

(b) Chronic

(1) One or more liquid to semiliquid stools per day for more than 2 weeks

(2) Intermittent or continuous episodes more than 3 weeks

■ **BOX 30-2**
■ **DIFFERENTIAL DIAGNOSES ASSOCIATED WITH NAUSEA AND VOMITING**

**INFECTIOUS/INFLAMMATORY**
- Acute gastroenteritis
- Sepsis
- Posttussive/allergy
- Otitis media
- Esophagitis/gastritis
- Ulcer disease
- Hepatitis
- Peritonitis
- Appendicitis
- Cholecystitis
- Pancreatitis
- Meningitis
- CNS abscess
- Subdural effusion
- Empyema
- Sexually transmitted infections

**CONGENITAL**
- Pyloric stenosis
- GI obstruction
- Imperforate anus
- Hirschsprung's disease
- Malrotation/volvulus
- Meconium ileus/plug
- Hydrocephalus

**PSYCHOLOGIC**
- Attention getting
- Hysterical/hyperventilation
- Conditioned
- Odors, visual stimuli

**NEOPLASTIC**
- GI tract
- Intracerebral

**TOXIC INGESTIONS**
- Salicylates
- Iron
- Lead
- Digitalis

**VASCULAR**
- Migraine
- Hypertensive encephalopathy

**ENDOCRINE/METABOLIC**
- Acidosis
- Diabetic ketoacidosis
- Uremia
- Inborn errors of metabolism
- Addison's disease

**MISCELLANEOUS**
- Cyclic vomiting syndrome (Bullard & Page, 2005)
- Incarcerated inguinal hernia
- Chalasia
- Ascites
- Pregnancy
- Epilepsy
- Hyperthermia
- Superior mesenteric artery syndrome

**TRAUMA**
- Concussion
- Subdural hematoma
- Foreign body
- Duodenal hematoma
- Ruptured viscus
- Subarachnoid hemorrhage
- Cerebral edema

   iii. Pathophysiology
     (a) Osmotic—excess fluid absorbed into intestine
     (b) Secretory—inhibition of ion absorption or stimulation of ion excretion
     (c) Motility disorders
     (d) Inflammatory processes
     (e) Dehydration may lead to acidosis, cardiovascular collapse, and death
   iv. Differential diagnoses for diarrhea (Box 30-3)
    v. Focused history and physical as shown in Chapter 8, with special attention to differential diagnoses
   vi. Treatment
     (a) Identify and eliminate the cause of diarrhea
     (b) Correction of dehydration and electrolyte imbalance is of primary concern with infants and children with diarrhea

■ **BOX 30-3**
■ **DIFFERENTIAL DIAGNOSES FOR DIARRHEA**

**ACUTE-ONSET DIARRHEA**
ACUTE GASTROENTERITIS
*Bacterial Pathogens*
- Salmonella
- Shigella
- *Campylobacter jejuni*
- *Escherichia coli*
- Shiga toxin-producing *E. coli*
- Yersinia
- Vibrio
- Aeromonas
- *Clostridium difficile*
- *Clostridium perfringens*
- *Listeria monocytogenes*

*Viral Pathogens*
- Rotavirus
- Norwalk
- Adenovirus
- Calicivirus
- Astrovirus
- Coronavirus

*Protozoal and Parasitic Pathogens*
- *Giardia lamblia*
- *Cryptosporidium parvum*
- *Entamoeba histolytica*
- *Clyclospora*
- *Isospora belli*
- *Strongyloides stercoralis*

**PERSISTENT AND/OR CHRONIC ONSET DIARRHEA**
FOOD ASSOCIATED
- Cow's milk or soy intolerance (allergic enterocolitis)
- Breast milk allergy
- Other food induced small bowel disturbances
- Celiac disease

**INTRACTABLE DIARRHEA OF INFANCY**
- Excessive fluids
- Low-fat, high-carbohydrate diet
- Stress and anxiety

**IRRITABLE BOWEL SYNDROME**

**INFLAMMATORY BOWEL DISEASE**
- Crohn's disease
- Ulcerative colitis

**HIRSCHSPRUNG'S DISEASE**

    (c) Bland, soft foods for 24 to 48 hours after rehydration; avoid fats, sweets

    (d) Antidiarrheal medications are not recommended

**g.** Dehydration and electrolyte imbalance

    **i.** Water and electrolyte balance is more tenuous in infants and young children for several reasons (Petersen-Smith, 2004)

        (a) Greater fluid intake and output relative to size

        (b) Greater amount of extracellular fluid (ECF) than intracellular fluid (ICF)

        (c) ECF has more sodium and chloride than ICF

    **ii.** Evaluate the extent of dehydration (Table 30-1)

        (a) Assessment of skin not very useful in children less than 2 years old

        (b) Percent of dehydration = (usual weight − current weight)/usual weight × 100

        (c) Lab tests to evaluate hydration and electrolyte balance (Table 30-2)

**h.** Treatment of fluid and electrolyte imbalance

    **i.** Rehydration

        (a) Calculation of fluid deficit volume

            (1) Total fluid deficit = child's ideal body weight in kilograms × 1000 × % dehydration

            (2) Give the first half of the fluid replacement over 8 hours and the second half over the next 16 hours

            (3) This fluid is given in addition to maintenance fluid requirements

■ **TABLE 30-1**
■ ■ **Intensity of Clinical Signs Associated with Varying Degrees of Isotonic Dehydration in infants**

| | Degree of Dehydration | | |
|---|---|---|---|
| | **Mild** | **Moderate** | **Severe** |
| Fluid volume loss | < 50 ml/kg | 50–90 ml/kg | ≥ 100 ml/kg |
| Skin color | Pale | Gray | Mottled |
| Skin elasticity | Decreased | Poor | Very poor |
| Mucous membranes | Dry | Very dry | Parched |
| Urinary output | Decreased | Oliguria | Marked oliguria and azotemia |
| Blood pressure | Normal | Normal or lowered | Lowered |
| Pulse | Normal or increased | Increased | Rapid and thready |
| Capillary filling time | < 2 seconds | 2–3 seconds | > 3 seconds |

From Hockenberry, M., Wilson, D., Winkelstein, M. L., et al. (2003). Wong's nursing care of infants and children (7th ed.),. p. 1178. Table 28-3.

   (b) Components of solutions occasionally used, but not recommended, for oral rehydration (Table 30-3)
   (c) Components of recommended oral rehydration solutions (Table 30-4)
      (1) Rehydrating solutions should be 75 to 90 mmol/L of sodium
      (2) Maintenance fluid should be 4 to 60 mmol/L of sodium
      (3) Recommended potassium concentration is 20 mEq/L
      (4) Carbohydrate to sodium ratios should not exceed 2:1 in maintenance or rehydration solutions (glucose ≤20 g/L)
      (5) Contraindications for oral rehydration include:
         a) Inability to take PO fluids
         b) Ongoing water losses more than 5 mL/kg/hr for more than 8 to 12 hours
         c) Severe metabolic acidosis (<16 mEq/L)
      (6) Child should be NPO for 1 to 2 hours before starting rehydration
   (d) Half of the fluid deficit should be replaced in the first 8 hours and the remainder over 16 hours
   (e) Mild dehydration
      (1) 5% fluid loss, or 50 mL/kg
      (2) Oral rehydrating solution 40 to 50 mL/kg over 4 hours (10 mL/k/hr)
      (3) Suggestion: give 5 to 15 mL every 5 to 10 minutes orally
   (f) Moderate dehydration
      (1) 5% to 10% fluid loss, or 100 mL/kg
      (2) Oral rehydrating solution 60 to 100 mL/kg over 4 to 6 hours (20 mL/kg/hr)
      (3) Suggestion: give 5 to 15 mL every 5 to 10 minutes orally
   (g) Severe dehydration
      (1) 11% to 15% fluid loss, or 150 mL/kg
      (2) Immediate hospitalization and IV fluids
 **ii.** Maintenance of balanced fluids and electrolytes
   (a) Calculation of maintenance fluid requirements
      (1) 100 mL/kg/day for the first 10 kg, 50 mL/kg/day for the next 10 kg
      (2) 20 mL/kg/day for each kg after 20 kg

■ **TABLE 30-2**
■ ■ **Laboratory and Other Diagnostic Tests for Differential Diagnosis of GI Signs and Symptoms**

| Test | Related Sign, Symptom, or Diagnosis |
|---|---|
| White blood cell count and differential | Infectious process |
| Erythrocyte sedimentation rate | Infectious process, Crohn's disease, ulcerative colitis |
| Hemoglobin | Crohn's disease, ulcerative colitis |
| Serum iron, total iron-binding capacity | Crohn's disease |
| Fecal protein | Crohn's disease |
| Hematocrit | Dehydration, vomiting, diarrhea |
| Serum electrolytes | Dehydration, vomiting, diarrhea |
|    Sodium | |
|    Potassium | |
|    Chloride | |
|    Glucose | |
|    Bicarbonate | |
| Urine specific gravity | Dehydration, vomiting, diarrhea |
| Blood urea nitrogen | Dehydration, vomiting, diarrhea |
| Stool cultures for ova and parasites | Vomiting, diarrhea, abdominal pain |
| Serum lead level | Abdominal pain—lead poisoning |
| Urine pregnancy test | Abdominal pain—pregnancy |
| Red blood cell count and differential | Abdominal pain—sickle cell disease |
| Abdominal flat plate | Abdominal pain, appendicitis, constipation, encopresis |
| Upper GI, lower GI barium tests | Abdominal pain, obstructions, strictures, Crohn's disease, ulcerative colitis, constipation, encopresis, Hirschsprung's disease |
| Stool guaiac | Bloody stools, black, tarry stools; viral AGE |
| Stool microscopy | Protozoal AGE |
| Stool WBCs | Bacterial AGE |
| Stool enzyme immunoassay | *G. lamblia* AGE |
| Stool antigen testing | Rotavirus AGE |
| Serum bilirubin, total and direct, conjugated, unconjugated | Jaundice |
| Liver function tests | Jaundice, hepatitis |
| Anti–hepatitis A antibody | Jaundice, hepatitis A antibodies |
| Enzyme immunosorbent assays | Jaundice, hepatitis C antibodies |
| Recombinant immunoblot assay | Confirms presence of hepatitis C antibodies |
| RNA amplification test | Detects circulating hepatitis C viruses |
| Serum albumin | Poor weight gain, failure to thrive, Crohn's disease |
| Esophageal pH | GERD |
| Endoscopy | GERD |
| *S. cerevisiae* antibodies | Crohn's disease, ulcerative colitis |
| Antineutrophil cytoplasmic antibodies | Crohn's disease, ulcerative colitis |
| Hydrogen ion breath testing | Abdominal pain, lactose intolerance |

■ **TABLE 30-3**
■ ■ **Components of Solutions Occasionally Used, but Not Recommended, for Oral Rehydration**

| Solution | Na+ mEq/L | K+ mEq/L | CL− mEq/L | Base | Glucose/CHO g/dL | Osmolality |
|---|---|---|---|---|---|---|
| Apple juice | 0.4 | 26 | 35 | NA | 12 | 700 |
| Ginger ale | 3.5 | 0.1 | 65 | NA | 9565 | |
| Milk | 22 | 36 | 45 | NA | 4.9 | 260 |
| Chicken broth | 2 | 3 | 80 | NA | 0330 | |

*NA,* Not available.

■ **TABLE 30-4**
■ ■ **Components of Recommended Oral Rehydration Solutions**

| Trade Name | Na+ mEq/L | K+ mEq/L | CL− mEq/L | Base | Glucose/CHO g/dL | Osmolality |
|---|---|---|---|---|---|---|
| Pedialyte (Ross) | 45 | 20 | 35 | 30 | 2.5 | 250 |
| Rehydralyte (Ross) | 75 | 20 | 65 | 30 | 2.5 | 310 |
| Enfalyte (Mead Johnson) | 50 | 25 | 45 | 30 | 3.0 | 200 |
| WHO rehydration formula | 90 | 20 | 80 | 30 | 2.0 | 310 |

    (b) Nursing mothers should be allowed to continue to nurse
    (c) Lactose-free, low-fat feedings are preferred following rehydration
        (1) If cow's milk formula is used check stools frequently for:
           a) Blood
           b) Reducing substances
           c) Leukocytes
        (2) No need to "rest the gut" after rehydration
        (3) Children can resume a normal diet as tolerated with emphasis on nonspicy, low-roughage foods (i.e., rice, crackers)
**i.** Prognosis
    **i.** Most episodes of nausea and vomiting are mild, self-limited illnesses
        (a) Knowledge of the specific etiology is usually not necessary
        (b) Follow-up is not routinely recommended
    **ii.** The emphasis of care should be rehydration as needed
    **iii.** For severe cases of vomiting, or recurrent episodes of vomiting, an etiology should be identified and treated
**j.** Pyloric stenosis (Kass & Sinert, 2006)
    **i.** Pathophysiology—diffuse hypertrophy of the smooth muscle of the antrum of the stomach and pylorus causes the channel to narrow and become easily obstructed
    **ii.** Etiology is unknown
    **iii.** Prevalence
        (a) 2 to 4/1000 live births; first born have higher risk
        (b) Less common in Hispanic, Black and Asian populations
        (c) Males more than females, 4:1
    **iv.** Signs and symptoms
        (a) Signs of gastric outlet obstruction appear at about 4 weeks of age
        (b) Nonbilious vomiting with increasing frequency
        (c) Becomes projectile vomiting
        (d) May have hematemesis
        (e) Otherwise healthy appearing, afebrile
        (f) Enlarged pylorus palpated in right upper quadrant (RUQ) of abdomen (feels like an olive)
           (1) Requires quiet, inactive infant
           (2) Stand on infant's left side, palpate liver edge near xiphoid process
           (3) Palpate downward, under liver to find pyloric "olive" on or to right of midline
           (4) Olive should be movable under fingers
    **v.** Diagnostic standard is ultrasound

        **vi.** Refer to pediatric surgery

      **vii.** Prognosis is excellent

  **k.** Gastroesophageal reflux disease (GERD) (Christensen & Gold, 2002; North American Society for Pediatric Gastroenterology, Hepatology and Nutrition, 2001)

       **i.** Definition of GERD—symptoms *and complications* from chronic gastric reflux

      **ii.** Etiology

        (a) Prolonged or frequent relaxation of the lower esophageal sphincter (LES) after swallowing such that gastric contents return to the esophagus

        (b) Reflux occurs when intragastric or intraabdominal pressure exceeds LES pressure

        (c) Aggravated by overeating, recumbent position, caffeine, high-fat foods, exposure to tobacco smoke

     **iii.** Incidence and prevalence

        (a) Occurs in 85% of premature infants

        (b) Occurs in 20% to 40% of infants ≤6 months of age

        (c) Persists in 10% to 20% of children ≥12 months of age

        (d) One of top three discharge diagnoses among 37 children's hospitals in 2000

     **iv.** Signs and symptoms

        (a) Intestinal symptoms—regurgitation, abdominal pain, heartburn, dysphagia

        (b) Other symptoms—chronic cough, sore throat, hoarseness, halitosis, dental erosion, pharyngitis, otitis media

      **v.** Diagnosis

        (a) Based on guidelines from North American Society for Pediatric Gastroenterology, Hepatology and Nutrition (2001) (current as of September, 2005)

        (b) History and physical findings consistent with GERD signs and symptoms is sufficient for diagnosis

        (c) Upper GI series is useful to detect abnormalities but not for diagnosis of GERD

        (d) Acute life-threatening episode (ALTE) of apnea, cyanosis, change in muscle tone (stiff or limp), and choking that requires immediate intervention

     **vi.** Referral to pediatric gastroenterology is recommended if GERD is diagnosed

        (a) Esophageal pH monitoring will be done to evaluate severity of GERD

        (b) Endoscopy and biopsy of esophageal mucosa may be done to detect serious complications

     **vii.** Treatment

        (a) Infants

          (1) Thickening infant formula with rice cereal may decrease vomiting episodes

          (2) Infant seat to elevate infants' head, with pillow under buttocks to prevent flexing of hips and increased abdominal pressure; supine for sleeping

        (b) Children

          (1) Avoid caffeinated foods and drinks

          (2) Elevate head of bed, position on left side for sleeping (children), or supine for infants

          (3) Avoid exposure to smoke (infants) and smoking (older children)

(c) Medications that may be prescribed by primary care providers
  (1) Histamine $H_2$-receptor antagonists inhibit gastric acid secretion caused by histamine
  (2) Proton pump inhibitors block gastric acid secretion caused by histamine, acetylcholine, or gastrin
(d) Surgery—Nissen fundoplicaton involves suturing folds in the fundus of stomach around the esophagus to increase LES pressure

  **viii.** Complications if not treated
  (a) Esophagitis, esophageal strictures
  (b) Barrett's esophagus—replacement of normal mucosa with potentially malignant epithelia

**l.** Acute gastroenteritis (AGE) (Berman, 2003)

  **i.** Pathophysiology—absorption ability of intestine is decreased by varied mechanisms
  (a) Viruses injure mature villous cells of the intestine
  (b) Bacteria invade the mucosa, damage the villous surface, or produce toxins
  (c) Parasites
  (d) May be secondary to other infections in body

  **ii.** Etiology
  (a) Oral-fecal route is most common
  (b) Inadequately cooked meats
  (c) Contaminated water

  **iii.** Prevalence
  (a) AGE is the leading cause of death for children worldwide, due to dehydration
  (b) Each U.S. child experiences 1.3 to 2.5 episodes of AGE per year

  **iv.** Rotavirus and adenovirus AGE (Berman, 2003)
  (a) Viruses are the leading cause of AGE
    (1) Rotavirus causes half of all AGE cases; adenovirus is second most common cause
    (2) Peaks in winter months
    (3) Primarily ages 4 to 24 months
  (b) 1- to 3-day incubation period with acute fever (moderate), vomiting, and watery diarrhea
  (c) Diarrhea resolves in 3 to 4 days
  (d) Ensure adequate rehydration and early return to feedings (see sections 3.g. and 3.h. above)
  (e) Avoid soup, broth, milk, tap water, undiluted juices

  **v.** Bacterial AGE (Berman, 2003)
  (a) Bacteria are the second leading cause of AGE
    (1) Salmonella most common bacterial pathogen
    (2) *Campylobacter* second most common bacterial pathogen
    (3) *Shigella*
    (4) *Escherichia coli* subspecies
  (b) Signs and symptoms
    (1) High fever, looks "sick" (septic)
    (2) Many small-volume stools, blood in stool
    (3) Known exposure to bacterial illness
    (4) White blood cells (WBCs) in stool
    (5) If *Shigella*, toxins produce fever spikes, bloody stools, febrile seizures
    (6) *E. coli* produces mild, loose stools

(c) Treatment
(1) Assure adequate rehydration and early return to feedings (see sections 3.g. and 3.h. above)
(2) Avoid soup, broth, milk, tap water, undiluted juices
(3) Salmonella—not very responsive to antibiotics
(4) Campylobacter—usually self-limiting; treat only severe cases with erythromycin or ciprofloxacin
(5) Shigella—treat all cases with trimethoprim-sulfamethoxazole (TMP-SMX)
(6) *E. coli* is usually self-limiting; duration shortened by TMP-SMX
vi. Parasitic AGE (Berman, 2003)
(a) *Giardia lamblia*
(1) Flagellate protozoan; most common parasitic cause of AGE
(2) Mild diarrhea, abdominal bloating, cramping
(3) Ensure adequate rehydration and early return to feedings (see sections 3.g. and 3.h. above)
(4) Avoid soup, broth, milk, tap water, undiluted juices
(5) Metronidazole is drug of choice
(b) *Cryptosporidium*
(1) Mild diarrhea
(2) Ensure adequate rehydration and early return to feedings (see sections 3.g. and 3.h. above)
(3) Avoid soup, broth, milk, tap water, undiluted juices
(4) Usually self-limiting
vii. Prevention is best treatment
(a) Cook ground meat and chicken thoroughly
(b) Cook eggs so that yolk is not runny
(c) Wash cutting boards and hands after cutting raw meat
(d) Exclude children with rotavirus, *E. coli* or shigella from daycare
(e) Note: two negative stool cultures required for *E. coli* and shigella before return to daycare
(f) Teach handwashing to children early
m. Irritable bowel syndrome (El Baba, 2004)
i. Presentation
(a) Diarrhea or constipation, or alternating diarrhea and constipation
(b) Chronic or recurrent abdominal pain, bloating
(c) Aggravated by stress, school-related problems, certain foods
ii. Pathophysiology
(a) Dysregulation of the brain-gut axis
(b) No known physiologic abnormality or cause
iii. Prevalence
(a) Among top 10 reasons for visits to primary care
(b) Irritable bowel syndrome (IBS) symptoms occur in 10% to 20% of adolescents and adults, 14% of high school students and 6% of middle school students, 16% of 11- to 17-year-olds
iv. Diagnosis
(a) Rome II criteria
(1) Children who can provide an accurate pain history of at least 12 weeks (not necessarily consecutive) in the preceding 12 months
(2) Abdominal pain has two out of three features:
a) Relief with defecation
b) Onset associated with a change in frequency of stool
c) Onset associated with a change in the form of stool

(3) No structural or physiologic cause
   v. Treatment
     (a) Avoid foods that aggravate symptoms
     (b) Ensure adequate fiber in diet, e.g., age in years + 5 = number of g of fiber/day
     (c) Education about mind-body relationships
     (d) Efficacy of antispasmodic medication for IBS has not been demonstrated

**n.** Inflammatory bowel disease (Petersen-Smith, 2004; Rowe, 2006)
  **i.** Crohn's disease
    (a) Definition—inflammation of mucosal lining of GI tract can occur at any point from mouth to anus; periods of flaring and remission
    (b) Presentation
      (1) Intestinal symptoms—abdominal pain, diarrhea (loose, bloody)
      (2) Other signs and symptoms in order of incidence, 90% to 1% to 3%: weight loss, fever, delayed growth and pubertal development, uveitis, conjunctivitis, arthritis, stomatitis, erythema nodosum, renal stones (oxalate), pyoderma gangrenosum
    (c) Pathophysiology
      (1) Probably an autoimmune response that results in inflammation of bowel
      (2) Triggers are unknown
      (3) Some areas of bowel are "skipped" (i.e., healthy bowel)
      (4) Chronic inflammation may lead to abscesses, fistulas, strictures
      (5) Long-term risk of malignancy
    (d) Etiology
      (1) Inherited susceptibility
      (2) Multifactorial
    (e) Laboratory findings: high sedimentation rate, microcytic anemia, low serum iron, low total iron-binding capacity, low serum albumin, high fecal protein loss, antineutrophil cytoplasmic antibodies present in 10% to 20%, *Saccharomyces cerevisiae* antibodies positive in 60%
    (f) Refer to pediatric or adult gastroenterology for a stepwise treatment
      (1) Symptom treatment: antidiarrheals, antispasmodics
      (2) Step I: oral aminosalicylates
      (3) Step IA: antibiotics
      (4) Step II: corticosteroids
      (5) Step III: immune modifiers
      (6) Step IIIA: anti–tumor necrosis factor agents
      (7) Step IV: experimental treatments
      (8) Surgery

**o.** Ulcerative colitis (Petersen-Smith, 2004; Rowe, 2006)
    (a) Definition—inflammation of mucosal lining of GI tract occurs only in the colon; periods of flaring and remission
    (b) Presentation
      (1) Intestinal symptoms—bloody diarrhea, abdominal pain, urgency, tenesmus
      (2) Other signs and symptoms in order of incidence, 68% to 4%: weight loss, fever, arthritis, renal stones (urate), delayed growth and pubertal development, pyoderma gangrenosum, sclerosis cholangitis, erythema nodosum, stomatitis
    (c) Pathophysiology
      (1) Probably an autoimmune response that results in inflammation of bowel

           (2) Triggers are unknown

           (3) Toxic megacolon is a life-threatening complication

           (4) Long-term risk of malignancy

        (d) Etiology

           (1) Inherited susceptibility

           (2) Multifactorial

        (e) Incidence

           (1) Occurs in 16 of every 100,000 people

           (2) Males = females

           (3) Primarily white

        (f) Laboratory findings: high SED rate, microcytic anemia, high WBC with shift to left, antineutrophil cytoplasmic antibodies present in 80%

        (g) Refer to pediatric or adult gastroenterology—same as for Crohn's-disease

4. Signs and symptoms: infrequent stools, straining and pain with stools, fecal soiling, bloody or black stools (Boynton, et al., 2003; Fox, 2003; Mason, et al., 2004; Mulligan, et al., 2003; Schwartz, 2003)

  a. Definitions

    i. Constipation

      (a) Stool frequency less than three times per week and a change in consistency

      (b) Lasts at least 2 weeks

      (c) Causes significant distress for child and/or family

    ii. Soiling—involuntary passage of stool

    iii. Encopresis

      (a) Voluntary or involuntary passage of stool in an inappropriate way

      (b) At regular intervals (at least 1 time/month)

      (c) After age 4, the usual age of toilet training

    iv. Hematochezia—bloody, red, or maroon stools

    v. Melena—black, tarry, and foul-smelling stools

  b. Pathophysiology

    i. Liquid chyme is passed from the small intestines into the large intestines, where the water is removed and fecal matter is concentrated

    ii. Passage of the fecal matter into the rectum stretches the rectal walls and stimulates the afferent nerves, which causes internal anal sphincter to relax

    iii. This is perceived as a sense of fullness and the need to defecate

      (a) Constipation results from any interruption or delay in that process

        (1) Fecal mass dries in colon, yielding hard, dry stools

        (2) Difficult expulsion of stool

        (3) Voluntary delay in defecation by contracting the external anal sphincter causes buildup of stool in rectum and pain

        (4) A vicious cycle of retention, pain, and further retention may occur

        (5) Retention may also be voluntary as a reaction to stress or need for control

    iv. Soiling may be a complication of constipation when external anal sphincter relaxes after long periods of contraction and stool seeps out

    v. Encopresis

      (a) Stool seeps out because a chronically impacted rectum prevents external anal sphincter from contracting appropriately

      (b) Child has no sensation of rectal fullness

  (c) Primary encopresis—occurs before child has been toilet trained

  (d) Secondary encopresis—occurs after child has been toilet trained

 **vi.** Bleeding from pathology in lower GI tract appears as frank blood in stools

 **vii.** Bleeding from pathology in upper GI tract appears as black, tarry, foul-smelling stools

**c.** Prevalence

 **i.** Approximately 5% of primary care pediatric visits are related to constipation

 **ii.** 25% of referrals to pediatric gastroenterologists involve constipation

 **iii.** Gender differences in constipation complaints vary with age

  (a) Toddlers, preschoolers: males equal to females

  (b) School-age: males more than females

  (c) Adolescents: females more than males

 **iv.** Soiling or encopresis affects 3 to 5% of 4-year-olds and 1.5% of 10-year-olds

**d.** Etiology

 **i.** 95% of cases are functional, i.e., no organic pathology

 **ii.** 5% are due to organic or anatomic abnormalities

**e.** Differential diagnoses for dry, hard, or infrequent stools and painful rectal area (Box 30-4)

**f.** Differential diagnoses for bloody or tarry stools (Box 30-5)

**g.** Focused history and physical as shown in Chapter 8, with special attention to differential diagnoses

**h.** Laboratory or diagnostic tests (see Table 30-1)

**i.** Treatment

 **i.** Goal of treatment is to achieve regular soft, formed stools without pain, and to eliminate fear of defecation

---

■ **BOX 30-4**

■ **DIFFERENTIAL DIAGNOSES FOR DRY, HARD, OR INFREQUENT STOOLS AND FOR PAINFUL RECTAL AREA**

**DIFFERENTIAL DIAGNOSES FOR DRY, HARD, OR INFREQUENT STOOLS**
Acute constipation
Chronic constipation
Encopresis
Hirschsprung's disease
Tethered cord
Anal stenosis
Mass or tumor
Hypothyroidism
Ingestion or medication use
Toxic ingestion (i.e., lead)

**DIFFERENTIAL DIAGNOSES FOR PAINFUL RECTAL AREA**
Chronic diarrhea
Hemorrhoids
Anal fissure
Cystic fibrosis
Proctitis
Perianal warts
Fistula
Crohn's disease
Ulcerative colitis

■ **BOX 30-5**
■ **DIFFERENTIAL DIAGNOSES FOR BLOODY RED OR BLACK TARRY STOOLS**

Swallowed blood
- Epistaxis
- Oropharyngeal trauma or bleeding

Esophagitis
- Ulceration
- GERD
- Ingestions of corrosives, Fe, or aspirin/ OTC NSAIDs
- Hiatal hernia

Esophageal tears
- Trauma or foreign bodies
- NG tube insertion
- Mallory-Weiss tear
- Esophageal varices

Gastritis
- Vomiting
- Viral infections
- Ulcer disease
- Eosinophilic gastroenteritis
- Pyloric stenosis

Enteritis
- Viral enteritis
- Bacterial enteritis
- Parasitic infection

Intestinal disorders
- Ulcerative colitis
- Crohn's disease
- Intussusception
- Obstruction
- Polyps
- Irritable bowel syndrome
- Diverticulitis
- Necrotizing enterocolitis
- Appendicitis
- Volvulus
- Meckel's diverticulum
- Anal fissure
- Hemorrhoids
- Sexual abuse

Neoplastic causes
- Zollinger-Ellison syndrome
- Leiomyosarcoma

Food allergy
- Milk, soy, eggs, peanuts, fish, e.g.

Blood and connective tissue disorders
- Hemosiderosis
- Henoch-Scholein purpura
- Systemic lupus erythematosus
- Hemolytic-uremic syndrome
- Bleeding disorder

    ii. Functional etiology
        (a) Generally takes 6 to 12 months; 20% failure rate
        (b) Clean out—using oral medications (preferable) or enemas; rectum must be empty before starting treatment
        (c) Maintenance management of constipation, with office visits at 2 weeks, and 1, 3, and 6 months at least
            (1) Oral laxatives
            (2) High-fiber diet (age in years + 5 = number of g of fiber/day)
            (3) Increased fluids
            (4) Behavior modification techniques
                a) Toilet-sitting schedule: start about 20 minutes after meal
                b) Two or three times per day for 10 to 15 minutes (use a timer that child can see)
                c) Feet flat on floor
                d) Private, unhurried, nonpunitive
            (5) Positive reinforcement for sitting and stooling in toilet; frequent reinforcement at first, decrease over time
        (d) Weaning
            (1) Gradual decrease in laxatives
            (2) Continue high-fiber and increased liquids

**5.** Symptom: abdominal pain, acute or chronic (Boynton, et al., 2003; Fox, 2003; Mulligan, et al., 2003; Schwartz, 2003)

   **a.** Prevalence

      **i.** Abdominal pain accounts for up to 40% of pediatric primary care visits

      **ii.** One of the leading three presenting complaints in the emergency department

      **iii.** Recurrent abdominal pain

         (a) Medically unexplained abdominal pain occurs in 1% to 30% of all children on a weekly basis

         (b) 90% of cases are functional, i.e., no identifiable organic cause (Gold, 2003)

      **iv.** Appendicitis

         (a) Most common surgical emergency in children (Smink, et al., 2004)

         (b) Occurs in 4 per 1000 children

         (c) Males more than females, 2:1 ratio

         (d) Typically at ages 6 to 10 years

         (e) Preschoolers most likely to have perforation (50% to 85%)

   **b.** Differential diagnoses (Box 30-6)

   **c.** Focused history and physical as shown in Chapter 8, with special attention to differential diagnoses

   **d.** Laboratory or diagnostic tests (see Table 30-2)

   **e.** Recurrent abdominal pain (RAP) (Gold, 2003)

      **i.** Pathophysiology

         (a) Brain-gut axis explains the stress response of abdominal pain

         (b) Child may have familial or genetic predisposition for GI system sensitivity to stress

         (c) Secondary gain may play a role in symptom maintenance, i.e., getting attention and being excused from normal responsibilities (Walker, 2003)

      **ii.** Additional notes related to history

         (a) Requires careful history taking to reveal that symptoms are stress related

         (b) Research shows that RAP is a multidimensional symptom with four major dimensions: pain intensity, nonpain symptoms, pain disability, and satisfaction with health (Malaty, et al., 2005)

         (c) Always inform parents that "functional" is included in your differential so that it may be easier to accept later (Rudolph & Miranda, 2004)

         (d) Providers find that parents do not like to accept the "functional" diagnosis, but want multiple tests to rule out or identify a definitive organic diagnosis and treatment

         (e) Providers must weigh the diagnostic need for tests versus parents' need for tests

         (f) In a research study, parents reported that they felt undermined and disrespected regarding their attempts to seek help for their children's RAP, and thus focused more on physical aspects of the symptoms than psychosocial (Smart & Cottrell, 2005)

      **iii.** Additional notes related to physical examination

         (a) Pain is typically periumbilical, does not wake child up at night

         (b) Child is physically normal, growing normally

      **iv.** Treatment

         (a) Cognitive-behavioral therapy (Youssef, et al., 2004)

            (1) Education of parents and child about mind-body interaction

            (2) Teach new coping skills to take the place of somatization, e.g., guided imagery, relaxation techniques, problem-solving

■ **BOX 30-6**
■ **DIFFERENTIAL DIAGNOSES FOR ABDOMINAL PAIN**

**ANATOMIC/CONGENITAL**
- Aortic aneurysm
- Incarcerated hernia
- Adhesions
- Intussusception
- Malrotation with volvulus
- Ovarian torsion
- Testicular torsion

**INFECTIOUS**
- Cystitis
- Fitz-Hugh-Curtis syndrome
- Epididymitis
- Gastroenteritis
- Hepatitis
- Herpes zoster
- *Helicobacter pylori*
- Kawasaki disease
- Mononucleosis
- Orchitis
- Peritonitis
- Pharyngitis
- PID
- Pneumonia
- Sepsis
- UTI
- Varicella

**TOXIC SUBSTANCES, DRUGS**
- Anticholinergic medications
- Caustic ingestions
- Foreign body
- Heavy metals (i.e., lead)

**TRAUMA**
- Child abuse
- Intestinal hematoma
- Liver/splenic contusion

**TUMOR**
- Wilms' tumor
- Neuroblastoma
- Leukemia
- Lymphoma
- Hepatoblastoma

- Ovarian tumor
- Teratoma
- Rhabdomyosarcoma

**METABOLIC**
- Diabetic ketoacidosis
- Collagen vascular diseases (i.e., SLE, polyarteritis nodosa)
- Inborn errors of metabolism
- Porphyria

**ALLERGIC/INFLAMMATORY**
- Appendicitis
- Cholecystitis
- Eosinophilic gastroenteritis
- Endometriosis
- HUS
- Henoch-Schonlein purpura
- IBD
- Mesenteric adenitis
- NEC
- Pancreatitis
- GERD

**FUNCTIONAL**
- Depression
- Recurrent abdominal pain

**MISCELLANEOUS**
- Abdominal migraine (cyclic vomiting syndrome)
- Cholelithiasis
- Colic
- Constipation
- Dysmenorrheal
- Ectopic pregnancy
- Ileus
- IBS
- Kidney stones
- Lactose intolerance
- Mittelschmerz
- Ovarian cyst
- Pregnancy
- Sickle cell disease

    (b) Psychology referral if stress seems unmanageable for child
  **f.** Appendicitis (Tucker, 2004)
    **i.** Pathophysiology
      (a) Appendix is a blind-ending diverticular structure arising from the cecum

        (b) A closed loop obstruction of the appendix leads to mucosal edema, increasing intraluminal pressure, and exudate from the appendix

        (c) When exudate touches the parietal peritoneum, pain is more intense and localized in right lower quadrant (RLQ)

        (d) Bacteria proliferate in obstructed appendix and stretch the lumen

        (e) Perforation of appendix releases bacteria into abdominal cavity

        (f) Peritonitis presents with more intense and generalized pain

    ii. Additional notes related to history

        (a) Diffuse periumbilical pain, often associated with anorexia

        (b) Nausea and vomiting develop shortly *after* onset of pain

        (c) After a few hours, pain shifts to the right lower quadrant, more intense, continuous, and more localized than the initial pain

        (d) Most are afebrile or have a low-grade fever

        (e) High fever may signal a perforation

    iii. Additional notes related to physical examination

        (a) Note child's facial expression during palpation of the abdomen to identify the location and intensity of abdominal pain

        (b) Signs of peritoneal irritation

            (1) Child prefers to lie still

            (2) Usually, maximal tenderness is at McBurney point in the RLQ

            (3) Rovsing's sign is pain in RLQ in response to left-sided palpation

            (4) Psoas sign is pain elicited by placing the child on the left side and hyperextending the right leg

            (5) Cough sign (sharp pain in RLQ after a voluntary cough)

        (c) Obturator sign is pain on internal rotation of the flexed right thigh (suggests an inflammatory mass overlying the psoas muscle)

        (d) A rectal examination should be done last and may reveal impacted stool, right-sided tenderness, or a mass

    iv. Immediate referral to pediatric surgery is required to minimize the chances of perforation of appendix or to prevent or treat peritonitis

6. Symptom: yellow tint of skin, eyes (Boynton, et al., 2003; Fox, 2003; Mulligan, et al., 2003; Schwartz, 2003)

  **a.** Pathophysiology

    i. Jaundice is yellow coloration of the skin and eyes that is apparent when the total serum bilirubin reaches 5 to 7 mg/dL

    ii. Liver damage is evident by: (Turner, 2004)

        (a) Viral infection causes injury to cells that elevates serum liver enzyme levels

        (b) Cholestasis, the decreased flow of bile from the liver into the common bile duct or into the small intestines that causes jaundice and hyperbilirubinemia

        (c) Inadequate liver function lowers serum albumin levels and prolongs the prothrombin time (PT)

  **b.** Differential diagnosis (Box 30-7)

  **c.** Hyperbilirubinemia (see Chapter 18)

  **d.** Physiologic jaundice (see Chapter 18)

  **e.** Hepatitis

    i. Hepatitis A, B, C, and E can cause acute viral illness lasting several weeks

    ii. Symptoms include jaundice of skins and eyes, dark urine, fatigue, nausea, vomiting, abdominal pain; sometimes enlarged liver; lymph nodes and spleen may also enlarge

    iii. Hepatitis A (Turner, 2004)

■ **BOX 30-7**
■ **DIFFERENTIAL DIAGNOSES FOR JAUNDICE**

Newborn hyperbilirubinemia
Physiologic jaundice
Idiopathic neonatal hepatitis
Hepatitis
Infection (STOURCH)
$\alpha_1$-antitrypsin deficiency
Extrahepatic biliary atresia
Alagille syndrome
Inherited syndromes (i.e., congenital hypothyroidism, galactosemia, glycogen storage disease, fructose intolerance, tyrosemia)
Thyroid disease
Sepsis
Gilbert's disease

    (a) Fecal-borne virus
    (b) Transmitted via poor handwashing techniques by an infected person who handles food or fluids consumed by others, contaminated water supplies, sexual contact
    (c) Symptoms range from asymptomatic to fulminating
    (d) Usually self-limiting; no specific treatment
    (e) Chronic illness, cirrhosis, or liver cancer is rare
    (f) May be given immune globulin within 2 weeks of exposure to someone with hepatitis A to prevent infection
    (g) A vaccine is available, but routine vaccination is not recommended for everyone, only those at highest risk
  **iv.** Hepatitis B (WHO, 2000a)
    (a) A serious global public health problem
    (b) Transmitted through mother to infant at birth, blood or body fluids of infected person, reuse of contaminated needles, and sexual contact
    (c) 50 to 100 times more infectious than HIV
    (d) Major occupational hazard for health care workers
    (e) Can become a chronic disease that may develop into cirrhosis or cancer of the liver in 25% of people who become infected during childhood
    (f) Treatment is very expensive; includes interferon or lamivudine therapy
    (g) Hepatitis B vaccine, in a series of three doses, is 95% effective in preventing chronic infections from developing
  **v.** Hepatitis C (WHO, 2000b)
    (a) Blood-borne virus transmitted primarily through transfusions and reuse of contaminated needles
    (b) May also transfer through sexual contact or mother to infant at birth
    (c) No evidence of transmission through breast milk (Mast, 2004)
    (d) AAP (2005) policy statement recommends breast-feeding unless nipples are cracked and bleeding
    (e) Usually asymptomatic or mild in childhood
    (f) Screening test—positive for antibodies in enzyme immunosorbent assay (EIA), but test is only 50% to 70% sensitive
    (g) Confirm positive EIA with recombinant immunoblot assay

(h) No vaccine is available for hepatitis C but research is ongoing

(i) Treatment includes combination of interferon and ribavirin (effective for about 30% to 50% of cases)

(j) Prevention includes infection control practices, sterilization of instruments, safer sex and injection practices

**vi.** Hepatitis E (WHO, 2005)

(a) A water-borne disease

(b) Transmitted by consumption of fecal-contaminated water or food (e.g., shellfish)

(c) Self-limiting infection; chronic infection does not occur

(d) Most common in 15- to 40-year-olds

(e) Frequent in children, but typically asymptomatic or mild and may be without jaundice

(f) No vaccine for hepatitis E is available

(g) No specific treatment is available

(h) Prevention is key: safe water supplies, properly cooked seafood, washed fruits and vegetables, good hygiene practices

---

# REFERENCES

American Academy of Pediatrics Section on Breastfeeding. (2005). Breastfeeding and the use of human milk. *Pediatrics, 115*(2), 496-506.

Ammaniti, M., Ambruzzi, A. M., Lucarelli, L., et al. (2004). Malnutrition and dysfunctional mother-child feeding interactions: Clinical assessment and research implications. *J Am Coll Nutr, 23*(3), 259-271.

Berman, J. (July 1, 2003). Heading off the dangers of acute gastroenteritis. *Contemp Pediatr.* Retrieved April 28, 2006, from www.contemporarypediatrics.com/contpeds/article/articleDetail.jsp?id=111759.

Boynton, R. W., Dunn, E. S., Stephens, G. R., & Pulcini, J. (2003). *Manual of ambulatory pediatrics* (5th ed.). New York: Lippincott Williams & Wilkins.

Bullard, J., & Page, N. E. (2005). Cyclic vomiting syndrome: A disease in disguise. *Pediatr Nurs, 31*(1), 27-29.

Christensen, M. L., & Gold, B. D. (2002). *Clinical management of infants and children with gastroesophageal reflux disease: Disease recognition and therapeutic options.* Monograph from the symposium presented at the American Society of Health-System Pharmacists in Atlanta, GA, Dec. 9, 2002.

El-Baba, M. F. (2004). *Irritable bowel syndrome.* Retrieved April 28, 2006, from www.emedicine.com/ped/topic1210.htm.

Fox, J. A. (2003). *Primary health care of infants, children, & adolescents* (2nd ed.). St. Louis: Mosby.

Gold, B. (2003). Recurrent abdominal pain in children. Presented at Digestive Disease Week 2003, May 17-22, Orlando, FL, and reported by J. Rusk, in *Infect Dis Child*, July, 2003, 39-40.

Hockenberry, M. J., Wilson, D., Winkelstein, M. L., & Kline, N. E. (2003). *Wong's nursing care of infants and children* (7th ed.). St. Louis: Mosby/Elsevier.

Kass, D. A., & Sinert, R. (2006). *Pediatrics: Pyloric stenosis.* Retrieved on April 28, 2006 from eMedicine at http://www.emedicine.com/EMERG/topic397.htm.

Krugman, S. D., & Dubowitz, H. (2003). Failure to thrive. *Am Fam Phys, 68*(5), 879-884.

Lobo, M. L., Kotzer, A. M., Keefe, Mm. R., et al. (2004). Current beliefs and management strategies for treating infant colic. *J Pediatr Health Care, 18*(3), 115-122.

Malaty, H. M., Abudayyeh, S., O'Malley, K. J., et al. (2005). Development of a multidimensional measure for recurrent abdominal pain in children: Population-based studies in three settings. *Pediatrics, 115*(2), 210-215.

Mason, D., Tobias, N., Lutkenhoff, M., et al. (2004). The APN's guide to pediatric constipation management. *Nurse Pract Am J Prim Health Care, 29*(7), 13-21.

Mast, E. E. (2004). Mother-to-infant hepatitis C virus transmission and breastfeeding. *Adv Exp Med Biol, 554*, 211-216.

Mulligan, S. A., Migita, D. S., Christakis, D. A., & Saint, S. (2003). *Saint-Frances guide to pediatrics.* New York: Lippincott Williams & Wilkins.

National Center for Shaken Baby Syndrome (2006). *Period of PURPLE Crying.* Retrieved April 28, 2006, from http://dontshake. com/Subject.aspx?categoryID=1.

North American Society for Pediatric Gastroenterology, Hepatology and Nutrition. (2001). Guidelines for evaluation and treatment of gastroesophageal reflux in infants and children. *J Pediatr Gastroenterol Nutr, 32*, Suppl 2.

O'Brien, L. M., Heycock, E. G., Hanna, M., et al. (2004). Postnatal depression and faltering growth: a community study. *Pediatrics, 113*, 1242-1247.

Petersen-Smith, A. M. (2004). Gastrointestinal disorders. In C. E. Burns, A. M. Dunn, M. A. Brady, et al. (Eds.). *Pediatric primary care: A handbook for nurse practitioners* (3rd ed.). Philadelphia: Saunders, pp. 839-883.

Rowe, W. A. (2006). *Inflammatory bowel disease.* Retrieved April 28, 2006, from www. emedicine.com/med/topic1169.htm.

Rudolph, C. D., & Miranda, A. (2004). Treatment options for functional abdominal pain. *Pediatr Ann, 33*(2), 105-112.

Sears, C. L. (2005). Proper evaluation necessary before treating diarrhea. Presentation at the Clinical Infectious Disease Meeting, March 31-April 3, 2005, Orlando, FL. Reported by C. A. Richards in *Infect Dis Child*, July, 2005, pp. 56, 58.

Schwartz, M. W. (2003). *Clinical handbook of pediatrics* (3rd ed.). New York: Lippincott Williams & Wilkins.

Smart, S., & Cottrell, D. (2005). Going to the doctors: The views of mothers of children with recurrent abdominal pain. *Child Care Health Dev, 31*(3), 265-273.

Smink, D. S., Finkelstein, J. A., Peña, B. M. G., et al. (2004). Diagnosis of acute appendicitis in children using a clinical practice guideline. *J Pediatr Surg, 39*(3), 458-463.

Tucker, J. (2004). *Pediatrics: appendicitis.* Retrieved April 28, 2006, from www. emedicine.com/ EMERG/topic361.htm.

Turner, L. C. (2004). *Hepatitis A.* Retrieved April 28, 2006, from www.emedicine. com/ped/topic977.htm.

Walker, L. S. (2003). Age and gender effects on GI symptoms and somatization. Presented at digestive Disease Week 2003, May 17-22, Orlando, FL, and reported by J. Rusk, in *Infect Dis Child*, July, 2003, pp. 41, 43.

World Health Organization (WHO). (2000a). Hepatitis B fact sheet no. 204. Retrieved April 28, 2006, from www.who.int/media centre/factsheets/fs204/en/index. html.

World Health Organization (WHO). (2000a). Hepatitis C fact sheet no. 164. Retrieved April 28, 2006, from www. who.int/mediacentre/factsheets/fs164/ en/index.html.

World Health Organization (WHO). (2005). Hepatitis e fact sheet no. 280. Retrieved April 28, 2006, from www.who.int/medi-acentre/factsheets/fs280/en/index. html.

Youssef, N. N., Rosh, J. R., Loughran, M., et al. (2004). Treatment of functional abdominal pain in childhood with cognitive behavioral strategies. *J Pediatr Gastroenterol Nutr, 39*, 192-196.

# Common Illness of the Reproductive and Urologic Systems

BARBARA VOLLENHOVER WISE, PhD, RN, AND BARBARA CARDINAL-BUSSE, MSN, CRNP

## SYMPTOMS: DYSURIA, FREQUENCY, URGENCY, HEMATURIA, OLIGURIA

1. History and symptom assessment
   a. Onset and duration of symptoms
   b. Pain: location, intensity, duration, onset
   c. Urine: color, odor
   d. History of voiding patterns
   e. Previous urinary tract infection (UTI)
   f. Gastrointestinal (GI): constipation, fecal soiling, diarrhea, anorexia, nausea, vomiting
   g. Skin: perineal rash, irritation, history of impetigo
   h. Hygiene practices and products
      i. Bowel movement remnants in perineal area
      ii. Retraction of foreskin in uncircumcised males
      iii. Use of bath oils, bubble bath commonly discouraged, but no research evidence supports this to date
   i. Sexual history: sexual practices, sexual abuse
   j. Recent streptococcal pharyngitis
   k. Preexisting medical conditions
   l. Trauma
   m. Slow physical growth
   n. Failure to thrive
2. Focused physical examination
   a. Blood pressure—hypotension in neonates
   b. Hydration status
   c. Periorbital edema
   d. Temperature
   e. Genitourinary system examination
   f. GI system examination
   g. Neurologic examination
      i. Sacral dimple or nevi
      ii. Hair tuft or indications of tethered cord syndrome
   h. Pelvic examination based on history

3. Differential diagnoses
   a. UTI
   b. Hemolytic-uremic syndrome
   c. Acute poststreptococcal glomerulonephritis
   d. Vesicoureteral reflux (VUR)
   e. Dysfunctional elimination syndrome
   f. Urethritis
   g. See also Box 31-1 and Table 31-1 for other potential diagnoses
4. Diagnostic tests
   a. Microscopic urinalysis
      i. Infants—optimal source is catheterized specimen
      ii. Older children—preferably first-voided urine, midstream, clean-catch
      iii. Pyuria ≥10 white blood cells (WBCs) in urine sediment per high-power field
      iv. Leukocyte esterase—positive for UTI and urethritis
      v. Hematuria = 5 or more red blood cells (RBCs) (Davis & Avner, 2004)
         (a) Upper urinary tract sources—glomerulus, tubules, interstitium
         (b) Lower urinary tract sources—pelvocalyceal system, ureter, bladder, urethra
      vi. Proteinuria
      vii. Gram stain of urine
         (a) Pink stain—gram-negative microorganisms (e.g., *E. coli*)
         (b) Blue stain—gram-positive microorganisms
         (c) ≥5 organisms per oil immersion field of centrifuged Gram-stained urine
   b. Enhanced urinalysis: use of hemocytometer to get accurate cell counts
   c. Urine culture – criteria for UTI diagnosis ranges from 50,000 to 100,000 culture-forming units (cfu)
   d. Urine specific gravity
   e. Urine glucose
   f. CBC with differential
      i. C-reactive protein
      ii. Sedimentation rate
      iii. Electrolytes, antistreptolysin O titer (ASO) or anti-DNAse B titers
   g. Cervical or urethral smear for presence of intracellular diplococci (*N. gonorrhoeae*)
   h. Cervical cultures or urethral cultures for chlamydia and gonorrhea

■ **BOX 31-1**
■ **CAUSES OF HEMATURIA IN CHILDREN**

---

**GLOMERULAR HEMATURIA**
Isolated renal disease
IgA nephropathy (i.e., Berger disease)
Alport syndrome (hereditary nephritis)
Thin glomerular basement membrane nephropathy
Postinfectious GN (i.e., poststreptococcal GN)
Membranous nephropathy
Membranoproliferative GN
Focal segmental glomerulosclerosis
Anti–glomerular basement membrane disease

■ **BOX 31-1**
■ **CAUSES OF HEMATURIA IN CHILDREN—cont'd**

**MULTISYSTEM DISEASE**
Systemic lupus erythematosus nephritis*
Goodpasture syndrome
Hemolytic-uremic syndrome
Sickle cell glomerulopathy
HIV nephropathy
Henoch-Schönlein purpura nephritis
Wegener granulomatosis
Polyarteritis nodosa

**EXTRAGLOMERULAR HEMATURIA**
**Upper Urinary Tract**
Tubulointerstitial
Calcium
Oxalate
Uric acid
Hemoglobinopathy (sickle cell trait/disease, SC hemoglobin)
Anatomic
Hydronephrosis
Cystic kidney disease
Polycystic kidney disease
Multicystic dysplasia
Tumor (Wilms, rhabdomyosarcoma, angiomyolipoma)
Trauma
Pyelonephritis
Interstitial nephritis
Acute tubular necrosis
Papillary necrosis
Nephrocalcinosis
Vascular
Arterial/venous thrombosis
Malformations (aneurysms, hemangiomas)
Nutcracker syndrome
Crystalluria

**Lower Urinary Tract**
Inflammation (infectious and noninfectious)
Cystitis
Urethritis
Urolithiasis
Trauma
Coagulopathy
Heavy exercise
   Munchausen/Munchausen-by-proxy syndrome

**COMMON CAUSES OF GROSS HEMATURIA**
Urinary tract infection
Meatal stenosis
Perineal irritation
Trauma
Urolithiasis/hypercalciuria
Coagulopathy
Tumor
Glomerular
   IgA nephropathy
   Alport syndrome (hereditary nephritis)
   Thin glomerular basement membrane disease
   Postinfectious glomerulonephritis
   Henoch-Schönlein purpura nephritis
   Systemic lupus erythematosus nephritis

Denotes glomerulonephritides presenting with hypocomplementemia. GN = glomerulonephritis
From Davis, I. D., & Avner, E. D. (2004). Nephrology. In R. E. Behrman, R. M. Kliegman, & H. B. Jenson (Eds.). *Nelson textbook of pediatrics* (17th ed.). Philadelphia: Saunders, p. 1736.

■ **TABLE 31-1**
■ ■ **Differential Diagnoses for Genitourinary Symptoms**

**Anatomic Abnormalities**

| | |
|---|---|
| Posterior urethral valves | Megaureter |
| Ectopic ureter | Renal lithiasis |
| Ureterocele | Duplication of the collecting system |
| Epispadias | Neurogenic bladder |
| Dysplastic kidney | Vesicoureteral reflux |
| Hydronephrosis | Bladder instability |
| Detrussor sphincter dyssynergia | Myelomeningocele |
| | Urethral stricture |

**Infectious Conditions**

| | |
|---|---|
| Urinary tract infection | Pyelonephritis |
| Sepsis/bacteremia | Meningitis |
| Pinworms | Vulvovaginitis |
| Varicella | Mononucleosis |
| Erythema multiforme | Scarlet fever |
| Kawasaki disease | HSV type 1 or 2 |
| Impetigo | Tinea cruris |
| Molluscum contagiosum | Measles |
| | Foreign object |

**Polyuria**

| | |
|---|---|
| Diabetes insipidus | Diabetes mellitus |
| Chronic renal failure | Renal tubular acidosis |
| Sickle cell disease | |

**Painful/Nonpainful Scrotal Mass or Swelling**

| | |
|---|---|
| Henöch-Schonlein purpura | Cellulitis |
| Hernia—incarcerated | Infected piercing |
| Acute idiopathic scrotal edema | Insect bite or sting |

**Dermatologic Symptoms**

| | |
|---|---|
| Seborrhea | Lichen sclerosus |
| Psoriasis | Eczema |
| Contact dermatitis | Diaper dermatitis |
| Behçet's syndrome | Aphthosis |
| Irritable bowel disease | Cervicitis |
| Endometriosis | Trichomoniasis |
| Urethritis | Allergy to contraceptive gel |
| Intrauterine device | |

**Abnormal Genital Bleeding**

| | |
|---|---|
| Trauma | Miscarriage |
| Ectopic pregnancy | Obstetric complications |
| Abortion | Autoimmune disorders |
| Pelvic inflammatory disease | Pregnancy |
| Bleeding disorders | Endocrine abnormalities |
| Renal or liver disease | Neuropsychiatric conditions |
| Infection (see above) | Ovarian tumor |
| Iron deficiency anemia | Thyroid abnormalities |
| Polycystic ovary syndrome | |

*Continued*

---

■ **TABLE 31-1**
■ ■ **Differential Diagnoses for Genitourinary Symptoms—cont'd**

---

**Gynecologic Causes of Pelvic Pain**

| | |
|---|---|
| Endometriosis | Pelvic adhesions |
| Ovarian cysts | PID |
| Uterine polyps | Cervical stricture or stenosis |

**Nongynecologic Causes of Pelvic Pain**

| | |
|---|---|
| Crohn's disease | Giardiasis |
| Chronic constipation | Henoch- Schönlein purpura |
| Meckel's diverticulum | Gastritis |
| Midgut volvulus | Esophagitis |
| Ureteropelvic junction obstruction | Musculoskeletal pain |

---

    i. Stool culture for Shiga toxin and Shiga toxin-producing *E. coli* (STEC)
    j. Flat plate abdominal x-ray
    k. Renal and bladder ultrasound
       i. Rule out hydronephrosis if febrile child less than 5 years
       ii. Assess for a postvoid residual
       iii. Initial examination with fluoroscopy, then ultrasound
    l. Standard voiding cystourethrogram (VCUG) to rule out VUR
       i. If febrile child less than 5 years
       ii. *And* history of one UTI
       iii. Provide 2 days of prophylactic antibiotics after study to prevent UTI
       iv. Dimercaptosuccinic acid (DMSA) renal scan is presently the technique of choice for assessing renal scars.
    m. Blood work to rule out other sources of infection
       i. HIV testing
       ii. Hepatitis B and C
       iii. Rapid plasma reagin (RPR) test for syphilis
5. Treatment appropriate for all urinary diagnoses
    a. Educate the child and family
    b. Specimen collection protocol
    c. Completion of antibiotics
    d. Side effects of medication
    e. Appropriate hygiene
    f. Prevention of constipation
    g. Adequate fluid intake
    h. Regular voiding schedules
    i. Avoid use of perfumed soaps and other personal hygiene products
    j. Review hygiene and safer sexual practices with adolescents
6. See Table 31-2 for when to refer
7. Signs, symptoms, prevalence, etiology, pathophysiology and treatment of specific diagnoses
    a. UTI
       i. Signs and symptoms differ according to age of child (Table 31-3)
       ii. See the American Academy of Pediatrics (1999) practice parameter for UTI (this is the latest edition as of May, 2006)
       iii. Types of UTI

■ **TABLE 31-2**
■ ■ **Referral Recommendations According to Diagnosis, Sign, or Symptom**

| Diagnosis: Sign or Symptom | Referral Recommendations |
| --- | --- |
| Enuresis, nonresponder | Pediatric urologist |
| 3 UTI in 6 months or 1 UTI in male | Pediatric urologist |
| VUR > grade 2 older than 5 years | Pediatric urologist |
| VUR > grade 3 | Pediatric urologist |
| Daytime incontinence if unresponsive to medical intervention | Pediatric urologist |
| Refer sexual contacts with positive STI | PCP, health department |
| Torsion (testicular or ovarian) | Pediatric urologist/general surgery/gynecologist |
| Epididymitis (nonsexually active male) | Pediatric urologist |
| Mumps orchitis—unresolved in 3 days | Pediatric urologist |
| Hydrocele if persists after 1–2 years of age | Pediatric urologist |
| Spermatocele: refer for unclear diagnosis | Pediatric urologist |
| Varicocele grade 3 or more, or testicular asymmetry, right unilateral | Pediatric urologist |
| Hernia—refer for repair | Pediatric urologist or general surgery |
| Undescended testicle | Pediatric urologist/endocrinologist |
| Unresolved phimosis > 3 years | Pediatric urologist |
| Unresolved balanitis | Pediatric urologist/dermatologist |
| Meatal stenosis | Pediatric urologist |
| Hypospadias | Pediatric urologist |
| Vulvovaginitis, if therapy fails, suspect abuse | Pediatric gynecologist/forensic pediatrician |
| Vaginal foreign body | Pediatric gynecologist |
| Unresolved labial adhesions | Pediatric urologist/gynecologist |
| Unresolved warts | Pediatric gynecologist |
| Incision and drainage if treatment fails | Pediatric surgeon/gynecologist |
| Gynecomastia > mild to moderate | Pediatric surgeon |
| Gynecomastia nonidiopathic | Pediatric endocrinologist |
| Fibroadenoma | Pediatric surgeon or breast specialist |
| Unclear diagnosis of fibrocystic changes | Pediatric breast specialist |
| Breast infections unresolved or abscess | Pediatric surgeon or breast specialist |
| PID with TOA or pregnancy | Gynecologist |
| Ectopic pregnancy suspected | Gynecologist |
| Ovarian cysts > 5 or 6 cm, persistent pain | Pediatric gynecologist/pediatric surgeon |
| DUB unresponsive to treatment 3–6 months | Pediatric gynecologist |
| Imperforate hymen | Pediatric surgeon or gynecologist |
| Unresolved or recurrent aphthosis | Pediatric dermatologist |
| DUB with persistent symptoms | Pediatric hematologist or gynecologist |
| Teen pregnancy | Gynecology/Planned Parenthood/social services |

    (a) Uncomplicated UTI = cystitis or pyelonephritis that develops in absence of structural abnormality, obstruction, or other disease
    (b) Complicated UTI = chronic cystitis or pyelonephritis that develops in presence of structural abnormality, obstruction, or other disease
  **iv.** Prevalence
    (a) Incidence inversely proportional to gestational age
    (b) In infants less than 3 months of age males at greater risk than females
    (c) 6.5% females and 3.3% males less than 1 year of age
    (d) 50% higher risk of recurrence in females
    (e) 8% females and 2% males more than 1 year of age
    (f) 13.6 % febrile infants less than 8 weeks of age

**■ TABLE 31-3**
**■ ■ Signs and Symptoms of Urinary Tract Infection According to Age**

| Neonates and Infants | Preschoolers | School Age | Adolescent |
|---|---|---|---|
| Fever >101.5° F (38° C) | Lethargy | Enuresis | Fatigue |
| Lethargy | Hematuria | Abdominal pain | Hematuria |
| Vomiting | Strong urine odor | Strong urine odor | Dysuria |
| Diarrhea | Abdominal pain | Fever | Urgency |
| Jaundice | Vomiting | Vomiting | Retention |
| Diaper rash | Diarrhea | Diarrhea | Frequency |
| Apnea | | | Flank pain |
| Irritability | | | Strong urine odor |
| | | | Chills |
| | | | Fever |

v. Etiology
  (a) Bacterial organisms
    (1) *Escherichia coli* accounts for:
      a) 80% to 90% of uncomplicated UTIs
      b) Only 20% of complicated UTIs
    (2) *Staphylococcus aureus* accounts for majority of organisms in complicated UTIs
    (3) *Enterobacter* species
    (4) *Pseudomonas aeruginosa*
    (5) *Actinobacter* species
    (6) *Proteus mirabilis* more common in males
    (7) *Staphylococcus saprophyticus* second-most common organism in adolescent female
    (8) Hemorrhagic cystitis
      a) Large quantities of blood in urine
      b) Due to acute bacterial infections
  (b) Viral pathogens, e.g., herpes
  (c) Fungal organisms unlikely except in immunocompromised patients
  (d) Sexually transmitted infections
    (1) Gonorrhea
    (2) Chlamydia
  (e) Congenital obstructive lesions
  (f) Acquired obstructive lesions
  (g) Nonobstructive causes
    (1) Voiding dysfunction
    (2) Neurogenic bladder
    (3) Ectopic kidney
  (h) Acquired nonobstructive causes
    (1) Poor hygiene
    (2) Constipation
    (3) Sexual intercourse
  (i) Metabolic abnormalities
vi. Pathophysiology
  (a) Short female urethra (3 to 4 cm)
  (b) Uncircumcised male in first 6 months

(1) 10 times higher incidence of UTI

(2) Periurethral organisms harbored behind foreskin

(c) Incomplete bladder emptying

(1) Urinary stasis

(2) Urethral high pressure enables microorganisms to ascend from the meatus or periurethral area to the bladder

(d) Bladder colonization with either gram-negative or gram-positive organism

(1) Increased adherence of bacteria to urothelial cells

(2) Rate of multiplication of bacteria in bladder (Moore, 2002)

vii. Treatment of UTI (See the American Academy of Pediatrics (1999) practice parameter for UTI (this is the latest edition as of May, 2006)

(a) First infection in males 6 to 15 years: refer to pediatric urologist for full evaluation

(b) Antibiotic therapy

(1) Oral medications in nontoxic infant younger than 2 months

(2) Hospitalize and manage with parenteral therapy for toxic or dehydrated infant (broad spectrum)

(3) Treat for 3 to 10 days (length of treatment depends on age)

a) Older than 2 months trimethoprim-sulfamethoxazole

b) Cephalosporins

(c) Reculture only if antimicrobial sensitivity not obtained

(d) Cranberry juice or tablets for prevention of UTI

(1) No clear evidence of efficacy

(2) Theoretically, it prevents bacteria from adhering to uroepithelial cells (Jepson, 2006)

(e) Pyridium for pain

viii. Follow-up

(a) Recurrent UTI (>3 in a 6-month period) consider prophylactic antibiotics

(b) Recurrent UTI in sexually active adolescent female consider postcoital antibiotics

ix. Prognosis

(a) 32% males reinfected

(b) 40% females reinfected

b. Hemolytic-uremic syndrome (HUS) (Davis & Avner, 2004)

i. Signs and symptoms

(a) Sudden onset of oliguria or anuria, acute hypertension

(b) Pallor

(c) Weakness, lethargy

(d) Watery diarrhea, changes to bloody diarrhea after 3 days, painful

(e) Systolic flow murmur

(f) Irritability

(g) Petechiae, purpura and bruising

(h) Mild hematuria

(i) Microangiopathic hemolytic anemia (5 to 9 g/dL)

(j) Thrombocytopenia (20,000-100,000/mm$^3$) in 90% of cases

ii. Prevalence

(a) Most common cause of acute renal failure in young children (atypical presentation < 1 yr)

(b) Most common in children younger than age 4 years

iii. Etiology

        (a) ≥80% cases due to acute diarrhea caused by Shiga toxin–producing *E. coli* 0157:H7

        (b) Present in undercooked meat and unpasteurized milk

        (c) Other cases due to many other bacterial (e.g., shigella, salmonella, *Streptococcus pneumoniae*) or viral (e.g., varicella, influenza) infections, no seasonal pattern

    **iv.** Pathophysiology

        (a) Toxin is absorbed from the intestine

        (b) Endothelial cell injury leads to intravascular coagulopathy

        (c) Microangiography results in hemorrhagic colitis

    **v.** Treatment (Davis & Avner, 2004)

        (a) Supportive care

        (b) Meticulous attention to:

            (1) Fluid and electrolyte levels

            (2) Control of hypertension

            (3) Hematologic support

            (4) Aggressive nutrition

            (5) Early institution of dialysis

            (6) Avoid nephrotoxic drugs

        (c) Antibiotics will increase risk of HUS if cause is *E. coli* 0157:H7

        (d) Antibiotics are appropriate for atypical HUS to treat infection caused by neuraminidase organisms

        (e) Education about food preparation and storage

    **vi.** Follow-up

        (a) Frequency during acute phase depends on signs and symptoms

        (b) Long-term follow-up required

    **vii.** Prognosis

        (a) Mortality is less than 10% with treatment described above

        (b) 9% develop end-stage renal disease

        (c) Hypertension, chronic renal insufficiency, or proteinuria may not appear for up to 20 years

  **c.** Acute poststreptococcal glomerulonephritis (Davis & Avner, 2004)

    **i.** Signs and symptoms

        (a) Sudden onset of gross hematuria and proteinuria

        (b) With or without oliguria

        (c) Periorbital edema

        (d) Hypertension (60% of cases)

        (e) Systemic symptoms—malaise, flank pain, fever

        (f) Renal insufficiency

        (g) Encephalopathy

    **ii.** Prevalence

        (a) One of most common glomerular causes of hematuria

        (b) Common in children ages 5 to 12; rare before age 3

    **iii.** Etiology

        (a) Nephritogenic strains of group A β-hemolytic streptococci

    **iv.** Pathophysiology

        (a) Enlargement and inflammation of glomeruli

        (b) Latency of 7 to 14 days after pharyngitis during cold months

        (c) Latency of 21 to 42 days after impetigo or pyoderma during warm months

    **v.** Treatment (Davis & Avner, 2004)

        (a) Treat acute effects of hypertension and renal insufficiency

(b) 10-day course of antibiotics to limit spread of nephritogenic organisms

(c) Sodium restriction

(d) Diuresis

(e) Culture family members for group A β-hemolytic streptococci and treat with antibiotics if positive

(f) Provide patient/family education about personal hygiene

   **vi.** Follow-up

(a) Every 2 weeks or more often depending on signs and symptoms

(b) Special attention to hematuria, proteinuria, hypertension

  **vii.** Prognosis

(a) Complete recovery in 6 to 8 weeks in 95% of cases

(b) Mortality can be avoided by proper management in acute stage

(c) Hematuria may persist for 1 to 2 years

(d) Recurrences are extremely rare

(e) Monitor blood pressure monthly for first 6 months

(f) Monitor electrolytes every three months for 1 year

**d.** Vesicoureteral reflux (VUR)

    **i.** Signs and symptoms

(a) UTI symptoms

(b) Bedwetting

(c) High blood pressure

(d) Protein in urine

(e) Kidney failure

   **ii.** Prevalence

(a) Children less than 1 year with a UTI, more than 50% diagnosed with VUR

(b) Reflux found in 34% to 50% of siblings

  **iii.** Etiology

(a) Primary

    (1) Short ureter due to congenital anomaly of the ureterovesical junction

    (2) Deficiency of longitudinal muscle of the intravesical ureter

    (3) Inadequate length of intravesical tunnel

(b) Secondary

    (1) Decompensation of the valvular mechanism as a result of elevated intravesical pressures

  **iv.** Pathophysiology (Gloor & Torres, 2001)

(a) Retrograde flow of urine from bladder through the ureter into the upper urinary potential tract

(b) Grading by International Grading System of Vesicoureteral Reflux

    (1) Grade I reflux involves only ureter

    (2) Grade II reflux reaches the renal pelvis

    (3) Grade III reflux extends into renal pelvis and calyces, mild to moderate

    (4) Grade IV reflux extends into renal pelvis and calyces

    (5) Grade V reflux with significant daytime enuresis dilatation of calyces

   **v.** Treatment

(a) Medical management

    (1) Prophylactic antibiotics to prevent renal scarring

      a) Bactrim, Macrodantin

b) Daily dose at night

c) Continue therapy until VUR resolves

(b) Surgical management

   (1) Patients with breakthrough infection

   (2) High-grade reflux or renal scarring

   (3) Ureteral reimplants

      a) Open procedure

      b) Laparoscopic procedure

      c) Collagen injection

vi. Follow-up

(a) Standard or nuclear medicine VCUG every 12 to 18 months until VUR resolves

(b) Continue antibiotic prophylaxis until VUR resolves

(c) Obtain urinalysis and culture with *all* febrile illnesses

(d) Screen siblings

   (1) Older than 5 years of age with standard or nuclear medicine VCUG

   (2) Siblings older than 5 years of age and no history of UTI screen with ultrasound

   (3) Siblings older than 5 years of age and history of UTI screen with VCUG of nuclear VCUG

vii. Prognosis

(a) Grades I and II, 80% to 82% in younger than 5 years of age resolve

(b) Grade III, 46% resolve

(c) Bilateral grade III, 10% resolve

(d) Conventional or laparoscopic repair, 95% of VUR corrected

(e) Potential long-term complications

   (1) Hypertension

   (2) Renal scarring in 48% to 54% with grades III through V dilating reflux

   (3) Pyelonephritis

   (4) End-stage renal disease

   (5) Pregnancy complications

e. Dysfunctional elimination syndrome

  i. Signs and symptoms (Shaikh, et al., 2003)

   (a) Bladder incontinence or withholding

   (b) 50% also have encopresis (see Chapter 30)

   (c) Previously toilet-trained children

   (d) No anatomic or neurologic abnormalities

  ii. Prevalence

   (a) 10% of children 4 to 6 years

   (b) 5% children 6 to 12 years

   (c) 4% of adolescents

   (d) Females at higher risk for dysfunctional voiding related to shorter urethra (13.3% vs. 9%)

  iii. Etiology

   (a) Constipation—mechanical pressure on bladder and pelvic musculature (Lucanto, et al., 2000)

   (b) Infrequent voiding

   (c) Small bladder capacity

   (d) Stress from anxiety-causing events

   (e) Structural abnormalities

(1) Labial adhesions
(2) Ectopic ureter
iv. Pathophysiology
   (a) Delayed or disturbed voluntary control of bladder or pelvic musculature
   (b) Overactive bladder
   (c) Filling phase defects
     (1) Detrusor hypertrophy—thickened bladder wall that alters the closure mechanism at the vesicoureteral junction
     (2) Bladder neck opens
     (3) Urine pushed into urethra
     (4) Contraction prevents bacteria from entering bladder
     (5) Lack of coordination between bladder and bladder outlet that results in inefficient bladder emptying
   (d) Voiding phase defects
     (1) Inappropriate contraction of the urethra and pelvic floor muscles during voiding rather than relaxation
     (2) Result is increased voiding pressure (Farhat, et al., 2000)
v. Treatment
   (a) Pharmacologic agents
     (1) Anticholinergic medications
     (2) Tricyclic antidepressants
     (3) Stool softener if constipated
     (4) Antibiotic treatment or prophylaxis if associated with recurrent UTI
   (b) Behavioral therapy
     (1) Timed voiding
     (2) Elimination of bladder irritants
     (3) Double voiding—urinate, wait a few minutes, urinate again
   (c) Referral for pelvic muscle retraining
     (1) Kegel exercises
     (2) Biofeedback (Porena, 2000)
vi. Follow-up
   (a) Reevaluate 6 months after treatment to assess continence results
   (b) Referral to urology if unresponsive to medical intervention
vii. Prognosis
   (a) 14% spontaneous cure rates in 5- to 9-year-olds
**f.** Urethritis
  i. Signs and symptoms
   (a) Dysuria
   (b) Males: urethral discharge
   (c) Females: usually asymptomatic
  ii. Prevalence and etiology
   (a) 14% to 20% prevalence in sexually active adolescents
   (b) Gonococcal urethritis due to *Neisseria gonorrhoeae*
   (c) Nongonococcal urethritis due to *Chlamydia trachomatis, Ureaplasma urealyticum, Mycoplasma hominis,* or *Trichomonas vaginalis*
  iii. Pathophysiology
   (a) Invasion of the urethral mucosa with gram-negative organism or protozoon
   (b) May be purulent or mucopurulent
  iv. Treatment (Terris, 2004)

        (a) Best to use antibiotic that is effective for gonococcal and nongonococcal etiology

        (b) Self-limiting without treatment, but prevention of morbidity and protection of partners is reason for treatment

        (c) Education about safer sexual practices

    **v.** Follow-up

        (a) Abstain from sexual intercourse until 7 days after treatment is initiated

        (b) Refer partners within past 60 days for evaluation and treatment

        (c) Report identifiable disease to the health department (CDC, 2002)

        (d) Reevaluate if symptoms persist

    **vi.** Prognosis

        (a) Cure rates high but risk of reinfection

        (b) 10% to 40% of females develop pelvic inflammatory disease

        (c) 1% to 2% of males develop urethral stricture or stenosis

## SYMPTOM: BEDWETTING

1. History and symptom assessment
   a. Onset, duration, frequency
   b. Family history, changes in family structure
   c. Psychosocial history, recent stressors
   d. Previous UTIs
   e. Allergies
   f. Associated daytime voiding problems: frequency, urgency, intermittent or weak stream, urge incontinence
2. Focused physical examination
   a. Abdominal examination
      i. Palpate kidneys
      ii. Rule out mass
      iii. Distended bladder
      iv. Fecal impaction
   b. Check for flank pain
   c. Neurologic examination
      i. Abnormalities are rare
      ii. Occult spinal dysraphism, a variant of spina bifida, may be present
         (a) Asymmetry of gluteal cleft
         (b) Pigmentation or hair tufts over lower spine
      iii. Check cerebellum function for subtle deficits (Thiedke, 2003)
      iv. Elicit the anal "wink" or have child stand on toes to test S2-S4 spinal reflex arc
   d. Genitourinary examination
      i. Structural abnormalities
3. Differential diagnoses
   a. UTI
   b. VUR
   c. Primary nocturnal enuresis
   d. Secondary nocturnal enuresis
   e. See also Table 31-1 for other potential diagnoses
4. Definition, prevalence and etiology
   a. UTI

    **b.** VUR

    **c.** Primary nocturnal enuresis (PNE)

        **i.** Defining characteristics

            (a) Involuntary passage of urine during sleep in child older than age 5 years

            (b) Child has never been dry for a period of at least 6 months

            (c) Not due to UTI

            (d) Physical examination usually normal

        **ii.** Prevalence

            (a) 7% of males and 3% of females at age 5 years

            (b) 28% of males and 11% of females with sickle cell disease (Barakat, 2001)

        **iii.** Etiology

            (a) Maturational delay in nocturnal secretion of the antidiuretic hormone, arginine vasopressin, resulting in urine overproduction (Thiedke, 2003)

            (b) Developmental delay—delayed functional maturation of central nervous system

            (c) Anatomic factors—small functional bladder capacity

            (d) Genetics (Eiberg, et al., 2001)

                (1) Family history

                    a) One parent with PNE: 40% risk in child

                    b) Two parents with PNE: 77% risk

                (2) Identified on chromosomes 4p16, 13q, 12q, 8, and 22

            (e) Sleep disorder

                (1) Enuresis is independent of sleep stages

                (2) Normal sleep patterns but difficulty awakening

            (f) Dyspnea—upper airway obstruction syndrome causes increased urine and sodium excretion (Sakai & Hebert, 2000)

    **d.** Secondary nocturnal enuresis (SNE) (Lane & Robson, 2005)

        **i.** Defining characteristics

            (a) Wetting during sleep that begins after at least 6 months of dryness

            (b) Not due to UTI

        **ii.** Etiology

            (a) Psychologic problems usually the cause

            (b) Comorbidity with behavioral problems two to five times higher with SNE than PNE

            (c) Sexual abuse

            (d) Depression (Brooks & Topol, 2003)

            (e) Attention deficit hyperactivity disorder—lack of attention to cues of full bladder

            (f) Dietary bladder irritants—insufficient research evidence

**5.** Diagnostic tests

**6.** Treatment and follow-up

    **a.** See Table 31-3 for when and to whom to refer

    **b.** UTI or VUR

    **c.** Primary nocturnal enuresis

        **i.** Treatment

            (a) Watchful waiting

                (1) Most appropriate for children less than 7 years

                (2) 15% of children outgrow nocturnal enuresis every year

            (b) Behavioral or motivational therapy

        (1) Limit fluids

        (2) Bladder-stretching exercises (holding urine)

        (3) Bladder fullness awareness

        (4) Sticker charts for increased responsibility

        (5) Nighttime awakening of child to void

           a) Parent awakening

           b) Self-awakening with alarm

    (c) Conditioning therapy: alarm systems

        (1) Liquid-sensitive alarm pad is worn in the underpants

        (2) Urine contact with the pad causes a bell to alarm and awaken the child

        (3) Requires prolonged family commitment

    (d) Pharmacotherapy

        (1) Desmopressin acetate (DDAVP)

           a) A synthetic analogue of the pituitary antidiuretic hormone, vasopressin

           b) Causes renal water conservation

           c) Uncommon side effect is headache ($\leq$3%)

        (2) Imipramine

           a) A tricyclic antidepressant

           b) Action related to enuresis is unknown

           c) Once was a common treatment; rarely used today

        (3) Most effective in children older than 10 years who fail other therapy

    (e) Hypnotherapy (Milling & Costantino, 2000)

        (1) Clinical trials show promising results for hypnosis

        (2) Hypnosis not labeled "efficacious" yet, according to stringent criteria

    (f) Psychotherapy

        (1) Brain-bladder connection is explained to child

        (2) Visual imaging of response to a full bladder

  ii. Follow-up (Glazener & Evans, 2006; Glazener, et al., 2006)

    (a) Phone contact with family in 2 to 4 weeks to assess response to treatment

    (b) For responders to medication, continue therapy for approximately 6 months

    (c) Withdraw medication for 1 week to assess response without treatment

    (d) Complicated history, nonresponders: refer to pediatric urologist

  iii. Prognosis (Lane & Robson, 2005; Redsell & Collier, 2001)

    (a) Psychologic treatments *and* a urine alarm treatment are superior to other treatment methods

    (b) Children who wet less frequently and who wet only at night have better outcome

    (c) Cure rates 60% to 80% long term

    (d) Most children relapse after withdrawal of medication

    (e) Drop-out rate of 30% with conditioning therapy (alarm systems)

    (f) 50% of children relapse after withdrawal of alarm system

    (g) Behavior problems are a result of bedwetting; rarely causal

    (h) Mixed evidence that children with bedwetting have lower self-esteem

   **d.** Secondary nocturnal enuresis
      **i.** Treatment
        **(a)** Identify and eliminate or minimize sources of stress
        **(b)** Referral for counseling or psychotherapy
      **ii.** Follow-up at each clinic visit
      **iii.** Prognosis: good with treatment; occasionally self-limiting

## SYMPTOMS: SCROTAL SWELLING, WITH OR WITHOUT PAIN

**1.** History and symptom assessment
  **a.** Age of onset
  **b.** Swelling: size, changes over time, discoloration
  **c.** Pain: location, severity, intermittent, constant, situations that aggravate pain, methods that alleviate pain
  **d.** Systemic symptoms: fever
  **e.** GI: abdominal pain, nausea, vomiting
  **f.** Dysuria
  **g.** Urologic history: previous episodes of scrotal swelling or urogenital diseases, recent urologic procedures
  **h.** Urethral discharge
  **i.** Trauma
  **j.** Recent physical or sexual activity
  **k.** Irritability in the neonate
  **l.** Family history
  **m.** Medications
  **n.** Hip or abdominal pain
**2.** Focused physical examination—see Chapter 9 for assessment details
  **a.** Frog-leg position
  **b.** Inspect
      **i.** Abdomen
      **ii.** Genitalia—supine and standing
      **iii.** Testes—supine and standing
      **iv.** Inguinal areas
      **v.** Classic blue dot sign (blue or purple discoloration of scrotum)
  **c.** Palpate
      **i.** Abdomen
      **ii.** Testicular surface
      **iii.** Epididymis
      **iv.** Spermatic cord
      **v.** Inguinal nodes
      **vi.** Silk glove sign
        **(a)** Feels like two fingers of a silk glove rubbing against each other
        **(b)** Could mean a hydrocele or hernia
  **d.** Check for presence or absence of specific signs
      **i.** Cremasteric reflex bilateral
        **(a)** Stroke thigh in downward direction
        **(b)** Contraction of cremasteric muscle
        **(c)** Pulls up the scrotum and testis on the side stroked
        **(d)** Tests nerve roots L1 and L2
      **ii.** Prehn's sign—elevation of scrotum relieves pain of epididymitis but not torsion

     **e.** Auscultate bowel sounds

**3.** Differential diagnoses

    **a.** Painful

       **i.** Testicular torsion

      **ii.** Epididymitis

    **iii.** Orchitis

    **b.** Nonpainful

       **i.** Hydrocele

      **ii.** Spermatocele

    **iii.** Varicocele

    **iv.** Hernia

     **v.** Undescended testicle

    **c.** See Table 31-1 for other potential diagnoses

**4.** Diagnostic tests

    **a.** Ultrasound to differentiate among diagnoses (Dogra & Resnick, 2002)

    **b.** Serum α-fetoprotein to rule out malignant tumor (Cooper et al., 2006)

    **c.** Transillumination of testicles

    **d.** Urinalysis

    **e.** Cultures

       **i.** Urine

      **ii.** Urethral discharge

    **f.** Gram stain of urethral discharge

    **g.** Bloodwork as indicated by differential diagnoses (Luzzi & O'Brien, 2001)

       **i.** HIV

      **ii.** Hepatitis B and C

    **iii.** RPR for syphilis

    **h.** Mumps titer IgG and IgM (if indicated; related to orchitis)

    **i.** Valsalva maneuver—no change in symptoms with spermatocele

    **j.** Abdominal flat and upright plain films (Marcozzi & Suner, 2001)

    **k.** Serial orchidometry measurements or ultrasound to measure testicular size

    **l.** Nonpalpable testicles require chromosome analysis to rule out female with adrenal hyperplasia

**5.** See Table 31-3 for when to refer

**6.** Signs, symptoms, prevalence, etiology, pathophysiology, and treatment

    **a.** Torsion (technically, torsion of spermatic cord or testicular appendix)

       **i.** Signs and symptoms

         (a) Torsion of spermatic cord

           (1) Sudden onset of acute pain

           (2) Diffuse tenderness

           (3) Negative cremasteric reflex

           (4) May be intermittent

           (5) May be associated with nausea and vomiting

           (6) Can usually be diagnosed on examination

         (b) Appendiceal torsion

           (1) Subacute onset

           (2) Pain, tenderness localized to upper portion of scrotum

           (3) Positive cremasteric reflex

      **ii.** Prevalence

         (a) Testicular torsion peaks at age 13 (12 to 20 years)

           (1) 1 per 4000 males younger than 25 years

           (2) Left testicle more than right

         (b) Appendiceal torsion typically prepubertal

      iii. Etiology

         (a) Anatomic risk factor 10 times greater with undescended testicle

         (b) Presence of "bell clapper" deformity or anomalous suspension of testicle

         (c) Additional weight of testicles during pubertal growth

         (d) Fetal remnant appendages of the testis and epididymis (mullerian polyps)

      iv. Pathophysiology

         (a) Twisting of testis, appendix testis, or epididymis on spermatic cord causes infarction of the testis

      v. Treatment

         (a) Testicular torsion

            (1) Manual de-torsion to relieve ischemia

            (2) Surgical emergency for exploration and correction

               a) Within 6 to 8 hours to salvage testicle

         (b) Appendiceal torsion of the testis or epididymis

            (1) Limit activity for 2 to 4 days

            (2) Nonsteroidal antiinflammatory drugs (NSAIDs) for pain management (see Table 55-5)

         (c) Unclear diagnosis—immediate referral

         (d) Persistent symptoms—refer to pediatric urology

      vi. Follow-up

         (a) Observe for recurrent signs and symptoms

         (b) Routine genital examination with annual physical examination

      vii. Prognosis

         (a) Testicular torsion

            (1) Good prognosis if surgery undertaken within 6 hours

            (2) If surgical repair greater than 12 hours from onset of symptoms 20% success rate in preserving testicle

            (3) May have decreased sperm count related to underlying testicular abnormality

         (b) Appendiceal torsion of the testis or epididymis

            (1) Usually self-limited with autoinfarction

            (2) Rare adverse outcome

   b. Epididymitis

      i. Signs and symptoms

         (a) Insidious onset of scrotal pain

         (b) Positive cremasteric reflex

         (c) UTI symptoms

         (d) Systemic symptoms, e.g., nausea, vomiting, fever, chills

         (e) Urethral discharge

      ii. Prevalence

         (a) Rare in children

         (b) Occurs in 1 per 1000 sexually active males

      iii. Etiology

         (a) Sexually transmitted enteric organism

         (b) Recent surgical procedures or trauma

         (c) Anatomic abnormalities

      iv. Pathophysiology

         (a) Spread of infection from the urethra or bladder to epididymis

         (b) 40% to 90% of patients have sterile urine (Luzzi, & O'Brien, 2001)

      v. Treatment

          (a) Appropriate antibiotic prophylaxis (CDC, 2002)

          (b) NSAIDs for pain

          (c) Scrotal support

          (d) Limit activity

             (1) Bed rest

             (2) No heavy lifting for 2 weeks

          (e) Treat sexual partners if sexually transmitted infection identified

      **vi.** Follow-up

          (a) Radiographic evaluation to rule out structural abnormalities if:

             (1) Nonsexually active males

             (2) *And* positive bacterial cultures

          (b) 2- to 3-week evaluation to assess for symptom resolution

          (c) Avoid sexual intercourse until 7 days posttreatment completion

          (d) Condom use education

      **vii.** Prognosis—compete recovery expected

  **c.** Orchitis (Mycyk & Moyer, 2004)

      **i.** Signs and symptoms

          (a) Scrotum tender, swollen, red, or purple

          (b) Systemic symptoms, e.g., nausea, vomiting, malaise

      **ii.** Prevalence

          (a) Occurs in 20% of prepubertal males who develop mumps

          (b) 70% unilateral testicle involvement

          (c) Develops in contralateral testicle in 1 to 9 days in 30%

      **iii.** Etiology

          (a) Rare prior to puberty unless due to mumps virus

          (b) If older than age 15 and sexually active, usually bacterial causes

          (c) Bacterial orchitis associated with epididymitis

      **iv.** Pathophysiology

          (a) Inflammation of the testis

          (b) May damage seminiferous tubules (Rowland & Herman, 2002)

          (c) Follows mumps parotitis in 4 to 7 days

      **v.** Treatment (Mycyk & Moyer, 2004)

          (a) If due to mumps virus

             (1) Resolves spontaneously in 3 to 10 days

             (2) NSAIDs for pain (see Table 55-5)

          (b) If bacterial

             (1) Appropriate antibiotic therapy

             (2) If severe pain, may require opioid analgesic

          (c) Bed rest

          (d) Scrotal support with a Bellvue bridge

          (e) Hot or cold packs

      **vi.** Follow-up

          (a) Reassess in 3 days if swelling or tenderness persists after antibiotic initiated

          (b) If due to sexually transmitted infection (STI), HIV testing is recommended

      **vii.** Prognosis

          (a) 60% have some testicular atrophy

          (b) Sterility is rare if unilateral; 7% to 13% if bilateral

  **d.** Hydrocele

      **i.** Prevalence

          (a) Apparent in 6% of males after full-term birth

    ii. Etiology
       (a) Communicating
         (1) Peritoneal fluid collection in abdomen and scrotum
         (2) Often associated with hernia
       (b) Noncommunicating
         (1) Fluid collection in scrotum
         (2) No connection to peritoneum
         (3) Acquired lesion
         (4) Results from inflammation of testis or epididymis
   iii. Pathophysiology
       (a) Fluid between the parietal and visceral layers of the tunica vaginalis, anterior to the testicle
       (b) Defect in processus vaginalis
       (c) Transillumination reveals a homogeneous glow, without internal shadows
       (d) High index of suspicion for malignant testicular tumor (Cooper et al., 2006)
         (1) 10% to 25% of children with tumor present with a hydrocele
    iv. Treatment
       (a) Referral for surgery if persistent after 1 to 2 years
     v. Follow-up
       (a) Reassurance about resolution that most hydroceles resolve in 1 year
       (b) Educate families about potential hernia
       (c) Surgical follow-up at 4 weeks postoperative
    vi. Prognosis (Schneck & Bellinger, 2002)
       (a) Spontaneous closure is likely to occur by age 2
       (b) Small potential recurrence rate

**e.** Spermatocele
    i. Prevalence
       (a) Benign, uncommon, 1%
       (b) Occurs in neonatal period, late childhood or early adolescence
       (c) Peak incidence in adolescence
    ii. Pathophysiology
       (a) Retention cyst containing sperm located in upper portion of epididymis
   iii. Diagnostic tests
       (a) Transillumination
       (b) Ultrasound if unable to differentiate (Dogra & Resnick, 2002)
    iv. Treatment
       (a) No treatment required
       (b) If large, refer for surgical evaluation
     v. Follow-up
       (a) Teach testicular self-examination
    vi. Prognosis—benign

**f.** Varicocele (Kogan, 2001)
    i. Prevalence
       (a) 5% to 15% adolescents
       (b) Peak age 10 to 20 years
       (c) 85% on left and 15% on right (isolated right sided requires further evaluation)
    ii. Etiology and pathophysiology
       (a) Incompetent venous valves in internal spermatic veins

(1) Increased venous pressure in left renal vein
(2) Collateral venous anastomoses
(b) Right internal spermatic vein enters vena cava at acute angle
(1) Creates too little backflow pressure
(c) Dilated and tortuous veins of the spermatic cord superior and posterior to testes
(d) Increased testicular blood flow exposes venous anomaly in adolescence
(e) Grading
(1) Grade 1—detected only with Valsalva
(2) Grade 2—palpable but not visible
(3) Grade 3—visible on inspection
iii. Treatment (Kogan, 2001)
(a) Refer to urology if:
(1) Testicular size discrepancy more than 3 mL, grade 3
(2) Symptomatic lesions
(3) Right unilateral or bilateral palpable varicoceles
iv. Follow-up
(a) Annual examination
(1) Evaluate testicular growth
(2) Varicocele grade
(3) Signs and symptoms
v. Prognosis
(a) 80% of men fertile
(b) Controversial whether surgical intervention alters fertility outcomes (Silber, 2001)
(c) 4.3% to 11% recurrence rate
g. Hernia
i. Prevalence
(a) 10 to 20 per 1000 live births
(b) Ratio 6:1 male to female
(c) 55% to 70% right-side hernia
(d) 10% to 40% have a subsequent contralateral hernia (other side)
(e) Increased incidence in younger children
(f) Increased incidence with premature birth (30%)
(g) 12% to 17% incarcerated
ii. Etiology and pathophysiology
(a) Processus vaginalis fails to obliterate
(b) Indirect (congenital)
(1) Bowel or omentum is forced into scrotum via the inguinal canal
(2) Hernia arises lateral to the inferior epigastric vessels
(3) Incarcerated or strangulated
(c) Direct
(1) Acquired
(2) Rare in children
(3) Increased incidence after age 3 (Marcozzi & Suner, 2001)
(4) May be related to obesity, weight-lifting, or family history
iii. Treatment
(a) Refer to surgery for repair
(b) Educate families about signs and symptoms of incarceration and strangulation

        **iv.** Follow-up

            (a) Routine genital examination with well child care

        **v.** Prognosis

            (a) 99% successful surgical repair

            (b) Overall recurrence rate 0.5% to 1%

            (c) Recurrence rate 3% to 6% with emergency repair

            (d) Recurrence 2% in premature infants

            (e) Recurrence highest in first 2 years postoperative

    **h.** Undescended testicle (cryptorchidism)

        **i.** Prevalence

            (a) Nonpalpable testicle 20% (Baker, Silver, Docimo, 2001)

            (b) Palpable testicle in inguinal area

                (1) Newborns 3% to 5%

                (2) By 1 year of age approximately 1%

                (3) Premature infants 30%

            (c) 95% are incompletely descended: intra-abdominal, in inguinal ring, or exiting the external ring

            (d) 3.3% are absent or atrophic as a result of perinatal torsion

        **ii.** Etiology and pathophysiology

            (a) Retractile testicle

                (1) Normal variant—testicles in inguinal canal

                (2) Due to hyperactive cremasteric reflex

                (3) Can be manually moved down to bottom of scrotum

                (4) Common (80% of males, ages 1 to 11 years)

                (5) Disappears by age 13

            (b) Canalicular testicle

                (1) Above scrotum, but outside abdominal cavity

                (2) Tension from external musculature prevents normal descent

            (c) Intra-abdominal testicle

                (1) Located along normal descent pathway

                (2) Hormonal abnormalities

                (3) At risk of becoming cancerous

            (d) Ectopic testicle

                (1) Outside the external inguinal ring

                (2) Misdirected attachment to the scrotum related to abnormal gubernaculum

            (e) Absent testicle

                (1) Due to in utero torsion, vascular insult, or agenesis

        **iii.** Treatment

            (a) Hormonal therapy—human chorionic gonadotropin (hCG)

                (1) Stimulates Leydig cells to produce male hormones

                (2) Better success with older children and retractile testicles

                (3) Approximately 20% respond

            (b) Surgical repair—orchiopexy

                (1) Definitive treatment before 1 year of age

            (c) Combination therapy

        **iv.** Follow-up

            (a) Routine testicular examination at well child visits

        **v.** Prognosis

            (a) Spontaneous descent in 70% to 77% of patients by 3 months of age

            (b) Bilateral undescended testicles (Lee & Coughlin, 2001)

                (1) 75% risk of abnormal semen

(2) Decreased fertility rates of 65.3%
(c) 89% normal paternity reported in patients with unilateral undescended testicles
(d) Increased risk of torsion or indirect inguinal hernia
(e) Orchiopexy success rate 92% below external ring, and 89% inguinal testes

## SYMPTOM: ALTERED URINARY STREAM, PAINFUL SWELLING OF FORESKIN, TIGHT OPENING

1. History and symptom assessment
   a. Circumcision
   b. Penis: erythema, swelling, discharge, pain
   c. Urination: dysuria, minimal or altered urinary stream, frequency
   d. Hematuria
2. Focused physical examination
   a. Abdominal examination
   b. Check for lymphadenopathy
   c. Genital examination
      i. Inspect the glans penis
      ii. Observe stream during voiding if possible
3. Differential diagnoses
   a. Phimosis
   b. Paraphimosis
   c. Balanitis
   d. Meatal stenosis, urethral stenosis, stricture
   e. Hypospadias
4. Diagnostic tests
   a. Cultures for sexually transmitted infections
   b. Visual inspection of urinary stream
   c. Karyotype if mid- or proximal hypospadias
   d. See Table 31-3 for when to refer
5. Prevalence, etiology, pathophysiology, and treatment
   a. Phimosis, paraphimosis (Cantu, 2006)
      i. Etiology and pathophysiology
         (a) Congenital phimosis—physiologic adherence of uncircumcised foreskin to glans
            (1) Prevalence—common in infancy through young adolescence
            (2) Normal variation
            (3) Should not cause problems with urine flow
            (4) Incomplete separation of epithelial layers causes nonretractile foreskin
         (b) Acquired phimosis—development of fibrotic ring near opening of prepuce
            (1) Forcible retraction of foreskin to clean the glans
            (2) Poor hygiene
            (3) Chronic infection
         (c) Paraphimosis—inability to reduce a retracted foreskin over the glans
            (1) Vigorous sexual activity
            (2) Trauma
            (3) Objects, e.g., penile rings

    **ii.** Treatment of phimosis and paraphimosis

        (a) Circumcision recommended if child is age 10 or older and ballooning while voiding is evident

        (b) Treatment of phimosis

            (1) Surgical release of scarred tissue or circumcision

            (2) Corticosteroid cream three times daily for 1 month (Elder, 2003) (see Table 54-5)

        (c) Treatment of paraphimosis

            (1) Topical analgesic, oral narcotic, or penile block before manipulation

            (2) Lubrication, gentle pressure, then compress glans while placing distal traction on foreskin

            (3) A urologic emergency if circulation is impaired

   **iii.** Follow-up (Elder, 2003)

        (a) Referral for development of adhesions or unresolved phimosis beyond 3 years

   **iv.** Prognosis

        (a) 90% of uncircumcised males retract by age 3

        (b) Most resolve with minimal intervention

**b.** Balanitis—inflammation of glans penis

   **i.** Prevalence

        (a) 4% of uncircumcised males (Cuckow & Nyirady, 2001)

        (b) 4% to 11% of adolescents with trichomoniasis

   **ii.** Etiology and pathophysiology (Jordan & Schlossberg, 2002)

        (a) Inflammation of the glans related to:

            (1) Nonretractile foreskin, which harbors bacteria

            (2) Contact allergy or irritation

            (3) Atopic dermatitis

            (4) Infection

            (5) Mechanical trauma (excessive masturbation)

   **iii.** Treatment

        (a) Topical antibiotic ointment or fungal cream

        (b) Oral antibiotics in severe cases

        (c) Education

            (1) Instruct families to avoid forceful reduction of foreskin of uncircumcised penis

            (2) Instruct about potential causes of balanitis

        (d) Sitz baths

   **iv.** Follow-up

        (a) As needed for recurrence of symptoms

        (b) If STI positive, provide partner treatment and monitor for reinfection in 3 months

        (c) Refer for evaluation for circumcision with repeated episodes

        (d) Referral to urology or dermatology as needed

   **v.** Prognosis

        (a) First episode is often self-limiting

**c.** Meatal stenosis, urethral stenosis, stricture

   **i.** Prevalence (Angel, 2004)

        (a) 9% to 10% of circumcised males

   **ii.** Etiology and pathophysiology

        (a) Incomplete separation of the endoderm from the proximal urethra

        (b) Urogenital membrane does not retract

(c) Narrow meatus or urethra resulting in altered urinary stream and dysuria

(d) Trauma—straddle injuries

(e) Neonatal circumcision secondary to denuded glans (Elder, 2003)

iii. Treatment

(a) Refer for surgical repair

iv. Follow-up

(a) Genital examination at well child visits

v. Prognosis

(a) Meatal stenosis—excellent outcome

(b) Urethral stricture or stenosis—high recurrence rate

d. Hypospadias

i. Prevalence

(a) 1 per 250 to 300 live births

(b) Endocrine or genetic factors involved

(c) Increased incidence in past 10 years related to environmental factors

(1) Pregnant mice exposed to synthetic estrogen resulted in male hypospadias in offspring (Kim, et al., 2004)

(d) Five times higher incidence in infants conceived in vitro

(e) Familial pattern (6% to 8% of fathers with offspring)

ii. Pathophysiology

(a) Incomplete development of the prepuce

(b) Hypoplasia of the ventral radius of the penis that results in ectopic opening of the meatus

(c) Hooded foreskin

(d) Ventral curvature of the penis (chordee)

(e) Usually an isolated anomaly but common in males with other congenital anomalies (undescended testis or inguinal hernia)

(f) 15% of proximal hypospadias associated with chordee

iii. Treatment

(a) Refer for surgical repair usually at 6 to 12 months

(b) If uncircumcised, foreskin used for repair

iv. Follow-up

(a) Reoperation for complications should be deferred for 6 months after initial repair

v. Prognosis

(a) Erection normal

(b) Fertility unaffected unless associated with undescended testis

## SYMPTOMS: VAGINAL DISCHARGE, VULVAR IRRITATION, ITCHING AND ODOR, GENITAL BUMPS

1. History and symptom assessment

   a. Onset

   b. Perineum: swelling, pruritus, pain, pain with urination, tingling sensation

   c. Vagina: change in vaginal secretions, pruritus, pain

   d. Urethra: discharge, pain with urination

   e. Menstrual cycle: last menstrual period, contraceptive method

   f. Sexual history: frequency and type of sexual activity, dyspareunia, masturbation, foreign

      i. Object insertion, history of sexually transmitted infections, sexual abuse

      **ii.** Trauma

      **iii.** Hygiene practices and products

  **g.** Exacerbation of symptoms

      **i.** Response to previous treatments

      **ii.** Antibiotic therapy

  **h.** Skin and mucous membranes: other skin lesions, oral lesions, conjunctivitis

  **i.** Family history of diabetes

  **j.** Other symptoms

      **i.** GI: diarrhea

      **ii.** Fever

      **iii.** Malaise

      **iv.** Headache

      **v.** Myalgia

      **vi.** Respiratory

  **k.** Family history of similar symptoms

  **l.** Chronic disease

  **m.** Drug or alcohol use

**2.** Focused physical examination

  **a.** Inspection of skin, scalp, conjunctiva, mucous membranes

  **b.** Palpate

      **i.** Abdomen

      **ii.** Inguinal area

      **iii.** Lymph nodes

      **iv.** Genitalia

         **(a)** External genitalia

         **(b)** Rectal examination

         **(c)** Bimanual examination if indicated

         **(d)** Vaginal speculum examination if indicated

**3.** Differential diagnosis

  **a.** Nonspecific vulvovaginitis (prepubertal)

  **b.** Bacterial specific vulvovaginitis (prepubertal)

  **c.** Pinworms

  **d.** Foreign bodies

  **e.** Candida vaginitis

  **f.** Trichomoniasis

  **g.** Bacterial vaginosis

  **h.** Mucopurulent cervicitis

  **i.** Nonpainful genital bumps

      **i.** Labial adhesions

      **ii.** Genital warts

  **j.** Painful genital bumps

      **i.** Herpes simplex virus

      **ii.** Aphthosis

  **k.** See Table 31-1 for other potential diagnoses

**4.** Diagnostic tests

  **a.** Bacterial vaginosis—Amsel criteria: three of the following

      **i.** Vaginal pH $\geq 4.5$

      **ii.** Whiff test for positive volatile amines (vaginal swab dipped in KOH)

      **iii.** Clue cells on saline wet prep, i.e., more than 20% of epithelial cells covered with bacteria

      **iv.** Thin, homogeneous discharge

  **b.** KOH wet prep to visualize yeast pseudohyphae

  c. Gram stain of vaginal fluid (CDC, 2002)
     i. Gram-negative intracellular diplococci suggest gonorrhea
     ii. 10 to 30 leukocytes per oil immersion field suggests chlamydia cervicitis (Myziuk, et al., 2001)
  d. Urinalysis
     i. Microscopy
     ii. Trichomoniasis associated with urine sediment in males
     iii. Culture
  e. Culture of discharge
  f. Urine culture
  g. Viral cultures—Gold standard
  h. RPR
  i. Pap smear
  j. HPV testing (Digene HPV)
  k. Biopsy may be indicated if diagnosis uncertain
  l. Stool cultures
  m. Test for pinworms
       i. Flashlight test
          (a) Visualize perineum during night
          (b) Reveals 1-cm-long thin white worms
       ii. "Scotch tape" test
          (a) Placed on perineum overnight
          (b) Pinworms stick to tape
          (c) Urinalysis
       iii. Screening for gonorrhea and chlamydia
       iv. Polymerase chain reaction (PCR) and ligase chain reaction (LCR) amplified probes
       v. Digital rectal examination to collect specimen for wet mount and microscopy (American Academy of Pediatrics, 2003; Patel & Kazura, 2003)
  n. See Table 31-3 for when to refer
5. Prevalence, etiology, pathophysiology, and treatment
  a. Vulvovaginitis (prepubertal) (Rau & Muram, 2001; Sanfilippo, 2004)
     i. Etiology
        (a) In childhood, 50% to 80% *nonspecific* etiology
        (b) Contact irritation
        (c) Most often associated with poor hygiene
        (d) Gastrointestinal pathogens
           (1) *Shigella*
           (2) *Yersinia entercolitica*
           (3) *E. coli*
        (e) More than 5% caused by *Candida*
        (f) 20% of girls with pinworms develop vulvovaginitis
        (g) Respiratory pathogens (i.e., Group A beta-hemolytic streptococcus (GABHS), *Haemophilus influenzae*) (Herbst, 2003)
        (h) Identified in sexual abuse cases
           (1) Chlamydia
           (2) Trichomonas
           (3) Gonorrhea
     ii. Pathophysiology
        (a) Inflammation of the vulva or vagina in response to a variety of stimuli
        (b) Prepubertal female susceptible to bacterial growth related to:

          (1) Low estrogen levels
          (2) Lack of labial fat pads
          (3) Small labia minora
          (4) Lack of protective labial hair
          (5) Neutral or alkaline pH

   iii. Treatment of prepubertal vulvovaginitis (Sanfilippo, 2004)
      (a) Improve personal hygiene, eliminate irritants
      (b) Sitz baths (Sanfilippo, 2003)
      (c) Oral antibiotics if due to microorganism
      (d) Short-term mild hydrocortisone creams to relieve pruritus
      (e) Referral to forensic medicine if sexual abuse suspected

   iv. Follow-up
      (a) Return to clinic if symptoms persist or recur in less than 2 months
      (b) Refer to pediatric gynecologist if therapy fails

   v. Prognosis
      (a) Recurrence common

**b.** Pinworms (enterobiasis) (American Academy of Pediatrics, 2003)
   **i.** Etiology
      (a) *Enterobius vermicularis,* roundworm

   **ii.** Pathophysiology
      (a) Inhaled eggs migrate to rectum
      (b) Oral ingestion of eggs carried on:
          (1) Fingernails
          (2) Clothing
          (3) Bedding
          (4) House dust
      (c) Incubation 1 to 2 months from ingestion of egg to gravid female in perianal area
      (d) Symptoms caused by:
          (1) Mechanical stimulation (scratching)
          (2) Irritation
          (3) Allergic reaction (Patel & Kazura, 2003)

   **iii.** Treatment (American Academy of Pediatrics, 2003)
      (a) Oral anthelmintic medications (see Table 54-3 in Chapter 54)
      (b) Wash bed linens and clothing in hot water
      (c) Treat household members (American Academy of Pediatrics, 2003)
      (d) Prevention with good handwashing

   **iv.** Prognosis
      (a) Fully treatable
      (b) Reinfestation possible
      (c) Complications—vaginitis, salpingitis

**c.** Foreign bodies
   **i.** Prevalence and etiology
      (a) Highest incidence females 3 to 9 years
      (b) 79% in this age group due to "balled up" toilet tissue
      (c) Most common object in adolescence is tampon (Haward & Shafer, 2002)

   **ii.** Pathophysiology
      (a) Chronic inflammatory response of vaginal mucosa
      (b) Presence of vaginal bleeding with discharge raises suspicion of foreign body by 18%; if no discharge 50% incidence (Smith, et al., 2002)

      **iii.** Treatment
         (a) Local anesthesia and vaginal lavage
         (b) Examination under anesthesia
         (c) Secondary infection treat with antibiotics
      **iv.** Prognosis and follow-up
         (a) Fully treatable
   **d.** Candida vulvovaginitis (CDC, 2002, Haward & Shafer, 2002)
      **i.** Prevalence
         (a) 25% of healthy women colonized
         (b) 75% of females have one episode
         (c) 40% to 50% of females have two or more episodes
      **ii.** Etiology and pathophysiology
         (a) Overgrowth of opportunistic fungal pathogens
         (b) 85% caused by *Candida albicans*
         (c) Reinfection through the GI tract or partners
         (d) Host factors
            (1) Pregnancy
            (2) Diabetes
            (3) Hormonal changes
            (4) Antibiotic or steroid use
            (5) Depressed cell-mediated immunity
     **iii.** Treatment (CDC, 2002; Watson, et al., 2003) (see Table 54-3 in Chapter 54)
         (a) Topical and intravaginal agents
         (b) Education about vaginal hygiene
      **iv.** Follow-up—return if symptoms persist or recur in 2 months
       **v.** Prognosis
         (a) Relief of symptoms in 80% to 90% of patients completing therapy
         (b) Recurrent in less than 5% of females
            (1) Defined as four or more episodes in 1 year
            (2) Manage with weekly suppressive therapy for 6 months
   **e.** Trichomoniasis
      **i.** Prevalence
         (a) 15% to 20% of cases of vulvovaginitis due to *T. vaginalis*
         (b) 90% of males and 25% to 50% of females with *T. vaginalis* are asymptomatic
      **ii.** Etiology and pathophysiology
         (a) Overgrowth of *T. vaginalis*
            (1) Protozoan that inhabits vagina and lower urinary tract
            (2) Often identified in extravaginal sites
               a) Urethra (82.5%)
               b) Periurethral glands (98%)
         (b) Alteration of the vaginal pH from acidic to alkaline
         (c) Reduced resistance to trichomonas infection if exposed or colonized but asymptomatic
         (d) Transmitted from one person to another
            (1) Usually sexually transmitted
            (2) Sharing contaminated items
            (3) Perinatal transmission has been described
     **iii.** Treatment (CDC, 2002) (see Table 54-3 in Chapter 54)
         (a) Treatment of choice is metronidazole, 2 g oral, single dose
         (b) Treat sexual partners
         (c) Recommend condom use and hygiene

        iv. Follow-up
          (a) None necessary if asymptomatic after treatment
          (b) Report resistant strains of trichomonas to CDC
        v. Prognosis
          (a) 90% to 95% cure rate

    f. Bacterial vaginosis (BV)
        i. Prevalence
          (a) 10% to 60% of females with vaginal symptoms have BV (Joesoef & Schmid, 2001)
        ii. Etiology
          (a) Host factors
             (1) Multiple sexual partners
             (2) Same-sex partners
             (3) Intrauterine device (IUD) use
             (4) Douching
             (5) Early age of sexual debut
        iii. Pathophysiology
          (a) Replacement of normal lactobacilli with anaerobic bacteria
          (b) Elevated vaginal pH with loss of lactobacilli
          (c) Overgrowth of bacteria
        iv. Treatment (CDC, 2002) (see Table 54-3 in Chapter 54)
          (a) Treatment of choice is metronidazole, oral or vaginal
          (b) No difference in cure rates between oral and/or vaginal routes
          (c) Education about condom use and hygiene
          (d) Sexual partner treatment not recommended
        v. Follow-up
          (a) Not necessary if asymptomatic after treatment
          (b) Risk for pelvic inflammatory disease (PID), salpingitis and postpelvic surgery infections
          (c) No maintenance therapy recommended (CDC, 2002)
        vi. Prognosis
          (a) Recurrence rates high
          (b) Spontaneous resolution possible
          (c) Increased risk of preterm delivery

    g. Mucopurulent cervicitis
        i. Prevalence
          (a) 77% cases in Black females (23 times higher than whites)
          (b) 5% to 14% of 15- to 20-year-old females have chlamydia (CDC, 2004)
          (c) 12% of 20- to 24-year-old females have chlamydia
          (d) Often coinfected with other pathogens
         ii. Etiology
          (a) *C. trachomatis* (2.5% to15%)
          (b) *N. gonorrhoeae* (3% to 15%)
          (c) Other microorganisms
         iii. Pathophysiology
          (a) Cervical plug has bacteriostatic properties
          (b) Loss of plug during menses may contribute to spread in upper genital tract
          (c) Pathogen invades mucosal and glandular structures lined by columnar or cuboidal noncornified epithelium
          (d) 70% of chlamydia infections are asymptomatic
          (e) 50% coinfection rate, may result in disseminated disease

      **iv.** Treatment

         **(a)** Appropriate antibiotic treatment depending on microorganism (see Table 54-3 in Chapter 54)

         **(b)** Treat presumptively if indicated

         **(c)** Patient should abstain from sexual intercourse

            **(1)** For 7 days after single-dose therapy

            **(2)** Until completion of 7 days of treatment

         **(d)** Quinolone resistance to gonococcus (GC) found in Hawaii and Southeast Asia

         **(e)** Preventive education (CDC, 2002)

      **v.** Follow-up

         **(a)** Return for reevaluation

         **(b)** Rescreen 3 to 4 months after treatment for reinfection if due to chlamydia or gonorrhea

         **(c)** Refer sex partners within past 60 days for evaluation and treatment

         **(d)** Surveillance screening in adolescents every 6 months

      **vi.** Prognosis

         **(a)** Increased incidence of PID with reinfection

**h.** Labial adhesions

    **i.** Prevalence

        **(a)** 33% of prepubertal females (2 to 6 years) develop fusion at vulva posterior fourchette

        **(b)** 1.4% of infants (Bacon, 2002)

    **ii.** Etiology and pathophysiology

        **(a)** Local irritation or inflammation removes external layers of epidermis

        **(b)** Irritation

           **(1)** Poor hygiene

           **(2)** Sexual abuse

        **(c)** Skin reepithelializes opposing skin agglutinates

    **iii.** Treatment

        **(a)** Treat only if adverse symptoms; surgical separation rarely required

        **(b)** Avoid traumatic separation in office

        **(c)** Topical estrogen applied twice daily for no longer than 2 weeks

        **(d)** Avoid irritation with periodic application of bland ointment (Bacon, 2002)

    **iv.** Follow-up in 2 to 3 weeks for resolution of symptoms

    **v.** Prognosis

        **(a)** Adhesion can reoccur

        **(b)** Resolves in puberty

**i.** Genital warts (condyloma acuminata)

    **i.** Prevalence

        **(a)** 1.5% of never sexually active females

        **(b)** 46% of sexually active females

        **(c)** Male incidence presumably similar to female

    **ii.** Etiology and pathophysiology

        **(a)** 30 types of human papillomavirus (HPV) can infect genital tract

        **(b)** Types 6 or 11 are usual cause of visible genital warts on penis, vulva, scrotum, perineum, perianal skin

        **(c)** Less visible infections of cervix, vagina, urethra, anus, mouth

        **(d)** Virus infects the basal layer of epithelial cells in areas where microtrauma or friction predominate

        **(e)** Vertical transmission from birth canal in children younger than 3 years can occur due to prolonged latency period of months to years

       iii. Treatment (CDC, 2002)

         (a) Children older than 2 years with genital warts should be evaluated for evidence of sexual abuse

         (b) Refer patients who are pregnant, immunodeficient, have squamous cell carcinoma in situ, or other pathology

         (c) Primary goal of treatment is removal of warts

           (1) Patient-applied topical solutions (see Table 54-3 in Chapter 54)

           (2) Provider-administered treatments

             a) Cryotherapy, repeated every 1 to 2 weeks

             b) Application of resin or acid preparations

             c) Surgical removal

           (3) Referral to urology or OB/GYN

             a) Intralesional interferon

             b) Laser surgery

         (d) Educate about safer sex practice and smoking cessation

       iv. Prognosis

         (a) Spontaneous resolution of virus possible

         (b) Usually within 1 to 2 years

         (c) 30% to 50% recurrence rate

         (d) Vaccine development promising for oncogenic HPV

       v. Follow-up

         (a) Routine examination and diagnostic testing for oncogenic screen

         (b) Refer partners with visible lesions for treatment

   **j.** Genital cysts—fluid-filled sacs

       i. Prevalence

         (a) Varies with location

           (1) Bartholin's most common

           (2) Occurs in 2% of females

       ii. Etiology and pathophysiology

         (a) May be developmental

         (b) Bacterial infection

         (c) Obstruction of duct or mucus secreting glands by:

           (1) Thickened mucus

           (2) Trauma

           (3) Epidermoid mass

       iii. Treatment

         (a) Without symptoms, none required

         (b) Antibiotics if appropriate

         (c) Sitz bath

         (d) Refer for incision and drainage if symptoms persist

         (e) Surgical repair

       iv. Follow-up if symptoms persist

       v. Prognosis

         (a) Bartholin's glands cysts increased risk for recurrent infection

   **k.** Herpes simplex virus (HSV)

       i. Etiology (Schack & Neinstein, 2002)

         (a) Two thirds caused by HSV-2 (type 2)

         (b) One third caused by HSV-1 (type 1)

       ii. Pathophysiology

         (a) Contagious infection of the skin and mucous membranes

         (b) Viral organism transmitted by close contact with person shedding the virus through:

(1) Skin

(2) Mucous membranes

(3) Body fluids

(4) Autoinoculation

(c) 8% to 50% orogenital route (CDC, 2002)

(d) Neonatal infection (Enright & Prober, 2002)

(1) Most commonly caused by HSV-2

(2) About 1000 cases per year in United States

iii. Treatment

(a) Initiate treatment early with symptoms

(b) Antiviral agents (see Table 54-3 in Chapter 54)

(c) Burows solution 1:40 on cool compress or sitz bath tid

(d) Bland barrier cream

(e) Catheterization and sedation as necessary

(f) Inform sex partners

(1) Avoid intercourse during outbreaks

(2) Encourage use of condoms

iv. Follow-up (CDC, 2002)

(a) Return to clinic in 1 week and include sexual partners

(b) Partners:

(1) 50% infection rate with exposure

(2) Treat same as patient if symptomatic

(3) Consider possibility of herpes-discordant relationship—partners have different types of herpes

(c) Six or more recurrences per year may require suppressive therapy

(d) Discontinue medication every 1 to 2 years to assess recurrence pattern

(e) If patient becomes pregnant, educate her to discuss history of HSV infection with provider

v. Prognosis

(a) No cure; infection is permanent

(b) Infection can be asymptomatic and in latent stage

(c) Viral shedding possible without active lesion

(d) Recurrence

(1) Less symptomatic and of shorter duration than initial exposure

(2) Risk of recurrence 80% with HSV-2

(3) 50% with HSV-1

(e) Neonatal mortality 50%

l. Aphthosis

i. Etiology and prevalence

(a) Unknown, may be associated with autoimmune disease, multifactorial

(b) Associated with oral lesions during periods of stress or anxiety

(c) Peak age late childhood to early adulthood

ii. Pathophysiology

(a) Painful red macule that evolves into ulcers within hours in moist area on genital mucosa

(1) White center similar to oral lesions

(2) Perimeter with erythematous ring

(b) Ulcers sharply marginated

(1) Deep

(2) Moderately to severely painful

       (c) Perianal lesions in both females and males
    **iii.** Treatment (McCarty, et al., 2003)
       (a) Burows solution 1:40 on wet compresses or sitz bath
       (b) Viscous lidocaine to lesions
       (c) Topical steroids twice daily
    **iv.** Follow-up
       (a) Referral to dermatology for recurrent or persistent disease
    **v.** Prognosis
       (a) Lesions heal in 2 to 4 weeks

## SYMPTOM: LOWER ABDOMINAL PAIN WITH OR WITHOUT MENSTRUATION

1. History and symptom assessment
   a. Pain: onset, location, duration, relation to menarche, exacerbating factors, measures that improve symptoms
   b. Menstruation: last menstrual period, regularity
   c. GI: bowel patterns, anorexia, nausea, vomiting
   d. Urinary tract complaints
   e. Vagina: cleansing practices, discharge
   f. Systemic symptoms: fever
   g. Sexual history: dyspareunia
   h. Excess bruising or bleeding
   i. Dizziness
   j. Eye, oral, or skin lesions
   k. Joint manifestations
   l. Hepatitis immunization status
   m. Family history of chronic illness or bleeding disorders
   n. Smoking history
   o. Medications
2. General examination
   a. Vital signs
   b. Inspect skin and extremities as indicated
   c. Auscultate lungs
   d. Abdominal examination
   e. Rectal examination
   f. Pelvic examination
3. Differential diagnosis
   a. Pelvic inflammatory disease
   b. Ectopic pregnancy
   c. Ovarian torsion
   d. Ovarian cyst
   e. Primary dysmenorrhea
   f. Imperforate hymen
4. Diagnostic tests
   a. Cervical cultures (Wiesenfeld, et al., 2002; 2003)
      i. GC
      ii. Trichomonas
      iii. Bacterial vaginosis
      iv. Chlamydia

    **b.** Wet prep and vaginal pH

    **c.** Urinalysis and culture

    **d.** Urine or serum hCG

    **e.** CBC with differential, C-reactive protein (CRP), sedimentation rate

    **f.** HIV testing

    **g.** Hepatitis B and C

    **h.** Abdominal flat plate (to rule out teratoma in younger child)

    **i.** Ultrasound (CDC, 2002)

**5.** See also Table 31-3 for when to refer

**6.** Prevalence, etiology, pathophysiology, and treatment

    **a.** Pelvic inflammatory disease (PID)

        **i.** Prevalence

            (a) Adolescents

                (1) 33% of cases

                (2) Compared with adults:

                    a) 10 times higher risk of PID

                    b) 3 times higher risk of chlamydia and GC

            (b) 2.3 times higher risk if previous history of PID

            (c) 4.6 times higher risk with multiple sex partners (Marks, et al., 2000)

            (d) 2.5 times higher risk in non-whites (Neinstein, 2002)

            (e) Increased risk during menstruation (Shrier, et al., 2003)

        **ii.** Etiology

            (a) 5% to 81% gonococcal

            (b) 6% to 68% chlamydial

            (c) Mixed bacteria present, may include anaerobes

        **iii.** Pathophysiology

            (a) Ascending spread of microorganism from the vagina and endocervix to:

                (1) Endometrium

                (2) Fallopian tubes

                (3) Contiguous structures

            (b) Affinity of STI to exposed columnar epithelium on adolescent cervix

            (c) Decreased levels of secretory cervical immunoglobulin A

        **iv.** Treatment (CDC, 2002)

            (a) Antibiotics

            (b) Immediate hospitalization if:

                (1) Disseminated disease

                (2) Pregnant

                (3) Tubo-ovarian abscess present

            (c) Analgesia

            (d) Sex partner treatment

        **v.** Follow-up

            (a) Hospitalize if no improvement in 48 to 72 hours

            (b) Repeated education aimed at prevention

            (c) Aggressive screening for STIs in adolescents (every 6 months or when symptoms occur)

        **vi.** Prognosis

            (a) Sequelae—25% of females develop sequelae after one episode

                (1) 4 times more likely to develop chronic pelvic pain

                (2) 6 to 10 times more likely to develop an ectopic pregnancy

                (3) 50% damage to fallopian tube from salpingitis

           (4) Potential for inflammation of liver capsule if bacteria travel along abdominal paracolic gutters (space between the kidney and the psoas muscle bilaterally) (CDC, 2002)

       (b) Infertility consequences

           (1) One episode, 11.4% incidence

           (2) Two episodes, 23%

           (3) More than three episodes, 54%

       (c) Subclinical PID (Wiesenfeld, et al., 2002)

           (1) Common among females with lower genital tract infections

           (2) Similar fertility outcomes to acute PID

**b.** Ectopic pregnancy

   **i.** Prevalence

      (a) 50% related to previous history of salpingitis and obstruction

      (b) 97% tubal, 1.4 % abdominal, less than 1 % ovarian or cervical

   **ii.** Hypothesized etiology (Coste, et al., 2000)

      (a) Defects in ovum

      (b) Endometrial abnormalities

      (c) Slow tubal motility

   **iii.** Pathophysiology

      (a) Delayed embryo passage to the uterus remaining in the oviduct at gestational age of implantation (7 days)

      (b) Trophoblast grows between lumen of tube and peritoneal covering

      (c) Invading vessels resulting in retroperitoneal hemorrhage

      (d) Leads to tubal rupture

   **iv.** Treatment

      (a) Emergency referral to gynecologist

   **v.** Follow-up

      (a) Routine gynecologic care

   **vi.** Prognosis (Nelson & Neinstein, 2002)

      (a) Major cause of maternal death related to hemorrhage

      (b) Death is 4 times more likely in Black females than white females

      (c) Death is 10 times more likely than death due to childbirth

      (d) Death is 50 times more likely than death due to abortion

**c.** Ovarian torsion

   **i.** Etiology

      (a) Complication of benign ovarian tumor

         (1) 25% incidence of torsion with ovarian mass

      (b) Complication of ovarian cyst

         (1) 50% to 60% females with torsion have cysts (Kokoska, et al., 2000)

         (2) Cyst usually 8 to 12 cm but may be smaller

         (3) 3:2 right ovary versus left ovary

      (c) Pregnancy

      (d) 10% have repeat episode on unaffected side

   **ii.** Pathophysiology

      (a) Adnexal structure rotates, obstructing venous flow

      (b) Mass enlarges

      (c) Obstructs arterial flow

   **iii.** Treatment

      (a) Immediate surgical referral

      (b) May perform plication of the contralateral adnexa

   **iv.** Follow-up

      (a) Routine gynecologic care
- v. Prognosis
  - (a) Early diagnosis
    - (1) Ovary spared
    - (2) Cyst or mass excised
  - (b) Laparoscopic detorsion may result in normal follicle development
  - (c) Delayed diagnosis and therapy
    - (1) Necrosis of fallopian tube
    - (2) Oophorectomy required
- **d.** Ovarian cyst (Kazzi & Roberts, 2004)
  - **i.** Prevalence
    - (a) 30% of females with regular menses
    - (b) 50% of females with irregular menses
    - (c) Also occur in infancy
    - (d) Less often in childhood
  - **ii.** Etiology
    - (a) Definition: fluid-filled sac of the graafian follicle or corpus luteum
    - (b) Follicular cysts most common (3 mm to 15 cm)
      - (1) Average to 3 cm
      - (2) First 2 to 3 weeks of menstrual cycle
      - (3) Not neoplastic
    - (c) Corpus luteal cyst (3 to 15 cm)
      - (1) Final 1 to 2 weeks of menstrual cycle
      - (2) Failure of corpus luteum degeneration to a corpus albicans
      - (3) Leads to prolonged secretion of progesterone
    - (d) Hemorrhagic cyst
      - (1) Prone to rupture with trauma, intercourse, or pelvic examination
      - (2) More clinically significant
      - (3) Rupture may occur during days 20 to 26 of cycle
    - (e) Smoking doubles the risk of follicular cysts
    - (f) Pathophysiology
      - (1) Dominant mature follicles fail to rupture
      - (2) Immature follicle fails to undergo atresia
      - (3) Secondary to torsion or rupture
        - a) Can occur during intercourse
        - b) Strenuous exercise
        - c) Trauma
  - **iii.** Treatment
    - (a) Conservative management
      - (1) 5- to 6-cm mass
      - (2) Observe for 6 weeks
    - (b) Refer to gynecology (Strickland, 2002)
      - (1) Masses that are stable and persist beyond 10 weeks
      - (2) Masses that are enlarging
      - (3) Oral contraceptives to decrease ovulation
    - (c) Refer to emergency department (ED) for episodes of acute pain
    - (d) Smoking cessation education
  - **iv.** Follow-up
    - (a) Ultrasound in 2 to months
  - **v.** Prognosis
    - (a) 40% recurrence rate after drainage of simple benign cysts
    - (b) 2% recurrence with surgical management (cystectomy)

           (c) Neonates (Kazzi & Roberts, 2004)
               (1) Ovarian cysts may complicate development
               (2) Associated with ascites, pulmonary hypoplasia, and renal insufficiency

**e.** Primary dysmenorrhea
    **i.** Incidence and prevalence
        (a) Overall incidence 79.6%
        (b) 39%, 12-year-olds
        (c) 72%, 17-year-olds
        (d) Peak incidence 1 to 3 years after menarche
    **ii.** Etiology
        (a) Psychologic
        (b) Prostaglandin and arachidonic acid production
        (c) Abnormal hypothalamic-pituitary adrenal axis response
        (d) Genetic factors
    **iii.** Pathophysiology
        (a) Prostaglandin released during ovulatory cycle causes uterine contractions
        (b) Grading system of dysmenorrhea
            (1) 0—menstruation not painful
            (2) 1—mild, painful menstruation, activities of daily living (ADLs) rarely affected
            (3) 2—moderate, interferes with ADLs , no systemic symptoms
            (4) 3—severe, restricts ADL for several days per month, associated with systemic symptoms
    **iv.** Treatment
        (a) NSAIDs (see Table 55-5 in Chapter 55)
        (b) Hormonal therapy (oral contraceptives)
        (c) Complementary therapies have little or no evidence-based research to support them
        (d) Exercise
    **v.** Follow-up
        (a) Reevaluate after three menstrual cycles
        (b) Refer to gynecology if no response in 3 to 6 months to:
            (1) NSAIDs
            (2) Oral contraceptives
    **vi.** Prognosis
        (a) 90% respond to hormonal therapy
        (b) 70% incidence of endometriosis in nonresponding patients

**f.** Imperforate hymen
    **i.** Definition
        (a) Anatomic abnormality obstructing flow of menstrual blood
    **ii.** Etiology
        (a) Presentation in newborn or at puberty with onset of menses
        (b) Failure of distal canalization of vaginal plate between the urogenital sinus and vagina
    **iii.** Treatment
        (a) No treatment required if microperforation is evident
        (b) Surgical intervention if completely imperforate
    **iv.** Follow-up
        (a) Routine gynecologic care
    **v.** Prognosis—excellent

## SYMPTOM: MENSES TOO MUCH, TOO LITTLE, TOO LONG, TOO LATE

1. History and symptom assessment
   a. Menstrual history
   b. Urinary tract
   c. Gastrointestinal symptoms
   d. Trauma
   e. Sexual history
   f. Skin and mucous membranes: acne, bruising, petechiae, bleeding from gums, epistaxis, skin or hair changes
   g. Symptoms of anemia, lethargy, temperature intolerance
   h. Medications
   i. Allergies
   j. Past medical history
   k. Exercise, diet, weight changes
   l. Psychosocial (HEADSS): H, Home; E, Education/employment; A, Activities; D, Drugs; S, Sexuality; S, Suicide/depression screen
   m. Family history
   n. Neurodevelopment
   o. Genetic abnormalities
2. Focused physical examination
   a. Height, weight
   b. Vital signs
   c. BP supine and standing
   d. Thyroid palpation
   e. HEENT
   f. Funduscopic examination
   g. Skin
   h. Auscultation of heart and lung
   i. Breast examination
   j. Abdomen
   k. Extremities, neurologic examination
   l. Rectal examination
   m. External genital
   n. Speculum bimanual pelvic examination dependent on history
   o. Sexual maturity (Tanner) staging
3. Differential diagnosis
   a. Dysfunctional uterine bleeding
   b. Amenorrhea secondary to pregnancy
   c. See also Table 31-1 for other potential diagnoses
4. Diagnostic tests
   a. Serum or urine hCG
   b. Blood work
      i. CBC with differential
      ii. Platelets
      iii. Prothrombin time (PT), partial thromboplastin time (PTT)
      iv. VW profile
      v. Thyroid stimulating hormone (TSH)
      vi. Liver function
      vii. Creatinine
      viii. BUN

ix. Prolactin levels (if amenorrhea precedes dysfunctional uterine bleeding [DUB])

c. Urinalysis

d. Sexually transmitted infection screen

e. Ultrasound

5. See also Table 31-3 for when to refer

6. Prevalence, etiology, pathophysiology and treatment

a. Anovulatory or dysfunctional uterine bleeding (DUB)

i. Etiology and prevalence

(a) Immaturity of HPA axis

(1) Associated with 50% to 80% of bleeding cycles during first 2 years after menarche

(2) 90% of dysfunctional uterine bleeding related to anovulation

(b) 10% structural pathology

(c) von Willebrand disease (VWD) (Woo, et al., 2002)

(1) Impaired platelet adhesion and aggregation

(2) 1% of population with VWD

(d) Endocrine disorders (25% of females with hypothyroidism)

(e) Primary ovarian dysfunction (Rimsza, 2002)

ii. Pathophysiology

(a) Excess estrogen stimulates endometrium without adequate progesterone levels to provide support and vasoconstriction

(b) Portions of lining slough at irregular intervals

(c) Impaired negative hormonal feedback

iii. Treatment

(a) Hemoglobin ≥12g/dL

(1) Multivitamin with iron

(2) Menstrual calendar monitoring

(3) Iron supplementation as appropriate

(b) Hemoglobin 10 to 12g/dL, hemodynamically stable, but moderate to heavy flow

(1) Oral contraceptive agents

(c) Hemoglobin 10 to 12g/dL, no active bleeding

(1) Oral contraceptives or progesterone only

(2) Iron supplementation

(d) Hemoglobin less than 10g/dL, active heavy bleeding

(1) Referral for probable hospitalization and management

(2) Fluid replacement

(3) Intravenous estrogen with progesterone therapy

(4) Transfusion if necessary

(5) Oral contraceptives when stable

(6) D&C rarely necessary (Rimsza, 2002)

(7) NSAIDs to reduce uterine bleeding (Lethaby, et al., 2006)

(8) Antiemetic

ii. Follow-up

(a) Based on therapy, every 3 to 6 months on oral contraceptive pills (OCPs)

(b) Referral to hematology, gynecology for persistent symptoms

iii. Prognosis

(a) 5% guarded, may have severe episodes of anovulatory bleeding

(b) 60% adolescents continued bleeding for 2 years after onset

(c) 50% adolescents continued bleeding for 4 years after onset

(d) 30% persistent problems 10 years later

(e) Patients with normal menses before onset of DUB and no bleeding problems have better outcome

b. Amenorrhea secondary to pregnancy

   i. Prevalence

      (a) 900,000 teen pregnancies annually

      (b) 85% unplanned

      (c) 50% occur within 6 months of first intercourse

      (d) U.S. highest rate of teen pregnancy rate in developed nations

      (e) Average age of first intercourse (MacKay, et al., 2000)

         (1) Females—age 17

         (2) Males—age 16

   ii. Pathophysiology

      (a) Hormones from corpus luteum and placenta feed back and suppress gonadotropin-releasing hormone to maintain the developing pregnancy

   iii. Treatment

      (a) Counseling about pregnancy options and appropriate referral

      (b) Prenatal vitamins

      (c) Self-care

      (d) Education about consequences of high risk behavior

   iv. Follow-up

      (a) Usual well child care

      (b) Pregnancy prevention

   v. Prognosis

      (a) Early pregnancy

         (1) May result in lower educational attainment

         (2) Prolonged welfare dependency and fewer employment opportunities

      (b) Teen fathers

         (1) Have low rates of marriage

         (2) High rates of divorce

         (3) May live with birth mother and child for short period of time after birth

      (c) Infant outcomes (MacKay, 2000)

         (1) Higher mortality rates

         (2) Increased incidence of placement in foster care

         (3) Cognitive development delays

         (4) Higher rates of repeating grades

         (5) Higher delinquency

         (6) Incarceration for boys

         (7) Early sexual activity

         (8) Prematurity

# SYMPTOM: BREAST LUMPS OR PAIN

1. History

  a. Breast lumps: onset, location

  b. Breast pain: onset, location, intensity, duration

  c. Nipple discharge or changes

  d. Breast swelling, redness, or heat

    **e.** Breast changes: size or symmetry, related to menses, cyclic

    **f.** Menstrual history

    **g.** Trauma

    **h.** Sexual abuse

    **i.** Fever

    **j.** GI: anorexia, nausea, vomiting

    **k.** Smoking

    **l.** Drug use (prescription or illicit), caffeine

    **m.** Pregnancy history

    **n.** Prior history of malignancy

    **o.** Radiation exposure

    **p.** Family history of breast cancer or disease

    **q.** Chronic illness

    **r.** Obesity

**2.** Focused physical examination

    **a.** Vital signs

    **b.** Breast examination (best if between days 3 and 10 of menstrual cycle)

    **c.** Lymph nodes

    **d.** Genital examination with sexual maturity rating (Tanner staging)

**3.** Differential diagnosis

    **a.** Nonpainful

        **i.** Gynecomastia

        **ii.** Fibroadenoma

        **iii.** Fibrocystic breast mass

    **b.** Painful

        **i.** Breast infection

        **ii.** Mastalgia

**4.** Diagnostic tests

    **a.** Ultrasound

    **b.** Culture of nipple discharge if present

        **i.** Do not squeeze nipples to obtain discharge

    **c.** Urine or serum hCG

**5.** See also Table 31-3 for when to refer

**6.** Prevalence, etiology, pathophysiology, and treatment

    **a.** Gynecomastia

        **i.** Prevalence

            (a) Idiopathic: peak prevalence at age 14 (64%)

            (b) Neonatal: 60% to 90% of newborns

            (c) 4% severe more than 4 cm diameter of breast tissue, bilateral in 77% to 95%

        **ii.** Etiology and pathophysiology

            (a) Idiopathic (Neinstein & Joffe, 2002)

                (1) Occurs with puberty

                (2) Breast tissue response to estrogen and androgen activity

                (3) Benign increase in glandular and stromal tissue

            (b) Increased maternal hormones postnatal period

            (c) Conditions that increase serum estrogen levels

            (d) Conditions that decrease androgen levels (Neinstein & Joffe, 2002)

            (e) Hypogonadisim, e.g., Klinefelter's syndrome

            (f) Medications and drugs

            (g) Obesity (Ersoz, et al., 2002)

        **iii.** Treatment

        (a) Watchful waiting with reexamination

        (b) Surgical referral if more than mild to moderate

        (c) If other pathology suspected refer to endocrinology (Khan & Blamey, 2003)

        (d) Referral to nutrition for management of obesity

   **iv.** Follow-up

        (a) With routine examinations

        (b) If symptoms worsen

   **v.** Prognosis

        (a) Most resolve in 12 to 24 months

        (b) 27% beyond 1 year

        (c) 7.7% greater than 2 years (Neinstein & Joffe, 2002)

        (d) No relationship to development of breast cancer

**b.** Fibroadenoma

   **i.** Prevalence

        (a) Highest prevalence in 15- to 16-year-olds

        (b) Account for 50% of breast masses in adolescent females

        (c) Twice as common in Black females

        (d) 90% of cases unilateral

        (e) 63% in upper quadrant (usually 2 to 3 cm)

   **ii.** Etiology and pathophysiology

        (a) Aberration of normal development, benign neoplasm

        (b) Stromal proliferation surrounding aggregate of compressed or uncompressed distorted ducts

        (c) If more than 5 cm, juvenile giant adenofibroma (Zacharia, et al., 2003)

   **iii.** Treatment

        (a) Watchful waiting

        (b) Refer

           (1) Pediatric surgery for surgical excision

           (2) Breast specialist (Osuch, 2002)

   **iv.** Follow-up

        (a) Every 6 months if conservative

        (b) If evidence of new mass

   **v.** Prognosis

        (a) 2% decrease in size with no intervention

        (b) 16% no change

        (c) 32% increase in size over 5 years

        (d) 20% recurrence rate with surgical excision

        (e) Unclear if increased risk of breast cancer

**c.** Fibrocystic breast mass—"cobblestone" consistency of breast tissue

   **i.** Prevalence

        (a) 50% of females in reproductive age have some percentage of proliferative breast changes

   **ii.** Etiology and pathophysiology

        (a) Cyclic levels of ovarian hormones

        (b) Increased levels of prolactin

        (c) Benign intense proliferation of stroma

        (d) May be related to imbalance between estrogen and progesterone

        (e) Adolescent disease

           (1) Found in upper outer quadrant

           (2) Commonly 1 week before menses

    iii. Treatment
        (a) Supportive bra
        (b) Analgesia
        (c) Teach regular self-breast examination
            (1) Watch for new, unusual, or dominant lump
        (d) Oral contraceptives
            (1) Progesterone on days 15 to 25 of cycle
            (2) 85% effective
        (e) Most popular remedies are unconfirmed in clinical trials, such as:
            (1) Reduce methylxanthines (caffeine and theobromine), e.g., coffee, tea, cola, chocolate
            (2) Reduce nicotine
            (3) Vitamin therapy (Horner & Lampe, 2000)
    iv. Follow-up
        (a) Determined by symptoms
    v. Prognosis
        (a) Subsides with menopause
  d. Breast infection (mastitis)
    i. Etiology and pathophysiology
        (a) 3% to 4 % related to inflammatory cause
        (b) Secondary to cutaneous bacteria introduced into the ductal system
        (c) Foreign body
        (d) Epidermal cyst
        (e) Trauma
        (f) Breast-feeding
    ii. Treatment
        (a) Antibiotics
        (b) Warm compress
        (c) Supportive bra
        (d) Analgesia
        (e) Education to avoid recurrence
        (f) Lactating adolescents
            (1) Encouraged to pump
            (2) Continue nursing
    iii. Follow-up
        (a) Refer to surgeon
            (1) If unresolved in 3 to 5 days
            (2) If abscess suspected
    iv. Prognosis—most cases resolve
  e. Mastalgia
    i. Prevalence
        (a) Prevalence unknown in adolescents
        (b) Cyclic—most common
        (c) 66% of females report symptoms
    ii. Etiology and pathophysiology
        (a) Symptoms not correlated to histologic changes (Millet & Dirbas, 2002)
        (b) May be associated with menstrual cycle
        (c) Premenstrual
    iii. Treatment
        (a) Analgesics
        (b) Supportive bra
        (c) Alternative therapies unconfirmed in U.S. clinical trials
            (1) Oral vitamin E, A, or B (Horner & Lampe, 2000; Osuch, 2002)

        (2) Evening primrose

        (3) Elimination of methylxanthines

    **iv.** Follow-up

        (a) Supportive care

        (b) Refer to endocrinologist for antigonadotropin therapy for cyclic mastalgia with disabling symptoms (Morrow, 2000)

    **v.** Prognosis—most cases resolve

## REFERENCES

American Academy of Pediatrics. (1999). Practice parameter: The diagnosis, treatment, and evaluation of the initial UTI in febrile infants and young children. *Pediatrics, 103*(4), 843-852. (Editor's Note: As of May 1, 2006, this practice guideline has not been revised. Check the AAP website periodically for updates).

American Academy of Pediatrics. (2003). Pinworm infection. In L. K. Pickering (Ed.). *Red Book: 2003 Report of the Committee on Infectious Diseases* (26th ed.). Elk Grove Village, IL: American Academy of Pediatrics, pp. 486-487.

Angel, C. A. (2004). Meatal stenosis. Retrieved May 1, 2006, from www.emedicine.com/ped/topic2356.htm.

Association for Genitourinary Medicine (AGUM), & Medical Society for the Study of Venereal Disease (MSSVD). (2002). National guideline on the management of vulvovaginal candidiasis. London: AGUM & MSSVD.

Bacon, J. L. (2002). Prepubertal labial adhesions: Evaluation of a referral population. *Am J Obstet Gynecol, 187*(2), 327-332.

Baker, L. A., Silver, R. I., & Docimo, S. G. (2001). Cryptorchidism. In J. P. Gearhart, R. C. Rink, & P. D. E. Mouriquand (Eds.). *Pediatric urology*. Philadelphia: Saunders, pp. 738-754.

Barakat, L. P., Smith-Whitley, K., Schulman, S., et al. (2001). Nocturnal enuresis in pediatric sickle cell disease. *J Dev Behav Pediatr, 22*(5), 300-305.

Brooks, L. J., & Topol, H. I. (2003). Enuresis in children with sleep apnea. *J Pediatr, 142*(5), 515-518.

Cantu, S. (2006). Phimosis and paraphimosis. Retrieved May 1, 2006, from www.emedicine.com/emerg/topic423.htm.

(CDC) Centers for Disease Control and Prevention (2004). Chlamydia screening among sexually active young female enrollees of health plans—United States, 1999-2001, *MMWR: Morb Mortal Wkly Rep, 53*(42), 983-985.

(CDC) Centers for Disease Control and Prevention (2002). Guidelines for treatment for sexually transmitted diseases. *MMWR Morb Mortal Wkly Rep, 51*, 1-80. (Editor's Note: Check the CDC website for the 2006 update that will be published in Spring, 2006).

Cooper, C. S., Gallagher, B. L., & Carson, M.R. (2006). Prepubertal testicular and paratesticular tumors. Retrieved from eMedicine on May 1, 2006, http://www.emedicine.com/ped/topic1423.htm

Coste, J., Fernandez, H., Joye, N., et al. (2000). Role of chromosome abnormalities in ectopic pregnancy. *Fertil Steril, 74*, 1259-1260.

Cuckow, P. M., & Nyirady, P. (2001). Foreskin. In J. P. Gearhart, R. C. Rink, & P. D. E. Mouriquand (Eds.). *Pediatric urology*. Philadelphia: Saunders, pp. 705-712.

Davis, I. D., & Avner, E. D. (2004). Nephrology. In R. E. Behrman, R. M. Kliegman, & H. B. Jenson (Eds.). *Nelson textbook of pediatrics* (17th ed.). Philadelphia: Saunders, pp. 1731-1775.

Dogra, V., & Resnick, M. I. (2002). Ultrasonography of the scrotum. *J Ultrasound Med, 21*(8), 848.

Eiberg, H., Shaumburg, H.L., Von Gontard, A., & Rittig, S. (2001). Linkage study of a large Danish 4-generation family with urge incontinence and nocturnal enuresis. *J Urol, 166*, 2401-2403.

Elder, J. S. (2004). Anomalies of the penis and urethra. In R E. Behrman., R. M. Kliegman, & H. B. Jenson (Eds.). *Nelson textbook of pediatrics* (17th ed.). Philadelphia: Saunders, pp. 1812-1817.

Enright, A. M., & Prober, C. G. (2002). Neonatal herpes infection: Diagnosis, treatment and prevention. *Semin Neonatol, 7*(4), 283-291.

Ersöz, H. O., Onde, M. E., Terekeci, H., et al. (2002). Causes of gynaecomastia in young adult males and factors associated with idiopathic gynaecoamastia. *Int J Androl, 25*(5), 312-316.

Farhat, W., Bagli, D. J., Capolicchio, G., et al. (2000). The dysfunctional voiding scoring system: Quantitative standardization of dysfunctional voiding symptoms in children. *J Urol, 164,* 1011-1015.

Glazener, C. M. A., & Evans, J. H. C. (2005). Alarm interventions for nocturnal enuresis in children. *Cochrane Database Syst Rev* (Online: Update Software), 2: CD003637. Retrieved on May 1, 2006, from http://www.cochrane.org/reviews/en/ab002911.html.

Glazener, C. M. A., Evans, J. H. C., & Peto, R. E. (2006). Tricyclic and related drugs for nocturnal enuresis in children. *Cochrane Database Syst Rev* (Online: Update Software), 3,: CD002117. Retrieved on May 1, 2006, from http://www.cochrane.org/reviews/en/ab002117.html.

Gloor, J. M., & Torres, V. E. (2001). Reflux and obstructive neuropathy. In R. W. Schrier (Series Ed.). *Atlas of diseases of the kidney* (Vol. 2, Ch. 8). CyberNephrology™ Center: Edmonton, Alberta, Canada. Retrieved May 1, 2006, from http://www.kidneyatlas.org/book2/adk2_08.pdf.

Haward, M., & Shafer, M. A. (2002). Vaginitis and cervicitis. In L. S. Neinstein (Ed.). *Adolescent health care: A practical guide* (4th ed.). Philadelphia: Lippincott Williams & Wilkins, pp. 1011-1030.

Herbst, R. (2003). Perineal streptococcal dermatitis/disease: Recognition and management. *Am J Clin Dermatol, 4*(8), 555-560.

Herrinton, L. J., Zhao, W., & Husson, G. (2003). Management of cryptorchidism and risk of testicular cancer. *Am J Epidemiol, 157*(7), 602-605.

Horner, N. K., & Lampe, J. W. (2000). Potential mechanisms of diet therapy for fibrocystic breast conditions show inadequate evidence of effectiveness. *J Am Dietetic Assoc, 100*(11), 1368-1380.

Jepson, R. G., Mihaljevic, L., & Craig, J. (2006). Cranberries for treating urinary tract infections. *Cochrane Database Syst Rev,* Cochrane Renal Group, 2. Retrieved on May 1, 2006, from http://www.cochrane.org/reviews/en/ab001322.html.

Joesoef, M.R., & Schmid, G. (2005). Bacterial vaginosis. *Clin Evidence.* Web publication.

Jordan, G. H., & Schlossberg, S. M. (2002). Surgery of the penis and urethra. In P. C. Walsh , A. B. Retik, E. D. Vaughan Jr., & A. J. Wein (Eds.). *Campbell's urology* (8th ed.). Philadelphia: Saunders, pp. 2983-2999.

Kazzi, A. A., & Roberts, R. (2004). Ovarian cysts. Retrieved December 20, 2004, from www.emedicine.com/EMERG/topic352.htm.

Khan, H. N., & Blamey, R. W. (2003). Endocrine treatment of physiological gynecomastia. *BMJ, 327*(7410), 301-302.

Kim, K. S., Torres, C. R., Yucel, S., et al. (2004). Induction of hypospadias in a murine model by maternal exposure to synthetic estrogens. *Environ Res, 94*(3), 267-275.

Kogan, S. J. (2001). The pediatric varicocele. In J. P. Gearhart, R. C. Rink, & P. D. E. Mouriquand (Eds.). *Pediatric urology*. Philadelphia: Saunders, pp. 763-776.

Kokoska, E. R., Keller, M. S., & Weber T. R. (2000). Acute ovarian torsion in children. *Am J Surg, 180*(6), 462-465.

Lane, W. M., & Robson, M. (2005). Enuresis. Retrieved from eMedicine on May 1, 2006, from www.emedicine.com/ped/topic689.htm.

Lee, P. A., & Coughlin, M. T. (2001). Fertility after bilateral cryptorchidisim, *Horm Res, 55,* 28-32.

Lethaby, A., Augood, C., & Duckitt, K. (2006). Nonsteroidal anti-inflammatory drugs for heavy menstrual bleeding. *Cochrane Database Syst Rev, (2)* CD000400. Retrieved on May 1, 2006 from http://www.cochrane.org/reviews/en/ab000400.html.

Lucanto, C., Bauer, S. B., Hyman, P. E., et al. (2000). Function of hollow viscera in children with constipation and voiding difficulties. *Dig Dis Sci, 45*(7), 1274-1280.

Luzzi, G. A., & O'Brien, T. S. (2001). Acute epididymitis. *Brit J Urol, 87*(8), 747-755.

MacKay, A. P., Fingerhut, L. A., & Duran, C. R. (2000). *Adolescent health chartbook. Health, United States, 2000.* Hyattsville, MD: National Center for Health Statistics,

Marcozzi, D. & Suner, S. (2001). Genitourinary emergencies: The nontraumatic acute scrotum. *Emerg Med Clin N Am, 19*(3), 547-568.

Marks, C., Tideman R. L., Estcourt, C. S., et al. (2000). Assessment of risk for pelvic inflammatory disease in an urban sexual health population. *Sex Transm Infect, 76*(6), 470-473.

McCarty, M. A., Garton, R. A., & Jorizzo, L. (2003). Complex aphthosis and Behcet's disease. *Dermatol Clin, 21*(1), 41-48.

Millet, A. V., & Dirbas, F. M. (2002). Clinical management of breast pain: A review. *Obstet Gynecol Surv, 57* (7), 451-461.

Milling, L. S., & Costantino, C. A. (2000). Clinical hypnosis with children: first steps toward empirical support. *Int J Clin Exper Hypnosis,* 48 (2), 113-137.

Moore, K. N., Day, R. A., & Albers, M. (2002). Pathogenesis of urinary tract infections: A review. *J Clin Nurs, 11*(5), 568-574.

Morrow, M. (2000). The evaluation of common breast problems. *Am Fam Phys, 61,* 2371-2378.

Mycyk, M., & Moyer, P. (2004). Orchitis. Retrieved May 1, 2006, from www.emedicine.com/EMERG/topic344.htm.

Myziuk, L., Romanowski, B., & Brown, M. (2001). Endocervical gram stain smears and their usefulness in the diagnosis of *Chlamydia trachomatis. Sex Transm Infect,* 77(2), 103-106.

Neinstein, L.S., & Joffe, A. (2002). Gynecomastia. In L. S. Neinstein. (ed.). *Adolescent health care: A practical guide* (4th ed.). Philadelphia: Lippincott Williams & Wilkins, pp. 264-272.

Nelson, A. L., & Neinstein, L. S. (2002). Ectopic pregnancy. In L. S. Neinstein (Ed.). *Adolescent health care: A practical guide* (4th ed.). Philadelphia: Lippincott Williams & Wilkins, pp. 1031-1044.

Osuch, J. R. (2002). Breast health and disease over a lifetime. *Clin Obstet Gynecol, 45*(4), 1140-1161.

Patel, S. S., & Kazura, J. W. (2004). Enterobiasis *(Enterobius vericularis).* In R. E. Behrman, R. M. Kliegman, & H. B. Jenson (Eds.). *Nelson textbook of pediatrics* (17th ed.). Philadelphia: Saunders, pp. 1159-1160.

Penna, C., Fambrini, M., & Fallani, M. G. (2002). $CO_2$ laser treatment for Bartholin's gland cyst. *Int J Gynaecol Obstet, 76*(1), 79-80.

Porena, M., Costantini, E., Rociola, W., & Mearini, E. (2000). Biofeedback successfully cures detrusor-sphincter dyssynergia in pediatric patients. *J Urol, 163,* 1927-1931.

Rau, F. J., & Muram, D. (2001). Vulvovaginitis in children and adolescents. In J. S. Sanfilippo, D. Muram, J. Dewhurst, & P. A. Lee (Eds.). *Pediatric and adolescent gyne-*

cology (2nd ed.). Philadelphia: Saunders, pp. 199-215.

Redsell, S. A., & Collier, J. (2001). Bedwetting, behavior and self-esteem: A review of the literature. *Child Care Health Devel, 27*(2), 149-162.

Rimsza, M. E. (2002). Dysfunctional uterine bleeding. *Pediatr Rev, 23,* 227-233.

Rowland, R. G., & Herman, J. R. (2002). Tumors and infectious disease of the testis, epididymis and scrotum. In J. Y. Gillenwater, J. T. Grayhack, S. S. Howard, & M. E. Mitchell (Eds.). *Adult and pediatric urology* (4th ed.). Philadelphia: Lippincott Williams & Wilkins, pp. 1887-1934.

Sakai, J., & Hebert, F. (2000). Secondary enuresis associated with obstructive sleep apnea. *J Am Acad Child Adolesc Psychiatry, 39*(2), 140-141.

Sanfilippo, J. S. (2004). Vulvovaginitis. In R. E. Behrman, R. M. Kliegman, & H. B. Jenson (Eds.). *Nelson textbook of pediatrics* (17th ed.). Philadelphia: Saunders, pp. 1828-1833.

Schack, L. E, & Nienstein, L. S. (2002). Herpes genitalis. In L. S. Neinstein (Ed.). *Adolescent health care: A practical guide* (4th ed.). Philadelphia: Lippincott, Williams & Wilkins, pp. 1189-1203.

Schneck, F. X., & Bellinger, M. F. (2002). Abnormalities of the testes and scrotum and their surgical management. In P.C. Walsh, A B. Retik, E. D. Vaughan, & A. J. Wein (Eds.). *Campbell's urology* (8th ed.). Philadelphia: Saunders, pp. 2353-2394.

Shaikh, N., Hoberman, A.., Wise, B., et al. (2003). Dysfunctional elimination syndrome: Is it related to early urinary tract infection or congenital vesicoureteral reflux? *Pediatrics 112*(5): 1134-1137, 2003.

Shrier, L. A., Bowman, F. P., Lin, M., & Crowley-Nowik, P. A. (2003). Mucosal immunity of the adolescent female genital tract. *J Adolesc Health, 32,* 183-186.

Silber, S. J. (2001). The varicocele dilemma. *Human Reproduction Update, 7*(1), 70-77.

Smith, Y. R., Berman, D. R., & Quint, E. H. (2002). Premenarchial vaginal discharge: findings of procedures to rule out foreign bodies. *J Pediatr Adolesc Gynecol, 15*(4), 227-230.

Strickland, J. L. (2002). Ovarian cysts in neonates, children and adolescents. *Curr Opin Obstet Gynecol, 14*(5), 459-465.

Terris, M. K. (2004). Urethritis. Retrieved December 20, 2004, from www.emedicine.com/med/topic2342.htm.

Thiedke, C. C. (2003). Nocturnal enuresis. *Am Fam Phys, 67*(7), 1499-1506.

Watson, M. C., Grimshaw, J. M., Bond, C. M., et al. (2003). Oral versus intravaginal imidazole and triazole anti-fungal treatment of uncomplicated vulvovaginal candidiasis. *BJOG Int J Obstet Gynaec, 109*(1), 85-95.

Wiesenfeld, H. C., Hillier, S. L., Krohn, M. A., et al. (2002). Lower genital tract infection and endometritis: Insight into subclinical pelvic inflammatory disease. *Obstet Gynecol, 100*(3), 456-463.

Wiesenfeld, H. C., Hillier, S. L., Krohn, M. A., et al. (2003). Bacterial vaginosis is a strong predictor of *Neisseria gonorrhoeae* and *Chlamydia trachomatis* infection. *HIV/AIDS, 36,* 663-668.

Woo, Y. L., White, B., Corbally, R., et al. (2002). Von Willebrand's disease: an important cause of dysfunctional uterine bleeding. *Blood Coagul Fibrinolysis, 13*(2), 89-93.

Zacharia, T. T., Lakhar, B., Ittoop, A., & Menachary, J. (2003). Giant fibroadenoma. *Breast J, 9* (1), 53.

# Common Illness of the Integumentary System

VICKI W. SHARRER, MS, RN, CPNP

1. Focused history and physical examination
   a. Symptom analysis
      i. Chief complaint—signs and/or symptoms described by parent or child
         (a) Skin abnormality
            (1) Single lesion or rash
            (2) Location—trunk, extremities, face
            (3) Color
            (4) Pruritus
            (5) Pain
            (6) Pattern
            (7) Body piercing (Thiem, 2005)
         (b) Hair abnormality
            (1) Location—head, face, pubic, axillary
            (2) Visible flakes, specks, insects
            (3) Pruritus of scalp
            (4) Pattern
         (c) Nail abnormality
            (1) Location—fingernails, toenails
            (2) Color
            (3) Pattern
      ii. Onset
         (a) Sudden, gradual
         (b) Duration—disappears within 24 hours; new lesions appear; last for days or weeks
         (c) Course—change in signs, symptoms over time
      iii. Precipitating and/or aggravating factors
         (a) Food allergies
            (1) Clinical history is accurate only about 50% of the time (Roberts & Lack, 2005)
            (2) 90% of food allergies due to cow's milk, soy, wheat, peanuts and tree nuts, and egg (Gold & Saavedra, 2004)
         (b) Medicines
         (c) Soaps, lotions
         (d) Cosmetics

        (e) Environmental exposures (AAP, 2003)
           (1) Grass
           (2) Weeds
           (3) Chemicals
           (4) Animals
           (5) Insects
           (6) Illness—daycare, school, work
        (f) Injury
      iv. Immunization status
      v. Other current signs or symptoms of illness
      vi. Medications or treatments given and their effectiveness

    **b.** Child and family past medical history related to integumentary system—see Chapter 10

    **c.** Focused physical examination related to the integumentary system
      **i.** See Chapter 10
      **ii.** Must examine the integument of the whole body
      **iii.** Allow for privacy and unnecessary uncovering of sensitive body parts
      **iv.** Use gloves only for wet or potentially infection lesions, and for genitals or oral cavity examination
      **v.** Pay particular attention to:
        (a) Description of skin lesions (Chapter 10, Table 10-1 and Figures 10-2 to 10-8)
        (b) Goldsmith, et al, 1977 text has excellent color photographs of skin lesions
           (1) Type
              a) Use free-standing lighting for examination
              b) Avoid intense lighting except for transillumination of cysts
              c) Wood's lamp accentuates hypopigmented areas and fluoresces
              d) Distinguish papule from macule by shining light on lesion from the side (darken the room); papule casts a shadow
           (2) Color
           (3) Does it blanche with pressure?
           (4) Abrupt or transient
           (5) Location at onset and over time
        (c) Configuration of skin lesions (Chapter 10, Figure 10-9)
           (1) Single or multiple
           (2) Circumscribed or diffuse

**2.** Diagnostic tests
    **a.** Diagnostic tests are rarely indicated for diagnosis of most skin, hair, or nail conditions
      **i.** See Chapter 53 for methods used to diagnose fungal and mite infections of the skin, hair and nails
      **ii.** Wood's lamp examination
      **iii.** KOH test of scrapings
      **iv.** Culture of exudates
      **v.** Tzanck test

**3.** Differential diagnoses
    **a.** See Boxes 32-1 to 32-11 for differential diagnoses according to the type of lesion, location of lesion, or presenting symptom
    **b.** Then refer to the specific diagnoses that are listed *alphabetically* in section 4 below for more details that will help distinguish among the potential diagnoses

■ **BOX 32-1**
■ **DIFFERENTIAL DIAGNOSES FOR MACULAR LESIONS**

| Characteristics | Diagnoses | Characteristics | Diagnoses |
|---|---|---|---|
| Brown macules | Ephelides (freckles) | Purple, blue, black macules | Ecchymosis: |
| | **Nevus**\* | | Trauma |
| | Drug-induced | | Clotting abnormalities |
| | hyperpigmentation | | Petechiae: |
| | **Rubeola** (3rd phase) | | Platelet abnormalities |
| | **Pityriasis versicolor** | | **Rocky Mountain spotted** |
| | Acanthosis nigricans, | | **fever** |
| | café-au-lait spots | | Dysproteinemia, e.g., |
| | (Albright's syndrome, | | Raynaud's phenomenon |
| | neurofibromatosis) | | **Mongolian spot** |
| | Becker's nevus | | Blue nevus |
| | Addison's disease | | Drug-induced lesion |
| | Urticaria pigmentosa | | Malignant melanoma |
| | Fanconi's anemia | | Tattoo |
| | **Scarlet fever** (last phase) | Red macules | Drug-induced lesion |
| | | | Coxsackievirus, |
| | | | enterovirus, echovirus |
| White macules | **Seborrheic dermatitis** | | **Actinic keratosis** |
| | **Pityriasis alba** | | **Erythema infectiosum** |
| | **Pityriasis versicolor** | | **Rubeola** |
| | **Tinea corporis** | | **Scarlet fever** |
| | **Postinflammatory** | | **Rocky Mountain spotted** |
| | **hypopigmentation** | | **fever** |
| | Melasma | | **Pityriasis rosea** |
| | Secondary syphilis | | **Stevens-Johnson** |
| | Vitiligo | | **syndrome** |
| | | | **Varicella** (1st phase) |
| | | | **Atopic dermatitis** |
| | | | **Cellulitis** |
| | | | **Intertrigo diaper dermatitis** |
| Red macules *and* | Infectious mononucleosis | | **Seborrheic dermatitis** |
| adenopathy | **Kawasaki disease** | | **Scarlet fever** |
| | **Rubella** | | Burns |
| | CMV | | |
| | HIV | Transient red macules | **Urticaria** |
| | Infectious hepatitis | (disappear in 24 hours) | Rheumatic fever |
| | Syphilis | | JRA |
| | **Rubeola** | | Raynaud's phenomenon |
| | **Lyme disease** (stage 1) | | Transient erythema of |
| | **Roseola infantum** | | newborn |

\*Diagnoses in **bold** are further described in section 4 of this chapter.

4. Common skin disorders (Schwartz, 2003)
   a. Acanthosis nigricans
      i. Brown macules that cause thickening and darkening of skin on neck and axillae
      ii. Indicator of insulin resistance and type 2 diabetes

■ **BOX 32-2**
■ **DIFFERENTIAL DIAGNOSES FOR PAPULAR LESIONS**

| Characteristics | Diagnoses | Characteristics | Diagnoses |
|---|---|---|---|
| Single blue-black papule | Blue nevus<br>Foreign body<br>Giant comedone<br>Malignant melanoma | Multiple brown papules | Acanthosis nigricans<br>**Nevus**<br>Histiocytosis<br>**Pityriasis versicolor** |
| Multiple blue-black papules | **Acne, comedonal*** | Single brown papule | Mastocytoma |
| Grouped, smooth, red papules; abrupt onset | **Contact dermatitis**<br>Folliculitis<br>Insect bites<br>**Miliaria rubra**<br>**Erythema toxicum**<br>**Impetigo** | Multiple smooth, red papules; abrupt onset | Drug-induced eruption<br>Allergic vasculitis<br>Erythema multiforme |
| | | Transient smooth, red papules; abrupt onset | **Urticaria**<br>Cholinergic urticaria<br>JRA |
| Single smooth, red papules; abrupt onset | Erysipelas | Flesh or light pink papules | **Acne comedone**<br>(whitehead)<br>**Nevus**<br>**Milia** |
| Smooth red papules with gradual onset | **Scabies**<br>**Lyme disease**<br>Granuloma annulare<br>Pyogenic granuloma<br>**Acne neonatorum**<br>**Kawasaki disease**<br>Granulomatous diseases:<br>cat scratch disease, TB<br>**Papular urticaria**<br>**Pediculosis corporis**<br>**Pityriasis rosea**<br>**Rubella**<br>**Rubeola (3rd phase)**<br>**Scarlet fever**<br>(late phase)<br>**Varicella (2nd stage)** | | Skin tags<br>**Verruca**<br>Granuloma annulare<br>**Keloids**<br>**Molluscum contagiosum**<br>Neurofibromatosis<br>Lymphangioma<br>circumscriptum<br>**Milia** |
| | | White papules | Molluscum contagiosum<br>Herpes simplex<br>**Acne neonatorum**<br>**Keratosis pilaris**<br>**Scarlet fever (early phase)** |

*Diagnoses in **bold** are further described in section 4 of this chapter.

 

    **b.** Acne neonatorum
      **i.** Presentation
        (a) Identical in appearance to adolescent acne
          (1) Open and closed comedones, erythematous papules and pustules
          (2) May occur over forehead, cheeks, chin
        (b) Lesions may be present at birth but usually appear at 4 to 6 weeks of age
      **ii.** Pathophysiology
        (a) Sebaceous gland hyperplasia in response to maternal androgens (typical)
        (b) A manifestation of a virilizing syndrome (rare)

■ BOX 32-3
■ DIFFERENTIAL DIAGNOSES FOR SCALE- OR PLAQUE-TYPE LESIONS

Drug reaction:
  Gold, nickel, drugs, e.g., barbiturates,
  penicillin, phenytoin, allopurinol
**Atopic dermatitis***
**Allergic dermatitis**
**Seborrheic dermatitis**
**Seborrheic diaper dermatitis**
**Candida diaper dermatitis**
**Contact dermatitis, chronic**
**Dry skin dermatitis**
**Primary irritant diaper dermatitis**
**Intertrigo diaper dermatitis**
**Infantile hemangioma**
**Kawasaki disease**
**Keratosis pilaris**

Nummular eczema
**Pityriasis rosea** (herald patch)
**Pityriasis alba**
**Pityriasis versicolor**
**Psoriasis**
**Psoriatic diaper dermatitis**
**Pediculosis capitis**
Secondary syphilis
**Scarlet fever**
**Tinea capitis**
**Tinea corporis**
**Tinea cruris**
**Tinea unguium**
**Verruca**
Condylomata
Lupus erythematosus
Cutaneous T-cell lymphoma

■ BOX 32-4
■ DIFFERENTIAL DIAGNOSES FOR VESICULAR LESIONS

Vesicles with red papules—multiple
  ■ **Allergic dermatitis***
  ■ **Contact dermatitis**
  ■ **Erythema multiforme**
  ■ **Genital herpes—primary**
  ■ **Genital herpes—recurrent**
  ■ **GIngivostomatitis**
  ■ Erythema toxicum
  ■ **Hand, foot, and mouth disease**
  ■ Insect bites
  ■ **Kawasaki disease**
  ■ **Pityriasis rosea**
  ■ Nummular eczema
  ■ **Scabies**
  ■ **Tinea corporis**

  ■ **Tinea cruris**
  ■ **Tinea pedis**
Umbilicated vesicles
  ■ **Herpes simplex**
  ■ **Varicella (3rd stage)**
Pinpoint vesicles
  ■ **Miliaria crystalline**
Large vesicles, bullae
Bullous impetigo
Burns
Drug eruptions
Epidermolysis bullosa
**Hand, foot, and mouth disease**
**Stevens-Johnson syndrome**

*Diagnoses in **bold** are further described in section 4 of this chapter.

■ BOX 32-5
■ DIFFERENTIAL DIAGNOSES FOR DESQUAMATION OF SKIN SURFACES

**Scarlet fever***
**Kawasaki disease**
Infectious mononucleosis
Toxic shock syndrome

Drug eruptions
**Rubeola** (4th phase)
**Erythema infectiosum** (3rd phase)
**Stevens-Johnson syndrome**

*Diagnoses in **bold** are further described in section 4 of this chapter.

■ **BOX 32-6**
■ **DIFFERENTIAL DIAGNOSES FOR PUSTULES OR ABSCESSES**

Pustules
- **Candida diaper dermatitis**\*
- Drug eruptions
- **Folliculitis**
- **Impetigo**
- **Pustular psoriasis**
- **Acne vulgaris**
- **Acne neonatorum**
- **Genital herpes—primary**
- **Pediculosis capitis**
- **Pediculosis corporis**
- **Erythema toxicum**

Abscesses
- Anthrax
- **Furuncle**
- Carbuncle

\*Diagnoses in **bold** are further described in section 4 of this chapter.

■ **BOX 32-7**
■ **DIFFERENTIAL DIAGNOSES FOR NODULAR LESIONS**

**Infantile hemangioma**\*
Rheumatic fever
Rheumatoid arthritis
Synovial cyst or ganglion

Carbuncle
**Keloid**
**Acne vulgaris**

\*Diagnoses in **bold** are further described in section 4 of this chapter.

■ **BOX 32-8**
■ **DIFFERENTIAL DIAGNOSES FOR PRURITIC LESIONS**

Drug eruptions
**Allergic dermatitis**\*
**Atopic dermatitis**
**Candida diaper dermatitis**
**Contact dermatitis**
**Dry skin dermatitis**
**Erythema infectiosum** (phase 1)
**Genital herpes—primary**
Insect bites
Nummular dermatitis
**Papular urticaria**
**Pediculosis capitis**

**Pediculosis corporis**
**Pityriasis rosea**
**Seborrheic dermatitis**
**Scabies**
**Tinea corporis**
**Tinea capitis**
**Tinea cruris**
**Tinea pedis**
**Scarlet fever**
**Urticaria**
**Varicella**

\*Diagnoses in **bold** are further described in section 4 of this chapter.

■ **BOX 32-9**
■ **DIFFERENTIAL DIAGNOSES FOR CRUSTY LESIONS**

**Actinic keratosis**\*
**Atopic dermatitis**
**Atopic diaper dermatitis**
**Genital herpes—primary**

**Impetigo**
**Seborrheic dermatitis**
**Tinea capitis**

\*Diagnoses in **bold** are further described in section 4 of this chapter.

■ **BOX 32-10**
■ **DIFFERENTIAL DIAGNOSES ACCORDING TO EXANTHEM SITE**

| Diagnosis | Scalp | Face | Oral | Neck | Trunk | Perineum | Arms/Legs | Generalized |
|---|---|---|---|---|---|---|---|---|
| Acne neonatorum | | X | | | | | | |
| Acne vulgaris | | X | | X | X | | | |
| Atopic dermatitis | | X (infants) | | X (children) | | X (infants) | X | |
| Candida dermatitis | | | X | | | X | | |
| Cellulitis | | X | | | X | | X | |
| Contact dermatitis | | X | | | X | X | X | |
| Erythema infectiosum | | X | | | X | | X | |
| Erythema neonatorum | | | | | X | X | | |
| Erythema subitum | | X | | | X | | X | |
| Erythema toxicum | | | | | X | X | | |
| Folliculitis | | | | | X | X | X | |
| Genital herpes | | | | | | X | | |
| Hand, foot, & mouth disease | | | X | | | | X | |
| Herpes labialis | | | | | | X | | |
| Herpes simplex, primary infection | | | X | | | | | |
| Impetigo | X | X | | | | | X | |
| Intertrigo diaper dermatitis | | | | | | X | | |
| Kawasaki disease | | | X | | X | | X + Soles/palms | |
| Keratosis pilaris | | X | | | | X | X | |
| Lyme disease | X | | | | X | | X | X |
| Milia | | X | | | | | | |
| Miliaria crystalline | | | | X | | | | |
| Miliaria rubra | | X | | | X | | | Intertriginous areas |
| Molluscum contagiosum | | X | | | X | | X | |
| Nevus simplex | | | X | X | | | | |
| Papular urticaria | | | | X (shoulder) | | X | X | |
| Pityriasis alba | | X | | | | | X | X (infants) |

*Continued*

■ **BOX 32-10**
■ **DIFFERENTIAL DIAGNOSES ACCORDING TO EXANTHEM SITE—cont'd**

| Diagnosis | Scalp | Face | Oral | Neck | Trunk | Perineum | Arms/Legs | Generalized |
|---|---|---|---|---|---|---|---|---|
| Pityriasis rosea | | | X | | X | | | |
| Primary irritant diaper dermatitis | | | | | | X | | |
| Psoriasis | X | Ears | | | X | X (infants) | X (infants) | |
| Rocky Mountain spotted fever | | | | | X (2nd phase) | | X (1st, 3rd phases) | |
| Roseola infantum | | X | | | X | | X | |
| Rubella | | X (1st phase) | | | X | X | X | X |
| Rubeola | | X | X | X | X | X | X | X |
| Scarlet fever | | | X | | X | X | X | |
| Scabies | X | | | X | X | X | X (flexor; <2 yr) | |
| Seborrheic dermatitis | X | X | | X | X | X (infants) | X (flexor) | |
| Stevens-Johnson syndrome | | X | X | | X | | X | |
| Telangiectatic nevus | | X | | X | | | | |
| Tinea | X | X | | | X | X | X | |
| Pityriasis versicolor | | X | | | X | | X | |
| Urticaria | | | | | | | | X |
| Varicella | X | X | | X | X | X | X | X |
| Vascular birthmarks | X | X | | | | | X | |

      **iii.** Treatment
        (a) No treatment required
        (b) Spontaneous resolution occurs over a period of 6 months to 1 year
  **c.** Acne vulgaris (Baldwin & Berson, 2005; Vernon, 2003)
      **i.** Presentation—lesions primarily on face; more than half of patients also have lesions on shoulders, neck, and back
      **ii.** Lesions (graded from mild to severe)
        (a) Mild: noninflammatory focal comedones
        (b) Moderate: inflammatory lesions; comedonal papules, possibly pustules
        (c) Moderate to severe: more severe localized inflammatory acne with comedones, papules, and pustules
        (d) Severe: generalized inflammatory nodules, pustules, and cysts

■ **BOX 32-11**
■ **NEUROCUTANEOUS DISORDERS AND THEIR CHARACTERISTIC LESIONS**

| Diagnosis | Characteristic Lesions |
| --- | --- |
| **Varicella zoster*** | Vesicles on an erythematous base on the trunk or face |
| Lyme disease | Erythema chronicum migrans (ECM): a small papule near tick bite |
| | Lesion progresses centrifugally over weeks and increases in size |
| | Central clearing in the lesion causes a bull's-eye appearance |
| | Secondary lesions may occur |
| | Multiple smaller erythematous macules with central clearing |
| | One bluish red nodule near the tick bite or near the ear, nose, scrotum, areola |
| | Atrophic, edematous, bluish red plaques on the extensor aspect of the legs and elbows, especially in women |
| Neurofibromatosis type 1 | 6 or more café-au-lait macules >5 mm in diameter (prepubertal) or >15 mm (postpubertal) |
| | Freckles in axillary or inguinal areas |
| | Two or more neurofibromas or 1 plexiform neurofibroma |
| Tuberous sclerosis | Hypopigmented macules (ash leaf, confetti) |
| | Connective tissue nevus |
| | Subungual or periungual fibromas |
| Nevoid basal cell carcinoma | Multiple basal cell carcinomas |
| | 2- to 3-mm erythematous pits in palms and soles |
| LEOPARD syndrome | LEOPARD = lentigines, electrocardiographic conduction abnormalities, ocular hypertelorism, pulmonary stenosis, abnormal genitalia in males, retardation of growth, and sensorineural deafness |
| | Lentigines—multiple 1- to 2-mm, flat, dark brown patches anywhere on body except mucous membranes |
| | Hypopigmentation where previous lentigines existed |
| Ataxia-telangiectasia | Telangiectasias develop on the bulbar conjunctivae and ears |
| | Later they appear on the flexor surface of the arms, eyelids, malar area of the face, and upper chest |
| | Granulomas, café-au-lait macules, graying hair, and progeria may occur |
| Sturge-Weber syndrome | Port-wine vascular lesion on face |
| | Involves ophthalmic and maxillary divisions of the trigeminal nerve |

*Diagnoses in **bold** are further described in section 4 of this chapter.
From Conologue, D., & Meffert, J. (2005). Dermatologic manifestations of neurologic disease. Retrieved on May 11, 2006 from http://www.emedicine.com/DERM/topic549.htm

 

   **iii.** Lesions (graded from 0 to 6)
     (a) 0 = none; skin clear
     (b) 1 = few comedones
     (c) 2 = mild comedones, few papules, minimal erythema
     (d) 3 = comedones, papules, pustules, erythema
     (e) 4 = moderate comedones, greater number of papules, pustules extending over wider area of face, chest shoulders, back; increasing erythema
     (f) 5 = comedones, increasing number of papules, pustules, nodules with erythema
     (g) 6 = comedones, papules, pustules, nodules, cysts; scarring may or may not be present with hyperpigmentation
  **iv.** Etiology and pathophysiology (Baldwin & Berson, 2005)
     (a) Four factors contribute to development of acne

(1) Increased size and activity of sebaceous glands

(2) Altered growth of follicles and abnormal differentiation of follicular keratinocytes, leading to formation of follicular plugs

(3) Proliferation of *Propionibacterium acnes*

(4) Inflammatory and immune responses

(b) Occurs in 85% of all adolescents and young adults

(c) Comedones in Black patients have a greater inflammatory response than in white patients (Trowers, 2005)

v. Treatment (Baldwin & Berson, 2005; Eichenfeld, et al., 2004; Parish, 2004)

(a) Goals

(1) Alter keratinization

(2) Decrease excess production of sebum

(3) Reduce production of *P. acnes*

(4) Minimize scarring and hyperpigmentation

(b) Patient education

(1) Avoid harsh soaps, grainy washes, picking lesions

(2) Moisturizers and makeup should be water based (avoid oil-based products)

(3) Discuss importance of consistent self-care

(4) Discuss time frame necessary for improvement (several months)

(5) Discuss need for sunscreen

(6) Tips to boost adherence to acne treatment (Zane, reported by Finn, 2003)

a) Simplify treatment regimen with fewest products possible

b) Minimize adverse effects (use retinoids before using benzoyl peroxide)

c) Set realistic expectations—may require 2 months to see benefit

d) Your clinical assessment of severity may not match the patient's assessment—how does the patient evaluate the acne?

e) Peer opinion is more important than scientific data—what do peers focus on more: acne on face or back?

f) Warn about behaviors that worsen acne—picking, squeezing, exfoliating, rubbing skin during sports or activities (helmets, violins), some cosmetics

(c) First-line therapy for all forms of acne, both noninflammatory (comedonal) and inflammatory (popular and pustular lesions) includes a retinoid product and a topic antimicrobial

(1) Topical retinoid agent (adapalene, tazarotene, tretinoin) (see Table 54-6 in Chapter 54)

a) Effects include:

i) Antiinflammatory

ii) Comedolytic

iii) Normalize follicular keratinization

iv) Prevent formation of new comedones

(2) Topical antimicrobial agent to reduce *P. acnes* bacteria (clindamycin, erythromycin, dapsone, sulfacetamide/sulfur) (see Table 54-6 in Chapter 54)

a) Effects include:

i) Antibacterial

ii) Antiinflammatory

b) Dapsone is also antineutrophilic

c) Sulfacetamide or sulfur is also keratolytic

        d) These can be obtained by prescription separately or in combination products

     (3) Oral antibiotics are recommended for moderate inflammatory or noninflammatory acne; e.g., subtherapeutic dosage regimen of tetracycline derivatives (see Table 54-6 in Chapter 54)

   (d) Some over-the-counter products may be effective

     (1) Benzoyl peroxide, which is bacteriostatic and has mild comedolytic activity

     (2) Salicylic acid, which inhibits comedone formation through desquamation of dead skin cells

     (3) Combination products of these two agents

   (e) Adjunctive measures

     (1) Hormone therapy for females

        a) Oral contraceptives suppress sebum production

        b) Antiandrogenic agents (spironolactone) inhibit androgen biosynthesis and bind androgen receptors in sebaceous glands

     (2) Nonablative laser treatments work by local heating at the sites of energy absorption; absorption of light by various structures in skin is wavelength dependent (Akita & Anderson, 2004)

  **vi.** Postinflammatory hyperpigmentation lasts longer in African Americans than in whites (see Postinflammatory hyperpigmentation description and management below)

**d.** Actinic keratosis (AK; solar keratosis) (Dohil, 2005; Norman & Wallace, 2005)

  **i.** Presentation

   (a) Area of increased vascularity, erythematous macules, and roughness of the epithelium

   (b) Lesions slowly develop a yellow adherent crust

  **ii.** Etiology

   (a) Years of exposure to sun and artificial tanning rays

   (b) Occurs especially in fair-skinned children and the elderly

  **iii.** Treatment

   (a) Cryotherapy is treatment of choice for isolated, superficial AK

   (b) Refer patients with malignant lesions to dermatology

   (c) Refer to dermatology for other treatments

  **iv.** Complications

   (a) 10% of AK become squamous cell carcinoma—indicated by induration and oozing

   (b) Risk of melanoma is 1 in 75 people by age 50, but initial solar injury was usually during childhood

   (c) Keratin may accumulate and form a cutaneous horn

  **v.** Prevention

   (a) ABCs—**A**void midday sun; **B**lock with sunscreen, hats and T-shirts; **C**over up and seek shade

   (b) Sunscreen

     (1) "Sun protection factor (SPF) is defined as the dose of UV radiation required to produce 1 minimal erythema dose (MED) on protected skin after the application of $2\,mg/cm^2$ of product divided by the UV radiation required to produce 1 MED on unprotected skin [Levy, 2005, Section 4 of 10]"

        a) A water-resistant product maintains the SPF level after 40 minutes of water immersion

b) A *very* water-resistant (formerly *waterproof*) product maintains the SPF level after 80 minutes of water immersion

(2) A broad-spectrum or full-spectrum sunscreen provides both ultraviolet-B (UVB) and ultraviolet-A (UVA) protection, ideally through the entire UVA I and UVA II range (Levy, 2005)

    a) Two mechanisms of action

        i) Chemical absorbers

        ii) Physical blockers

    b) Apply 15 to 30 minutes before sun exposure

        i) Apply liberally—1 ounce may be needed to cover entire body

        ii) Reapply after prolonged swimming or vigorous activity

        iii) Most vulnerable spots include back of the neck, the ears, and scalp if hair is thin

(3) For infants, a physical sunscreen barrier such as zinc oxide or titanium oxide is best

(4) A telephone survey of 505 teen boys and girls revealed that 81% are aware that sunburns increase risk of cancer but only 53% of girls and 33% of boys use sunscreen (Opinion Research Corporation, 2005)

(5) Boys wear hats outside more often than do girls

(c) Avoid tanning beds

(1) UV rays reduce the effectiveness of the immune system

(2) Longer wavelength UVA rays (314 to 400 nm) used in tanning beds penetrates skin more deeply than ultraviolet (UV) rays from sun

(3) WHO recommends that no one younger than 18 years use a tanning bed; see report at www.who.int/mediacentre/news/notes/2005/np07/en

(d) Sunless tanning products—FDA-approved color additive is dihydroxyacetone; remember that these products are *not* sunscreens

e. Allergic dermatitis (Darmstadt & Sidbury, 2004)

  i. Presentation

    (a) Acute reaction—erythematous, intensely pruritic, eczematous dermatitis

    (b) Severe reaction—edematous, vesiculobullous

    (c) Chronic—looks similar to eczema; lichenification, scaling, fissuring, hyperpigmentation

  ii. Etiology

    (a) Antigen (i.e., allergen) that makes contact with the skin surface

    (b) Allergens include foods, medications, metals, plants (rhus dermatitis)

      (1) In a study of peanut allergy (Roberts & Lack, 2005)

        a) Safer and less expensive method than oral food challenge to detect food allergy in children was recently reported

        b) Positive test criteria were:

          i) Skin prick test with a wheal of $\geq 8\,mm$

          ii) *Or* immunoglobulin E (IgE) test of at least $15\,kU_A/L$

  iii. Pathophysiology

    (a) Antigen penetrates skin, then conjugates with a cutaneous protein

    (b) These hapten-protein complexes are transported to lymph nodes by antigen-presenting Langerhans cells

    (c) Primary contact with the antigen causes a local response in the nodes, with dissemination of sensitized T cells over several days

(d) Second contact with the antigen causes a contact dermatitis

(e) Generalized reaction may occur because of sensitized T cells

    iv. Treatment

      (a) Avoidance of allergen

      (b) Medications (see Tables 54-4 and 54-5 in Chapter 54)

        (1) Antihistamines for pruritus

        (2) Fluorinated topical corticosteroids for antiinflammatory effect can be used in areas other than the face, axilla, or groin for 1 to 2 weeks

        (3) Use weak steroid cream, e.g., hydrocortisone, on face, axilla, or groin to prevent side effects of skin atrophy, striae

        (4) New topical immunomodulators (tacrolimus, pimecrolimus) are available

          a) For use where potent topical steroids should be avoided, e.g., around the eye, groin

          b) No steroidal side effects such as striae and skin thinning

      (c) Oatmeal, cornstarch, or baking soda baths and lotions may soothe skin

**f.** Atopic dermatitis (AD) (Dohil & Eichenfield, 2005; Hansen, 2003; Shwayder, 2003)

    **i.** Definition: general term for chronic superficial inflammation of the skin

    **ii.** Clinical presentation

      (a) Often marks the beginning of an "atopic march" of atopic dermatitis in infancy, followed by food allergies, allergic rhinitis, and asthma between ages 2½ and 6 years (Tharp, 2005)

      (b) Pruritus is primary symptom; AD is known as "the itch that rashes"

      (c) Secondary changes in skin result from trauma of scratching

        (1) Enhanced transepidermal water loss

        (2) Impaired skin barrier, which increases its permeability

      (d) May present with acute edema, erythema and oozing with crusting; mild erythema alone, or lichenification

      (e) Lichenification: thickening of the skin with a shiny surface and exaggerated, deepened skin markings (response of chronic rubbing or scratching)

    **iii.** Three clinical phases

      (a) Phase 1: infantile eczema

        (1) Dermatitis begins on cheeks and scalp and frequently with oval patches on the trunk; later involving the extensor surfaces of the extremities

        (2) Usual age at onset is 2 to 3 months

        (3) Spontaneous remission occurs by age 3

        (4) One third of infants progress to phase 2—childhood or flexural eczema

      (b) Phase 2

        (1) Predominant involvement is in the antecubital and popliteal fossae, the neck, wrists, and sometimes the hands or feet

        (2) Lasts from age 2 years through adolescence

        (3) Some children just have cracked, red painful soles of feet (atopic feet)

      (c) Phase 3: adolescent eczema

        (1) Usually manifested by hand dermatitis only

      (d) Atopic dermatitis is unusual after age 30

**iv.** Pathophysiology (Shwayder, 2003)

    (a) AD requires the atopic gene(s) *and* antigenic or environmental stimulation

    (b) An antigen trigger encounters an antigen-presenting cell on skin surface

        (1) Stimulates Th-2 cells to send chemical signals that cause Th-0 cells to become Th-2 cells

        (2) Inflammatory pathways are then stimulated

        (3) Food allergies and aeroallergens are rarely the cause of AD

    (c) Prevalence

        (1) Affects 10% to 20% of children younger than age 14 years at some time during childhood

        (2) Condition worse in winter and improved in summer

        (3) 30% also have asthma and hay fever

        (4) 70% of families have allergic symptoms

**v.** Treatment

    (a) See Dohil and Eichenfield (2005) and Eichenfield (2004) for a severity-based treatment algorithm

    (b) Teach parents and child about chronic nature of AD, how to manage symptoms and avoid irritants

    (c) Emotional support for child and family

        (1) Chronic itching from AD often causes psychologic, behavioral, and social problems for the child

        (2) Family disruptions are also common

        (3) Emphasize importance of consistent skin care and medication use

        (4) Educational resources

            a) National Eczema Society: www.eczema.org

            b) Talk Eczema: www.eczema.com

    (d) Goals

        (1) Control pruritus to interrupt the itch-scratch cycle

        (2) Hydrate skin

        (3) Reduce inflammation

        (4) Repair and maintain the skin barrier

        (5) Prevent secondary infections

            a) Usually due to *Staphylococcus aureus*

            b) Topical mupirocin if excessive crusting is evident

            c) Or a course of oral antibiotic, e.g., dicloxacillin sodium or cephalexin

    (e) Acute stages (weeping)

        (1) Wet dressings—replace wet dressings and do not let dry out

        (2) Avoid chilling (keep room warm)

        (3) Medications

            a) Topical corticosteroids (see Table 54-5 in Chapter 54)

            b) Systemic antibiotics for secondary bacterial infections (see Table 54-3 in Chapter 54)

            c) Antihistamines to control itching (see Table 54-4 in Chapter 54)

        (4) Cover hands of infants periodically to deter scratching

        (5) Keep nails trimmed to avoid skin damage from scratching

    (f) Chronic stages

        (1) Two philosophies: wet method versus dry method

a) Wet method: frequent warm (not hot) baths up to four per day, followed by a lubricant while the skin is wet to trap moisture; either no soap or a mild or nonperfumed soap, e.g., Dove, Neutrogena; oil or oatmeal baths may be used with light drying

b) Dry method: baths are infrequent; skin is cleansed with a nonlipid, hydrophilic agent, e.g., Cetaphil, followed by moisturizing

  (2) Hydration

a) Restore hydration to the skin daily: apply moisturizers frequently, e.g., tid

b) The thicker and greasier the better (Shwayder, 2003)

c) Moisturizers containing urea or lactic acid improve binding of water in the skin and prevent evaporation

  (3) Avoid irritants

a) Harsh soaps and shampoos

b) Synthetic or wool clothing—recommend 80% to 100% cotton

c) Overheating and sweating.

  (4) Control pruritus

a) Oatmeal, cornstarch, or baking soda baths and lotions may soothe skin

b) Oral antihistamines (see Table 54-4 in Chapter 54)

  (g) Flare-ups

    (1) Apply topical steroids alternated with moisturizers to decrease inflammation and symptoms (see Table 54-5 in Chapter 54)

    (2) Phototherapy (Dohil & Eichenfield, 2005)

a) Broadband UVA and psoralen plus ultraviolet A (PUVA) rays produce an immunologic response through Langerhans cells and eosinophils

b) Broadband and narrowband UVB rays have immunosuppressive effects by inhibiting Langerhans cells and altering keratinocyte production

  (h) Complications

    (1) Secondary bacterial infections

**g.** Cellulitis (Darmstadt & Sidbury, 2004)

  **i.** Characteristic signs and symptoms: inflammation (heat), erythematous macules; may be scattered, edema, pain

  **ii.** May be accompanied by fever, malaise, chills, headache

  **iii.** Septicemia is common

  **iv.** Etiology

    (a) Appears at site of prior trauma or infection, insect bite, varicella

    (b) Inflammation and infection of the skin or subcutaneous tissue

    (c) Most common organisms

      (1) Group A β-hemolytic streptococci (tend to spread more rapidly)

      (2) Coagulase-positive staphylococci (usually more localized with a purulent center)

      (3) Rarely pneumococci and *Haemophilus influenzae*

  **v.** Diagnostic tests

    (a) If lesion is present, Gram stain, culture and sensitivity of exudate before initiating antibiotics

    (b) Obtain CBC and blood cultures if cellulitis is extensive or evidence of systemic toxicity

  **vi.** Treatment

    (a) Refer for hospitalization and IV antibiotics if child appears toxic

      (b) Oral antibiotics, e.g., amoxicillin-clavulanate, cephalexin, or erythromycin (see Table 54-3 in Chapter 54)

  vii. Contact dermatitis (Darmstadt & Sidbury, 2004)

 viii. Allergic dermatitis (see section 4.e. above)

   ix. Primary irritant dermatitis—nonallergic types

      (a) Diaper dermatitis (see section 4.h. below)

      (b) Skin contact with alkaline or acidic agent

         (1) Common sources of irritation

            a) Saliva from drooling, licking lips

            b) Citrus juices, bubble bath, proprietary medications

         (2) Usually clears after removal of the irritant and temporary treatment with a topical corticosteroid (see Table 54-5 in Chapter 54)

   h. Diaper dermatitis (Shwayder, 2003)

     i. Types of diaper dermatitis

      (a) Primary irritant diaper dermatitis

         (1) Glazed, red plaques; may develop into erosions

         (2) Mostly on convex surface of perineum

         (3) Pathophysiology

            a) Fecal enzymes (lipase, protease) are activated by contact with alkaline urine

            b) Fecal enzymes cause skin damage

            c) Diaper rash is NOT caused by ammonia from urine

      (b) Candida diaper dermatitis

         (1) Due to primary or secondary infection by *Candida albicans*

         (2) Occurs in 80% of cases of diaper rash

         (3) Classic picture is beefy red, sharply marginated scaly plaques

         (4) Also, small papules and pustules

         (5) Satellite lesions, usually on trunk

         (6) Found on convex surfaces and folds of perineum

      (c) Atopic diaper dermatitis

         (1) Seen in conjunction with atopic dermatitis

         (2) Excoriations, crusting, and lichenification

         (3) Mostly on convex surfaces of perineum

      (d) Intertrigo diaper dermatitis

         (1) Sharply demarcated red plaques in the folds of perineum

         (2) Few scales

      (e) Seborrheic diaper dermatitis

         (1) Salmon-colored scaly plaques with some yellowish scale

         (2) Asymptomatic—no pain, itch, discomfort from rash

         (3) Seen in conjunction with similar rash on scalp, ear folds, neck folds, axilla, umbilicus, knee, and arm folds

      (f) Psoriatic diaper dermatitis

         (1) Clearly delineated red plaque with slight scale

         (2) Occurs in an exact line along midline, from clitoral hood to gluteal cleft in girls; base of penis, inner folds and gluteal cleft in boys

    ii. Diagnostic tests

      (a) If lesion is scaly or pustular, do a KOH microscopic exam to identify candida or dermatophytes

   iii. Treatment

      (a) Change diapers as soon as they become wet or soiled

      (b) Cleanse skin with soap and water with *each* diaper change (baby wipes are okay if skin is not sensitive to the ingredients)

      (c) Use disposable diapers rather than cloth diapers to reduce incidence of diaper rash

         (1) An agent in disposable diapers combines with liquid urine or stool to form a gel that keeps liquid away from infant's skin

         (2) Some diapers have petroleum lining to protect skin

      (d) Avoid occlusive clothing, e.g., plastic pants

      (e) Expose rash to air as much as possible to facilitate healing

    iv. Antifungal topical ointment, cream or powder for candida and intertrigo diaper dermatitis

      (a) Apply bid if powder, or qid if cream or ointment until rash is resolved (see Table 54-3 in Chapter 54)

      (b) Cover the entire diaper area with zinc oxide paste or Triple Paste ointment; mineral oil helps remove these products

    v. Topical steroids (low potency, 1% hydrocortisone cream) if the skin is red (see Table 54-5)

    vi. Instruct parents to *alternate* application of antifungals and topical steroids

i. Dry skin dermatitis (asteatotic eczema, xerosis)

    i. Presentation

      (a) Abnormal dryness of skin, mucous membranes, or conjunctiva

      (b) Often characterized by fine lines in skin—accentuation of skin markings

      (c) Scaling skin

      (d) Itching

      (e) Large cracked scales with erythematous borders

    ii. Etiology

      (a) Arid climates

      (b) Inherited disorder

      (c) Families with history of atopy

    iii. Pathophysiology

      (a) Epidermis lacks moisture or sebum

      (b) Cracks in epidermal barrier allow loss of water and invasion of irritating substances, predisposing patient to dermatitis

    iv. Treatment

      (a) Rehydrate the stratum corneum

         (1) House humidifiers

         (2) Two 5-minute baths per day followed by immediate application of products to help retain water in skin

            a) Emollients that contain urea or lactic acid (e.g., Eucerin, Lubriderm)

            b) Ointments (petrolatum)

            c) Oils

      (b) Avoid products and situations that cause loss of water from skin

         (1) Soaps

         (2) Harsh deodorants

         (3) Alcohol-based products

         (4) Over zealous hygiene measures

         (5) Long, frequent baths or showers

j. Erythema infectiosum (fifth disease)

    i. Prodrome—fever, headache, malaise for 7 to 10 days

    ii. Clinical phase

      (a) Symptoms—about 1 week after prodrome, a rash appears; some children develop a persistent arthritis

(b) Rash (appears in three stages)
    (1) Stage 1
        a) Intensely red maculopapular lesions appear first on face
        b) Lesions coalesce on cheeks to form a "slapped face" appearance (circumoral area is spared)
        c) Lesions are warm, nontender, sometimes pruritic
        d) Facial lesions fade in 1 to 120 days
    (2) Stage 2
        a) A day after facial lesions appear, a rash appears on the proximal extensor surfaces of the extremities and spreads distally symmetrically (palms and soles usually spared)
        b) 1 day later, rash invades flexor surfaces and trunk
        c) Lesions last 1 week or more
    (3) Stage 3
        a) Lesions fade from center outward, giving a lacelike appearance to rash
        b) Fine desquamation may occur
        c) Rash may be precipitated by trauma, sunlight, hot, or cold
iii. Etiology
    (a) Exposure to parvovirus B19
    (b) Transmission—from contact with respiratory tract droplets; percutaneous exposure to blood or blood products, and vertical transmission from mother to fetus
    (c) Communicability—time period is uncertain; mildly contagious; not believed to be infectious after rash appears
    (d) Incubation period: 4 to 14 days; up to 21 days
iv. Diagnostic tests
    (a) Mild leucopenia occurs early in some patients followed by a leukocytosis and lymphocytosis
    (b) Specific IgM and IgG serum antibody tests are available
    (c) Antigen and nucleic acid detection tests are available
v. Treatment
    (a) Supportive (antipyretics and analgesics)
    (b) Avoid contact with pregnant women
    (c) Return to school as soon as rash appears
vi. Immunity—none
vii. Complications are rare; however teratogenic for a fetus (occasional hydrops fetalis) when susceptible pregnant women are infected
k. Erythema toxicum (erythema neonatorum) (Darmstadt & Sidbury, 2004)
    i. Blotchy erythematous, evanescent, papular rash frequently superimposed with vesicles or pustules
    ii. Covers thorax, but can also appear on abdomen, back, diaper area
    iii. Appears in 50% of newborns within 24 to 48 hours after birth; rare after 4 to 5 days
    iv. Etiology
        (a) Unknown
        (b) Smear of papules and pustules shows eosinophils
    v. Treatment—none
    vi. Benign self-limiting rash spontaneously disappears after several days
l. Folliculitis
    i. Pustule at site of hair follicle opening
    ii. Due to bacterial infection, usually staphylococci and streptococci

      iii. Associated with use of hot tubs

      iv. Diagnostic test—may culture exudates to verify antibiotic choice

      v. Treatment

        (a) Cool, wet compresses

        (b) Antibiotics (see Table 54-3 in Chapter 54)

        (c) Keratolytics (see Table 54-6 in Chapter 54)

**m.** Genital herpes—primary infection (Lutwick & Seenivasan, 2005)

      i. *Primary* infection with herpes simplex virus type 1 or 2 (HSV-1, HSV-2) can manifest as genital herpes (*see also* Section 4.t.iii and iv above)

      ii. 70% to 80% of seropositive individuals have no history of symptomatic genital herpes

      iii. Incubation period is 3 to 7 days (range = 1 day to 3 weeks)

      iv. Presentation—severe and prolonged systemic and local symptoms

        (a) Systemic symptoms: fever, headache, malaise, myalgia (especially in the first 3 to 4 days)

        (b) Local symptoms: pain, itching, dysuria, vaginal and urethral discharge, tender lymphadenopathy

      v. Physical examination

        (a) Women have more severe symptoms than men

          (1) Herpetic vesicles appear on the external genitalia, labia majora, labia minora, vaginal vestibule, and introitus

          (2) Vesicles in moist areas may rupture and form painful ulcers

          (3) Vaginal mucosa is inflamed and edematous

          (4) Ulcerative or necrotic cervical mucosa in 70% to 90% of patients (may be the only sign of infection in some patients)

        (b) Men

          (1) Herpetic vesicles appear in the glans penis, the prepuce, the shaft of the penis, and sometimes on the scrotum, thighs, and buttocks

          (2) Vesicles in dry areas progress to pustules and then crust

          (3) Herpetic urethritis with severe dysuria and mucoid discharge occurs in 30% to 40% of patients

        (c) Men and women

          (1) New lesions occur in 75% of patients, forming in 4 to 10 days from the primary lesion

          (2) Lesions last from 4 to 15 days, while crusting and reepithelialization occurs

          (3) Viral shedding lasts about 12 days (median length)

      vi. Treatment

        (a) Symptomatic treatment for pain, fever

        (b) Antiviral medications—acyclovir, valacyclovir can be used for current treatment and for suppression of recurrences (see Table 54-3 in Chapter 54)

      vii. Immunity

        (a) Preexisting antibodies to HSV-1 minimizes disease severity caused by HSV-2

        (b) Preexisting orolabial HSV-1 antibodies protects against genital HSV-1 but not HSV-2

      viii. Complications

        (a) Recurrent genital herpes (see section 4.n. below)

        (b) Bacterial and fungal superinfections

        (c) Autoinoculation—ocular, fingers, hands, skin

        (d) Aseptic meningitis, herpes simplex encephalitis

      **ix.** Prevention

        (a) Handwashing

        (b) Safer sexual practices, e.g., condoms

**n.** Genital herpes—recurrent infection (Lutwick & Seenivasan, 2005)

    **i.** Reactivation of genital herpes simplex infection may be subclinical or symptomatic

      (a) Both are more common with primary genital HSV-2 infection (60%) than with HSV-1

      (b) The more severe the primary infection, the more frequent and longer the recurrences

    **ii.** Note: subclinical reactivation with viral shedding may occur in the 70% to 80% of seropositive individuals who had no symptoms from the primary HSV-1 or HSV-2 infection; thus *they are an unwitting source of infection*

    **iii.** Prodromal symptoms

      (a) Tenderness, pain, and burning at the site of eruption (may last from 2 hours to 2 days)

      (b) Some patients may have severe ipsilateral sacral neuralgia

    **iv.** Clinical phase

      (a) Women have more severe symptoms than men

        (1) Painful vesicles on the labia majora, labia minora, or perineum

        (2) Viral shedding lasts 5 days (average)

        (3) Lesions heal in 8 to 10 days

      (b) Men

        (1) One or more patches of grouped vesicles on the shaft of the penis, prepuce, or glans

        (2) Pain is mild

        (3) Lesions heal in 7 to 10 days

        (4) Frequency and severity of recurrences decrease with time

    **v.** Treatment

      (a) Symptomatic treatment for pain, fever

      (b) Antiviral medications—acyclovir, valacyclovir can be used for current treatment and for suppression of recurrences (see Table 54-3 in Chapter 54)

    **vi.** Complications

      (a) Bacterial and fungal superinfections

      (b) Autoinoculation—ocular, fingers, hands, skin

      (c) Aseptic meningitis, herpes simplex encephalitis

    **vii.** Prevention

      (a) Handwashing

      (b) Safer sexual practices, e.g., condoms

**o.** Genital warts (Rakel, et al., 2005) (*see also* Chapter 31)

**p.** Hair loss (Table 32-1)

**q.** Hand, foot, and mouth disease

    **i.** Symptoms

      (a) Abrupt onset of fever (101° F) and malaise

      (b) Sore throat, anorexia, occasional headache, and abdominal pain

      (c) Rash

        (1) Vesicles or red papules on the tongue, oral mucosa, hands, and feet

        (2) Rash may appear when fever abates, simulating roseola

    **ii.** Etiology

      (a) Coxsackievirus A (A5, A10, A 16—an enterovirus)

■ **TABLE 32-1**
■ ■ **Characteristics, Diagnoses and Etiology of Conditions That Cause Hair Loss**

| Characteristics | Diagnosis | Etiology and Treatment Recommendations |
|---|---|---|
| Nonscarring, asymptomatic hair loss; coin-shaped bald spots; 2- to 4-mm "exclamation point" hairs on the perimeter have dark, thick tops, and light, thin bottoms; easily plucked with fingers | Alopecia areata | Antigen-antibody reaction at the root of a hair follicle shuts down hair growth<br>Refer to dermatologist |
| Diffuse hair loss, no broken off or "exclamation point" hairs | Telogen effluvium | Hair loss from a traumatic stimulus, e.g., too tight braids, chemicals treatment<br>Eliminate source of trauma |
| Diffuse hair loss; hairs are of all different lengths | Trichotillomania | Compulsive hair pulling<br>Refer to psychologist or psychiatrist |
| Circular bald patches, black dots of hair protruding from hair shafts near scalp; scales, pustule, itch | **Tinea capitis** | *Trichophyton tonsurans*<br>*Microsporum canis* (ringworm infection)<br>Tinea antiinfectives (Table 54-7) |

*Diagnoses in **bold** are further described in section 4 of this chapter.
Reprinted with permission from Shwayder, T. (2003). Five common skin problems—and a string of pearls for managing them. *Contemp Pediatr* July, 20:34, a copyrighted publication of Advanstar Communication Inc. All rights reserved.

    (b) Communicability: highly infectious
    (c) Transmission: fecal-oral route and possibly by respiratory route; virus can remain active for days at room temperature
    (d) Incubation period: 3 to 6 days
    (e) Seen mainly in summer
  iii. Treatment: symptomatic
    (a) Hydration
    (b) Antipyretics
    (c) Warm saline mouth rinses
  iv. Immunity: to infecting strain is generally conferred after one attack
  v. Complications: dehydration, febrile convulsions
**r.** Henoch-Schönlein purpura (HSP) (see Chapter 33)
**s.** Herpes simplex infections (Lutwick & Seenivasan, 2005)
  i. Genital herpes (see Section 4.n above)
  ii. Genital herpes—recurrent (see section 4.o above)
  iii. Gingivostomatitis
    (a) *Primary* infection with HSV-1 produces antibodies and is asymptomatic in about 80% of cases
    (b) In others, it appears as an acute herpetic gingivostomatitis
    (c) Typical age is 6 months to 5 years
    (d) Presentation
      (1) Lesions
        a) Abrupt onset
        b) Painful, grouped vesicles and ulcers on an erythematous base on the buccal mucosa, lips, tongue, palate, tonsillar facets
        c) Irritability and drooling in infants
        d) Lesions occasionally extend to pharynx, especially in older children and adolescents
        e) Diffusely swollen red gums are friable and bleed easily

(2) Tender anterior cervical lymphadenopathy

(3) Fever (104° to 105° F), anorexia and malaise

(e) Etiology

(1) HSV-1–infected saliva from an adult or another child

(2) Incubation period is 3 to 6 days

(3) Acute disease lasts 5 to 7 days, and the symptoms subside in 2 weeks

(4) Communicability: greatest early in course of infection

(5) Saliva may shed virus for 3 weeks or more

(f) Treatment

(1) Pain relief, maintain hydration with nonacidic, cool fluids

(2) Older children: Kaopectate and viscous lidocaine mixture (equal parts) may be used as mouthwash (do not swallow)

(3) Topical acyclovir may be used during recurrent episodes (see Table 54-3 in Chapter 54)

(g) Complications

(1) Dehydration, malnourishment

(2) Recurrent HSV-1 virus infections typically appear as herpes labialis

(3) Bacterial and fungal superinfections

(4) Autoinoculation—ocular, fingers, hands, skin

(5) Aseptic meningitis, herpes simplex encephalitis

(h) Immunity

(1) Immunity to primary herpes response is gained after one incident

(2) No immunity to recurrent herpes infections; virus lies dormant in body until activated by stress, sun exposure, fever, other illness, or menstruation

(i) Prevention

(1) Handwashing

(2) Safer sexual practices, e.g., condoms

iv. Herpes labialis (Lutwick & Seenivasan, 2005)

(a) Most common *recurrent* infection from HSV-1 (see Gingivostomatitis above)

(b) Prodromal symptoms

(1) Pain, burning, and tingling on labia

(2) Erythematous papules that rapidly develop into tiny, thin-walled, intraepidermal vesicles that become pustular and ulcerate

(c) Communicability—most viral shedding occurs in first 24 hours; may last 5 days

(d) Recurrence—typically 1 or 2 per year; but monthly for some individuals

(e) Treatment

(1) Symptomatic treatment for pain, fever

(2) Antiviral medications—acyclovir, valacyclovir can be used for current treatment and for suppression of recurrences (see Table 54-3 in Chapter 54)

(f) Complications

(1) Bacterial and fungal superinfections

(2) Autoinoculation—ocular, fingers, hands, skin

(3) Aseptic meningitis, herpes simplex encephalitis

(g) Prevention

(1) Handwashing

(2) Safer sexual practices, e.g., condoms

**t.** Impetigo (Darmstadt & Sidbury, 2004)
- **i.** Presentation
  - (a) Characterized by focal erythema, a papule that vesiculates and breaks, leaving an eroded, denuded area covered with honey-colored crusts
  - (b) May also appear as a large vesicle with an erythematous border and filled with clear fluid (called bullous impetigo)
  - (c) Usually begins on face and spreads locally
- **ii.** Etiology
  - (a) Trauma to skin (abrasion or insect bite) provides entry site for bacteria, usually Group A streptococci and *S. aureus*
  - (b) Highly contagious; transmitted through contact with exudates from lesions
  - (c) Incubation period: 2 to 5 days
- **iii.** Treatment
  - (a) Wash lesions daily with soap and water
  - (b) Topical mupirocin (Bactroban) tid for 10 days if affected area is small
  - (c) Oral antibiotics; β-lactamase–resistant antibiotics for 7 to 10 days (see Table 54-3 in Chapter 54)
    - (1) First-line choices: cephalexin or erythromycin ethylsuccinate
    - (2) Second-line choices: dicloxacillin, clindamycin, amoxicillin-clavulanate, or azithromycin

**u.** Infantile hemangioma (Miller & Frieden, 2005)
- **i.** Subtypes stratified by risk (all are more common in females than in males)
  - (a) Localized
    - (1) Nodules more often than plaques
    - (2) Focal or with clear spatial containment
    - (3) Relatively benign unless in periorbital area
  - (b) Multifocal
    - (1) More than five to eight noncontiguous lesions of any type
    - (2) Likely to be associated with morbidity and other abnormalities
  - (c) Segmental
    - (1) Plaque-like, linear or geographic localization
    - (2) Often unilateral
    - (3) High likelihood of morbidity and associated abnormalities
- **ii.** Presentation
  - (a) Often present at birth as a blanched area of skin
  - (b) 2 to 4 weeks of age, red rubbery nodules with roughened surfaces appear
  - (c) Proliferative phase is followed by slow, spontaneous involution
  - (d) Strawberry hemangiomas: bright red elevated lesions ranging from 0.5 to 4 cm
  - (e) Cavernous hemangiomas: located deep beneath surface of skin and appear bluish
- **iii.** Etiology—two theories
  - (a) Originate from embolized placental tissue
  - (b) Somatic mutation may have caused improper differentiation of fetal vascular precursor cells
  - (c) Organic involvement in order of frequency: liver, GI tract, brain, mediastinum, lung
- **iv.** Diagnostic tests
  - (a) Ultrasound useful to identify visceral involvement
  - (b) MRI with contrast-enhanced and gradient sequences

    **v.** Treatment

        (a) Spontaneous resolution occurs in 50% of cases by age 5 and 100% by adolescence

        (b) Refer to dermatology if hemangioma is a multifocal or segmental type

        (c) Pulsed-dye laser treatment may help if lesions are bleeding or ulcerated

    **vi.** Complications that may require immediate treatment

        (a) Thrombocytopenia from platelet trapping

        (b) Airway obstruction from subglottic hemangiomas

        (c) Visual disturbances, cardiac decompensation

**v.** Kawasaki disease (KD, mucocutaneous lymph node syndrome)

    **i.** See Chapter 29 for complete description of KD

    **ii.** See also, www.circulationaha.org for a copy of the American Heart Association guidelines for diagnosis, treatment, and long-term management of KD

    **iii.** Delayed diagnosis of KD is a significant risk factor in the development of coronary abnormalities in children (Pannaraj, et al., 2004)

        (a) More than 50% of pediatricians reported that they do not consider KD in children younger than 6 months of age or older than 8 years of age

        (b) A higher index of suspicion is required to avoid missed or late diagnosis of KD in these age-groups

**w.** Keloid (Darmstadt & Sidbury, 2004)

    **i.** Presentation

        (a) Sharply demarcated, benign, dense growth of connective tissue

        (b) Firm, raised, pink, rubbery nodule

        (c) May be tender or pruritic

        (d) Particularly on the face, earlobes, neck, shoulders, upper trunk, lower legs

    **ii.** Etiology

        (a) Forms in the dermis after trauma

        (b) Familial tendency

        (c) Blacks are more predisposed to keloid formation than other racial groups

    **iii.** Refer to dermatology for treatment and potential removal

**x.** Keratosis pilaris (Darmstadt & Sidbury, 2004)

    **i.** Presentation

        (a) Noninflammatory

        (b) Follicular papules containing a white scale

        (c) Discrete, individual lesions may be erythematous; lesions may also coalesce

        (d) Prominent on extensor surfaces of the upper arms and thighs and buttocks and cheeks; in severe cases may be generalized

    **ii.** Associated with dry skin, atopic dermatitis, ichthyosis vulgaris

    **iii.** Treatment is primarily palliative

        (a) Avoid frequent bathing

        (b) Hypoallergenic soaps and lotions

        (c) Lubricants applied immediately after bathing

        (d) Moderate to severe forms: use keratolytics, e.g., retinoic acid, lactic acid, or urea creams

    **iv.** May continue until age 30 or more

**y.** Lyme disease
  **i.** Symptoms—three stages
   (a) Stage 1: early localized
      (1) 7 to 10 days after inoculation
      (2) Erythema migrans rash—round red macule or papule that enlarges over time, forming a large annular, erythematous lesion that is ≥5 cm in diameter, sometimes with central clearing; may have one or several lesions
      (3) Center may be intensely erythematous and indurated in early lesions
      (4) Nonpruritic, nonpainful
      (5) Chills, fever, headache, mild neck stiffness, backache, malaise, myalgia, arthralgia, regional or generalized lymphadenopathy
   (b) Stage 2: early disseminated
      (1) Occurs 3 to 5 weeks after tick bite
      (2) Secondary migratory annular lesions are smaller; centers are not indurated
      (3) May occur anywhere but generally spare palms, soles, and mucous membranes
      (4) Systemic symptoms: arthralgia, myalgia, headache, fatigue (common)
      (5) Palsies of cranial nerves (especially cranial nerve VIII), meningitis and conjunctivitis may occur
      (6) Carditis occurs rarely in children
   (c) Stage 3: late disease
      (1) Weeks to years after onset if untreated
      (2) Recurrent pauciarticular arthritis (particularly knees)
      (3) Less commonly: memory loss, mood swings, inability to concentrate
  **ii.** Etiology
   (a) *Borrelia burgdorferi* spirochete, transmitted by a tiny deer tick (*Ixodes dammini*)
   (b) Primarily occurs in Northeast, Midwest, and western United States
   (c) Incubation period: 3 to 31 days; typically 7 to 14 days
  **iii.** Diagnostic tests
   (a) Diagnosis most readily made by evaluation of rash, history of associate flulike symptoms, epidemiologic date, and serologic testing
   (b) Lyme titer not accurate until 3 weeks after exposure
  **iv.** Treatment
   (a) Medications
      (1) Early localized disease, age 8 years and older: doxycycline is treatment of choice
      (2) For all ages: amoxicillin or erythromycin if penicillin allergy
   (b) Referral for hospitalization and IV therapy if persistent arthritis, carditis, meningitis, or encephalitis
  **v.** Complications
   (a) Cardiac complications in approximately 8% of untreated cases
   (b) Lyme arthritis
   (c) Bell's palsy
   (d) Guillain-Barré syndrome
   (e) Polyradiculitis

    **z.** Milia (Darmstadt & Sidbury, 2004)
        **i.** Presentation
            (a) Multiple white papules 1 mm in diameter, pearly, opalescent white
            (b) Scattered over forehead, nose, cheeks
            (c) Present in up to 40% of newborns
        **ii.** Etiology
            (a) Superficial epidermal inclusion cysts in the papillary dermis filled with keratinous material
            (b) Associated with the developing pilosebaceous follicle
            (c) Intraoral counterparts are called Epstein's pearls (common)
        **iii.** Treatment
            (a) No treatment required
            (b) Papules will rupture spontaneously and exfoliate
  **aa.** Miliaria crystalline (heat rash)
        **i.** Occurs frequently in neonates (compare with miliaria rubra)
        **ii.** Tiny superficial grouped vesicles without erythema over intertriginous areas and adjacent skin of neck and/or upper chest
        **iii.** Prolonged exposure to heat and high humidity causes obstruction of eccrine sweat ducts of the stratum corneum
        **iv.** Treatment
            (a) Keep child cool and well ventilated in hot weather
            (b) Baking soda baths
  **bb.** Miliaria rubra (heat rash)
        **i.** Most common form of miliaria (compare with miliaria crystalline)
        **ii.** Erythematous, grouped papules
        **iii.** Prolonged exposure to heat and high humidity causes obstruction of eccrine sweat ducts deeper in the epidermis of the forehead, upper trunk, and intertriginous areas
        **iv.** Tingling and prickling sensations are common
        **v.** Treatment
            (a) Keep child cool and well ventilated in hot weather
            (b) Baking soda baths
  **cc.** Molluscum contagiosum (Crowe, 2005; Smolinski & Yan, 2005)
        **i.** Presentation
            (a) Rash consists of 1- to 5-mm diameter flesh-colored to translucent papules, some with central umbilication, on trunk, face, or extremities
            (b) A benign, usually asymptomatic skin disease with no systemic manifestations
        **ii.** Etiology
            (a) Molluscum contagiosum virus (MCV), a large DNA poxvirus
            (b) Transmission: direct contact, autoinoculation, contaminated objects, swimming pools
            (c) Communicability: low infectivity
            (d) Incubation period: 2 to 7 weeks, but may be as long as 6 months
            (e) Common in infants and preschool children
            (f) Considered a sexually transmitted disease when it occurs in adolescents and adults
        **iii.** Pathophysiology
            (a) Virus infects skin's epithelial cells and replicates in the cytoplasm
            (b) Produces large cytoplasmic viral inclusions

      **iv.** Treatment:
         (a) Benign, asymptomatic, self-limiting—spontaneous regression usually occurs in 2 to 3 years
         (b) Removal of lesions is curative
            (1) Curettage—removal of entire wart or central core under local anesthesia
            (2) Peeling agents (salicylic and lactic acid)
            (3) Electrocautery
            (4) Cryotherapy—liquid nitrogen drops on warts; repeat at 2- to 4-week intervals
            (5) Pulsed-dye laser treatments—refer to dermatology
         (c) Check for other STIs in adolescents and adults
         (d) Medications (Crowe, 2005)
            (1) 17% topical salicylic acid leads to desquamation and inflammation
            (2) Cantharidin topical solution is a strong vesicant
            (3) Imiquimod 5% cream; action unknown; pediatric dose not established
            (4) Antivirals only for immunocompromised patients
      **v.** Complications
         (a) Local inflammatory reaction to treatment
         (b) Secondary infection

**dd.** Mongolian spot (congenital dermal melanocytosis) (see Chapter 18)

**ee.** Nevus (often called a mole)
      **i.** Brown pigmented macule
      **ii.** Congenital
      **iii.** Usually benign, but may become cancerous

**ff.** Nevus simplex (salmon patch; nevus flammeus) (Darmstadt & Sidbury, 2004)
      **i.** Small, pale pink, ill-defined vascular macule
         (a) Occur on glabella, eyelids, upper lip, nuchal area of 30% to 40% of normal newborns
         (b) Become more visible when crying or during environmental temperature changes
      **ii.** Benign—no treatment required
      **iii.** Lesions on face usually fade; those on neck and occiput may persist

**gg.** Papular urticaria
      **i.** Groups of pruritic erythematous papules surrounded by an urticarial flare
      **ii.** Typically located on shoulders, upper arms, and buttocks in infants
      **iii.** May last 4 to 6 months
      **iv.** Etiology: delayed hypersensitivity reactions to stinging or biting insects (fleas, mosquitoes, lice, scabies, mites)
      **v.** Treatment: oral antihistamines and topical corticosteroids (see Tables 54-4 and 54-5 in Chapter 54)

**hh.** Pediculosis (lice) (Shwayder, 2005)
      **i.** Types
         (a) Pediculosis capitis—infestation of scalp
         (b) Pediculosis corporis—infestation of skin of body
      **ii.** Clinical presentation
         (a) Small white flecks on hair shaft, behind ears or nape of neck (nits or lice eggs)
         (b) Do not confuse these with dandruff, which flakes off easily

(c) Nits may be found in seams of underwear or crawling on scalp or body
(d) Excoriated papules and pustules
(e) Severe pruritus at night (suggests pediculosis corporis)
iii. Treatment
(a) Pediculosis capitis
(1) Permethrin 1% cream rinse
a) Available over the counter
b) Apply to scalp and hair for 10 minutes
c) Low potential for toxic side effects
d) High cure rate
e) Also available as a shampoo
(2) Lindane 1% (Kwell)
a) 4-minute shampoo
b) Requires prescription
c) Indicated primarily for failure of other therapies
d) Repeated application in 7 to 10 days often recommended
e) Many contraindications—see product reference
(3) Malathion 0.05% lotion
a) Requires prescription
b) Highly effective—has the best kill rate
c) 8- to 12-hour application with repeat application in 7 to 9 days if still present
d) Contraindicated in neonates and infants
(4) Comb hair with fine-tooth comb to remove all nits
a) AAP states that manual removal of nits is not necessary (Frankowski & Weiner, 2002)
b) Others recommend removal of nits for two reasons:
i) 5% to 35% of treated nits will still hatch
ii) Some schools have a "no nit" policy for return to school
c) Vinegar hair rinse may help loosen nits before combing
(5) Household and other close contacts need to be examined for infestation
(6) Fomites do not have a major role in infestation; environmental disinfecting is often unnecessary
(b) Pediculosis corporis
(1) Lindane cream or lotion applied to the body for 4 hours
(2) Improve hygiene
(3) Wash clothes and bedding in boiling water followed by ironing seams with hot iron to remove organisms
(4) Pediculicides are not necessary if materials are laundered at least weekly
ii. Pityriasis alba
i. White, scaly macular lesions with indistinct borders
ii. Blotchy areas of hypopigmentation (decreased melanin in skin)
iii. Appears over cheeks and extensor surfaces of extremities in children; more generalized in infants
iv. Etiology
(a) Unknown
(b) Probably a postinflammatory hypopigmentation
(c) Regarded as a mild form of eczema
v. Diagnostic tests—test skin scrapings with KOH to rule out tinea versicolor

      vi. Treatment
        (a) Mild topical steroids may facilitate return of normal skin color
        (b) Moisturizers to control scaling
        (c) Loss of pigment is temporary; tends to improve after puberty

**jj.** Pityriasis rosea (Darmstadt & Sidbury, 2004)
    i. Prodromal symptoms: mild; headache, malaise, sore throat
    ii. Clinical symptoms
        (a) May be asymptomatic until rash appears
        (b) Mild regional lymphadenopathy
        (c) Rash
            (1) Herald patch is initial lesion; scaly with central clearing; salmon colored; round or oval plaque 3 to 6 cm in diameter with erythematous border
            (2) Rash appears 3 to 10 days after initial lesion; salmon colored, oval lesions; smaller than herald patch; vary in size; scaly macular and papular; vcsicular lesions may be present; axes of lesions are along cleavage lines, parallel to ribs and a "Christmas tree" configuration may be seen on the back
            (3) Pruritus of varying degrees
            (4) Mucous membranes, palms, and soles are spared
            (5) Duration of rash can be 3 to 4 months
    iii. Etiology
        (a) Unknown; thought to be viral
        (b) Communicability: low
    iv. Diagnostic tests
        (a) Venereal Disease Research Laboratory (VDRL) test or rapid plasma regain (RPR) test to rule out syphilis
        (b) Diagnosis made by appearance and distribution of rash
    v. Treatment
        (a) Cool compresses
        (b) Diphenhydramine (Benadryl) or hydroxyzine hydrochloride (Atarax) for marked pruritus
        (c) Exposure to sunlight may relieve itching and enhance resolution of rash
    vi. Immunity: recurrences are uncommon
    vii. Complications: secondary bacterial infection from scratching lesions

**kk.** Pityriasis versicolor (tinea versicolor)
    i. Superficial skin infection characterized by multiple hypopigmented connected macules and very fine scales in areas of sun-induced pigmentation (tanned skin)
    ii. Lesions may be brown or orange in winter and hypopigmented in summer upon exposure to sun
    iii. A common noninflammatory superficial fungal infection of the skin
    iv. Etiology
        (a) Lipophilic yeast
        (b) *Pityrosporum orbiculare (Malassezia furfur)*—a yeastlike fungus
    v. Diagnostic tests—infected areas are fluorescent yellow under a Wood's light
    vi. Treatment
        (a) Application of selenium sulfide (Selsun) as 2.5% lotion or 1% shampoo; leave product on skin for 30 minutes daily for 1 week; followed by monthly applications for 3 months to prevent recurrence

        (b) Small focal infections may be treated with topical antifungals applied twice a day for to 4 weeks (see Table 54-7 in Chapter 54)

        (c) Oral antifungal therapy may be administered but is expensive and associated with greater risk of adverse reactions (see Table 54-7 in Chapter 54)

        (d) Relapses are common because *M. furfur* is part of normal flora of skin

**ll.** Port-wine stain

    i. A type of hemangioma

    ii. Dark red or bluish red macule

    iii. May appear anywhere on body

    iv. Refer to dermatology for pulsed-dye laser treatment that can begin in infancy

    v. Large, bilateral port-wine stain, or one covering entire half of face associated with Sturge-Weber syndrome (seizures, mental retardation, glaucoma, hemiplegia)

    vi. Port-wine stain over an extremity associated with Klippel-Trenaunay syndrome (hypertrophy of the extremity's soft tissue and bone)

**mm.** Postinflammatory hyperpigmentation (Darmstadt & Sidbury, 2004; Trowers, 2005)

    i. Occurs after acne, bites, traumatic injuries to skin

    ii. Lasts longer in Black patients than in whites

    iii. Recommended treatments

        (a) Treat with 6% hydroquinone preparations (by prescription)

        (b) Sunscreen used simultaneously will hasten healing of lesions

        (c) Chemical peels (salicylic acid)

        (d) UV protective clothing; or use Sun Guard, a laundry addition made by Rit dye that increases the SPF of clothing

**nn.** Psoriasis (Darmstadt & Sidbury, 2004)

    i. Presentation

        (a) Circumscribed erythematous patches covered by thick, dry, silvery, adherent scales

        (b) Lesions appear anywhere on body but more common on extensor surfaces, body prominences, scalp, ears, genitalia, and perianal area

        (c) Pustular psoriasis is associated with fever, malaise, and anorexia

        (d) Exacerbations and remissions typical

    ii. Etiology—a common, chronic, inherited skin disease

    iii. Pathophysiology—unknown, except for excessive development of epithelial cells

    iv. Diagnostic tests

        (a) Elevated uric acid level is common

        (b) Other lab tests are generally within normal limits

        (c) In severe cases, CBC reveals anemia, elevated erythrocyte sedimentation rate, and decreased albumin levels

        (d) Pustular psoriasis associated with leukocytosis and hypocalcemia

    v. Treatment

        (a) Therapy aimed at diminishing time of epidermal regeneration

            (1) Sunlight or artificial ultraviolet light (UVL)

            (2) Coal tar enhances effect of UVL and hastens disappearances of lesions

            (3) 10% liquor carbonis detergens in petrolatum applied after bath (Estar Gel, psoriGel) applied bid for 6 to 8 weeks

        (b) Topical corticosteroids may be preferred by patients to messy tar therapy
- (1) Potent preparations must be used to penetrate enlarged epidermal barrier, e.g., Lidex, Aristocort, Kenalog bid or tid
- (2) A combination of fluocinolone and peanut oil is extremely moisturizing (oil is purified, so patients with peanut allergy are not at risk) (Paller, et al., 2003)

**oo.** Rocky Mountain spotted fever
- **i.** Clinical presentation
  - (a) Systemic symptoms: high fever of abrupt onset; severe and persistent headache, general toxicity, myalgia, nausea, vomiting, anorexia, diarrhea
  - (b) Systemic small-vessel vasculitis with characteristic rash occurs in 80% to 95% of patients
    - (1) Appears before the sixth day of illness
    - (2) Erythematous macules later become maculopapular and often petechial
    - (3) Rash appears first on wrists and ankles, often spreading within hours proximally to the trunk; often palms and soles are involved
- **ii.** Etiology
  - (a) *Rickettsia rickettsii* arthropod
  - (b) Bite from, or fecal contact with arthropod for 4 hours or longer
- **iii.** Clinical phase
  - (a) History of contact may be absent in children
  - (b) Rarely occurs in West; most common eastern seaboard, southeastern states, and Arkansas, Texas, Missouri, Kansas, Oklahoma
  - (c) Incubation: 2 to 14 days (usually about 1 week)
- **iv.** Diagnostic tests:
  - (a) Laboratory findings are nonspecific
  - (b) Serologic diagnosis achieved with indirect fluorescent or latex agglutination antibody methods (generally only 7 to 10 days after onset of illness)
- **v.** Treatment (CDC, 2006)
  - (a) Drug of choice is doxycycline for children of any age (doxycycline less likely than other tetracyclines to stain teeth)
    - (1) Initiate treatment immediately upon suspicion of RMSF—do not wait for laboratory confirmation
    - (2) Continue for at least 3 days after fever subsides and until clinical improvement is evident (usually 5 to 10 days)
  - (b) Alternative is chloramphenicol, but has many side effects
- **vi.** Complications
  - (a) Refer patients with prominent central nervous system, cardiac, pulmonary, gastrointestinal tract and/or renal symptoms

**pp.** Roseola infantum (exanthem subitum)
- **i.** Symptoms
  - (a) First symptom is high fever (104° to 105° F)
  - (b) Infants may be irritable and anorexic but rarely appear ill (usually appear alert and playful)
  - (c) Pharynx may be slightly inflamed
  - (d) Lymphadenopathy may be present (occipital, cervical, postauricular)
  - (e) After 3 or 4 days, fever falls abruptly and distinctive rash appears

    **ii.** Rash—hallmark is its appearance after a fever
- (a) Discrete rose-pink macules approximately 2 to 3 mm in size; fade with pressure; most prominent on trunk; lasts 1 to 2 days

    **iii.** Etiology and prevalence
- (a) Exposure to human herpesvirus 6 (HHV-6)
- (b) Generally occurs in children 6 months to 3 years
- (c) Occurs mainly spring and fall
- (d) Transmission method is unknown
- (e) Communicability occurs during febrile period
- (f) Incubation period: 10 to 14 days

    **iv.** Diagnostic tests
- (a) Laboratory tests not helpful in diagnosis
- (b) WBC count usually decreased; lymphocytes increased

    **v.** Treatment
- (a) Primarily symptomatic and supportive
- (b) Acetaminophen or ibuprofen for fever
- (c) Baking soda baths or antihistamines for pruritus

    **vi.** Immunity
- (a) Having the disease offers lasting natural immunity
- (b) No artificial immunity is available

    **vii.** Complications
- (a) Usually benign
- (b) May have febrile seizure

**qq.** Rubella (German measles; 3-day measles)

    **i.** Prodromal symptoms: nonspecific upper respiratory symptoms, ocular pain, pharyngitis and generalized lymphadenopathy (postauricular, cervical, and occipital)

    **ii.** Clinical phase
- (a) Illness symptoms: fever, arthralgia, and characteristic rash
  - (1) Diffuse, fine erythematous maculopapular rash
  - (2) Begins on face and rapidly spreading to entire body
  - (3) Disappears by the fourth day in same order that it appeared
- (b) Etiology
  - (1) Exposure to rubella virus
  - (2) History of rubella vaccination usually absent; therefore no antibodies against virus
  - (3) Transmission: spreads by direct and indirect contact with respiratory droplets
  - (4) Incubation: 14 to 23 days (usually 16 to 18 days)
  - (5) Communicability
    - a) A few days before, to approximately 7 days after the rash appears
    - b) Exclude child from school or daycare for 7 days after onset of rash
    - c) A small number of infants with congenital rubella shed virus in nasopharyngeal secretions and urine for 1 year or more
    - d) Congenital rubella cases are considered contagious until at least 1 year of age unless repeated cultures are negative
- (c) Congenital rubella infection is also associated with growth retardation, cardiac anomalies, ocular anomalies, deafness, cerebral disorders, hematologic disorders

(d) Immunity
(1) Contracting disease offers lasting natural immunity; a high rubella titer reveals infection has occurred
(2) Active artificial immunity obtained from live attenuated measles vaccine
(3) Passive artificial immunity can be obtained from immune serum globulin; consider this for exposed pregnant women
iii. Diagnostic tests
(a) Virus may be isolated from nasal, throat, urine, blood, or cerebrospinal fluid
(b) A fourfold or greater rise in specific rubella antibodies, IgG, or a single IgM is diagnostic
iv. Treatment is symptomatic and supportive
**rr.** Rubeola (regular measles, 7-day measles, brown or black measles)
i. Prodromal symptoms: 11- to 12-day prodrome of fever, cough, conjunctivitis (with photophobia), coryza, lymphadenopathy
ii. Clinical phase
(a) Koplik's spots
(1) Small irregular, bright red spots with a blue-white center point on buccal membranes
(2) A hallmark of the disease, although they may be absent
(b) Rash
(1) Appears by fourth day of fever
(2) Deep red maculopapular rash begins at hairline on forehead, behind ears, and at back of neck
(3) Spreads down from face and hairline over 3 days and later becoming confluent
(4) After several days red rash (fades with pressure) becomes brown (does not fade with pressure)
(5) Rash fades after 5 to 6 days followed by fine desquamation (spares hands and feet)
iii. Etiology
(a) Exposure to measles (rubeola) virus
(b) History of rubeola vaccination usually absent; therefore no antibodies against virus
(c) Transmission: spread by direct or indirect contact with respiratory droplets
(d) Incubation: 7 to 14 days
(e) Communicability: fifth day of incubation period through first few days of rash
(f) Complications
(1) Respiratory bacterial superinfections (lung, middle ear, sinus, cervical nodes)
(2) Encephalitis
(3) Other: thrombocytopenia, appendicitis, keratitis, myocarditis, optic neuritis, reactivation or progression of tuberculosis in untreated children, jaundice and premature delivery or stillbirth
iv. Diagnosis
(a) Positive serologic result for measles immunoglobulin (Ig) M antibody
(b) Isolation of measles virus from specimens of urine, blood, nasopharyngeal secretions

     **v.** Treatment

        (a) Symptomatic and supportive

        (b) Antimicrobials for secondary bacterial infection

        (c) Vitamin A supplementation

           (1) For children 6 months to 2 years who are hospitalized with measles and one or more of its complications (croup, pneumonia, diarrhea)

           (2) And for children older than 6 months who have risk factors such as immunodeficiency, vitamin A deficiency, impaired intestinal absorption, moderate to severe malnutrition and recent immigration from areas where high mortality rates from measles have been observed.

        (d) Immunity:

           (1) Contracting disease offers lasting natural immunity; a high rubella titer reveals infection has occurred

           (2) Active artificial immunity obtained from live attenuated measles vaccine

           (3) Passive artificial immunity obtained from immune serum globulin

**ss.** Scabies (Shwayder, 2003)

     **i.** Lesions

        (a) Erythematous papular and/or vesicular eruption that forms shallow serpiginous burrows directly beneath the stratum corneum

        (b) Intensely pruritic in most individuals

        (c) Location

           (1) Older children and adolescents—anterior axillary lines, areolae, inner aspect of the upper arm, wrists and interdigital webs, ankles, penis, groin

           (2) Children younger than 2 years—eruption is vesicular and often occurs on the head, neck, palms, and soles

     **ii.** Etiology

        (a) *Sarcoptes scabiei* subspecies hominis (human scabies mite); an 8-legged arachnid

        (b) Transmission: prolonged, close, personal contact

        (c) Mite dries up and dies quickly if it is not on a human body

        (d) Incubation

           (1) If no previous exposure: 3 to 4 weeks

           (2) If history of previous infestation: 1 to 4 days

     **iii.** Diagnostic test

        (a) *Always* verify the diagnosis before treating—the diagnosis of scabies carries significant psychosocial distress for families

        (b) Drop mineral oil on the top of primary lesion, scrape gently, place on glass slide, add more mineral oil, then microscopically examine for presence of mites, feces, or eggs

     **iv.** Treatment

        (a) Scabicide cream or lotion

           (1) Cover entire body below head in children and adults

           (2) Cover head, neck and body in infants and young children

        (b) Drug of choice: permethrin 5 % cream (Elimite)

           (1) Remove medication by bathing after 8 to 14 hours

        (c) Second line of therapy: 1% lindane cream or lotion (Kwell)

           (1) Remove medication by bathing after 8 to 12 hours

           (2) FDA health advisory about its neurotoxicity

(d) Oral ivermectin is a newer treatment method

(e) One treatment usually clears infestation

(f) Check for infestation about 2 weeks later to determine if a second treatment is necessary

(g) Treat all family members (usually one treatment is sufficient)

(h) Wash all bedding, towels, and worn clothes with soap and hot water

(i) If items cannot be washed, but can be heated, place in dryer at high temperature for 20 minutes

(j) Items that cannot be washed or heated, place in sealed plastic bag for 1 week

(k) Postscabetic eczema—pruritus may persist for several weeks following successful treatment; use 1% hydrocortisone cream and/or oral antihistamine

(l) Complications

(1) Secondary bacterial infection

(2) Untoward reaction to scabicide treatment

**tt.** Scarlet fever

   **i.** Symptoms

(a) Fever (103° to 104° F), chills, headache, malaise

(b) Sore throat, tonsils inflamed, enlarged and may have white exudate

(c) Palate usually covered with erythematous punctiform macular lesions and perhaps scattered petechiae

(d) Circumoral pallor

(e) Rash

(1) Appears 12 to 48 hours after onset of pharyngeal symptoms

(2) Both enanthematous (mucous membrane) and exanthematous (skin)

(3) Tongue rash

   a) First 2 days: white and appears furry

   b) Day 3: papillae enlarge and protrude through white coat, giving a "white strawberry" appearance

   c) Days 4 to 5: white coat disappears and the prominent papillae of tongue give it a red "strawberry" appearance; distinctive sign of scarlet fever

(4) Skin rash

   a) Pinpoint erythematous lesions that blanch on pressure

   b) Sandpapery texture

   c) Most lesions are on trunk and in skinfolds; few lesions appear on face

   d) Hyperpigmentation in folds of joints (Pastia's sign) may be present

   e) Rash persists for 1 week, then desquamates with large areas of skin peeling off in fine flakes

   **ii.** Etiology

(a) Exposure to group A β-hemolytic streptococci (GABHS) causes the illness

(b) Rash is caused by GABHS toxin

(c) Transmission occurs by direct contact with large respiratory droplets

(d) Communicability is greatest during acute phase (1 to 7 days)

(e) Incubation period: 2 to 5 days

   **iii.** Diagnostic tests

(a) Laboratory confirmation is recommended for group A streptococcal (GAS) infections using a tonsillar swab for culture on sheep blood agar

(b) Several rapid tests are available; negative results should be followed up by culture

iv. Treatment

    (a) Medications (see Table 54-3 in Chapter 54)

        (1) Penicillin V is drug of choice

        (2) May use penicillin G benzathine

        (3) Or erythromycin if there is a penicillin allergy

        (4) Alternatives may be macrolides, e.g., clarithromycin or azithromycin; or first-generation cephalosporin

        (5) Rash may be pruritic—use antihistamines, baking soda baths

        (6) Analgesics and antipyretics for pain and fever (see Table 55-5 in Chapter 55)

    (b) Soft or liquid diet until throat soreness diminishes

v. Complications: acute rheumatic fever (see Chapter 29) or acute glomerulonephritis (see Chapter 31)

vi. Immunity—one episode of the disease gives lasting immunity to scarlet fever toxin

**uu.** Seborrheic dermatitis (Darmstadt & Sidbury, 2004)

  **i.** Presentation

    (a) Characterized by dry or moist greasy scales and yellowish crusts

    (b) Affects areas of high sebum production

    (c) Common sites are scalp, eyelids (seborrheic blepharitis), face, external surfaces of ears and ear canals (otitis externa), axillae, breasts, groin, and gluteal folds

    (d) Appears in neonate as "cradle cap," aggravated by caretaker's reluctance to wash infant's head

    (e) Appears in young infant as dermatitis of scalp and diaper area

    (f) Appears in adolescent as dandruff or dermatitis of midsternum, upper midback and head

  **ii.** Etiology

    (a) Unknown cause

    (b) Reactivated by stressful situations, poor hygiene, excessive perspiration

    (c) May be associated with paralysis agitans (Parkinson's disease), diabetes mellitus, malabsorption disorders, epilepsy, or an allergic reaction to gold or arsenic

  **iii.** Treatment

    (a) Involved area must be kept clean, dry, cool, and free from irritation

    (b) Parental education

        (1) Proper hygiene of infant scalp using daily shampooing

        (2) Removal of crusts: leave shampoo on for several minutes to loosen crusts; rinse thoroughly; use fine-tooth comb or soft brush after shampooing to remove crusts from strands of hair

    (c) Selenium sulfide shampoos may be necessary; use several times per week initially; decreasing to once or twice weekly

    (d) Corticosteroids (topical/oral) for acute inflammation (see Table 54-5 in Chapter 54)

    (e) Avoid sweating and irritants

    (f) Treat underlying disorders when present

**vv.** Stevens-Johnson Syndrome (Darmstadt & Sidbury, 2004)

  **i.** Prodrome—flulike URI with severe mucosal ulceration (often not painful)

  **ii.** Presentation

(a) Erythematous macules; rapidly develop central necrosis and form vesicles, bullae and denuded areas

(b) Appears on face, trunk, and extremities

(c) Two or more mucosal surfaces are involved—eyes, oral cavity, upper airway, esophagus, GI tract, anogenital tract

(d) Burning sensation, erythema, edema of lips are often presenting signs

(e) Most serious sign: toxic epidermal necrolysis and desquamation of mucous membranes and skin

iii. Etiology

(a) *Mycoplasma pneumoniae*

(b) Side effect of some drugs, especially sulfonamides, NSAIDs, phenytoin, salicylates, pyrazolines, ibuprofen

iv. Laboratory findings

(a) Leukocytosis

(b) Elevated erythrocyte sedimentation rate (ESR)

(c) Elevated liver transaminase levels

(d) Decreased serum albumin

v. Treatment

(a) Topical anesthetics

(b) Cleans denuded skin lesions with saline or Burow's solution compresses

(c) Antibiotic therapy if secondary infections—not necessary as prophylactic

(d) May need to refer to pediatrician for admission to ICU

vi. Complications

(a) Superinfection of lesions

(b) Sepsis

ww. Telangiectasia—a permanent group of superficial, dilated capillaries

xx. Telangiectatic nevus

i. Flat, deep pink localized areas of capillary dilatation

ii. Occur predominantly on back of neck ("stork bite"), lower occiput, upper eyelids, upper lip, and bridge of nose

iii. Common condition of neonates

iv. Disappear by about 2 years of age

yy. Tinea capitis (ringworm of scalp) (Roberts & Friedlander, 2005)

i. Presentation

(a) Characterized by circular bald patches with slight erythema, scaling, and crusting

(b) Hair is thickened and broken off

(c) Pruritus is common

(d) May have a noninflammatory presentation with dandruff-like scale, minimal itching and little hair loss

ii. Etiology

(a) *Trichophyton tonsurans* (90%)

(b) *Microsporum canis* (10%)

iii. Diagnostic tests

(a) KOH wet mount examination of scrapings from moistened area of scalp

(b) Fungal culture of scrapings should always be done

iv. Treatment

(a) Medications—a systemic treatment is necessary to kill the organism (see Table 54-7 in Chapter 54)
  (1) Griseofulvin is the only FDA-approved oral treatment for tinea capitis
    a) Microsize or ultramicrosize preparations must be taken for 6 to 12 weeks
    b) Take with high-fat food such as whole milk or ice cream to enhance absorption
  (2) Several clinical trials show promising results with terbinafine, itraconazole, fluconazole, and oral antifungal agents (see Roberts & Friedlander [2005] article for details)
(b) Topical antifungal medications will not kill the organisms, but products such as selenium sulfide shampoo 1% or 2.5% (twice per week for 2 weeks) may reduce infectivity and decrease fungal shedding
(c) Frequent hair-washing is not typical of some cultural groups (ask how often child washes his/her hair) (Trowers, 2005)
  (1) Recommend the treatment shampoo once per week
  (2) Use Nizoral cream twice a week on the scalp
(d) Haircuts, shaving of head, or wearing a cap during treatment is *unnecessary*
(e) If no improvement after 2 weeks of therapy, consult physician
(f) Child may return to school if using topical treatment, e.g., selenium sulfide shampoo to decrease shedding
(g) Examine family siblings and educate family not to share combs, ribbons, etc.

**zz.** Tinea corporis (ringworm of the body and face)
  **i.** Circular, erythematous, well-demarcated with a raised scaly, vesicular border
  **ii.** Central area becomes hypopigmented and less scaly as the active border progresses outward
  **iii.** Pruritus is common
  **iv.** Occurs in all age-groups
  **v.** Etiology
    (a) *Trichophyton rubrum, Trichophyton mentagrophytes, Trichophyton tonsurans*
    (b) *Microsporum canis*
  **vi.** Diagnostic tests
    (a) KOH wet mount examination of scrapings from lesions
    (b) Fungal culture of scrapings
    (c) Wood's lamp is helpful but may not fluoresce with all tinea infections (Burns, et al, 2004, p. 999)
  **vii.** Treatment (see Table 54-7 in Chapter 54)
    (a) Topical antifungal cream gently rubbed into affected areas and surrounding skin once or twice daily or for 4 to 6 weeks
    (b) A minimum duration of treatment is 4 weeks even with earlier resolution
    (c) If lesions are extensive or unresponsive to topical therapy, griseofulvin is administered orally for 4 weeks (see Tinea capitis)

**aaa.** Tinea cruris (ringworm of the inguinal area)
  **i.** Presentation
    (a) Symmetric, sharply marginated red, raised, scaly patches; appearance of a ring

(b) Pruritic; may also blister and ooze

(c) In inguinal area and upper thighs

ii. Etiology

(a) *T. rubrum*

(b) *T. mentagrophytes*

(c) *Epidermophyton floccosum*

iii. Diagnostic tests—same as tinea corporis

iv. Treatment (see Table 54-7 in Chapter 54)

(a) Antifungals—same as tinea corporis

(b) Teach patient after bathing to dry groin before drying feet to avoid inoculating dermatophytes of tinea pedis into groin area

(c) If tinea pedis present, treat concurrently

(d) If unimproved after 2 weeks of therapy, consult physician

**bbb.** Tinea pedis (ringworm of the feet)

i. Pruritic vesicles on the instep of foot; fissures between toes

ii. Most commonly seen in postpubertal males

iii. In younger age-groups, rash is more likely due to contact dermatitis or atopic dermatitis than due to tinea pedis

iv. Etiology—same as tinea cruris

v. Diagnostic tests—same as tinea cruris

vi. Treatment (see Table 54-7 in Chapter 54)

(a) Same as tinea cruris

(b) If acute vesicular lesions are present, apply intermittent open wet compresses, e.g., with Burow's solution, 1:80

(c) If tinea cruris is present, treat concurrently

**ccc.** Tinea unguium (onychomycosis)

i. Yellow discoloration of one or two nails is the presenting sign

ii. Progresses to thickened distal nail plate and loosening of nail plate from nail bed

iii. Scaling and crumbly appearance of entire nail plate surface

iv. Etiology

(a) *T. rubrum*

(b) *T. mentagrophytes*

v. Differential diagnosis

(a) If all nails involved, consider psoriasis or lichen planus versus fungal infection

vi. Diagnostic tests—same as tinea corporis

vii. Treatment

(a) Topical antifungals are ineffective

(b) *No* oral therapies are approved for children

(c) Oral therapy for adolescents is rarely successful even after 6 to 12 months of treatment

(d) Consult physician regarding risks and benefits of treatment

**ddd.** Tinea versicolor (see section 4.kk)

**eee.** Urticaria

i. Presentation

(a) Well-circumscribed, localized or generalized erythematous raised wheals or welts of various sizes (often called "hives")

(b) Tend to appear quickly, spread irregularly, and fade within a few hours

(c) Intensely pruritic

ii. Etiology

(a) Common allergic skin disorder that may occur in response to:

(1) Foods—seafood, nuts, eggs, food additives

(2) Medications—penicillin, sulfa, aspirin

(3) Direct contact—plants

(4) Injected agents—medications, blood products, insect stings and bites (Elston, 2005)

(5) Infectious agents—virus (hepatitis, Epstein-Barr virus [EBV]), bacteria, fungus, parasite

(6) Physical factors—cold, pressure, sun exposure, water exposure

(7) Psychologic factors—stress, anxiety

(8) Systemic diseases—collagen-vascular, serum sickness, malignancy, hyperthyroidism, anaphylaxis

iii. Diagnostic tests may be done to identify suspected cause

(a) Throat culture

(b) Titers for hepatitis, EBV, etc.

(c) ANA, RF, ESR, CBC

(d) Thyroid studies

(e) Skin tests to confirm IgE mediated urticaria

iv. Treatment

(a) Remove or avoid known allergens

(b) Usually self-limiting and benign

(c) Oral antihistamines (see Table 54-4 in Chapter 54)

(d) Chronic urticaria recurs frequently or lasts longer than 6 weeks

(1) Combination $H_1$- (Benadryl & Atarax) and $H_2$-receptor antagonists (ranitidine, cimetidine)

(2) Corticosteroids (see Table 54-5 in Chapter 54)

(3) Referral to allergist or immunologists if underlying etiology not identified and persistent symptoms more than 6 weeks

v. Complications: airway compromise; a medical emergency

fff. Varicella (chickenpox)

i. Prodromal symptoms: 1 to 3 days of fever and respiratory symptoms

ii. Clinical phase

(a) Mild systemic symptoms

(b) Followed by rash

(1) Development of rash progresses from crop of red macules to papules and finally a vesicle that first becomes umbilicated and then forms a crust

(2) All four stages of lesions are seen at one time (macule, papule, vesicle, crust)

(3) Rash is highly pruritic

(4) Most lesions are found on trunk, may also involve face, scalp, palate, neck

(5) Appear in three separate series or crops, each moving through the three stages

iii. Etiology

(a) Exposure to varicella-zoster virus

(b) Transmission: highly contagious; spread by direct or indirect contact with fluid from saliva or vesicles

(c) Communicability: 1 day before rash to when all vesicles have crusted (about 5 to 6 days after their appearance)

(d) Incubation: 10 to 21 days

iv. Diagnosis

(a) Rash is distinctive

(b) Can be isolated from scrapings of a vesicle during first 3 to 4 days of therapy

(c) Direct fluorescent antibody test, enzyme immunoassay, latex agglutination test, indirect immunofluorescent antibody test, fluorescent antibody to membrane assay, complement fixation test, polymerase chain reaction assay

v. Treatment

(a) Symptomatic and supportive

(1) Hydration

(2) Acetaminophen

(3) Cool soaks or oral antipruritics for itching (see Table 54-4 in Chapter 54)

(b) Acyclovir (Zovirax)

(1) Not recommended for routine use in otherwise healthy children with varicella

(2) Administration within 24 hours of onset results in only modest decrease in symptoms

(3) Should be considered for otherwise healthy people at increased risk of moderate to severe varicella, e.g., more than 12 years of age, chronic cutaneous or pulmonary disorders, receiving long-term salicylate therapy, and those receiving short, intermittent, or aerosolized courses of corticosteroids

vi. Immunity

(a) Disease almost always results in lifelong immunity (95%)

(b) Virus remains latent in sensory ganglia and reappears as herpes zoster in 10% to 15% of individuals (increased rate in immunosuppressed individuals)

(c) Active artificial immunity obtained with attenuated live virus vaccine

(d) Passive artificial immunity obtained with varicella-zoster immune globulin (VZIG); may prevent or modify chickenpox in immunosuppressed children if given within 72 hours of exposure

vii. Complications: secondary bacterial infections (staphylococci or group A streptococci) presenting as impetigo, cellulitis, abscess, scarlet fever, sepsis, varicella pneumonia (immunocompromised, pregnant, or older and may be fatal)

ggg. Verruca (warts)

i. Types (Smolinski & Yan, 2005)

(a) Common warts—verruca vulgaris

(1) Flesh-colored scaly, keratotic papules from 1 to 10 mm in diameter

(2) Most common on hands and knees

(3) Asymptomatic

(b) Flat warts—verruca plana

(1) Flat, smooth, 1 to 5 mm in diameter

(2) Most common on face, hands, and shins

(3) Asymptomatic

(c) Palmoplantar warts—myrmecia (Cooper, 2005; Smolinski & Yan, 2005)

(1) Rough, scaly, hyperkeratotic plaques with tiny pinpoint petechiae centrally

          (2) Most common on weight-bearing areas of feet; may also be on palms and periungual areas

          (3) Painful when on weight-bearing surfaces

          (4) Difficult to differentiate from corns, calluses, foreign body, keratoses

      (d) Genital warts (Rakel, 2005) (see Chapter 31)

   ii. Etiology

      (a) Human papillomavirus (HPV)—more than 150 serotypes

   iii. Immunity: recurrences are reported in more than 30% of cases

   iv. Treatment

      (a) Most spontaneously resolve within several months to years

      (b) Emphasize that recurrence rate is about 30% despite treatment

      (c) First-line therapy

          (1) Active nonintervention

          (2) Salicylic acid (see Table 54-6 in Chapter 54)

          (3) Occlusion or adhesiotherapy—plain duct tape applied every morning and removed at night for 6 days per week for 2 months had success rate of 85% compared with 60% with cryotherapy (Norman & Wallace, 2005)

          (4) Heat

      (d) Second-line therapy

          (1) Cryotherapy with liquid nitrogen

          (2) Cantharidin, imiquimod, tretinoin, cimetidine (see Table 54-6 in Chapter 54)

      (e) Third-line therapy (requires referral to dermatology)

          (1) Podophyllin, 5-fluorouracil

          (2) Laser therapy surgical excision

          (3) Contact sensitization

          (4) Immunotherapy

## REFERENCES

Akita, H., & Anderson, R. R. (June, 2004). Laser treatments in dermatology, CME #119. Retrieved May 9, 2006, from www.hmpcommunications.com/sa/displayArticleaa.cfm?articleID=article2755.

American Academy of Pediatrics Committee on Infectious Diseases (2003). *Red book*. Elk Grove Village, IL: American Academy of Pediatrics.

Baldwin, H. E., & Berson, D. S. (2005). *New perspectives in the management of acne, photo damage, and wound healing*. Cherry Hill, NJ: Elsevier.

Burns, C. E., Dunn, A. M., Brady, M. A., et al. (2004). *Pediatric primary care – a handbook for nurse practitioners* (3rd ed.). Philadelphia: Elsevier.

Conologue, D., & Meffert, J. (2005). Dermatologic manifestations of neurologic disease. Retrieved on May 11, 2006 from http://www.emedicine.com/DERM/topic549.htm.

Cooper, J. S. (2005). Warts, plantar. Retrieved May 9, 2006, from www.emedicine.com/emerg/topic641.htm.

Crowe, M. A. (2005). Molluscum contagiosum. Retrieved on May 5, 2006 from http://www.emedicine.com/PED/topic1759.htm.

Darmstadt, G. L., & Sidbury, R. (2004). The skin. In R. E. Behrman, R. M. Kliegman, & H. B. Jenson (Eds.). *Nelson textbook of pediatrics* (17th ed.). Philadelphia: Saunders, pp. 2153-2250.

Dohil, M. A. (2005). Moles, skin care and sun safety. Presentation at the Pediatric Dermatology for the Practitioner meeting in San Diego, March 18-19, 2005. Reported by L. J. Chamberlain in *Infect Dis Child, 6,* 48-49.

Dohil, M. A., & Eichenfield, L. F. (2005). A treatment approach for atopic dermatitis. *Pediatr Ann, 34*(3), 201-210.

Eichenfield, L. F. (2004). Consensus guidelines in diagnosis and treatment of atopic dermatitis. *Allergy, 59*(Suppl 78), 86-92.

Eichenfield, L., Honig, P. J., Harper, J., & Bikowski, J. B. (2004). Advances in the treatment of teenage acne. *Infect Dis Child, 9*(Suppl.), 4-13.

Elston, D. M. (2005). Bites and stings: Be ready to respond quickly. *Clin Adv,* July 20, 24-32.

Frankowski, B. L., & Weiner, L. B. (2002). Head lice: American Academy of Pediatrics Clinical Report. *Pediatrics, 110,* 638-643.

Gold, B., & Saavedra, J. (2004). Allergies are on the rise; focus on prevention. Reported by L. Riley in *Infect Dis Child,* November, 53.

Goldsmith, L. A., Lazarus, G. S., & Tharp, M. D. (1997). *Adult and pediatric dermatology: A color guide to diagnosis and treatment.* Philadelphia: F. A. Davis. [Editor's note: This classic text has not been revised, but serves as an excellent resource for photographs and basic descriptions of lesions and photographs.]

Hansen, R. C. (2004). Atopic dermatitis: Taming the "itch that rashes." *Contemp Pediatr Online.* July. Retrieved on May 9, 2006 from http://contpeds.adv100.com/contpeds/article/articleDetail.jsp?id=111753.

Levy, S. B. (2005). Sunscreens and photoprotection. Retrieved May 9, 2006, from www.emedicine.com/derm/topic510.htm.

Lutwick, L. I., & Seenivasan, M. (2005). Herpes simplex. Retrieved May 9, 2006, from www.emedicine.com/med/topic1006.htm.

Miller, T., & Frieden, I. J. (2005). Hemangiomas: New insights and classifications. *Pediatr Ann, 34*(3), 179-187.

Norman, R., & Wallace, K. (2005). A quick guide to five common skin diseases. *Clin Adv,* March, 24-30.

Opinion Research Corporation. (2005). TEEN CARAVAN® survey conducted in collaboration with the American Academy of Dermatology. *Infect Dis Child,* June, p. 50.

Paller, A. S., Nimmagadda, S., Schachner, L., et al. (2005). Fluocinolone acetonide 0.01% in peanut oil: therapy for childhood atopic dermatitis, even in patients who are peanut sensitive. *J Am Acad Dermatol, 48*(4), 569-577.

Pannaraj, P. S., Turner, C. L., Bastian, J. F., & Burns, J. C. (2004). Failure to diagnose Kawasaki disease at the extremes of the pediatric age range. *Pediatr Infect Dis J, 23*(8), 789-791.

Parish, T. G. (2004). Inflammatory acne: Management in primary care. *Clin Rev, 14*(7), 40-45.

Rakel, R. E., Ault, K. A., Bocchini, J. A., Jr., et al. (2005). Combating human papillomavirus infection: Update on treatment and prevention. *Consultant, 45*(3), S5-S29.

Roberts, B. J., & Friedlander, S. F. (2005). Tinea capitis: A treatment update. *Pediatr Ann, 34*(3), 191-200.

Roberts, G., & Lack, G. (2005). Diagnosing peanut allergy with skin prick and specific IgE testing. *J Allergy Clin Immunol, 115*(6), 1291-1296.

Paller, A. S. (2005). New tools for managing pediatric psoriasis. Reported by M. Rosenthal in *Infect Dis Child,* April, 36, 39.

Schwartz, M. W. (Ed.). (2003). *The 5 minute pediatric consult.* Philadelphia: Lippincott Williams & Wilkins.

Shwayder, T. (2003). Five common skin problems—and a string of pearls for managing them. *Contemp Pediatr, Online,* July. Retrieved on May 11, 2006 from, http://www.contemporarypediatrics.com/contpeds/article/articleDetail.jsp?id=111757.

Smolinski, K. N., & Yan, A. C. (2005). How and when to treat molluscum contagiosum and warts in children. *Pediatr Ann, 34*(3), 211-221.

Tharp, M. D. (2005). Atopic dermatitis today: A brief overview. *Pediatr News* (Suppl), 4-5.

Thiem, L. J. (2005). Body piercing: Clinical considerations. *Clin Rev, 15*(1), 30-35.

Trowers, A. (2005). Ethnicity in pediatric dermatology. Reported by M. Rosenthal in *Infect Dis Child,* April, 42-43.

Vernon, P. (2003). Acne vulgaris: Current treatment approaches. *Adv Nurse Pract, 11*(2), 59-62.

Zane, L. T. (2003). Tips to boost adherence to acne treatment. Reported by R. Finn in *Pediatr News,* September, 46.

# Common Illness of the Hematologic and Lymphatic Systems

SHEILA JUDGE SANTACROCE, PhD, APRN, CPNP

1. Symptoms: pallor, fatigue, light-headedness, dyspnea on exertion, irritability
   a. Focused history
      i. Family history
         (a) Hematologic disorders
             (1) Anemia
             (2) Thalassemia
             (3) Others
         (b) Ethnicity and racial group—Mediterranean, Southeast Asian, Black
      ii. Child's history
         (a) Prematurity
         (b) Hyperbilirubinemia
         (c) Acute or chronic infections
         (d) Recent illnesses
         (e) Medications
             (1) OTC
             (2) Prescription, e.g., trimethoprim-sulfamethoxazole
             (3) Herbs; alternative or complementary treatments
         (f) Injury
             (1) Physical trauma
             (2) Loss of blood
         (g) Behavioral changes
             (1) Decreased attention span
             (2) Pica (eating nonfood substances such as dirt)
         (h) Dietary patterns
             (1) Recent changes
             (2) Anorexia
             (3) Consumption of large amounts of cow's milk
             (4) Iron-poor diet
             (5) Pica
         (i) Gastrointestinal patterns
             (1) Constipation
             (2) Diarrhea
             (3) Abdominal pain
             (4) Old blood in stools (tarry)
             (5) Emesis (coffee grounds)

(j) Heavy menstruation
(k) Environment—child's home, school, daycare
    (1) Estimated age of building
    (2) Location
    (3) Condition
    (4) Recent renovations
    (5) Exposures
        a) Inhaled
        b) Ingested
        c) Puncture (ask about footwear when outside)
(l) Travel
    (1) To other states or countries
    (2) Exposure to individuals from other states or countries

**b.** Focused physical examination (Bickley & Szilagyi, 2004) (see also Chapter 11)
  **i.** Inspection
    (a) Evaluate weight and linear growth; determine percentiles
    (b) Apparent nutritional status
    (c) Assess the skin
        (1) Pallor
        (2) Jaundice
    (d) Inspect eyes
        (1) Blue sclera
        (2) Icteric sclera
    (e) Mental status
        (1) Attention span
        (2) Alertness
        (3) Cooperation
  **ii.** Auscultation
    (a) Heart
        (1) Tachycardia
        (2) Systolic murmur
  **iii.** Palpation
    (a) Abdomen
    (b) Spleen

**c.** Laboratory tests (Carley, 2003b; Corbett, 2004; Hermiston & Mentzer, 2002)
  **i.** Screening recommendations for anemia in children (AAP, 2000)
    (a) Hemoglobin and hematocrit at 6-, 9-, and 12-month visit for *all* infants
  **ii.** See Table 33-1 for age-specific blood test standards (Irwin & Kirschner, 2001)
  **iii.** CBC with differential
    (a) Hemoglobin
    (b) Hematocrit
    (c) Red blood cell (RBC) count
    (d) White blood cell (WBC) count
    (e) Peripheral smear
        (1) Color—hypochromic, hyperchromic
        (2) Size—microcytosis, macrocytosis, megaloblasts
        (3) Age—nucleated
        (4) Shape—sickled, Heinz bodies, poikilocytosis
    (f) Reticulocytes—immature RBCs
    (g) Mean corpuscular volume (MCV) indicates RBC size; microcytic, macrocytic, megaloblastic

**TABLE 33-1**
**Age-Specific Blood Test Standards**

| Coagulation tests | Preterm infant 30-36 wk, day of life #1 | Term infant, day of life #1 | 1-5yr | 6-10yr | 11-16yr | Adult |
|---|---|---|---|---|---|---|
| PT (sec) | 15.4 (14.6-16.9) | 13.0 (10.1-15.9) | 11 (10.6-11.4) | 11.1(10.1-12.1) | 11.2 (10.2-12.0) | 12 (11.0-14.0) |
| INR | — | — | 1.0 (0.96-1.04) | 1.0 (0.91-1.11) | 1.02 (0.93-1.10) | 1.10 (1.0-1.3) |
| aPTT (sec) | 108 (80-168) | 42.9 (31.3-54.3) | 30 (24-36) | 31 (26-36) | 32 (26-37) | 33 (27-40) |
| Fibrinogen (g/L) | 2.43 (1.50-3.73) | 2.83 (1.67-3.09) | 2.76 (1.70-4.05) | 2.79 (1.57-4.0) | 3.0 (1.54-4.48) | 2.78 (1.56-4.0) |
| Bleeding time (min) | — | — | 6 (2.5-10) | 7 (2.5-13) | 5 (3-8) | 4 (1-7) |
| Thrombin time (sec) | 14 (11-17) | 12 (10-16) | — | — | — | 10 |
| II (U/mL) | 0.45 (0.20-0.77) | 0.48 (0.26-0.70) | 0.94 (0.71-1.16) | 0.88 (0.67-1.07) | 0.83 (0.61-1.04) | 1.08 (0.70-1.46) |
| V (U/mL) | 0.88 (0.41-1.44) | 0.72 (0.43-1.08) | 1.03 (0.79-1.27) | 0.90 (0.63-1.16) | 0.77 (0.55-0.99) | 1.06 (0.62-1.50) |
| VII (U/mL) | 0.67 (0.21-1.13) | 0.66 (0.28-1.04) | 0.82 (0.55-1.16) | 0.85 (0.52-1.20) | 0.83 (0.58-1.15) | 1.05 (0.67-1.43) |
| VIII (U/mL) | 1.11 (0.50-2.13) | 1.00 (0.50-1.78) | 0.90 (0.59-1.42) | 0.95 (0.58-1.32) | 0.92 (0.53-1.31) | 0.99 (0.50-1.49) |
| vWF (U/mL) | 1.36 (0.78-2.10) | 1.53 (0.50-2.87) | 0.82 (0.47-1.04) | 0.95 (0.44-1.44) | 1.00 (0.46-1.53) | 0.92 (0.50-1.58) |
| IX (U/mL) | 0.35 (0.19-0.65) | 0.53 (0.15-0.91) | 0.73 (0.47-1.04) | 0.75 (0.63-0.89) | 0.87 (0.59-1.22) | 1.09 (0.55-1.63) |
| X (U/mL) | 0.41 (0.11-0.71) | 0.40 (0.12-0.68) | 0.88 (0.58-1.16) | 0.75 (0.55-1.01) | 0.79 (0.50-1.17) | 1.06 (0.70-1.52) |
| XI (U/mL) | 0.30 (0.08-0.52) | 0.38 (0.10-0.66) | 0.97 (0.56-1.50) | 0.86 (0.52-1.20) | 0.74 (0.50-0.97) | 0.97 (0.67-1.27) |
| XII (U/mL) | 0.38 (0.10-0.66) | 0.53 (0.13-0.93) | 0.93 (0.64-1.29) | 0.92 (0.60-1.40) | 0.81 (0.34-1.37) | 1.08 (0.52-1.64) |
| PK (U/mL) | 0.33 (0.09-0.57) | 0.37 (0.18-0.69) | 0.95 (0.65-1.30) | 0.99 (0.66-1.31) | 0.99 (0.53-1.45) | 1.12 (0.62-1.62) |
| HMWK (U/mL) | 0.49 (0.09-0.89) | 0.54 (0.06-1.02) | 0.98 (0.64-1.32) | 0.93 (0.60-1.30) | 0.91 (0.63-1.19) | 0.92 (0.50-1.36) |
| XIIIa (U/mL) | 0.70 (0.32-1.08) | 0.79 (0.27-1.31) | 1.08 (0.72-1.43) | 1.09 (0.65-1.51) | 0.99 (0.57-1.40) | 1.05 (0.55-1.55) |
| XIIIs (U/mL) | 0.81 (0.35-1.27) | 0.76 (0.30-1.22) | 1.13 (0.69-1.56) | 1.16 (0.77-1.54) | 1.02 (0.60-1.43) | 0.97 (0.57-1.37) |
| d-Dimer | — | — | — | — | — | Positive titer = 1:8 |
| FDPs | — | — | — | — | — | Borderline titer = 1:25<br>Positive titer = 1:50 |

**Coagulation inhibitors**

| | | | | | |
|---|---|---|---|---|---|
| ATIII (U/mL) | 0.38 (0.14–0.62) | 0.63 (0.39–0.97) | 1.11 (0.82–1.39) | 1.11 (0.90–1.31) | 1.05 (0.77–1.32) | 1.0 (0.74–1.26) |
| $\alpha_2$-M (U/mL) | 1.10 (0.56–1.82) | 1.39 (0.95–1.83) | 1.69 (1.14–2.23) | 1.69 (1.28–2.09) | 1.56 (0.98–2.12) | 0.86 (0.52–1.20) |
| $C_1$-Inh (U/mL) | 0.65 (0.31–0.99) | 0.72 (0.36–1.08) | 1.35 (0.85–1.83) | 1.14 (0.88–1.54) | 1.03 (0.68–1.50) | 1.0 (0.71–1.31) |
| $\alpha_2$-AT (U/mL) | 0.90 (0.36–1.44) | 0.93 (0.49–1.37) | 0.93 (0.39–1.47) | 1.00 (0.69–1.30) | 1.01 (0.65–1.37) | 0.93 (0.55–1.30) |
| Protein C (U/mL) | 0.28 (0.12–0.44) | 0.35 (0.17–0.53) | 0.66 (0.40–0.92) | 0.69 (0.45–0.93) | 0.83 (0.55–1.11) | 0.96 (0.64–1.28) |
| Protein S total (U/mL) | 0.26 (0.14–0.38) | 0.36 (0.12–0.60) | 0.86 (0.54–1.18) | 0.78 (0.41–1.14) | 0.72 (0.52–0.92) | 0.81 (0.60–1.13) |

**Fibrinolytic system**

| | | | | | |
|---|---|---|---|---|---|
| Plasminogen (U/mL) | 1.70 (1.12–2.48) | 1.95 (+/−0.35) | 0.98 (0.78–1.18) | 0.92 (0.75–1.08) | 0.86 (0.68–1.03) | 0.99 (0.7–1.22) |
| TPA (ng/mL) | — | — | 2.15 (1.0–4.5) | 2.42 (1.0–5.0) | 2.16 (1.0–4.0) | 4.90 (1.40–8.40) |
| $\alpha_2$-AP (U/mL) | 0.78 (0.4–1.16) | 0.85 (+/−0.15) | 1.05 (0.93–1.17) | 0.99 (0.89–1.10) | 0.98 (0.78–1.18) | 1.02 (0.68–1.36) |
| PAI (U/mL) | — | — | 5.42 (1.0–10.0) | 6.79 (2.0–12.0) | 6.07 (2.0–10.0) | 3.60 (0–11.0) |

Data from Andrew[9,11]

HMWK, high-molecular-weight kininogen; PK, prekallikrein; VIII, factor VIII procoagulant.

$\alpha_2$-AP, $\alpha_2$-antiplasmin; $\alpha_2$-AT, $\alpha_2$-antitrypsin; $\alpha_2$-M, $\alpha_2$-macroglobulin; ATIII, antithrombin III; PAI, plasminogen activator inhibitor; TPA, total plasminogen activator.

Reprinted with permission from Siberry, G.K., Iannone, R. (2000). *The Harriet Lane handbook: A manual for pediatric house officers* (15th ed.). St. Louis: Mosby, Table 15.10.

     **iv.** Coombs' test—detects the presence of antibody and potential immune etiology

     **v.** Hemoglobin electrophoresis—analyzes globin chains that are components of hemoglobin, e.g., $\alpha$- or $\beta$-thalassemia

     **vi.** Serum ferritin levels—indicate iron storage

     **vii.** Serum lead levels

     **viii.** Serum $B_{12}$ and folate levels

     **ix.** Stool

        (a) Test for frank and occult blood

        (b) Parasites

     **x.** Urine—test for RBCs

     **xi.** Bone marrow biopsy (by oncology specialists)

**d.** Normal physiology of RBC development and pathophysiology of anemia (Carley, 2003b)

     **i.** Major role of RBC is to carry oxygen to the tissues

     **ii.** Kidneys produce and release erythropoietin in response to low oxygen levels

     **iii.** Erythropoietin stimulates RBC precursors in the bone marrow to mature

     **iv.** RBCs live about 120 days

        (a) Normally destroyed in spleen

        (b) Heme and globulin components of hemoglobin are reused

        (c) Abnormally shaped RBC are destroyed more quickly

     **v.** Anemia definition—imbalance between RBC production and RBC destruction

**e.** Prevalence of anemia (Irwin & Kirchner, 2001)

     **i.** Before age 18 years, 20% of children in the United States become anemic

     **ii.** Up to 80% of children in developing countries will become anemic

**f.** Differential diagnoses for anemia—two methods (Carley, 2003b)

     **i.** Diagnosis based on RBC characteristics (Table 33-2)

        (a) RBC mass, amount of hemoglobin, and/or volume of packed RBCs less than normal

        (b) Hematocrit or hemoglobin concentration greater than 2 standard deviations (SDs) below the normal mean for age

     **ii.** Diagnosis based on suspected etiology (Box 33-1)

        (a) Blood loss → loss of RBC volume

        (b) RBC hemolysis → premature loss of RBC from circulation

        (c) RBC underproduction → lack of stimulation of RBC production or lack of RBC precursors

**g.** Transient erythroblastopenia of childhood (Huang & Miller, 2003)

     **i.** Signs and symptoms

        (a) A gradual onset of pallor in skin and mucosa

        (b) Usually no other symptoms

        (c) May have fatigue, low energy

        (d) Physical examination usually normal

        (e) May have tachycardia, cardiac flow murmur

     **ii.** Etiology

        (a) Etiology is unknown

        (b) May be viral or immunologic

        (c) Not a lack of erythropoietin

        (d) Bone marrow shows absence of RBC precursors

     **iii.** Prevalence

        (a) Unknown prevalence

■ **TABLE 33-2**
■  ■ **Differential Diagnosis for Anemia Based on Laboratory Values**

| Laboratory values | Potential Diagnosis or Mechanism |
| --- | --- |
| **Peripheral Smear** | |
| Hypochromia and microcytosis | Chronic blood loss and iron depletion |
| Numerous nucleated RBC | Active hematopoiesis due to hemolysis |
| Abnormal cell forms | |
|   Howell-Jolly bodies, sickling | Sickle cell anemia |
|   Heinz bodies | G6PD deficiency |
| **Reticulocyte (Retic) Count** | |
| Elevated retic count | Active hematopoiesis due to hemolysis |
| | Acute blood loss, hemorrhage |
| Low retic count | Underproduction or release of RBC |
| **MCV** | |
| Low MCV—microcytic | Iron deficiency anemia |
| | $\beta$-Thalassemia trait |
| | Lead poisoning |
| | Anemia from chronic illness |
| | Sideroblastic anemia (rare) |
| High MCV | |
| Macrocytic | Vitamin $B_{12}$ deficiency |
| | Folic acid deficiency |
| Megaloblasts | Chemotherapy |
| **Normal MCV + Normal Retics** | Chronic inflammation |
| **Normal MCV + Low Retics** | Bone marrow failure |
| | Red cell aplasia |
| | Aplastic anemia |
| | Erythropoietin deficiency |
| **Normal MCV + High Retics** | Acute blood loss, hemorrhage |
| | Rapid RBC loss, hemolysis |
| **High MCV + Low Retics** | Hereditary hyporegenerative anemias |
| | Drug suppression (chemotherapy) |
| | Vitamin $B_{12}$ deficiency (pernicious anemia) |
| | Folic acid deficiency |
| | Inborn errors of metabolism |
| | Chronic liver disease |
| | Hypothyroidism |
| | Myelodysplasia |
| **Low MCV + High Retics** | $\beta$-Thalassemia |
| **Low MCV + Low Retics** | Iron deficiency anemia |
| | Lead poisoning |
| **Coombs' Test—Positive** | Rh incompatibility |
| **Serum Ferritin Level** | |
| Normal ferritin | Thalassemia |
| | Transient erythroblastopenia of childhood |
| Low ferritin | Iron deficiency anemia |
| High ferritin | Anemia of inflammation |
| Normal to high ferritin | Lead poisoning |
| **Serum Lead Level** | |
| High lead level | Lead poisoning |

From Carley, A. (2003b). Anemia: When is it not iron deficiency? *Pediatr Nurs, 29*(3), 205–211.

■ **BOX 33-1**
■ **DIFFERENTIAL DIAGNOSIS OF ANEMIA BASED ON SUSPECTED ETIOLOGY**

**BLOOD LOSS**
Perinatal
- Abruptio placentae
- Placenta abnormalities
- Umbilical cord accidents

Neonatal
- Ruptured liver or spleen
- Intracranial bleeding
- Hematomas
- Excess blood sampling for testing

Infants
- Excess whole milk consumption

Children, adolescents, and young adults
- Hookworm
- Heavy menstruation
- GI ulcer or diverticulum

**RBC HEMOLYSIS**
Perinatal
- Intrauterine infection

Neonatal
- Rh, ABO incompatibility
- Hyperbilirubinemia

Infant and child
- Hereditary spherocytosis
- G6PD deficiency
- α- or β-thalassemia

**RBC UNDERPRODUCTION**
- Anemia of prematurity
- Congenital bone marrow failure (rare)
- Breast-fed infants of strict vegan mothers or mothers with pernicious anemia
- Acute lymphoblastic leukemia
- Anemia of inflammation
- Transient erythroblastopenia of childhood
- Iron deficiency
- Lead poisoning
- Folic acid, vitamin $B_{12}$ deficiency

From Carley, A. (2003b). Anemia: When is it not iron deficiency? *Pediatr Nurs, 29*(3), 205–211.

  (b) Males more than females, 1.4 : 1
  (c) Median age of 18 to 26 months
 iv. Laboratory findings
  (a) Peripheral smear—normochromic normocytic
  (b) MCV
   (1) Usually normal on diagnosis
   (2) May increase on recovery due to reticulocytosis
  (c) Hemoglobin is usually 5 to 7 g/dL but may be as low as 2 g/dL
  (d) Neutropenia may be as high as 64%
  (e) Reticulocyte count
   (1) Less than 0.1% at diagnosis
   (2) Spontaneous increase indicates the recovery phase
  (f) Serum iron
   (1) No indication of iron deficiency
   (2) May be elevated because of underuse of iron stores
  v. Treatment
  (a) Typically resolves spontaneously within 1 to 2 months, but may take a year
  (b) If severe anemia is symptomatic, packed RBCs may be necessary
  (c) Iron supplements are not indicated and will have no effect on the anemia
 vi. Follow-up
  (a) Frequent examinations and CBC and checks are critical to detect significant drops in hemoglobin and to rule out other more serious diagnoses, e.g.:
   (1) Diamond-Blackfan anemia

   (2) Aplastic anemia

   (3) Drug-induced anemia

   (4) Leukemia

   (5) Hemolytic anemia

**h.** Iron deficiency anemia due to insufficient dietary iron (see also Chapter 16)

 **i.** Definition and prevalence (Carley, 2003a, 2003b; Glader, 2004; Tender & Cheng, 2002)

  (a) Iron deficiency—insufficient iron stores for growth

   (1) Affects 9% of children younger than 2 years of age

   (2) 9% to 11% of adolescent females

   (3) Less than 1% of adolescent boys

  (b) Iron deficiency anemia—anemia due to insufficient iron for RBC formation

   (1) Affects 3% of children younger than 2 years of age

   (2) Up to 3% of adolescent females

   (3) Less than 1% of adolescent males

 **ii.** Pathophysiology

  (a) In first months of life

   (1) Most of a newborn's iron is in circulating hemoglobin

   (2) Hemoglobin reduced

   (3) Iron reclaimed and stored in liver, spleen, and bone marrow

    a) Iron stores support erythropoiesis for the first 6 to 9 months

     i) Fewer iron stores with prematurity and low birth weight

     ii) Fewer iron stores with perinatal blood loss

  (b) 3 phases

   (1) Iron depletion—iron stores in bone marrow decrease; asymptomatic

   (2) Iron deficiency

    a) Inadequate *dietary* iron causes further depletion of iron stores

    b) Hemoglobin synthesis is affected

    c) Asymptomatic

   (3) Iron deficiency anemia

    a) Insufficient iron stores for hemoglobin synthesis

    b) Evidenced by low hemoglobin and low hematocrit (H&H)

    c) NOTE—unless H&H screening is done routinely or on suspicion of anemia, the iron stores became significantly depleted

     i) Impaired RBC production

     ii) Impaired hemoglobin transport

 **iii.** Etiology

  (a) Most common in children ages 9 to 24 months who consume:

   (1) Large amounts of cow's milk

   (2) Foods lacking iron

  (b) Adolescents are especially prone to iron deficiency anemia because of:

   (1) Poor nutritional choices

   (2) Growth spurts

   (3) Menstrual blood loss

 **iv.** Treatment

  (a) Children with very severe anemia should be referred to hematology or oncology specialist

  (b) Oral administration of iron

   (1) Daily total of 6 mg/kg of elemental iron in three divided doses or daily doses

   (2) Administer with vitamin C product to enhance absorption

        (3) Do not administer with meals or with dairy products because calcium inhibits absorption

        (4) Side effects and recommendations

          a) Unpleasant taste—try once-daily dosing

          b) Stains teeth

            i) Administer in back of mouth for infants

            ii) Use a straw for older children

            iii) Wipe teeth after dosing

    (c) Limit intake of cow's milk

    (d) Increase intake of dietary sources of iron

    (e) Educate parents about iron-rich foods (Box 33-2)

  **v.** Follow-up

    (a) Expected course if anemia is due to iron deficiency

      (1) RBC count increases within 3 to 10 days

      (2) Reticulocyte count increases within in 3 to 4 days

      (3) Hemoglobin values increase within 2 to 4 weeks

    (b) Continue oral iron therapy

      (1) Continue for 8 weeks after blood values return to normal for age

      (2) Not more than 6 months

    (c) Lack of expected response can be due to:

      (1) Poor adherence to oral iron therapy

      (2) Poor absorption

      (3) Incorrect diagnosis

  **vi.** Prognosis

    (a) Excellent

**i.** Lead poisoning (see Chapter 19, section 7.n.iii and Chapter 22, section 4.i. for detailed information on lead poisoning)

**j.** Iron deficiency anemia due to lead toxicity

---

■ **BOX 33-2**
■ **SOURCES OF DIETARY IRON**

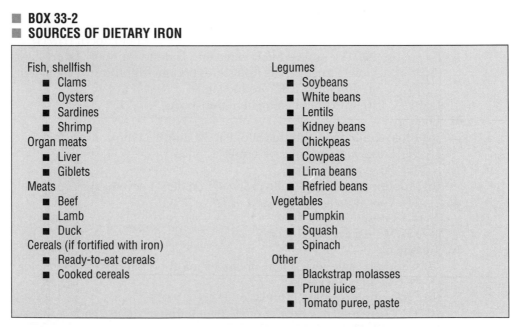

Fish, shellfish
- Clams
- Oysters
- Sardines
- Shrimp

Organ meats
- Liver
- Giblets

Meats
- Beef
- Lamb
- Duck

Cereals (if fortified with iron)
- Ready-to-eat cereals
- Cooked cereals

Legumes
- Soybeans
- White beans
- Lentils
- Kidney beans
- Chickpeas
- Cowpeas
- Lima beans
- Refried beans

Vegetables
- Pumpkin
- Squash
- Spinach

Other
- Blackstrap molasses
- Prune juice
- Tomato puree, paste

From Health and Human Services (HHS) and U. S. Department of Agriculture (USDA).(2005). *Dietary guidelines for Americans 2005*. Washington, DC: Government Printing Office. [Appendix B-3.]

    **i.** Signs and symptoms
      (a) Often there are no symptoms
      (b) Listlessness
      (c) Loss of appetite
      (d) Irritability
      (e) Problems with coordination, balance
      (f) Behavioral changes
      (g) Developmental delays
      (h) Growth delays
    **ii.** Pathophysiology (Habal, 2004; Marcus, 2005)
      (a) 99% of absorbed lead binds to erythrocytes
        (1) Interferes with critical phases of heme synthesis
        (2) Heme is essential for oxygenation of cells
        (3) Decreased heme production results in anemia
      (b) 1% of absorbed lead is deposited in soft tissues (brain) and rapidly growing bone
      (c) Diets low in calcium and high in fat increase GI lead absorption
    **iii.** Etiology and prevalence (see Chapter 22)
    **iv.** Laboratory findings, treatment, follow-up and prognosis (see Chapter 22)
**k.** Iron deficiency anemia due to hookworm infestation (American Academy of Pediatrics, 2003; Tam & Hexdall, 2006)
    **i.** Signs and symptoms
      (a) Early stages
        (1) Usually asymptomatic
        (2) "Ground itch"—itchy papules where infestation occurred
        (3) Low-grade fever
        (4) Mild cough, wheeze
      (b) Later stages
        (1) GI discomfort
        (2) Fatigue
        (3) Dyspnea
        (4) Pallor
        (5) Tachycardia
    **ii.** Pathophysiology
      (a) Hookworms are small off-white parasites
      (b) Eggs release larvae in fecal-contaminated soil within 24 hours
      (c) Larvae then molt to form infective filariform larvae within 24 hours
      (d) Filariform larvae penetrate the skin and enter bloodstream
      (e) Larvae lodge in pulmonary capillaries
      (f) After 3 to 4 days larvae travel into bronchi, trachea, and pharynx
      (g) Larvae are swallowed and attach themselves to intestinal wall
      (h) Survive on blood from the intestinal wall
      (i) Loss of blood leads to anemia
      (j) Eggs appear in stool after 4 to 6 weeks
    **iii.** Etiology and prevalence
      (a) Two types of hookworm
        (1) *Ancylostoma duodenale*—life span is up to 1 year
        (2) *Necator americanus*—life span is up to 5 years
      (b) Hookworm is endemic in tropical areas of the developing world
        (1) Sanitation is poor
        (2) Water and soil are contaminated with human feces
        (3) Exposure is primarily from walking barefoot on contaminated soil

          (4) Immigration from tropical countries is increasing the incidence of hookworm in the United States

    iv. Diagnostic tests

        (a) Stool examination for ova and parasites

    v. Treatment

        (a) Anthelmintics (see Table 54-13 in Chapter 54)

        (b) Iron supplementation for correction of the anemia (see section 1.h. above)

    vi. Prognosis—excellent with proper treatment

l. Pernicious anemia (Conrad, 2005; McCance & Huether, 2006)

    i. Signs and symptoms

        (a) Usually discovered as a result of lab tests for other conditions

        (b) Slow and insidious onset

        (c) May have anorexia and weight loss

        (d) White patients often have a lemon yellow waxy pallor with premature whitening of the hair

        (e) Appear flabby, with a bulky frame

        (f) Hematocrit of about 15% is often well tolerated by patients

        (g) Beefy red, sore tongue with loss of papillae and taste

        (h) Neurologic symptoms—paresthesia, unsteady gait

        (i) Tachycardia

    ii. Pathophysiology

        (a) Vitamin $B_{12}$ is obtained primarily from dietary meat and milk

        (b) Intrinsic factor (IF) in gastric secretions is necessary to absorb vitamin $B_{12}$

        (c) Vitamin $B_{12}$ (cobalamin) is necessary for erythropoiesis

        (d) $B_{12}$ deficiency causes abnormalities in deoxyribonucleic acid (DNA) and ribonucleic acid (RNA) of the erythroblasts

        (e) RBC destruction is the cause of anemia

    iii. Etiology

        (a) Acquired

           (1) Inadequate intake of vitamin $B_{12}$

           (2) Inadequate absorption of vitamin $B_{12}$

        (b) Congenital

           (1) Probably autoimmune and some genetic predisposition for deficiency of IF in gastric secretions

    iv. Prevalence

        (a) Usually occurs in adults older than age 40, but can occur in younger people

        (b) Occurs in all racial and ethnic groups

        (c) Higher in Celtic or Scandinavian groups

        (d) 10 to 20 cases per 100,000 people occur per year in these groups

    v. Laboratory findings

        (a) Macrocytic, normochromic RBC

        (b) Poikilocytosis—abnormally shaped RBCs

        (c) Normal hemoglobin levels

    vi. Treatment

        (a) Refer to hematology specialist

        (b) May receive loading IV doses of vitamin $B_{12}$

        (c) Followed by supplementary vitamin $B_{12}$ therapy—oral tablet of 100 to 200 mcg taken weekly

1. Hemolytic anemias
   i. Neonatal
      (a) Hemolytic disease of the newborn (Wagle & Deshpande, 2003)
         (1) Etiology
            a) Rh-positive fetus of an Rh-negative mother (more common in whites [15%] than in blacks [5%]; rare in Asians)
            b) Type A or B fetus of a Type O mother
            c) Kell system antibodies
         (2) Pathophysiology
            a) Maternal response to the foreign antigens results in production of antibodies of the IgG isotype that cross the placental barrier
            b) Antibodies attach to the fetal RBCs
            c) Lysosomal enzymes released by macrophages and natural killer lymphocytes cause hemolysis of fetal RBCs
         (3) Signs
            a) Jaundice appears in the first 24 hours after birth
            b) Rapid increase in unconjugated bilirubin level
            c) Anemia due to destruction of antibody-coated RBCs by the reticuloendothelial system
            d) Intravascular destruction may occur in some infants
         (4) Treatment and Prognosis
            a) Mild hemolytic disease (50% of cases)
               i) Usually have no anemia, minimal hemolysis
               ii) Treat with early phototherapy
               iii) At risk for development of severe late hyporegenerative anemia of infancy and low reticulocyte count at age 3-6 weeks
               iv) Monitor hemoglobin levels frequently after hospital discharge
            b) Moderate hemolytic disease (25% of cases)
               i) Often have hepatosplenomegaly
               ii) At risk of developing bilirubin encephalopathy if not treated early
               iii) Treat with exchange transfusion with type-O Rh-negative fresh RBCs
               iv) Intensive phototherapy usually required
               v) At risk of developing late hyporegenerative anemia of infancy at age 6 weeks
      (b) Hyperbilirubinemia (see Chapter 18)
   ii. Infant and child
      (a) Refer to pediatric hematology immediately
         (1) Hereditary spherocytosis
         (2) G6PD deficiency
         (3) α- or β-thalassemias (see Chapter 47)
2. Symptoms: excessive or unusual bruising and bleeding
   a. Focused history
      i. Family history
         (a) Bleeding disorders
      ii. Child's history
         (a) Previous history of unusual bleeding
            (1) Cord separation
            (2) Circumcision
            (3) Immunization sites

    (4) Shedding of teeth

    (5) Minor falls

    (6) Surgery

   (b) Symptom assessment

    (1) Location

     a) Mucosal

      i) Epistaxis

      ii) Menstrual

     b) Tissues

     c) Joints

    (2) Onset

     a) Spontaneous

     b) After injury

    (3) Duration

   (c) Detailed drug use history

   (d) Use of herbs or complementary therapies

 **b.** Focused physical examination (see also Chapter 11)

  **i.** Inspect

   (a) Skin

    (1) Purpura

     a) Platelet disorder

     b) Vasculitis

    (2) Bruises can indicate a factor deficiency

     a) Nodular centers present

     b) Hematoma

     c) Poorly healed scars

   (b) Mucosa—nose, throat, vaginal

   (c) Joints

  **ii.** Palpate

   (a) Lymph nodes for enlargement

   (b) Abdomen for hepatosplenomegaly

   (c) Joints

 **c.** Normal physiology

  **i.** Platelets (thrombocytes) (see Chapter 11)

   (a) One third of total platelets are in the spleen

  **ii.** Platelets control bleeding after a vessel wall injury by:

   (a) Adhering to the endothelium to form a plug

   (b) Releasing substances that attract other platelets to the site

   (c) Releasing serotonin, which causes vasoconstriction

  **iii.** Coagulation factors on platelet surface are activated by hormones to form a fibrin clot through a coagulation cascade (American Association of Clinical Chemistry, 2004; King, 2005)

 **d.** Differential diagnoses (Montgomery & Scott, 2004a, 2004b, 2004c)

  **i.** NOTE: refer patients to hematology or oncology for most of the conditions below

  **ii.** Platelet disorders (Leung & Chan, 2001)

   (a) *Quantitative* platelet disorders—reduced numbers of platelets due to:

    (1) Inadequate production due to:

     a) Bone marrow suppression due to viral and bacterial infections

     b) Bone marrow infiltration, e.g., leukemia, other malignancies

     c) Drug reactions, e.g., alkylating agents, antimetabolites, anticonvulsants, chlorothiazide diuretics, and estrogens

      d) Thrombocytopenia absent radii (TAR) syndrome, an autosomal recessive disorder

      e) Fanconi's anemia, an autosomal recessive disorder

      f) Wiskott-Aldrich syndrome, an X-linked recessive disorder

    (2) Increased destruction

      a) Idiopathic (immune) thrombocytopenic purpura

    (3) Sequestration

      a) Splenomegaly

      b) Giant hemangioma

  (b) *Qualitative* platelet disorders—defective platelet functioning despite adequate numbers of platelets due to:

    (1) Drug effects, e.g., aspirin, furosemide (Lasix), nitrofurantoin, heparin, sympathetic blockers, clofibrate, and some nonsteroidal antiinflammatory drugs (NSAIDs)

    (2) Congenital syndromes

  iii. Coagulation factor deficiencies (Leung & Chan, 2001)

    (a) Coagulation factor VIII deficiency—hemophilia type A, X-linked recessive

    (b) Coagulation factor IX deficiency—hemophilia type B, X-linked recessive

    (c) von Willebrand disease

      (1) Type I is most common

      (2) Types I, II are autosomal dominant

    (d) Type III is autosomal recessive

  iv. Vascular disorders

    (a) Henoch-Schönlein purpura

    (b) Congenital syndromes

    (c) Infections

    (d) Psychogenic

e. Idiopathic (immune) thrombocytopenic purpura (ITP) (Leung & Chan, 2001; Thiagarajan, 2004)

  i. Characteristics

    (a) Most common acquired form of platelet disorder

    (b) Autoantibodies directed against platelet surface are produced

    (c) Autoantibodies destroy platelets and thereby reduce their number

  ii. Etiology and presentation

    (a) Acute ITP

      (1) History of recent viral illness

      (2) Response to an infectious agent or autoimmunity

      (3) Drugs such as heparin

      (4) Acute onset of generalized purpura and petechiae

        a) Purpura results from the extravasation of blood from the vasculature into the skin or mucous membranes (Leung & Chan, 2001)

      (5) Otherwise normal exam

    (b) Underlying systemic disease

      (1) Insidious onset in an older child

      (2) Lymphadenopathy

      (3) Hepatosplenomegaly

  iii. Laboratory findings

    (a) No definitive test for ITP

    (b) CBC

      (1) WBC and differential are normal

(2) Hgb may be low in the presence of significant bleeding

(3) Platelet count is commonly less than 20,000/mL

(4) Prothrombin time (PT) and partial thromboplastin time (PTT) should be normal

(c) Other tests as indicated by history and physical

(d) HIV testing in sexually active teens to eliminate HIV infection as cause of ITP

iv. Treatment

(a) Avoid aspirin

(b) Avoid contact sports

(c) Other treatment planned in collaboration with a hematologist

(1) For mild ITP—platelets greater than 20,000/mL, no bleeding other than purpura

a) Watchful waiting is indicated

(2) If high risk for internal hemorrhage—platelets less than 20,000/mL, extensive mucosal bleeding

a) There are no data that treatment affects the course, but it can address the immediate crisis

b) Raise the platelet count to a safe level with transfusions

c) Prednisone—can suppress immune attack on platelets but also can have long term side effects

d) IV immune globulin (IVIG)

i) 0.8 to 1 g/kg for 2 days

ii) Difficult to administer and quite costly

e) Non-splenectomized children with $Rh_o(D)$ positive blood receive IV anti-D immune globulin

i) Onset of effect of IV anti-D can be slower than with IVIG

ii) Easier to administer, safe and effective, less costly but still expensive

iii) Side effects include fever, chills, headache, decrease in hemoglobin

v. Prognosis

(a) Prognosis is excellent

(b) Illness course is benign

(c) More than 50% recover within 4 weeks without treatment

(d) 80% recover within 6 months

(e) Most serious complication is intracranial hemorrhage (<1%)

vi. Follow-up

(a) Platelet count is followed until recovery established

(b) Counsel parents to protect child from falls or other trauma that can cause bleeding

(c) Acute ITP does not tend to recur

f. Hemophilia

i. Symptoms

(a) Deep soft-tissue bleeding and hemarthrosis are hallmarks

(1) Become evident when child starts to walk

(2) Knees, elbows, ankles most common sites

(3) Central nervous system bleed most feared

(b) Surface bleeding and purpura can be seen

(1) Mucus membrane bleeds in mouth and bruises common in infancy

ii. Pathophysiology

(a) After injury to blood vessel, platelet plug forms fibrin clot

        (b) In hemophilia
           (1) Clot formation is slow
           (2) Clot is not strong

  **iii.** Etiology and prevalence
        (a) X-linked recessive trait
        (b) Some cases are attributable to spontaneous mutation
        (c) Occurs in about 1:5000 males
        (d) About 85% have hemophilia type A (classic; factor VIII deficiency)
        (e) Remaining have hemophilia type B (Christmas disease; factor IX deficiency)

  **iv.** Laboratory findings
        (a) Platelet count, PT, and bleeding time normal
        (b) PPT is two to three times normal
        (c) Diagnosis confirmed by deficient factor VIII or IX and normal von Willebrand factor (vWf) assay
        (d) Severity classified by baseline level of affected factor
           (1) Severe hemophilia is less than 1% of specific factor
           (2) Moderate is 1% to 5%
           (3) Mild is more than 5%

  **v.** Treatment
        (a) Continuous prophylaxis with recombinant factor from ages 2 to 18 years can reduce disability in people with hemophilia
           (1) Prevents spontaneous bleeds
           (2) Prevents development of joint deformity
           (3) Removes risk of transmission of potentially infectious agents
        (b) With minor bleeds, replacement factor is given to achieve 35% to 40% (hemostatic) levels
        (c) With major bleeds (iliopsoas muscle, CNS, upper airway), factor replacement is given to achieve 100% levels
        (d) Infants with hemophilia should be immunized against hepatitis B
        (e) People with hemophilia who receive plasma-derived factor or other blood product should be screened regularly for:
           (1) Transfusion-acquired infections
           (2) Liver disease

  **vi.** Prognosis and expected course
        (a) Chronic illness
        (b) Long-term complications include:
           (1) Joint destruction
           (2) Transfusion-borne infectious diseases in patients who receive human blood-derived factor or other blood products
           (3) Immune response (inhibitors) can develop and hamper the effect of replacement factor
        (c) Best outcomes and reduced costs can be achieved through comprehensive care at a regional hemophilia center
           (1) Best available medical treatment
           (2) Family centered, multi-disciplinary approach
           (3) Health education and anticipatory guidance for prevention of common complications
           (4) Regular monitoring for early recognition of complications

**g.** von Willebrand disease
  **i.** Most common hereditary coagulation disorder; also involves a clotting-factor deficiency

    ii. Symptoms

      (a) Gingival bleeding

      (b) Epistaxis

      (c) Hemorrhage after dental extraction, surgery, trauma

      (d) Melena and excessive menstrual bleeding

   iii. Pathophysiology

      (a) von Willebrand factor (vWf) adheres to subendothelial cells, then changes formation so that platelets adhere to vWf

      (b) Platelets become activated, which attracts other platelets

      (c) Initiates key steps in the coagulation cascade

      (d) Because vWf carries factor VIII, secondary factor VIII deficiency can be seen when vWf is lacking

   iv. Etiology and prevalence

      (a) Inherited autosomal dominant trait with variable clinical manifestations

        (1) Occurs in 1% to 2% of population

        (2) Males and females can be affected

        (3) More women are reported as having the disease probably because menorrhagia causes women to seek medical attention

    v. Laboratory findings

      (a) Platelet count usually normal but can be low

      (b) PT normal

      (c) Bleeding time and PTT usually prolonged

      (d) When history and exam suggest von Willebrand disease, specific tests include:

        (1) vWf quantitative assay

        (2) vWf (ristocetin cofactor) activity

        (3) vWf multimers (structure)

        (4) Plasma factor VIII activity

   vi. Treatment

      (a) Not required in mild cases

      (b) In type I (classic) von Willebrand disease (mild quantitative deficiency of vWf and factor VIII:C), DDAVP (Desmopressin) can induce release of vWf from endothelial cells.

        (1) Test for efficacy before therapeutic use.

      (c) Some people with type II disease (qualitative abnormalities) respond to (DDAVP)

      (d) Not all responders release functional vWf and responses are transient

      (e) People for whom DDAVP is not effective and those with type III disease (severe quantitative abnormalities) require vWf and factor VIII replacement therapy

      (f) Parents and child education

        (1) Apply pressure to the anterior nasal septum with the finger and thumb to control epistaxis

        (2) Adolescent females taught how to manage excessive menstrual blood flow

**h.** Henoch-Schönlein (anaphylactoid) purpura (vasculitis) (Bossart, 2005)

   i. Signs and symptoms

      (a) Purpura—a hallmark rash (95% to 100%)

        (1) Crops of maculopapules

        (2) Most often on legs, buttocks

        (3) Progress to petechiae or purpura

        (4) Lesions are nonpruritic

    (5) Change in color over time

    (6) New crops arise as others fade

  (b) Fever

  (c) Joint pain, mostly knees and ankles (60% to 80%)

  (d) Abdominal pain or tenderness, vomiting (85%)

  (e) GI bleeding

  (f) Hematuria

  (g) Periorbital swelling

  (h) Painful nonpitting edema in hands, feet, scalp, ears (20% to 50%)

  (i) Scrotal edema (2% to 35%)

  (j) Hepatomegaly

 **ii.** Pathophysiology

  (a) A small vessel vasculitis

  (b) Etiology unknown

    (1) Preceding URI in 50% of cases

  (c) Immunoglobulin A (IgA), C3, and immune complex deposit in arterioles, capillaries, and venules of the skin, connective tissues, GI tract, joints, scrotum, and kidneys

 **iii.** Prevalence

  (a) 14 cases occur per 100,000 school-aged children

  (b) Male more than female, 2:1

 **iv.** Specific laboratory findings

  (a) Elevated serum IgA levels

 **v.** Differential diagnoses

  (a) Disseminated intravascular coagulation

  (b) Meningitis, encephalitis

  (c) Testicular torsion

  (d) Systemic lupus erythematosus

  (e) Rickettsia

  (f) Thrombocytopenic purpura

 **vi.** Treatment

  (a) Most patients recover without treatment

  (b) Symptom management

    (1) NSAIDs for joint pain (see Table 55-5 in Chapter 55)

    (2) Monitor in collaboration with physician

     a) Effects of corticosteroids on abdominal pain, edema, and nephritis

      1) No effect on renal outcomes but can relieve symptoms

     b) IV immune globulin

     c) Effect of factor VIII administration on symptoms or course of Henoch-Schönlein purpura not established

  (c) Hospital admission for monitoring indicated with clinically significant changes in signs and symptoms

 **vii.** Prognosis and expected course

  (a) Relatively benign disease

  (b) Children younger than 2 years compared with older children

    (1) Milder

    (2) Shorter course

    (3) Fewer recurrences and complications

  (c) Symptoms persist for 4 weeks on average

  (d) Recurrence in 10% to 20% of patients

  (e) 5% become chronic

  (f) 1% progress to end-stage renal failure

3. Symptom: swollen lymph nodes (Leung & Robson, 2004)
   a. Focused history
      i. Symptom analysis
         (a) Location of enlarged nodes
         (b) Painful or painless
         (c) Fever
            (1) Presence
            (2) Pattern
            (3) Duration
      ii. Headache
      iii. Fatigue
      iv. Nausea
      v. Abdominal discomfort
      vi. Joint pain
         (a) Which joints
         (b) Patterns of pain
      vii. Unintended weight loss
      viii. Night sweats to the extent that the sheets need to be changed
      ix. Chest pain
      x. Difficulty breathing
      xi. Exposure to cats
      xii. Drug history
      xiii. Adolescents—sexual activity
      xiv. Family members or friends have or had similar symptoms
   b. Focused physical examination
      i. Inspection
         (a) Assess weight loss relative to previously recorded information
         (b) Note shortness of breath
         (c) Inspect skin
            (1) Petechiae
            (2) Purpura
            (3) Bruising
            (4) Rash
            (5) Facial flushing or swelling
         (d) Neck vein engorgement
         (e) Throat
            (1) Pharyngitis
            (2) Tonsillar enlargement
            (3) Exudates
            (4) Petechiae on soft palate
      ii. Palpation
         (a) All lymph nodes
            (1) Determine pattern of distribution of enlarged nodes
            (2) Visualize the body in the area of nodal enlargement for signs of infection
         (b) Palpate abdomen
            (1) Liver enlargement
            (2) Spleen enlargement
         (c) Joints
            (1) Assess motion
            (2) Swelling
            (3) Warmth
            (4) Rheumatoid nodules

a) Extensor aspect of elbows

b) Over Achilles tendons

iii. Auscultation

(a) Listen for pericardial rub

(b) Cardiac murmur

c. Pathophysiology

  i. Lymph nodes enlarge as they filter lymph and collect immune system cells and debris from destruction of infectious agents

  ii. Anterior cervical lymphadenopathy considered more suggestive of malignancy than posterior cervical or supraclavicular

d. Differential diagnosis (American Academy of Pediatrics, 2003)

  i. Viral infection: primary Epstein-Barr virus (EBV) (infectious mononucleosis)

  ii. Bacterial infection: *Bartonella henselae* infection (cat scratch disease)

  iii. Connective tissue disease (juvenile rheumatoid arthritis) (see Chapter 48)

  iv. Leukemia, lymphoma, Hodgkin's lymphoma (see Chapter 38)

e. Primary EBV (infectious mononucleosis) (CDC, 2002)

  i. Signs and symptoms

(a) Viral infection—slow onset

(b) Most common findings

(1) Lymphadenopathy

(2) Severe pharyngitis

(3) Tonsillar enlargement with exudates

(4) Soft palate petechiae

(5) Splenomegaly

(c) Fever

(d) Headache

(e) Fatigue

(f) Abdominal pain

(g) Nausea

(h) Myalgia

  ii. Etiology

(a) EBV, a member of the herpesvirus family and one of the most common human viruses (CDC, 2002)

(b) Most individuals have been previously infected with EBV, but were asymptomatic

(c) Humans are the only source of EBV; found in saliva of most people

(d) Close contact with saliva of infected person is required for transmission

(e) Not transmitted through air or blood

(f) Intrafamilial spread is common

(g) Incubation period is 4 to 6 weeks

(h) Although infected people can spread the virus, no special precautions are recommended because EBV is found in saliva of most healthy people

  iii. Laboratory findings (CDC, 2002)

(a) Paul-Bunnell heterophile antibody test—positive finding is diagnostic

(1) Antibodies are highest during first 4 weeks

(2) False positives found in a few patients

(3) False negatives in 10% to 15% of patients, usually those younger than 10 years of age

(b) "Mono spot" test is positive if EBV

(c) If mono spot or heterophile test is negative, additional testing needed to differentiate EBV infections from similar illness due to:

(1) Cytomegalovirus

          (2) Adenovirus

          (3) *Toxoplasma gondii*

      (d) Specific antibody tests such as viral capsid antibody (VCA) can distinguish:

          (1) No infection

          (2) Acute infection

          (3) Recent infection

          (4) Past infection

      (e) Normal to moderately elevated WBC of 10,000 to 20,000 cells/mm$^3$

      (f) Increased total number of lymphocytes

          (1) 20% to 40% of these atypical

      (g) Because HIV antibody does not develop until 6 to 12 weeks after infection, sexually active adolescents should have HIV DNA polymerase chain reaction (PCR) test to rule out acute HIV infection

    iv. Treatment

      (a) Referral to hematology oncology to rule out leukemia is indicated if:

          (1) Child is acutely ill with markedly high or low WBC

          (2) Low platelets

          (3) Hemolytic anemia

      (b) Supportive care

          (1) Rest if fatigue is debilitating

          (2) Avoid contact sports until spleen not palpable

      (c) Corticosteroids

          (1) Used in consultation with physician only when:

             a) Marked tonsil enlargement

             b) Massive spleen

             c) Myocarditis

             d) Thrombocytopenia with hemorrhage

             e) Hemolytic anemia

          (2) Caution—EBV is a human tumor virus (oncovirus) and corticosteroid-induced immunosuppression may promote oncogenesis

    v. Prognosis and expected course

      (a) Prognosis for complete recovery is excellent if no complications

      (b) Symptoms last about 2 to 4 weeks

          (1) Followed by gradual recovery

          (2) Fatigue occasionally persists for years

      (c) EBV remains dormant or latent in the throat and blood for life

      (d) The virus can reactivate without symptoms of illness, but individual can transmit the virus to others

      (e) Complications include

          (1) Spleen rupture

          (2) Airway impairment

          (3) Neurologic involvement

          (4) Guillain-Barré syndrome

          (5) Hemolytic anemia

      (f) Heart problems or involvement of the CNS occurs only rarely

      (g) Infectious mononucleosis is almost never fatal

    vi. Follow-up

      (a) People with recent EBV should not donate blood

  f. *B. henselae* infection (cat scratch disease or CSD)

    i. Distinctive physical findings

      (a) Inoculation site—bite marks

    (b) Lymph nodes in one or more of the sets that drain the site are:
- (1) Warm
- (2) Red
- (3) Tender
- (4) Indurated

  **ii.** History of recent contact with a cat or kitten (bite)

 **iii.** Etiology
- (a) *B. henselae* is most common bacterial cause of chronic regional lymph-adenitis
- (b) Spread by cutaneous inoculation
- (c) Most patients are younger than 20 years old

  **iv.** Laboratory findings
- (a) Indirect fluorescent antibody test (IFA)
  - (1) Detects serum antibody to antigens of the *Bartonella* species
  - (2) Test reagents are available at state health departments
  - (3) Test is available through CDC
  - (4) NOTE: results of IFA done at commercial laboratories not reliable

   **v.** Treatment
- (a) Symptom management
  - (1) No studies show clear benefit of any specific treatment
  - (2) Antibiotics considered for patients:
    - a) With acute systemic symptoms such as hepatosplenomegaly or large painful adenopathy
    - b) Who are immunocompromised

  **vi.** Prognosis and expected course
- (a) Excellent in otherwise normal hosts
- (b) Often resolves on its own in 2 to 4 months
- (c) Encephalopathy occurs in about 5% of cases
  - (1) 1 to 3 weeks after onset of lymphadenitis
- (d) Potential complications
  - (1) Osteolytic bone lesions
  - (2) Granulomatous hepatitis

 **vii.** Follow-up
- (a) Discourage rough play with cats
- (b) Immunocompromised children should avoid contact with:
  - (1) Cats that bite or scratch
  - (2) Kittens
- (c) Wash cat bites or scratches
- (d) Do not allow cats to lick child's open wounds

---

# REFERENCES

American Academy of Pediatrics Committee on Nutrition. (2004). *Pediatric nutrition handbook* (5th ed.). Elk Grove Village, IL: American Academy of Pediatrics.

American Academy of Pediatrics Committee on Practice and Ambulatory Medicine (2000). Recommendations for Preventative Pediatric Health Care, *Pediatrics, 105*(3), 645-646.

American Academy of Pediatrics (2003). *Red book: Report of the Committee on Infectious Diseases* (26th ed.). Elk Grove Village, IL: American Academy of Pediatrics.

American Association for Clinical Chemistry. (2004). The coagulation cascade. Retrieved May 11, 2006, from www.labtestsonline. org/understanding/analytes/coag_cascade/coagulation_cascade.html.

Bickley, L., & Szilagyi. P. (2004). *Bates' guide to physical examination & history taking* (8th ed.). Philadelphia: Lippincott.

Bossart, P. (2005). Henoch-Schönlein purpura. Retrieved May 11, 2006, from www.emedicine.com/emerg/topic845.htm.

Carley, A. (2003a). Anemia: When is it iron deficiency? *Pediatr Nurs, 29*(2), 127-133.

Carley, A. (2003b). Anemia: When is it not iron deficiency? *Pediatr Nurs, 29*(3), 205-211.

Centers for Disease Control and Prevention (CDC), National Center for Infectious Diseases. (2002). Epstein-Barr virus and infectious mononucleosis. Retrieved September 9, 2005, from www.cdc.gov/ncidod/diseases/ebv.htm.

Conrad, M. E. (2006). Anemia. Retrieved on May 12, 2006 from eMedicine at http://www.emedicine.com/med/topic132.htm.

Corbett, J. V. (2004). *Laboratory tests and diagnostic procedures with nursing diagnoses* (6th ed.). Stamford, CT: Appleton & Lange.

Glader, B. (2004). Iron deficiency anemia. In R. E. Behrman, R. M. Kliegman, & H. B. Jenson (Eds.). *Nelson textbook of pediatrics* (17th ed.). Philadelphia: Saunders, pp. 1614-1616.

Health and Human Services (HHS) and U.S. Department of Agriculture (USDA). (2005). *Dietary guidelines for Americans 2005*. Washington, DC: Government Printing Office.

Habal, R. (2004). Toxicity, lead. Retrieved May 11, 2006, from www.emedicine.com/MED/topic1269.htm.

Hermiston, M. L., & Mentzer, W. C. (2002). A practical approach to the evaluation of the anemic child. *Pediatr Clin N Am, 49*(5), 877-891.

Hockenberry, M., Wilson, D., Winkelstein, M., & Kline, N. (2003). *Wong's nursing care of infants and children* (7th ed.). St. Louis: Mosby.

Huang, L., & Miller, R. (2003). Transient erythroblastopenia of childhood. Retrieved September 9, 2005, from www.emedicine.com/ped/topic2279.htm.

Irwin, J. J., & Kirchner, J. T. (2001). Anemia in children. *Am Fam Phys, 64*(8), 1379-1386.

King, M. W. (2005). Medical biochemistry: Blood coagulation. Retrieved May 11, 2006, from http://web.indstate.edu/thcme/mwking/blood-coagulation.html.

Leung, A. K. C., & Chan, K. W. (2001). Evaluating the child with purpura. *Am Fam Phys, 64*(3), 419-428.

Leung, A. K. C., & Robson, W. L. M. (2004). Childhood cervical lymphadenopathy. *J Pediatr Health Care, 18*(1), 3-7.

Marcus, S. (2005). Toxicity, lead. Retrieved May 12, 2006, from www.emedicine.com/emerg/topic293.htm.

McCance, K. L., & Heuther, S. C. (2006). *Pathophysiology: The biologic basis for disease in adults and children* (5th ed.). St. Louis: Mosby.

Montgomery, R. R., & Scott, J. P. (2004). Hereditary clotting factor deficiencies (bleeding disorders). In R. E. Behrman, R. M. Kliegman, & H. B. Jenson (Eds.). *Nelson textbook of pediatrics* (17th ed.) Philadelphia: Saunders, pp. 1657-1662.

Montgomery, R. R., & Scott, J. P. (2004). Platelet and blood vessel disorders. In R. E. Behrman, R. M. Kliegman, & H. B. Jenson (Eds.). *Nelson textbook of pediatrics* (17th ed.) Philadelphia: Saunders, pp. 1670-1675.

Montgomery, R. R., & Scott, J. P. (2004). von Willebrand disease. In R. E. Behrman, R. M. Kliegman, & H. B. Jenson (Eds.). *Nelson textbook of pediatrics* (17th ed.) Philadelphia: Saunders, pp. 1662-1664.

Tam, A. B., & Hexdall, A. (2006). Hookworm. Retrieved on May 12, 2006 from eMedicine at http://www.emedicine.com/emerg/topic841.htm.

Tender, J., & Cheng, T.L. (2002). Iron deficiency anemia. In F.D. Burg., J.R. Ingelfinger, R.A. Polin, & A.A. Gershon (Eds.), *Gellis & Kagan's current pediatric therapy* (pp. 633-637). Philadelphia: Saunders.

Thiagarajan, P. (2004). Platelet disorders. Retrieved May 12, 2006, from www.emedicine.com/emerg/topic845.htm.

Wagle, S., & Deshpande, P. G. (2003). Hemolytic disease of newborn. Retrieved on May 12, 2006 from eMedicine at http://www.emedicine.com/med/topic987.htm.

# Common Illness of the Musculoskeletal System

BARBARA HOYER SCHAFFNER, PhD, RN, CPNP

1. "Growing pains"
   a. Characteristics
      i. Pain is usually reported:
         (a) In the lower limbs
         (b) Bilateral
         (c) Intermittent
         (d) Localized to the muscles of the leg
      ii. Begins after age 5 years
      iii. Associated with a rapid growth spurt
   b. Etiology
      i. Normal growth
      ii. Idiopathic
      iii. Increased incidence of migraines in children's families
      iv. No evidence of vascular perfusion changes in painful areas as occurs in migraines (Hashkes, et al., 2004)
   c. Differential diagnoses
      i. Neurologic disorders such as:
         (a) Paralysis
         (b) Spinal disease
         (c) Ataxia
      ii. Psychologic disorders such as:
         (a) Hysteria
         (b) Anxiety
   d. Focused assessment (Seidel, et al., 2003)
      i. Symptom analysis
      ii. Musculoskeletal assessment (Chapter 12)
      iii. Neurologic assessment (Chapter 13)
   e. Diagnosis
      i. A diagnosis of exclusion
         (a) No history of trauma
         (b) No systemic illness
         (c) No swelling
         (d) No erythema

    **f.** Treatment

        **i.** Education and reassurance that it is typical and will resolve spontaneously

        **ii.** Massage

        **iii.** Application of heat can be helpful

        **iv.** Avoid unnecessary use of medication

        **v.** If severe, nonsteroidal antiinflammatory drugs (NSAIDs) may be used (see Chapter 55, Table 55–5)

    **g.** Prognosis

        **i.** Excellent after rapid growth spurts

        **ii.** No residual deficits occur

**2.** Signs: knock-knees, bowlegs, intoeing, foot abnormalities

    **a.** Focused assessment

        **i.** Symptom analysis

        **ii.** Musculoskeletal assessment (Chapter 12)

        **iii.** Neurologic assessment (Chapter 13)

    **b.** Differential diagnoses

        **i.** Most cases are physiologic variants of normal

            (a) Genu varum

            (b) Genu valgum

            (c) Intoeing

            (d) Congenital talipes equinovarus

            (e) Metatarsus adductus

        **ii.** Genu varum—alignment of the knee with the tibia medially deviated (varus) in relation to the femur (Brady & Burns, 2004)

            (a) Bowlegged appearance

            (b) Normally infants begin life with 10- to 15-degree bowlegs as a result of uterine position

            (c) Measure distance between knees with feet together—should be less than 5 inches

            (d) An angular deformity

                (1) Physiologic: normal up to age 3

                (2) Pathologic if:

                    a) More than 15 degrees in infants

                    b) Does not begin to decrease in second year

                    c) Asymmetric

                    d) Associated with short stature

                    e) Rapidly progressing

             (e) Etiology

                (1) Physiologic—uterine positioning, normal development

                (2) Pathologic

                    a) Blount disease

                    b) Rickets

                    c) Tumor

                    d) Neurologic problems

                    e) Infection

                    f) Fracture

            (f) Treatment

                (1) Physiologic

                    a) Explanation and reassurance that it usually corrects itself over time

                    b) Splints are not useful

                    c) Observe leg position over time (photos in chart are helpful)

(2) Pathologic
    a) Refer to orthopedics if deformity is unilateral, painful, or very asymmetric, or has pathologic characteristics
    b) Blount disease
      i) Blount brace will reverse the condition if applied early
      ii) Later, surgical osteotomy may be necessary
        *a)* If not treated, may lead to knee deformity and degeneration

**iii.** Genu valgum—alignment of the knee with the tibia laterally deviated (valgus) with relation to the femur (Brady & Burns, 2004)
    (a) Knock-kneed in appearance
    (b) An angular deformity
    (c) Etiology
      (1) Physiologic or developmental
        a) Over first 3 years, bowlegs straighten and progress to 10- to 15-degree knock-kneed appearance by age 3
        b) Girls more pronounced than boys
        c) By age 7 to 8 years, normal appearance is a mild valgum
      (2) Pathologic
        a) Development of knock-knees before the age of 2 years
        b) Valgus angle greater than 15 degrees
        c) Increasing in severity
        d) Associated with short stature, obesity, or asymmetry
        e) Potential causes
          i) Developmental disorder
          ii) Metaphyseal dysplasia or injury
          iii) Cerebral palsy
          iv) Tumor
          v) Osteochondrodysplasia
    (d) Treatment
      (1) Physiologic
        a) Braces for angles more than 15 degrees
        b) Resolves spontaneously by age 6
        c) Explanation and reassurance that it usually corrects itself over time
        d) Observe leg position over time (photos in chart are helpful)
      (2) Refer to orthopedics if suspected pathologic cause
        a) Surgical intervention may be needed

**iv.** Tibial torsion or femoral anteversion (Brady & Burns, 2004)
    (a) Foot turns in during walking and running
    (b) "Pigeon-toed" appearance
    (c) Awkward appearance when running
    (d) A rotational, torsional deformity in three potential areas:
      (1) Foot—distinguish between metatarsus adductus and clubfoot
      (2) Between knee and ankle—tibial torsion; most common younger than age 3
      (3) Between hip and knee—femoral anteversion medial femoral torsion; most common older than age 3
    (e) Etiology and incidence
      (1) Some degree of femoral anteversion (intoeing) occurs in everyone (10 to 15 degrees by ages 10 to 12 years)
      (2) May be congenital from uterine positioning
      (3) May be acquired from increased load on the femur while in torsion, e.g., "W" sitting position

(4) May be a family history of intoeing

(5) Diagnostic tests

    a) Usually a clinical diagnosis

    b) Leg or hip x-rays may be done

(f) Treatment

    (1) Explanation and reassurance that it usually corrects itself over time

    (2) Braces, special shoes, and casts offer no benefit

    (3) Refer to orthopedics if deformity is severe, unilateral, painful or very asymmetric, or if bowlegs persist after ages 3 to 4 years

(g) Prognosis is excellent with normal growth for most children

(h) Follow-up

    (1) Assessment of leg development at 3 to 6 months intervals is necessary

**v.** Pes planus (flatfoot) (Brady & Burns, 2004)

  (a) Physiologic

    (1) Common in infants and toddlers

    (2) Due to a fat pad in the arch

    (3) Resolves by ages 2 to 3

    (4) If it persists into adulthood

      a) Note abnormal wear of shoe on inner side

      b) Arch is *flexible*, i.e., can be achieved with pressure on the arch

      c) Usually familial

      d) Usually painless

      e) May be due to lax soft tissue, muscle weakness, or tight Achilles tendon

      f) May lead to bunions and abnormal pronation of feet over time if not treated

    (5) Treatment—refer to orthopedics for:

      a) Arch supports (orthotics) for shoes

      b) Achilles tendon stretching exercises

  (b) Pathologic

    (1) Flatness is *rigid* and an arch cannot be achieved with pressure

    (2) Rocker-bottom appearance may be a congenital vertical talus or calcaneovalgus foot

      a) This must be referred to orthopedics immediately for early treatment

    (3) Associated with:

      a) Marfan's syndrome

      b) Down syndrome

      c) Myelodysplasia

      d) Cerebral palsy

      e) Overweight

    (4) Treatment

      a) Weight management if cause is due to overweight

      b) Refer to orthopedics for arch supports (orthotics) for shoes

      c) Refer to appropriate specialist for underlying conditions

**vi.** Congenital talipes equinovarus (clubfoot) (Gore & Spencer, 2004)

  (a) Characteristics usually obvious at birth

    (1) Adduction of forefoot

    (2) Foot plantar flexed at the ankle (equines)

    (3) Forefoot curves in (varus)

(4) Inability to passively straighten the foot
(b) Etiology and incidence
(1) A congenital deformity of the foot
(2) Exact cause is unknown
(3) May be caused by postural induced compression in utero
(4) Present in approximately 1 per 1000 births
a) Male/female ratio is 1:2
b) Risk in siblings rises to 1:50
(5) Consequences may include vascular, cartilage, neurologic or muscular growth disturbances
(c) Diagnostic tests
(1) Clinical observations as described above
(2) X-ray will demonstrate aberrant bony or anatomic relationships
(d) Treatment
(1) Refer to orthopedics
(2) Nonsurgical treatment
a) Serial manipulation and casting
b) Most successful if begun very early
(3) Surgical correction at ages 6 to 9 months necessary for severe cases and when residual deformity exists
(e) Prognosis is excellent with early diagnosis and treatment
vii. Metatarsus adductus (Gore & Spencer, 2004)
(a) Characteristics
(1) Foot has a turned-in appearance
(2) Range of motion (ROM) of the ankle, hindfoot, and midfoot is normal
(3) Flexibility of the forefoot may range from flexible to rigid
(b) Etiology and incidence
(1) A positional foot deformity believed to be caused by in utero positioning
(2) The feet wrap around the posterolateral aspect of the thighs, producing forefoot adduction
(3) Occurs in 1 per 1000 live births
(4) Affects boys and girls equally
(5) Bilateral in 50% of the children affected
(6) Common in first-born children
(c) Diagnostic tests
(1) Clinical observations as described above
(2) If the forefoot is rigid, AP and lateral x-rays are needed
(d) Treatment
(1) Observation is usually sufficient if forefoot is flexible
(2) Passive ROM of the foot through all planes
(3) A corrective shoe may hasten correction
(4) Surgery is infrequently required but may be necessary if forefoot adduction is still present by age 6 years
(e) Prognosis is excellent with minimal to no disability as an adult
3. Symptoms: painless or painful limp, gait disturbance
a. Characteristics of limp
i. A limp in a child is never normal
ii. Categorized as painless or painful
iii. Screening of extremities for abnormalities in first year of life is important
iv. Early diagnosis and treatment lead to best prognosis

    **b.** Focused history

        **i.** Family history

           (a) Arthritis

           (b) Any other hip disorders, acute or chronic

        **ii.** Child's history

           (a) Developmental milestones

           (b) Symptom analysis

           (c) Acute or chronic onset

           (d) Position of birth, e.g., breech

           (e) Injury

           (f) Risk factors for the development of a limp

              (1) Participation in sports

              (2) Low birth weight

              (3) Growth delay

              (4) Delayed bone age

              (5) Overweight greater than 90th percentile

  **c.** Focused physical assessment (Box 34-1)

  **d.** Differential diagnoses (Box 34-2)

      **i.** Painless limp

          (a) Developmental dysplasia of the hip (DDH), previously known as "congenital hip dysplasia"

              (1) See Ganel & Grogan (2003) for a 5-minute orthopedic examination for infants

---

■ **BOX 34-1**
■ **FOCUSED ASSESSMENT FOR MUSCULOSKELETAL SIGNS AND SYMPTOMS**

**INSPECTION**
- General posture, resting position
- Gait
- Symme    try of body parts
- Symmetry of movements
- Spinal alignment
- Muscle tone

**PALPATION**
- Joints for heat, tenderness, swelling, crepitus, laxity

**RANGE OF MOTION (ROM) OF ALL JOINTS**
- Active
- Passive
- Goniometer measurements

**MUSCLE STRENGTH**
- Grade muscle strength 0–5
  - 0 = no evidence of contractility
  - 1 = slight contractility, no movement
  - 2 = full range of motions, gravity eliminated
- 3 = full range of motion against gravity
- 4 = full range of motion against gravity, some resistance
- 5 = full range of motion against gravity, full resistance

**LIMB MEASUREMENTS**
- Circumference
- Length

**LOWER SPINE**
- Bragard stretch
  - Extend and externally rotate the tibia
  - If a meniscal lesion is present, it will be displaced forward
  - Tenderness with palpation along the anterior medial joint line decreases with flexion and internal rotation
- Sitting knee extension test
  - Patient sits with back straight and knee dangling at 90° angle and extends leg
  - Using a goniometer, measure range of motion (ROM) angle

## ■ BOX 34-1
## ■ FOCUSED ASSESSMENT FOR MUSCULOSKELETAL SIGNS AND SYMPTOMS—cont'd

- Normal is 80° (170° minus 90°)
- Limited ROM suggests sciatic nerve tenderness or shortened hamstring
- Femoral stretch test
  - Patient lies prone with the knee flexed
  - Lift the hip into extension
  - Pain felt in the front of the thigh and the back indicates inflammation of the nerve root at L1, L2, L3

### KNEE
- Ballotement
  - With patient supine, force fluid from suprapatellar pouch
  - Firmly grasp just above patella with one hand
  - Force *joint* fluid between patella and femur
  - Pushes patella downward into femur
  - A palpable click from patella striking femur indicate knee joint effusion
- Bulge sign
  - Place ball of hand over medial patella
  - Milk fluid distally from suprapatellar pouch
  - Repeat several times
  - Press behind patella lateral margin
  - Reappearance of swelling indicates knee joint effusion
- The following tests for anterior and posterior cruciate ligament (ACL, PCL) injuries are best done by an orthopedic specialist
  - McMurray test—torn meniscus
  - Drawer test—ACL or PCL rupture
  - Lachman test—ACL rupture
  - Varus and valgus stress test—medial or lateral collateral ligament instability

### HIP
- Thomas test
  - While patient lies supine, flex both hips simultaneously to their limit
  - Hold one hip in position and lower the other leg
  - Normally, leg will lie flat on table
  - Positive Thomas test is when leg will not lie flat
  - Indicates flexion contracture or deformity

- Trendelenburg test
  - While patient stands unassisted on one leg, place fingers on the anterior superior iliac spines and ask patient to bend the knee on the contralateral leg
  - Normally, the gluteus medius stabilizes the contralateral hip
  - Positive Trendelenburg sign is when the pelvis drops on the unsupported side and supported hip is painful
  - Indicates weak gluteus medius hip abductor muscles
- Barlow's maneuver (for infants <2 months of age)
  - Position infant supine, knees flexed
  - Grasp the thigh and adduct it while applying downward pressure
  - Positive Barlow's test is palpable dislocation of femoral head
  - Clicks during these maneuvers are considered to be benign
- Ortolani's maneuver (for infants <2 months of age)
  - Position infant supine with knees flexed bilaterally
  - Support hip with thumb forefinger and place pad of second finger on bony prominence of greater trochanter, and thumb near lesser trochanter
  - With abduction of thighs, pressure to greater trochanter causes unstable hip to move from unreduced to reduced position
  - Positive Ortolani's sign is a "clunk" during the maneuver
  - Indicates hip dislocation
- Allis sign
  - When patient is standing, one knee is higher than the other
  - Suggests hip dislocation, shortened femur

### FOOT
- In resting position, observe the position of the front of the foot
- If front of foot is bent inward (toward the midline) at the instep
- And flexible, indicates metatarsus adductus
- And not flexible, indicates clubfoot

From Family Practice Notebook.com, retrieved on May 13, 2006 at http://www.fpnotebook.com and GP Notebook.com, retrieved at http://www.gpnotebook.co.uk.

■ BOX 34-2
■ **DIFFERENTIAL DIAGNOSES FOR COMMON MUSCULOSKELETAL SIGNS AND SYMPTOMS**

**PAINLESS LIMP**
- Development dysplasia of the hip (DDH)
- Leg length discrepancy
  - Genu varus (bowlegged)
  - Genu valgus (knock-kneed)

**PAINFUL LIMP**
- Trauma
- Fractures
- Septic arthritis
- Osteomyelitis
- Toxic synovitis
- Juvenile rheumatoid arthritis (JRA)
- Slipped capital femoral epiphysis
- Aseptic necrosis/osteochondritis (Osgood-Schlatter)
- Legg-Calvé-Perthes disease
- Torsion
- Malignancies
- Sickle cell disease

**LEG LENGTH DISCREPANCY**
- Wilms' tumor
- Arteriovenous malformation
- Neurofibromatosis
- Development dysplasia of the hip
- Legg-Calvé-Perthes disease
- Osteomyelitis

- Osteogenesis imperfecta
- Tumors
- Scoliosis

**BACK PAIN/DEFORMITY**
- Scoliosis
- Torticollis
- Trauma (spondylolisthesis/spondylolysis)
- Functional—heavy backpacks, high heels

**ARM PAIN**
- Brachial plexus injuries
- Subluxation of radial head (nursemaid's elbow)
- Little League elbow
- Fractures
- CNS injuries or lesions

**FOOT ABNORMALITIES**
- Congenital talipes equinovarus (clubfoot)
- Metatarsus adductus
- Femoral anteversion
- Cerebral palsy

**MUSCULOSKELETAL DEVELOPMENTAL DELAY**
- Muscular dystrophy
- Nonmusculoskeletal origins

(2) Pathophysiology
    a) A congenital condition involving abnormal development or dislocation of the hip resulting in:
        i) Limited abduction of the hip
        ii) Thigh fold asymmetry
        iii) Leg length inequality
    b) A painless limp noted when child begins to walk
(3) Etiology
    a) Unknown
    b) Associated with intrauterine position; incidence is 14 times higher with breech births
    c) 4 times more common in females
    d) Left hip affected 10 times more often than right hip
(4) Diagnostic tests
    a) Physical assessment or manipulation of hip joint can identify DDH in infants less than 3 months of age.
        i) Positive Barlow's maneuver—abnormal hip dislocates on adduction of the affected hip
        ii) Positive Ortolani's maneuver—an audible "clunk" felt in 10% of infants when femoral head slides into the acetabulum

iii) Positive Allis sign—unequal knee heights when supine with knees flexed

b) Ultrasound imaging

   i) Most useful imaging in infants younger than 4 months of age

   ii) Ultrasound should not be done on infants less than 2 weeks of age because of the chance of false-positive findings due to the expected hip joint laxity of newborns

c) X-ray: AP view of pelvis is recommended at older ages

(5) Treatment

a) Pavlik harness (Figure 34-1)

   i) Maintains a flexed adducted position of the hip in infants less than 6 months of age

b) Surgical reduction if harness not effective

(6) Prognosis is excellent, especially when correction begins in infancy

(b) Leg length discrepancy

(1) Characteristics—can occur at the level of the femur, tibia, or both

(2) Etiology

a) Multiple causes including:

   i) Traumatic growth disruption

   ii) Infection

   iii) Inflammation

b) Most cases are mild and clinically insignificant

(3) Differential diagnoses (see Box 34-2)

(4) Diagnostic tests

a) X-ray examination of extremity is indicated if discrepancy is large

(5) Treatment

a) Conservative treatment involves a shoe lift on the affected side

b) Initiated for leg length discrepancies greater than 2 cm when leg growth is complete

c) For larger defects, surgery may be necessary

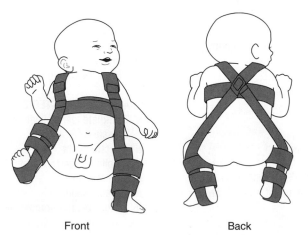

Front                    Back

FIGURE 34-1 ■ Child in a Pavlik harness for developmental dysplasia of the hip (DDH). (From Wong, et al. [2001]. *Wong's essentials of pediatric nursing* (6th ed.). St. Louis: Mosby, Figure 31-15, p. 1223.)

          (6) Prognosis

             a) Expected outcome with treatment is elimination of noticeable limp

    **ii.** Painful limp

        (a) Characteristics

           (1) Abrupt onset

           (2) May have history of trauma

        (b) Etiology

           (1) Trauma

             a) Trauma is the leading cause of painful limp and can occur at any age

                i) Fracture—a break in the continuity of a bone

                   *a)* Most common fractures in children occur in the epiphyseal plate (growth plate) because this is the weakest part of the growing bone

                ii) Sprain—a stretch or tear injury involving a ligament

                   *a)* Graded from I to III (see Box 34-3)

                   *b)* Ankle sprains are most common in children (Wolfe, et al., 2001)

                iii) Strain—a stretch or tear involving a muscle or its tendon

             b) Diagnostic testing

                i) Consistent with extent and location of injury

                ii) Usually involves x-ray of affected area

                iii) CT scan or MRI is usually not necessary

        (c) Treatment

           (1) Refer to orthopedics if fracture is noted

           (2) Goal of treatment for sprains and strains:

             a) Achieve pain-free movement

             b) Achieve pain-free weight bearing

           (3) Immediately following trauma (in first 24 to 48 hours) follow the PRICE protocol (Table 34-1)

---

■ **BOX 34-3**
■ **GRADING SCALE FOR SPRAINS**

**GRADE I CHARACTERISTICS**
- Mild stretching of ligament, tendons, or muscle
- Stable joint
- No feeling of looseness
- Full ROM
- Minimal pain
- Minimal swelling
- Normal weight bearing

**GRADE II CHARACTERISTICS**
- Partial tear of ligament, tendon, or muscle
- Stable joint
- Decreased active ROM
- Moderate pain
- Moderate swelling
- Weight bearing difficult

**GRADE III CHARACTERISTICS**
- Complete tear of ligament, tendon, or muscle
- Unstable joint
- Inability to perform active ROM
- Severe pain
- Severe swelling
- Weight bearing impossible

From Foot & Ankle Institute (2006). Retrieved on May 12, 2006 from http://www.footankleinstitute.com/Anklesprain.html.

■ **TABLE 34-1**
■ ■ **PRICE Protocol for Management of Sprains and Strains**

| | Action | Comment |
|---|---|---|
| P | Protection | Ensure that area is fully protected from further injury using splints, elastic, wrap, or brace |
| R | Rest | Allow injured area to rest<br>Use splint/crutches as necessary<br>Allow limited or no activity |
| I | Ice | Apply ice to area immediately after injury<br>Place ice on injured area for 15 minutes, then remove<br>Repeat three times/day and after any activity<br>Continue ice for the first 24 to 48 hours |
| C | Compression | Apply an elastic bandage/wrap to help decrease swelling<br>Do not allow patient to sleep with elastic bandage/wrap on |
| E | Elevation | Elevate to decrease swelling |

(4) Use NSAIDs for pain and swelling, particularly the first 72 hours after injury (see Chapter 55, Table 55-5 for details)
(5) Rehabilitation can begin 48 hours after injury if no fracture documented
(d) Prognosis depends on the extent and severity of injury, and timeliness of treatment
(e) Follow-up
(1) Any change in pain or sensation pattern requires an immediate return visit
(2) Return visit should be scheduled approximately 1 week after injury
(3) If injury affects athletic activity, review the sport-specific "return to play" criteria (Rimando, 2005)
a) Full pain-free active and passive ROM
b) No pain or tenderness
c) Strength of ankle muscles 70% to 80% of the uninvolved side
d) Balance on one leg for 30 seconds with eyes closed
iii. Slipped capital femoral epiphysis (Brady & Burns, 2004)
(a) Characteristics
(1) Displacement of the femoral head from the femoral neck in a downward and backward position relative to the neck of the femur
(2) Varied levels of pain
(3) Frequently located:
a) Anterior thigh
b) Knee
(4) Hip is held in:
a) External rotation
b) Abduction
(5) Flexion of the hip is limited
(6) In acute cases

a) History of injury or strain precedes complaints of pain (Santarlasci, 2000)

b) Usually will not bear weight on affected side

c) Holds limb in external rotation

d) Passive ROM is painful

(b) Etiology and incidence

(1) May be caused by severe trauma

(2) Most often due to a *gradual* slip from chronic, abnormal forces or overuse

(3) Most common hip disorder in 9- to 15-year-old adolescents

a) Before epiphyseal plate closes

b) Occurs in boys later than girls due to later maturity

c) Occurs in boys more than girls, 2:1 to 3:1

(4) Overweight more than 90th percentile is a risk factor

(5) Higher incidence in African Americans and Pacific Islanders

(6) Associated with many endocrine and systemic disorders

(c) Diagnostic tests

(1) X-ray is most common diagnostic measure

a) AP pelvis—anteroposterior

b) "Frog-leg lateral"—frog-leg position

c) True lateral view of pelvis

(2) Early radiologic changes will indicate irregularity and widening of growth plate of femur

(3) Later, more chronic changes include displacement of femoral head and widening of the epiphysis

(d) Treatment

(1) Immediate referral to orthopedics

(2) Usually followed by surgical fixation of the epiphysis

(e) Prognosis

(1) Good with early identification and repair

(2) Can result in limb shortening

iv. Septic arthritis

(a) Characteristics

(1) Affects children of any age

(2) A sudden onset of symptoms that include:

a) Pain of the affected joint

b) Occurrence most often in hip, ankles, and knees

c) Painful limp

d) Fever

e) Limited ROM

f) Unwillingness or inability to bear weight on the affected joint

g) Joint effusion

(b) Etiology

(1) *Haemophilus influenzae* infection

(2) *Staphylococcus aureus* infection

(c) Diagnosis

(1) Clinical findings as described above

(2) Laboratory tests

a) Elevated serum WBC

b) Elevated erythrocyte sedimentation rate (ESR)

i) Rises 24 or more hours after onset of symptoms

ii) Returns to normal in approximately 1 month

iii) C-reactive protein elevated in approximately 95% of cases (peaks in 48 hours)
  (d) Treatment
    (1) Immediate referral to a physician is necessary for further examination and testing
    (2) Children with septic arthritis are immediately hospitalized for intravenous antibiotics
    (3) Analgesics given every 6 to 8 hours
    (4) Rest
  (e) Prognosis
    (1) Child will be ill for 3 to 5 days
    (2) Length of hospitalization will depend on child's response to the antibiotic therapy
    (3) With appropriate treatment, illness is benign
v. Osteomyelitis
  (a) Characteristics
    (1) An infection primarily of a long bone, but can develop in any bone
    (2) Presents with:
      a) Redness
      b) Tenderness over involved bone and decreased ROM in the adjacent joint
      c) Swelling at site
      d) Unwillingness or inability to use affected limb
      e) Guarding of area
  (b) Systemic symptoms follow
    (1) Fever
    (2) Chills are common
    (3) Lethargy
    (4) Irritability
  (c) Etiology
    (1) Infection most commonly caused by *S. aureus*
    (2) Usually spreads from another primary site such as:
      a) Skin trauma
      b) Ear
      c) Throat infection
  (d) Prevalence
    (1) Occurs most commonly in children:
      a) Less than 1 year of age
      b) Between 3 and 10 years of age
    (2) More common in boys
  (e) Diagnosis
    (1) Clinical findings as described above
    (2) Gold standard is aspiration to identify the organism
    (3) Laboratory findings
      a) Leukocytosis with shift to left
      b) Elevated erythrocyte sedimentation rate (ESR) in most children
      c) Elevated C-reactive protein
      d) Positive blood cultures (~50% of cases)
    (4) X-rays
      a) Usually negative for first 10 to 14 days
      b) Bone destruction and lysis may be evident later

(5) MRI

(6) CT scan

(7) Ultrasound can detect fluid collection and abnormal bone surfaces

(f) Treatment

    (1) Immediate referral to physician

    (2) Initial hospitalization for intravenous antibiotics

        a) Continued for 4 to 6 weeks

        b) Home IV therapy is common

(g) Prognosis

    (1) Excellent with proper prompt treatment

    (2) Occasional failure to respond to antibiotic therapy may result in permanent bone damage

  **vi.** Toxic, transient synovitis (Whitelaw & Schilkler, 2004)

    (a) Characteristics

      (1) A transient, nonspecific, common, unilateral, inflammatory arthritis of the hip

      (2) Presents with:

        a) Acute onset of hip pain not associated with trauma

        b) Diminished active and passive ROM (decreased hip extension and internal rotation)

        c) Painful limp

        d) Crying at night

      (3) Frequently follows a history of an upper respiratory infection

    b) Prevalence and incidence

      (1) The most common cause of nontraumatic painful limp in children.

      (2) Incidence increases in young boys

      (3) Occurs twice as often in boys

      (4) Peaks between 3 and 6 years of age

    (c) Diagnosis

      (1) Clinical findings as described above

      (2) May have slight leukocytosis with an elevated ESR

      (3) Diagnosis of exclusion

        a) Hip x-ray usually demonstrates a normal hip

        b) No other obvious cause

    (d) Treatment

      (1) Bed rest

      (2) No weight bearing on painful limb

      (3) NSAIDs for pain relief (see Chapter 55, Table 55-5 for details)

    (e) Prognosis

      (1) Usually self-limiting with recovery in 3 to 5 days

      (2) Good prognosis—a benign disorder

 **vii.** Juvenile rheumatoid arthritis (JRA) (Calmbach & Hutchens, 2003; Hong, 2003) (see Chapter 48)

**viii.** Osgood-Schlatter disease, aseptic necrosis of tibial tubercle, tibial apophysitis

    (a) Characteristics

      (1) A painful swelling of tibial tubercle

      (2) Painful limp

      (3) Intermittent pain over period of months

(b) Etiology and prevalence
    (1) Considered an overuse injury during adolescence
    (2) Associated with athletic activity during times of rapid growth
    (3) Usually develops during periods of rapid growth of the tibial tubercle
    (4) Caused by detachment of cartilage fragments from the tibial tuberosity
    (5) Pain and limp can be aggravated by extension of knee against resistance
        a) Pressure over the tibial tubercle
        b) Worsened by activity, especially squatting, stair walking, forceful contraction of the quadriceps
        c) Relieved by rest
    (6) Occurs in males more than in females
(c) Diagnosis
    (1) Clinical observations as described above
    (2) A diagnosis of exception by ruling out other disorders
    (3) May be visualized on x-ray
    (4) MRI should be used if osteochondral lesion is suspected
(d) Treatment
    (1) Activity modification
    (2) Activity restriction may be necessary in severe cases
    (3) Athletes can continue to play but need to adjust training or participation in relation to pain
    (4) Ice
    (5) NSAIDs (see Chapter 55, Table 55-5 for details)
    (6) Quadriceps strengthening and stretching is helpful to minimize recurrence
    (7) A tibial band may be used during periods of activity
(e) Prognosis
    (1) Excellent—condition is self-limiting
    (2) In rare cases, atrophy of the quadriceps muscles may occur

ix. Legg-Calvé-Perthes disease (avascular necrosis of the femoral head epiphyses) (Nochimson, 2005)
  (a) Characteristics
    (1) Insidious onset of a painful limp
    (2) Thigh, hip and/or knee pain that is worse with activity and relieved by rest
    (3) Restriction of voluntary motion
    (4) Limited and painful passive motions
    (5) Limited abduction and rotation of affected hip
    (6) May see atrophy of thigh or calf muscle
  (b) Etiology
    (1) An idiopathic avascular necrosis of the femoral head
    (2) May be associated with:
        a) Trauma
        b) Transient synovitis
        c) Coagulation abnormalities
  (c) Prevalence
    (1) Relatively uncommon, 1 in 1200 children younger than age 15
    (2) Boys, ages 4 to 10 years, are affected four times more often than girls

(3) Associated with:
a) Low birth weight
b) Low socioeconomic status
c) White race
(d) Diagnosis
(1) Hip x-ray
(2) MRI
a) Should be conducted on any child with persistent limp and limited motion
b) Will reveal femoral head necrosis
(e) Treatment
(1) An abduction brace or long leg cast can effectively contain the hip in the socket
(2) Surgery may be needed if compliance with bracing or casting is inconsistent or bone reconstruction is necessary
(f) Prognosis
(1) Generally good for children younger than the age of 6 years
(2) Children older than 8 years typically do very poorly, with lifelong sequelae
x. Malignancies (Goyal, et al., 2004)
(a) Bone cancer accounts for 6% of all total cases of childhood cancer
(b) Characteristics
(1) Limb pain
(2) Pain with activity
(3) May or may not be a visible, palpable lump
(c) Requires immediate referral to oncology specialists
(1) Delay in diagnosis and referral was studied in 115 patients with newly diagnosed osteosarcoma and Ewing's sarcoma (Goyal, et al., 2004)
(2) Delay from first report of symptom to referral was 3.8 months (range 1 to 46 months)
(3) Patients older than 12 years had a longer delay
(4) However, the delay did not influence overall progress or survival in this sample
(5) Metastases to lungs and other organs may occur
(d) Osteosarcoma (Mehlman & Cripe, 2005)
(1) Rapidly growing malignant tumor of the bone
a) Originates from osteoblasts
b) Found in areas of active skeletal growth such as:
i) Humerus—most common site in children
ii) Distal femur
iii) Proximal tibia
(2) Prevalence
a) Most common (but still rare) malignant bone tumor in adolescents and young adults ages 10 to 25 years
b) Occurs more often in males (5.2/million males per year) than females (4.5/million females per year)
c) More common in Black than white children
(3) Risk factors
a) Radiation exposure
b) Rapid bone growth
c) Genetic predisposition

        (4) Diagnostic tests
          a) Frequently made by x-ray
          b) Confirmed by bone biopsy
        (5) Treatment
          a) Surgical removal of tumor
          b) Amputation is frequently necessary
          c) Limb salvage may be an option
          d) Chemotherapy
        (6) Prognosis is dependent on:
          a) Location of tumor
          b) Extent of surgery needed
          c) Presence of metastatic lesions
     (e) Ewing's sarcoma
        (1) Most lethal type
        (2) Second most common malignant bone tumor
          a) Round-cell tumor of the bone
          b) Originates in myelogenic cells of bone marrow
        (3) Found in:
          a) Pelvis
          b) Humerus
          c) Femur
          d) Clavicle
          e) Fibula
        (4) Prevalence
          a) Occurs mostly in adolescents and young adults ages 10 to 30 years
          b) Males are affected twice as often as females
        (5) Diagnostic tests
          a) Frequently made by x-ray
          b) Confirmed by bone biopsy
          c) Laboratory findings may include:
            i) Leukocytosis with a left shift
            ii) Increased ESR
        (6) Treatment
          a) Treated with chemotherapy
          b) Radiation, depending on tumor location
        (7) Prognosis
          a) Dependent on location of tumor
          b) Extent of surgery needed
          c) Presence of metastatic lesions

**4.** Symptom and sign: back pain, neck pain, back or neck deformity
  **a.** Back pain or deformity may develop:
    **i.** After an acute illness
    **ii.** Over time during periods of growth
    **iii.** From repeated trauma to the spine
  **b.** Early detection through screening and early management is important to minimize deformities
  **c.** Focused assessment
    **i.** Symptom analysis
    **ii.** Inspection
      (a) Gait
      (b) Movement from various positions

        (1) Sitting
        (2) Lying
        (3) Standing
     (c) Muscle movement, including:
        (1) Coordination
        (2) Spontaneity of movement
        (3) Symmetry
     (d) Swelling, redness
     (e) Scoliometry
   iii. Palpation
     (a) Tenderness
     (b) Deep tendon reflexes
     (c) Generalized muscle tone
        (1) Symmetry
     (d) Strength of:
        (1) Spine movement
        (2) Upper and lower extremity
        (3) Grasp
     (e) Spine
        (1) Passive ROM
        (2) Active ROM
     (f) Sensation
     (g) Circulation
 **d.** Differential diagnosis
   **i.** Trauma—spondylisthesis, spondylosis
   **ii.** Kyphosis
   **iii.** Lordosis
   **iv.** Scoliosis—functional, structural
   **v.** Torticollis
 **e.** Trauma (spondylolisthesis, spondylosis)
   **i.** The most common disorders leading to back pain in children include:
     (a) Stress fractures
     (b) Infection
     (c) Tumors
   **ii.** Typical back injuries in children occur between the lowest lumbar vertebra (L5) and the sacrum (S1)
   **iii.** A forward slip of the upper vertebral body (spondylolisthesis) or acute fracture (spondylosis) can occur
   **iv.** Etiology
     (a) Significant injury is usually the cause of acute trauma
        (1) Can occur at any age
        (2) Most common in young athletes in early adolescence with a higher incidence in:
          a) Ballet
          b) Gymnastics
          c) Skating
          d) Wrestling
          e) Football
     (b) Heredity plays a significant role
     (c) Spondylolysis is associated with an increased incidence of other congenital spinal defects (Huether & McCance, 2004)
   **v.** Diagnostic tests (Jarvik & Deyo, 2002)

(a) X-ray is frequently diagnostic

(b) Bone scan may be required to identify an acute process

(c) MRI and CT are usually reserved for patients who are considering surgery or those who are suspected of having systemic disease

  **vi.** Treatment

(a) Short-term rest

(b) NSAIDs for pain control (see Chapter 55, Table 55-5 for details)

(c) Bracing during the acute stages.

(d) Surgery is rarely needed, only if the pain is disabling or chronic.

  **vii.** Prognosis

(a) Depends on severity of illness and effectiveness of treatment

(b) Recurrence of back pain may occur and is usually muscular in origin

 **viii.** Follow-up

(a) Frequent

(b) Necessary if pain continues

(c) Monitor for any change in neurologic status

    (1) Sensation

    (2) Tingling

    (3) Numbness of extremities

(d) Continued follow-up into adulthood is needed, especially with vertebral slip

 **f.** Kyphosis (Brady & Burns, 2004)

  **i.** Definition—anteroposterior (AP) curve of thoracic spine (Figure 34-2)

  **ii.** Characteristics

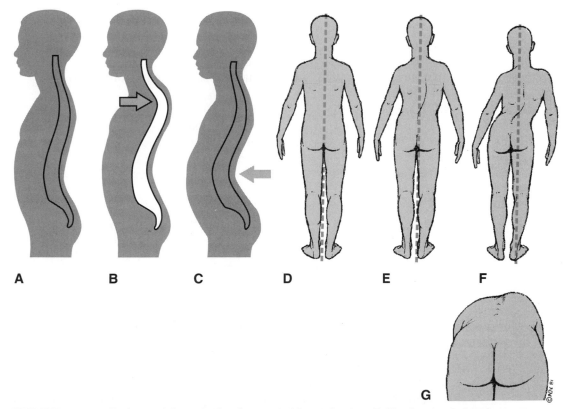

**A**      **B**      **C**      **D**      **E**      **F**

**G**

FIGURE 34-2 ■ Defects of the spinal column. **A,** Normal spine. **B,** Kyphosis. **C,** Lordosis. **D,** Normal spine in balance. **E,** Mild scoliosis in balance. **F,** Severe scoliosis not in balance. **G,** Rib hump flank asymmentry seen in flexion caused by rotary component (From Wong, et al. [2001]. *Wong's essentials of pediatric nursing* (6th ed.). St. Louis: Mosby, Figure 31-18, p. 1230.)

(a) Round back

(b) Poor posture

iii. Etiology

(a) Familial

(b) Congenital

(c) Secondary to tumor, trauma

(d) Postural (not a true kyphosis)

iv. Treatment

(a) Refer to orthopedics

(b) Physical therapy

g. Lordosis (Brady & Burns, 2004)

i. Definition—AP curve of lumbar spine (see Figure 34-2)

ii. Characteristics

(a) Protruding abdomen and buttocks

iii. Etiology

(a) Hip contractures (lordosis disappears when sitting)

(b) Typical of some family and racial groups

(c) Physiologic (lordosis disappears when bending forward)

iv. Treatment

(a) No treatment for physiologic lordosis

(b) Refer to orthopedics if lordosis is fixed

h. Scoliosis (Huether & McCance, 2004; Taft & Francis, 2004)

i. Definition—lateral curvature of spine (see Figure 34-2)

ii. Incidence

(a) Incidence is as high as 1 per 200 children

(b) Greater incidence for adolescent girls

(c) Boys tend to have a more aggressive course

(d) Onset usually during pubertal growth

iii. Etiology

(a) Idiopathic etiology in 80% of cases

(b) May be associated with familial and some genetic influences

iv. Treatment

(a) Functional scoliosis

(1) Curvatures between 5 to 10 degrees are considered to be functional spinal asymmetry and not true scoliosis

(2) Monitored over time in primary care setting

(b) Structural scoliosis

(1) Mild cases

a) Curvatures less than 20 degrees

b) Requires close observation for evidence of progression

c) Follow-up every 3 to 4 months during growth spurts

(2) More serious cases are curves that progress to 25 to 40 degrees

a) Refer to orthopedic specialists

b) Milwaukee brace

i) Bracing slows the curvature process

ii) Usually needed 23 hours per day

(c) Back exercises as prescribed by orthopedist

(d) Spinal fusion surgery may be necessary if bracing does not slow curvature progression, or for severe curves

(e) Primary care providers should recognize that bracing and spinal fusion surgery can create significant psychologic and social issues in the adolescent (LaMontagne, et al., 2004)

        (1) Psychosocial issues

          a) Negative body image

          b) Depression

          c) Limitations in mobility and therefore ability to participate in sports, group activities

          d) Decreased independence

        (2) LaMontagne et al. (2004) compared the effects of three cognitive-behavioral interventions with a control group on adolescents' physical and social activities after spinal fusion surgery:

          a) Groups

            i) Concrete objective information about the surgery and post-surgical self-care

            ii) Coping-only intervention taught coping strategies for pre- and postoperative self-care

            iii) Concrete objective information and coping strategies

            iv) Control group—usual care

          b) Group 1 showed a significant increase in activities from 3 to 6 months postop

          c) For younger adolescents, groups 3 and 4 engaged in more social activities than group 2; no differences among groups for older adolescents

          d) Additional interventions that address return to social activities are needed

          e) Emphasize the temporary nature of these treatments

          f) Encourage participation in school and community activities, especially clubs, etc. that do not require vigorous movement

  **v.** Prognosis

    (a) Functional scoliosis is self-limiting

    (b) Prognosis for moderate to severe structural scoliosis is good with successful bracing and back exercises

    (c) Progressive structural scoliosis produces prominent scapula and ribs, uneven shoulders, and an asymmetric waistline

    (d) Untreated scoliosis can cause pressure on internal organs, leasing to respiratory distress and heart problems

    (e) Structural scoliosis most likely leads to long-term back pain

  **vi.** Follow-up

    (a) During treatment is per orthopedic specialist

    (b) Annual well child exams, with scoliosis assessment necessary during adolescence

**i.** Torticollis (see Chapter 35)

  **i.** Characteristics

    (a) Flexed neck that deviates toward side that has a shortened sternocleidomastoid muscle

    (b) A palpable mass over the muscle may be felt, especially in infants during the first month of life

  **ii.** Incidence and etiology

    (a) Incidence is unknown

    (b) A congenital or acquired condition

    (c) May be a self limiting *muscular* problem due to minor soft tissue trauma

    (d) May be self-limiting due to an *inflammatory* process (Note: may be a *sign* of these processes as well)

(1) Adenitis

(2) Pharyngitis

(3) Retropharyngeal abscess

iii. Diagnostic tests

(a) X-ray may be needed to identify disorder of the spine or disks

(b) CT scan may be necessary to exclude vertebral anomalies

iv. Treatment

(a) Accurate diagnosis is critical to prevent neurologic damage from vigorous manipulation or physical therapy

(b) Treatment of the underlying inflammatory processes

(c) Early therapy for muscular torticollis involves:

(1) Gentle, stretching exercises and positioning

(2) Brace or surgical correction may be necessary in severe cases

(d) NSAIDs for pain management (see Chapter 55, Table 55-5 for details)

v. Prognosis is excellent with accurate diagnosis and appropriate treatment

5. Symptom and sign: arm pain, limited mobility of arm

a. Decreased movement of the arm is never normal

b. Focused assessment

i. Symptom analysis

ii. Inspection

(a) Swelling or redness of arm, shoulder, hand, fingers

(b) Passive arm position

(c) Spontaneous arm movement

(d) Active ROM

(e) Symmetry

iii. Palpation

(a) Circulation, warmth of extremity

(b) Passive ROM

(c) Strength of arm movement

(d) Muscle tone

(e) Symmetry

c. Differential diagnosis

i. Brachial plexus injuries

ii. Subluxation of radial head (nursemaid's elbow)

iii. Overuse injuries

(a) "Little League" elbow

d. Brachial plexus injuries (Brady & Burns, 2004)

i. Characteristics

(a) Found mostly in newborns: 0.28 to 2.6 of 100 full-term newborns

(b) Paralysis or limited movement of the limb

(c) Absent or incomplete reflexes on affected side: biceps, Moro, grasp

ii. Etiology

(a) Damage to brachial plexus and nerves C5 to C7 and T1 due to:

(1) Traumatic stretching of neck and shoulder during birth

(2) Unknown injury in utero

(b) Labeled as types I to IV based on increasing level of nerve involvement

iii. Diagnostic tests

(a) X-ray to rule out fractures

(b) Electromyography

iv. Treatment and prognosis

(a) Refer to pediatric orthopedics

(b) Recovery ranges from complete (types I, II) to variable (type III) and complete paralysis (type IV)

**e.** Subluxation of radial head

  **i.** Characteristics

  (a) History of sudden onset of elbow pain after the arm has been pulled

  (b) Refusal to move the arm

  (c) Arm held in slight flexion with the forearm pronated

  (d) Limited supination

  (e) Flexion and extension remains normal

  (f) No swelling, ecchymosis, or other signs of injury

  **ii.** Etiology

  (a) Most common in children less than 4 years of age

  (b) Immature radial head and annular ligament

  (c) Dislocation of radial head

  **iii.** Diagnostic tests

  (a) Clinical observations as noted above

  (b) X-rays should only be taken after one or two attempts at closed reduction

  **iv.** Treatment

  (a) Reduction of subluxation

   (1) Apply pressure to head of radius, and supinate arm in 90-degree flexion

   (2) If successful, provider may feel a "clunk" and note freer and less painful rotation of the forearm

   (3) Dramatic relief of pain if conducted shortly after injury

  (b) Instruct parents not to lift child by the arm in the future

  (c) If dislocation occurs frequently, bracing or short-term casting may be necessary

  (d) If dislocation occurs in children older than 3 or 4 years, surgical reconstruction of the ligamentous structure may be necessary

  **v.** Prognosis is typically excellent with no sequelae

  **vi.** Follow-up only as needed for pain or decreased ROM

**f.** Overuse injury, "Little League elbow" (Boyarski & Rank, 2004)

  **i.** Characteristics

  (a) Primary presenting symptom is pain in elbow

  (b) May also have:

   (1) Decreased elbow ROM

   (2) Mild flexion contracture

   (3) Point tenderness

   (4) Swelling

   (5) Decreased performance in throwing a ball

  **ii.** Etiology and incidence

  (a) An overuse injury of the elbow, usually from excessive overhand throwing of a baseball

  (b) The physical stress of throwing overhand produces exceptional forces in and around the elbow

  (c) During the throwing motion, valgus stress is placed on the elbow

  (d) Valgus stress results in tension on the medial structures

  (e) Repetition of this action causes pathologic changes in and about the elbow joint when tissue damage exceeds the rate of tissue repair

  (f) Annually, an estimated 4.8 million children ages 5 to 14 years participate in baseball and softball

(g) Incidence of all baseball-related injuries is 2% to 8% per year

(h) Highest incidence in the adolescent age group: 30% to 50% of all injuries are due to overuse

(i) Prevalence should decrease with Little League policy changes

(1) Decreased number of games per week

(2) Young pitchers pitch no more than six innings per week with 3 days off between games

(3) Managers must constantly observe the technique of young pitchers and monitor their fatigue levels

iii. Diagnosis

(a) Clinical observations as described above

(b) X-ray

iv. Treatment

(a) See PRICE protocol (Table 34-1)

(b) Initially, ice can be applied to painful elbow specifically over any noticeable swelling, tenderness

(c) Resting the pitching arm

(d) Progressive rehabilitation once healing has occurred (usually 3 to 4 weeks)

(e) Ibuprofen can be used to help with pain control (see Chapter 55, Table 55-5)

v. Prognosis is good with proper treatment and prevention

6. Sign: musculoskeletal developmental delay

a. Characteristics

i. Any developmental delay, musculoskeletal activity that is behind what would be normally expected for the age of the child should be considered abnormal

ii. Either a slow or rapid onset

b. Differential diagnosis—delay due to:

i. Acute illness

ii. Lengthy chronic illness

iii. Neurologic disorders such as spinal cord injury, paralysis

iv. Congenital syndromes

v. Muscular dystrophy

vi. Social issues

(a) Neglect

(b) Abuse

(c) Nonorganic failure to thrive (FTT)

(d) Psychologic disorders such as hysteria, anxiety

vii. Organic FTT due to disorders such as malabsorption, malnutrition

c. Focused assessment

i. Compare child's musculoskeletal abilities to standardized developmental norms

ii. The Denver II is a standardized tool that assesses fine and gross motor activities of children ages birth through 6 years (see Chapter 4)

d. Muscular dystrophy

i. Characteristics (El-Bohy & Wong, 2005)

(a) Newborn (congenital muscular dystrophy) (Mercuri & Longman, 2005)

(1) Hypotonia

(2) Muscle weakness

(3) Contractures

      (4) Motor delay

    (b) Older infants to preschoolers

      (1) Previously acquired motor skills gradually disappear between ages 2 to 4 years

      (2) Parent report of child "walking funny," clumsy, persistent toe-walking, unusual method of getting from the floor to a standing position (Gower's maneuver)

      (3) Muscle weakness appears first in lower extremities

        a) Progressive involvement of other skeletal muscles

      (4) Eventually involves muscles of the:

        a) Upper extremities

        b) Chest wall

        c) Heart

**ii.** Etiology and incidence (El-Bohy & Wong, 2005; Mercuri & Longman, 2005; Wong, 2005)

    (a) A heterogeneous group of inherited muscle disorders

      (1) Congenital muscular dystrophy (MD)—six types, with and without CNS involvement

      (2) X-linked recessive

        a) Transmitted by unaffected female carriers through the dystrophin gene

        b) Absence of dystrophin in the muscle membrane leads to progressive skeletal and cardiac muscle damage

        c) Duchenne's MD is the most common and the most severe

        d) Duchenne's MD affects approximately 1 in 3500 males

        e) Becker's MD is a milder variation that manifests as muscle aches after exercise

        f) Occur more typically in males

        g) The average age of diagnosis of MD is 3 to 5 years

      (3) There are about six other types

**iii.** Focused assessment (El-Bohy & Wong, 2005)

    (a) Detailed antenatal and birth history

    (b) History of motor milestones

    (c) Musculoskeletal assessment (see Chapter 12)

    (d) Neurologic assessment (see Chapter 13)

    (e) Increasing incidence of Gower's maneuver in rising from a sitting to standing position is especially suspicious

**iv.** Diagnostic tests (El-Bohy & Wong, 2005)

    (a) Diagnosis is based on classic clinical findings described above

    (b) Elevated serum creatine kinase is a good screening test for MD

    (c) Immediate referral to orthopedic specialists is necessary; tests they will conduct:

      (1) Muscle biopsy, which will demonstrate characteristic MD changes in muscle tissue

      (2) MRI

      (3) Electromyography, which will show classic myopathic characteristics

      (4) Genetic

**v.** Treatment

    (a) The use of a multidisciplinary health care team is necessary to balance to lifelong and ever increasing needs of the patient and family (Weidner, 2004)

    (b) No effective treatment

    (c) The goal of therapy is maintenance of maximal function for as long as possible

    (d) Corticosteroids slow the rate of progression by at least 2 to 4 years (Wong, 2005)

    (e) Supportive therapies are helpful

        (1) Physical therapy

        (2) Nutritionist (for weight control)

        (3) Orthotics may be helpful

  **vi.** Prognosis

    (a) Poor with progressing decrease in muscle strength and action over time

    (b) Eventually the chest wall muscle and heart become affected, causing death

# REFERENCES

American Academy of Pediatrics, Committee on Infectious Disease (2003). *Red book: 2003 Report of the Committee on Infectious Diseases* (26th ed.). Elk Grove Village, IL: American Academy of Pediatrics.

Boyarsky, I., & Rank, C. (2004). Little League elbow syndrome. Retrieved from eMedicine on May 12, 2006, at www.emedicine.com/sports/topic62.htm.

Brady, M. A., & Burns, C. E. (2004). Musculoskeletal disorders. In C. E. Burns, A. M. Dunn, M. A. Brady, et al. (Eds.). *Pediatric primary care: A handbook for nurse practitioners* (3rd ed.). Philadelphia: Saunders, pp. 1047-1082.

Calmbach, W. L., & Hutchens, M. (2003). Evaluation of patients presenting with knee pain; Part II: Differential diagnosis. *Am Fam Phys, 68*(5), 917-922.

El-Bohy, A. A., & Wong, B. L. (2005). The diagnosis of muscular dystrophy. *Pediatr Ann, 34*(7), 525-530.

Family Practice Notebook.com. Retrieved on May 13, 2006 at *http://www.fpnotebook.com.*

Foot & Ankle Institute (2006). Retrieved on May 12, 2006 from http://www.footankleinstitute.com/Anklesprain.html.

Ganel, A., Dudkiewicz, I., & Grogan, D. P. (2003). Pediatric orthopedic physical examination of the infant: A 5-minute assessment. *J Pediatr Health Care, 17*(1), 39-41.

Gore, A. I., & Spencer, J. P. (2004). The newborn foot. *Am Fam Phys, 69*(4), 865-872.

Goyal, S., Roscoe, J., Ryder, W. D., et al. (2004). Symptom interval in young people with bone cancer. *Eur J Cancer, 40*(15), 2280-2286.

GP Notebook.com. Retrieved on May 13, 2006 at http://www.gpnotebook.co.uk.

Hashkes, P. J., Gorenberg, M., Oren, V., et al. (2004). "Growing pains" in children are not associated with changes in vascular perfusion patterns in painful regions. *Clin Rheumatol, 24*(4), 342-345.

Hong, E. (2003) An approach to knee pain. Patient care for the nurse practitioner. Retrieved on May 12, 2006 from www.patientcarenp.com/be_core/content/journals/n/data/2003.html.

Jarvik, J. B., & Deyo, R. T. (2002) Diagnostic evaluation of low back pain with emphasis on imaging. *J Intern Med, 137*, 586-597.

LaMontagne, L. L., Hepworth, J. T., Cohen, F., & Salisbury, M. H. (2004). Adolescent scoliosis: Effects of corrective surgery, cognitive-behavioral interventions, and age on activity outcomes. *Appl Nurs Res, 17*(3), 168-177.

Mayo Clinic. (2005). Sprains and strains. Retrieved on May 12, 2006 from http://www.mayoclinic.com/health/sprains-and-strains/DS00343/DSECTION=9.

Mehlman, C. T., & Cripe, T. P. (2005). Osteosarcoma. Retrieved May 12, 2006, from www.emedicine.com/orthoped/topic531.htm.

Mercuri, E., & Longman, C. (2005). Congenital muscular dystrophy. *Pediatr Ann, 34*(7), 560-568.

Nochimson, G. (2005). Legg-Calve-Perthes disease. Retrieved from eMedicine on May 12, 2006, at www.emedicine.com/emerg/topic294.htm.

Rimando, M. P. (2005). Ankle sprain. Retrieved from eMedicine on May 12, 2006 at http://www.emedicine.com/pmr/topic11.htm.

Santarlasci, P. R. (2000). Weekend warrior: Common injuries in recreational athletes. *Adv Nurse Pract, 8*(4), 42-46.

Seidel, H. M., Ball, J., Dains, J. E., & Benedict, G. W. (2003). *Mosby's guide to physical examination* (5th ed.). St. Louis: Mosby.

Taft, E., & Francis, R. (2003). Evaluation and management of scoliosis. *J Pediatr Health Care, 17*(1), 42-44.

Weidner, N. J. (2005). Developing an interdisciplinary palliative care plan for the patient with muscular dystrophy. *Pediatr Ann, 34*(7), 547-552.

Whitelaw, C. C., & Schikler, K. N. (2004). Transient synovitis. Retrieved from eMedicine on May 12, 2006, at www.emedicine.com/ped/topic1676.htm.

Wolfe, M. W., Uhl, T. L., & McCluskey, L. C. (2001) Management of ankle sprains. *Am Fam Phys, 63*(1), 93-104.

Wong, B. L. (2005). Muscular dystrophies. *Pediatr Ann, 34*(7), 507-510.

# Common Illness of the Neurologic System

RITAMARIE JOHN, RN, DrNP, PNP

1. Signs: unusual size and/or shape of the head
   a. Embryologic development of the skull (Larsen, 2001; Moore & Persaud, 2003)
      i. Skull derives from mesenchyme around the developing brain
         (a) Neurocranium—a protective case for the brain
            (1) Several cartilages fuse
            (2) Endochondral ossification forms bones at base of skull
         (b) Viscerocranium—jaw bones
            (1) Intramembranous ossification forms the premaxilla, maxilla, zygomatic and squamous temporal bones, mandible
      ii. Osteoblasts from the mesoderm manufacture bone
      iii. Flexible fibrous sutures that separate plates of bone accommodate growth of the brain (Figure 35-1)
   b. Normal skull growth patterns (Sheth & Iskandar, 2005)
      i. Five bones (skull plates) join to form the skull
      ii. Four sutures separate the skull plates at birth
         (a) Sutures contain osteogenic cells, blood vessels, connective tissue
         (b) Sutures fuse at predictable rates that allow for brain growth and normal shaping of the head
         (c) Recent studies show that *noggin,* a bone morphogenetic protein antagonist, is involved in closure of sutures (Warren, et al., 2003)
         (d) Growth of the sagittal suture increases the width of the skull
      iii. Fontanelles are two fibrous areas at the junction of the skull plates that allow for growth and molding of the skull
      iv. *Craniotabes* is a term that refers to the skull's ability to indent under pressure, then spring back
      v. Skull ossification continues through puberty until mid-20s
   c. Focused assessment
      i. Focused family history
         (a) Appearance and shape of mother's and father's head
         (b) Family history of neurologic disorders
         (c) History of craniofacial abnormalities
         (d) Developmental delays
         (e) Prenatal and perinatal history of mother
            (1) Familial relationship to father (metabolic disorders are higher among consanguineous parents)

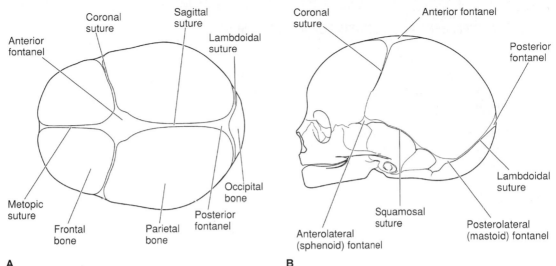

FIGURE 35-1 ■ Normal sutures. (From Goldbloom, R. B. (2003). *Pediatric clinical skills* [3rd ed.]. Philadelphia: Saunders).

        (2) Diet
        (3) Drug use
        (4) Trauma
        (5) Infections
  ii. Focused infant history
     (a) Delivery history—vaginal, C-section, breech, etc.
        (1) Gestational age
        (2) Shape of head at birth
        (3) Presence of cephalhematoma, caput succedaneum
        (4) Fontanelles
     (b) Timing of change in head shape—present at birth, sudden or gradual
     (c) Sleeping position
     (d) Pattern of repositioning during the day
     (e) Recent illness or injury
     (f) Change in level of consciousness, e.g., lethargy, stupor
     (g) Irritability
     (h) Change in feeding patterns
     (i) Chronology of attainment of normal developmental milestones
 iii. Focused physical assessment
     (a) Pattern of changes in head circumference (percentiles)
     (b) Pattern of changes in fontanelle shape and size
     (c) Examine and describe the head shape
        (1) From above (bird's-eye view)
        (2) Side view
        (3) Rear view
        (4) Face forward
     (d) Macrocephaly
        (1) A descriptive term, not a diagnosis
        (2) Head circumference more than 2 standard deviations above the mean for age and sex
        (3) Differential diagnoses for macrocephaly (Box 35-1)

■ **BOX 35-1**
■ **DIFFERENTIAL DIAGNOSIS FOR MACROCEPHALY**

**BIRTH TO 6 MONTHS**
- Hydrocephalus
- External hydrocephalus
- Megalencephaly
  - Familial
  - Cellular proliferation
  - Storage of metabolites
- Achondroplasia (skeletal dysplasia)
- Craniostenosis and associated syndromes
- Brain lesions
- Subdural effusion
- Intrauterine infection
- Peri- or postnatal hemorrhage

**OLDER THAN AGE 6 MONTHS**
- Megalencephaly
  - Cerebral gigantism (Sotos syndrome)
  - Neurocutaneous syndromes
  - Porencephaly
  - Metabolic CNS disease
    - Aminoaciduria
    - Leukodystrophies
    - Lysosomal storage disorder
- Hydrocephalus (arrested or progressive)
- Brain lesion
- Primary skeletal cranial dysplasia
- Increased intracranial pressure due to pseudotumor cerebri, cyanotic heart disease, hypoparathyroidism, lead, steroids
- Postbacterial meningitis
- Trauma or vascular malformation

From Johnston, M. V., & Kinsman, S. (2004). Microcephaly. In R. E. Behrman, R. M. Kliegman, & H. B. Jenson (Eds.). *Nelson textbook of pediatrics* (17th ed.). Philadelphia: Saunders, pp. 1988–1999, and others.

  (e) Transilluminate head with light
  (f) Listen for cranial bruits
  (g) Look for signs of increased intracranial pressure
      (1) Extraocular movement, particularly upward gaze
      (2) Bulging fontanelle
  (h) Plagiocephaly—flattening of a portion of the head
  (i) Bald spot at the back of head—if unilateral, evaluate for flattening on that side (Biggs, 2003)
  (j) Palpate for overriding sutures by feeling for a ridge over sutures (see Figure 35-1 for normal sutures)
  (k) Facial symmetry and structure
      (1) Evaluate for possible syndromes
          a) Eyes
              i) Not on same horizontal plane
              ii) Extraocular eye movement
              iii) Cover-uncover test at 6 months reveals muscle weakness
              iv) Evaluate fundi for retinal hemorrhages (abuse)

        v) Strabismus may cause the child to adopt an abnormal head posture, resulting in an abnormal head shape (Gupta, et al., 2003)

     b) Ears (Adams & Hugkins, 2003)

        i) Assymmetry in the position of ears

        ii) Low-set ears

        iii) One ear set posterior to the other

  (l) Neck

    (1) Weblike attachment of neck to shoulders suggests a syndrome

    (2) Limited range of motion

    (3) Evaluate for torticollis—with infant sitting on the mother's lap, infant should be able to follow an interesting object or a face that is moving from side to side (Persing, et al., 2003)

  (m) Other skeletal abnormalities

    (1) Limb abnormalities, i.e., short extremities

    (2) Examine spine for scoliosis

    (3) Developmental hip dysplasia is associated with abnormalities of head shape

    (4) Short extremities

  (n) Other major organ abnormalities

  (o) Evaluate muscle tone

  (p) Inspection of skin to consider neurocutaneous disorders (Conologue & Meffert, 2005), e.g., café-au-lait spots, multiple epidermal nevi, hypopigmented macules

**d.** Differential diagnoses for abnormal size and/or shape of the head (Shin & Persing, 2003)

  **i.** Megalencephaly—also called macrencephaly; head circumference greater than 98th percentile for age and sex

    (a) Primary megalencephaly

      (1) Present at birth; not due to disease

      (2) Autosomal dominant and familial

      (3) Associated with low intelligence level and mental retardation

    (b) True megalencephaly—a disturbance in cell regulation and reproduction leading to an abnormality of migration and organization within the brain, and abnormal neurologic development

    (c) Microcephaly (Johnston & Kinsman, 2004)

      (1) Head circumference more than three standard deviations below the mean for age and sex

      (2) Differential diagnoses for microcephaly (Box 35-2)

        a) Primary—genetic

        b) Secondary—not genetic

    (d) Nonsynostosis plagiocephaly

    (e) Craniosynostosis (also called craniostenosis) (Sargent, 2000)

      (1) Primary craniosynostosis

        a) Premature closure of one or more cranial sutures due to a defect in ossification

        b) Growth stops in direction that is perpendicular to the closed suture but continues in the direction parallel to the closed suture

        c) Terminology is based on the sutures that close early

          i) Scaphocephaly—sagittal suture; boat-shaped skull

          ii) Anterior plagiocephaly—1 coronal suture; flat skull

■ **BOX 35-2**
■ **DIFFERENTIAL DIAGNOSIS FOR MICROCEPHALY**

**PRIMARY: GENETIC FACTORS**
- Familial microcephaly—autosomal recessive
- Autosomal dominant
- Trisomy 18
- Trisomy 21
- Genetic deletion syndromes
- Ring chromosomes
- Nonchromosomal hereditary syndromes

**PRENATAL FACTORS**
- Maternal infection—CMV, rubella, toxoplasmosis
- Maternal radiation
- Maternal hyperthermia
- Maternal hypertension
- Maternal malnutrition
- Maternal diabetes
- Maternal hyperphenylalaninemia
- Placental insufficiency
- Intrauterine growth retardation
- Maternal radiation exposure
- Maternal smoking
- Maternal alcohol use
- Maternal drug use (cocaine and crack)

**PERINATAL INSULTS**
- Vascular damage to the developing brain from:
  o Neonatal stroke
  o Thrombosis of the vessel
  o Hypoxic-ischemic encephalopathy
  o Intracranial hemorrhage
  o Congenital infection
- Trauma

**POSTNATAL FACTORS**
- Meningitis
- Hypoxic-ischemic encephalopathy
- Intracranial hemorrhage
- CNS infections
- HIV infection
- Craniosynostosis
- Degenerative diseases
- Aminoacidurias
- Endocrine dysfunction
  o Hypothyroidism
  o Hypopituitarism
- Severe malnutrition
- Shaken baby syndrome

From Johnston, M. V., & Kinsman, S. (2004). Microcephaly. In R. E. Behrman, R. M. Kliegman, & H. B. Jenson (Eds.). *Nelson textbook of pediatrics* (17th ed.). Philadelphia: Saunders, pp. 1988–1999, and others.

        iii) Brachycephaly—bilateral coronal sutures; short skull
        iv) Posterior plagiocephaly—1 lambdoid suture; flat skull
        v) Trigonocephaly—metopic suture; triangular skull
    (2) Secondary craniosynostosis
       a) Premature closure of sutures due to failure of brain growth
       b) Usually accompanied by microcephaly
  **e.** Brief descriptions of common diagnoses
    **i.** Hydrocephalus
      (a) Pathophysiology (Zitelli & Davis, 2002)
        (1) Normally, cerebrospinal fluid (CSF) production and absorption are in equilibrium
        (2) CSF travels throughout ventricular system, surrounds brain, and is reabsorbed into venous system by arachnoid villi
        (3) Impaired absorption is the most common cause of hydrocephalus
        (4) Other causes are excessive production of CSF or obstructed circulation of CSF
        (5) CSF production can increase threefold when there is increased intracranial pressure
      (b) Signs and symptoms
        (1) Infant

   a) Progressively enlarging head
   b) Bulging fontanelles
   c) Enlarged scalp veins
(2) Child
   a) Headache
   b) Drowsiness
   c) Decreased cognitive ability
   d) Blurred vision
(c) Treatment—immediate referral to neurosurgeon for diagnostic testing and treatment
   (1) A ventriculoperitoneal (VP) shunt is inserted into the ventricles to release pressure of CSF and drain it into the abdominal cavity
   (2) VP shunt is associated with scaphocephaly (Cohen, 2000)
      a) The drop in intracranial pressure from the shunt signals the overlying sutures to close
      b) Skull thickens and the skull base changes, causing premature closure of the sagittal suture
   (3) Surgical correction of the abnormally shaped skull is possible
ii. External hydrocephalus
   (a) Pathophysiology—a benign enlargement of subarachnoid space in the frontal or frontoparietal region (Sarnat & Menkes, 2000)
   (b) Signs
      (1) Macrocephaly—head size rapidly increases to approximately the 90th percentile, then parallels the growth curve
      (2) Infant presents with a full but pulsatile anterior fontanelle with normal ventricles
   (c) Prevalence
      (1) 16% of infants with hydrocephalus have the external, benign type
      (2) Boys more than girls
   (d) Diagnostic tests
      (1) Cerebral ultrasound
      (2) MRI
   (e) Treatment—none, but referral to neurology for validation of diagnosis is wise
   (f) Prognosis
      (1) The condition resolves by 2 to 3 years
      (2) Large proportion of the children are developmentally normal (Handique, et al., 2002; Sarnat & Menkes, 2000)
iii. Familial microcephaly
   (a) Pathophysiology
      (1) MRI reveals lesions of gray and white matter, abnormal myelination pattern and disorders of neuronal migration, sulci, and gyri
   (b) Etiology and prevalence
      (1) Autosomal dominant form of familial microcephaly is milder and associated with normal intelligence or mild mental retardation
      (2) Autosomal recessive form in which the parents have normal head is associated with more severe mental retardation
   (c) Treatment—none, but referral to neurology for validation of diagnosis is wise
   (d) Prognosis (Berman, 2003)
      (1) Excellent if other family members are functioning normally

    (2) If the head is 3 standard deviations below the mean, there is higher incidence of developmental delay with cognitive impairment

  **iv.** Nonsynostotic (positional) plagiocephaly (Persing, et al., 2003)

   (a) Pathophysiology

    (1) Progressive craniofacial growth asymmetry due to positioning of head and neck

    (2) Normal closure of sutures

    (3) Flattening of the occipital area will cause frontal and temporal prominence (bossing)

    (4) Supine infant positioning causes external pressure on the skull, resulting in flattening (Biggs, 2003)

    (5) May be preceded by a sternocleidomastoid mass

     a) A benign fibrotic mass that can be palpated in the body of the muscle

     b) If mass is untreated, can lead to shortening of the muscle on the affected side (torticollis) and/or progressive craniofacial growth asymmetry

   (b) Prevalence

    (1) Prevalence has increased since 1992 when the "Back to Sleep" campaign was started by American Academy of Pediatrics (Biggs, 2003; Habal, et al., 2003)

    (2) A cohort study of 200 infants by Hutchison, et al. (2004) showed the following prevalence data

     a) Age 6 weeks: maximum range of head shape deformity was observed in cohort

     b) Age 4 months: greatest point prevalence at nearly 30% of the cohort

     c) Age 2 years: most infants improved over time, with a point prevalence of 3.3%

   (c) Diagnostic tests

    (1) If there is no improvement with exercise and positioning evaluate carefully for overriding or fused suture

    (2) If deformity is severe and craniosynostosis is suspected, radiographs or CT may be helpful

    (3) Refer to neurosurgeon, neurologist, or craniofacial team for further evaluation

   (d) Treatment (Persing, et al., 2003)

    (1) Position child's head on unaffected side

    (2) Exercise the neck side to side three times with each diaper change

     a) Turn the head toward the right shoulder, allowing chin to touch shoulder and hold it for 10 seconds and repeat on opposite side

     b) Then tilt the entire head toward the shoulder so the ear touches the shoulder for 10 seconds and repeat this exercise on the opposite side

    (3) Allow for supervised time on the child's abdomen

    (4) Helmet or headband therapy if no improvement; this must be done before 15 months in order to improve the head shape (Shin & Persing, 2003)

   (e) Prevention

    (1) During the newborn period teach the parents to position the infant's head from side to side on alternating days

(2) Encourage the family to gently move the infant's head from side to side

(3) After the infant is able to raise its own head, place the infant in a prone position during supervised "tummy time," which can avoid need for later intervention (Habal, 2003)

(f) Follow-up

(1) Congenital torticollis may occur if the there is stretching of the sternocleidomastoid muscle with a localized hematoma

(2) Routine well child visits if mild and compliance is excellent

(3) If the child fails to improve after 4 to 8 weeks of physical therapy, consider obtaining a three-dimensional CT and/or refer to surgeon

v. Positional scaphocephaly of prematurity

(1) Positional deformity from placement of the premature infant on a flat mattress and infant's inability to move head from side to side

(2) No premature closure of the sutures; head shape is long and narrow

(3) Recommend a waterbed or similar mattress and careful repositioning of the infant

2. Symptom: headache

a. Focused assessment

i. Symptom assessment

(a) Ask parent or child to describe a headache episode with attention to time of day, intensity, location and description of pain

(b) Prodromal signs or symptoms

(c) Aura (visual, auditory, olfactory, kinesthetic)

(d) Factors that precede, elicit, or aggravate the headache

(e) Does headache wake child from a sound sleep?

(f) Acute or chronic?

(g) Medications, dosage and effectiveness

(h) Related symptoms—sensory, motor, somatic

(i) Recommend a headache diary to identify the above factors

ii. Family history

(a) Migraine

(b) Other headaches

iii. Child history

(a) New onset of seizures

(b) Head trauma

(c) Change in headache history

b. Focused physical assessment

i. Blood pressure

ii. Measure child's head circumference if younger than age 3

iii. Thorough eye assessment (see Chapter 5)

iv. Teeth—signs of dental disease

v. See Box 35-3 for worrisome signs and symptoms of headache

c. Red flags in the diagnosis of headache that require immediate referral (Lipton, et al., 2004)

i. Sudden onset of headache

ii. Worsening pattern of headache

iii. Headache with systemic illness

iv. Focal neurologic signs other than typical aura

v. Papilledema

vi. Headache triggered by Valsalva, cough, or exertion

■ **BOX 35-3**
■ **WORRISOME SIGNS AND SYMPTOMS OF HEADACHE**

- Early morning headaches
- Progressive headache
- Persistent vomiting
- Changes in language skills
- Changes in motor skills
- Headaches that get worse with sneezing, coughing, or straining
- Diplopia (double vision)
- Visual field defects
- Impaired school performance

- Ataxia
- Macrocephaly
- Neurocutaneous lesions
- Difficulties with upward gaze
- Changes in mental status
- Growth abnormalities including precocious puberty
- Nuchal rigidity
- Hemiparesis
- Seizures

    **vii.** Headache during pregnancy or postpartum
   **viii.** New headache in patient with cancer, Lyme disease, HIV
 **d.** Prevalence (Lewis, et al., 2002 )
    **i.** A common pediatric symptom, particularly in adolescents
   **ii.** Prevalence: 37% to 51% in 7-year-olds and as high as 82% in 15-year-olds
 **e.** Differential diagnoses
    **i.** 2004 classification of headaches (Haslam, 2005; Headache Classification Subcommittee of the International Headache Society; Lipton, et al., 2004)
      **(a)** Primary headaches
        **(1)** Tension-type headaches
        **(2)** Migraine
        **(3)** Cluster headache and other trigeminal autonomic cephalgias (Lampl, 2002)
        **(4)** Other primary headaches
      **(b)** Secondary headaches—due to variety of injuries, illnesses, and disorders
    **ii.** Acute headache (Box 35-4)
   **iii.** Chronic, recurrent headache (Box 35-5)

■ **BOX 35-4**
■ **DIFFERENTIAL DIAGNOSIS FOR ACUTE HEADACHE**

**SYSTEMIC DISORDERS**
- Fever
- Viral illness
- Hypertension
- Electrolyte disturbances
- Hypoglycemia
- Exertion

**DISORDERS INVOLVING THE HEAD**
- Orbital infection
- Sinusitis
- Dental disease

**DISORDERS OF CNS**
- First migraine
- Postictal state
- First cluster headache
- Acute trauma
- Central nervous system bleed
- Pseudotumor cerebri
- Postinfectious hydrocephalus

**TOXINS AND DRUGS**
- Carbon monoxide poisoning
- Exposure to lead
- Drug use

■ **BOX 35-5**
■ **DIFFERENTIAL DIAGNOSES FOR CHRONIC RECURRENT HEADACHE**

- Migraine headache
- Cluster headache
- Tension headache
- Depression
- Sinusitis
- Allergies
- Tension and stress
- Conversion disorder
- Pseudotumor cerebri

- Increased intracranial pressure
- Oral contraceptives
- Withdrawal from steroids
- Brain tumor
- Environmental factors
- Sleep apnea
- Postconcussive syndrome
- Vascular malformations

 

 

**f.** Tension-type headache (Lipton, et al., 2004)
  **i.** Definition
    (a) Described as a tightening feeling (nonpulsating) with or without associated photophobia or phonophobia, but without nausea, vomiting, or exacerbation with activity
    (b) In children, it may be difficult to distinguish between migraine and tension headache due to their limited vocabulary for describing symptoms (Olness, 1999)
    (c) In the absence of other symptoms, recurrent headaches of more than 3 months' duration are rarely due to an organic cause
  **ii.** Pathophysiology
    (a) Most common type of headache; now believed to have a neurobiologic basis
    (b) Central pain mechanisms play a role in frequent tension headaches
    (c) Peripheral pain mechanisms play a role in infrequent episodic tension headaches
  **iii.** Prevalence
    (a) General prevalence is between 30% and 78% in the general population
    (b) More common in older girls
  **iv.** Diagnostic tests—no specific tests are required
  **v.** Treatment
    (a) Nonpharmacologic—avoid precipitating factors
    (b) Pharmacologic—nonsteroidal antiinflammatory drugs (NSAIDs) (see Chapter 55, Table 55-5)
  **vi.** Prognosis—no negative sequelae
**g.** Migraine headache (Haslam, 2004; Headache Classification Subcommittee, 2004; Hershey & Winner, 2005; Mack, 2006)
  **i.** Signs and symptoms
    (a) In children a migraine headache is a recurrent headache with symptom-free intervals and at least three of the following signs or symptoms:
      (1) Visual, sensory, or motor aura
      (2) Abdominal pain
      (3) Nausea or vomiting
      (4) Throbbing headache
      (5) Unilateral location

(6) Relief after sleeping

(7) Positive family history

(b) Usually frontotemporal and bilateral in children

(c) Occipital headaches are rare and require immediate evaluation

(d) School-aged children may also present without headaches, but with temporal or visual aura lasting 10 minutes and resolving within 1 hour

ii. Migraine classified into five categories (Haslam, 2004)

(a) Common migraine—most common type of migraine in children; no aura, 90% positive family history, signs and symptoms in numbers 2, 3, 4, 5, and 7 as listed above

(b) Migraine with aura (classic migraine)—visual auras are rare; may have vertigo, light-headedness, perioral paresthesia, numbness of hands and feet; symptoms during migraine include those listed above

(c) Migraine variants—e.g., cyclic vomiting, acute confusional states, benign paroxysmal vertigo (Li & Howard, 2002)

(d) Cluster headaches (rare in children)

(e) Complicated migraine—neurologic signs that occur during headache persist; suggests an underlying structural lesion

iii. Pathophysiology (Mack, 2006; Millichap & Yee, 2003)

(a) A neurovascular phenomenon in which a migraine generator in the trigeminal vascular complex acts as a relay station for signals that the thalamus and cortex perceive as pain

(b) The initial neuronal sensitization of trigeminal nerve ganglia is followed by a secondary phase of vasoconstriction, vasodilation, and vascular inflammation

(c) In the blood vessels, release of neurokinin, substance, and calcitonin gene reactive peptide (CGRP) cause dilatation, with subsequent pain

(d) Serotonin receptors in blood vessels play a prominent role

iv. Etiology

(a) Most common triggers are psychologic: stress, fatigue, anxiety (Haslam, 2004)

(b) See Box 35-6 for dietary factors in migraine headache

(c) See Box 35-7 for chronic periodic syndromes that are migraine precursors

v. Prevalence

(a) Migraine headaches start at age 6 to 7 in females and males equally

(b) Occurs in 5% to 10% of school-aged children (Mack, 2006)

(c) Most disabling headache disorder (Headache Classification Subcommittee, 2004; Millichap & Yee, 2003)

(d) At puberty, spontaneous remission occurs in many children, and the female/male ratio becomes 2:1

vi. Diagnostic tests (Lewis, et al., 2002)

(a) Guidelines show no value in routine lumbar puncture or electroencephalogram (EEG)

(b) EEG is recommended if there are motor or sensory components to the headache

(c) Guidelines do not recommend neuroimaging for patients with recurrent headaches and normal neurologic exams

(d) Neuroimaging is recommended if there are the following changes in headache history:

### ■ BOX 35-6
### ■ DIETARY FACTORS IN MIGRAINE

**FOOD TRIGGERS**
- Cheese
- Chocolate
- Citrus fruits
- Hot dogs, ham, cured meats
- Dairy products, yogurt, ice cream
- Fatty and fried foods
- Asian foods
- Coffee, tea, cola
- Food dyes, additives
- Artificial sweeteners
- Wines, beers
- Nuts
- Fasting

**CHEMICAL TRIGGERS**
- Tyramine
- Phenylethylamine
- Nitrites, nitric oxide
- Caffeine or caffeine withdrawal
- Linoleic and oleic fatty acids
- Monosodium glutamate
- Allergenic proteins
- Sulfites and tartrazine
- Aspartame
- Histamine, tyramine
- Stress hormone
- Hypoglycemia

Adapted from Millichap, J. G., & Yee, M. (2003). The diet factor in pediatric and adolescent migraine. *Pediatr Neurol, 28*(1), 1–14; and Mack, K. J. (2006). Episodic and chronic migraine in children. *Semin Neurol, 26*(2), 223–231.

### ■ BOX 35-7
### ■ CHILDHOOD PERIODIC SYNDROMES THAT ARE MIGRAINE PRECURSORS

**BENIGN PAROXYSMAL TORTICOLLIS**
- Age: infants to 8 months
- Primary symptom: torticollis
- Associated symptoms: pallor, vomiting, changes in behavior
- Time: episodic and nonprogressive
- Resolves by ages 2 to 5 with decreasing intervals

**CYCLIC VOMITING**
- Age: 4 to 10 years
- Primary symptom: severe vomiting
- Associated symptom: pallor
- Time: occurs frequently and regularly and can last for several hours

**ABDOMINAL MIGRAINE**
- Age: school-aged children
- Primary symptom: cramping abdominal pain located in periumbilical or epigastric areas
- Associated symptoms: vague headaches, motion sickness
- Time: self-limiting; resolves within 2 to 3 years

**BENIGN PAROXYSMAL VERTIGO**
- Primary symptom: vertigo
- May evolve from benign paroxysmal torticollis

From: Headache Classification Subcommittee of the International Headache Society. (2004). The International Classification of Headache Disorders (2nd ed.). *Cephalgia, 24*(Suppl. 1). Retrieved May 17, 2006, from http://216.25.100.131/ihscommon/guidelines/pdfs/ihc_II_main_no_print.pdf.

(1) Worsening headaches
(2) Changes in types of headaches
(3) Changes in neurologic function including changes in school performance
(4) Onset of severe headaches

  **vii.** Treatment (Wright, 2004)

    (a) Help patients understand that while medications can help, they work only 60% to 70% of the time

    (b) Nonpharmacologic treatments

      (1) Regular schedule
        a) Regular mealtimes
        b) Sleep pattern
        c) Regular exercise
      (2) Identify migraine triggers by keeping a headache diary of events that precede headaches
      (3) Avoid known triggers
        a) Foods—an estimated 50% of children with migraine have food triggers (Mack, 2006)
        b) Medication
        c) Activity
        d) Environmental
        e) Stress, anxiety
          i) Headaches may be worse at start of school
          ii) Identify and make efforts to decrease sources of stress
          iii) Relaxation techniques, e.g., yoga, meditation, mental imagery, breath control
      (4) Universal avoidance of the common triggers of migraine headaches can be recommended if the patient is noncompliant with keeping a headache diary
      (5) Behavioral therapy or counseling may be helpful to enhance:
        a) Self-esteem
        b) Feelings of personal mastery
        c) Coping skills
      (6) Biofeedback, self-hypnosis
    (c) Pharmacologic treatments
      (1) Acute treatments
        a) Ibuprofen, acetaminophen (see Chapter 55, Table 55-5 for details)
        b) Antiemetics for nausea and vomiting
        c) None of the triptans are currently approved for use in children and adolescents; therefore, their use is off label
      (2) Preventive treatments
        a) β-adrenergic–blocking agents
        b) Off-label use of the following drugs:
          i) Cyproheptadine
          ii) Calcium channel blockers
          iii) Antidepressants
          iv) Antiepileptics
  **viii.** Prognosis
    (a) Spontaneous remission is possible
    (b) May be a chronic condition throughout life
**3.** Symptom: closed head trauma
  **a.** Note: This section refers to cases that are likely to be brought to a primary care office, not multiple trauma, cervical spine injury, suspected shaken baby syndrome, or bleeding diathesis
  **b.** Identification of the mechanism of injury provides cues for focused assessment, but interview must be conducted carefully, without assumption of blame
  **c.** Mechanism of injury (Schutzman & Greenes, 2001)
    **i.** Is the mechanism of injury developmentally appropriate, i.e., plausible?
    **ii.** Was the head trauma witnessed, and by whom?

      **iii.** What happened between the time of the injury and when parents brought the child to the office?

      **iv.** Does the history vary from caretaker to caretaker?

      **v.** Does the history change over time?

      **vi.** Are there signs that the child might suffer from an inflicted head injury?

        (a) History is of minor injury but examination points to more serious injury

        (b) Delay in seeking medical advice

        (c) Repeated injuries

        (d) History of previous head injuries or concussions

        (e) Signs of other injury on the body in same or different stages of healing

        (f) Lack of explanation for what happened

**d.** Focused assessment of the child

    **i.** Signs and symptoms after the incident

      (a) Loss of consciousness at any time following the event

      (b) Glasgow Coma Scale score (if possible)

      (c) Vomiting, headache

      (d) Is the child acting like his or her usual self?

      (e) Changes in affect or memory (based on age)

        (1) Judgment

        (2) Orientation

        (3) Memory

        (4) Affect

        (5) Calculation

    **ii.** Does the child have pain anywhere at present?

    **iii.** Physical assessment

      (a) Bruising

      (b) Periorbital ecchymosis

      (c) Clear fluid or sanguineous fluid from nose or ears

      (d) Salty taste at back of throat

      (e) Point tenderness anywhere on body

      (f) Skull—bony or soft tissue abnormalities

    **iv.** Neurologic examination (see Chapter 13)

      (a) Evaluate for neck pain along the cervical spine

      (b) Facial expression

        (1) Symmetry

        (2) Dazed look with vacant stare following a concussion suggests basilar fracture and cranial nerve VII damage (Schutzman & Greenes, 2001)

      (c) Mental status

        (1) If the child is old enough, does the child have retrograde amnesia, i.e., failure to remember events that happened prior to the injury; may indicate a more severe injury

        (2) Does the child have antegrade amnesia, i.e., failure to remember the injury or events after the injury?

        (3) Is the child slow to answer questions?

        (4) Does the speech sound different to you or the parent?

      (d) Ear

        (1) Signs of middle ear hematoma may indicate basilar skull fracture (Schutzman & Greenes, 2001)

        (2) Hearing—use acoustic reflex or hearing screen including higher frequency of 4000, 6000, and 8000 Hertz (cycles per second) to evaluate for sensorineural loss

    **v.** Gross motor—if the child can walk, evaluate gait

**e.** Diagnostic testing—most tests will be conducted by specialists, but PNP should be familiar with the types of diagnostic tests and their purposes

    **i.** Plain radiograph of skull—94% to 99% sensitive for assessing linear or depressed skull fracture (Schutzman & Greenes, 2001)

    **ii.** Plain radiograph of neck—limited usefulness

    **iii.** Cranial ultrasound—only useful if fontanelles are open to detect ventricular size and intraventricular hemorrhage

    **iv.** Ultrasound of sacral spine—useful before age 3 months to evaluate spinal dysraphism

    **v.** CT scan of head—to evaluate calcifications, ventricle size, bleeding, bone structure

       **(a)** Only 47% to 94% sensitive for identifying fractures

       **(b)** Does not reveal the posterior fossa or brainstem as well as magnetic resonance imaging (MRI)

    **vi.** Three-dimensional CT of head—to evaluate craniofacial abnormalities and atlant-axial rotary subluxation

    **vii.** MRI—for detection of intraaxial pathology, congenital malformation of brain and spine; the only diagnostic tool for proper evaluation of posterior fossa

    **viii.** Functional MRI (MRI)—dynamic image measures oxygen consumption by visual, motor, or speech areas of brain; evaluates tumors and seizure foci

    **ix.** Magnetic resonance spectroscopy (MRS)—imaging of specific chemistry of brain to determine cell apoptosis related to epilepsy, tumor, and congenital malformations

    **x.** Magnetic resonance angiography (MRA)—images cerebral vascular pathology including aneurysm, AV malformation, and stroke

    **xi.** Myelogram—to identify spinal cord pathology

    **xii.** Conventional angiography—only used for intervention neuroradiology, i.e., embolization of aneurysm or arteriovenous malformation

    **xiii.** Positron emission tomography (PET)—using tagged radioactive isotopes, measures cerebral metabolic activity via glucose utilization

    **xiv.** Single photon emission computed tomography (SPECT)—to measure cerebral perfusion

    **xv.** EEG—records brain activity; used to diagnose epilepsy, sleep disorder, change in mental status, coma, differentiate pseudoseizures from seizures

    **xvi.** Brainstem auditory evoked potential (BAER)—determines level of hearing impairment and identifies lesion in the auditory pathway

    **xvii.** Visual evoked potential (VER)—identifies pathology of the visual pathway including cortical blindness

    **xviii.** Somatosensory evoked potential (SSEP)—identifies pathology between peripheral nerve and sensory cortex including spinal cord and brainstem lesions; differentiates hysteria versus pathologic blindness

    **xix.** Electromyography and nerve conduction velocity (EMG/NCV)—evaluates peripheral nerve, neuromuscular junction, and muscle pathology

    **xx.** Muscle or nerve biopsy—used in conjunction with immunohistochemistry for evaluation of muscular dystrophies such as dystrophin

**f.** Differential diagnoses for closed head trauma (Box 35-8)

■ **BOX 35-8**
■ **DIFFERENTIAL DIAGNOSES FOR CLOSED HEAD TRAUMA**

**BONE**
- Concussion and contusion
- Closed head trauma without concussion or fracture
- Linear fracture
- Depressed fracture
- Basilar fracture
- Compound fracture
- Diastasis (wide separation of bone)

**SKIN**
- Lacerations

**VASCULAR**
- Ecchymosis
- Subacute and chronic subdural hematoma
- Acute epidural hematoma
- Acute subdural hematoma

**NECK**
- Atlantoaxial dislocation or subluxation

g. Concussion
   i. Definition (Demorest & Landry, 2003; Perriello & Barth, 2000, Schutzman & Greenes, 2001)
      (a) There is no one definition or set of criteria for concussion
      (b) Loss of consciousness is not a requirement for the diagnosis of concussion (Demorest & Landry, 2003: Perriello & Barth, 2000; Schutzman & Greenes, 2001)
      (c) If loss of consciousness occurs, associated underlying injury is likely
   ii. Concussions are graded I through IV (see Chapter 24)
   iii. Pathophysiology
      (a) When the head hits an object at rest, deceleration of the brain can cause direct injury to delicate brain tissue
      (b) Deceleration can cause an injury to the opposite side of the brain due to countercoup forces
      (c) Animal studies show a disturbance in brain autoregulation with an increased glucose need by the neurons (Demorest and Landry, 2003)
   iv. Etiology and prevalence (Demorest & Landry, 2003 )
      (a) 4.5% of high school and college sport injuries are head injuries
      (b) Concussion rates in NCAA athletes vary from 9% to 13%
      (c) Concussions are more common in adolescents due to size of the players generating more force
      (d) Encourage car seat safety, seat belts, helmets during sports and other hazardous activities
   v. Diagnostic tests
      (a) Not routinely done unless there are deficits in cognition, mental status, memory, attention, or coordination or evidence of depressed skull fracture, large nonfrontal scalp hematoma, or persistent symptoms (Perriello & Barth, 2000)
      (b) Clear fluid or sanguineous fluid from nose or ears
         (1) Drop some fluid on filter paper (CSF separates from blood and forms a single or double ring or halo)
         (2) Use a glucose strip to test glucose (CSF is ≈25 mg)
      (c) Skull radiographs are sensitive for diagnosing skull fractures but do not give adequate information about cerebral injuries (Schutzman & Greenes, 2001)
      (d) CT of the head

(1) If signs of abnormal mental status, focal neurologic deficits or evidence of depressed or basilar skull fracture

(2) In children younger than age 2, if evidence of a nonfrontal scalp hematoma, or a large skull hematoma

(e) Functional MRI (Perriello & Barth, 2000)

(1) For patients with mild head injury and persistent symptoms

(2) May show changes in neurobiochemistry of the brain

(f) Ophthalmologic referral if there a suspicion of inflicted head injury

vi. Neurologic referral is indicated if any symptoms persist beyond 2 weeks (Demorest & Landry, 2003)

vii. Treatment

(a) See CDC Concussion Tool Kit for High School Coaches (CDC, 2005)

(b) Immediate referral to local Child Protective Services if abuse is suspected

(c) Analgesia such as acetaminophen for pain (see Chapter 55, Table 55-5)

(d) Close observation for any changes

(e) Avoid straining

(f) Do not pack nose or ears (if CSF leak will increase risk of infection)

(g) Cold compresses if there is a subcutaneous hematoma

(h) See also Chapter 24 for treatment recommendations based on concussion levels I to IV

(i) Encourage use of helmets for prevention of sports and activity head injuries

viii. Prognosis

(a) Excellent if treatment and prevention guidelines are followed and patient is honest about symptoms

(b) Postconcussion syndrome (Demorest & Landry, 2003)

(1) Headache, dizziness, fatigue, and personality changes

(2) Incidence is not known

(3) Children may have continued lingering neurologic symptoms

(4) Educate parent and child (particularly the teen who may want to return to a contact sport immediately) about post-concussion syndrome

ix. Follow-up

(a) Monitor every 1 to 2 weeks for increasing symptoms until completely well for 1 month

(b) Refer for neuropsychologic testing if neurologic symptoms persist

**h.** Linear skull fracture (Schutzman & Greenes, 2001)

i. Prevalence

(a) Skull fractures are more common on the parietal bone (60% to 70%)

(b) Occipital, frontal, and temporal bone fractures are the next most common; more common in children younger than 2

(c) Because infants have a thinner skull, there is a higher incidence of skull fractures from falls of 3 to 4 feet than in older children

ii. Diagnostic tests

(a) Plain radiographs

(b) CT of head

(1) For more accurate visualization of fractures of calvaria, face, and skull base

(2) Intracranial blood can be detected on noncontrast-enhanced CT

iii. Treatment—none

      **iv.** Follow-up

      **v.** Prognosis

        (a) Linear skull fractures almost always heal without complications

        (b) Monitor for growing linear skull fractures that may become evident months to years after injury (Schutzman & Greenes, 2001)

          (1) May observe a skull defect or swelling

          (2) Neurologic changes

          (3) Enlargement of the skull fracture on x-ray

**i.** Depressed or basilar skull fractures (Schutzman & Greenes, 2001)

    **i.** Prevalence and pathophysiology

      (a) Basilar skull fractures are the third most common skull fractures in children

      (b) Depressed skull fractures can present with bony abnormalities of the skull

      (c) If the mechanism of injury is significant, depressed fracture should be considered

      (d) A depressed fracture may:

        (1) Lacerate the dura

        (2) Compress the underlying brain parenchyma

        (3) Result in intraparenchymal bone fragments that may also cause lacerations or compression

        (4) Produce an obvious cosmetic deformity

      (e) Basilar fractures that occur through the temporal bone

        (1) Can disrupt the mastoid air cells or paranasal sinuses

        (2) A dural tear can occur following the fracture causing a CSF leak with resultant CSF otorrhea or rhinorrhea in 15% to 30% of children

        (3) Hearing loss and cranial nerves VI, VII, or VII impairment can follow basilar skull fractures

    **ii.** Diagnostic tests—same as in concussion described above

    **iii.** Treatment—refer immediately to neurosurgery to lift depressed skull fracture

    **iv.** Prognosis—excellent if no complications from surgery

    **v.** Follow-up should be maintained with neurosurgery until discharged

**4.** Symptoms: neck stiffness and pain

  **a.** Focused assessment

    **i.** Symptom assessment

      (a) New symptom

      (b) Recent illness

      (c) Change in level of:

        (1) Alertness

        (2) Responsiveness

        (3) Cry

        (4) Consolability

      (d) Measures taken at home and their effectiveness

        (1) Application of heat, cold

        (2) Medications

        (3) Complementary therapies

      (e) Fever

    **ii.** Focused history

      (a) Recent history of seizures

      (b) History of torticollis

    **iii.** Focused physical assessment
        (a) Inspection
            (1) Toxic appearance may indicate meningitis
            (2) Interest in environment
            (3) Irritability
            (4) Consolability
            (5) Eye contact
            (6) Level of alertness
            (7) Quality of cry, e.g., high pitched, weak
            (8) Throat
            (9) Skin
                a) Mild papular exanthema
                b) Petechiae
        (b) Vital signs
            (1) Fever
            (2) Tachycardia
        (c) Palpation
            (1) Neck (Hunstad, 2002)
                a) Range of motion
                b) Neck and back stiffness are considered clinical signs of meningitis
                c) Examine the sternocleidomastoid muscle for tightness
            (2) Lymph nodes of the cervical region that may indicate abscess or adenitis
  **b.** Differential diagnosis for neck stiffness and pain (Box 35-9)
  **c.** Diagnostic tests

---

■ **BOX 35-9**
■ **DIFFERENTIAL DIAGNOSIS FOR NECK PAIN OR NECK RIGIDITY**

**INFECTION**
- Meningitis
- Nasopharyngeal infections
- Postinfectious torticollis

**GI DISEASE**
- Gastroesophageal reflux resulting in Sandifer's syndrome

**CENTRAL NERVOUS SYSTEM ABNORMALITIES**
- Chiari malformation
- Brain tumor, particularly of posterior fossa
- Spinal tumor
- Syringomyelia

**TORTICOLLIS**
- Acquired torticollis
- Congenital muscular torticollis
- Paroxysmal torticollis
- Spasmodic torticollis
- Idiopathic torticollis

**SKELETAL ABNORMALITIES**
- Fetal deformation
- Cervical bony abnormalities

**OCULAR ABNORMALITIES**
- Strabismus
- Nystagmus
- Fourth cranial nerve palsy

From Gupta, P., Foster, J., Crowe, S., et al. (2003). Ophthalmologic findings in patients with nonsyndromic plagiocephaly. *J Craniofac Surg, 14*(4), 529–532.

      **i.** If symptom presents in a school-aged child with no history of trauma or fever, and the onset is mild, with an otherwise normal neurologic exam, the child can be observed without diagnostic testing

      **ii.** If torticollis is noted in an infant with normal sternocleidomastoid muscle, order radiographs of the cervical spine to rule out congenital scoliosis and Klippel-Feil syndrome

      **iii.** If the x-rays are normal and the torticollis persists, an ophthalmologic exam should be done to rule out ocular torticollis

      **iv.** Neurologic referral for further testing if there are no abnormalities identified on cervical films or ophthalmologic exam

**d.** Neck spasm

      **i.** The child presents with torticollis but will otherwise be well appearing

      **ii.** Following upper respiratory infection, there may a spontaneous subluxation from retropharyngeal edema, which causes minor malposition on the atlas

      **iii.** Most common in school-aged children 6 to 12

      **iv.** Treatment—warm compresses and ibuprofen (see Chapter 55, Table 55-5)

      **v.** Prognosis—condition should resolve within 5 days

      **vi.** Follow-up

        (a) Close follow-up

        (b) If the child is not improving, refer to neurology for further evaluation

**e.** Torticollis (see Chapter 34)

**f.** Benign paroxysmal torticollis

      **i.** Occurs in infants between 2 and 8 months of age

      **ii.** Considered to be a migraine precursor

**g.** Ocular torticollis

      **i.** The child tilts the head to one side to correct double vision

      **ii.** Seen in:

        (a) Fourth cranial nerve palsy

        (b) Congenital nystagmus

        (c) Refractive errors

        (d) Strabismus

      **iii.** Prevalence is not known

      **iv.** Diagnostic tests

        (a) Cover and uncover tests

        (b) Extraocular movements

      **v.** Treatment—refer to ophthalmology

**h.** Meningitis (Prober, 2004)

      **i.** Signs and symptoms—headache, fever, and stiff neck

      **ii.** Pathophysiology (Kumar, 2004)

        (a) A diffuse infection of the central nervous system

        (b) Caused by growth of bacteria, fungi, or parasites within the subarachnoid space, or by growth of bacteria or viruses within the meningeal or ependymal cells

        (c) Results in release of inflammatory mediators, interleukin-1, tumor necrosis factor-$\alpha$ and enhanced nitric oxide production

        (d) This inflammatory response causes:

          (1) Neurologic damage

          (2) Swelling of the arterioles and veins

          (3) Brain edema due to an increase of sodium and water

      **iii.** Etiology, prevalence, and incidence (Kumar, 2004)

(a) Bacterial meningitis
  (1) Major bacterial causes are *Haemophilus influenzae, Streptococcus pneumoniae,* and *Neisseria meningitidis*
  (2) More common younger than the age 5
  (3) 70% of those cases occur younger than age 2
  (4) Since the HIB vaccine, there is a marked decrease in bacterial meningitis
(b) Viral meningitis
  (1) Major viral causes are enteroviruses, mumps virus and lymphocytic choriomeningitis virus
  (2) Enteroviruses cause more than 80% of all cases of meningitis (Prober, 2004)

iv. Diagnostic tests (Hunstad, 2002)
  (a) CT of head may be ordered before doing lumbar puncture if there are signs of increased intracranial pressure or neurologic deficits such as:
    (1) Language abnormality
    (2) Abnormal eye examination, including gaze palsy
    (3) Changes in level of consciousness
  (b) Lumbar puncture—note opening pressure recording, glucose, protein, cell count
  (c) Laboratory studies
    (1) CBC with WBC differential
    (2) Electrolytes (may find low serum sodium)

v. Treatment
  (a) Refer immediately to pediatrician or neurologist for hospital admission
  (b) Empiric treatment is started depending on likely infecting organism, patient's history, clinical manifestations including rash, initial lab results, and age of child (Hunstad, 2002)
  (c) Chemoprophylaxis of family members, close contacts, and staff may be needed depending on the infecting organism

vi. Prognosis (Kanegaye, et al., 2001)
  (a) Mortality rate is 4% to 15% depending on the infecting organism
    (1) Untreated bacterial meningitis is usually fatal
    (2) Viral meningitis is benign
  (b) Hearing loss can occur in 2% to 28%

vii. Follow-up (Kumar, 2004)
  (a) Will need neurology follow-up
  (b) Long term audiology follow-up referral

i. Brain tumor—may present with hypertonia and flexion of neck (see section 5.1. below)

5. Signs—clumsiness, low muscle tone, muscle weakness
  a. Definitions
    i. Clumsiness—a lack of dexterity and speed in motor task (Ellison, 2003)
      (a) A normal variation in the normal population
      (b) Clumsiness can be seen with children with attention deficit hyperactivity disorder (ADHD)
      (c) If clumsiness is progressive, further investigation is indicated
    ii. Ataxia—inability to regulate the body's posture and the strength and direction of movements
    iii. Joint laxity—joint hypermobility due to looseness or stretching of tendons

    **iv.** Muscle weakness—a lack of ability to resist against pressure

    **v.** Myotonia—failure of immediate muscle relaxation after voluntary contraction has stopped

        (a) Inability to release a smile

        (b) Inability to release a contracted hand

        (c) Myotonia can be elicited by percussion on a muscle

    **vi.** Hypotonia—severely reduced muscle tone; reduced amount of tension or resistance to movement in a muscle (NINDS, 2005)

        (a) Head lag; little or no head control

        (b) Poor tone when being carried in arms

        (c) Paucity of movement

        (d) Diminished resistance to passive movement

        (e) Hypermobility with doughy feeling in older children

        (f) Children hang their arms and legs by their sides rather than flexing elbows and knees when at rest

**b.** Associated signs and symptoms

    **i.** Mobility problems

    **ii.** Poor posture

    **iii.** Breathing and speech difficulties

    **iv.** Lethargy

    **v.** Ligament and joint laxity

    **vi.** Poor reflexes

    **vii.** Hypotonia does not affect intellect unless associated with some syndromes

    **viii.** Child may take longer to develop social, language, and reasoning skills

**c.** Pathophysiology

    **i.** Normally, motor impulses come from the precentral gyrus in the cerebral cortex and travel through the cerebral white matter on the ipsilateral side until they reach the lower medulla where they cross over to the contralateral side

    **ii.** Impulses travel the lateral corticospinal tracts in the spinal cord until they synapse with the anterior horn cell

    **iii.** The synapse is the area of transition from the upper motor neuron to the lower motor neuron

    **iv.** Diseases of the anterior horn cell, peripheral nerves, and neuromuscular junction are considered lower motor neuron diseases

    **v.** Upper motor neuron disease includes hydrocephalus, malformation of the brain, abnormalities of the spinal cord such as transverse myelitis, dysraphism, and Chiari malformation (Gupta & Appleton, 2001)

        (a) Real muscle weakness indicates some involvement of peripheral neuromuscular system including (Gupta & Appleton, 2001):

            (1) Anterior horn cell disorder

            (2) Peripheral neuropathy

            (3) Myopathy

**d.** Focused assessment

    **i.** Symptom assessment

        (a) Timing of onset and progression; periodic or continuous; since birth

            (1) Acute onset of hypotonia or weakness suggests CNS hemorrhage or trauma

            (2) Evident with gross motor activities: walking, running

            (3) Evident with fine motor activities: writing, coloring

(b) Associated pain
(c) Location
    (1) Proximal—implies myopathy
    (2) Distal—implies neuropathy, spinal cord origin
    (3) Symmetric—implies brain or spinal lesions
    (4) Asymmetric—implies anterior horn lesion or nerve root compression
(d) Change in the child's motor skills
    (1) At onset
    (2) Present
(e) Relieving and exacerbating factors
    (1) Hot bath may cause weakness if multiple sclerosis
    (2) Cramps and weakness on exertion occurs with Becker's muscular dystrophy
(f) Associated signs and symptoms
    (1) Tenderness in the muscle as well as a rash implies dermatomyositis
    (2) Vision changes
        a) Diplopia
        b) Blurred vision
        c) Problems with accommodation
    (3) Weight loss, fatigue, or pain implies neoplastic disease
    (4) Change in bowel or bladder habits
    (5) Exposure to poisons or toxins
    (6) Other systemic symptoms
    (7) Fatigue worse at the end of the day
ii. Focused history
  (a) Family history
    (1) Other children with delayed motor or cognitive development
    (2) Family members who had weakness or neurologic or muscle disorders
    (3) Consanguineous couple—evaluate for rare recessive gene disorders
  (b) Child's history
    (1) Prenatal and perinatal history, e.g., difficult delivery, neonatal asphyxia, infection
    (2) Consider botulism if infant was exposed to honey
    (3) Ingestion of drugs such as benzodiazepines, alcohol, carbamazepine, clonazepam, phenobarbital, dilantin, or primidone
iii. Focused physical examination
  (a) See Chapter 12 for details on muscle assessment
  (b) Hands
    (1) Check for proximal strength of the hand by asking the child to spread open the hand and not allow you to close it (Ellison & Berman, 2003)
    (2) Examine hand grasp for equality in appearance and strength
  (c) Legs and feet
    (1) In infant older than 8 months observe:
        a) Child reaching above head for an object
        b) The parachute reflex for symmetry
    (2) If toddler or older, watch as the child rises from the floor to standing position

(3) Pseudohypertrophy of the calf muscles with a rubbery and firmer feeling than normal implies myopathy

(4) Atrophy of the calf muscle

(5) Positive Gower's sign implies myopathy (see Chapter 12)

(6) A high foot arch and contractures of the toes imply spinal cord or peripheral neuropathy

(d) Gait

(1) Weakness greater in the legs or generalized

(2) Waddling or toe walking

(3) Pattern of arm swing when walking

(4) Ataxia

(e) Assess developmental milestones

(f) Reflexes

(1) Strength and symmetry of the reflexes

(2) With central hypotonia, the deep tendon reflexes (DTRs) may be normal

(3) With peripheral hypotonia, DTRs are likely to be depressed

(4) Evaluate spinal cord function with anal reflex and cremasteric reflex

(g) Spine

(1) Sacral dimples more than 2.5 cm from the anus indicate higher rate of underlying malformation in the spine (Williams & Wessel, 2002)

(2) Skin tag, hairy patch, port-wine stain, hemangioma, lipoma, sinus tract, or cutis aplasia along spine indicates spinal dysraphism

(3) Excessive lordosis with proximal weakness implies myopathy

(h) Looseness of the joint ligaments but without weakness implies connective tissue disorder, e.g., Ehlers-Danlos syndrome, Marfan's syndrome, osteogenesis imperfecta

(i) Evaluate cognitive level—usually normal with peripheral hypotonia, but may be abnormal with central hypotonia

  **e.** Differential diagnoses

  **i.** Clumsiness

(a) Neurologic soft sign

(b) ADHD

(c) Learning disabilities

(d) Familial clumsiness

(e) Myotonic dystrophy

(f) Neurogenerative disease of white or gray matter

  **ii.** Hypotonia with or without muscle weakness (Box 35-10)

  **iii.** Ataxia (Box 35-11)

 **f.** Floppy baby syndrome

  **i.** Signs

(a) Poor muscle tone in an infant or young toddler; the infant with hypotonia will form a U when held in hand, belly down (Williams & Wessel, 2002).

(b) Hypotonia in the neonate tends to be central

(1) Associated with a weak cry, poor sucking reflex, decreased body movement, respiratory problems

(2) If the hypotonia is central, other neurologic abnormalities are common, such as lack of interest in the environment, delayed development seizures

■ **BOX 35-10**
■ **DIFFERENTIAL DIAGNOSIS FOR HYPOTONIA AND MUSCLE WEAKNESS**

**DISORDERS OF CENTRAL NERVOUS SYSTEM**
- Static encephalopathies due to congenital malformation, perinatal or postnatal
- Acquired encephalopathy
- Congenital brain abnormalities: Dandy-Walker cyst, Arnold-Chiari
- Malformation, hydrocephalus
- Inborn errors of metabolism: amino acid disorder, organic acid disorder, urea cycle disorder, lysosomal disorder

**GENETIC SYNDROMES**
- Trisomy 21
- Ehlers-Danlos syndrome
- Prader-Willi syndrome
- Fragile X syndrome
- Laurence-Moon-Biedl syndrome

**ENDOCRINOPATHIES**
- Congenital hypothyroidism
- Disorders of parathyroid

**NO KNOWN CAUSE**
- Essential hypotonia
- Conversion reaction

**DISORDERS OF PERIPHERAL NERVOUS SYSTEM**
Anterior Horn Cell
- Spinal muscular atrophies
- Congenital myasthenia
- Congenital muscular dystrophy
- Polio
- Metabolic defects
- Congenital myopathies
- Metabolic myopathies

Peripheral Nerves
- Guillain-Barré syndrome
- Heavy metal poisoning
- Charcot-Marie-Tooth disease

Neuromuscular Junction
- Botulism
- Myasthenia
- Tick paralysis
- Organophosphate poisoning
- Nerve gas

**CELLULAR PROLIFERATION**
- Tumor

From Ellison, P., & Berman, S. (2003). Childhood weakness and paralysis. In S. Berman (Ed.). *Pediatric decision making* (4th ed.). Philadelphia: Mosby, pp. 620–623; and Williams, S., & Wessel, H. (2002). Neurology. In B. Zitelli & H. Davis (Eds). *Atlas of pediatric physical diagnosis* (4th ed.). Philadelphia: Mosby, pp. 502-559.

    ii. Etiology
        (a) The majority do not have a congenital myopathy
        (b) Hypotonia can also be the response of a sick infant to illness
        (c) Mostly unknown etiology
    iii. Diagnostic tests
        (a) Electrolyte studies including calcium and magnesium
        (b) Thyroid studies to rule out hypothyroidism
        (c) CBC with differential
        (d) C-reactive protein
        (e) Blood and urine cultures to rule out infection
        (f) Lumbar puncture (LP) if meningitis is suspected.
        (g) Toxin screen if ingestion or heavy metal poisoning is suspected
        (h) Chromosomes if genetic problem is suspected
        (i) Stool sample for *Clostridium botulinum* (Cox & Hinkle, 2002)
        (j) Refer to neurology for muscle testing
    iv. Treatment—refer to appropriate specialist depending on suspected etiology
  g. Spinal cord tumor
    i. Spinal cord mass is divided into intramedullary and extramedullary
        (a) Intramedullary tumors

■ **BOX 35-11**
■ **DIFFERENTIAL DIAGNOSIS FOR ATAXIA**

**GENETIC ABNORMALITIES**
- Angelman's syndrome
- Ataxia telangiectasia
- Niemann-Pick disease type C
- X-linked spinocerebellar ataxia

**NEOPLASTIC ABNORMALITIES**
- Tumors of the cerebellum
- Posterior fossa tumors
- Neuroblastoma

**CONGENITAL CNS ABNORMALITIES**
- Chiari malformation
- Dandy-Walker malformation

**TOXIC INGESTIONS**
- Drugs
- Lead

**INFECTION**
- Varicella
- Coxsackie
- Rubeola
- Mononucleosis
- *Mycoplasma pneumoniae*
- Postmeningitis

**METABOLIC CONDITIONS**
- Aminoaciduria
- Organoaciduria
- High ammonia levels
- Transport chain defects

**HEREDITARY ATAXIAS**
- Friedreich's ataxia
- Ataxia-telangiectasia
- Spinocerebellar ataxia

**VASCULAR ABNORMALITIES**
**PRIMARY PSYCHOGENIC ATAXIA**

 

       (1) Comprise about 30% to 40% of tumors and a large percentage of astrocytomas or gangliogliomas (Jallo, et al., 2003)
       (2) Gliomas are the most common
       (3) May present with low back pain, weakness, gait changes, sensory changes, or disturbances of bowel or bladder (Henson, 2001)
     (b) Extramedullary tumors
       (1) Pain and weakness are the common presentations
       (2) Motor deficits include weakness, increased falling, or clumsiness as well as motor regression
       (3) Toddler may present with weakness or loss of a previous motor ability
       (4) Bowel and bladder problems also are common, and in the younger child may be attributed to behavior problems
   ii. Painful spinal deformities can be a sign of spinal tumor
   iii. Refer to neurosurgery or oncology for further diagnosis and management
**h.** Spinal dysraphism (see Chapter 51 for spina bifida and other myelodysplasias)
 **i.** Myopathies (see Chapter 34)
 **j.** Ataxia (DiNolfo, 2001)
   i. Definition—muscle weakness that causes balance problems and an altered gait
   ii. Assessment
     (a) If the child is old enough to walk, carefully evaluate gait
     (b) If older than age 4 years, evaluate:

          (1) Tandem gait

          (2) Hop in place

          (3) Walk on heel and toes

          (4) Heel-to-shin maneuver

      (c) High stepping gait and a positive Romberg sign suggest posterior column damage

      (d) Dysarthria or slow, weak, imprecise, and uncoordinated speech due to lack of coordination of the muscles of speech

      (e) Truncal ataxia causes swaying, reduced balance, and occasional falls (Pandolfo, 2003)

      (f) Ataxia and areflexia suggest Guillain-Barré syndrome

   **iii.** Signs of cerebellar dysfunction

      (a) Head and neck titubations—tremor resulting from demyelination in the cerebellum

      (b) Head nodding

      (c) Nystagmus

      (d) Wide-based gait

      (e) Intentional or action tremor

      (f) Hypotonia

      (g) Does the child have poor balance during sitting and standing?

   **iv.** Etiology

      (a) Hereditary ataxia is an autosomal recessive trait

      (b) Ataxia may be secondary to infection or drug toxicity

   **v.** Refer to neurology for further evaluation, diagnosis, and treatment cause

  **k.** Vertigo (Isaacson & Vora, 2003)

   **i.** Definition

      (a) Sensation of dizziness

      (b) May be associated with:

          (1) Acute hearing changes, ringing in the ear

          (2) Positional changes

          (3) Nausea or vomiting

   **ii.** Focused history

      (a) Recent head trauma

      (b) Trauma to the eardrum

      (c) Recent infections

      (d) Medication history or illicit drug use

      (e) Ingestions, especially salicylic acid

   **iii.** Focused physical assessment

      (a) Check eyes for nystagmus

      (b) Torticollis

      (c) Tandem Romberg test

          (1) Have the child stand with one foot in front of the other

          (2) Eyes closed and arms out in front

          (3) The child with unilateral labyrinthine disease will fall to the affected side

   **iv.** Differential diagnosis for vertigo (Box 35-12)

      (a) Benign paroxysmal vertigo

          (1) Child experiences severe vertigo that lasts for minutes or hours

          (2) May have nystagmus during attacks

          (3) No neurologic signs between attacks; normal EEG

          (4) No hearing impairment

■ **BOX 35-12**
■ **DIFFERENTIAL DIAGNOSIS FOR VERTIGO**

| VERTIGO WITH HEARING LOSS | VERTIGO WITHOUT HEARING LOSS |
|---|---|
| ■ Labyrinthitis | ■ Seizures |
| ■ Perilymphatic fistula | ■ Paroxysmal positional vertigo |
| ■ Acoustic neuroma | ■ Headache-migraine or tension |
| ■ Posterior fossa tumor | ■ Panic disorder |
| ■ Cholesteatoma | ■ Depression |
| ■ Temporal bone fracture | ■ Hyperventilation |
| ■ Vascular occlusion from sickle cell disease or stroke | ■ Vestibular neuronitis |
| ■ Demyelinating disease | |

From Ellison, P., & Berman, S. (2003). Childhood weakness and paralysis. In S. Berman (Ed.). *Pediatric decision making* (4th ed.). Philadelphia: Mosby, pp. 620-623.

        (5) A condition that starts in toddlers and spontaneously resolves by ages 4 to 6 years

        (6) A group of disorders that is now classified as a form of migraine headache (Headache Classification Subcommittee, 2004)

    (b) No treatment is recommended

l. Brain tumor

    **i.** Incidence

        (a) 2.4 to 3.3 new cases per 100,000 children per year

        (b) Brain and spinal cord tumors cause more deaths than either leukemia or lymphoma

    **ii.** Pathophysiology

        (a) The brain is divided into an upper and lower section by the tentorium, a fibrous sheet

            (1) Supratentorial tumors are in the cerebrum, pituitary gland, hypothalamus, basal ganglia, and pineal region

            (2) Infratentorial tumors are in the cerebellum, brainstem, or fourth ventricular region

        (b) Brain tumors are the most common pediatric tumor; divided into five major classes based on cell type (Kieran, 2000)

            (1) Glial cells—gliomas comprise two thirds of all childhood brain tumors

               a) Ependymoma

                  i) Arise from the cells that line the ventricles, mostly the fourth ventricle affecting the cerebellum and pons

                  ii) Third most common childhood brain tumor

                  iii) Displace brain tissue rather than invade brain tissue

                  iv) Present with ataxia when the tumors are in the floor or roof of the fourth ventricle

                  v) Other signs include headache, vomiting, head tilt, torticollis, clumsy movements, dysmetria, and dysphonia

               b) Astrocytoma

                  i) CNS neoplasm that arises from astrocytes

                  ii) Causes compression, invasion, and destruction of brain parenchyma.

  c) Oligodendroglioma
   i) Oligodendrocytes
    *a*) Normally produce the sheaths of myelin that cover axons and astrocytes
    *b*) Contain neurotransmitter receptors
   ii) Create the blood-brain barrier
  (2) Neural cells
  (3) Choroid plexus cells
  (4) Craniopharyngial cells
  (5) Germ cells
 (c) Another class of common brain tumors in children is the embryonal or primitive neuroectodermal tumor (PNET) group (Jallo & Marcovici, 2005
  (1) Medulloblastomas are the most common; comprise 30% of brain tumors
  (2) Usually arise in the fourth ventricle
  (3) Present with unsteady gait, vomiting, and other signs of increased intracranial pressure
 (d) See Box 35-13 for clinical presentation of brain tumors
 (e) Certain genetic diseases have a higher incidence of brain tumors, including neurofibromatosis, tuberous sclerosis, multiple endocrine neoplasia (type 1), and retinoblastoma
 **iii.** Immediate referral to pediatric oncology or neurosurgery for further evaluation, diagnosis, and treatment
**m.** Facial weakness
 **i.** Symptom assessment
  (a) Timing—when did the symptom start?

---

■ **BOX 35-13**
■ **LOCATION OF BRAIN TUMOR AND RELATED CLINICAL MANIFESTATIONS**

**SUPRATENTORIAL**
Cerebrum
- Intellectual changes, seizures, contralateral hemiparesis

Midline region
- Endocrinopathies, e.g., diabetes insipidus, growth retardation
- Decreased vision, visual field defects

Hypothalamic region
- Growth retardation with precocious puberty
- Visual field defects, headache, seizure
- Developmental disabilities

Optic nerve and pineal region
- Ptosis, paralysis of upward gaze

Ependymomas
- Focal headache, seizures, hyperreflexia, focal signs

**INFRATENTORIAL**
Posterior fossa
- Hydrocephalus, headache, vomiting, papilledema
- Torticollis, clumsiness, ataxia, multiple cranial nerve signs

Brainstem
- Ptosis, eye movement defects, peripheral facial weakness
- Cranial nerve VII, IX, X abnormalities
- Pyramidal tract signs, abnormal gait, one hand preference

Cerebellum
- Ataxia of extremities, abnormalities in finger-to-nose testing, rapid alternating movement, and heel-to-shin maneuver
- Truncal ataxia, gait ataxia, titubation

Ependymomas
- Nystagmus, papilledema, meningismus, dysmetria, vomiting

        (b) Associated weakness

        (c) Ear pain near the mastoid—occurs in half of the cases of Bell's palsy

        (d) Is the child having difficulty with drinking and eating?

        (e) Decreased lacrimation on the affected side

        (f) Signs of hypothyroidism or hyperparathyroidism

    ii. Focused physical assessment

        (a) Can the child close the eye, move the forehead?

        (b) Is the nerve palsy localized to the lower one half of the face?

        (c) Other neurologic signs

    iii. Differential diagnoses for facial weakness

        (a) Genetic syndrome

        (b) Congenital structural disorder

        (c) Infectious or inflammatory causes

        (d) Trauma causing nerve compression

        (e) Neoplasm

        (f) Vascular

        (g) Myasthenia gravis

        (h) Metabolic condition

        (i) Idiopathic

    iv. Refer to neurology for further evaluation, diagnosis, and treatment

6. Symptoms: awkward, stereotypic, or uncontrollable movements

  a. Symptom assessment

    i. Characteristics of the movements

        (a) Part of the body involved

        (b) Purposeful, uncontrollable, repetitive

        (c) Does it cause the body part to adopt an abnormal or twisting configuration?

    ii. Timing of movements

        (a) Sudden onset

        (b) Frequency—repetitive, random

        (c) Duration

        (d) During sleep

        (e) While awake

    iii. Child's ability to control the movements

    iv. Precipitating factors, e.g., stress

    v. Factors that decrease or stop the movements

  b. Focused family history

    i. Movement or neurologic disorders

  c. Focused child's history

    i. Recent systemic infection

    ii. Drug use

    iii. Caffeine intake

    iv. Weight loss

  d. Focused physical assessment

    i. See Chapter 13 for detailed neurologic assessment

    ii. Evaluate size of thyroid

    iii. Evaluate gait

  e. Differential diagnosis for movement disorders (Box 35-14)

  f. Tremors (Smaga, 2003)

    i. Resting tremor occurs when the limb is stationary

    ii. Action tremor occurs when the limb is voluntarily moving or extended for a prolonged period

      **iii.** Postural tremor occurs when the person maintains a position against gravity

      **iv.** Kinetic tremor

        (a) Intentional tremor

          (1) Occurs as the limb approaches the target

          (2) Accompanied by ataxic gait or cerebellar signs (nystagmus or slurred speech)

        (b) Simple kinetic tremor

          (1) A mild tremor at end of targeted movement

          (2) Not accompanied by cerebellar signs

**g.** Familial essential tremor (Burke & Hauser, 2001)

    **i.** Tremor is involuntary trembling in part of the body

    **ii.** Essential tremor is associated with purposeful movement (e.g., holding a glass to drink)

      (a) Usually affects upper extremities

      (b) Slowly progressive

      (c) Not associated with any other signs or symptoms

    **iii.** Etiology

      (a) First becomes apparent in late adolescence, early adulthood, or in elderly

      (b) Autosomal dominant hereditary trait linked to chromosome 3q13 and chromosome 2p2-22

    **iv.** Diagnostic tests are not necessary if there is a family history of essential tremor

    **v.** Treatment consists of β-adrenergic blocker: propranolol 1 to 4 mg/kg/day

**h.** Tic (Black & Webb, 2005; Schlaggar & Mink, 2003)

    **i.** A sudden, rapid, recurrent, nonrhythmic, stereotyped motor movement or vocalization

      (a) Simple motor tics include eye blinking, grimacing, shoulder elevation, teeth grinding, or abdominal tensing

      (b) Verbal tics include sniffing, throat clearing, grunting, blowing, or sucking

---

■ **BOX 35-14**
■ **DIFFERENTIAL DIAGNOSIS FOR MOVEMENT DISORDERS**

**TICS**
- Stereotypic behavior, habits, mannerisms
- Sporadic tics
- Tourette syndrome
- Tuberous sclerosis
- Wilson's disease
- Drug-induced tics

**TREMORS**
- Posttraumatic tremor
- Familial essential tremor
- Resting, action, postural, kinetic tremors

**DYSTONIA**
- Idiopathic generalized torsion dystonia
- Dopa–responsive dystonia
- Transient dystonia
- Torticollis
- Sandifer's syndrome
- Drugs
- Rett's syndrome

From Bressman, S. B. (2004). Dystonia genotypes, phenotypes, and classification. *Advances in Neurology, 94*, 101–107.

      ii. Neurologic examination is otherwise normal

     iii. Treatment

         (a) Tics must interfere with quality of life to consider pharmacologic treatment

         (b) Pharmacologic treatment includes use of clonidine or neuroleptics

     iv. Prognosis—many tics tend to improve with time

i. Dystonia (Krauss & Jankovic, 2002)

      i. Signs and symptoms

         (a) Involuntary, sustained, patterned muscle contraction resulting in twisting movement or posturing due to the action of opposing muscle groups

         (b) Forces the body into an abnormal, sometimes painful position

         (c) May have accompanying tremor or myoclonic movements

         (d) Typically occurs during voluntary movements

      ii. Etiology

         (a) An autosomal dominant condition with onset around age 12 years (Schlaggar & Mink, 2003)

         (b) Secondary to brain lesions of the basal ganglia and putamen

            (1) Dopa-responsive dystonia

               a) Presents at about age 6 with gait disturbance

               b) Symptoms worsen by the end of the day

               c) Progressive

            (2) Myoclonus dystonia

         (c) Acute dystonia may be secondary to neuroleptic or antipsychotic drugs that are dopamine receptor antagonists

            (1) Present emergency department with anticholinergic medication

     iii. Refer to pediatric neurology for further evaluation, diagnosis, and treatment

j. Myoclonus

      i. Very short, jerky movements associated with contractions of muscles

      ii. Myoclonic jerks in infancy are associated with sleep and are normal

     iii. Other types of myoclonus should be referred to pediatric neurologist for further evaluation, diagnosis, and treatment

k. Tourette syndrome (Black & Webb, 2005; Jankovic, 2001)

      i. Signs and symptoms

         (a) A spectrum of neurobehavioral signs, including tics

         (b) Associated with behavioral disorders such as obsessive-compulsive disorders, attention deficit disorder, anxiety and mood disorder, conduct disorder, self- injurious behavior, sleep disorder, and oppositional defiant behavior

      ii. Etiology

         (a) A genetic disorder of synaptic neurotransmission

         (b) An imbalance of the striate cortex and thalamic circuitry

         (c) The caudate nucleus and inferior prefrontal cortex of the basal ganglia is the area in the brain where Tourette syndrome, obsessive-compulsive disorder, and attention deficit disorder arise

     iii. Prevalence

         (a) Tourette syndrome affects males three to five times more often than females

         (b) The prevalence is about 0.7% of children

   iv. Diagnostic criteria
      (a) Must demonstrate multiple motor tics and one or more phonic tics
      (b) Occurring multiple times a day during a period of 1 year
      (c) No tic-free period of more than 3 consecutive months
      (d) Onset must be before age 21 years
   v. Refer to neurology for evaluation, diagnosis, and treatment
      (a) Treatment is primarily symptomatic
      (b) Family education and support is key; refer to the National Tourette Syndrome Association (www.tsa-us.org) and local support groups
      (c) Medications are needed if symptoms interfere with the quality of life
      (d) Prognosis—symptoms may wax and wane, but generally persist throughout life
l. Febrile seizure (Baumann, 2005; Gill & Gieron-Korthals, 2002)
   i. Most common seizure disorder in children
   ii. Three types
      (a) Simple febrile seizure (70% to 75%)
         (1) Fever in a child ages 6 months to 5 years
         (2) Single seizure is generalized and lasts less than 15 minutes
         (3) Child is otherwise neurologically healthy
         (4) Fever (and seizure) is not caused by meningitis, encephalitis, or other illness affecting the brain
      (b) Complex febrile seizure (20% to 25%)
         (1) Fever in a child ages 6 months to 5 years
         (2) Seizure is either focal or prolonged (>15 minutes), or multiple seizures in succession
      (c) Symptomatic febrile seizure (5%)
         (1) Fever in a child ages 6 months to 5 years
         (2) Child has a preexisting neurologic abnormality or acute illness
   iii. Pathophysiology
      (a) A unique form of "epilepsy" that occurs in early childhood and only in association with an elevation of temperature
      (b) Genetic predisposition
      (c) Occurs in 2% to 4% of children before age 5 years
      (d) Occurs in males slightly more often than females
      (e) About one third of children will have a second febrile seizure
   iv. Differential diagnosis for febrile seizure
      (a) Meningitis (see section 4.h. above)
      (b) Epilepsy (see Chapter 46)
      (c) Shaking or shivering associated with fever
      (d) Other paroxysmal disorder
   v. Diagnostic testing
      (a) LP in children younger than 12 months is strongly recommended because the signs and symptoms of bacterial meningitis may be minimal or absent in this age group
      (b) Consider LP in other age-groups depending on level of suspicion of bacterial meningitis
   vi. No specific treatment for the seizure is recommended, but antipyretics are suggested
   vii. Teach parents about management of child during a seizure
   viii. Prognosis is excellent—no neurologic sequelae are expected

# REFERENCES

Adams, M., & Hugkins, L. (2003). The importance of minor anomalies in the evaluation of the newborn. *NeoRev, 4*(4), 99-104.

Baumann, R. (2005). Febrile seizures. Retrieved May 17, 2006, from www.emedicine.com/neuro/topic134.htm.

Berman, S. (2003). Abnormal head: size and shape. In S. Berman (Ed.). *Pediatric decision making* (4th ed.). Philadelphia: Mosby, pp. 604-610.

Biggs, W. (2003). Diagnosis and management of positional head deformity. *Am Fam Phys, 67*(9), 1953-1956.

Black, K. J., & Webb, H. (2005). Tourette syndrome and other tic disorders. Retrieved October 15, 2005, from www.emedicine.com/neuro/topic664.htm#targetL.

Bressman, S. B. (2004). Dystonia genotypes, phenotypes, and classification. *Advances in Neurology, 94*, 101-107.

Burke, D., & Hauser, R. A. (2001). Essential tremor. Retrieved October 15, 2005, from www.emedicine.com/NEURO/topic129.htm.

Centers for Disease Control and Prevention. (2005). Notice to readers: Concussion tool kit for high school coaches, *MMWR Morb Mortal Wkly Rep, 54*(37), 934. See also: www.cdc.gov/ncipc/tbi/Coaches_Tool_Kit.htm.

Cohen, M. M. (2000). Sutural pathology. In M. M. Cohen, & R. E. MacLean, eds. *Craniosynostosis: Diagnosis, evaluation and management* (2nd ed.).(pp. 51-68). New York: Oxford University Press.

Conologue, T., & Meffert, J. (2005). Dermatologic manifestations of neurologic disease. Retrieved October 24, 2005, from www.emedicine.com/derm/topic549.htm.

Cox, N., & Hinkle, R. (2002). Infant botulism. *Am Fam Phys, 65*(7), 1388-1392.

Demorest, R., & Landry, G. (2003). A football player with a concussion, *Pediatr Case Rev, 3*(3), 127-140.

Dinolfo, E. (2001). Ataxia. *Pediatrics in Review, 22*(5), 177-78.

Ellison, P. (2003). The clumsy child. In S. Berman (Ed.). *Pediatric decision making* (4th ed.). Philadelphia: Mosby, pp. 624-625.

Ellison, P., & Berman, S. (2003). Childhood weakness and paralysis. In S. Berman (Ed.). *Pediatric decision making* (4th ed.). Philadelphia: Mosby, pp. 620-623.

Gill, J., & Gieron-Korthals, M. (2002). What pediatricians and parents need to know about febrile convulsions. *Contemp Pediatr, 19*(5), 139-150.

Goldbloom, R. B. (2003). *Pediatric clinical skills* (3rd ed.). Philadelphia: Saunders.

Gupta, R., & Appleton, R. E. (2001). Cerebral palsy: not always what it seems. *Arch Dis Child, 85*, 356-360.

Gupta, P., Foster, J., Crowe, S., et al. (2003). Ophthalmologic findings in patients with nonsyndromic plagiocephaly. *J Craniofac Surg, 14*(4), 529-532.

Habal, M., Leimkuehler, T., Chambers, C., et al. (2003). Avoiding the sequela associated with deformational plagiocephaly. *J Craniofac Surg, 14*(3), 430-437.

Handique, S., Das, R., Barua, N., et al. (2002). External hydrocephalus in children. *Indian J Radiol Imag, 12*(2), 197-200.

Haslam, R. H. A. (2005). Headaches. In R. E. Behrman, R. M. Kliegman, & H. B. Jenson (Eds.). *Nelson textbook of pediatrics* (17th ed.). Philadelphia: Saunders, pp. 2012-2019.

Headache Classification Subcommittee of the International Headache Society. (2004). The International Classification of Headache Disorders (2nd ed.). *Cephalgia, 24*(Suppl. 1). Retrieved May 17, 2006, from http://216.25.100.131/ihscommon/guidelines/pdfs/ihc_II_main_no_print.pdf.

Henson, J. (2001). Spinal cord gliomas. *Current Opinion in Neurology, 14*, 679-682.

Hershey, A. D., & Winner, P. K. (2005). Pediatric migraine: Recognition and treatment. *J Am Osteopath Assoc, 105*(Suppl. 4), 2S-8S.

Hunstad, D. (2002). Bacterial meningitis in children. *Pediatric Case Reviews, 2*(4), 195-202.

Hutchison, B. L., Hutchison, L. A. D., Thompson, J. M. D., & Mitchell, E. A. (2004). Plagiocephaly and brachycephaly in the first two years of life: A prospective cohort study. *Pediatrics, 114*(4), 970-980.

Isaacson, J. E., & Vora, N. M. (2004). Differential diagnosis and treatment of hearing loss. *Am Fam Phys, 68*(6), 1125-1132.

Jallo, G. I., Freed, D., & Epstein, F. (2003). Intramedullary spinal cord tumors in children. *Childs Nerv Syst, 19*(9), 641-649.

Jallo, G. & Marcovici, A. (2005). Medulloblastoma. Retrieved on May 17, 2006 at http://www.emedicine.com/neuro/topic624.htm.

Jankovic, J. (2001). Medical Progress: Tourette syndrome. *New England Journal of Medicine, 345*(16), 1184-1192.

Johnston, M. V., & Kinsman, S. (2004). Microcephaly. In R. E. Behrman, R. M. Kliegman, & H. B. Jenson (Eds.). *Nelson textbook of pediatrics* (17th ed.). Philadelphia: Saunders, pp. 1988-1999.

Kanegaye, J. T., Soliemanzadeh, P., & Bradley, J. S. (2001). Lumbar puncture in pediatric bacterial meningitis: defining the time interval for recovery of cerebrospinal fluid pathogens after parenteral antibiotic pretreatment. *Pediatrics, 108*, 1169-1174.

Kieran, M. (2000). Advances in pediatric neurooncology. *Current Opinion in Neurology, 13*, 627-634.

Krauss, J., & Jankovic, J. (2002). Head injury and posttraumatic movement disorders. *Neurosurgery, 50*(5), 927-939.

Kumar, A. (2004). Meningitis, bacterial. Retrieved October 15, 2005, from www.emedicine.com/PED/topic198.htm.

Lampl, C. (2002). Childhood-onset cluster headaches, *Pediatr Neurol 27*(2), 138-140.

Larsen, W. J. (2001). *Human embryology*. New York: Churchill Livingstone.

Lewis, K., Ashwal, S., Dahl, G., et al. (2002). Practice parameter: Evaluation of children and adolescents with recurrent headaches: Report of the Quality Standards Subcommittee of the American Academy of Neurology and the Practice Committee of the Child Neurology Society. *Neurology, 59*, 490-498. [Editor's note: This practice guideline is current as of October, 2005.]

Li, B. U. K., & Howard, J. C. (2002). New hope for children with cyclic vomiting syndrome. *Contemp Pediatr, 19*(3), 121-130.

Lipton, R. B., Bigal, M. E., Steiner, T. J., et al. (2004). Classification of primary headaches. *Neurology, 63*(3), 427-435.

Mack, K. J. (2006). Episodic and chronic migraine in children. *Semin Neurol, 26*(2), 223-231.

Menkes, J. H., & Sarnat, H. B. (2000). *Child Neurology* (6th ed.). Philadelphia: Lippincott Williams & Wilkins.

Millichap, J. G., & Yee, M. (2003). The diet factor in pediatric and adolescent migraine. *Pediatr Neurol, 28*(1), 1-14.

Moore, K. L., & Persaud, T V. N. (2003). *The developing human: Clinically oriented embryology*. Philadelphia: Saunders.

National Institute of Neurological Disorders and Stroke (NINDS). (2005). NINDS infantile hypotonia information page. Retrieved October 15, 2005, from www.ninds.nih.gov/disorders/hypotonia/hypotonia.htm.

Olness, K. (1999). Managing headaches without drugs. *Contemp Pediatr,16*, 101-110.

Pandolfo, M. (2003). Friedreich's ataxia. In H. R. Jones, D. De Vivo, & B. Darras, *Neuromuscular disorders of infancy, childhood, and adolescence: A clinician's approach*. Amsterdam: Butterworth-Heinemann, pp. 1141-1165.

Perriello, V. A., & Barth, J. T. (2000). Sports concussions: coming to the right conclusions. *Contemp Pediatrics, 17*(2), 132-142.

Persing, J., James, H., Swanson, J., Kattwinkel, J., and the American Academy of Pediatrics Committee on Practice and Ambulatory Medicine, Section on Plastic Surgery and Section on Neurological Surgery. (2003). Clinical report: Prevention and management of positional skull deformities in infants. *Pediatrics, 112*(1), 199-202.

Prober, C. G. (2004). Central nervous system infections. In R. E. Behrman, R. M. Kliegman, & H. B. Jenson (Eds.). *Nelson textbook of pediatrics* (17th ed.). Philadelphia: Saunders, 2038-2047.

Sargent, L. A. (2000). *Tennessee Craniofacial Center Textbook*. Chattanooga, TN: Erlanger Health Systems. Available at www.craniofacialcenter.com.

Sarnat, H. & Menkes, J. (2000). Neuroembryology, genetic programming and malformation of the nervous system. In J. Menkes & H. Sarnat (Eds.). *Child Neurology* (pp. 241-305), Philadelphia: Lippincott, Williams and Wilkins.

Schlaggar, B., & Mink, J. (2003). Movement disorders in children. *Pediatr Rev, 24*(2), 39-51.

Schutzman, S. A., & Greenes, D. S. (2001). Pediatric minor head trauma. *Ann Emerg Med, 37*(1), 65-74.

Sheth, R. D., & Iskandar, B. J. (2005). Craniosynostosis. Retrieved on May 17, 2006 from eMedicine at www.emedicine.com/neuro/topic80.htm.

Shin, J., & Persing, J. (2003). Asymmetric skull shapes: Diagnostic and therapeutic considerations. *J Cranio Surg, 14*(5), 696-699.

Smaga, S. (2003). Tremor. *Am Fam Phys, 68*(8), 15445-1552.

Warren, S. M., Brunet, L. J., Harland, R. M., et al. (2003). *Nature, 422*(6932), 625-629.

Williams, S., & Wessel, H. (2002). Neurology. In B. Zitelli & H. Davis (Eds.). *Atlas of pediatric physical diagnosis* (4th ed.). Philadelphia: Mosby, pp. 502-559.

Wright, W. (2004). Impact of the nurse practitioner in the management of migraine. *Am J Nurse Pract, 8*(6), 64-76.

Zitelli, B. J., & Davis, H. W. (2002). *Atlas of pediatric diagnosis* (4th ed.). St. Louis: Mosby.

# Diagnosis and Management of Chronic Conditions in Children and Adolescents

# Asthma

TERRY A. BUFORD, RN, PhD, CPNP

## DEFINITION

A common chronic condition in childhood characterized by persistent airway inflammation, bronchial hyperresponsiveness and periodic obstruction of airflow; an immunologic response to a variety of stimuli (Liu, Spahn, & Leung, 2004)

1. Incidence and prevalence
   a. Asthma is the most common chronic condition of childhood
   b. Prevalence—affects 6,213,000 children in the United States (CDC, 2006b)
   c. The overall prevalence of asthma in children 17 and younger was 8.5% in 2003 according to the National Health Survey (CDC, 2006a)
      i. 9.5% of boys less than age 18
      ii. 7.2% of girls less than age 18
      iii. Boys more than girls in white non-Hispanic, Black non-Hispanic, Hispanic, Mexican, Mexican-American
      iv. Girls more than boys in Puerto Rican children
   d. An estimated 9 million (12.5%) children younger than age 18 in the United States have had asthma diagnosed *at some time in their lives* (CDC, 2006c)
   e. Asthma care (CDC, 2003)
      i. More than 10 million office visits for children per year
      ii. More than 700,000 emergency department visits
   f. Children miss an estimated 14 million school days per year due to asthma (CDC, 2003)
   g. Prevalence not associated with ethnicity or income
   h. Black children have three times more hospitalization and mortality than white children
2. Etiology and precipitating factors
   a. Believed to be the effect of interactions between genetic predisposition and environmental factors
   b. Genetic factors may determine the direction of T-lymphocyte cytokine production tendency causing an imbalance between Th-1 and Th-2 lymphocytes (Busse & Busse, 2002; Leonard & Sur, 2003)

       **i.** Th-2 lymphocytes release cytokines that regulate the inflammatory response

       **ii.** Th-1 lymphocytes release cytokines that counteract this response

    **c.** Risk factors for onset of asthma

       **i.** Parental asthma

       **ii.** Male gender

       **iii.** Low birth weight

       **iv.** Exposure to tobacco smoke prenatally and/or postnatally

       **v.** Severe lower respiratory tract infection

         (a) Pneumonia

         (b) Bronchiolitis

       **vi.** Wheezing in absence of colds

       **vii.** Exposure to allergens (Samet, Wiesch, & Ahmed, 2001)

    **d.** Risk factors (Liu, 2004; Martinez, 2002)

       **i.** Atopic dermatitis

       **ii.** Food allergy

       **iii.** Inhalant allergen sensitization

       **iv.** Food allergen sensitization

**3.** Pathophysiology

    **a.** Airway obstruction

       **i.** Constriction of smooth muscle in small bronchial airways restricts airflow

       **ii.** Inflammation damages the airways

       **iii.** Cellular infiltrate contains eosinophils, neutrophils, monocytes, lymphocytes

       **iv.** Excess production of mucus and edema of tissues also block the airways

    **b.** Tissues of asthmatic airways contain cells that produce preallergic, preinflammatory cytokines and chemokines

       **i.** Mast cells

       **ii.** Activated eosinophils

       **iii.** Activated helper T lymphocytes

    **c.** Inflammation of airways is linked to:

       **i.** Airway hyperresponsiveness to allergen exposures—reversible

       **ii.** Airway *remodeling*

         (a) Thickening of basement membrane

         (b) Subepithelial collagen deposition

         (c) Smooth muscle and mucous gland hypertrophy and hyperplasia

    **d.** Phases of airflow obstructive processes due to allergen exposure

       **i.** Early phase—within 15 to 20 minutes

       **ii.** Bronchoconstriction hyperresponsiveness that can last weeks

         (a) Inflammation

         (b) Immune cellular infiltration into airways

         (c) Airway edema

         (d) Excess mucus production

         (e) Peak at night (midnight to 8:00 AM)

    **e.** Airflow obstructions can be life threatening

       **i.** Complications include atelectasis and air leaks in chest

    **f.** Ongoing exposure to asthma triggers and late phase reactions are the major factors contributing to disease chronicity

**4.** Presentation, focused assessment, and differential diagnoses

    **a.** Signs and symptoms

       **i.** Vary in presentation from well appearing, to chronic, to acute respiratory distress (Box 36-1)

■ **BOX 36-1**
■ **SYMPTOMS AND COMPONENTS OF A FOCUSED ASSESSMENT FOR THE CHILD WITH A SUSPECTED ASTHMA DIAGNOSIS**

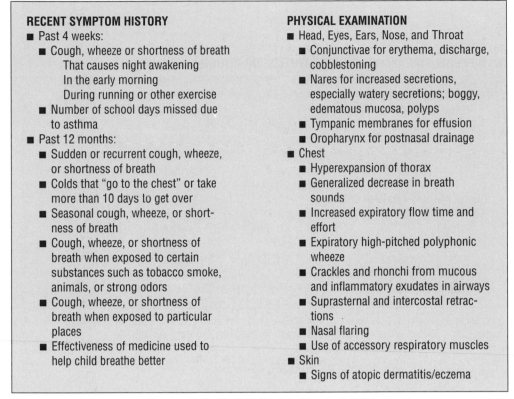

**RECENT SYMPTOM HISTORY**
- Past 4 weeks:
  - Cough, wheeze or shortness of breath
    That causes night awakening
    In the early morning
    During running or other exercise
  - Number of school days missed due to asthma
- Past 12 months:
  - Sudden or recurrent cough, wheeze, or shortness of breath
  - Colds that "go to the chest" or take more than 10 days to get over
  - Seasonal cough, wheeze, or shortness of breath
  - Cough, wheeze, or shortness of breath when exposed to certain substances such as tobacco smoke, animals, or strong odors
  - Cough, wheeze, or shortness of breath when exposed to particular places
  - Effectiveness of medicine used to help child breathe better

**PHYSICAL EXAMINATION**
- Head, Eyes, Ears, Nose, and Throat
  - Conjunctivae for erythema, discharge, cobblestoning
  - Nares for increased secretions, especially watery secretions; boggy, edematous mucosa, polyps
  - Tympanic membranes for effusion
  - Oropharynx for postnasal drainage
- Chest
  - Hyperexpansion of thorax
  - Generalized decrease in breath sounds
  - Increased expiratory flow time and effort
  - Expiratory high-pitched polyphonic wheeze
  - Crackles and rhonchi from mucous and inflammatory exudates in airways
  - Suprasternal and intercostal retractions
  - Nasal flaring
  - Use of accessory respiratory muscles
- Skin
  - Signs of atopic dermatitis/eczema

From Liu, A. H., Spahn, J. D., & Leung, D. Y. M. (2004). Childhood asthma. In R. E. Behrman, R. M. Kliegman, & H. B. Jenson (Eds.). *Nelson textbook of pediatrics* (17th ed.). Philadelphia: Saunders, pp. 760–774.

    **b.** History (see Box 36-1)
        **i.** History of recurrent symptoms is important
    **c.** Focused assessment (see Box 36-1)
    **d.** When asthma is not symptomatic, the physical examination may be entirely normal
    **e.** Diagnostic criteria (NHLBI, 1997)
        **i.** Asthma is primarily a clinical diagnosis
        **ii.** Reversible or partially reversible lower airway obstruction
        **iii.** Cough or wheeze that improves with bronchodilator therapy
        **iv.** Rule out other potential diagnoses (Box 36-2)
**5.** Diagnostic tests
    **a.** Diagnostic testing may be useful to confirm clinical findings and rule out alternative diagnoses
    **b.** Spirometry (Table 36-1)
        **i.** Important diagnostic test used to confirm the presence of obstructive lung disease consistent with asthma
        **ii.** Should be attempted in children ages 4 and older
        **iii.** Children up to age 7 may not be able to perform a reliable test

    c. Children less than 4 years old and older children who cannot cooperate with testing are diagnosed based on clinical assessment and response to bronchodilator therapy

---

■ **BOX 36-2**
■ **DIFFERENTIAL DIAGNOSES FOR WHEEZE OR COUGH IN CHILDREN**

**UPPER AIRWAY DISEASE**
  Allergic rhinitis
  Chronic rhinitis
  Sinusitis
  Hypertrophy of adenoids or tonsils
  Nasal foreign body

**LARGE AIRWAY OBSTRUCTION**
  Laryngotracheobronchomalacia
  Pertussis
  Tracheal stenosis
  Bronchostenosis
  Vascular rings or tracheal webs
  Foreign body aspiration

Vocal cord dysfunction or paralysis
Chronic bronchitis
Toxic inhalations

**SMALL AIRWAY OBSTRUCTION**
  Bronchopulmonary dysplasia
  Viral bronchiolitis
  Cystic fibrosis
  Gastroesophageal reflux
  Congenital heart disease
  Tuberculosis
  Pneumonia
  Pulmonary edema

From Liu, A. H., Spahn, J. D., & Leung, D. Y. M. (2004). Childhood asthma. In R. E. Behrman, R. M. Kliegman, & H. B. Jenson (Eds.). *Nelson textbook of pediatrics* (17th ed.). Philadelphia: Saunders, pp. 760-774.

---

■ **TABLE 36-1**
■ ■ **Office-Based Spirometry for the Child with a Suspected Asthma Diagnosis**

| Test | Meaning of Results | Precision | Cost $, $$, $$$ |
|---|---|---|---|
| $FEV_1$ (forced expiratory volume over 1 second) | Reduced in the presence of asthma in most cases | Equipment and technique should meet or exceed American Thoracic Society (1995) recommendations | $$ |
| $FEV_1$ before and 15 minutes after administering a short-acting inhaled bronchodilator | ≥12% improvement in value between the first and second test confirms diagnosis of asthma, even if initial $FEV_1$ is >80% of expected | Precision of test also depends on the child's technique and effort | |
| FEV 25–75 (mean expiratory flow volume over the middle half of the FVC) | Reduced values are indicative of small airway obstruction | | |
| FVC (forced vital capacity) | May be normal or reduced in asthma | | |
| $FEV_1$/FVC | Used to assess overall lung function | | |
| PEFR (peak expiratory flow rate) | May be normal or reduced in asthma | | |

### ■ TABLE 36-2
### ■ ■ Additional Diagnostic and Monitoring Tests for the Child with a Suspected Asthma Diagnosis

| Test | Purpose | Relative Cost $, $$, $$$ |
|---|---|---|
| Portable peak expiratory flow rate (PEFR) meter | Not a diagnostic test due to lack of standardization, but helpful to provide objective home measure of lung function over time; also used to assess diurnal variation over 1–2 weeks | $ |
| Chest x-ray | Normal findings consistent with asthma | $$ |
| | Can be used to rule in pneumonia, vascular ring, congenital heart disease | |
| Oxygen saturation | Monitor severity of an exacerbation | $ |
| Additional pulmonary function studies including methacholine provocation test or exercise test | Ordered by pulmonary or allergy specialist | $$$ |
| | Indicated when symptoms are atypical or child does not respond to treatment; or symptoms persist despite normal or near-normal spirometry | |
| Allergy testing | Identify specific triggers for asthma and determine need for immunotherapy | $$ |
| Upper GI, pH probe test, sleep test | Evaluate for gastroesophageal reflux disease | $$$ |
| CT scan of the sinuses | Evaluate for chronic rhinosinusitis | $$$ |

    **d.** Additional tests (Table 36-2)
        **i.** Used to rule out alternative diagnoses
        **ii.** Assess the degree of respiratory compromise of a child with acute symptoms
        **iii.** Indicated in the presence of specific signs and symptoms
        **iv.** When the child does not respond to asthma therapy
**6.** Treatment
    **a.** Goals of childhood asthma management (CDC, 2003; Liu, et al., 2004)
        **i.** Minimal or no chronic asthma symptoms, day or night
        **ii.** No limitations in activity, including sports participation
        **iii.** No missed school or work because of asthma
        **iv.** Normal or near-normal lung function
        **v.** Minimal or no adverse side effects from medications
        **vi.** Satisfaction with asthma care
            (a) Plan for asthma management
                (1) Developed in collaboration with family and child as appropriate
                (2) Direct responses to changes in asthma symptoms and condition
                (3) Written plans are recommended
                (4) May use a green, yellow, red designation to distinguish among treatment options (NHLBI, 2002)
                    a) "Green" plan includes daily control medications and quick relief medications for use during healthy, relatively asymptomatic times
                    b) "Yellow" plan indicates how to intensify therapy in the presence of predetermined symptom patterns or decreases in peak expiratory flow rate PEFR rates

       c) "Red" plan indicates what is to be done in an acute asthma exacerbation

    (b) Two approaches to prescribing (AAAAI, 2004, 2000; NHLBI, 1997, 2002)

      (1) Preferred approach

        a) Begin treatment at a step higher than the child's disease classification

        b) Or with a short course of oral steroids

        c) Then step down when symptoms are controlled

      (2) Alternate approach

        a) Begin treatment consistent with the child's level

        b) Then step up if control is not achieved

        c) Once control is achieved, therapy can be maintained or stepped down as needed

      (3) Step up therapy

        a) Asthma symptoms are increasing

        b) Child cannot play and exercise normally

        c) Gradual decrease in PEFR values (about 20%)

      (4) Step down therapy

        a) 25% every 2 to 3 months

**b.** Guidelines—*Pediatric Asthma: Promoting Best Practice* (AAAAI, 2004)

    **i.** Established by collaboration of three organizations:

      (a) American Academy of Asthma, Allergy and Immunology (AAAAI)

      (b) National Heart, Lung and Blood Institute (NHLBI)

      (c) American Academy of Pediatrics (AAP)

    **ii.** Individual patient response and clinical judgment should ultimately be used to guide decision making

    **iii.** Data on asthma management for infants are limited (AAAAI, 2004; NHLBI, 2002)

**c.** Four components of optimal asthma management (CDC, 2003)

    **i.** Regular assessment and monitoring—see Follow-up, section 8 below

    **ii.** Control of environmental factors contributing to asthma severity

      (a) Important aspect of management

      (b) Reduced exposure to allergens and irritants can decrease:

        (1) Asthma symptoms

        (2) Need for medications

        (3) Airways hyperresponsiveness

      (c) Exposures to cats, cockroaches, and house dust mites are strongly associated with exacerbations (Institute of Medicine, 2000)

      (d) A recent meta-analysis failed to demonstrate significant effects from reducing exposure to house dust mite antigens in homes of people with mite-sensitive asthma, using chemical, physical or combined measures (Gotzsche, Johansen, Schmidt, & Burr, 2004).

      (e) Nevertheless, the following strategies are currently recommended to reduce or eliminate exposure to known or suspected triggers (Kieckhefer & Ratcliff, 2004)

        (1) Remove carpets

        (2) Change bedding frequently—as often as daily for severe cases

        (3) No pets if allergic to dander

        (4) Avoid use of aspirin—check labels on over-the-counter products for aspirin content

        (5) Nonsteroidal antiinflammatory drugs (NSAIDs) are asthma triggers for some individuals

        (6) Avoid smoking in the home

        (7) If family member must smoke, do it outside and wear a jacket that can be removed after returning inside

**iii.** Asthma pharmacotherapy

    (a) Selection of pharmacologic therapy is based on the severity of the individual child's asthma

    (b) Severity levels (NHLBI, 2002)

        (1) Mild intermittent—symptoms during day $\leq 2$ days per week; symptoms during night $\leq 2$ nights per month

        (2) Mild persistent—symptoms during day more than two per week but less than one per day; symptoms during night more than 2 nights per month

        (3) Moderate persistent—symptoms during day occur daily; symptoms during night more than 1 night per week

        (4) Severe persistent—symptoms during day continual; symptoms during night frequent

    (c) A stepwise approach is used to gain and maintain control of asthma symptoms

    (d) Two categories of pharmacologic treatment are important in asthma treatment (NHLBI, 1997, 2002)

        (1) Control therapy (Table 36-3 and Table 36-4)

           a) Children with persistent asthma symptoms should always receive control therapy

           b) Reduce chronic airway inflammation, the primary pathophysiologic mechanism of asthma

        (2) Quick-relief therapy (Table 36-5)

           a) Control medications are aimed at reducing chronic airway inflammation, the primary pathophysiologic mechanism of asthma

    (e) Inhaled corticosteroids (ICS) (Table 36-3)

        (1) Most effective and preferred class of medications for reducing airway inflammation

        (2) Shown to improve prebronchodilator FEV1

        (3) Reduce airway hyperresponsiveness

        (4) Reduce need for supplemental bronchodilator and oral steroid use

        (5) Reduce hospitalizations for asthma (Aronson, et al., 2001; NHLBI, 2002)

        (6) ICS has been shown to be safe for children, based on studies lasting from 1 to 6 years.

           a) Studies that compare growth in children receiving ICS at recommended doses to controls show an average difference in height to be 1 cm, whether measured for 1 year or 4 to 6 years

           b) Cumulative effects of ICS therapy in later life are not known at present

           c) Available evidence shows that ICS has minimal effects on adult bone mineral density, risk of cataract formation and function of the hypothalamic-pituitary-adrenal axis (Aronson, et al., 2001; NHLBI, 2002)

    (f) Long-acting $\beta_2$-agonists are used to enhance the effect of ICS therapy (Table 36-4)

        (1) Provide effective 12-hour bronchodilation

■ **TABLE 36-3**
■ ■ **Long-Term Control Medications Used for Children with Asthma: Inhaled Corticosteroids**

| Generic Name | Trade Name(s) | Low Daily Dose(mcg) | | Medium Daily Dose(mcg) | | High Daily Dose(mcg) | | Relative Cost $,$$,$$$ |
|---|---|---|---|---|---|---|---|---|
| | | Child | Adult | Child | Adult | Child | Adult | |
| Beclomethasone CFC 42 or 84 mcg/puff | Beclovent, Vanceril, Vanceril DS | 84–336 | 168–504 | 336–672 | 504–840 | >672 | >840 | $$ |
| Beclomethasone HFA 40 or 80 mcg/puff | | 80–160 | 80–240 | 160–320 | 240–480 | >320 | >480 | $$ |
| Budesonide DPI 200 mcg/inhalation | Pulmicort Turbihaler | 200–400 | 200–600 | 400–800 | 600–1200 | >800 | >1200 | $$ |
| Budesonide inhalation suspension | Pulmicort Respules | 0.5 | | 1 | | 2 | | $$ |
| Flunisolide 250 mcg/puff | AeroBid AeroBid-M | 500–750 | 500–1000 mcg | 1000–1250 | 1000–2000 | >1250 | >2000 | $$ |
| Fluticasone MDI 44, 110 or 220 mcg/puff | Flovent Generic available | 88–176 | 88–264 | 176–440 | 264–660 | >440 | >660 | $$ |
| Fluticasone DPI 50, 100, or 250 mcg/inhalation | Flovent Rotadisk | 100–200 | 100–300 | 200–400 | 300–600 | >400 | >600 | $$ |
| Triamcinolone acetonide 100 mcg/puff | Azmacort | 400–800 | 400–1000 | 800–1200 | 1000–2000 | >1200 | >2000 | $$ |

(2) Synergistic with ICS to suppress airway inflammation (Aronson, et al., 2001; Bisgaard, 2000; Markham & Jarvis, 2000; Shewsbury, et al., 2000)

(3) Addition of a long-acting $\beta_2$-agonist to low to medium doses of ICS has improved lung function and is recommended when asthma therapy needs to be increased or when there is a need to decrease the dosage of ICS (NHLBI, 2002; Ni Chroinin, et al, 2005).

■ **TABLE 36-4**
■ ■ **Long-Term Control Medications Used for Children with Asthma: Noncorticosteroids**

| Class and Indication | Generic Name | Trade Name(s) | Dosage Regimen | | Relative Cost $, $$, $$$ |
|---|---|---|---|---|---|
| Long-acting $\beta_2$-agonists Used to augment effectiveness of inhaled corticosteroids and for exercised induced asthma | Salmeterol MDI: 21 mcg/puff DPI 50 mcg/blister | Serevent | 1 or 2 puffs q12h 1 blister q12h | 2 puffs q12h 1 blister q12h | $$ |
| Combined medication Works synergistically to enhance antiinflammatory effect of corticosteroid | Fluticasone/salmeterol DPI 100 mcg fluticasone/ 50 mcg salmeterol 250 fluticasone/ 50 salmeterol 500 flucticasone/ 50 salmeterol | Advair Diskus | 1 inhalation bid; dose depends on asthma severity | 1 inhalation bid; dose depends on asthma severity | $$ |
| Cromolyn and nedocromil NSAIDs: Primary advantage is safety. Use for exercise-induced asthma or when inhaled corticosteroids are contraindicated | Cromolyn MDI 1 mg/puff Nebulizer solution 20 mg/ampule Nedocromil MDI 1.75 mg/puff | Intal Tilade | 1 or 2 puffs 10–15 minutes before exercise 1 or 2 puffs tid or qid 1 ampule tid or qid 1 or 2 puffs 30 minutes before exercise 1 or 2 puffs bid to qid | 2–4 puffs 10–15 minutes before exercise 2–4 puffs tid or qid 1 ampule tid or qid 2–4 puffs 30 minutes before exercise 2–4 puffs bid to qid | $ $ $ |
| Leukotriene modifiers | Montelukast 4- or 5-mg chewable tablet 10-mg tablet Zafirlukast 10- or 20-mg tablet Zileuton 300- or 600-mg tablet | Singulair Accolate Zyflo | 4 mg at bedtime (2–5 years) 5 mg at bedtime (6–14 years) 10 mg (>14 years) 10 mg bid (7–11 yrs) 2400 mg daily divided qid for >12 years | 10 mg at bedtime 20 mg bid 2400 mg daily divided qid | $$ $$ $$ |
| Methylxanthines | Theophylline | Various | Starting 10 mg/kg/day For infants less than 1 year, maximum dose is 0.2 × age in weeks + 5. For children ≥ 1 year old, maximum dose is 16 mg/kg/day up to 800 mg/day | Starting 10 mg/kg/day up to maximum dose of 800 mg/day | $ |

■ **TABLE 36-5**
■ ■ **Quick-Relief Medications Used for Children with Asthma**

| Indication and Class | Generic Name | Trade Names | Dosage Regimen | | Relative Cost |
|---|---|---|---|---|---|
| | | | *Child* | *Adult* | *$,$$,$$$* |
| Short-acting β₂-agonist | Albuterol | Accuneb Proventil Proventil HFA Ventolin Ventolin HFA Ventolin Roto- caps Volmax | Nebulization: 2.5 mg (3 mL of a 0.083% solution) q 20 minutes for 3 doses, then 0.15–0.3 mg/kg (up to 10 mg) q 1–4 hr as needed MDI: 4–8 puffs every 20 minutes for 3 doses, then q 1–4 hr | Nebulization: 2.5–5 mg q 20 minutes for 3 doses, then 2.5–5 mg q 1–4 hr MDI: 4–8 puffs q 20 minutes for 3 doses then 4–8 puffs q 1–4 hr; maximum inhala- tion 12 puffs/day | Generic—$ Brand name—$$ |
| | Bitolterol | Tomalate | — | 2 or 3 puffs tid-qid; maximum dose 3 puffs q6h or 2 puffs q4h | $ |
| | Levalbuterol | Xopenex | Nebulized: 1.6– 1.25 mg tid | Nebulized: 0.63 mg tid | $$ |
| | Pirbuterol | Maxair Maxair auto- haler | | 1 or 2 puffs or inha- lations q 4–6 hr up to 12 per day | $$ |
| Oral cortico- steroids for acute exacerba- tions or for severe asthma un- controlled by other means | Methylpren- isolone 2-, 4-, 8-, 16-, 32-mg tablets | Medrol | 0.25–2 mg/kg/daily as single dose in AM or every other day as needed for control | 7.5–60 mg daily in a single dose in AM or every other day as needed for control | $$ |
| | Prednisolone 5-mg tablets 5 mg/5 mL 15 mg/5 mL | Prelone, Pedia- pred | Short-course "burst": 1–2 mg/ kg/day up to 60 mg/day maxi- mum, given for 3–10 days | Short-course "burst": 40–60 mg/day as single or 2 divided doses for 3–10 days | Generic—$ Brand name—$$ |
| | Prednisone 1-, 2.5-, 5-, 10-, 20-, 50-mg tablets 5 mg/mL 5 mg/5mL | Prednisone Deltasone Orasone Liquid Pred Prednisone Intensol | | | Generic—$ Brand name—$$ |
| Anticholinergics | Ipratropium bromide | Atrovent | Nebulization: 250 mcg q 20 minutes for 3 doses, then q 2–4 hr as needed MDI: 4–8 puffs as needed | Nebulization: 500 mcg q 20 minutes for 3 doses, then q 2–4 hr as needed MDI: 4–8 puffs as needed | $$ |

(4) Should not be used alone as control medications or to treat acute asthma symptoms (NHLBI, 2002; Taketomo, et al., 2005)

(5) Should not be used alone as control medications or to treat acute asthma symptoms (NHLBI, 2002)

(6) When used alone, may reduce responsiveness to short-acting 2-agonists and have been associated with asthma deaths (Bisgaard, 2000; Taketomo et al, 2005)

(g) Combined medications

(1) Ease of administration when an inhaled steroid and 2-agonist are to be routinely administered

(2) Cost less and require less patient time

(3) Have been shown to be equally effective (Kavru et al, 2000; Markham & Jarvis, 2000; O'Byrne, et al., 2001)

(h) Cromolyn and nedocromil (Table 36-4)

(1) Two NSAIDs used because of their excellent safety profile

(2) Large, long-term study by the Child Asthma Management Group (CAMP) (Szefler, Weiss, & Tonascia, 2000) showed no differences in lung function or symptom outcomes between nedocromil and placebo

(3) Based on this study and others, the recommended use of cromolyn and nedocromil is for infants and children with mild asthma as an alternative treatment when ICSs are not tolerated (Aronson, et al., 2001; NHLBI, 2002)

(i) Leukotriene modifiers (Table 36-4)

(1) Inhibit one of the inflammatory pathways involved in asthma pathogenesis

(2) Montelukast is most often used

a) Approved for children as young as 2 years

b) Dosed once daily

c) No known interactions with other medications or food

(3) Indicated as alternative treatment alone for mild persistent asthma and in combination with ICS for moderate persistent asthma (Aronson, et al., 2001; NHLBI, 2002)

(4) Less effective and more expensive as combination therapy than combination ICS and long-acting 2-agonist (Stempel, O'Donnell, & Meyer, 2002)

(5) Benefit in the treatment of allergic rhinitis, which is a common cormorbid condition that must be controlled in order to optimize response to asthma treatment (AAAAI, 2000)

(6) Adherence to leukotriene modifiers has been shown to be better than to ICS, an important factor in clinical outcomes (Jones, et al., 2003)

(j) Theophylline a methylxanthine (Table 36-4)

(1) Provides sustained bronchodilation for asthma

(2) Used as an adjunct in cases of moderate to severe asthma; current evidence does not support larger role in moderate asthma (Suessmuth, Freihorst, & Gappa, 2003)

(3) Most effective for nocturnal asthma symptoms

(4) Narrow therapeutic index

(5) Interacts with many other medications

    (6) Therapeutic drug monitoring needed with desired serum concentrations of 10 to 20 mcg/mL (NHLBI, 1997; Taketomo, Hodding, & Kraus, 2005)

  (k) Omalizumab (Xolair) for injection

    (1) Recently approved by the U.S. Food and Drug Administration (FDA)

    (2) Use with moderate to severe asthma uncontrolled by ICS

    (3) Used primarily by asthma specialists for a select population of patients 12 years and older to help achieve asthma control

    (4) Acts by disabling IgE and therefore inflammation

  (l) Quick relief therapy (see Table 36-5)

    (1) All children with asthma should have relief therapy on hand

    (2) Quick relief medications

     a) General

      i) Designed to manage asthma symptoms

       *a)* Chest tightness

       *b)* Cough

       *c)* Wheezing

      ii) Used in advance of exposure to a known asthma trigger

       *a)* Animal dander

       *b)* Exercise

      iii) Frequent or increasing use of quick relief medications is an indication of asthma exacerbation

     b) Short-acting $\beta_2$-agonists

      i) Primary medications used for quick relief of symptoms

      ii) Albuterol is available for inhalation

       *a)* Metered-dose inhaler

       *b)* Nebulized solution

       *c)* Available in a generic form

       *d)* Most cost effective of the drugs in this class

      iii) Levalbuterol (Xopenex)

       *a)* Alternate agent used for quick relief

       *b)* Derivative of albuterol

       *c)* Fewer effects on the 2-receptors in the heart

       *d)* Useful when tremulousness and tachycardia are uncomfortable or dangerous adverse effects

       *e)* Available only in nebulized form

       *f)* Much more expensive

      iv) Oral steroids

       *a)* Quick relief medication

       *b)* Use as a short burst during asthma exacerbations

      v) Anticholinergic drugs

       *a)* Such as ipratropium

       *b)* Adjunct treatment primarily during acute exacerbations

 (m) Aerosol delivery devices for asthma medications

    (1) Selection based on:

     a) Delivery system

     b) Particular drug desired

    (2) Correct technique

     a) Essential to ensure consistent medication delivery

     b) Parents and children receive instruction

    c) Technique should be assessed periodically, preferably at each follow-up visit (Marguet, et al., 2001)

(3) Metered-dose inhalers (MDIs)
    a) Most commonly used delivery system
    b) Technique
      i) Require the child to coordinate actuation of the inhaler with a slow (3 to 5 seconds) inhalation
      ii) Followed by breath holding for 10 seconds
    c) Spacers
      i) Come in a variety of forms and materials
      ii) Required for use with ICS
      iii) Minimize systemic absorption of medication
      iv) Help provide consistent medication delivery
      v) Most hard spacers are appropriate for children older than 4 years.
      vi) For younger children, spacers with face mask allow drug delivery using tidal breathing
      vii) Can cause thrush—teach children to use mouthwash afterward, swish it around, and spit it out
    d) Breath-actuated MDI
      i) Used with children 5 years and older
      ii) Avoid the need to coordinate actuation of the MDI with inhalation
      iii) Require that the inhalation be strong enough to effectively actuate the device
    e) Dry powder inhalers (DPIs)
      i) Useful for children 5 years and older
      ii) Avoid the use of propellants
      iii) May deliver the drug more consistently than traditional MDIs
    f) Nebulizers
      i) Offer an alternative to MDIs and DPIs
      ii) Do not require as much cooperation from the child
      iii) Useful in exacerbations
      iv) When inspiratory volumes decreased due to chest tightness
      v) Unable or unwilling to cooperate with treatment
      vi) Variations in technique and positioning of the nebulized flow can result in reductions of medication actually received by the child

(n) Nonpharmacologic treatment
  (1) Herbal remedies
    a) Not recommended
    b) Popular in some families
    c) Large lay body of literature about herbal remedies
    d) Lack of controlled studies that document their effectiveness (Huntley & Ernst, 2000)

**iv.** Patient education should address the following topics:
  (a) Identification and avoidance of asthma triggers
  (b) Recognition of impending asthma episode
  (c) Appropriate use of peak flowmeters

(d) Appropriate use of asthma inhalers

(e) Medication adherence

(f) Control of asthma exacerbations maximizes child's:

(1) School performance

(2) Self-esteem

(3) Activity tolerance

7. Influence on growth and development

a. Children with asthma can be expected to live a normal life

b. Regular school attendance is essential (Halterman, et al., 2001)

i. Children who have poor asthma control miss more school than well children

ii. May have more difficulty concentrating because they do not feel well

iii. May interfere with academic performance

iv. Young children may be less prepared for the demands of school than well children

c. Routine health maintenance including anticipatory guidance for age (Kieckhefer & Ratcliff, 2004)

i. Age-appropriate immunizations are recommended

ii. If child is receiving systemic or long-term steroids, avoid immunizations with live virus

iii. Annual influenza vaccine for infants older than 6 months of age

iv. Regular assessment of height, weight, head circumference, and body mass index (BMI) using standardized growth charts

(a) Children with more severe asthma are at higher risk for decreased growth velocity due to (AAAAI, 2004; Aronson, et al., 2001; NHLBI, 2002):

(1) Poor lung function

(2) Higher doses of inhaled steroids

v. Children with food allergies may need specific advice about managing dietary restrictions

d. Active exercise participation is recommended

i. Active lifestyle should be encouraged, including participation in normal childhood activities and sports

ii. Severe allergies or asthma triggers might make it necessary to avoid certain experiences

iii. Families should be encouraged to seek other activities that will provide similar social and developmental experiences

iv. Some evidence that children who begin wheezing very early in life (Martinez, 2002):

(a) May have smaller lung volumes

(b) May persist into adulthood

(c) May be more at risk for asthma exacerbations and decline in lung function

e. Sexual development may be delayed due to (Kieckhefer & Ratcliff, 2004):

i. Poorly controlled asthma

ii. Frequent, long-term use of corticosteroids

iii. Consider potential for drug interactions if sexually active adolescent requires oral contraceptives

f. Psychosocial development (Knafl, et al., 1996)

i. Asthma poses a disruption to any family

ii. Child's psychosocial development may be affected by the family's management style (FMS)

■ **TABLE 36-6**
■ ■ **When to Refer Children with Asthma**

| Diagnosis, Sign, or Symptom | Referral Recommendations |
|---|---|
| • Atypical signs and symptoms | Comanage with pediatrician or appropriate pediatric subspecialist if other comorbid conditions complicate diagnoses or treatment |
| • Testing for alternative diagnoses (see Box 36-1)<br>• Child less than 3 years old and has moderate or severe persistent asthma<br>• Goals of therapy are not being met within 6 months of appropriate treatment; earlier if child is not responding to treatment<br>• Allergy testing and possible immunotherapy needed<br>• Use of long-term oral corticosteroid therapy, high-dose inhaled corticosteroid therapy, or more than 2 bursts of oral corticosteroids within 12 months | Refer to asthma specialist |
| • Life-threatening asthma exacerbation | Refer to emergency department |

    iii. Families who demonstrate a thriving FMS find ways to integrate asthma management into their lives in a way that minimizes the degree of disruption caused by the disease and its treatment

    iv. Development of self-care is an essential part of growing up with asthma

    v. As children grow and mature, their participation in treatment should increase accordingly with a shift in parental role from caregiving to care supervision and coaching (Kieckhefer & Trahms, 2000)

  g. Preparation for transition to adult providers should considered when child is in late teens

8. Follow-up

  a. Criteria for referral (Table 36-6)

    i. Most children are managed effectively in the primary care setting

    ii. Comanagement is appropriate with younger children or when asthma is more severe or does not respond as expected to treatment plans

  b. Monitoring and follow-up are essential aspects of care

  c. Parents of young children should be taught to recognize symptoms of worsening asthma

  d. Older children and their parents may use symptom monitoring or monitoring PEFR

    i. Compare daily PEFRs with the child's "personal best" PEFR

    ii. "Personal best" PEFR is the highest PEFR that the child can achieve over a 2 to 3 week period when the asthma is under control

  e. Follow-up office visits

    i. Scheduled every 1 to 6 months

    ii. Depending on the child's symptoms and condition

    iii. Closer follow-up when changes in therapy are made

    f.  Follow-up assessment should include the following:
        i.  Recent (past 2 weeks) symptom history
        ii.  History of exacerbations since the last visit
        iii.  Monitoring of quality of life
        iv.  Past 2 week history of PEFRs if used at home
    g.  Spirometry
        i.  Initially, once therapy is stabilized
        ii.  At least annually
        iii.  When evaluating a change in treatment
    h.  Use recommendations for adjusting therapy for day-to-day changes in their child's condition (AAAAI, 2004; NHLBI, 1997)
        i.  Depending on the reliability of the child's symptoms
        ii.  Frequency and duration of exacerbations
    i.  Review of the action plan, medications, and techniques for MDI and PEFR as appropriate
9.  Long-term implications
    a.  The natural history for any particular child is difficult to predict (Peat, Toelle, & Mellis, 2000)
    b.  Most children begin experiencing wheeze or cough in the first year of life
        i.  A proportion of these will continue to have symptoms after 3 years of age
        ii.  Others will totally resolve (Martinez, 2002)
    c.  The Tucson Children's Respiratory Study (Taussig, et al., 2003)
        i.  Large prospective study of children spanning more than 20 years
        ii.  Identified three distinct wheezing syndromes in early childhood
        iii.  Found that children who wheezed frequently during the first 3 years of life and either had a parent with physician-diagnosed asthma or eczema or had two of the following three historical factors:
          (a)  Physician-diagnosed allergic rhinitis
          (b)  Wheezing in the absence of an upper respiratory infection (URI)
          (c)  Eosinophilia
        iv.  These children were also likely to continue having asthma symptoms at school age (Castro-Rodriguez, et al., 2000)
        v.  Mortality
          (a)  Relatively low, although it does occur (CDC, 2003)
          (b)  Factors that increase children's risk for death
             (1)  A previous intensive care unit admission for asthma
             (2)  Required intubation
             (3)  Have poor control
             (4)  Rely on excessive use of $\beta_2$-agonists for control (NHLBI, 1997)

## REFERENCES

American Academy of Allergy, Asthma & Immunology (AAAAI). (2004). *Pediatric asthma: Promoting best practice.* Milwaukee: American Academy of Allergy, Asthma & Immunology.

American Academy of Allergy, Asthma & Immunology (AAAAI). (2000). *The allergy report: Diseases of the atopic diathesis* (vol. 2). Milwaukee: American Academy of Allergy, Asthma & Immunology, p. 164.

Aronson, N., Lefervre, F., Piper, M., et al. (2001). Management of chronic asthma. Evidence report/technology assessment number 44 (AHRQ Publication No. 01-E044). Rockville, MD: Agency for Health-care Research and Quality.

Bisgaard, H. (2000). Long-acting beta(2) agonists in the management of childhood asthma. A critical review of the literature. *Pediatr Pulmonol, 29*(3), 221-234.

Busse, P., & Busse, W. (2002). Pathogenesis of asthma. In R. Slavin & R. Reisman (Eds.). *Asthma*. Philadelphia: American College of Physicians.

Castro-Rodriguez, J., Holberg, C., Wright, A., & Martinez, F. (2000). A clinical index to define risk of asthma in young children with recurrent wheezing. *Am J Respiratory Crit Care Med, 162*, 1403-1406.

Centers for Disease Control and Prevention. (2006a). Current asthma prevalence percents by age: National Health Interview Survey, 2003. Retrieved April 17, 2006, from www.cdc.gov/asthma/NHIS/2003_5able3-1.htm.

Centers for Disease Control and Prevention. (2006b). Lifetime asthma population estimates by age: National Health Interview Survey, 2003. Retrieved April 17, 2006, from www.cdc.gov/asthma/NHIS/2003_table4-1.htm.

Centers for Disease Control and Prevention (2006c). Lifetime asthma population estimates by age: National health Interview Survey, 2003. Retrieved April 17, 2006, from www.cdc.gov/asthma/NHIS/2003_table1-1.htm.

Centers for Disease Control and Prevention. (2003). Key clinical activities for quality asthma care: Recommendations of the National Asthma Education and Prevention Program. *MMWR Morb Mortal Wkly Rep, 52*(RR6), 1-8. Retrieved June 5, 2005, from www.cdc.gov/mmwr/preview/mmwrhtml/rr5206a1.htm.

Gotzsche, P. C., Johansen, H. K., Schmidt., L. M., & Burr, M. L. (2004). House dust mite control measures for asthma. *Cochrane Database of Systematic Reviews (4)*: CD001187. Retrieved April 17, 2006 from OVID Medline database.

Halterman, J., Montes, G., Aligne, C., et al. (2001). School readiness among urban children with asthma. *Ambu Pediatr, 1*(4), 201-205.

Huntley, A., & Ernst, E. (2000). Herbal medicines for asthma: A systematic review. *Thorax, 55*, 925-929.

Institute of Medicine (IOM). (2000). *Clearing the air: asthma and indoor air exposures*. Washington, DC: National Academy Press.

Jones, C., Santanello, N. C., Boccuzzi, S. J., et al. (2003). Adherence to prescribed treatment for asthma: Evidence from pharmacy benefits data. *J Asthma, 40*(1), 93-101.

Kavuru, M., Melamed, J., Gross, G., et al. (2000). Salmeterol and fluticasone propionate combined in a new powder inhalation device for the treatment of asthma: a randomized, double-blind, placebo-controlled trial. *Journal of Allergy & Clinical Immunology, 105*(6 Pt 1): 1108-16.

Kieckhefer, G., & Ratcliffe, M. (2004). Asthma. In P. L. Jackson & J. C. Vessey (Eds.). *Primary care of the child with a chronic condition* (4th ed.). St. Louis: Mosby, pp. 174-197.

Kieckhefer, G., & Trahms, C. (2000). Supporting development of children with chronic conditions: From compliance toward shared management. *Pediatr Nurs, 26*(4), 354-363.

Knafl, K., Breitmayer, B., Gallo, A., & Zoeller, L. (1996). Family response to childhood chronic illness: Description of management styles. *J Pediatr Nurs, 11*(5), 315-326. (Older reference, but still salient to today's families)

Leonard, P., & Sur, S. (2003). Interleukin-12: potential role in asthma therapy. *BioDrugs, 17*(1), 1-7.

Liu, A. H., Spahn, J. D., & Leung, D. Y. M. (2004). Childhood asthma. In R. E. Behrman, R. M. Kliegman, & H. B. Jenson (Eds.). *Nelson textbook of pediatrics* (17th ed.). Philadelphia: Saunders, pp. 760-774.

Marguet, C., Couder, L., Le Roux, P., et al. (2001). Inhalation treatment: Errors in application and difficulties in acceptance of the devices are frequent in wheezy infants and young children. *Pediatr Allergy Immunol, 12*(4), 224-230.

Markham, A., & Jarvis, B. (2000). Inhaled salmeterol/fluticasone propionate combination: a review of its use in persistent asthma. *Drugs, 60*(5): 1207-33.

Martinez, F. (2002). Development of wheezing disorders and asthma in preschool children. *Pediatrics, 2*, 362-367.

National Heart, Lung, and Blood Institute NHLBI (1997). Expert panel report II: Guidelines for the diagnosis and management of asthma (97-4051). Bethesda, MD: National Institutes of Health.

National Heart, Lung, and Blood Institute NHLBI (2002). NAEPP expert panel report: Guidelines for the diagnosis and management of asthma—update on selected topics 2002. Bethesda, MD: National Heart Lung and Blood Institute.

Ni Chroinin, M., Greenstone, I., R., Danish, A., Magdolinos, H., Masse, V, Zhang, X., & DuCharme, F. M. (2005). Combination of inhaled long-acting beta2-agonists and inhaled steroids versus higher dose of inhaled steroids in children and adults with persistent asthma, *Cochrane Database of Systematic Reviews, 4*: CD005533. Retrieved April 17, 2005 from OVID Medline database.

O'Byrne, P. M., Barnes, P. J., Rodriquez-Roisin, R., et al. (2001). Low dose inhaled budesonide and formoterol in mild persistent asthma: The OPTIMA randomized trial. *Am J Respir Crit Care Med, 164*(8), 1392-1397.

Peat, J., Toelle, B., & Mellis, C. (2000). Problems and possibilities in understanding the natural history of asthma. *J Allergy Clin Immunol, 106*, S144-S152.

Samet, J., Wiesch, D., & Ahmed, I. (2001). Pediatric asthma: Epidemiology and natural history. In C. K. Naspitz, S. J. Szefler, D. G. Tinkelman, & J. O. Warner (Eds.). *Textbook of pediatric asthma: An international perspective.* London: Martin Dunitz, pp. 35-66.

Shrewsbury, S., Pyke, S., & Britton, M. (2000). Meta-analysis of increased dose of inhaled steroid or addition of salmeterol in symptomatic asthma (MIASMA). *British Medical Journal, 320*(7246): 1368-73.

Stempel, D. A., O'Donnell, J. C., & Meyer, J. W. (2002). Inhaled corticosteroids plus salmterol or montelukast: effects on resource utilization and costs. *J Allergy Clin Immunol, 109*(3), 433-439.

Suessmuth, S., Freihorst, J., & Gappa, M. (2003). Low-dose theophylline in childhood asthma: a placebo-controlled, double-blind study. *Pediatric Allergy & Immunology, 14*(5), 394-400.

Szefler, S. J., Weiss, S., & Tonascia, J. (2000). Long-term effects of budesonide or nedocromil in children with asthma. *N Engl J Med, 343*(15), 1054-1106.

Taketomo, C. K., Hodding, J. H., & Kraus, D. M. (2005). *Pediatric dosage handbook.* (9th ed.). Hudson, OH: Lexicomp.

Taussig, L., Wright, A., Holberg, C., et al. (2003). Tucson children's respiratory study: 1980 to present. *J Allergy Clin Immunol, 111*(4), 661-675.

# Cerebral Palsy

WENDY M. NEHRING, PhD, RN, FAAN

## DEFINITION

Cerebral palsy (CP) is a collection of motor syndromes resulting from disorders of early brain development, or acquired insult to the central nervous system (CNS). Although CP is believed to be a nonprogressive disorder, there is evidence that the abnormal posture and/or movement features of CP often change over time (Griffin, Fitch, & Griffin, 2002; Johnston, 2004; National Institute of Neurological Disorders and Stroke [NINDS], 2001; Rosenbaum, et al., 2002).

1. Incidence and prevalence
   a. First described by George Little in 1861
   b. Most common and costly form of chronic motor disability that begins in childhood (Johnston, 2004)
   c. Approximately 10,000 infants are born each year with CP (Centers for Disease Control and Prevention, National Center for Birth Defects and Developmental Disabilities, 2002)
   d. Incidence in the United States has remained stable or has slightly increased since 1970 (Griffin et al., 2002; Winter et al., 2002) due to:
      i. Increase in number of premature and very low birth weight infants
      ii. Increase in incidence in infants of normal birth weight
      iii. Decrease in incidence of kernicterus
      iv. Increase in incidence of multiple births
   e. 8000 to 12,000 children diagnosed with this condition each year (Schendel, Schuchat, & Thorsen, 2002; Winter et al., 2003)
   f. Prevalence of cerebral palsy in the United States is 1.5 to 2 per 1000 live births
   g. Prevalence rates vary by country
      i. From a low of 1.34 per 1000 in 6-year-olds in Shiga Prefecture, Japan from 1977 to 1991 (Suzuki & Ito, 2002)
      ii. To 1.6 to 2.3 per 1000 in northeastern England from 1970 to 1994 (Drummond & Colver, 2002)
   h. Recurrence risks in subsequent births are rare

2. Etiology
   a. Pathogenesis of cerebral palsy is complicated by multifactorial causes and much remains unknown
   b. Possible causes are grouped by the developmental period when the neurologic insult may have occurred (Demott, 2001; Dizon-Townson, 2001; Griffin, et al., 2002; NINDS, 2001; Schendel, 2001)
   c. Antenatal factors (insults) that cause abnormal brain development account for 80% of cases (Johnston, 2004)
      i. Maternal
         (a) Bleeding
         (b) Diabetes
         (c) Hyperthyroidism
         (d) Exposure to radiation or toxins
         (e) Genetic abnormalities
         (f) Incompetent cervix
         (g) Infections
            (1) Maternal Group B streptococcus triples risk (Demott, 2001; Schendel, et al., 2002)
         (h) Inflammatory response
         (i) Malnutrition
         (j) Medication use (e.g., thyroid or hormone replacement)
         (k) Mental retardation
         (l) Polyhydramnios
         (m) Previous child with developmental disabilities
         (n) Previous fetal loss
         (o) Previous premature birth
         (p) Seizure disorder
         (q) Severe proteinuria
   d. Congenital abnormalities external to the CNS
      i. Chorioamnionitis
      ii. Chromosomal abnormalities
      iii. Congenital malformations
      iv. Fetal development problems
      v. Genetic syndromes
      vi. Hereditary fetal thrombophilias (Gibson, et al., 2003)
      vii. Inflammatory response
      viii. Problems in placental functioning
      ix. Rh incompatibility
      x. Teratogens
   e. Perinatal factors
      i. Labor and delivery
         (a) Abnormal presentations
         (b) Intrapartum asphyxia accounts for less than 10% of cases
         (c) Fetal heart rate depression
         (d) Preeclampsia
         (e) Premature delivery
         (f) Prolonged labor
         (g) Prolonged membrane rupture
      ii. Neonate
         (a) Cystic periventricular leukomalacia (Wu & Colford, 2000)
         (b) Days on mechanical ventilation
         (c) Intrauterine growth restriction

        (d) Intraventricular hemorrhage (IVH)

        (e) Low birth weight

        (f) Meconium aspiration

        (g) Periventricular leukomalacia (PVL)

        (h) Persistent pulmonary hypertension during newborn period

        (i) Prematurity

           (1) Mechanisms of pathogenesis for preterm and term causes of CP are different

        (j) Low birth weight, less than 1000 g

        (k) Seizures

        (l) Sepsis and/or CNS infection

    **f.** Postnatal and childhood factors

        **i.** Brain injury

        **ii.** Infections

        **iii.** Meningitis or encephalitis

        **iv.** Stroke

        **v.** Toxins

        **vi.** Traumatic brain injury

    **g.** Socioeconomic deprivation (Dolk, Pattenden, & Johnson, 2001).

    **h.** Unknown factors

**3.** Pathophysiology

    **a.** Brain insults cause alterations in:

        **i.** Primitive reflexes

        **ii.** Muscle stretch reflexes

           (a) Spasticity is at least partially a result of the defective release of gamma-aminobutyric acid (GABA) in the spinal cord

           (b) GABA causes overstimulation of alpha motor neurons that create spasticity

           (c) More research is needed to fully understand the pathophysiology of spasticity

        **iii.** Muscle tone

        **iv.** Postural reactions

    **b.** Major secondary conditions resulting from the CNS insult may include:

        **i.** Mental retardation

        **ii.** Seizures

        **iii.** Vision and hearing problems

        **iv.** Medical complications

    **c.** A structural abnormality in the brain

**4.** Presentation

    **a.** Symptoms

        **i.** Irritability

        **ii.** Weak cry

        **iii.** Poor sucking ability with tongue thrust

        **iv.** Excessive sleep patterns

        **v.** Lack of interest in environment

        **vi.** May sleep in "rag doll" or extended and arched position

        **vii.** Difficulty diapering

    **b.** Focused assessment for a child with suspected CP or diagnosis of CP (Box 37-1)

    **c.** Signs associated with CP can appear on one or both sides

        **i.** Poor head control

        **ii.** Clenched hands present after 3 months of age

        **iii.** Side protective reflexes absent after 5 months of age

■ **BOX 37-1**
■ **FOCUSED ASSESSMENT OF A CHILD WITH SUSPECTED OR DIAGNOSED CP**

**HEALTH HISTORY**
- Prenatal and perinatal history. Review Apgar scores and medical complications before, during, and after birth.
- Developmental history. Review age for attainment of milestones, especially motor. Assess parent's opinion and concerns about child's growth and development.

**PHYSICAL EXAMINATION**
- Height and weight. Assess height for age.
- Assess primitive and protective reflexes. Assess hand preference.
- Assess motor behaviors, e.g., midline reaching, crawling ("bunny hopping"), or walking (toe walking).
- Assess muscle tone.
- Assess hip and knee flexion and extension.
- Assess for scissoring of legs.
- Complete neurologic examination.
- Check for specific attributes of specific types of cerebral palsy.

Adapted from Nehring, W. M. (2004). Cerebral palsy. In P. L. Jackson & J. A. Vessey (Eds.). *Primary care of the child with a chronic condition* (4th ed.). St. Louis: Mosby, pp. 327–344; and Thorogood, C., & Alexander, M. A. (2005).

    iv. Extended atonic neck and Moro reflexes after 6 months of age
    v. Parachute reflex absent after 10 months of age
    vi. Crosses midline to obtain objects before 12 months of age
    vii. Hand preference noted between 6 and 18 months of age
    viii. Leg scissoring noted between late infancy and early toddlerhood (NINDS, 2001)
    ix. Cramped synchronized general movements in premature infants
       (a) Described as simultaneous muscle relaxation and contraction in a "monotonous sequence" (Ferrari, et al., 2002, p. 464)
    x. Presence of abnormal muscle tone
  d. Later signs include "bunny hopping" when crawling and "W sitting"
  e. Additional signs may include: (Nehring, 2004)
    i. Crouched gait
    ii. Unequal leg length
    iii. Flat foot
    iv. Foot deformity
    v. Toe walking
    vi. Walking on outer parts of the feet
5. Differential diagnoses (Box 37-2)
  a. The most important determinants of a diagnosis include:
    i. Child's mental, motor, and functional abilities
    ii. Child's medical history
  b. Diagnostic criteria
    i. Motor deficit with static signs and symptoms
    ii. Failure to obtain developmental motor milestones
    iii. CNS abnormality
  c. Diagnosis is often not made until 2 years of age to rule out any other neurodevelopmental disorder

■ **BOX 37-2**
■ **DIFFERENTIAL DIAGNOSES**

| | |
|---|---|
| Acute poliomyelitis | Hypotonia |
| Adrenoleukodystrophy | Lesch-Nyhan disease |
| Arginase deficiency | Metachromatic leukodystrophy |
| Dopa-responsive dystonia | Mitochondrial cytopathies |
| Duchenne's or Becker's muscular | Niemann-Pick disease type C |
| dystrophy | Rett's syndrome |
| Heredity progressive spastic paraplegia | |

Adapted from Raymond, G. V. (2002). Abnormal mental development. In D. L. Rimoin, J. M. Connor, R. E. Pyeritz, & B. R. Korf (Eds.). *Emery and Rimoin's principles and practice of medical genetics* (4th ed.). New York: Churchill Livingstone, pp.1046–1065; and Thorogood, C., & Alexander, M. A. (2005).

6. Diagnostic tests
   a. Computed tomography (CT) of head to reveal undeveloped areas of brain, cysts in brain
   b. Magnetic resonance imaging (MRI) of head to detect abnormal structures or areas of brain
   c. Ultrasonography of the brain to reveal cysts and abnormal structures
   d. Electroencephalogram (EEG) to rule out seizure disorder
   e. Intelligence tests to detect mental retardation and/or learning disabilities
   f. Motor delays
      i. Bayley Scales of Infant Development II (BISD II)
      ii. Motor tests
         (1) BSID II
         (2) Gross Motor Function Measure (GMFM) (Rosenbaum, et al., 2002)
         (3) Severity of CP determined by the Gross Motor Function Classification System (CMGCS) (Rosenbaum, et al., 2002)
            a) Level I—walks without restrictions; limitations in more advanced gross motor skills
            b) Level II—walks without assistive devices; limitation in walking outdoors
            c) Level III—walks with assistive mobility devices; limitations in walking outdoors
            d) Level IV—self-mobility with limitation; transported or uses power mobility outdoors
            e) Level V—self-mobility is severely limited even with use of assistive technology
      iii. Vision and hearing tests as needed to rule out vision and hearing deficits (NINDS, 2001)
      iv. Laboratory studies to rule out metabolic and genetic disorders
         (1) Thyroid
         (2) Lactate level
         (3) Pyruvate level
         (4) Organic and amino acids
         (5) Chromosomes
         (6) Protein levels

7. Types and characteristics of cerebral palsy (Sanger, et al., 2003)
  a. Commonly used categories of CP are pyramidal (spastic) and extrapyramidal (dystonic and athetoid types)
    i. Most children with CP actually have both pyramidal and extrapyramidal features, so those categories are not always useful
    ii. To encourage a more consistent use of terms associated with the features of CP, the Task Force on Childhood Motor Disorders (Sanger, et al., 2003) has defined the terms and recommended methods to evaluate them clinically
      (a) Tone (p. e89)
        (1) State of active muscle contraction while muscle is at rest and subjected to external force
          a) Palpate the muscle to estimate resting tone
          b) Test the muscle's resistance to passive range of motion (ROM)
        (2) Tone is perceived by the examiner, but not by the child
      (b) Hypertonia—abnormally increased resistance to externally-imposed movement about a joint (p. e89)
      (c) Spasticity (p. e90)
        (1) A velocity-dependent resistance of a muscle to stretch
        (2) Hypertonia that increases as speed of passive ROM increases
        (3) Resistance increases rapidly once a threshold for stretch is reached; sometimes called the "spastic catch"
      (d) Upper motor neuron syndrome is spasticity plus one of the following (p. e90):
        (1) Hyperreflexia with or without clonus
        (2) Reflex overflow
        (3) Positive Babinski reflex
        (4) Leg flexor or arm extensor weakness
      (e) Dystonic hypertonia (p. e91)
        (1) Involuntary alteration in the pattern of muscle activation during voluntary movement or maintenance of posture
        (2) Observed as abnormal twisted posture or repetitive movements
        (3) Triggered by voluntary movements
        (4) Varies in intensity and quality
      (f) Rigidity—hypertonia that meets four criteria (p. e92):
        (1) Resistance to externally imposed joint movement
          a) Is present at very low speeds of movement
          b) Does not depend on imposed speed
          c) Does not exhibit a speed or angle threshold
        (2) Immediate resistance to a reversal of the direction of movement about a joint
        (3) Limb does not tend to return toward a particular fixed posture or extreme joint angle
        (4) Voluntary activity in distant muscle groups does not lead to involuntary movements about the rigid joints, although rigidity may worsen
  b. Traditional categories of CP are still used in practice and will be described below
    i. Pyramidal (spastic) CP
      (a) Characteristics of this form of CP include:
        (1) Ankle clonus
        (2) Exaggerated stretch reflexes
        (3) Prolonged primitive reflexes
        (4) Positive Babinski reflex

      (5) Rigidity

      (6) Scoliosis

      (7) Later development of contractures

  (b) Accounts for 70% to 80% of cases of CP

  (c) Damage occurs in pyramidal tracts in the brain and to the motor cortex (Task Force on Childhood Motor Disorders, 2001)

  (d) Different types of spastic CP affect different extremities

      (1) Spastic diplegia

         a) Affects all extremities, with the lower extremities affected more than the upper

         b) More prominent in low birth weight and premature infants

         c) Cause is related to cerebral asphyxia with or without intraventricular hemorrhage and hydrocephalus

         d) May not be diagnosed until school years

         e) Occurs in 25% to 35% of cases of CP

      (2) Spastic quadriplegia

         a) Affects all extremities, and often the musculature circumventing the mouth, pharynx, tongue, and trunk

         b) Sometimes the lower extremities are more affected

         c) In rare situations, only three extremities (triplegia) are affected

         d) Most common form of CP, occurring in 40% to 45% of all cases

         e) Diagnosed in premature and low birth weight infants who have had an asphyxial insult

         f) Secondary conditions often include medical complications, mental retardation, and sensory impairments

         g) Spastic hemiplegia

         h) Affects one side of the body, with the upper extremities more affected than the lower

         i) Characterized by motor dysfunction

         j) Often found in low birth weight infants who have experienced:

           i) An episode of asphyxiation

           ii) A congenital vascular malformation

           iii) An embolism that resulted in postnatal brain damage

         k) Secondary conditions include growth retardation, medical complications, and sensory impairments

         l) Occurs in 30% to 40% of all cases

      (3) Double hemiplegia

         a) Affects both sides of the body, with the upper extremities more affected than the lower

         b) Caused by insults or damage to each brain hemisphere (Nehring, 2004)

 **ii.** Extrapyramidal (dyskinetic) CP

  (a) Dysfunctional involuntary movements *after* a voluntary movement is initiated

  (b) Characteristics include rigid muscle tone during daytime hours and normal or hypotonic muscle tone when sleeping

  (c) Due to abnormal regulation of muscle tone by the CNS resulting from cerebral insult to the extrapyramidal tracts or the basal ganglia

  (d) Occurs in 10% to 15% of cases of CP

  (e) Two main forms of dyskinetic CP:

    (1) Athetoid
     a) Results from damage to the basal ganglia
     b) Movements are purposeless, rapid, and jerky (chorea) and slow and writhing (athetosis)
    (2) Dystonic
     a) Characterized by abnormal twisting and slow, rhythmic movements of the extremities and/or trunk
     b) The Task Force on Childhood Motor Disorders (Sanger, et al., 2003) prefers the term "dystonic hypertonia" to describe this form of dyskinetic CP
  iii. Ataxic CP
   (a) Characterized by the degree of movement and balance coordination and muscle tone
   (b) Muscle tone can range from atonic to hypotonic to hypertonic
   (c) Children with ataxia present with a wide-based and unstable walk and have difficulty voluntarily moving their hand or arm or planning for such movement
   (d) Caused by damage to the cerebellum
   (e) Occurs in 5% to 10% of cases of CP (NINDS, 2001)
  iv. Mixed CP
   (a) More than one motor pattern is identified due to various neurologic insults
**8.** Refer child to a pediatric neurologist if any of the above signs and symptoms suggest CP or other central nervous system disorder
**9.** Specialized treatment
 **a.** Goals of individualized treatment (Rosenbaum, 2003)
  **i.** Promote function
  **ii.** Optimize health and development
  **iii.** Prevent or diminish secondary conditions
 **b.** An interdisciplinary team is mandatory for optimal management (Johnston, 2004)
 **c.** Cerebral palsy clinics exist in many urban settings, often in University Centers for Excellence in Developmental Disabilities (UCEDD)
 **d.** Pharmacologic treatment
  **i.** Spasticity (see Table 37-1)
   (a) See the Consensus Statement on Pharmacotherapy for Spasticity (Tilton & Maria, 2001)
   (b) Medications help to reduce spasticity and increase function
   (c) Decision making in choice of treatment for spasticity includes age, adverse effects, comorbidity, compliance, costs, degree of spasticity, prior health history and drug allergies
   (d) Choose muscles for injection in which the resulting weakness will not affect function
   (e) Continuous intrathecal baclofen infusion most helpful to reduce spasticity in the lower extremities and enhance ambulation (Edgar, 2001)
   (f) Effectiveness is individual and more research is needed to fully understand the efficacy and adverse effects of these medications (Boyd & Hays, 2001; Butler & Campbell, 2000; Murphy, Irwin, & Hoff, 2002)
   (g) Greater effectiveness has been found with the use of multiple treatment options (Desloovere, et al., 2001; Graham, 2001; Molenaers, et al., 2001)
   (h) Monitor medications for spasticity closely if adolescent with CP is pregnant
   (i) Seizure control can be altered with use of diazepam (Valium) and baclofen

■ **TABLE 37-1**
■ ■ **Medications for Muscular Symptoms in Children with CP**

| Symptom | Generic Name | Examples of Trade Names | Recommended Route, Pediatric Dosages, Regimen | Relative Cost: $, $$, $$$ |
|---|---|---|---|---|
| Muscle spasms | Baclofen | Lioresal oral (PO) | PO: 2-7 years: 10-15 mg/day divided q8h; may increase by 5-15 mg/day q 3 days (max: 40 mg/day) | $$ |
| | ≥≤ | intrathecal (after 4 years of age) | ≥8 years: 10-15 mg/day divided q8h; may increase by 5-15 mg/day q 3 days (max: 60 mg/day) No pediatric dose given for intrathecal | |
| Anxiety, muscle spasm | Diazepam | Apo-Diazepam Diastat Diazemuls Novodipam Valium Valrelease Vivol | PO: ≥6 months: 1-2.5 mg bid or tid Not recommended for infants less than 6 months of age | $ |
| Spasticity | Dantrolene sodium | Dantrium | PO: 0.5 mg/kg, increase tid/qid at 4- to 7-day intervals, then increase dose by 0.5 mg/kg Not to exceed 3 mg/kg/dose bid/qid or 400 mg/day | $$ |
| Spasticity | Botulinum A toxin | BOTOX Dysport | 1–6 units/kg per bodyweight per muscle | $$ |
| Extrapyramidal reactions | Benztropine mesylate | Apo-Benztropine Besylate Cogentin PMS Benztropine | PO/IM/IV: >3 years, 0.02–0.05 mg/kg, 1 or 2 times/day | $$ |

Adapted from Koman, L. A., Smith, B. P., & Balkrishnan, R. (2003). Spasticity associated with cerebral palsy in children: Guidelines for the use of botulinum A toxin. *Pediatr Drugs, 5*(1), 11–23; and Wilson, B. A., Shannon, M. T., & Stang, C. L. (2005). *Nurse's drug guide 2005.* Upper Saddle River, NJ: Prentice-Hall.

       (j) Alcohol can also influence the effectiveness of baclofen (Dantrium) and dantrolene

       (k) Dantrolene also warrants careful monitoring of bowel function and respiratory problems (Wilson, Shannon, & Stang, 2003)

    ii. Pain

       (a) Find out how the child communicates pain

       (b) NSAIDs are needed (see Chapter 55, Table 55-5)

       (c) The use of botulinum toxin A and intrathecal baclofen to treat spasticity has also been found to reduce pain associated with spasticity

          (1) More research on this is warranted (Nolan, et al., 2000)

  **e.** Nonpharmacologic treatment

    **i.** Therapies

       (a) First line of treatment includes physical and occupational therapy

       (b) Goal—to provide optimal motor development, prevent weakening and deterioration of the muscles, and reduce incidence of contractures (NINDS, 2001)

          (1) Physical therapy

          (2) Occupational therapy

          (3) Speech therapy

          (4) Behavioral therapy or counseling

          (5) Neuromuscular electrical stimulation

    ii. Adaptive equipment

       (a) Standing boards

       (b) Computers

       (c) Functional equipment (e.g., for feeding)

       (d) Scooters and tricycles

       (e) Switches

       (f) Wheelchairs, often individually molded

    iii. Orthotic devices accompany therapy (White, et al., 2002).

       (a) Help to maintain optimal range of motion to the joints

       (b) Prevent occurrence or worsening of contractures

       (c) Stabilize the joints

       (d) Control involuntary motion

       (e) Braces

       (f) Casting

       (g) Splints

  f. Surgery—not an early choice for treatment.

    i. Corrective orthopedic surgery (e.g., muscle lengthening)

    ii. Usually not performed until the child is 6 years old (Flynn & Miller, 2002; NINDS, 2001)

    iii. Degree of spasticity important to consider when weighing surgical options (Boop, Woo, & Maria, 2001)

    iv. Selective dorsal rhizotomy (Kim, et al., 2001; McLaughlin, et al., 2002; Steinbok, 2001)

       (a) Involves cutting nerves that influence spasticity in the legs

       (b) Short-term efficacy has been found

       (c) Additional research is needed to ascertain long-term effects and quality of life versus the cost of the surgery

    v. Neurologic (e.g., for seizure control)

10. Education

  a. Parental education (Johnston, 2004)

    i. Methods to handle child's daily activities in ways that limit the effects of abnormal muscle tone

    ii. Exercises to prevent development of contractures

    iii. Age-appropriate discipline and limit-setting to minimize behavior problems

  b. Special education

    i. Developmental screening and diagnostic testing from infancy is recommended

    ii. In addition to mental and motor tests, assess functional independence

       (a) Functional Independence Measure for Children (WeeFIM)

    iii. Attention to emotional development is important

    iv. Early intervention programs

       (a) Need for individual family service plan (IFSP) and interdisciplinary involvement

    v. Specialized preschool and school programs

       (a) Need for individualized education plan (IEP) and interdisciplinary involvement

       (b) Plan for as much integration as possible

       (c) Parents need to be advocates for their child

11. Complementary and alternative therapies for CP (Liptak, 2005)
    a. Liptak (2005) reviewed the research evidence for nine alternative therapies and made the following assessment of the evidence
    b. Evidence is promising
        i. "Hippotherapy"—therapeutic horseback riding
            (a) Demonstrated beneficial effects on body structures and functioning
            (b) Few risks
            (c) More research is needed to evaluate benefit to balance, tone and range of motion, self-esteem, and confidence building
    c. More evidence required
        i. Hyperbaric oxygen—oxygen reactivates "dormant" cells in the brain
        ii. Electrical stimulation—stimulation of muscle increases blood flow and increases the bulk of the muscle
        iii. Acupuncture
    d. Inconclusive evidence
        i. Adeli suit—specially-made clothing that provides resistance across muscle groups
        ii. Conductive education—promotes independence; discourages learned helplessness
    e. No evidence, i.e., no research at all
        i. Craniosacral therapy—light touch and pressure is used to remove "impediments" to the flow of cerebrospinal fluid from the head to the sacrum
        ii. Feldendrais—relaxation therapy to improve movement, posture and functioning
    f. Not recommended
        i. Patterning—passively and repetitively putting child through motions of normal motor tasks
    g. Research does not support the efficacy of the following treatments for children with CP
        i. Neurodevelopmental treatment
            (a) Also known as NDT, patterning, or the Bobath method
        ii. Hyperbaric oxygenation
    h. Massage therapy and aquatherapy (Hurvitz, et al., 2003)
        i. Reported by parents to be helpful
        ii. More research in this area is warranted
12. Influence of having CP on growth and development
    a. Physical
        i. Gross motor
            (a) Universally delayed and more obvious as child ages
            (b) Delays in all gross motor milestones
            (c) Prolonged primitive reflexes
            (d) Lack of protective reflexes
            (e) Hip dislocation and subluxation
            (f) Contractures
            (g) Scoliosis
            (h) Balance and gross movement problems
            (i) Dyspraxia
        ii. Fine motor
            (a) Tactile hyposensitivity or hypersensitivity
            (b) Stereognosis
            (c) Speech articulation deficits

      (d) Vocal strength and quality deficits
      (e) Chewing, swallowing, and sucking problems
      (f) Drooling
      (g) Fatigue
   iii. Vision and hearing
      (a) Amblyopia
      (b) Cataracts
      (c) Cortical blindness
      (d) Homonymous hemianopsia (25% with hemiplegia)
      (e) Refractive errors
      (f) Retinopathy of prematurity
      (g) Strabismus
      (h) Conductive hearing loss
      (i) Sensorineural hearing loss
   iv. Respiratory
      (a) Aspiration
      (b) Asthma
      (c) Hypoxemia
      (d) Respiratory infections
      (e) Pneumonia
   v. Gastrointestinal
      (a) Gastroesophageal reflux
      (b) Constipation
      (c) Encopresis
   vi. Urinary
      (a) Bladder control
      (b) Incontinence
      (c) Urinary tract infections
      (d) Urine retention
   vii. Integumentary
      (a) Latex allergy
      (b) Decubitus ulcers
   viii. Other
      (a) Under- or overweight
      (b) Dental problems, such as malocclusions, caries, and enamel defects (dos Santos, et al., 2003)
      (c) Decreased bone mineral density leading to risk of fractures and/or osteopenia (Henderson, et al., 2002; Tasdemir, et al., 2001)

**b.** Cognitive
   **i.** Intelligence
      (a) Mental retardation (MR)
         (1) Many children with CP have normal intelligence
         (2) 50% to 60% of children with spastic quadriplegia, diplegia, and mixed type of cerebral palsy have MR (Fennell & Dikel, 2001)
      (b) Learning disabilities
   **ii.** Neurologic disorders
      (a) Seizure disorders
         (1) Most common in children with spastic quadriplegia and hemiplegia
      (b) Language processing
      (c) Proprioception difficulties

    c. Psychologic
        i. Behavioral problems
           (a) Behavioral disorders
           (b) Attention disorders, with and without hyperactivity
           (c) Self-injurious behaviors
           (d) Autism spectrum disorders
        ii. Emotional problems
           (a) Depression
        iii. Social (Feldman-Winter, et al., 2002; Nehring, 2004; NINDS, 2001)
           (a) Stigma of condition
               (1) Appearance of "being different"
               (2) Difficulty moving about
               (3) Want to "fit in" (normalization)
               (4) Language problems and difficulty in communication
           (b) Self-esteem and self-concept
           (c) Need for support systems and role models
    d. Sexuality (Worley, et al., 2002)
        i. Compared with white children in the general population:
           (a) Puberty begins earlier but ends later in white children with CP
           (b) Menarche occurs later in white girls with CP
           (c) More advanced sexual maturation is associated with more body fat in girls but less body fat in boys
13. Primary care follow-up
    a. The care of the child with CP must be continual and involve an interdisciplinary team
    b. The American Academy of Pediatrics recommends a primary care medical home (Cooley, 2004)
        i. From which care is initiated, coordinated, and monitored
        ii. With which families can form a reliable alliance for information, support, and advocacy through transition to adulthood
    c. Anticipate that all office visits will require extra time
    d. Health care maintenance
        i. Growth
           (a) If height cannot be measured with the child standing, take upper arm length (UAL) and lower leg length (LLL) measurements
           (b) Triceps and subscapular skinfold measurements
           (c) See the North American Growth in Cerebral Palsy Project's website—www.healthsystem.virginia.edu/Internet/NAGCePP/healthcare/home.cfm—for directions on measuring extremity lengths and other anthropometric measures
        ii. Nutritional status and feeding problems need to be consistently assessed and corrected as needed
           (a) Spasticity and disordered movement increases metabolism, and thus increases nutritional needs
           (b) Problems with chewing, swallowing, and gastroesophageal reflux interfere with adequate caloric intake
           (c) Almost half of all children with CP are significantly undernourished
           (d) Eventually a feeding tube may be needed, especially for the child with spastic quadriplegia
           (e) Avoid excessive weight gain that is often associated with feeding tubes
        iii. Injury prevention—the child with CP is at risk for injury
           (a) Use seizure precautions

    (b) Specially designed car seats

    (c) Safety precautions around the home

    (d) Adaptive equipment in the home as needed

    (e) Local police and fire departments should be made aware of the special needs of the child in case of an emergency

  iv. Immunizations

    (a) Children with CP should receive the normal schedule of immunizations unless they have a seizure disorder

    (b) See Chapter 15 for details on all immunizations

  v. Vision

    (a) Annual assessment by a pediatric ophthalmologist

    (b) Contact lenses are contraindicated

  vi. Hearing

    (a) Regular assessments by a pediatric audiologist

    (b) In some cases, a pediatric otolaryngologist may be needed to assess hearing loss

    (c) If a hearing aid is needed, a speech therapist may also assist in treating this child

  vii. Dental

    (a) Children with CP tend to have many dental problems

    (b) Refer to a developmental dentist who has experience in caring for children with motor and developmental problems

    (c) Dental visits should take place every 6 months, especially if the child is taking phenytoin (Dilantin)

  viii. Elimination

    (a) Adequate fluid intake is difficult to maintain, which contributes to constipation and risk for urinary tract infections (UTI)

    (b) Referral to a pediatric urologist may be needed for recurrent UTI

    (c) A pattern for bowel elimination is needed

      (1) If diet and exercise do not maintain such a pattern, then a bowel management program may be needed

      (2) An interdisciplinary team effort is warranted

  ix. Sexuality

    (a) Developmental age-appropriate education

    (b) Encourage parents not be overprotective

    (c) Address child's increased risk for victimization if child has mental retardation

    (d) Help parents to assist their child to develop normally in this area

    (e) Adolescent may need assistance to position tampon or menstrual pad

    (f) Begin gynecologic care for females with CP when pubertal development occurs

      (1) Evaluate the need for pelvic examinations on an individual basis

      (2) Depending on degree of spasticity and contractures, the Sims' position may be better than the lithotomy position

  x. Psychosocial

    (a) Referral to a psychologist or psychiatrist may be needed for behavioral and/or emotional problems

  xi. Transition to adulthood

    (a) The child with CP will need assistance with making a successful transition to adulthood

    (b) Involves transition to adult health care, work, living arrangements, transportation, education, and social opportunities

(c) Independence, rather than learned helplessness, should be encouraged

**14.** Long-term implications

    **a.** Prognosis

        **i.** Depends on severity and type of CP

            (a) The more extremities involved, the more severe the involvement, the greater the nutritional and developmental problems, the worse the prognosis (Liptak, et al., 2001; NINDS, 2001)

            (b) Functional status, informal and formal support networks, and perceived quality of life greatly influence prognosis (Bjornson & McLaughlin, 2001; Houlihan, et al., 2004)

        **ii.** Mortality studies

            (a) Mortality affected by degree of physical, cognitive, and sensory limitations (Pharoah & Hutton, 2002)

            (b) Pneumonia most common cause of death in Victoria, Australia, between 1970 and 1995 (Reddihough, Baikie, & Walstab, 2001)

            (c) More research needed in this area

        **iii.** Research that evaluates outcomes of CP should focus on 5 areas (Sanger, et al., 2003)

            (a) Pathophysiology—underlying disease

            (b) Impairment—clinically observable abnormality

            (c) Functional limitations—effect on task performance (Rosenbaum, 2003)

            (d) Disability—effect on daily living

            (e) Societal limitations—effect on lifetime opportunities

            (f) Optimize health and development (Rosenbaum, 2003)

# REFERENCES

American Academy of Pediatrics, Committee on Infectious Diseases. (2000). *2000 Red book: Report of the committee on infectious diseases* (25th ed.), Elk Grove Village, IL: American Academy of Pediatrics.

Bjornson, K. F., & McLaughlin, J. F. (2001). The measurement of health-related quality of life (HRQL) in children with cerebral palsy. *Eur J Neurol, 8*(Suppl. 5), 183-193.

Boop, F. A., Woo, R., & Maria, B. L. (2001). Consensus statement on the surgical management of spasticity related to cerebral palsy. *J Child Neurol, 16*, 68-69.

Boyd, R. N., & Hays, R. M. (2001). Current evidence for the use of botulinum toxin type A in the management of children with cerebral palsy: A systematic review. *Eur J Neurol, 8*(Suppl. 5), 1-20.

Butler, C., & Campbell, S. (2000). Evidence of the effects of intrathecal baclofen for spastic and dystonic cerebral palsy. *Dev Med Child Neurol, 42*, 634-645.

Centers for Disease Control and Prevention, National Center for Birth Defects and Developmental Disabilities. (2002). *Cerebral palsy among children*. Retrieved May 20, 2006, from www.cdc.gov/ncbddd/factsheets/cp.pdf.

Cooley, W. C., & American Academy of Pediatrics Committee on Children with Disabilities. (2004). Providing a primary care medical home for children and youth with cerebral palsy. *Pediatrics, 114(4)*, 1106-1113.

Demott, K. (2001). *E. coli* infection quadruples risk of cerebral palsy. *OB GYN News, 36*(18), 1.

Desloovere, K., Molenaers, G., Jonkers, I., et al. (2001). A randomized study of combined botulinum toxin type A and casting in the ambulant child with cerebral palsy using objective outcome measures. *Eur J Neurol, 8*(Suppl. 5), 75-87.

Dizon-Townson, D. S. (2001). Preterm labour and delivery: A genetic predisposition.

*Paediatr Perinat Epidemiol, 15*(Suppl. 2), 57-62.

Dolk, H., Pattenden, S., & Johnson, A. (2001). Cerebral palsy, low birthweight and socioeconomic deprivation: Inequalities in a major cause of childhood disability. *Paediatr Perinat Epidemiol, 15*, 359-363.

dos Santos, R., Masiero, D., Novo, N. F., & Simionato, M. R. (2003). Oral conditions in children with cerebral palsy. *ASDC J Dent Child, 70*(1), 40-46.

Drummond, P. M., & Colver, A. F. (2002). Analysis by gestational age of cerebral palsy in singleton births in northeast England 1970-94. *Paediatr Perinat Epidemiol, 16*, 172-180.

Edgar, T. S. (2001). Clinical utility of botulinum toxin in the treatment of cerebral palsy: Comprehensive review. *J Child Neurol, 16*, 37-46.

Feldman-Winter, L. B., Krueger, C. J., Neyhart, J. M., & McAbee, G. N. (2002). Public perceptions of cerebral palsy. *J Am Osteopath Assoc, 102*, 471-475.

Fennell, E. B., & Dikel, T. N. (2001). Cognitive and neuropsychological functioning in children with cerebral palsy. *J Child Neurol, 16*, 58-63.

Ferrari, F., Cioni, G. E., Roversi, C., et al. (2002). Cramped synchronized general movements in preterm infants as an early marker for cerebral palsy. *Arch Pediatr Adolesc Med, 156*, 460-468.

Flynn, J. M., & Miller, F. (2002). Management of hip disorders in patients with cerebral palsy. *J Am Acad Orthop Surg, 10*, 198-209.

Gibson, C. S., MacLennan, A. H., Goldwater, P. N., & Dekker, G. A. (2003). Antenatal causes of cerebral palsy: Associations between inherited thrombophilias, viral and bacterial infection, and inherited susceptibility to infection. *Obstet Gynecol Surv, 58*, 209-220.

Graham, H. K. (2001). Botulinum toxin type A management of spasticity in the context of orthopaedic surgery for children with spastic cerebral palsy. *Eur J Neurol, 8*(Suppl. 5), 30-39.

Griffin, H. D., Fitch, C. L., & Griffin, L. W. (2002). Causes and interventions in the area of cerebral palsy. *Infant Young Child, 14*(3), 18-24.

Henderson, R. C., Lark, R. K., Gurka, M. J., et al. (2002). Bone density and metabolism in children and adolescents with moderate to severe cerebral palsy. *Pediatrics, 110*(1, Pt 1), e5.

Henderson, R. C., Kairalla, J., Abbas, A., & Stevenson, R. D. (2004). Predicting low bone density in children and young adults with quadriplegic cerebral palsy. *Dev Med Child Neurol, 46*(6), 416-419.

Houlihan, C. M., O'Donnell, M., Conaway, M., & Stevenson, R. D. (2004). Bodily pain and health-related quality of life in children with cerebral palsy. *Dev Med Child Neurol, 46*(5), 305-310.

Johnston, M. V. (2004). Cerebral palsy. In R. E. Behrman, R. M. Kliegman, & H. B. Jenson (Eds.). *Nelson textbook of pediatrics* (17th ed.). Philadelphia: Saunders, pp. 2024-2025.

Kim, D. S., Choi, J. U., Yang, K. H., & Park, C. I. (2001). Selective posterior rhizotomy in children with cerebral palsy: A 10-year experience. *Childs Nerv Syst, 17*, 556-562.

Koman, L. A., Smith, B. P., & Balkrishnan, R. (2003). Spasticity associated with cerebral palsy in children: Guidelines for the use of botulinum A toxin. *Pediatr Drugs, 5*(1), 11-23.

Liptak, G. S., O'Donnell, M., Conaway, M., et al. (2001). Health status of children with moderate to severe cerebral palsy. *Dev Med Child Neurol, 43*, 364-370.

McLaughlin, J., Bjornson, K., Temkin, N., et al. (2002). Selective dorsal rhizotomy: Meta-analysis of three randomized controlled trials. *Dev Med Child Neurol, 44*, 17-25.

Molenaers, G., Desloovere, K., De Cat, J., et al. (2001). Single event multilevel botulinum toxin type A treatment and surgery similarities and differences. *Eur J Neurol, 8*(Suppl. 5), 88-97.

Murphy, N. A., Irwin, M. C., & Hoff, C. (2002). Intrathecal baclofen therapy in children with cerebral palsy: Efficacy and complications. *Arch Phys Med Rehab, 83*, 1721-1725.

National Institute of Neurological Disorders and Stroke (NINDS). (2001). Cerebral palsy: Hope through research. Retrieved May 20, 2006, from www.ninds.nih.gov/disorders/cerebral_palsy/detail_cerebral_palsy.htm.

Nehring, W. M. (2004). Cerebral palsy. In P. L. Jackson & J. A. Vessey (Eds.). *Primary care of the child with a chronic condition* (4th ed.). St. Louis: Mosby, pp. 327-344.

Nolan, J., Chalkiadis, G. A., Low, J., Olesch, C. A., Brown, T. C. (2000). Anaesthesia and pain management in cerebral palsy. Anaesthesia, 55(5), 32-41.

Pharoah, P. O. D., & Hutton, J. L. (2002). Effects of cognitive, motor, and sensory disabilities on survival in cerebral palsy. *Arch Dis Child, 86,* 84-71.

Raymond, G. V. (2002). Abnormal mental development. In D. L. Rimoin, J. M. Connor, R. E. Pyeritz, & B. R. Korf (Eds.). *Emery and Rimoin's principles and practice of medical genetics* (4th ed.). New York: Churchill Livingstone, pp.1046-1065.

Reddihough, D. S., Baikie, G., & Walstab, J. E. (2001). Cerebral palsy in Victoria, Australia: Mortality and causes of death. *J Paediatr Child Health, 37,* 183-186.

Rosenbaum, P. (2003). Cerebral palsy: What parents and doctors want to know. *BMJ, 326,* 970-974.

Rosenbaum, P. L., Walter, S. D., Hanna, S. E., et al. (2002). Prognosis for gross motor function in cerebral palsy: Creation of motor development curves. *JAMA, 288*(11), 1357-1363.

Sanger, T. D., Delgado, M. R., Gaebler-Spira, D., Hallett, M., & Mink, J. W. (2003). Classification and definition of disorders causing hypertonia in childhood. *Pediatrics, 111*(1), e89-e97.

Schendel, D. E. (2001). Infection in pregnancy and cerebral palsy. *J Am Womens Assoc, 56,* 105-108.

Schendel, D. E., Schuchat, A., & Thorsen, P. (2002). Public health issues related to infection in pregnancy and cerebral palsy. *Ment Retard Dev Disabil Res Rev, 8,* 39-45.

Steinbok, P. (2001). Outcomes after selective dorsal rhizotomy for spastic cerebral palsy. *Childs Nerv Syst, 17,* 1-18.

Suzuki, J., & Ito, M. (2002). Incidence patterns of cerebral palsy in Shiga Prefecture, Japan, 1977-1991. *Brain Dev, 24,* 39-48.

Tasdemir, H. A., Buyukavci, M., Akcay, F., et al. (2001). Bone mineral density in children with cerebral palsy. *Pediatr Int, 43,* 157-160.

Thorogood, C., & Alexander, M. A. (2005). Cerebral palsy. Retrieved from eMedicine on May 20, 2006, at www.emedicine.com/pmr/topic24.htm.

Tilton, A. H., & Maria, B. L. (2001). Consensus statement on pharmacotherapy for spasticity. *J Child Neurol, 16,* 66-67.

White, H., Jenkins, J., Neace, W. P., et al. (2002). Clinically prescribed orthoses demonstrate an increase in velocity of gait in children with cerebral palsy: A retrospective study. *Dev Med Child Neurol, 44,* 227-232.

Wilson, B. A., Shannon, M. T., & Stang, C. L. (2005). *Nurse's drug guide 2005.* Upper Saddle River, NJ: Prentice-Hall.

Winter, S., Autry, A., Boyle, C., & Yeargin-Allsopp, M. (2002). Trends in the prevalence of cerebral palsy in a population-based study. *Pediatrics, 111,* 1220-1225.

Worley, G., Houlihan, C. M., Herman-Giddens, M. E., et al. (2002). Secondary sexual characteristics in children with cerebral palsy and moderate to severe motor impairment: a cross-sectional survey. *Pediatrics, 110*(5), 897-902.

Wu, Y. W., & Colford, J. M., Jr. (2000). Chorioamnionitis as a risk factor for cerebral palsy: A meta-analysis. *JAMA, 284,* 1417-1429.

# Childhood Cancer

SHARRON L. DOCHERTY, PhD, CPNP-AC

## DEFINITION

A group of congenital or acquired childhood diseases characterized by the uncontrolled growth and spread of abnormal cells. Characterized as very fast-growing and highly metastatic diseases

1. Classification of childhood cancers
   a. International Classification of Childhood Cancer with Surveillance, Epidemiology, and End Results (SEER) Modifications (National Cancer Institute, 2005a; 2005c)
      i. Based on recommendations from the International Agency for Research on Cancer (IARC), the International Association of Cancer Registries (IACR), and the International Society of Paediatric Oncology (SIOP)
      ii. With modifications to the classification of nervous system and bone tumors by the SEER Committee of the National Cancer Institute
   b. 12 groups classified by *histology,* as compared with the anatomic site classification used for adult populations
      i. Leukemia
         (a) Acute lymphoblastic leukemia (ALL)
         (b) Acute nonlymphoblastic leukemia, also known as:
            (1) Acute myelogenous leukemia
            (2) Acute myelocytic leukemia
            (3) Acute myeloblastic leukemia
            (4) AML
         (c) Chronic myeloid leukemia
         (d) Other specified and unspecified leukemias
      ii. Lymphomas and reticuloendothelial neoplasms
         (a) Hodgkins lymphoma
         (b) Non-Hodgkins lymphoma
         (c) Burkitts lymphoma
         (d) Miscellaneous lymphoreticular neoplasms
         (e) Unspecified lymphomas

iii. CNS and miscellaneous intracranial and intraspinal neoplasms
  (a) Ependymoma
  (b) Astrocytoma
  (c) Primitive neuroectodermal tumors
  (d) Other gliomas
  (e) Medulloblastoma
  (f) Miscellaneous specified and unspecified intracranial and intraspinal neoplasms
  iv. Sympathetic nervous system tumors
  (a) Neuroblastoma
  (b) Ganglioneuroblastoma
  (c) Other nervous system tumors
  v. Retinoblastoma
  vi. Renal tumors
  (a) Wilms' tumor
  (b) Rhabdoid and clear cell sarcoma
  (c) Renal carcinoma
  (d) Unspecified malignant renal tumors
  vii. Hepatic tumors
  (a) Hepatoblastoma
  (b) Hepatic carcinoma
  (c) Unspecified malignant hepatic tumors
  viii. Malignant bone tumors
  (a) Osteosarcoma
  (b) Chondrosarcoma
  (c) Ewings sarcoma
  (d) Other specified and unspecified malignant bone tumors
  ix. Soft tissue sarcomas
  (a) Rhabdomyosarcoma and embryonal sarcoma
  (b) Fibrosarcoma
  (c) Neurofibrosarcoma
  (d) Kaposi's sarcoma
  (e) Primitive neuroectodermal tumors
  (f) Other specified and unspecified soft tissue sarcomas
  x. Germ-cell, trophoblastic, and other gonadal neoplasms
  (a) Intracranial and intraspinal germ-cell tumors
  (b) Gonadal germ-cell tumors
  (c) Gonadal carcinomas
  (d) Other specified and unspecified malignant gonadal and nongonadal tumors
  xi. Carcinomas and other malignant epithelial neoplasms
  (a) Adrenocortical carcinoma
  (b) Thyroid carcinoma
  (c) Nasopharyngeal carcinoma
  (d) Malignant melanoma
  (e) Skin carcinoma
  (f) Other and unspecified carcinomas
  xii. Other and unspecified malignant neoplasms
2. Etiology and precipitating factors
  a. Childhood cancer is a label given to wide group of neoplastic diseases with highly variable pathophysiologic processes (Kassner, Alcoser, & Hockenberry, 2002)

i. Most childhood cancers originate from the mesodermal germ layer, which is responsible for the development of:
   (a) Connective tissue
   (b) Bone
   (c) Cartilage
   (d) Muscle
   (e) Blood
   (f) Blood vessels
   (g) Gonads
   (h) Kidney
   (i) Lymphatic system
   ii. Some types originate from molecular pathogenesis in which mutations to specific oncogenes and tumor suppressor genes occur
   iii. For most types of childhood cancer, the cause is unknown
   iv. Childhood cancer can be considered *genetic* because it occurs at the molecular level, but most childhood cancers are not *hereditary*

b. Genetic factors are associated with higher risk for developing childhood cancer
   i. Children can inherit an increased susceptibility to certain cancers through transmission of a cancer-associated gene mutation that is passed from parent to child (Ganjavi & Malkin, 2002)
   ii. But, less than 10% of newly diagnosed childhood cancers cases can be attributed to inherited cancer susceptibility (Plon & Malkin, 2002)
      (a) Important role of PNP is to recognize major cancer genetic syndromes and refer families for genetic counseling and testing (Pakakasama & Tomlinson, 2002)
      (b) Familial cancer syndromes bring an increased susceptibility to certain types of cancer (Pakakasama & Tomlinson, 2002)
   iii. Autosomal dominant disorders associated with childhood cancer
      (a) Retinoblastoma
         (1) Some children inherit a mutation in the *Rb* tumor suppressor gene
      (b) Li-Fraumeni syndrome
         (1) Inheritance of a mutation in the *p53* tumor suppressor gene
         (2) An early onset cancer predisposition syndrome associated with soft tissue sarcoma, breast cancer, leukemia, osteosarcoma, melanoma, and cancer of the colon, pancreas, adrenal cortex, and brain
      (c) Von Hippel–Lindau disease—multiple organ malignancies (Gulani, 2006)
         (1) Multiple endocrine neoplasia
         (2) Familial adenomatous polyposis
         (3) Familial Wilms' tumor
   iv. Autosomal recessive disorders associated with childhood cancer
      (a) Ataxia-telangiectasia is associated with acute lymphocytic leukemia or lymphoma (Joswiak, et al., 2005)
      (b) Bloom syndrome
   v. Chromosomal abnormalities associated with childhood cancer:
      (a) Down syndrome (Hasle, Clemmensen, & Mikkelsen, 2000)
         (1) Associated with increased risk of leukemia
         (2) High level of tumor suppressor cells on chromosome 21 may be responsible for decreased risk of other cancers such as breast cancer
      (b) Turner syndrome (occurs only in females) increases child's risk for Wilms tumor and ovarian cancer (Postellon, 2005)

        (c) Klinefelter syndrome (occurs only in males) increases child's risk for breast cancer 20 times higher than for the average male (Chen, 2005)

        (d) WAGR syndrome—a combination of Wilms' tumor, aniridia, GU malformations, and mental retardation (Bergstrom, 2002)

        (e) Beckwith-Wiedemann syndrome increases child's risk for Wilms tumor (Ferry & Cohen, 2005)

  **c.** Children with AIDS have an increased risk of developing non-Hodgkins lymphoma and Kaposis sarcoma and leiomyosarcoma

  **d.** Environmental factors (National Cancer Institute, 2005b)

    **i.** Ionizing radiation

      (a) Radiation therapy

        (1) For certain childhood cancers, such as Hodgkins disease, brain tumors, sarcomas

        (2) May lead to development of a second primary malignancy

      (b) Nonmedical sources—no clear associations with childhood cancers

    **ii.** Nonionizing radiation, e.g., cell phones, power lines, etc.—no clear association with childhood cancers

    **iii.** Drugs

      (a) Chemotherapy with alkylating agents or topoisomerase II inhibitors may cause increased risk of leukemia

      (b) Treatment with chemotherapy for certain cancers, such as Hodgkins disease, brain tumors, sarcomas may lead to development of a second primary malignancy

      (c) Anabolic steroids are linked to liver cancer

**3.** Incidence and prevalence (National Cancer Institute, 2005b)

  **a.** After accidents, cancer is the second leading cause of death in children, yet cancer is relatively rare

  **b.** In 2005, approximately 9510 children younger than the age 15 will be diagnosed with cancer

  **c.** The *peak age* at diagnosis varies with the type of cancer (Figure 38-1) (Reis, et al., 2005)

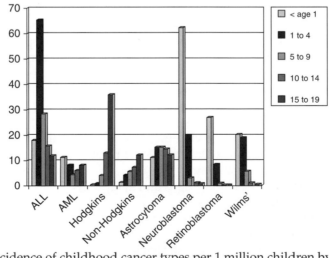

FIGURE 38-1 ■ Incidence of childhood cancer types per 1 million children by age-group. (Ries, L. A. G., Harkins, D., Krapcho, M., et al. (Eds). (2006). *SEER Cancer Statistics Review, 1975–2003*, National Cancer Institute. Bethesda, MD, http://seer.cancer.gov/csr/1975_2003/based on November 2005 SEER data submission, posted to the SEER web site, 2006)

        i. Younger than age 1
           (a) Acute myelocytic leukemia (AML)
           (b) Neuroblastoma
           (c) Retinoblastoma
           (d) Wilms' tumor
       ii. Ages 1 to 4 years
           (a) Acute lymphocytic leukemia (ALL)
      iii. Ages 15 to 19 years
           (a) Hodgkin's
           (b) Non-Hodgkin's
      iv. Fairly evenly distributed across age-groups
           (a) Astrocytoma
    d. Gender differential (National Cancer Institute, 2006)
        i. Male incidence: 15.4/100,000/year
       ii. Female incidence: 13.8/100,000/year
    e. More common in white than Black children
    f. Leukemias—3.7 to 4.8 cases per 100,000
    g. Brain tumors—3.5 per 100,000
    h. Cure
        i. Five years of disease-free survival is considered a cure for childhood cancer
       ii. Currently 75% of children are cured (Jemal, et al., 2004)
    i. Mortality
        i. Steadily decreased since 1977
       ii. In 2005, about 1585 children will die from the disease
      iii. Survival rate remains low for some forms of childhood cancer (Jemal, et al., 2004; Reaman, 2002)
           (a) AML
           (b) Relapsed ALL
           (c) ALL with specific structural chromosomal abnormalities
           (d) Some types of neuroblastoma
4. Presentation
    a. Diagnosing a child with possible cancer is complex
    b. The relative rarity of most types of childhood cancer and the lack of specificity of signs and symptoms contribute to a low index of suspicion
    c. Research shows a small likelihood that any single primary care provider will be involved in the diagnosis and referral of a child resulting in a confirmed diagnosis of cancer (Feltbower, et al., 2004)
    d. Thus the diagnostic priorities shift to identifying *suspicious cases* and making appropriate, prompt referrals
    e. See Table 38-1 for the possible presentation of common childhood cancers in primary care (Baggott & Dragone, 2004; Young, et al., 2000)
        i. Possible chief complaint
       ii. Associated presenting signs and symptoms
      iii. Differential diagnoses
           (a) Oncologic diagnoses
           (b) Other diagnoses
      iv. Appropriate first diagnostic tests
    f. Role of primary care practitioner
        i. Recognize potential signs and symptoms of oncologic disease in children (see Table 38-1)

**■ TABLE 38-1**
**■ ■ Oncologic and Other Differential Diagnoses for Observations Typically Made in Pediatric Primary Care**

| Type of Cancer | Peak Age | Possible Chief Complaint | Possible Presenting Signs/ Symptoms | Differential Diagnoses | Appropriate First Test |
|---|---|---|---|---|---|
| Leukemia:<br>ALL (acute lymphocytic leukemia)<br>AML (acute myelocytic leukemia) | 4 years—ALL<br>10 years—AML | Low grade fever for 1 to 2 weeks; bruising, mucous membrane bleeding, bone pain, headache, pallor | Pancytopenia: fatigue, pallor, mucosal bleeding, petechiae, purpura<br>Lymphadenopathy<br>Splenomegaly: abdominal swelling, pain<br>Mediastinal mass: dyspnea, cough | Oncologic dx:<br>ALL<br>AML<br>Myelodysplasia<br>Lymphoma<br>Neuroblastoma<br>Other dx: Infection<br>JRA—juvenile rheumatoid arthritis<br>Mononucleosis<br>ITP—idiopathic thrombocytopenia purpura<br>Aplastic anemia | CBC (complete blood count) with differential<br>ESR (erythrocyte sedimentation rate)<br>Chemical panel |
| Lymphoma:<br>Hodgkin's<br>Non-Hodgkin's | 10 to 20 years | Painless lump<br>Recurrent fevers<br>Cough and sweating at night<br>Dysphagia<br>Weight loss | 2- to 3-month history of lymphadenopathy, nontender lymph nodes; fever<br>Mediastinal mass: dyspnea, superior vena cava syndrome; swelling of neck, face, upper extremities<br>Abdominal disease: intussusception, obstruction, hepatosplenomegaly, jaundice | Oncologic dx: Leukemia<br>Hodgkin's lymphoma<br>Non-Hodgkin's lymphoma<br>Burkitts lymphoma<br>Other dx: Infection<br>JRA<br>Mononucleosis | Chest x-ray<br>CBC with differential<br>ESR<br>Chemical panel |
| Wilms' tumor | 2 to 3 years unilateral<br><3 years bilateral | Swollen abdomen<br>Diaper doesn't fit<br>Blood in urine (<25%) | Nontender, easily palpable abdominal mass<br>Hypertension<br>Hematuria<br>Rare: fever, diarrhea, weight loss, dyspnea | Oncologic dx: Neuroblastoma<br>Wilms' tumor<br>Lymphoma<br>Rhabdomyosarcoma<br>Other dx: Hydronephrosis<br>Hepatomegaly<br>Intussusception | Abdominal ultrasound (documents organomegaly, vascular involvement)<br>CBC with differential<br>ESR<br>Chemical panel |

*(Continued)*

**TABLE 38-1**
**Oncologic and Other Differential Diagnoses for Observations Typically Made in Pediatric Primary Care—cont'd**

| Type of Cancer | Peak Age | Possible Chief Complaint | Possible Presenting Signs/ Symptoms | Differential Diagnoses | Appropriate First Test |
|---|---|---|---|---|---|
| Neuroblastoma | 2 years | Signs and symptoms reflect location of primary disease: abdominal or thoracic<br>Swollen abdomen; tired; not eating well<br>Difficulty breathing, upper respiratory infection | Abdominal mass: spinal cord compression symptoms<br>Thoracic mass: Horners syndrome, dyspnea, edema of upper and lower extremities<br>Cervical mass: paresis, paralysis, bowel/bladder dysfunction, hypertension, diarrhea, nystagmus, cerebellar ataxia, proptosis, orbital ecchymosis, hepatosplenomegaly | Oncologic dx: Wilms' tumor<br>Rhabdomyosarcoma<br>Ewings sarcoma<br>Lymphoma<br>Renal mass<br>Other dx: Bowel obstruction | Abdominal ultrasound<br>Urine test for catecholamines (urinary VMA [vanillylmandelic acid] & homovanillic acid [HVA])<br>CBC with differential<br>ESR<br>Chemical panel |
| Bone tumor<br>Osteosarcoma<br>Ewings sarcoma | 15 to 25 years: osteosarcoma<br>10 to 20 years: Ewings | Limp, localized persistent pain, swelling of bone, low-grade fever, fatigue, weight loss | Pain and swelling at site<br>Limitation of range of motion | Oncologic dx: Ewings sarcoma<br>Osteosarcoma<br>Other dx: Osteomyelitis<br>JRA<br>Physical activity<br>Trauma<br>Growth pain | X-ray of involved limb<br>CBC with differential<br>ESR<br>Chemical panel |

| | | | | |
|---|---|---|---|---|
| Brain Tumor: Infratentorial Supratentorial Posterior fossa | 2 to 12 years: infratentorial <2 or >13 years: supratentorial or posterior fossa | Headaches, morning or persistent vomiting Falls Behavioral changes Sensory changes Decreased school performance Lethargy Loss of developmental milestones | Signs and symptoms of increased intracranial pressure: Papilledema Cerebellar signs: truncal ataxia, dysmetria (over- or under-shooting motor movements), vomiting, unsteady gait Cranial nerve alterations: gaze palsies, setting sun sign Upper motor neuron signs: hemiparesis, asymmetric hyperreflexia, clonus Midbrain signs: Parinauds syndrome Seizures, diabetes insipidus | Oncologic dx: Medulloblastoma Ependymoma Astrocytoma Primitive neuroectodermal tumor Other dx: Hydrocephalus Encephalitis Hematoma Atrioventricular malformation Migraine headaches | Computed tomography (CT) scan CBC with differential ESR Chemical panel |
| Retinoblastoma | 2 years | White eye reflex in photographs; crossed eyes | Leukokoria Proptosis Strabismus | Oncologic dx: Neuroblastoma Other dx: Strabismus | CT scan |

    ii. Prompt referral to pediatric cancer center, who has the primary responsibility for diagnosis, initiation, and monitoring of treatment

5. Treatment
   a. Role of PNP
      i. Understand the basic principles underlying childhood cancer treatment
      ii. Provide primary, preventive, health maintenance, and care of common acute illnesses to child and family throughout and following cancer treatment
      iii. Acquire information from pediatric oncologist regarding cancer treatment, possible late effects and guidance for appropriate follow-up care
      iv. Counseling and education of child and family regarding:
         (a) Effects of cancer and treatment
         (b) Use of nonconventional therapies (Jankovic, et al., 2003)
         (c) Long-term effects of cancer treatment (Oeffinger & Hudson, 2004)
      v. Recognition of oncologic emergencies while child is undergoing treatment
         (a) Tumor lysis syndrome
         (b) Fever and neutropenia
         (c) Mediastinal mass or tumor
         (d) Coagulopathy and bleeding, e.g., DIC
   b. Childhood cancer treatment
      i. Greater than 70% of children receive cancer treatment at pediatric cancer treatment centers (Liu, et al., 2003)
      ii. Centers use a multidisciplinary team approach to meet the biopsychosocial needs of the child and family
      iii. In the United States, more than 90% of children are prescribed a treatment plan protocol that is designed, implemented, and studied by the national cooperative, Children's Oncology Group (COG)
      iv. Treatment is a combination of modalities
         (a) Based on specific cytogenics of the cancer
         (b) Type and stage of cancer
         (c) Variables related to the child
            (1) Age
            (2) Symptoms
            (3) General health
      v. Treatment stages
         (a) Induction
            (1) Intensive therapy used to:
               a) Remove bulk of disease
               b) Obtain remission
         (b) Post-remission consolidation and intensification
            (1) Consisting of a variable number of courses of chemotherapy or other therapy
            (2) Designed to eradicate subclinical disease
         (c) Maintenance therapy
            (1) Long-term therapy included as treatment for some types of childhood cancer
            (2) Designed to eliminate all residual cancer
            (3) Can continue for 2 to 3 years
      vi. Goals of treatment (Alcoser & Rodgers, 2003)
         (a) Improve survival
         (b) Minimize toxicity

(c) Preserving quality of life

**c.** Treatment modalities

**i.** Surgery—used for multiple purposes:
  (a) Placement of indwelling central venous catheter that will be used for long-term treatment
  (b) Biopsy of tumor for diagnosis and treatment design
  (c) Removal of tumor
  (d) "Second look" to evaluate effect of treatment

**ii.** Chemotherapy (Alcoser & Rodgers, 2003)
  (a) Primary treatment modality
  (b) Used singly or as component of multimodal therapy such as radiation and/or surgery
  (c) Multiple chemotherapy agents are often used together
  (d) Used to reduce the primary tumor size, destroy cancer cells, and prevent metastases
  (e) Vascular access (Baggott & Dragone, 2004)
    (1) Long-term indwelling catheters often placed to reduce trauma of frequent needlesticks
    (2) Requires strict attention to:
      a) Patency of lumen
      b) Education of family members about catheter care
      c) Prevention of infection at catheter site
      d) Prompt treatment of infection at catheter site

**iii.** Radiation (Alcoser & Rodgers, 2003)
  (a) Used as adjuvant treatment for specific types of childhood cancer
    (1) Medulloblastoma
    (2) Germ-cell tumors
    (3) Hodgkins disease
    (4) Retinoblastoma
    (5) Wilms' tumor
    (6) Ewings sarcoma
  (b) Used as palliative therapy to control pain for cancers that are not responsive to other pain modalities (Tarbell & Kooy, 2002)

**iv.** Issues related to chemotherapy and radiation (Baggott & Dragone, 2004)
  (a) Side effect of nausea and vomiting lasts up to 48 hours
    (1) Use antiemetics and adjunctive methods for prevention
    (2) Continue antiemetics until symptoms subside
  (b) Side effects of anorexia and weight loss may occur during therapy
    (1) Give nutritional supplements as needed or may need total parental nutrition for a period of time
  (c) Hair loss
    (1) Loss is usually temporary
    (2) Regrowth is often different in texture and color
  (d) Bone marrow suppression
    (1) Occurs with radiation therapy
    (2) Begins within 7 to 10 days after drug administration
  (e) Prevention of infection is critical due to bone marrow suppression

**v.** Corticosteroids
  (a) High-dose steroids often used with acute lymphocytic leukemia
  (b) Used to decrease intracranial pressure with brain tumor

**vi.** Stem cell transplantation
  (a) Therapy of choice for some highly resistant childhood cancers

(b) Second-line treatment after first-line treatment has failed

(c) Very high doses of chemotherapy and radiation are used to eradicate resistant cancers

   (1) This destroys the cancer and the bone marrow as well

   (2) The bone marrow is replaced by either:

      a) Autologous bone marrow transplant—reinfusing some of the child's own bone marrow that had been removed before treatment

      b) Allogenic bone marrow transplant from a related or unrelated donor

      c) Stem cells from umbilical cords

  **vii.** Other therapies

    (a) Some childhood cancers remain resistant to standard therapies and/or require very high doses and toxic drug combinations

    (b) Research and development are ongoing in the design of childhood cancer therapies to treat the highly resistant cancers while minimizing harm to normal tissue

      (1) Biologic response modifiers (Areci & Cripe, 2002)

        a) Therapy directed at innate biologic systems that are designed to destroy cells

        b) Modify normal immunologic defense mechanisms to target cancer cells instead of microorganisms

        c) Examples are immunotherapy (e.g., monoclonal antibodies) and immunostimulatory vaccines

      (2) Molecular intervention (Areci & Cripe, 2002)

        a) Uses agents that disrupt growth and division of cancer cells at a very early molecular stage, such as development of nucleic acids, genes, and proteins

    (c) Use of these therapies is limited to supplementation of dose-intensive chemotherapy to target microscopic disease not susceptible to traditional therapy (Cheung & Rooney, 2002)

**6.** Influence on growth and development

  **a.** Childhood cancer and its treatment have a profound effect on the biopsychosocial development of the child and family

    **i.** In the acute period

    **ii.** During treatment

    **iii.** Up to 3 months following cessation

    **iv.** Long-term effects

  **b.** Physical growth

    **i.** Treatment exerts a more profound effect on growth than the cancer itself

    **ii.** Decreased growth during treatment has been well documented

      (a) Depending on the timing of the treatment, short stature may be permanent

      (b) If chemotherapy is given alone

        (1) It may contribute to slowing of growth

        (2) Usually temporary

        (3) Most children will experience catch-up growth once treatment is complete

    **iii.** Radiation therapy has a direct effect on the growth of bones in the radiation field

        (a) Radiation can cause damage to the epiphyseal plates of long bones

        (b) More critically, cranial radiation may damage glands responsible for growth-related hormone production

        (c) In a study on prepubertal growth of children who had undergone bone marrow transplant (Arvidson, et al., 2000):

            (1) Prepubertal growth was suppressed only in those children who received cranial irradiation

            (2) Normal prepubertal growth was found in those with no cranial radiation therapy CRT

    iv. Childhood cancer treatment indirectly contributes to growth alterations because of effects on the nutritional status

        (a) The child's desire to eat is affected by treatment side effects:

            (1) Mucositis

            (2) Anorexia

            (3) Nausea and vomiting

            (4) Altered taste and smell

    v. Growth curves

        (a) While in treatment, primary care providers should use standardized height, weight, and BMI curves to closely document and follow growth

        (b) Every 2 months during therapy and for first year after therapy

        (c) Head circumferences should be documented and followed in children younger than 3 years of age

    vi. Reproductive effects

        (a) Dose and age related

        (b) Overall, less risk for infertility in girls who are treated before puberty versus after puberty

        (c) Boys as well as girls may experience delayed or arrested pubertal development while in treatment

        (d) Postpubertal girls may experience:

            (1) Delayed menarche

            (2) Oligomenorrhea

            (3) Amenorrhea

        (e) Boys (Bottomley & Kassner, 2003)

            (1) Radiation treatment to the pelvic area or alkylating chemotherapy agents may lead to temporary or permanent azoospermia

            (2) Recovery of sperm production may occur within 5 to 10 years following treatment

**c.** Cognitive development

    i. It is well documented that children with cancer and other chronic illnesses often find understanding what is happening to them a challenge

        (a) They struggle with their part in having caused the illness

            (1) Children who have not reached the formal operational stage of cognitive development may confuse their condition with a form of justice for bad behavior

            (2) For example, cancer is retribution for a rule they have broken or for having unacceptable thoughts

        (b) They struggle with their inability to control painful symptoms, treatments, or procedures

    ii. Ask children what they think is making them ill

    iii. Correct their misconceptions at an appropriate cognitive level

    iv. Assure them that it is not their fault

    **d.** Socioemotional development

        **i.** In infancy and toddler period, the parent often treats the child as special or vulnerable, and this vulnerability may persist for years

        **ii.** The childhood cancer experience

            (a) May slow the development of independence for all age-groups

            (b) May limit their development of sense of competence and mastery

        **iii.** Adolescents must struggle with body image and developing a new sense of identity (Baggott & Dragone, 2004)

        **iv.** Overall, researchers have documented the critical importance of assisting the family to "keep the spirit alive" by continuing to engage in the processes that gave the child and family their identity (Woodgate & Degner, 2003)

**7.** Follow-up and late effects

    **a.** PNP role

        **i.** Once the child has completed therapy the PNP takes on a more centralized role

            (a) In continuing to provide health maintenance and preventive care

            (b) Assessing for potential late effects

        **ii.** It is essential that the PNP collect up to date information from the cancer care team regarding: (Institute of Medicine, 2003)

            (a) Treatment exposures

            (b) Complications that occurred during the acute treatment period

            (c) Possible late effects

    **b.** Late effects (Baggott & Dragone, 2004; National Cancer Institute, 2006)

        **i.** Definition—long-term consequences of childhood cancer treatment that occur several years after cessation of treatment

        **ii.** Types of late effects

            (a) Highly variable and dependent on many factors including:

                (1) Age of the child during treatment

                (2) Type of cancer and the type of treatment

            (b) In general, the younger child is at greatest risk

            (c) Researchers have found evidence that relates some of the following problems to treatment for childhood cancer (Bottomley & Kassner, 2003; Oeffinger & Hudson, 2004)

                (1) Secondary malignancies

                (2) Learning disabilities

                (3) Vision problems

                (4) Hearing problems

                (5) Growth and physical maturity

                (6) Fatigue

                (7) Cardiovascular and pulmonary function

                (8) Sexual development and reproduction in girls

                (9) Sexual development and reproduction in boys

    **c.** Posttreatment surveillance and follow-up care by specialty clinic

        **i.** While the child will be monitored closely by the pediatric oncologist for at least 3 years following treatment, lifelong follow-up is ideal

        **ii.** Some children will be followed through comprehensive long-term follow clinics at the cancer treatment center

        **iii.** Follow-up care will focus on:

            (a) Screening for and treatment of short- and long-term complications of treatment

            (b) Monitoring for recurrent and secondary cancers

    (c) Anticipatory guidance related to health behaviors that may cause secondary cancers in adulthood
      (1) Smoking
      (2) Sun exposure
      (3) Nutrition
    (d) Assessment of psychosocial adjustment and quality of life (Institute of Medicine, 2003)

**d.** Psychosocial support
   **i.** The first several years after completion of therapy are a very difficult and anxiety ridden time for children and their families (Nagel, et al., 2002)
    (a) In one study, 17% of survivors of childhood cancer had depressive, somatic, or anxious symptoms (Hudson, et al., 2004)
    (b) Even though nearly 50% reported significant changes to their health status including physical impairments and limitations, only 10% thought that their health was fair or poor
    (c) Therefore, even though survivors experienced posttraumatic stress, concurrently, they were feeling resilience and enhanced quality of life (Zebrack & Zeltzer, 2003)

**e.** Neuropsychologic testing should be done within first 2 years after completion of therapy for children who received cranial radiation or those younger than 8 years of age at time of diagnosis (Baggott & Dragone, 2004)

**f.** Immunizations
   **i.** Immune suppression that results from the treatment generally lasts for 3 to 6 months following treatment
   **ii.** Immunizations with live viruses should not be given until at least 6 months following treatment
    (a) Measles
    (b) Rubella
    (c) Mumps
    (d) Polio
  **iii.** Household contacts of children being treated with cancer should not be given oral polio vaccine (CDC, 2006)
  **iv.** Killed vaccines schedules may resume 6 months following the completion of therapy
  **v.** Consider testing for immunity to MMR following treatment; otherwise revaccinate 6 months after treatment
  **vi.** Children who have been treated for Hodgkins disease should be given:
    (a) Meningococcal
    (b) Pneumococcal vaccine

# REFERENCES

Alcoser, P. W., & Rodgers, C. (2003). Treatment strategies in childhood cancer. *J Pediatr Nurs, 18*(2), 103-112.

Areci, R. J., & Cripe, T. P. (2002). Emerging cancer-targeted therapies. *Pediatr Clin North Am, 49*(6), 1339-1368.

Arvidson, J., Lonnerholm, G., Tuvemo, T., et al. (2000). Prepubertal growth and growth hormone secretion in children after treatment for hematological malignancies, including autologous bone marrow transplantations. *Pediatr Hematol Oncol, 17,* 285-297.

Baggott, C., & Dragone, M. A. (2004). Cancer. In P. L. Jackson, & J. A. Vessey (Eds.). *Primary care of the child with a chronic condition* (4th ed.). St. Louis: Mosby, pp. 299-326.

Bergstrom, S. K. (2006). WAGR syndrome. eMedicine. Retrieved April 18, 2006, from http://http://www.emedicine.com/ped/topic2423.htm.

Bottomley, S. J., & Kassner, E. (2003). Late effects of childhood cancer therapy. *J Pediatr Nurs, 18*(2), 126-132.

Center for Disease Control and Prevention. (2006). National immunization program. Retrieved April 18, 2006 from http://www.cdc.gov/nip/home-hcp.htm.

Chen, H. (2005). Klinefelter syndrome. Retrieved May 20, 2006, from www.emedicine.com/ped/topic1252.htm.

Cheung, N. K., & Rooney, C. M. (2002). Principles of immune and cellular therapy. In P. A. Pizzo & D. G. Poplack (Eds.). *Principles and practice of pediatric oncology* (4th ed.). Philadelphia: Lippincott Williams & Wilkins, pp. 381-408.

Feltbower, R. G., Lewis, I. J., Picton, S., et al. (2004). Diagnosing childhood cancer in primary care—A realistic expectation? *Brit J Cancer, 90*, 1882-1884.

Ferry, R. J., & Cohen, P. (2005). Beckwith-Wiedemann syndrome. Retrieved May 15, 2005, from www.emedicine.com/ped/topic218.htm.

Ganjavi, H., & Malkin, D. (2002). Genetics of childhood cancer. *Clin Orthop Rel Res, 401*, 75-87.

Ghosh, S., & Jichici, D.. (2005). Primitive neuroectodermal tumors of the central nervous system. Retrieved May 20, 2006, from http://www.emedicine.com/NEURO/topic326.htm.

Gulani, A. (2006). Von Hippel-Lindau disease. Retrieved May 20, 2006, from http://www.emedicine.com/OPH/topic354.htm.

Hasle, H., Clemmensen, I. H., & Mikkelsen, M. (2000). Risks of leukaemia and solid tumours in individuals with Down's syndrome. *Lancet, 355*, 165-169.

Hudson, M. M., Mertens, A. C., Yasui, Y., et al. (2003). Health status of adult long-term survivors of childhood cancer: A report from the Childhood Cancer Survivor Study. *JAMA, 290*, 1583-1592.

Institute of Medicine. (2003). *Childhood cancer survivorship: Improving care and quality of life.* The National Academies Press: Washington, DC.

Jankovic, M., Spinetta, J. J., Martins, A. G., et al. (2004). Non-conventional therapies in childhood cancer: Guidelines for distinguishing non-harmful from harmful therapies. *Pediatr Blood Cancer, 42*, 106-108.

Jemal, A., Clegg, L. X., Ward, E., et al. (2004). Annual report to the nation on the status of cancer, 1975-2001, with a special feature regarding survival. *Cancer, 101*(1), 3-27.

Joswiak, S., Janniger, C. K., Kmiec, T., & Bernatowska, E. (2005). Ataxia-telangiectasia. Retrieved May 20, 2006, from www.emedicine.com/DERM/topic691.htm.

Kassner, E., Alcoser, P. W., & Hockenberry, M. J. (2002). Cancer in children. In K. L. McCance & S. E. Huether (Eds.). *Pathophysiology. The biologic basis for disease in adults and children* (4th ed.). Philadelphia: Mosby, pp. 357-362.

Liu, L. Krailo, M., Reaman, G. H., & Bernstein, L. (2003). Childhood cancer patients' access to cooperative group cancer programs: A population based study. *Cancer, 97*, 1339-1345.

Nagel, K., Eves, M., Waterhouse, L., et al. (2002). The development of an off-therapy needs questionnaire and protocol for survivors of childhood cancer. *J Pediatr Oncol Nurs, 19*(6), 229-233.

National Cancer Institute. (2005a). International classification of childhood cancer (ICCC). International Agency for Research on Cancer (IARC) Technical Report No. 29. Retrieved May 20, 2006, from http://seer.cancer.gov/iccc/iarciccc.html.

National Cancer Institute. (2005b). National Cancer Institute research on childhood cancers. Retrieved May 20, 2006, from http://cis.nci.nih.gov/fact/6_40.htm.

National Cancer Institute. (2005c). Surveillance, epidemiology and end results (SEER) modifications of the ICCC. Retrieved May 20, 2006, from http://seer.cancer.gov/iccc/seericcc.html.

National Cancer Institute. (2006). Late effects of childhood cancer therapies (PDQ®) Health Professional Version. Retrieved May 20, 2006, from www.nci.nih.gov/cancertopics/pdq/treatment/lateeffects/healthprofessional.

Oeffinger, K. C., & Hudson, M. M. (2004). Long-term complications following childhood and adolescent cancer: Foundations for providing risk-based health care for survivors. *CA Cancer J Clin, 54*, 208-236.

Pakakasama, S., & Tomlinson, G. E. (2002). Genetic predisposition and screening in pediatric cancer. *Pediatr Clin North Am, 49*(6), 1393-1413.

Plon, S. E., & Malkin, D. (2002). Childhood cancer and heredity. In P. A. Pizzo & D. G. Poplack (Eds.). *Principles and practice of pediatric oncology* (4th ed.). Philadelphia: Lippincott Williams & Wilkins, pp. 21-44.

Postellon, D. (2005). Turner syndrome. Retrieved May 20, 2006, from www.emedicine.com/ped/topic2330.htm.

Reaman, G. H. (2002). Pediatric oncology: current views and outcomes. *Pediatr Clin North Am, 49*(6), 1305-1318, vii.

Ries, L. A. G., Harkins, D., Krapcho, M., et al. (Eds). (2006). *SEER Cancer Statistics Review, 1975-2003*, National Cancer Institute. Bethesda, MD, http://seer.cancer.gov/csr/1975_2003/, based on November 2005 SEER data submission, posted to the SEER web site, 2006.

Tarbell, N. J., & Kooy, H. M. (2002). General principles of radiation oncology. In P. A. Pizzo & D. G. Poplack (Eds.). *Principles and practice of pediatric oncology* (4th ed.). Philadelphia: Lippincott Williams & Wilkins, pp. 369-380.

Woodgate, R. L., & Degner, L. F. (2003). A substantive theory of keeping the spirit alive: The spirit within children with cancer and their families. *J Pediatr Oncol Nurs, 20*(3), 103-119.

Young, G., Toretsky, J. A., Campbell, A. B., & Eskenazi, A. E. (2000). Recognition of common childhood malignancies. *Am Fam Phys, 61*(7), 2144-2154.

Zebrack, B. J., & Zeltzer, L. K. (2003). Quality of life issues and cancer survivorship. *Curr Prob Cancer, 27*, 198-211.

# Cleft Lip and Palate

MARY TEDESCO-SCHNECK, RN, MSN, CPNP

1. Pathophysiology
   a. Definition: a failure of fusion between one or more of the five primordial prominences of the developing embryo between 3 and 12 weeks of gestation (Sandberg, Magee, & Denk, 2002)
      i. Single frontonasal prominence
      ii. Bilateral maxillary prominences
      iii. Bilateral mandibular prominences
      iv. Frontonasal prominences
      v. Medial and lateral nasal prominences
   b. Cleft lip and cleft palate are embryologically distinct disorders (Thigpen & Kenner, 2003)
   c. Early stages of facial development in 30- to 32-day-old embryo (Figure 39-1)
   d. Sequence of embryologic development of the face (Figure 39-2) and palate (Figure 39-3)
2. Classification
   a. Figure 39-4 illustrates the parts of palate, lip, and nose that may be affected by inadequate fusion during embryologic development
   b. Developmental classification of clefting system—most widely used by primary care providers
      i. General terms
         (a) Unilateral—one side
         (b) Bilateral—both sides
      ii. Cleft lip
         (a) Complete—extends into nasal cavity
         (b) Incomplete—extends from vermilion-cutaneous junction to two thirds the height of the lip
      iii. Cleft palate (Moore & Persaud, 2003)
         (a) Primary palate—anterior to the incisive foramen
         (b) Secondary palate—posterior to the incisive foramen
         (c) Primary and secondary
   c. Palindromic system—primarily used by surgeons (Kirschner & LaRossa, 2000; Kreins, 1989)

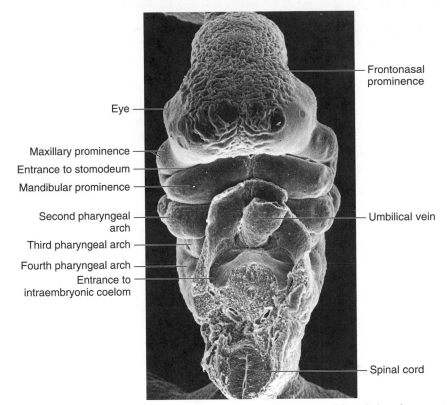

Eye

Maxillary prominence

Entrance to stomodeum

Mandibular prominence

Second pharyngeal arch

Third pharyngeal arch

Fourth pharyngeal arch

Entrance to intraembryonic coelom

Frontonasal prominence

Umbilical vein

Spinal cord

**FIGURE 39-1** ■ Electron micrograph illustrating early stages of facial development in an embryo at 30 to 32 days.

      **i.** Uses the letters LAHSHAL

      **ii.** S in the center represents the soft palate, H refers to the right and left sides of the hard palate, A refers to the alveolus (gum) on each side, and L represents the two sides of the lip

     **iii.** Upper- and lowercase letters denote complete and incomplete clefts, respectively

     **iv.** Example: LAHSHAL = complete bilateral clefts of the lip and palate; lAHSHAL = bilateral clefts of lip and palate with an incomplete cleft lip on the right

**d.** Subjective findings

      **i.** Not all infants born with cleft palate are identified in the immediate neonatal period

     **ii.** A submucous cleft is a split in the hard and/or soft palate that is covered by the mucous membrane of the roof of the mouth

        (a) Often associated with a cleft uvula

        (b) Has same genetic risk as an obvious cleft

**e.** Index of suspicion should increase with history of: (Curtin & Boekelheide, 2004)

      **i.** Feeding difficulties

        (a) Ineffective suck

        (b) Prolonged feeding

        (c) Nasal regurgitation

        (d) Aspiration

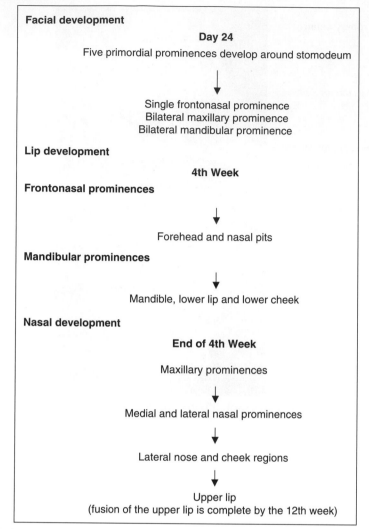

**Facial development**

**Day 24**

Five primordial prominences develop around stomodeum

Single frontonasal prominence
Bilateral maxillary prominence
Bilateral mandibular prominence

**Lip development**

**4th Week**

**Frontonasal prominences**

Forehead and nasal pits

**Mandibular prominences**

Mandible, lower lip and lower cheek

**Nasal development**

**End of 4th Week**

Maxillary prominences

Medial and lateral nasal prominences

Lateral nose and cheek regions

Upper lip
(fusion of the upper lip is complete by the 12th week)

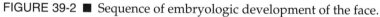

FIGURE 39-2 ■ Sequence of embryologic development of the face.

    (e) Malocclusion of newly erupted teeth
    (f) Dehydration
  **ii.** Nasal speech quality first noted in older children (submucous cleft likely)
  **iii.** Slow speech development
  **iv.** Poor hearing
  **v.** Frequent infections
    (a) Upper respiratory infections
    (b) Otitis media
  **vi.** Sleep disruption, especially for 6 weeks after surgery due to edema
**f.** Objective findings
  **i.** Inspection
    (a) Face
      (1) Inspect face for dysmorphic features or other anomalies
      (2) See Table 39-1 for syndromes associated with cleft lip, cleft palate, and/or isolated cleft palate

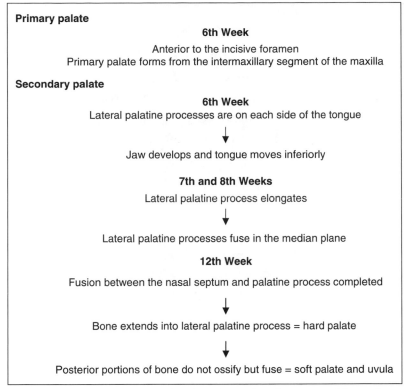

> **Primary palate**
> ### 6th Week
> Anterior to the incisive foramen
> Primary palate forms from the intermaxillary segment of the maxilla
>
> **Secondary palate**
> ### 6th Week
> Lateral palatine processes are on each side of the tongue
>
> ↓
>
> Jaw develops and tongue moves inferiorly
>
> ### 7th and 8th Weeks
> Lateral palatine process elongates
>
> ↓
>
> Lateral palatine processes fuse in the median plane
>
> ### 12th Week
> Fusion between the nasal septum and palatine process completed
>
> ↓
>
> Bone extends into lateral palatine process = hard palate
>
> ↓
>
> Posterior portions of bone do not ossify but fuse = soft palate and uvula

FIGURE 39-3 ■ Sequence of embryologic development of the palate.

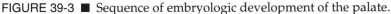

      (b) Oropharynx
         (1) With good lighting, inspect oropharynx for obvious cleft
         (2) Bifid uvula can be a normal variant or associated with a submucous cleft
         (3) Check translucence of soft palate
   **ii.** Palpation
      (a) Presence of notch in the posterior border of the hard palate can signify a submucous cleft
 **g.** Diagnostic tests
   **i.** Ultrasound in utero can detect clefts as early as 14 to 16 weeks
   **ii.** MRI will detect presence of a submucous cleft (Kuehn, et al., 2001)
 **h.** Differential diagnosis (Thigpen & Kenner, 2003)
   **i.** Major condition to consider is van der Woude's syndrome
      (a) Inherited as autosomal dominant trait
      (b) Appearance can be:
         (1) A minor, single lower lip depression
         (2) Pairs of pits or fistulas on the vermilion of the lower lips
         (3) Clefting of the lip with or without cleft palate
**3.** Incidence
 **a.** Incidence of cleft lip and cleft palate
   **i.** General
      (a) Estimates of the U.S. prevalence of orofacial defects (CDC, 2006)
         (1) Cleft palate: 6.39 per 10,000 live births
         (2) Cleft lip with or without cleft palate: 10.68 per 10,000 live births
      (b) 68% percent of unilateral cleft lips are associated with cleft palate

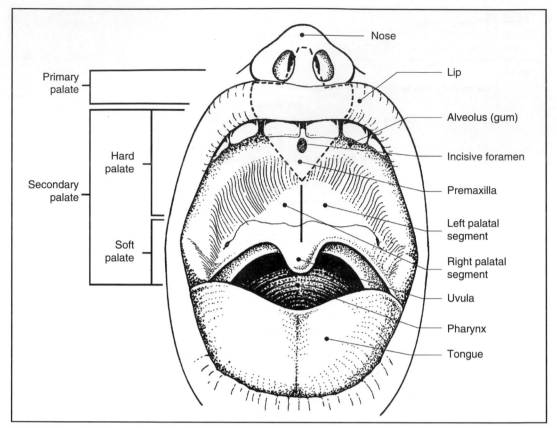

**FIGURE 39-4** ■ Parts of palate, lip, and nose that may be affected by inadequate fusion during embryologic development. Dotted lines show the portion of the lip and palate that develops separately from the hard and soft palate. Unilateral clefts occur along the dotted line. Bilateral clefts include the incisive foramen and premaxillary area. (From Jackson, P. L., & Vessey, J. A. [2000]. *Primary care of children with a chronic condition* [3rd ed.]. St. Louis: Mosby, p. 332.)

        (c) Left unilateral clefts occur twice as frequently as right unilateral clefts
        (d) Incidence of submucous cleft palate constitutes 3% of all clefts (Lidral & Moreno)
        (e) Isolated bilateral cleft lips are very uncommon
        (f) One third of all are associated with fetal alcohol syndrome
        (g) 60% to 80% occur in males
    **ii.** Racial differences
        (a) Native American—1 in 300 live births
        (b) Asian—1 in 500 live births
        (c) Hispanic—1 in 500 live births
        (d) White—1 in 1000 live births
        (e) Black—0.3 to 0.4 in 1000 live births
  **4.** Etiology
    **a.** Multifactorial etiology
    **b.** Genetics
      **i.** Syndromic clefts (Jones, 2005)
        (a) Associated with malformations involving other developmental regions
        (b) 50% of children with isolated cleft palate have other birth defects

■ **TABLE 39-1**
■ ■ **Syndromes Frequently Associated with Cleft Lip and/or Palate, and Their Genetic Inheritance Pattern**

| Syndrome | Genetic Inheritance Pattern | Cleft Lip with/ without Cleft Palate | Isolated Cleft Palate |
|---|---|:---:|:---:|
| 4p-5 | Sporadic | | X |
| Cerebro-costo-mandibular | Autosomal recessive | | X |
| Ectrodactyly-ectodermal dysplasia | Autosomal dominant | X | |
| Escobar | Autosomal recessive | | X |
| Femoral hypoplasia | Sporadic | | X |
| Hays-Wells | Autosomal dominant | X | X |
| Kneist's dysplasia | Sporadic; possibly autosomal dominant | X | X |
| Meckel-Gruber | Autosomal recessive | | X |
| Miller's | Autosomal recessive | X | |
| Nager's | Sporadic | | X |
| Oro-facial-digital (type I) | Possibly X-linked | X | X |
| Oro-facial-digital (type II) | Autosomal recessive | X | X |
| Oto-palato-digital (type I) | X-linked semidominant | | X |
| Oto-palato-digital (type II) | X-linked | | X |
| Partial trisomy 10q | Sporadic | | X |
| Pierre Robin | Sporadic | | X |
| Popliteal pterygium | Autosomal dominant | X | X |
| Rapp-Hodgkin ectodermal dysplasia | Autosomal dominant | X | |
| Roberts-SC phocomelia | Autosomal recessive | X | |
| Spondyloepiphyseal dysplasia congenita | Autosomal dominant | | X |
| Stickler's | Autosomal dominant | | X |
| Treacher Collins | Autosomal dominant | | X |
| Trisomy 13 | Sporadic | X | |
| Van der Woude's | Autosomal dominant | X | X |

Adapted from Jones, L. L. (2005). *Smith's recognizable patterns of human malformation* (6th ed.). Philadelphia: Saunders.

    ii. Nonsyndromic clefts may be *isolated* anomalies (Kirschner & LaRossa, 2000, p. 1195)

    iii. Table 39-2 shows familial risks (Kirschner & LaRossa, 2000, p. 1196)

  c. Gene and environment interactions—factors that alter gene expression and interrupt facial and palatal development

    i. Anticonvulsants

      (a) Phenytoin

      (b) Valproic acid

    ii. Lithium

    iii. Retinoids

    iv. Vitamin A

    v. Thalidomide

    vi. Steroids

    vii. Penicillin

■ **TABLE 39-2**
■ ■ **Familial Risks for Nonsyndromic Cleft Lip and Palate**

| Family History | Cleft Lip ± Cleft Palate | Cleft Palate |
|---|---|---|
| No family history of cleft lip or cleft palate | 0.1% | 0.04% |
| Unaffected patients with: | | |
| One previously affected child | 4% | 2% |
| Two previously affected children | 9% | 1% |
| One affected parent | 4% | 6% |
| One affected parent and one previously affected child | 17% | 15% |

± = with or without (From Kirschner, R. E., & LaRossa, D. [2000]. Syndromic and other congenital anomalies of the head and neck: Cleft lip and palate. *Otolaryngol Clin North Am, 33*[6], 1191–1215.)

    **viii.** Benzodiazepines
    **ix.** Salicylates
    **x.** Opiates
    **xi.** Pesticides—dioxin
    **xii.** Substance use
        (a) Maternal alcohol consumption
        (b) Maternal cigarette smoking (Bender, 2000)
            (1) More than 20 cigarettes per day results in a twofold increase in risk
            (2) Fewer than 20 cigarettes per day results in a 1.5 increase in risk
  **d.** Other associated factors during pregnancy
    **i.** Infectious diseases; viruses
    **ii.** Folic acid deficiency
    **iii.** Uncontrolled maternal diabetes mellitus (Bender, 2000; Spilson, Kim, & Chung, 2003)
  **e.** Low socioeconomic status
**5.** Influence on growth and development
  **a.** Slow or retarded growth
    **i.** Infants born with clefts have a higher incidence of low birth weight and very low birth weight without prematurity (Wyszynski, et al., 2003)
    **ii.** Poor growth may be related to the associated syndrome
  **b.** Poor feeding
    **i.** Ineffective suck
        (a) Inability of the levator palatine muscles to lift the soft palate and close off the posterior pharynx
        (b) Ability to lift soft palate and close off posterior pharynx is necessary to create increased intraoral pressure required for sucking
        (c) Poor sucking may be related to the associated syndrome
  **c.** Speech delays
    **i.** Speech includes pronunciation of sounds, voice, resonance quality, and fluency of sound production
    **ii.** Speech delays result from structural deficiencies, specifically:
        (a) Velopharyngeal insufficiency
        (b) Oronasal fistulas
        (c) Dental and occlusal problems
        (d) Impaired hearing acuity

        iii. Speech problems
          (a) Hypernasality (most common)
          (b) Articulation problems
          (c) Disturbed voice quality

  **d.** Language delays
      **i.** "Understanding and use of words and sentences and the organization of conversation is essential for social interaction and learning" (Balasubrahmanyam, et al., 1998, p. 133)
     **ii.** Language delays may result from
        (a) Impaired hearing ability
        (b) Cognitive delays secondary to associated syndromes
    **iii.** Impaired hearing
        (a) Increased incidence of otitis media with effusion
        (b) Increased incidence of chronic otitis media
        (c) Increased incidence of hearing loss
        (d) Pathophysiology
          (1) Abnormal insertion of the tensor and levator palate muscles
          (2) Failure of the eustachian tube to open
          (3) Functional eustachian tube obstruction
          (4) Negative middle-ear pressure
        (e) Other suggested contributory factors include (Sheahan & Blayney, 2003):
          (1) Failure of the eustachian tube to close
          (2) Abnormal eustachian tube compliance
          (3) Associated abnormalities of the craniofacial skeleton
            a) Reduced mastoid depth and height

  **e.** Dental problems
      **i.** Malocclusions
     **ii.** Increased incidence of caries in children with cleft lip and palate (Chapple & Nunn, 2001)

  **f.** General development delays related to associated syndromes

  **g.** Cognitive delays
      **i.** Cognitive delays are evident at age 5 months
     **ii.** Increased incidence of ADHD
    **iii.** Increased incidence of reading difficulties
     **iv.** Impaired hearing can have a negative effect on learning

  **h.** Psychosocial issues
      **i.** Parental "feelings of fear, guilt, resentment, inadequacy, shame, and grief are common" (Sandberg, et al., 2002, p. 490)
     **ii.** These feelings lead to risk for impaired parent-infant relationship
    **iii.** Children with craniofacial abnormalities experience more teasing by their peers (Broder, Smith, & Strauss, 2001)
        (a) Risk for poor self-esteem of child
        (b) Risk for impaired socialization

**6.** Treatment
  **a.** Role of the PNP in management and primary care
      **i.** Coordinate comprehensive, multidisciplinary services
        (a) Referral to reputable, experienced, craniofacial team that includes nurse, plastic surgeon, speech therapist, dentist, orthodontist, otolaryngologist, social worker, geneticist
        (b) Primary care providers who refer parents to craniofacial teams versus individuals were (Grow & Lehman, 2002):

(1) Three times more likely attend cleft lip and cleft palate–related conferences

(2) Four times more likely to have a protocol for management of infants with cleft lip or palate

ii. Request copy of craniofacial team's recommendations

iii. Facilitate implementation of recommendations in the child's home and community

iv. Promote optimal growth

    (a) Monitor growth parameters

    (b) Encourage breast-feeding

    (c) Children with cleft lip are likely to be successful breast-feeders because the breast fills the defect

    (d) Otitis media may occur more often after breast-feeding is stopped (Sheahan & Blayney, 2003)

    (e) Encourage feeding expressed breast milk via bottle when breast-feeding is not feasible

    (f) Teach strategies to minimize feeding difficulties

        (1) Parents want this information early in the newborn period (Young, et al., 2001)

        (2) Feed in a semi-upright position to prevent nasal regurgitation

        (3) Use adaptive feeding equipment (Figure 39-5)

            a) Palatal obturators are used by some cleft palate teams

            b) Adaptive nipples can compensate for a weak suck

v. Promote optimal development

    (a) Evaluate developmental milestones at each office visit, especially language, hearing, and cognition

    (b) Provide anticipatory guidance for each stage of development, particularly when the cleft lip or palate may cause delays or difficulties

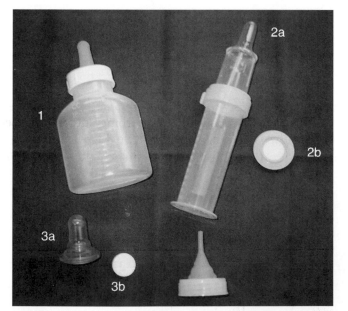

FIGURE 39-5 ■ Adaptive feeding equipment for cleft lip and/or cleft palate.

        (c) Refer to subspecialties as needed
     **vi.** Promote optimal health and prevention of illness
        (a) Ensure timely immunizations
        (b) Teach strategies to prevent dental caries
          (1) Brushing *all* teeth, recognizing that with cleft palate they are often oddly distributed
          (2) Flossing
          (3) Fluoride supplementation for children with unfluoridated water
          (4) Regular dental care
        (c) Teach strategies to minimize the risk of upper respiratory tract infections and otitis media
          (1) Handwashing
          (2) Eliminating exposure to secondhand smoke
          (3) Smaller daycare settings when feasible
    **vii.** Promote optimal psychologic development (Kapp-Simon, 2004)
        (a) Adults should demonstrate positive attitudes and belief in child's ability to cope with challenges of treatment
        (b) Child's ability to cope with these challenges leads to self-efficacy
  **b.** Surgery
     **i.** Timing of surgical repair of cleft lip and palate can vary among craniofacial teams (Anastassov & Joos, 2001; Kirschner & LaRossa, 2000)
        (a) Can be done during the neonatal period due to advances in neonatology and pediatric anesthesia (Sandberg, et al., 2002, p. 492)
        (b) Cleft lip repair
          (1) Usually between 2 and 6 months of age
        (c) Cleft palate repair
          (1) Usually between 6 and 18 months of age
          (2) May require further staged reconstruction
    **ii.** Rule of 10s: at least 10 weeks, 10 pounds, hemoglobin of 10 (Curtin & Boekelheide, 2004)
    **iii.** Ventilation tubes often inserted at time of surgery
    **iv.** Postoperative care for the child with cleft lip and palate includes:
        (a) IV hydration until oral intake is sufficient, usually within 24 hours
        (b) Pain management
        (c) Sutures
          (1) Care of suture line of lip usually consists of gentle cleansing with diluted (half-strength) hydrogen peroxide or saline
          (2) For cleft lip repair, if nonabsorbing sutures are used, removal of sutures is within 5 postoperative days.
        (d) Feeding methods may include breast, bottle, syringe feeding
        (e) To prevent the child from manually disrupting the repair, soft elbow restraints may be used
**7.** Prognosis
  **a.** Long-term prognosis is excellent (Curtin & Boekelheide, 2004)
  **b.** Goals of team management are to achieve:
     **i.** Good speech articulation
    **ii.** Functional dental occlusion
    **iii.** Normal hearing acuity
    **iv.** An acceptable appearance
    **v.** Positive self-regard

# REFERENCES

Anastassov, G. E., & Joos, U. (2001). Comprehensive management of cleft lip and palate deformities. *J Oral Maxillofac Surg, 59,* 1062-1075.

Balasubrahanyam, G., Scherer, N.J., Martin, J., Michael, M. (1998). Cleft lip and palate: Keys to successful management. *Contemporary Pediatrics, 15,* (ii), 133.

Bender, P. L. (2000). Genetics of cleft lip and palate. *J Pediatr Nurs, 15,* 242-249.

Broder, H. L., Smith, T. B., & Strauss, R. P. (2001). Developing a behavioral rating scale for comparing teachers' rating of children with and without craniofacial anomalies. *Cleft Palate Craniofac J, 38,* 560-565.

Centers for Disease Control and Prevention (CDC). (2006). Improved National Prevalence Estimates for 18 Selected Major Birth Defects—United States, 1999-2001. *MMWR, 54*(51&52), 1301-1305.

Chapple, J. R., & Nunn, J. H. (2001). The oral health of children with clefts of the lip, palate, or both. *Cleft Palate Craniofac J, 38,* 525-528.

Curtin, G., & Boekelheide, A. (2004). Cleft lip and palate. In P. L. Jackson & J. A. Vessey (Eds.). *Primary care of the child with a chronic condition* (4th ed.). St. Louis: Mosby, pp. 347-363.

Grow, J. L., & Lehman, J. A. (2002). A local perspective on the initial management of children with cleft lip and palate by primary care physicians. *Cleft Palate Craniofac J, 39*(5), 535-540.

Jones, K. L. (2005). *Smith's recognizable patterns of human malformation* (6th ed.). Philadelphia: Saunders.

Kapp-Simon, K. A. (2004). Psychological issues in cleft lip and palate. *Clin Plast Surg, 31*(2), 347-352.

Kirschner, R. E., & LaRossa, D. (2000). Syndromic and other congenital anomalies of the head and neck: Cleft lip and palate. *Otolaryngol Clin North Am, 33,* 1191-1215.

Kreins, O. (1989). lAHSHAL. A concise documentation system for cleft lip, alveolus, and palate diagnoses. In O. Kriens (Ed.). *What is a cleft lip and palate? A multidisciplinary update.* Stuttgart, Germany: Thieme.

Kuehn, D. P., Ettema, S. L., Goldwasser, M. S., et al. (2001). Magnetic resonance imaging in the evaluation of occult submucous cleft palate. *Cleft Palate Craniofac J, 38,* 421-431.

Lidral, A. C., & Moreno, L. M. (2005). Progress toward discerning the genetics of cleft lip. *Curr Opin Pediatr, 17*(6), 731-739.

Moore, K. L., & Persaud, T. V. N. (2003). *The developing human: Clinically oriented embryology* (6th ed.). Philadelphia: Saunders.

Sandberg, D. J., Magee, W. P., & Denk, M. P. (2002). Neonatal cleft lip and cleft palate repair. *AORN J, 75,* 490-499.

Sheahan, P., & Blayney, A. W. (2003). Cleft palate and otitis media with effusion: a review. *Rev Laryngol Otol Rhinol, 124*(3), 171-177.

Spilson, S. V., Kim, H. J., & Chung, K. C. (2001). Association between maternal diabetes mellitus and newborn oral cleft. *Ann Plast Surg, 47,* 477-481.

Thigpen, J. L., & Kenner, C. (2003). Assessment and management of the gastrointestinal system In C. Kenner & J. W. Lott (Eds.). *Comprehensive neonatal nursing: A physiologic perspective.* Philadelphia: Saunders, pp. 448-485.

Wyszynski, D. J., Sarkozi, A., Vargha, P., & Czeilel, A. E. (2003). Birth weight and gestational age of newborns with cleft lip with or without cleft palate. *J Pediatr Dentist, 27,* 185-190.

Young, J. L., O'Riordan, M., Goldstein, J. A., & Robin, N. H. (2001). What information do parents of newborns with cleft lip, palate, or both want to know? *Cleft Palate Craniofac J, 38,* 55-58.

# Common Genetic Conditions in Children

SUSAN M. HEIGHWAY, MS, APRN, BC-PNP, APNP

## GENETIC PRINCIPLES

1. See Chapter 14 for review of the following material required to fully appreciate the causes and effects of genetic conditions in children
   a. Human genome
   b. Human variation and pedigree
   c. General information about chromosomal and genetic disorders

## INBORN ERRORS OF METABOLISM (IEM)

1. Pathophysiology
   a. IEM are also called metabolic disorders
   b. A classic IEM is caused by a defect in the activity of a specific enzyme involved in either amino acid, carbohydrate, or lipid metabolism
   c. Autosomal dominant or recessive inheritance patterns
2. Presentation (Weiner & Wilkes, 2005)
   a. Most important clue is progressive deterioration in the newborn after an initial period of apparent good health
      i. Developmental delay or loss of developmental milestones
      ii. Onset after change in diet
      iii. Unusual food aversions, such as protein or carbohydrate
   b. A high index of suspicion is required to diagnose these conditions early
3. Newborn screening
   a. Most states screen for various metabolic disorders at 24 to 48 hours of age
   b. All states screen blood for phenylketonuria (PKU)
   c. Other IEM commonly included in newborn screening:
      i. Galactosemia
      ii. Biotinidase deficiency
      iii. Maple syrup urine disease
      iv. Homocystinuria
   d. For majority of other IEM, blood or urine is tested for elevations in blocked metabolites or their associated derivatives
   e. More definitive tests
      i. Direct enzyme analysis

  **ii.** Skin or muscle cells biopsy and analysis

**4.** Incidence and prevalence

 **a.** Individually, these disorders are rare

 **b.** Total reported incidence at birth varies from 1% to 2% (but probably underestimated)

 **c.** As a group they impose a considerable burden to the patient, family, community, and society

 **d.** Diagnostic accuracy is compromised by delayed appearance of mutant gene effects and failure to diagnose inherited disorders in newborns that die suddenly

**5.** Etiology

 **a.** Most IEM are single gene defects

 **b.** 3500 metabolic disorders have been identified

  **i.** Basic molecular defect has been identified in less than 10%

  **ii.** Remainder are characterized by:

   (a) Pathophysiologic consequence

   (b) Clinical manifestations

   (c) Secondary biochemical alterations

   (d) Mode of inheritance

 **c.** Caused by a heritable permanent change (mutation) occurring in the DNA

 **d.** Results in defective or deficient function of the gene product

  **i.** Gene products are usually polypeptide chains composed of amino acid sequences

  **ii.** Form an entire molecular or subunit of a structural protein, a membrane receptor, a transport protein, or an enzyme

 **e.** Most are inherited by autosomal recessive (mendelian) inheritance

  **i.** Both parents must each pass the defective gene to the offspring for the disease to be manifested

  **ii.** Carrier parents have a 25% chance of having an affected child with each pregnancy

**6.** Diagnostic criteria based on results of specialized diagnostic testing are available through specialty genetics centers

**7.** Follow-up of IEM

 **a.** Management of IEM is usually directed by a metabolic specialty clinic

  **i.** At least yearly clinical evaluations or consultations at genetic specialty clinics

  **ii.** Monitor appropriate laboratory studies specific to the disorder

  **iii.** Make treatment adjustments

 **b.** Children with IEM require the same primary care same as other children without metabolic disorders

 **c.** PNPs need periodic continuing education to keep up with the rapid changes in knowledge about genetic conditions (Williams, 2002)

 **d.** See the Genetics & Your Practice CD-ROM, Version 2.0

  **i.** Designed for health care professionals working with patients from preconception/prenatal, infant/children to adolescent/adult

  **ii.** Curriculum provides practical information and resources to integrate genetics into primary patient care

  **iii.** Obtained from the March of Dimes (call 1-800-367-6630, use order number 09-1177-99)

 **e.** Family support

  **i.** Refer child and family to support groups

  **ii.** Identify and refer family to community, state, or national support services

8. Incidence, pathophysiology, signs, influence on growth and development, and treatment of selected IEM
    a. PKU (March of Dimes, 2004)
        i. 1 in 14,000 births, an autosomal recessive trait
        ii. Inability of the body to utilize phenylalanine, one of the eight essential amino acids, and convert it to tyrosine
        iii. Missing enzyme is phenylalanine hydroxylase that is expressed only in the liver
        iv. Signs of untreated PKU (extremely rare in the U.S. for children)—skin rashes, spasticity, tremors, hand posturing, "mousy" odor of urine and sweat, microcephaly, unusually light coloration of hair, eyes, skin
        v. Treatment
            (a) Classic manifestations of the disorder are avoided with early diagnosis and compliance with dietary treatment
            (b) A lifetime diet of protein restriction is required, although after the first year of age when brain growth is rapid, small amounts of phenylalanine may be tolerated
            (c) Infant with PKU can be breastfed, but phenylalanine amounts in breast milk must be calculated
            (d) Avoid high-protein foods, e.g., milk, eggs, products with NutraSweet (aspartame)
            (e) Provide a measured amount of whole protein from foods
            (f) Use phenylalanine-free medical food (in the form of Lofenalac formula) for main source of amino acids, nutrients and calories in the diet
            (g) Monitor efficacy of dietary treatment with periodic plasma phenylalanine levels
        vi. Prognosis
            (a) If untreated in the first years, leads to mental retardation, delayed developmental skills, seizures, and autistic-like behaviors
            (b) Generally beginning in adolescence, treated individuals with persistent elevated phenylalanine levels may experience some neurological symptoms—tremors, impaired executive function, psychiatric disorders (e.g., depression, anxiety, obsessive-compulsive disorder)
    b. Galactosemia (Anadiotis & Berry, 2003)
        i. Galactose-1-phosphate-uridyl transferase (GALT) deficiency
        ii. An autosomal recessive trait
        iii. 1 in 40,000 to 60,000 births
        iv. Pathophysiology—the accumulation of galactose-1-phosphate causes inability of the body to metabolize the simple sugar galactose
        v. Signs
            (a) Feeding intolerance within a few days of birth
            (b) Vomiting, low blood sugar, lethargy, irritability, convulsions
            (c) Enlarged liver, jaundice
        vi. Treatment (Roth, 2005)
            (a) Strictly avoiding all milk and milk-containing products throughout life
            (b) Infants can be fed soy formula, meat-based formula, Nutramigen, or other lactose-free formula
            (c) Calcium supplementation is important because soy products are not rich in calcium
            (d) Some lactose-free foods still contain free galactose

(e) A helpful tip is to suggest that parents shop for kosher foods that by kosher law must be clearly marked "dairy" and "meat" or "neither"

vii. Prognosis

(a) If treated, prognosis is excellent

(b) Small, frequent intake of galactose will manifest in development of cataracts

(c) Despite adherence to dietary treatment, developmental problems may occur

(1) Speech/language (i.e., verbal dyspraxia, expressive language deficits)

(2) Cognitive functioning problems and visual perceptual problems leading to poor school performance

(3) Ovarian failure

(d) If untreated, leads to cirrhosis of the liver, cataracts, mental retardation

c. Biotinidase deficiency (Difazio & Davis, 2006)

i. 1 in 61,067 births, an autosomal recessive trait

ii. Complete or partial absence of the enzyme biotinidase

iii. Due to gene mutation

iv. Pathophysiology

(a) Biotinadase is a cell enzyme present in the liver, serum, and kidney, and found in many natural foods

(b) Biotin is bound to the four human carboxylases, which, when metabolized, provide free biotin to maintain the normal cycle of metabolism

(c) Deficiency of biotin causes abnormalities in fatty acid synthesis, amino acid catabolism, and gluconeogenesis

v. Signs—hypotonia, eczematous rash, alopecia, intractable seizures, acidosis, failure to thrive, chronic fungal infections, breathing abnormalities

vi. Treatment—administer oral biotin, usually 10 mg/day although some may require higher doses up to 40 mg/day

vii. Prognosis

(a) Excellent prognosis with treatment; child can grow to adulthood and lead a normal lifestyle

(b) If untreated, leads to mental retardation, seizures, coma, and death

d. Maple syrup urine disease (MSUD) (Bodamer & Lee, 2006)

i. A disorder of branched chain amino acid metabolism in which elevated quantities of leucine, isoleucine, and valine and their corresponding oxoacids accumulate in body fluids

ii. 1 in 180,000 newborns, an autosomal recessive trait

iii. Pathophysiology

(a) Deficient in an enzyme complex that is a catalyst for normal metabolism of branched chain amino acids

(b) Accumulation of leucine causes neurological symptoms

(c) Accumulation of plasma isoleucine produces the maple syrup odor

iv. Signs

(a) Signs present as soon as the infant is fed protein (within 4 to 7 days, or 2 weeks if breastfed)

(b) Poor feeding, vomiting, poor weight gain, and increasing lethargy

(c) Urine smells like maple syrup or burnt sugar

v. Treatment

(a) Long-term management involves dietary restriction of the three branched-chain amino acids (leucine, isoleucine, and valine)

    (b) Feed infant/child a special medical formula to ensure adequate calories and nutrients
  vi. Prognosis
    (a) With early initiation of treatment and avoidance of metabolic crises, child can develop typically
    (b) Periodic metabolic decompensation episodes require referral, but practitioner may begin intravenous glucose infusions (5 to 8 mg/kg/minute for infants) as rapidly as possible
    (c) If untreated, leads to developmental delay and death within a few months
  e. Homocystinuria (Baloghova & Schwartz, 2005)
    i. Deficiency in cystathionine synthase leading to a multisystemic disorder of connective tissue, muscles, CNS, and cardiovascular system
    ii. 1 in 344,000 newborns worldwide
    iii. An autosomal recessive trait, more in males than females
    iv. Pathophysiology—accumulation of homocysteine in serum and urine due to:
      (a) Various levels of Vitamin $B_6$ resistance
      (b) Insufficient Viamin $B_{12}$ synthesis
      (c) Deficiency in methyltetrachlorofolate reductase enzyme
    v. Signs
      (a) Macules on buccal surfaces, large pores, coarse hair, hyperhydrosis, acrocyanosis, muscle weakness, aggression
    vi. Treatment
      (a) Methionine-restricted diet, i.e., limited amounts of protein (1 g/kg/day)
      (b) Cysteine supplements from medical food, formula and other supplements that are amino acid mixtures, free of protein hydrolysate to a maximum of 500 mg/day
      (c) Vitamins $B_6$ or $B_{12}$, folic acid, or pyridoxine in some cases
    vii. Prognosis
      (a) Even with treatment, about 25% of patients die before age 30
      (b) If untreated, leads to developmental delay noted at 2 to 3 years of age, severe myopia, osteoporosis, long thin extremities and fingers, thromboembolic events

## SPECIFIC GENETIC CONDITIONS

# Down Syndrome (AAP, 2001; Bosch, 2003)

1. Pathophysiology
  a. First described by Esquirol in 1838 and made known to the public by Down in 1866
  b. Chromosomal aberration—karyotype 47XY or XX+21, also known as trisomy 21
  c. Recognizable grouping of congenital physical anomalies and mental retardation
2. Incidence and prevalence
  a. 1/800 to 1000 live births
  b. Affects males and females equally
  c. Increased risk with advanced maternal age

    **d.** Most infants with Down syndrome are born to younger mothers due to higher birth rates among younger women

**3.** Etiology or precipitating factors

    **a.** Caused by extra chromosome 21 material

    **b.** Referred to as trisomy 21, with differing inheritance patterns

        **i.** 92% to 95% of cases from nondisjunction

            (a) Failure of two homologous chromosomes to separate during cell division

            (b) Results in abnormal number of chromosome 21 in gametes or cells

            (c) Not an inherited form

            (d) Occurs in meiosis, which is before fertilization

        **ii.** 2% to 3% occurs from mosaicism

            (a) Presence in the same individual of two or more cell lines that differ in number of chromosome 21

            (b) Derived from a single zygote

            (c) Nondisjunction occurs in mitosis, which is after fertilization

        **iii.** 4% to 6% from translocation

            (a) Transfer of all or part of a chromosome to another chromosome

            (b) Inherited

            (c) Parents have translocation that is balanced or unbalanced

**4.** Presentation

    **a.** Diagnostic criteria

        **i.** Confirmed by chromosomal analysis

        **ii.** Presence of critical lower region of a third 21 chromosome

    **b.** Signs

        **i.** Inspection

            (a) Typical phenotypic signs

                (1) Flat facial profile with flattened nasal bridge

                (2) Small nose

                (3) Epicanthal folds

                (4) Prominent lips

                (5) Small mouth

                (6) Protruding tongue

                (7) Small short ears

                (8) Single transverse palmar crease

                (9) Fifth finger with one flexion crease instead of two

                (10) Excessive space between the first and second toes

                (11) Widened internipple space

        **ii.** Diagnostic tests

            (a) Chromosomal karyotyping to determine an accurate genetic diagnosis is necessary as soon as Down syndrome is suspected

            (b) Evaluation by clinical geneticist

            (c) Genetic counseling with the family

    **c.** Associated problems

        **i.** Congenital heart disease seen in 40% to 60%

            (a) Most common

                (1) Atrioventricular septal defect

                (2) Atrial or ventricular septal defect alone

                (3) Persistent ductus arteriosus

                (4) Tetralogy of Fallot

        **ii.** Feeding problems

            (a) Failure to thrive

          (b) Muscular hypotonia

          (c) Gastroesophageal reflux

    **iii.** Gastrointestinal problems seen in 10%

          (a) Duodenal atresia

          (b) Hirschsprung disease (can be corrected surgically)

    **iv.** Visual problems seen in 50%

          (a) Crossed eyes

          (b) Near- or farsightedness

          (c) Cataracts

    **v.** Hearing problems are common

    **vi.** Increased risk for thyroid problems and leukemia

    **vii.** Tend to have more respiratory infections

          (a) Colds

          (b) Bronchitis

          (c) Pneumonia

    **viii.** Ligamentous laxity present in 100%

    **ix.** Obesity by early childhood present in 50%

**5.** Influence on growth and development

    **a.** Developmental

       **i.** General

          (a) Perform as other children walking, talking, reading, and writing

          (b) Takes them longer to develop these skills

      **ii.** Mental retardation

          (a) Degree of mental retardation varies widely

          (b) Most fall within mild to moderate range

          (c) Cannot predict the mental development based on physical features

      **iii.** Other developmental issues arise related to the associated conditions, such as congenital heart disease, feeding problems, and obesity

**6.** Treatment

    **a.** There is no specific medical treatment for the primary genetic problem

    **b.** Developmental delays

       **i.** Educational programming is primary treatment; usually begins with early intervention program

          (a) Occupational

          (b) Physical

          (c) Speech language therapist

          (d) Developmental

          (e) Behavioral specialists

          (f) Progress to school with individualized special education services

    **c.** Associated health problems (Roizen, 2002)

       **i.** Early detection and treatment of health problems are essential, with a few specialized screenings

      **ii.** Referral for specialty care as needed

          (a) Ophthalmologist

          (b) Audiologist

          (c) Cardiologist

          (d) Health care guidelines for individuals with Down syndrome (Anonymous, 1999)

    **d.** Preventive care

       **i.** Same as for any other child

          (a) Vaccinations

          (b) Dental care

          (c) Medical care

          (d) Reproductive issues at puberty should be addressed

  **e.** Nutritional support to avoid obesity

  **f.** Genetic counseling

     **i.** Family members

     **ii.** Individual

  **g.** Family support

     **i.** Refer child and family to support groups

     **ii.** Community support services

7. Follow-up

  **a.** Monitor health needs

  **b.** Provide appropriate primary health care (Bosch, 2003)

  **c.** Pre-sports participation—obtain cervical spine x-rays for atlantoaxial instability

8. Long-term implications

  **a.** With medical advances, early diagnosis and treatment can prolong the life span

  **b.** Refer for Supplemental Social Security income

  **c.** Average life span is 55 years

# Fetal Alcohol Syndrome (FAS) (AAP, 2000)

1. Pathophysiology

  **a.** A group of physical and mental birth defects due to the teratogenic effect of maternal prenatal alcohol ingestion

2. Incidence and prevalence

  **a.** FAS occurs in approximately 1 to 2 out of every 1000 births

  **b.** The most common cause of mental retardation in the United States

3. Etiology or precipitating factors

  **a.** No amount of alcohol is considered safe to be ingested during pregnancy

  **b.** It is not known whether alcohol itself causes the fetal effects or whether they are caused by some intermediate metabolite of the alcohol, such as acetaldehyde

  **c.** Factors that play a role in the extent of the fetal consequences of alcohol ingestion include differences in the metabolism of alcohol, the timing of fetal exposure, maternal nutritional status, and dose of alcohol

  **d.** Totally preventable cause of mental retardation

4. Presentation

  **a.** Diagnosis

     **i.** Need for accurate diagnosis by well-trained physician

     **ii.** Known exposure of fetus to alcohol ingestion by the mother during pregnancy can strengthen evidence, but is not necessary for diagnosis

     **iii.** Confirmed absence of prenatal exposure to alcohol would rule out FAS

  **b.** Diagnostic criteria—must exhibit an abnormality in each of the following three general categories to meet criteria for FAS:

     **i.** Documentation of growth deficits

         (a) Confirmed prenatal or postnatal height and weight growth at or below the 10th percentile

         (b) Corrected for gestational age, documented at any one time

     **ii.** Documentation of central nervous system abnormality

         (a) Structural

            (1) Head circumference at or below the 10th percentile

(2) Clinically significant brain abnormalities observable through imaging
- (b) Neurological
    - (1) Not due to a postnatal insult or fever
    - (2) Other soft neurological signs outside normal limits
- (c) Functional
    - (1) Performance substantially below that expected for an individual's age, schooling, or circumstances
    - (2) In either global cognitive deficits or functional deficits in 3 out of 6 domains
    - (3) Documentation of all three facial abnormalities
        - a) Smooth philtrum
        - b) Thin vermillion border
        - c) Small palpebral fissures

5. Influence on growth and development
   a. Developmental problems
      i. Wide variation in intellectual abilities
      ii. Problems in learning and information processing
   b. Physical and health problems
      i. Cardiac anomalies
      ii. Limb, joint, and other skeletal anomalies
      iii. Neurologic problems
         (a) Increased incidence
            (1) Seizures
            (2) Cerebral palsy
         (b) Problems in sensory regulation affecting:
            (1) Sleep
            (2) Activity level
            (3) Behavior
      iv. Failure to thrive
         (a) Associated with poor suck

6. Treatment
   a. No definitive, single treatment for FAS
      i. Variety of treatments to help minimize the symptoms
      ii. Individualized educational programming is primary treatment
         (a) Physical
         (b) Occupational
         (c) Physical therapies as needed
         (d) Behavioral specialists
   b. Medications
      i. May be used to treat the symptoms or conditions associated with FAS; for example, for behavioral issues such as attention problems, or seizures
   c. Associated health problems
      i. Early detection and treatment of health problems are essential
      ii. Referral for specialty care as needed
   d. Preventive care
      i. Same as for any other child
         (a) Vaccinations
         (b) Dental care
         (c) Medical care
   e. Nutritional support to avoid obesity

    **f.** Genetic counseling
        **i.** Family members
        **ii.** Individual
    **g.** Family support
        **i.** Child and family support groups
        **ii.** Community support services
**7.** Follow-up
    **a.** Monitor health needs
    **b.** Provide appropriate health care
**8.** Long-term implications
    **a.** Prognosis is improved because of improved health care to individuals with disabilities

# Fragile X Syndrome (AAP, 1996)

**1.** Pathophysiology
    **a.** Caused by a mutation in the gene called the fragile X mental retardation 1 gene (FMR1) on the X chromosome at X127.3
    **b.** Derives its name from the presence of a fragile site or break in the X chromosome at a specific site, which is identifiable by chromosome analysis
**2.** Incidence and prevalence
    **a.** Most common cause of inherited mental retardation (MR)
    **b.** Second most common genetic cause of MR
    **c.** Affected individuals
        **i.** Approximately 1 per 1250 males
        **ii.** 1 per 2500 females
    **d.** Carrier females
        **i.** 1 in 239 females in general population carries the permutation
**3.** Etiology or precipitating factors
    **a.** Atypical X-linked recessive inheritance pattern
    **b.** No spontaneous mutations have been found for fragile X syndrome
**4.** Presentation
    **a.** Diagnostic criteria
        **i.** DNA analysis from whole blood in approved laboratory to confirm diagnosis
        **ii.** Prenatal testing from chorionic villus or amniocentesis sample
        **iii.** Confirmed by presence of genetic mutation
    **b.** Signs
        **i.** Individuals share a phenotype
            (a) Much variability
            (b) Phenotype may not suggest fragile X syndrome in all children
        **ii.** Males
            (a) Three classic physical features (1 or more seen in 80% of males)
                (1) Long, narrow face
                (2) Prominent or large ears (in about 50%)
                (3) Enlarged testicles postpubescence (seen in 70% to 90%)
            (b) Majority of younger males may have no abnormal characteristics
        **iii.** Females
            (a) Overall, tend to display milder phenotypic features than males
            (b) Physical characteristics are less obvious than in males

(1) Including prominent ears
(2) Long, narrow face
(3) Prominent forehead and jaw
(4) Hyperextensible finger joints
5. Influence on growth and development
   **a.** Developmental problems
      **i.** Males
        (a) Majority have IQs in the mild to moderate range of mental retardation
        (b) Delayed onset of speech or language
          (1) Often exhibit speech characteristics
            a) Perseveration
            b) Echolalia
            c) Repetitive speech
        (c) Behavioral concerns
          (1) Hyperactivity (occurs in 70% prepubertal age, then disappears after puberty)
          (2) Poor attention span, often with impulsivity (occurs regardless of cognitive functioning)
          (3) Poor eye contact (seen in 90%)
          (4) Unusual hand mannerisms (60% to 70%)
      **ii.** Females
        (a) Carriers of permutation are usually unaffected intellectually
        (b) Carriers of full mutation are affected to mild or severe degree
          (1) Mental retardation (seen in 25%)
          (2) Borderline intellectual abilities (seen in 25%)
          (3) Normal intellectual abilities, but commonly with learning difficulties (seen in 50%)
        (c) Speech or language problems (Philofsky, et al., 2004)
   **b.** Physical and mental health problems
      **i.** Seizures in 20%
      **ii.** Vision problems
        (a) Strabismus in 30% to 56%
      **iii.** Recurrent otitis media in 45% to 60%
      **iv.** Dental malocclusion caused by high-arched palate
      **v.** Connective tissue problems, joint laxity, scoliosis, hernias
   **c.** Neurodevelopmental
      **i.** Social anxiety in both males and females
      **ii.** Autistic-like tendencies
      **iii.** Sensory integration difficulties
6. Treatment
   **a.** There are no known specific medical treatments for the primary genetic defect
   **b.** Educational
      **i.** Enroll in early intervention program as soon as delays are recognized
        (a) Speech or language therapy
        (b) Sensory or motor integration therapy
      **ii.** Ensure appropriate educational placement with necessary supports throughout school-age years, including:
        (a) Communication
        (b) Social skills
        (c) Behavioral supports
   **c.** Genetic counseling

    **i.** All family members should undergo genetic testing to identify:
      (a) Transmitting males
      (b) Carrier females
      (c) Affected individuals
  **d.** Medical
    **i.** Regular well-child examinations
  **e.** Refer to specialty care as appropriate
    **i.** Ophthalmology
    **ii.** ENT
    **iii.** Cardiologist
    **iv.** Psychiatrist
**7.** Follow-up
  **a.** Monitor health and medical needs
  **b.** Refer as appropriate for specialty care
**8.** Long-term implications
  **a.** Prognosis is improved because of improved health care services to individuals with fragile X syndrome

---

## REFERENCES

American Academy of Pediatrics (AAP) Committee on Genetics. (2001). Policy Statement: Health supervision for children with Down syndrome. *Pediatrics, 107*(2), 442-449.

American Academy of Pediatrics (AAP) Committee on Genetics. (1996). Policy Statement: Health supervision for children with fragile X syndrome. *Pediatrics, 98*(2), 297-300.

American Academy of Pediatrics (AAP) Committee on Substance Abuse and Committee on Children with Disabilities. (2000). Policy Statement: Fetal alcohol syndrome & alcohol related neurodevelopmental disorders. *Pediatrics, 106* (2), 358-361.

Anadiotis, G. A., & Berry, G. T. (2006). Galactose-1-phosphate uridyltransferase deficiency (galactosemia). Retrieved May 21, 2006, from www.emedicine.com/ped/topic818.htm.

Anonymous. (1999). Health care guidelines for Down syndrome. *Down Synd Quart, 4*(3), 1-16.

Baloghova, J., & Schwartz, R. A. (2005). Homocystinuria. Retrieved May 21, 2006, from www.emedicine.com/ped/topic708.htm.

Bodamer, O. A., & Lee, B. (2006). Maple syrup urine disease. Retrieved May 21, 2006, from www.emedicine.com/ped/topic1368.htm.

Bosch, J. J. (2003). Health maintenance throughout the life span for individuals with Down syndrome. *J Am Acad Nurse Pract 15*(1), 5-17.

Difazio, M. P., & Davis, R. G. (2006). Biotinidase deficiency. Retrieved May 21, 2006, from www.emedicine.com/ped/topic239.htm.

March of Dimes. (2004). PKU. Retrieved May 21, 2006, from www.marchofdimes.com/professionals/681_1219.asp.

National Coalition for Health Professional Education in Genetics (NCHPEG). (2005). *Core competencies in genetics essential for all health-care professionals* (2nd ed.). Lutherville, MD: NCHPEG.

Philofsky, A., Hepburn, S. L., Hayes, A., et al. (2004). Linguistic and cognitive functioning and autism symptoms in young children with fragile X syndrome. *Am J Ment Retard AJMR, 109*(3), 208-218.

Roizen, N. J. (2002). Medical care and monitoring for the adolescent with Down syndrome. *Adolesc Med (Philadelphia), 13*(2), 345-358.

Roth, K. S. (2005). Galactokinase deficiency. Retrieved from eMedicine on May 21, 2006 at http://www.emedicine.com/ped/topic815.htm.

Weiner, D. L., & Wilkes, G. (2005). Inborn errors of metabolism. Retrieved from eMedicine on May 21, 2006 at http://www.emedicine.com/emerg/topic768.htm.

Williams, J. (2002). Education for genetics and nursing practice. *AACN Clin Issues, 13*(4), 492-500.

# Common Mental Health Disorders in Children and Adolescents

ZENDI MOLDENHAUER, PhD, RN-CS, PNP/NPP AND
BERNADETTE MAZUREK MELNYK, PhD, RN, CPNP/NPP, FAAN, FNAP

1. Assumptions about common mental health disorders in children and adolescents
   a. In general, children's emotional and behavioral symptoms vary along a continuum from normal variations to problems to disorders
   b. Children's environments have a significant impact on their mental health
   c. Some children have genetic or familial predispositions for symptoms
   d. PNPs can manage the more serious disorders with special training and collaborative relationships with child psychiatrists and child psychologists
2. Assessment (See also, Chapter 23)
   a. Value the child's/adolescent's report of symptoms, especially worries (Melnyk, et al., 2002) and sense of functional impairment
   b. Evaluate onset and context in which symptoms develop and are sustained
   c. Identify psychosocial stressors (peers, school, family, environment)
   d. Coping behaviors and styles
   e. Academic, athletic, social, and behavioral functioning
   f. Potential versus actual achievements
   g. Separations/losses
   h. Comorbid psychopathology
   i. Identify biological stressors (puberty, chronic illness)
   j. Impact of symptoms on activities of daily living and the family
   k. Medical visits/hospitalizations (e.g., trauma, recurrent pain syndromes)
   l. Medications (e.g., seizure medications, thyroid medications)
   m. Medical disorders that may mimic depression (e.g., hypothyroidism, anemia, chronic illness, mononucleosis and chronic fatigue syndrome, CNS lesions, mitral valve prolapse, failure to thrive, eating disorders)
   n. Family medical, mental health, and medication history
   o. Evaluate pattern of symptoms according to diagnostic criteria (see below)
   p. Use interview, observation and other assessment tools
      i. Depending on developmental level, use play, drawing, or other artistic expressions as assessment tools (Ryan-Wenger, 2001)
      ii. Children's Depression Inventory for ages 7 to 17 years
      iii. Beck II Depression Inventory for ages 13 years through adult

      iv. Child Behavior Checklist and Youth Self-report Checklist (Achenbach CBCL)

      v. Behavioral Assessment System for Children (BASC)

      vi. Revised Children's Manifest Anxiety Scale (RCMAS)

      vii. State-Trait Anxiety Inventory for Children (STAIC)

      viii. Beck Anxiety Inventory (BAI)

      ix. School Refusal Assessment Scale

      x. Children's Post-traumatic Stress Disorder Inventory

      xi. Pediatric Symptom Checklist

      xii. Adolescent Psychopathology Scale

3. Diagnosing mental health disorders

    **a.** PNPs with advanced training in psychiatric mental health can diagnose mental health disorders

    **b.** The American Psychiatric Association (1994) *Diagnostic and statistical manual of mental disorders (DSM-IV™)*, 4th edition, includes diagnostic criteria for mental health disorders

    **c.** All PNPs should understand the classification system used to define mental health diagnoses (American Psychiatric Association DSM-IV Multiaxial Classification System)

      i. Axis 1: Psychological disorders, e.g.,

        (a) Major depressive disorder

        (b) Generalized anxiety disorder

      ii. Axis 2: Personality disorders, e.g., borderline personality (mental retardation)

      iii. Axis 3: General medical conditions (e.g., asthma, diabetes)

      iv. Axis 4: Psychosocial and environmental problems, including problems with:

        (a) Primary support group

        (b) Social environment

        (c) Educational problems

        (d) Occupational problems

        (e) Housing

        (f) Economic

        (g) Access to health care services

        (h) Interaction with the legal system

      v. Axis 5: Global assessment of functioning (GAF) (i.e., psychological, social, and work functioning)

        (a) A score is given on a scale of 100 (superior functioning) to 0 (inadequate information)

        (b) A score of 21–50 would indicate serious symptoms or serious impairment in social, occupational, or school functioning (DSM-IV)

4. Symptoms: sadness, apathy, loss of interest in normally pleasurable activities, irritability, agitation, crying, decreased energy, decreased concentration, sleep disturbance, low self-esteem

    **a.** Differential diagnoses (Box 41-1) (APA, 1994)

      i. Sadness variation or bereavement

        (a) Does not interfere with development; developmentally appropriate

        (b) Infancy: evident at about age 9 months; crying, brief withdrawal, transient anger

        (c) Early childhood: transient withdrawal and sad affect after losses

        (d) Middle childhood: transient loss of self-esteem, sadness

        (e) Adolescence: same as middle childhood, and fleeting thoughts of death

■ **BOX 41-1**
■ **DIFFERENTIAL DIAGNOSES FOR MOOD AND BEHAVIORAL SYMPTOMS**

| SYMPTOMS | DIFFERENTIAL DIAGNOSES |
|---|---|
| ■ Sadness<br>■ Apathy<br>■ Loss of interest in normally pleasurable activities<br>■ Irritability<br>■ Agitation<br>■ Crying<br>■ Decreased energy<br>■ Decreased concentration<br>■ Sleep disturbance<br>■ Low self-esteem | ■ Sadness variation, developmentally appropriate[1]<br>■ Bereavement[1]<br>■ Sadness problem[1]<br>■ Dysthymic disorder[1]<br>■ Major depressive disorder[1]<br>■ Bipolar disorder[1]<br>■ Thoughts of death variation, developmentally appropriate<br>■ Thoughts of death problem<br>■ Suicidal ideation and attempts[1]<br>■ Endocrine or metabolic abnormalities<br>■ Malignancies<br>■ Malnutrition<br>■ Chronic fatigue syndrome<br>■ Neurologic disorders<br>■ Autoimmune disorders<br>■ Substance abuse |
| ■ Anxiety<br>■ Fear<br>■ Nervousness<br>■ Worry about future events<br>■ Wariness<br>■ Avoidant behavior<br>■ Hypersensitivity<br>■ Sense of "going crazy"<br>■ Sense of impending death<br>■ Motor tension<br>■ Tremulousness<br>■ Autonomic hyperactivity<br>■ Palpitations<br>■ Dizziness<br>■ Shortness of breath<br>■ Tachycardia<br>■ Sleep difficulties | ■ Anxious variation, developmentally appropriate[1]<br>■ Anxiety problem[1]<br>■ Separation anxiety disorder[1]<br>■ Phobia[1]<br>■ Social phobia[1]<br>■ Adjustment disorder[1]<br>■ Post-traumatic stress disorder[1]<br>■ Generalized anxiety disorder[1]<br>■ Panic disorder[1]<br>■ ADHD[2]<br>■ Hyperthyroidism<br>■ Hypoglycemia<br>■ Pheochromocytoma<br>■ Acute bronchospasm<br>■ Mitral valve prolapse<br>■ Substance-related anxiety symptoms |
| ■ Rituals<br>■ Obsessions<br>■ Compulsions | ■ Ritual variation or repetitive behavior variation, developmentally appropriate[1]<br>■ Ritual, obsessive, compulsive problem<br>■ Repetitive behaviors problem<br>■ Stereotypic movement disorder<br>■ Obsessive-compulsive disorder[1]<br>■ Cocaine, amphetamine abuse<br>■ Autistic disorder<br>■ Mental retardation<br>■ Blindness, deafness<br>■ Fragile X syndrome<br>■ Hypochondriasis<br>■ Trichotillomania<br>■ Scalp infestations<br>■ Chorea |

*Continued*

■ **BOX 41-1**
■ **DIFFERENTIAL DIAGNOSES FOR MOOD AND BEHAVIORAL SYMPTOMS—cont'd**

| SYMPTOMS | DIFFERENTIAL DIAGNOSES |
|---|---|
| ■ Negative emotional behaviors<br>Anger<br>Frustration<br>Irritation<br>Whining<br>Temper tantrums<br>Screaming<br>Swearing | ■ Head injury<br>■ Substance-related symptoms<br>■ Negative emotional behavior variation, developmentally appropriate[1]<br>■ Negative emotional behavior problem[1]<br>■ Oppositional defiant disorder[1]<br>■ Conduct disorder[1]<br>■ Any illness that results in anger, loss of self-esteem<br>■ Severe physical injury<br>■ Prolonged illness, fatigue<br>■ Illness affecting central nervous system<br>■ Encephalitis<br>■ Systemic lupus erythematosus<br>■ Seizure disorders<br>■ Degenerative disorders<br>■ Tumor or injury affecting limbic system<br>■ Substance abuse (alcohol, opioids, withdrawal of stimulants) |
| Poor social skills | ■ Social interaction variation, developmentally appropriate<br>■ Social withdrawal problem<br>■ Pervasive developmental disorder[1]<br>■ Autistic disorder[1] |
| Antisocial behaviors<br>Lying<br>Cheating<br>Stealing<br>Destroying property | ■ Secretive, antisocial behaviors variation, developmentally appropriate<br>■ Adjustment disorder[1]<br>■ Oppositional defiant disorder[1]<br>■ Conduct disorder[1]<br>■ Substance abuse |

Source: American Psychiatric Association. (1994). *Diagnostic and statistical manual of mental disorders (DSM-IV™)*, 4th edition. Washington, DC: American Psychiatric Association.
[1]Topics that are covered in this chapter.
[2]See Chapter 49.

    ii. Sadness problem
      (a) Infancy: developmental regressions, fearfulness, anorexia, sleep disturbances, social withdrawal, irritability, increased dependency; all responsive to caregiver soothing
      (b) Early childhood: similar to infancy; sad affect, increase in temper tantrums; constipation, secondary enuresis, encopresis
      (c) Middle childhood: sadness and brief suicidal ideation but no plan; apathy, boredom, low self-esteem, headache, stomachache
      (d) Adolescence: decreased motivation, disinterest in school work, apathy, boredom
    iii. Dysthymic disorder (DD)
      (a) Not diagnosed in infancy; rare in early childhood
      (b) Middle childhood and adolescence: depressed mood or irritability for most of the day, for more days than not, either by subjective account or by observation, for one year

(c) Also the presence of two (or more) of the following:
  (1) Poor appetite or overeating
  (2) Insomnia or hypersomnia
  (3) Low energy or fatigue
  (4) Poor concentration or difficulty making decisions
  (5) Feelings of hopelessness
(d) Precedes major depressive disorder in 10% to 25% of cases
iv. Major depressive disorder (MDD)
  (a) Symptoms are present during the same 2-week period and represent a change from previous functioning
  (b) At least one symptom is either (1) depressed mood or (2) loss of interest or pleasure (anhedonia)
  (c) Also, five (or more) of the following symptoms:
    (1) Weight loss or gain
    (2) Insomnia or hypersomnia
    (3) Psychomotor agitation or retardation
    (4) Fatigue or energy loss
    (5) Feelings of worthlessness
    (6) Diminished ability to think or concentrate
    (7) Recurrent thoughts of death and suicidal ideation
v. Bipolar disorder
  (a) Depressive symptoms are similar to MDD
  (b) Manic symptoms include:
    (1) Severe changes in mood compared to others of the same age and background—either unusually happy or silly, or very irritable, angry, agitated, or aggressive
    (2) Unrealistic highs in self-esteem—for example, a teenager who feels all powerful or like a superhero with special powers
    (3) Great increase in energy and the ability to go with little or no sleep for days without feeling tired
    (4) Increase in talking—talks too much, too fast, changes topics too quickly, and cannot be interrupted
    (5) Increased distractibility
    (6) Repeated high-risk–taking behavior; such as abusing alcohol and drugs, reckless driving, or sexual promiscuity
b. Epidemiology of depression-related diagnoses
  i. MDD occurs in 5% of children, 10% to 20% of adolescents; higher rates for DD
  ii. Strong genetic component: risk increased in children of depressed parents
  iii. Male: female ratio: children 1:1; adolescent/young adult 1:2
  iv. MDD mean age of onset is 14 years; DD mean age of onset is 8 years
  v. Detection is low, less than 20% of cases, even fewer are effectively treated
  vi. Average length of untreated episode of MDD is 7 to 9 months
  vii. Reoccurrence rate 60% to 70% by 5 years; commonly reoccurs as adults
  viii. Depression is a risk factor for high risk behaviors
  ix. MDD precedes substance abuse by about 4.5 years in some children
  x. 40% to 70% of children and adolescents have comorbid diagnoses
c. Risk factors for depression
  i. Parental depression or family dysfunction
  ii. Societal, family, or personal history of violence or abuse
  iii. Acute or chronic illness, life stressors and changes, trauma and/or losses
  iv. Low self-esteem, attachment issues, and lack of social or peer support

  **v.** Substance abuse and other psychopathology

 **d.** Management of depression (Melnyk & Moldenhauer, 1999)

  **i.** Education about the depressive condition and support of the child and family

  **ii.** See NAPNAP's KySS (Keep Your Children/Yourself Safe and Secure Campaign) for helpful resources at www.napnap.org)

  **iii.** Teach healthy self-care behaviors

  **iv.** Referral for psychotherapy: individual, cognitive-behavioral therapy, and/or family therapy

  **v.** Teach about suicide warning signs and contract for safety; remove drugs, alcohol, weapons

  **vi.** Interdisciplinary collaboration with child psychiatrist, psychologists, therapist, teachers, after-school care directors

  **vii.** PNP can coordinate this care

  **viii.** Medications are reserved for severe depression (Melnyk & Moldenhauer, 1999; Moldenhauer & Melnyk, 2000; Nemeroff & Vale, 2005; Ryan, 2005; Scahill, et al., 2005; Wagner, 2005)

   (a) Selective serotonin reuptake inhibitors (SSRIs: Celexa, Paxil, Zoloft, Prozac, Effexor) are the recommended first line treatment

   (b) In September 2004, a U.S. Food and Drug Administration advisory committee called for the labels of all antidepressants to get a "black box" warning about the risk of increased suicidal tendencies in young people; such warnings are used to signal extremely serious side effects for a prescription drug (FDA, 2004)

   (c) These medications should be ordered only by PNPs with specific training in diagnosis and management of these conditions

   (d) This type of training for PNPs is encouraged

    (1) Few child psychiatrists are available for large number of children who need these services

    (2) Specially trained PNPs can solve some of the access to care issues

    (3) Requires close consultative relationships with child psychiatrists and child psychologists

   (e) See Table 54-8 in Chapter 54 for details about SSRI medications

   (f) Start antidepressant medication at LOW doses in children and adolescents and increase dosage SLOWLY

   (g) 8-week trial is recommended; takes 4 to 6 weeks to see effect

   (h) Antidepressants should be used for 6 to 9 months

   (i) Wean off drug slowly; NEVER stop abruptly

   (j) Monitor weekly somatic symptoms, heart rate, and blood pressure

   (k) Assess therapeutic levels when initiating and increasing dosage

 **e.** Suicide ideations or attempts

  **i.** Epidemiology (AACAP, 2001; Pelkonen & Martunen, 2003; Pompili, et al., 2005)

   (a) Over 90% of children and adolescents who commit suicide have a mental disorder before their death

   (b) About 2 million U.S. teenagers attempt suicide annually, almost 700,000 receive medical attention for their attempt

   (c) 3rd leading cause of death in teenagers, about 2000 deaths annually in U.S. adolescents

   (d) Suicide increases with age

   (e) Females make more attempts, males are more successful

**ii.** Assessment of suicidal ideation (AACAP, 2001)

    (a) Ideation: e.g., "Have you ever felt like you wanted to kill yourself?"

    (b) Method: e.g., "Have you ever thought about how you would do it?" "Is [method] available to you?"

    (c) Plan: e.g., "Have you made a plan for how or when you would do it?"

    (d) Intent: e.g., "Do you intend to kill yourself?"

    (e) Obtain information from several sources: child, parent; get release of information to speak to teacher, grandparent

**iii.** Risk factors for suicide (AACAP, 2001)

    (a) Hopelessness (the number one predictor)

    (b) Sudden change in behavior (e.g., giving away treasured items)

    (c) Sudden change in mood (e.g., sudden upswing in mood)

    (d) Depressive or pessimistic thinking (e.g., preoccupation with death)

    (e) Major life changes (e.g., death of a loved one, loss)

    (f) Preexisting psychiatric disorder (e.g., depression, panic attacks, psychosis, separation anxiety, disruptive and aggressive disorders, adjustment disorder)

    (g) History of self-harming behavior

    (h) Impulsivity of adolescence, i.e., permanent solution to a temporary problem

    (i) Disciplinary troubles in school or with the law, academic or family difficulties, relationship trouble, poor parent-teen communication

    (j) Drug and alcohol use/abuse

    (k) Not future-oriented

    (l) Suicide method available (e.g., firearm)

    (m) Family violence, family pathology, family history of suicide, or recent suicide in school or community

    (n) Isolation, runaway behavior

    (o) Serious medical illness

    (p) Gay, lesbian, and bisexual youth

    (q) History of abuse

**iv.** Management of suicidal ideation (AACAP, 2001)

    (a) Depending on seriousness of suicidal ideation and community resources, refer child or adolescent to:

        (1) Emergency room, in-patient hospitalization, in-home crisis intervention program, residential program, outpatient mental health professionals

        (2) Establish a "no-suicide contract" between the child and PNP, parent

        (3) Mobilize social supports and continuous supervision

        (4) Remove from the home firearms, sharp objects, and all medications that can be used for overdose

        (5) Identify and manage underlying cause of suicidal ideation (e.g., depression, loss, abuse, stress, exposure to violence) with appropriate interventions

        (6) Close follow-up and support

        (7) 24-hour availability of clinical support to the family in the acute period

        (8) Educate children about crisis hotlines

**5.** Symptoms: Anxiety, fear, nervousness, worry about future events, wariness, avoidant behavior. Hypersensitivity, sense of "going crazy," sense of impending death, motor tension, tremulousness, sleep difficulties, autonomic hyperactivity (palpitations, dizziness, shortness of breath, tachycardia), obsessions, compulsions

  **a.** Differential diagnoses (Box 41-1) (APA, 1994; Brookman & Sood, 2006)

   **i.** Anxious variation

    (a) Developmentally appropriate fear and anxiety; does not interfere with normal development

    (b) Infancy: normal fears include fear of heights, noises; fear of separation from parents and fear of strangers (which peaks at 8 to 9 months)

       (1) Anxiety is evident in infancy with changes in feeding or sleeping routines, nightmares, transient developmental regressions

    (c) Early childhood: specific fears may develop (dogs, thunder, darkness)

    (d) Middle childhood (Sharrer & Ryan-Wenger, 2002)

       (1) Anxiety is evidenced by motor responses (nail biting, thumb sucking); somatic symptoms (headache, stomachache, limb pain, breathlessness, vomiting)

       (2) Transient fears relieved by reassurance

    (e) Adolescence

       (1) Anxiety is evidenced by reluctance to engage in typical but new experiences

       (2) Risk-taking behaviors (drugs, alcohol, sex) may be a compensatory response to anxiety

   **ii.** Anxiety problems

    (a) Symptoms similar to above, but more pronounced and more prolonged

    (b) Excessive fear or anxiety is maladaptive if it interferes with daily functioning or attainment of developmental milestones or if it cannot be relieved by reassurance or appeal to reason or logic

    (c) Other symptoms

       (1) Feeling lonely

       (2) Excessive crying

       (3) Irritability

       (4) Nervousness

       (5) Self-consciousness

       (6) Suspiciousness

       (7) Afraid of failure/mistakes

       (8) Withdrawal (overly shy, refusing to talk, school refusal, peer avoidance)

   **iii.** Separation anxiety disorder

    (a) Developmentally inappropriate age for separation anxiety

    (b) Excessive worry about being away from home or from the attachment figure(s)

    (c) Avoidance of situations that require separation

    (d) At least 4 weeks duration

    (e) Clinically significant distress or social or academic impairment

   **iv.** Specific phobia

    (a) Excessive and unreasonable fear

    (b) Exposure to the stimulus will provoke an immediate anxiety response

    (c) Symptoms must be present for 6 months or greater

    (d) Children may not recognize the fear as excessive; adolescents typically will acknowledge it as an excessive fear

    (e) Fear is cued by the presence or anticipation of a specific object or situation

    (f) Avoidance of fearful stimulus interferes with normal developmental activities

  v. Social phobia

    (a) Child has capacity for age-appropriate social relationships

    (b) Marked and persistent fear of acting in an embarrassing or humiliating way in social or performance situations with peers, not just adults

    (c) Occurs when child is exposed to unfamiliar people or to possible scrutiny of others

  vi. Obsessive compulsive disorder (OCD)

    (a) Obsessions are unwanted, repetitive, persistent, intrusive, inappropriate thoughts, impulses or images that cause marked anxiety or distress

    (b) Child recognizes obsessions as products of his/her own mind

    (c) Not simply excessive worries about real life problems

    (d) Child tries to ignore or suppress the obsessions

    (e) Or, child tries to neutralize obsessions, prevent or reduce distress, or prevent some dreaded event or situation with some *other* thought or action (compulsions)

    (f) Compulsions are repetitive stereotyped behaviors or mental acts performed according to rigidly applied rules (e.g., handwashing, open and close door three times)

    (g) Child feels compelled to perform compulsions in response to obsessions

    (h) Note: some infants need rigid bedtime rituals, and many young children engage in bedtime rituals, but these are short-lived and do not interfere with normal development

  vii. Generalized anxiety disorder

    (a) Excessive anxiety and worry about a number of activities or events

    (b) Occurs more days than not for at least 6 months

    (c) Accompanied by at least three of the following symptoms in adolescents or one symptom in children:

      (1) Restlessness or feeling on edge

      (2) Easily fatigued

      (3) Difficulty concentrating or mind going blank

      (4) Irritability

      (5) Muscle tension

      (6) Sleep disturbance

  viii. Panic disorder

    (a) Characterized by panic attacks: discrete periods of intense fear or discomfort; symptoms develop abruptly and peak within 10 minutes

    (b) Recurrent and *unexpected*

    (c) At least one attack followed by 1 month or more of one of the following:

      (1) Persistent concern about having additional attacks

      (2) Worry about the implications or consequences of the attack (e.g., "going crazy, "dying")

      (3) Worry about a significant change in behavior related to the attacks

    (d) Terrified about leaving the home for fear of being alone or as an avoidance tactic for further panic attacks (agoraphobia)

    ix. Adjustment disorder
      (a) Emotional or behavioral symptoms occurring within 3 months of an identifiable stressor
      (b) Symptoms are in excess of what would be expected from exposure to the stressor
      (c) Or, significant impairment in social or occupational/academic functioning
      (d) Presentation does not meet diagnostic criteria for bereavement or other disorder
      (e) Not merely an exacerbation of a preexisting disorder
      (f) Acute: if the disturbance lasts less than 6 months
      (g) Chronic: if disturbance lasts greater than 6 months
      (h) Once the stressor (or its consequences) has terminated, the symptoms do not persist for more than an additional 6 months

    x. Posttraumatic stress disorder (PTSD) (APA, 1994; Melnyk, et al., 2002)
      (a) Child experienced, witnessed, or was confronted with event(s) that involved actual or threatened death or serious injury to self or others
      (b) Initial response involved intense fear, helplessness, or horror
      (c) Children may respond with disorganized or agitated behavior
      (d) Traumatic event is persistently re-experienced as:
        (1) Recurrent and intrusive distressing recollections of the event, including images, thoughts, or perceptions
        (2) In young children, themes or aspects of the trauma are expressed in repetitive play
        (3) Recurrent distressing dreams (without recognizable content for young children)
        (4) A sense of reliving the experience, illusions, hallucinations, and dissociative flashback episodes
      (e) Cues that symbolize the event cause intense distress, physiologic reactivity
      (f) Numbing of general responsiveness
      (g) Persistent avoidance of stimuli associated with the trauma, indicated by three or more of the following:
        (1) Avoidance of trauma-related thoughts, feelings, or conversations
        (2) Avoidance of activities, places, or people associated with the trauma
        (3) Inability to recall important aspects of the trauma
        (4) Diminished interest in significant activities
        (5) Feelings of detachment from others
        (6) Restricted range of affect
        (7) Sense of foreshortened future
      (h) Persistent symptoms of increased arousal for more than 1 month, as indicated by two of the following:
        (1) Sleep difficulties
        (2) Irritable, angry outbursts
        (3) Difficulty concentrating
        (4) Hypervigilance
        (5) Exaggerated startle response
      (i) PTSD causes clinically significant distress or impairment in social, academic, or other important areas of functioning

    xi. Medication reactions that may mimic anxiety (e.g., thyroid medications, antihistamines, antiasthmatics, sympathomimetics, steroids, haloperidol, pimozide, SSRIs, antipsychotics, diet pills, cold medications, caffeine, illegal drugs)

    **xii.** Medical disorders that may mimic anxiety disorders (e.g. hypoglycemic episodes, hyperthyroidism, cardiac arrhythmias, pheochromocytoma, seizure disorders, migraine, central nervous system disorders)

  **b.** Epidemiology of anxiety-related disorders

    **i.** The combined prevalence of anxiety disorders affects 6% to 18% of children and adolescents

    **ii.** Highest prevalence compared to other pediatric mental health disorders

    **iii.** Age at onset: separation anxiety (young children); social phobia (mid-teens), phobias (under 6); acute stress (all ages, often after a trauma); PTSD (delayed after a trauma); generalized anxiety (child/adolescent onset), OCD (males 6 to 15, females 20 to 29); panic or agoraphobia (late teens)

    **iv.** Females are twice as likely to have an anxiety disorder, especially separation anxiety, phobias, generalized anxiety disorder, and panic attacks

    **v.** High co-morbidity with depression, ADHD, and conduct disorder

    **vi.** Research shows PTSD prevalence rates after trauma such as abuse, motor vehicle accident: 3% to 100%

  **c.** Risk factors for anxiety or trauma response

    **i.** Parental anxiety, depression, or family dysfunction

    **ii.** Trauma, exposure to violence, natural disaster, loss, abuse, or major stressor

    **iii.** May be learned by repeated exposure to unpleasant events

    **iv.** Learned vicariously by observing others reacting fearfully, including media exposure

    **v.** Attachment and parenting issues

    **vi.** Genetic predisposition

  **d.** Management (Emslie & Mayes, 2001; James, et al., 2005; Lyons, et al., 2006; Waslick, 2006)

    **i.** Multimodal and interdisciplinary approach

    **ii.** Education about anxiety condition and promotion of coping skills

    **iii.** Support the child and family, and help family mobilize supports (e.g. "you are not alone; others have similar problems; it's not your fault, we can help you")

    **iv.** Referral for full mental health and/or psychopharmacology evaluation

    **v.** Referral for psychotherapy: individual, cognitive-behavioral therapy, grief counseling, and/or family therapy

    **vi.** Relaxation training, biofeedback, and self-regulation strategies

    **vii.** Behavioral modification and minimizing of secondary gains

    **viii.** Pharmacotherapy

      (a) See Table 54-9 in Chapter 54 for details about medications for anxiety disorders

      (b) Adjunctive therapy to psychiatric or behavioral interventions

      (c) Anxiolytics are less commonly prescribed for children

      (d) May help manage arousal responses to severe anxiety

      (e) As child develops coping skills and mastery of anxiety or stressors, medicine can often be withdrawn

    **ix.** Effective treatment of co-morbid disorders is essential

**6.** Symptoms: negative emotional behaviors, anger, frustration, irritation, whining, temper tantrums, screaming, cursing

  **a.** Differential diagnoses (Box 41-1) (APA, 1994)

    **i.** Negative emotional behavior variation
- (a) Developmentally normal behaviors that decrease with age as self-control and adoption of social norms improves
- (b) Infancy: cries in response to any frustration, or for no apparent reason, especially in late afternoon and evening
- (c) Early childhood: whines, easily frustrated, hits and bites when angry, temper tantrums
- (d) Middle childhood: fewer temper tantrums, pounds fists, screams
- (e) Adolescence: hits objects, slams doors, screams

   **ii.** Negative emotional behavioral problem
- (a) More frequent and more intense symptoms
- (b) Begin to interfere with normal developmental tasks

  **iii.** Oppositional defiant disorder (ODD) (Frick, 2006; Karnik, et al., 2006)
- (a) Pattern of negative, hostile, and defiant behavior
- (b) Exceeds that seen in other children of the same age
- (c) Appears between 3 to 7 years; manifests fully by 8 years
- (d) Precursors include social aggression, defiance, negativism, harsh or abusive parenting
- (e) Family dysfunction
- (f) Epidemiology
  - (1) One of the most common behavioral diagnoses in children/adolescents
  - (2) 2% to 14% prevalence rate
  - (3) Boys (14%) > girls (10%) in childhood
  - (4) Girls (12% to 15%)> boys as adolescents
  - (5) Greater incidence in lower socioeconomic status

  **iv.** Conduct disorder (CD)
- (a) Repetitive, persistent pattern of aggressive behavior
- (b) Basic rights of others or major age-appropriate societal norms and rules are violated
- (c) Onset of aggressive behavior is observed during toddler period
- (d) Early onset at 4 to 6 years
- (e) Formal diagnosis made at age 7 years or older
- (f) Typically diagnosed in late childhood or early adolescence
- (g) Precursors: chronic negative circumstances (e.g., poverty, child abuse and neglect), harsh parenting practices, dysfunctional family or chaos, chronic illness and disability
- (h) Associated with witnessing violence, including via media
- (i) Related to difficult temperament
- (j) Epidemiology
  - (1) Children age 10 to 13 years: 4% girls, 16% boys
  - (2) Adolescents age 14 to 16 years: 9% girls, 16% boys
  - (3) Adolescents age 17 to 20 years: 7% women, 9.5% men

**b.** Management
- **i.** Multi-modal and interdisciplinary
- **ii.** Referral for individual, group, and/or family therapy
- **iii.** Peer intervention, social skills groups
- **iv.** School intervention
- **v.** Juvenile justice system intervention
- **vi.** Social services referral
- **vii.** Other community resources (e.g., Big Brother, Big Sister)
- **viii.** Out-of-home placement

    **ix.** Job and independent-living skills training

    **x.** Education about disorder and medications

    **xi.** Parenting books/classes/support groups

    **xii.** Discuss fundamental parenting principles

    **xiii.** Increasing positive attention for appropriate behavior, incentives versus punishments, reducing attention for inappropriate behavior, removing attention through the use of time-out, avoiding punitive discipline, and avoiding accidentally rewarding misbehavior

    **xiv.** Choose battles wisely, avoid power struggles

    **xv.** Logical consequences close in time with behavior

    **xvi.** Active listening, encourage positive autonomy and responsibility

    **xvii.** Firm, empathetic limits on behaviors, not feelings

    **xviii.** All feelings are okay and teens are responsible for behavior chosen to reflect feelings; teach "I feel" messages

    **xix.** Limit setting strategies "if… then…" statements

    **xx.** Structure and consistency, give effective instructions

    **xxi.** Medications: Collaboration with experienced psychiatric health care providers is essential, especially for the prescribing of psychoactive medication

        (a) Lack rigorous studies for use with children

        (b) Stimulants for co-morbid attention deficit hyperactivity disorder

        (c) Neuroleptics for aggression (e.g., haloperidol, risperidone)

        (d) Mood stabilizers (e.g., lithium carbonate)

        (e) Anticonvulsants both for seizure disorders and for aggression (e.g., Carbamazepine)

        (f) Antidepressants for mood and anxiety disorders (e.g., trazodone, imipramine)

        (g) Alpha agonists for behavioral control (e.g., clonidine, guanfacine)

        (h) Low-dose tranquilizers for paranoid ideation with aggression (e.g., benzodiazepines: diazepam, clonazepam)

        (i) Atypical anxiolytics (e.g., buspirone)

---

# REFERENCES

Academy of Child and Adolescent Psychiatry (AACAP). (2001). Summary of the practice parameters for the assessment and treatment of children and adolescents with suicidal behavior. *J Acad Child and Adolecs Psy, 40,* 495-499.

American Psychiatric Association. (1994). *Diagnostic and statistical manual of mental disorders (DSM-IV™),* 4th edition. Washington, DC: American Psychiatric Association.

Brookman, R. R., & Sood, A. A. (2006). Disorders of mood and anxiety in adolescents. *Adolesc Med Clin, 17*(1):79-95.

Emslie, G.J. & Mayes, T.L. (2001). Mood disorders in children and adolescents: Psychopharmacological treatment. *Biological Psychiatry, 49, 1082-1090.*

Frick, P. J. (2006). Developmental pathways to conduct disorder. *Child Adolesc Psychiatr Clin N Am, 15*(2):311-331, vii.

James, A., Soler, A., & Weatherall, R. (2005). Cognitive behavioural therapy for anxiety disorders in children and adolescents. *Cochrane Database Syst Rev,* (4):CD004690.

Karnik, N. S., McMullin, M. A., & Steiner, H. (2006). Disruptive behaviors: conduct and oppositional disorders in adolescents. *Adolesc Med Clin, 17*(1):97-114.

Lyons, R. K, Dutra, L., Schuder, M. R., et al. (2006). From infant attachment disorganization to adult dissociation: relational adaptations or traumatic experiences? *Psychiatr Clin North Am, 29*(1):63-86, viii.

Melnyk, B.M., Feinstein, N.F., Tuttle, J., Moldenhauer, Z., Herendeen, P., Veenema, T.G., Brown, H., Gullo, S., McMurtrie, M., & Small, L. (2002). Mental health worries, communication, and needs of children, teens, and parents during the year of the nation's terrorist attack: Findings from the national KySS survey. *J Ped Health Care, 16,* 222-234.

Melnyk, B. M., & Moldenhauer, Z. (February/1999). Current approaches to depression in children and adolescents. *ADVANCE for Nurse Practitioners, 7*(2) 24-29, 97.

Melnyk, B.M., Moldenhauer, Z., Veenema, McMurtrie, M., T., Gullo, S., O-Leary, E., Small, L., Tuttle, J. (2001). The KySS (Keep your children/yourself Safe and Secure) campaign: A national effort to decrease psychosocial morbidities in children and adolescents. *J Ped Health Care, 15,* 31A-34A.

Moldenhauer, Z., & Melnyk, B. M. (2000). Use of anti-depressants in the treatment of child and adolescent depression: Are they effective? *Pediatric Nursing, 25,* 643-646.

Nemeroff, C. B., & Vale, W. W. (2005). The neurobiology of depression: inroads to treatment and new drug discovery. *J Clin Psychiatry, 66,* Suppl 7:5-13.

Pelkonen, M., & Marttunen, M. (2003). Child and adolescent suicide: epidemiology, risk factors, and approaches to prevention. *Paediatr Drugs, 5*(4):243-265.

Pompili, M., Mancinelli, I., Girardi, P., et al. (2005). Childhood suicide: a major issue in pediatric health care. *Issues Compr Pediatr Nurs, 28*(1): 63-68.

Ryan, N. D. (2005). Treatment of depression in children and adolescents. *Lancet, 366*(9489): 933-940.

Ryan-Wenger, N. A. (2001). Use of children's drawings for measurement of developmental level and emotional status. *Journal of Child and Family Nursing, 4* (2), 139-149.

Scahill, L., Hamrin, V., & Pachler, M. E. (2005). The use of selective serotonin reuptake inhibitors in children and adolescents with major depression. *J Child Adolesc Psychiatr Nurs, 18*(2):86-9.

Sharrer, V. W., & Ryan-Wenger, N. A. (2002). School-age children's self-reported stress symptoms. *Pediatric Nursing, 28,* 21-27.

Wagner, K. D. (2005). Pharmacotherapy for major depression in children and adolescents. *Prog Neuropsychopharmacol Biol Psychiatry, 29*(5): 819-826.

Waslick, B. (2006). Psychopharmacology interventions for pediatric anxiety disorders: a research update. *Child Adolesc Psychiatr Clin N Am, 15*(1):51-71.

1. Congenital heart disease
   a. A group of congenital malformations that result from abnormal structural development of the heart and/or vessels in utero
   b. MedlinePlus, a service of the National Library of Medicine and the National Institutes of Health, has excellent illustrations of each type of congenital malformation; see http://www.nlm.nih.gov/medlineplus/mplusdictionary.html
   c. Congenital heart disease (CHD) is categorized on the basis of the presence or absence of cyanosis (Table 42-1) (Allen, et al., 2001)
       i. Acyanotic
          (a) Left-to-right shunt due to communication between two sides of the heart
          (b) 82% to 90% of CHD diagnoses
       ii. Cyanotic
          (a) Obstruction of pulmonary blood flow or mixing of oxygenated and unoxygenated blood
          (b) 10% to 18% of CHD diagnoses
   d. Etiology
       i. Genetic—chromosomal abnormality
       ii. Multifactorial—genetic and environmental trigger
   e. Incidence
       i. Affects less than 1% of all children
       ii. One of the most common birth defects
       iii. No gender differences
   f. Fetal development of the heart and major vessels
       i. See Chapter 7 for details on first 8 weeks of embryonic development
       ii. Critical period of cardiac development is from days 20 to 50
       iii. Placenta responsible for delivering oxygen and removal of waste during fetal development
       iv. Fetal lungs do not deliver oxygen to the fetus
   g. Fetal circulation and the origin of some congenital heart defects
       i. Ductus arteriosus
          (a) Physiologic shunt between pulmonary artery and aorta
          (b) Allows fetal blood to bypass the lungs
          (c) Normally closes at the first breath or shortly after birth

TABLE 42-1

**Characteristics of Acyanotic and Cyanotic Congenital Heart Disease Lesions**

| Diagnosis | Description | Signs and Symptoms | Heart Sounds and Observations | Treatment | Notes |
|---|---|---|---|---|---|
| **Acyanotic—left-to-right shunt due to communication between two sides of the heart** | | | | | |
| Ventricular septal defect (VSD) | A hole in the septum that divides the right and left ventricles | May be asymptomatic if holes are small CHF symptoms | Holosystolic murmur heard best at LLSB May not be heard until 2 to 6 weeks of age | 90% close by age 8 years If not, surgically repaired with a synthetic patch | Most common cardiac defect Females > males |
| Patent ductus arteriosus (PDA) | Ductus arteriosus fails to close after birth; aortic blood shunted into pulmonary artery | May be asymptomatic Increasing signs of CHF | Birth—soft systolic murmur Later—grades 2 to 5/6 harsh, rumbling, continuous murmur and a thrill at the base | Indomethacin or ibuprofen (prostaglandin inhibitor) to medically close the PDA Surgically ligated if necessary | Common cause is rubella in mother Females > males, 2:1 Premature > full term |
| Atrial septal defect (ASD) | Hole in atrial septum classified by its location: Primum = low in septum Ostium secundum = midsection of septum Sinus venosus = high in septum | May be asymptomatic Fatigue easily Exertional dyspnea Physically underdeveloped | Grades 1 to 3/6 systolic, widely radiating, medium-pitch murmur Low intensity, heard best in upper left sternal border. Often confused with innocent murmur Sometimes a diastolic murmur heard | 80% will close spontaneously by 18 months If not, repaired either by cardiac catheterization or surgical placement of a synthetic patch | Ostium type more common in females than males, 2:1 If untreated, child may develop pulmonary hypertension as an adult |
| **Cyanotic—right-to-left shunt due to obstruction of pulmonary blood flow or mixing of oxygenated and unoxygenated blood** | | | | | |
| Coarctation of the aorta (COA) | Narrowing of the aorta at the ductus arteriosus | May not be evident until PDA closes | Higher pulse rate and BP in the upper than lower extremities Sometimes a murmur | Urgent surgical repair if there are symptoms Prostaglandin therapy to keep PDA open, then surgical repair | Typical age of diagnosis is 10 years |
| Aortic valve stenosis (AVS) | Obstruction to outflow from the left ventricle due to constriction at or near the aortic valve | Syncope Angina with activity | Midsystolic ejection murmur heard best over URSB with radiation into the right neck | If mild may not need treatment; otherwise need surgery Valves may calcify, requiring surgery as adult | May be congenital or acquired from rheumatic heart disease |

| Defect | Pathology | Symptoms | Physical findings | Treatment | Comments |
|---|---|---|---|---|---|
| Tetralogy of Fallot (TOF or TET) | Four defects: VSD, pulmonary stenosis, overriding aorta with right-to-left shunt, right ventricular hypertrophy | Cyanosis<br>Hypercyanotic periods, called "TET spells"<br>Poor weight gain<br>Squatting when fatigued<br>Clubbing<br>Irritability<br>Syncope | Grades 3 to 5/6 harsh systolic ejection murmur at LUSB<br>Palpable thrill and holosystolic murmur at LLSB<br>Observable sternal lift | Prostaglandins used to keep PDA open for oxygenation<br>Surgical repair at about age 6 months | Most common cyanotic CHD diagnosis<br>During "TET spell" immediately hold child in knee-chest position until symptoms subside |
| Transposition of the great arteries (TGA) | Pulmonary artery leaves left ventricle; aorta leaves right ventricle<br>Right-to-left shunt and systemic blood gets no oxygen<br>Associated with ASD, VSD, PDA | Cyanosis at birth<br>CHF symptoms | Heart murmur usually absent for first 2 weeks<br>Murmur due to associated lesions | Prostaglandin therapy to keep PDA open, then surgical repair to switch the arteries | Males > females: 6–7:1<br>Often LGA but grow poorly after birth |
| Truncus arteriosus (TA) | Failure of normal separation of aorta and pulmonary arteries | Cyanosis | | Medications to control heart failure<br>Surgical repair | |
| Hypoplastic left heart syndrome (HLHS) | Underdevelopment of left side of heart<br>Hypoplastic left ventricle, aortic atresia, PDA | Cyanosis | | Three-stage reconstruction: at birth, ages 4 to 6 months, ages 2 to 3 years | |
| Tricuspid pulmonary atresia with VSD | No communication between right ventricle and pulmonary artery | Cyanosis<br>Dyspnea on exertion<br>Fatigue after feeding or crying<br>Hypoxic episodes<br>FTT | Grade 3 to 5/6 harsh, holosystolic murmur along middle LSB | Prostaglandin therapy to keep PDA open, then surgical repair | Frequent surgeries and hospitalizations throughout life |
| Pulmonic stenosis | Narrowing of pulmonic valve with increased right-sided pressure | Usually asymptomatic<br>Increasing fatigue and dyspnea<br>Cyanosis | Grades 2 to 4/6 harsh, mid- to late systolic ejection murmur at ULSB with radiation throughout<br>Intermittent systolic ejection click | Balloon valvuloplasty or surgical valvulotomy | Stenosis may progress during periods of rapid growth |

From Burns, C. E., Dunn, A. M., Brady, M. A., et al. (2004). *Pediatric primary care: A handbook for nurse practitioners* (3rd ed.). St. Louis: Saunders.

(d) In premature infants and hypoxic infants it may remain open much longer

(e) Oxygen is the most important factor in controlling closure in full-term infants

(f) Closure is also mediated by bradykinin, a substance released by the lungs on initial inflation

ii. Ductus venosus

(a) Fetal blood vessel connecting umbilical vein to inferior vena cava

(b) Shunts oxygenated blood from the placenta via umbilical vein

(c) Vasoconstriction occurs at first or subsequent breaths; then the ductus normally closes

iii. Foramen ovale

(a) Opening between right and left atrium

(b) Allows shunting of oxygenated blood from the right to left atrium

(c) Right ventricle does all of the work for fetal circulation

(d) Normally closes at birth due to:

(1) Decreased flow from placenta to hold it open

(2) Increased pulmonary blood flow, which causes:

a) Increased pulmonary venous return to left heart

b) Increased pressure in the left atrium

c) Pressure in left atrium is higher than in the right atrium

(3) Output from the right ventricle flows into the pulmonary circulation

h. Signs and symptoms

i. Newborns and infants (Harris & Valmorida, 2000)

(a) Rapid breathing

(b) Difficulty feeding

(c) Cyanosis

(d) Failure to thrive

ii. Child or adolescent

(a) Fatigue

(b) Squatting

(c) Difficulty exercising or doing physical activity

(d) Chest pain

(e) Syncope

(f) Diaphoresis

(g) Palpitations

i. Focused history

i. Maternal history (risk factors for CHD)

(a) Maternal age (>40 years)

(b) Rubella infection

(c) Drugs—medications, e.g., trimethadione, retinoic acid

(d) Illegal drug use

(e) Alcohol

(f) Smoking

(g) Diabetes

(h) PKU

(i) Exposure to radiation, toxins

ii. Neonatal history

(a) Cyanosis

(1) Timing of cyanosis: 48 to 72 hours suggests ductal-dependent lesion

    (2) Intermittent cyanosis suggests neurologic or metabolic disorders
   (b) Dyspnea
    (1) Was infant in NICU?
    (2) Oxygen or ventilator required?
    (3) Tachypnea
   (c) Congenital syndrome or dysmorphism, e.g., Down syndrome
  iii. Family history
   (a) CHD more common with positive family history of CHD
   (b) Genetic or dysmorphic syndromes
   (c) Connective tissue disorder (Marfan's syndrome)
   (d) Inborn error of metabolism
   (e) Other congenital defects
  iv. Child's past medical history
   (a) Hospitalizations, surgeries
   (b) Frequent use of the ED
   (c) Poor growth, poor feeding
   (d) Easily fatigued, exercise intolerance
   (e) Chronic cough, asthma symptoms
   (f) Rheumatic fever or Kawasaki disease
   (g) Immunizations
   (h) Medication history
   (i) Attainment of developmental milestones
  v. Social history
   (a) Socioeconomic status
   (b) Members of the household
   (c) Pets
   (d) Smokers in the home
j. Focused physical examination
  i. Inspection
   (a) Observe for dysmorphic features
   (b) Height and weight for age and sex
    (1) Plotted on growth chart
    (2) BMI for children > 2 years of age
   (c) Pulse, blood pressure (see Chapter 7)
   (d) Color (Harris & Valmorida, 2000)
    (1) Cyanotic newborn
     a) Normal newborns have a $PaO_2$ of 50 mm Hg within 5 to 10 minutes after delivery
     b) Central cyanosis correlates better with hypoxia than does peripheral cyanosis
     c) An anemic patient must be severely hypoxic to appear cyanotic
     d) If an infant is acidotic or febrile or has more adult than fetal hemoglobin, cyanosis will occur more readily
     e) Because a patient can be hypoxemic without cyanosis, arterial blood gases must be done to obtain oxygen tension ($PaO_2$)
    (2) Cyanosis for CHD is classified into two basic categories
     a) Decreased pulmonary blood flow caused by right-sided obstruction (i.e., tetralogy of Fallot [TOF])
     b) Abnormal intracardiac mixing, i.e., transposition of great arteries (TGA)
   (e) Clubbing (Box 42-1) (Schwartz, Richards, & Goyal, 2006)

■ **BOX 42-1**
■ **TECHNIQUE TO EVALUATE CLUBBING OF FINGERS**

---

1. Observe the distal end of fingers in profile. A Lovibond angle is the angle made by the proximal nail fold and nail plate
**Normal**
Less than or equal to 160 degrees
**Clubbing**
Angle flattens out and increases
An angle between 160 and 180 degrees may indicate early stages of clubbing or "pseudoclubbing"
An angle ≥180 degrees is considered to be clubbing
2. Ask the patient to place the nails of opposing fingers on the right and left hand together, e.g., left index fingernail next to right index fingernail
**Normal**
Diamond-shaped "window" is visible at the base of the nail beds
**Clubbing**
The diamond window is absent
3. Press on the nail beds
**Normal**
Nail does not move
**Clubbing**
The nail moves more freely
Note a spongy sensation as the nail is pressed toward the nail plate
Skin at the base of the nail may be smooth and shiny

---

From Schwartz, R. A., Richards, G. M., & Goyal, S. (2006). Clubbing of the nails. Retrieved June 28, 2006, from www.emedicine.com/DERM/topic780.htm.

    (f) Edema
    (g) Chest
        (1) Contour
        (2) Respiratory effort
  **ii.** Cardiac auscultation
    (a) Difficult to auscultate cardiac sounds in a 1- to 2-year-old child
        (1) Perform cardiac auscultation first before child becomes upset
        (2) Child needs to be quiet enough for a good examination to be performed
        (3) Have child sit in the lap of a parent
        (4) Play "games" during examination
        (5) Use distraction techniques
    (b) Always auscultate in the four listening areas with *both* the bell and the diaphragm to hear the high- and low-pitched sounds (Figure 42-1)
        (1) Upper right sternal border (URSB)
        (2) Upper left sternal border (ULSB)
        (3) Lower left sternal border (LLSB)
        (4) Apex
        (5) Erbs' point
    (c) Murmurs (Poddar & Basu, 2004)
        (1) Audible sound waves in the range of 20 to 2000 Hz
        (2) Caused by turbulent blood flow from the heart and surrounding vessels
    (d) Evaluation of murmurs (Blosser & Frietas-Nichols, 2004)
        (1) *Grade* murmurs according to their loudness (intensity) and associated sounds (Box 42-2)

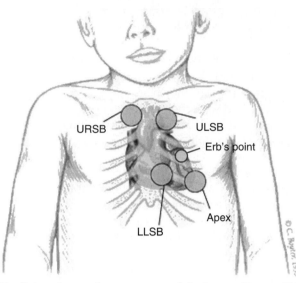

FIGURE 42-1 ■ Traditional auscultatory areas of the heart. (Burns, C. E., Dunn, A. M., Brady, M. A., et al. [2004]. *Pediatric primary care: A handbook for nurse practitioners* [3rd ed.]. Philadelphia: Saunders, Figure 31-2, p. 776.)

          a) Intensity is not necessarily related to severity of the defect

  (2) Describe the *pitch* of the sound

          a) Low

          b) Medium

          c) High

  (3) Describe the *quality* of the sound

          a) Harsh—high-velocity blood flow from higher to lower pressure

          b) Whooping or blowing

          c) Flow murmur—a crescendo/decrescendo murmur

          d) Vibratory or musical

  (4) Note the *timing* within the heartbeat cycle

          a) Early systolic

          b) Middle systolic

          c) Late systolic

          d) Holosystolic—throughout systole

          e) Diastolic

          f) Continuous

■ **BOX 42-2**
■ **GRADING CRITERIA FOR MURMURS BASED ON INTENSITY AND ASSOCIATED SOUNDS**

| | |
|---|---|
| Grade 1 | Barely audible |
| Grade 2 | Louder |
| Grade 3 | Louder but not accompanied by a thrill |
| Grade 4 | Loud and associated with a palpable thrill |
| Grade 5 | Associated with a thrill; heard with the stethoscope partially off the chest |
| Grade 6 | Audible without a stethoscope |

    (5) Note if sound *radiates* toward other areas
      a) Back
      b) Apex
      c) Carotids
    (6) Note effect of change in child's *position*
      a) After the supine examination, the examination should be repeated with the patient standing
      b) Helpful in differentiating functional (change) and pathologic (no change) murmurs
(e) Heart sounds
    (1) S1 is the first heart sound
      a) Normally a single sound heard at the LLSB
      b) Caused by closure of the mitral and tricuspid valves
      c) Murmurs that obscure S1 are also known as "holosystolic" murmurs, and suggest pathology
        i) Ventricular septal defect (VSD)
        ii) Atrioventricular valve regurgitation
        iii) Patent ductus arteriosus (PDA)
        iv) Severe pulmonary valve stenosis in a young child
    (2) Click
      a) High-pitched sounds
      b) S1 is audible but appears to have two components at some spots in the precordium
      c) Clicks originate from any valve in the heart
      d) Clicks have different identifying characteristics depending on what valve is affected
        i) Ejection clicks
          *a)* Originate from the pulmonic valve
          *b)* Best heard at the middle to upper LSB
          *c)* Begin shortly after the atrioventricular valves closes
          *d)* Vary with respiration
        ii) Aortic valve ejection clicks
          *a)* Begin shortly after S1
          *b)* Best heard at the apex
          *c)* Do not vary with respiration
        iii) Systolic clicks
          *a)* Originate from the mitral valve
          *b)* Best heard at the apical area URSB
          *c)* Loudest when the patient is standing
    (3) Second heart sound (S2)
      a) Double sound best heard at ULSB
      b) Caused by closure of the aortic and pulmonic valves
      c) Single S2 heard with:
        i) TOF
        ii) TGA
        iii) Hypoplastic left heart syndrome (HLHS)
        iv) Tricuspid atresia
    (4) Systolic murmur
      a) Caused by blood flow across an outflow tract (pulmonary or aortic)
      b) Functional murmur (innocent), e.g., Still's murmur
        i) No symptoms are present

ii) S1 is normal
iii) S2 splits, is of normal intensity, and moves with respiration
iv) Normal precordial activity
v) No clicks are heard
vi) Vibratory or musical
vii) Grade 1 or grade 2
viii) Decreases in intensity when patient stands
c) If grade 3 or higher, may indicate:
    i) VSD
    ii) Atrioventricular valve regurgitation
    iii) PDA
    iv) Atrial septal defect (ASD)
(5) Venous hum
  a) Common functional murmur—benign, not pathologic
    i) Caused by the flow of venous blood from the head and neck into the thorax
    ii) Heard continuously when the child is sitting but disappears when:
      *a)* Light pressure is applied over the jugular vein
      *b)* Child's head is turned
      *c)* Child is lying supine
    iii) Does not require pediatric cardiology referral
  b) All other diastolic murmurs are pathologic and warrant referral
(6) Other sounds that are always pathologic and indicate need for referral
  a) Friction rub is a sound that increases and decreases with systole and diastole
  b) Gallop is a triple or quadruple sound at S3 or S4
  c) Radiation—if a murmur radiates to the axilla or back, then it is a grade 3 murmur or greater

**iii.** Respiratory auscultation
  (a) Equal breath sounds
  (b) Respiratory rate for age (see Chapter 6, Table 6-1)
  (c) Adventitious sounds

**iv.** Palpation
  (a) Note increased precordial activity
    (1) Caused by increased right or left ventricular stroke volume
    (2) Increases the possibility that auscultatory findings may be pathologic
      a) Atrial septal defect
      b) Moderate to large VSD
      c) PDA
    (3) Other causes of increased precordial activity
      a) Anxiety
      b) Anemia
      c) Hyperthyroidism
  (b) Pulses
    (1) Brachial pulses should be equal and strong
    (2) Compare brachial and femoral pulses simultaneously
      a) Timing and intensity of the two pulses should be equal

        (c) Thrill
            (1) Vibration felt in combination with a murmur
            (2) Caused by blood flowing rapidly from high pressure to lower pressure
            (3) VSD causes a thrill at the LLSB
            (4) Pulmonary valve stenosis causes a thrill at the ULSB
            (5) Aortic stenosis causes a thrill at the suprasternal notch
        (d) Palpate the liver (see Chapter 8)

    k. Diagnostic testing (Danford, 2000)
       i. See Table 42-2 for details on diagnostic tests for congenital cardiac disorders

    l. Differential diagnoses
       i. See Box 42-3 for characteristics of innocent murmurs
      ii. See Table 42-1 for characteristics of CHD diagnoses categorized on the basis of acyanotic versus cyanotic
     iii. Consultation with a pediatrician or pediatric cardiologist is recommended before making a CHD diagnosis (Danford, 2000)

    m. Referral (Box 42-4)

■ **TABLE 42-2**
■ ■ **Diagnostic Tests for Congenital Heart Disease**

| Diagnostic Test | Invasiveness | Purpose | Sensitivity | Specificity | Cost |
|---|---|---|---|---|---|
| Pulse oximetry | Noninvasive | Level of oxygen saturation<br>Arm—preductal<br>Leg—postductal | High | High | Low |
| Arterial or capillary blood gases | Invasive | pH of blood<br>$Pao_2$<br>$Paco_2$ | High | High | Low |
| Chest x-ray | Noninvasive | Heart enlargement, position<br>Lung vascularity<br>Lung congestion | Low | Low | Low |
| Electrocardiogram | Noninvasive | Cardiac rhythm disturbance | Low | Intermediate | Low |
| Echocardiogram | Noninvasive | Graphic outline of heart and its movement<br>Size of chambers<br>Blood shunting<br>Valves opening/closing<br>Obstruction of valves | High | High | High |
| Doppler studies | Noninvasive | Estimates the degree of obstruction | Intermediate | Intermediate | Low |
| Exercise stress test | Noninvasive | Effect of exercise on heart function | High | Intermediate | High |
| Cardiac catheterization | Invasive | Quantifies the degree of disease present<br>Oxygenation and pressure measurements<br>Observe obstruction of flow<br>Can be used for treatment or correction | High | Intermediate | High |

■ **BOX 42-3**
■ **CHARACTERISTICS OF INNOCENT (FUNCTIONAL) MURMURS IN CHILDHOOD**

**Vibratory Still's Murmur** (most common innocent murmur in children; noted most often between ages 2 and 6 years)
- Early systolic, grades 1 to 3, usually 2
- Low to medium pitch
- Heard at LLSB and extends to apex
- Loudest in supine position, decreases upon sitting or standing
- Musical sound, like a vibratory "twang"

**Pulmonary Flow Murmur** (heard in children, adolescents, and young adults)
- Ejection systolic murmur
- Crescendo-decrescendo in character
- Low intensity (grades 2 and 3)
- Heard at the left sternal border in the second and third intercostal spaces
- "Rough" in character
- Best heard in the supine position
- Increases in intensity with expiration
- Decreases in intensity with inspiration and sitting or standing

**Peripheral Pulmonary Arterial Stenosis Murmur** (common in neonates and infants)
- Ejection systolic murmur, grades 1 and 2
- Low pitch, extends until or beyond S2
- Best heard in the axillae or on the back
- Louder in association with viral URI and asthma

**Aortic Systolic Murmur** (commonly heard during fever, anemia, anxiety, hyperthyroidism; may be heard in trained athletes)
- Ejection systolic flow murmur
- Heard at URSB

**Supraclavicular/Brachiocephalic Systolic Murmur** (heard in children and young adults)
- Crescendo-decrescendo early systolic murmur
- Low- to medium-pitched and brief
- Best heard above the clavicles with radiation to the neck
- No change with supine or sitting position
- Diminishes with hyperextension of the shoulders

**Venous Hum** (most common continuous murmur in children)
- Varies widely in intensity, from faint to grade 6
- Heard in the neck near sternocleidomastoid
- Louder on right side
- Heard best when sitting up and head turned away
- Decreased by gentle compression over the jugular vein or turning the head toward the side of the murmur

Adapted from Poddar, B., & Basu, S. (2004). Approach to a child with a heart murmur. *Ind J Pediatr, 71,* 63-66.

    **i.** Note: many normal children have innocent heart murmurs
        (a) These children do not require referral to a pediatric cardiologist
        (b) Referral may be made primarily to reassure child and parents that condition is a variation of normal and is not serious
**2.** Influence of CHD on child's growth and development and primary care implications (Jackson & Vessey, 2004; Park, 2002; Smith, 2001)
    **a.** Primary care concerns after surgery
        **i.** Assess that a continuous murmur is present after a Blalock-Taussig shunt procedure; an indication that the shunt is open

■ **BOX 42-4**
■ **WHEN TO REFER A CHILD TO A PEDIATRIC CARDIOLOGIST**

**SIGNS, SYMPTOMS**
- Physical findings (clusters of the following signs and symptoms)
  - Rapid breathing
  - Difficulty feeding
  - Cyanosis
  - Failure to thrive
  - Child or adolescent
  - Fatigue
  - Squatting
  - Difficulty exercising or doing physical activity
  - Chest pain
  - Syncope
  - Diaphoresis
  - Palpitations
    - Increased precordial activity
    - Decreased femoral pulses
    - Abnormal second heart sound
    - Clicks/thrills/gallops
    - Murmurs
    - Any murmur grade 3 or louder
    - Any harsh murmur
    - Diastolic murmurs
    - A murmur that *increases* in intensity with standing

**INFANTS WITH MURMURS AND THESE ASSOCIATED FINDINGS:**
- Poor feeders or failure to thrive
- Unexplained respiratory symptoms
- Cyanosis
- Family history of Marfan's syndrome or sudden death

**OLDER CHILDREN WITH MURMURS AND THESE ASSOCIATED FINDINGS:**
- Chest pain (especially with exercise)
- Syncope
- Exercise intolerance
- Family history of early sudden death

    ii. Administer immunizations according to usual schedule, especially yearly flu vaccine

   iii. Assess growth and development at least yearly

   iv. Nutritional assessment

    v. Check for and prevent development of anemia

   vi. Subacute bacterial endocarditis prophylaxis (see ACC/AHA 1997 guidelines on website)

      (a) Procedures that require antibiotic prophylaxis

        (1) Dental, oral procedures

        (2) Surgical procedures

      (b) Dosages (see Chapter 54, Table 54-3 for prophylaxis dosages of antibiotics)

   vii. Do not restrict activity if possible (see section 2.e. below)

**b.** Physical effects
 **i.** Increased workload of the heart increases energy demands on the body
 **ii.** Children with CHD often grow slowly
  (a) Body needs more calories to grow
  (b) Breast-feeding is encouraged
  (c) May need supplements to increase calories
   (1) Symptomatic children need 150 kcal/kg/day
   (2) May need 24 to 30 kcal/oz formula
   (3) May need additional gavage feedings to conserve energy
 **iii.** Tire easily, physical stamina varies with each child
 **iv.** Developmental milestones may be delayed
 **v.** Children with abnormal cardiac examination need frequent follow-up with the PNP
**c.** Cognitive
 **i.** Inadequate nutrition can influence brain development during first year
 **ii.** Speech and learning ability can be negatively affected
 **iii.** Additional stimulation may be needed
 **iv.** Physical, occupational, and speech therapy are often helpful
**d.** Psychosocial
 **i.** Infants and children may have frequent and prolonged hospitalizations
 **ii.** Encourage family visits during hospitalizations
  (a) Encourage talking, touching, and holding child
 **iii.** The unique needs of a chronically ill child can interfere with family dynamics
 **iv.** Family members as well as the child may feel angry, fearful, or resentful
 **v.** Child's body image may be an issue from surgical scars, cyanosis
**e.** Social and physical activity
 **i.** Most children with CHD play normally with other children unless physical stamina is an issue
 **ii.** Most can play sports and participate in physical education
  (a) May require referral for exercise testing
  (b) Contact sports may be limited especially for children with pacemakers
  (c) Ask parent and/or child to report any irregularities of blood pressure, heart rate, or physical performance during activity
 **iii.** Participation in all sports in general is permitted:
  (a) For children with ASD
  (b) For children with VSD
  (c) For children with PDA
  (d) Especially those who have undergone surgical correction of their defect
 **iv.** Participation in sports is limited for those with high pressures in the arteries to the lungs or heart rhythm irregularities
 **v.** Participation in sports if no symptoms are present is normally permitted in the following patients with CHD
  (a) Children with *mild* narrowing of the valves from the right-sided pumping chamber from the pulmonary artery to the lungs
   (1) Children with a narrowing of the aortic valve need closer supervision
   (2) Those with mild or medium narrowing of the valve can participate in low to moderate dynamic noncontact sports
   (3) If there is severe narrowing across the aortic valve, children should not participate in competitive sports

    **vi.** Individual exercise prescriptions are recommended for the following:
- (a) Children with cyanotic heart defect, whether it has been corrected surgically or not, usually can participate only in low-intensity competitive sports
- (b) Some children with Marfan's syndrome should engage in only low-intensity competitive sports

    **vii.** All athletes with CHD need to pay particular attention to hydration
- (a) Avoid dehydration by drinking water while exercising
- (b) Prevent problems with hyperviscosity

## REFERENCES

Allen, H. D., Clark, E. B., Gutgesell, H. P., & Driscoll, D. J. (2001). *Moss and Adams' heart disease in infants, children, and adolescents: Including the fetus and young adult* (Vol 1 & 2). Philadelphia: Lippincott Williams & Wilkins.

American College of Cardiology (ACC) and American Heart Association (AHA) (1997). Endocarditis prophylaxis information. Retrieved June 30, 2006, from www.americanheart.org/presenter. jhtml?identifier=11086. [Editor's note: these guidelines are still in use, despite their development in 1997.]

Blosser, C. G., & Freitas-Nichols, J. (2004). Cardiovascular disorders. In C. E. Burns, A. M. Dunn, M. A. Brady, et al. (Eds.). *Pediatric primary care: A handbook for nurse practitioners* (3rd ed.). Philadelphia: Saunders, pp. 769-810.

Burns, C. E., Dunn, A. M., Brady, M. A., et al. (2004). *Pediatric primary care: A handbook for nurse practitioners* (3rd ed.). Philadelphia: Saunders.

Harris, M., & Valmorida, J. (2000). Neonates with congenital heart disease: An overview. *Neonat Network, 19*(5), 37-41.

Jackson, P., & Vessey, J. (2004). *Primary care of the child with a chronic condition* (4th ed.). St. Louis: Mosby, Inc.

Park, M. (2002). *Pediatric cardiology for practitioners* (4th ed.). St. Louis: Mosby.

Poddar, B., & Basu, S. (2004). Approach to a child with a heart murmur. *Ind J Pediatr, 71*, 63-66.

Schwartz, R. A., Richards, G. M., & Goyal, S. (2006). Clubbing of the nails. Retrieved May 21, 2006, from www.emedicine.com/derm/topic780.htm.

Smith, P. (2001). Primary care in children with congenital heart disease. *J Pediatr Nurs, 16*(5), 308-319.

# Cystic Fibrosis

JEANNE WEILAND, MS, CPNP

## DEFINITION

Cystic fibrosis is an autosomal recessive disorder in which defective epithelial cell chloride transport affects the exocrine gland tissues of the body. Cystic fibrosis is a chronic multisystem disorder characterized by recurrent endobronchial infections, progressive obstructive pulmonary disease, and pancreatic insufficiency with intestinal malabsorption (Sharma, 2006).

1. Presentation
   a. The most likely clinical manifestations vary with age (Davis, 2001)
      i. Neonates—meconium ileus or generalized swelling, meconium peritonitis, jaundice
      ii. Infants younger than 1 year—wheezing, coughing, frequent respiratory infections, hypochloremic alkalosis, failure to thrive
      iii. Early infancy—steatorrhea, failure to thrive, fat soluble vitamin deficiencies
      iv. Childhood, adulthood—chronic productive cough, recurrent or persistent pneumonia
   b. Symptoms
      i. Respiratory
         (a) Chronic or acute sinusitis
            (1) Nasal congestion
            (2) Postnasal drip
            (3) Frontal headaches, pressure
         (b) Chronic cough
         (c) Thick, purulent mucus
         (d) Shortness of breath
         (e) Dyspnea on exertion
         (f) Wheeze
      ii. Gastrointestinal
         (a) Viscid meconium
         (b) Failure to thrive
         (c) Weight loss in spite of high calorie intake
         (d) Frequent bulky, greasy, foul-smelling stools

        (e) Excessive flatus
        (f) Abdominal pain and/or distention
     iii. Other
        (a) Excessively salty sweat
        (b) Delayed puberty
        (c) Infertility

2. Etiology and pathophysiology
    **a.** Genetics
        i. Autosomal recessive inheritance pattern
        ii. Caused by a defect in the CF gene, cystic fibrosis transmembrane conductance regulator (CFTR) (Sharma, 2006)
            (a) Located on long arm of chromosome 7
            (b) More than 1400 mutations of CF gene identified (Cystic Fibrosis Consortium, 2006)
            (c) CFTR encodes for a protein that functions as a chloride channel
            (d) Regulated by cyclic adenosine monophosphate (cAMP)
            (e) Mutations in the gene for CFTR result in abnormalities of cAMP-regulated chloride transport across epithelial cells on mucosal surfaces
    **b.** Pathophysiology (Sharma, 2006)
        i. Lungs are normal in utero, at birth, and shortly after birth
        ii. An acquired lung infection causes an inflammatory response
        iii. A repeating cycle of infection and neutrophilic inflammation occurs
        iv. Failure of epithelial cells to conduct chloride
        v. Associated water transport abnormalities
        vi. Result in viscid secretions and hallmark problems in:
            (a) Respiratory tract
            (b) Pancreas
            (c) Gastrointestinal tract
            (d) Sweat glands
            (e) Other exocrine tissues
        vii. Increased viscosity of these secretions makes them difficult to clear
        viii. Pulmonary disease is chronic and progressive
            (a) Characterized by airway infection and inflammation
            (b) Results in irreversible bronchiectasis
            (c) 95% of patients die from end-stage lung disease
        ix. Pancreatic insufficiency is seen in 85% to 95% of patients with CF

3. Incidence
    **a.** Carrier frequency is 1 per 30 among whites
    **b.** Racial prevalence of CF in the United States (Gibson, 2003)
        i. White—1900 to 3700
        ii. Black—1 in 15,000
        iii. Hispanic—1 in 9000
        iv. Asian—1 in 31,000
    **c.** Gender
        i. Males with CF are typically less affected than females with CF
        ii. In females pulmonary function deteriorates faster with increasing age
        iii. Females have a younger mean age at death
    **d.** Age at time of diagnosis
        i. One third of patients are diagnosed at less than 2 months of age by:
            (a) Positive family history
            (b) Meconium ileus
            (c) Neonatal screening

      **ii.** Median age at diagnosis is 14 months, with a range of prenatal to more than 40 years

**4.** Physical examination

  **a.** Respiratory system

    **i.** Nasal polyps

    **ii.** Evidence of airway obstruction on pulmonary function test

    **iii.** Chest x-ray shows:

      (a) Air trapping

      (b) Infiltrates

      (c) Bronchial wall thickening

      (d) Atelectasis

    **iv.** Increased work of breathing

      (a) Compliance work—force to expand lung against its elastic properties

      (b) Force to overcome viscosity of lung and chest wall

      (c) Airway resistance work—force to move air through airways

    **v.** Adventitious breath sounds

      (a) Crackles

      (b) Wheeze

      (c) Rhonchi

      (d) Decreased breath sounds

    **vi.** Airway infection

  **b.** Gastrointestinal system

    **i.** Abdominal distention

    **ii.** Hepatosplenomegaly (fatty liver and portal hypertension)

    **iii.** Rectal prolapse

    **iv.** Dry skin (vitamin A deficiency)

    **v.** Cheilosis (cracking at corners of mouth, vitamin B complex deficiency)

  **c.** Skeletal system

    **i.** Digital clubbing

    **ii.** Scoliosis

    **iii.** Kyphosis

**5.** Differential diagnosis

  **a.** Associated with nasal polyps (Sharma, 2006)

    **i.** Nasal polyposis (rare in absence of CF)

    **ii.** Severe allergic rhinitis

    **iii.** Inflammation associated with Samter's triad

      (a) Asthma

      (b) Aspirin insensitivity

      (c) Nasal polyposis

    **iv.** Other immunologic disorders

  **b.** Associated with respiratory symptoms (Murray & Brown, 2005)

    **i.** Allergic bronchopulmonary aspergillosis

    **ii.** Asthma

    **iii.** Bronchiectasis

    **iv.** Bronchiolitis

    **v.** Sinusitis

    **vi.** Frequent respiratory infections due to immunodeficiency

      (a) *Staphylococcus aureus*

      (b) *Haemophilus influenzae*

      (c) *Pseudomonas aeruginosa*

      (d) *Burkholderia cepacia*

      (e) *Atypical mycobacterium*

       **vii.** Pneumothorax

     **viii.** Massive hemoptysis

       **ix.** Cor pulmonale

        **x.** Bronchiectasis

  **c.** Associated with gastrointestinal symptoms

        **i.** Celiac disease

       **ii.** Meconium ileus

      **iii.** Rectal prolapse

      **iv.** Distal intestinal obstruction syndrome

       **v.** Intussusception

      **vi.** Fat-soluble vitamin deficiency

     **vii.** Zinc deficiency

    **viii.** Hyponatremic, hypochloremic dehydration

      **ix.** Osteopenia, osteoporosis

       **x.** Liver disease and portal hypertension

     **xi.** Essential fatty acid deficiency

    **xii.** Iron deficiency

   **xiii.** Gastroesophageal reflux disease

   **xiv.** Glucose intolerance

  **d.** Associated with skeletal system

        **i.** Failure to thrive

       **ii.** Short stature

      **iii.** Hypertrophic pulmonary osteoarthropathy

  **e.** Diagnostic criteria for cystic fibrosis (CF)

        **i.** One or more characteristic phenotypic features and/or

       **ii.** CF in sibling and/or positive newborn screen PLUS evidence of CFTR defect by:

          **(a)** Elevated sweat chloride (>60 mEq/L) by pilocarpine iontophoresis, or

          **(b)** Identification of two CF mutations, or

          **(c)** Abnormal nasal epithelial ion transport

      **iii.** Several factors may be associated with false-positive sweat chloride results (see section 6.b.vii)

      **iv.** False-negative results are typically due to laboratory error (see section 6.b.viii)

**6.** Diagnostic tests and procedures

  **a.** Newborn screening for CF recommended by CDC on October 15, 2004 (Grosse, et al., 2004)

  **b.** Pilocarpine iontophoresis test (sweat test)

        **i.** A chemical analysis of the chloride content of sweat

       **ii.** The "gold standard" for diagnosing CF when conducted according to guidelines of the Cystic Fibrosis Foundation (2006)

      **iii.** Recommended that it be conducted in a CF Foundation–accredited care center

      **iv.** Requires 75 to 100 mg of sweat

          **(a)** Pilocarpine, a colorless, odorless chemical is applied to an area of arm or leg

          **(b)** Electrode attached to the area

          **(c)** Weak current stimulates sweating for 5 minutes (patient may feel tingling or warmth)

          **(d)** Sweat is collected with a special device

          **(e)** Specimen sent to lab in 30 minutes

      **v.** Results

         (a) Normal sweat chloride level: less than 40 mEq/L

         (b) Borderline: 40 to 60 mEq/L

         (c) Diagnostic of CF: more than 60 mEq/L

      **vi.** Repeat test to confirm positive results

      **vii.** False positives

         (a) Occur in ≤10%

         (b) Caused by a variety of conditions, including anorexia nervosa, atopic dermatitis, malnutrition, nephrosis, metabolic enzyme deficiencies (Murray & Brown, 2005; Peckham & Littlewood, 2003)

      **viii.** False negatives occur less than 1%

         (a) Repeat negative test if clinical presentation suggests CF

         (b) Some individuals with CF have normal or borderline sweat chloride levels

  **c.** Chest x-ray

  **d.** Sinus x-ray

  **e.** Genotyping

  **f.** Pulmonary function test

  **g.** Bronchoalveolar lavage

  **h.** Sputum microbiology

**7.** Referral and treatment

  **a.** When to refer (Box 43-1)

  **b.** Treatment managed by CF specialists (Gibson, Burns, & Ramsey, 2003)

      **i.** Pharmacologic treatment

         (a) Upper airway

            (1) Hypertonic saline nasal washes

            (2) Nasal steroids

         (b) Lower airway

            (1) Bronchodilators

            (2) Mucus modifying agents

■ **BOX 43-1**
■ **INDICATIONS OF WHEN TO REFER PATIENTS**

Refer patient to the pediatrician or appropriate specialist when the following diagnoses or observations are made, and/or treatment trials have failed:

Failure to thrive

Malabsorption: steatorrhea, frequent, bulky, foul-smelling stools

Recurrent pneumonia

Chronic cough/wheezing

Meconium ileus

Rectal prolapse

Symptoms of cystic fibrosis (CF) in the presence of a family history of CF (sibling, parent, first cousin)

Nasal polyps

Pansinusitis

Digital clubbing

Pancreatitis

Hypochloremic, hyponatremic dehydration

Unexplained cirrhosis

Bronchiectasis

Positive sweat test

a) rhDNAse—aerosolized recombinant human dornase alfa

b) Nebulized hypertonic saline, 3% to 7%

(3) Antimicrobials

a) Oral—clinical trials suggest that azithromycin may reduce sputum viscosity and airway adhesion of *Pseudomonas aeruginosa (PA)*, the most common infectious agent in CF (Abbott & Hart, 2005)

b) Inhaled

c) Intravenous

(4) Antiinflammatory medications—high-dose ibuprofen is given to decrease inflammation of airways

(5) Oxygen as needed

(c) Gastrointestinal

(1) Pancreatic enzymes with all meals and snacks

(2) $H_2$ receptor blockers

a) To improve efficacy of enzymes

b) For gastroesophageal reflux disease (GERD)

(3) Proton pump inhibitors for GERD

(4) Colonic lavage solution for distal intestinal obstruction syndrome

(5) Insulin for CF-related diabetes

(6) Ursodiol for CF-associated liver disease

c. Nonpharmacologic

i. Respiratory

(a) Airway clearance

(1) Chest physiotherapy: percussion and drainage

(2) Huff cough—low pressure, multiple coughs with gottis open

(3) Therapy vest

(4) Positive expiratory pressure

(5) Oscillating flow device

(b) Functional endoscopic sinus surgery

(c) Exercise (as an adjunct to airway clearance)

(d) Lung transplantation

ii. Gastrointestinal/nutrition (McMullen & Bryson, 2004)

(a) High-calorie diet (high fat, high protein)

(b) High-calorie supplements

(1) Oral

(2) Nasogastric overnight feeds

(3) Gastrostomy tube overnight feeds

(c) Vitamins A, D, E, and K replacement

(d) Calcium, iron, zinc, and sodium supplements as needed

8. Influence on growth and development

a. Physical

i. Increased caloric need (120% of RDA for calories) due to increased caloric demands and malabsorption

ii. Delayed puberty (likely due to chronic lung disease and/or poor nutrition)

iii. Most children with CF are expected to lead a normal life with respect to developmental milestones

b. Cognitive—no effect on cognitive development

9. Follow-up and primary care of children with cystic fibrosis

a. CF center care (interdisciplinary approach) that follows the Cystic Fibrosis Foundation (2006) minimum guidelines for care:

  **i.** Outpatient visits—four times per year

  **ii.** Pulmonary function tests—two or more per year

  **iii.** Respiratory cultures—at least one per year

  **iv.** Creatinine level every year

  **v.** Glucose level every year after age 13

  **vi.** Liver enzymes every year

**b.** Primary care (CF Foundation, 2006; McMullen & Bryson, 2004)

  **i.** Strongly encourage good nutrition

   (a) CF Foundation (2005) patient registry data show a strong relationship between good nutrition and survival

   (b) Proper nutrition is a constant challenge for children with CF

    (1) Keep up with increases in energy requirements that are related to activity, normal physiologic changes, and disease progression

   (c) Monitor growth percentiles—head circumference in infants, height, weight, BMI after age 2

   (d) Monitor pubertal development—usually delayed by 2 to 4 years

  **ii.** Monitor for complications of CF

   (a) Salt depletion, hyponatremia, dehydration

   (b) Constipation

   (c) Hemoptysis

    (1) Usually small amounts, self-limiting

    (2) Massive hemoptysis requires immediate referral to CF team

   (d) Rectal prolapse

    (1) Occurs in 20% to 25% of individuals with CF

    (2) A frightening experience when it first occurs

    (3) Child or parent can learn to manually reduce the prolapse with a glove and sterile lubricant

   (e) Gastroesophageal reflux (see Chapter 30)

   (f) Decreased lung function

   (g) Respiratory infections

    (1) Teach prevention methods (Saiman & Siegel, 2004)

    (2) Immediate treatment (Rosenfeld, et al., 2001; Saiman, et al., 2003)

   (h) CF-related diabetes

   (i) Bone fractures

   (j) Depression (see Chapter 41)

    (1) Low self-esteem may develop due to rigors of medication and treatment and realities of this progressive disease

    (2) Quality of life measure for children with CF (Modi & Quittner, 2003)

  **iii.** Immunizations

   (a) There is no evidence to support delay in administering routine immunizations

   (b) Annual influenza vaccine is recommended (defer if high doses of corticosteroids are being given)

   (c) Immunize all household contacts against influenza

   (d) Immunize infants with the 23-valent pneumococcal conjugate vaccine

  **iv.** Routine screening for vision, hearing, dental, hematocrit, BP

  **v.** Sleep patterns may be altered due to more frequent nighttime awakenings (Amin, 2005)

  **vi.** Discipline

        (a) Parents often feel guilty about their genetic contribution to the child's illness

        (b) Children with CF need limits and responsibilities

        (c) Sibling rivalry—siblings may feel left out because of the time commitment required of parents to provide daily therapy to child with CF

        (d) May also have sibling with CF or sibling who has died due to CF complications

    **vii.** Self-care—parents need to be helped to allow children to increasingly monitor their own health and adherence to medications and treatment

    **viii.** School represents new issues of coordination of medications and treatments

        (a) Symptoms may be distracting to classmates and embarrassing to child with CF

        (b) Full participation in school activities is encouraged

        (c) No evidence of impairment in intellectual or academic performance compared with peers

        (d) Absenteeism due to symptoms may contribute to problems in school performance

    **ix.** Sexuality

        (a) 98% of males are sterile due to obstruction or absence of the vas deferens

        (b) Females can have successful pregnancies but need management as a high-risk pregnancy

        (c) Frequent antibiotics may cause frequent fungal vaginitis

        (d) Puberty may be delayed 1 to 2 years as a result of poor nutrition or chronic lung disease

**10.** Long-term implications

  **a.** Transition to adulthood requires transition to adult providers

    **i.** Difficult for patient and family due to the long relationship established with pediatric providers

    **ii.** CF centers are developing programs to ease this transition

  **b.** Prognosis

    **i.** Average life expectancy is 36.8 years as of 2005 (CF Foundation, 2005)

    **ii.** Females with CF have successfully delivered healthy infants (CF Foundation, 2004)

    **iii.** 95% of patients die from respiratory failure

  **c.** Research—CF Foundation supports basic science research and clinical trials aimed at finding better treatments, as well as a cure for CF (see http://www.cff.org/home/)

---

## REFERENCES

Abbott, J., & Hart, A. (2005). Measuring and reporting quality of life outcomes in clinical trials in cystic fibrosis: a critical review. *Health Qual Life Outcomes, 3*, 19. Available at http://www.pubmedcentral.gov/articlerender.fcgi?artid=1079915.

Amin, R., Bean, J., Burklow, K., & Jeffries, J. (2005). The relationship between sleep disturbance and pulmonary function in sta-ble pediatric cystic fibrosis patients. *Chest, 128*, 1357-1363.

Cystic Fibrosis Consortium. (2006). Database on CFTR gene. Retrieved on May 21, 2006 from http://www.genet.sickkids.on.ca/cftr/.

Cystic Fibrosis Foundation (2006). Clinical practice guidelines for cystic fibrosis—cystic fibrosis outpatient treatment map for patients, parents, and professionals. Retrieved on June 26, 2006 from http://www.rain.org~medmall/cysticfibrosis/index.html.

Cystic Fibrosis Foundation (2005). Patient registry annual data report, 2005. Retrieved May 21, 2006, from www.cff.org/publications/files/2002%20CF%20Patient%20Registry%20Report.pdf.

Davis, P. (2001). Cystic fibrosis. *Pediatr Rev, 22*(8), 257-263.

Gibson, R.L., Burns, J. L., & Ramsey, B. W. (2003). Pathophysiology and management of pulmonary infections in cystic fibrosis. *Am J Resp Crit Care Med, 168*(8), 918-951.

Grosse, S., Boyle, C. A., Botkin, J. R., et al. (2004). Newborn screening for cystic fibrosis: Evaluation of benefits and risks and recommendations for state newborn screening programs. *MMWR Morb Mortal Wkly Rep, 53*(RR13), 1-36.

Kulich, M., Rosenfeld, M., Goss, C. H., & Wilmott, R. (2003). Improved survival among young patients with cystic fibrosis. *J Pediatr, 142*(6), 631-636.

McMullen, A. H., & Bryson, E. A. (2004). Cystic fibrosis. In P. L. Jackson, & J. A. Vessey (Eds.). *Primary care of the child with a chronic condition* (4th ed.). St. Louis: Mosby, pp. 404-425.

Modi, A. C., & Quittner, A. L. (2003). Validation of a disease-specific measure of health-related quality of life for children with cystic fibrosis. *J Pediatr Psychol, 28*(8), 535-545.

Murray, N., & Brown, K. R. (2005). Cystic fibrosis. Retrieved June 26, 2006, from www.emedicine.com/ent/topic515.htm.

Peckham, D., & Littlewood, J. (2003). The sweat test. Retrieved on May 21, 2006 from http://www.cysticfibrosismedicine.com/htmldocs/CFText/sweat.htm.

Rosenfeld, M., Gibson, R. L., McNamara, S., et al. (2001). Early pulmonary infection, inflammation, and clinical outcomes in infants with cystic fibrosis. *Pediatric Pulmonol, 32*(5), 356-366.

Saiman, L., & Siegel, J. (2004). Infection control in cystic fibrosis. *Clin Microbiol Rev, 17*(1), 57-71.

Saiman, L., Marshall, B. C., Mayer-Hamblett, N., et al. (2003). Azithromycin in patients with cystic fibrosis chronically infected with *Pseudomonas aeruginosa. JAMA, 290*(13), 1749-1756.

Sharma, G. (2006). Cystic fibrosis. Retrieved June 26, 2006, from www.emedicine.com/PED/topic535.htm.

# 44 Diabetes Types 1 and 2

STEPHANIE BONNEY, MS, RN, CPNP

## TYPE 1 DIABETES

Metabolic disorder resulting from a reduction in insulin secretion; originally called insulin-dependent diabetes mellitus or juvenile diabetes

1. Incidence and prevalence (Gale, 2002)
   a. 60% to 70% of all children with diabetes have Type I (Boland & Grey, 2004)
   b. In children younger than the age of 18 years, 150,000 have Type I diabetes (CDC)
   c. Incidence is 1.7/1000 children (CDC, 2005)
   d. More than 13,000 children are diagnosed with Type I diabetes each year (CDC, 2005)
   e. Occurs more in whites than blacks (Votey & Peters, 2006)
   f. Equal prevalence in boys and girls (Votey & Peters, 2006)
   g. Global increase in Type 1 diabetes is projected to be 40% from 1998 to 2010
2. Etiology or precipitating factors (Boland & Grey, 2004)
   a. Polygenic heredity component
      i. Note that about 85% of newly diagnosed children have no family history of the disease (Morales, et al., 2004)
   b. Genetic susceptibility is a necessary precursor
      i. Histocompatibility leukocyte antigen (HLA) genes are elevated
      ii. Some HLA genes are associated with autoimmunity
   c. Autoimmune response
      i. Process may have been ongoing for up to 9 years before symptoms appear
   d. Other factors
      i. Stress
      ii. Infectious agents
3. Pathophysiology (Votey & Peters, 2006)
   a. Autoimmune destruction of beta cells of the pancreas

    i. Leads to a decrease in the amount of insulin produced by the pancreas
      (a) Hyperglycemia
        (1) Glucose unavailable to cells
        (2) Carbohydrates unavailable for energy
        (3) Leads to osmotic diuresis
          a) Polyuria from diuresis
          b) Polydipsia from body's attempt to regain homeostasis
      (b) Cells use alternative sources of energy
        (1) Fatty acids from body fat stores
        (2) Amino acids from body protein
        (3) Polyphagia is body's reaction to "starvation"
      (c) Ketosis results from breakdown of fat
      (d) Ketoacidosis
  **b.** Nonautoimmune destruction of pancreatic beta cells (Alemzadeh & Wyatt, 2004)
    i. Occurs in some African and Asian populations
    ii. Destruction due to drugs, chemicals, viruses mitochondrial gene defects, ionizing radiation
    iii. Present with ketoacidosis
    iv. Extensive periods of remission
4. Presentation
  **a.** Symptoms (Silverstein, et al., 2005; Votey & Peters, 2006)
    i. Polydipsia
    ii. Polyphagia
    iii. Polyuria
      (a) Increased urine volume
      (b) Colorless urine
    iv. Abdominal pain
    v. Vomiting
    vi. Fatigue
  **b.** Signs
    i. Most common in slender, prepubertal child (Silverstein, et al., 2005)
    ii. Dehydration
      (a) Poor skin turgor
      (b) Dry mucous membranes
      (c) Irritability
      (d) Lethargy
      (e) Weakness
    iii. Incontinence
      (a) Daytime or nighttime enuresis in a previously continent child
    iv. Frequent infections
      (a) Perineal skin infections including candida
    v. Weight loss
      (a) Evidence of low or decreased height, weight, or BMI
      (b) Ask parents about weight loss or loose clothing
    vi. Random plasma glucose greater than 200 mg/dL
    vii. Presence of islet cell and anti-insulin autoantibodies within first 6 months of disease
    viii. Ketonuria indicates high risk for diabetic ketoacidosis
5. Differential diagnosis (Table 44-1)
  **a.** Refer to an endocrinologist to differentiate among:
    i. Prediabetes—impaired glucose tolerance

■ **TABLE 44-1**
■ ■ **Differential Diagnosis for Diabetes Symptoms**

| Differential Diagnoses | Diagnostic Criteria |
|---|---|
| Prediabetes | Fasting plasma glucose: 110–125 mg/dL<br>2-hour plasma glucose during oral glucose tolerance test (OGTT): 140–200 mg/dL |
| Type 1 diabetes | Classic symptoms of polydipsia, polyuria, polyphagia, and weight loss<br>Random plasma glucose ≥200 mg/dL, *or*<br>Fasting plasma glucose level ≥126 mg/dL, *or*<br>2-hour plasma glucose during OGTT: ≥200 mg/dL |
| Type 2 diabetes | Presence of obesity<br>Acanthosis nigricans<br>Absence of antibodies to pancreatic beta cells<br>New onset, plasma glucose >750–1000 mg/dL and no ketosis |
| Diabetes insipidus (DI)<br>Central DI<br>Nephrogenic DI | Urine output suppressed by a dose of ADH<br>Urine output not suppressed by a dose of ADH<br>Evidence of kidney damage |

Alemzadeh, R., & Wyatt, D. T. (2004). Diabetes mellitus in children. In R. E. Behrman, R. M. Kliegman, & H. B. Jenson (Eds.). *Nelson textbook of pediatrics* (17th ed.). Philadelphia: Saunders, pp. 1947–1972; Boland, E. A., & Grey, M. (2004). Diabetes mellitus (types 1 and 2). In P. J. Allen, & J. A. Vessey (Eds.). *Primary care of the child with a chronic condition*. St. Louis: Mosby, pp. 426–444; and Votey, S. R., & Peters, A. L. (2006). Type 1 diabetes: A review. Retrieved June 30, 2006, from www.emedicine.com/EMERG/topic133.htm#target1.

      ii. Type 1 diabetes—reduction in insulin secretion
     iii. Type 2 diabetes—peripheral insulin resistance
     iv. Diabetes insipidus—inability of kidneys to conserve water
  6. Screening and diagnostic tests
    a. Screening for type 1 diabetes
      i. Primary autoantibody screening is recommended for children with first degree relatives with Type 1 diabetes
     ii. Free testing program available through TrialNet, funded by NIH
    iii. Call 1-800-425-8361 for more information
    iv. Benefits
      (a) Possible early diagnosis
      (b) Avoidance of severe diabetic ketoacidosis
     v. Risks
      (a) Anxiety on part of child and parents
      (b) No effective method to prevent the onset of diabetes (yet)
    b. Diagnostic tests for differential diagnoses (Alemzadeh & Wyatt, 2004)
      i. Random plasma glucose
     ii. Fasting plasma glucose
    iii. 2-hour plasma glucose during oral glucose tolerance test
    iv. Urinalysis for color, presence of sugar, ketones
     v. HLA
    vi. Autoantibodies to:
      (a) Islet cell cytoplasm (ICA, ICA512)
      (b) Insulin (IAA)
      (c) Glutamic acid decarboxylase (GADA, GAD65) is a test that distinguishes between Type I and Type II diabetes; may also serve as a screening test to predict Type I diabetes before diagnosis

7. Referral and treatment
   a. Diabetic ketoacidosis (DKA)
       i. A pediatric emergency—refer to emergency department (ED)
       ii. IV insulin
       iii. IV fluid and electrolyte replacement
   b. New or suspected diagnosis of Type 1 diabetes
       i. Requires immediate action
           (a) Refer to ED if child appears ill or toxic
           (b) Refer to endocrinologist immediately if child meets these criteria:
               (1) Nontoxic
               (2) Able to tolerate fluids and food
           (c) Endocrinologist often able to see child the next day
           (d) Inform parents that ED or endocrinologist may admit child to hospital
   c. Education (Roemer, 2004; Silverstein, et al., 2005)
       i. See Box 44-1 for recommended websites for patients and providers
       ii. Education should be child centered, directed to both family and child
       iii. Age and culturally appropriate
       iv. Effective educational interventions
           (a) Use methods that are continuous
               (1) Frequent telephone contact
               (2) In-person education
               (3) Telephone availability
           (b) Content should include:
               (1) Prevention of and screening for the microvascular and macrovascular complications of diabetes
               (2) Optimizing blood glucose
               (3) Lipid and blood pressure treatment
               (4) Avoidance of smoking
               (5) Wearing medical identification band
               (6) Age-appropriate self-management (Table 44-2)

## ■ BOX 44-1
## ■ RECOMMENDED WEBSITES FOR PATIENTS AND PROVIDERS

**INFORMATION**

| | |
|---|---|
| American Diabetes Association | www.diabetes.org |
| Centers for Disease Control and Prevention | www.cdc.gov/diabetes |
| About Diabetes | www.diabetesabout.com |
| Juvenile Diabetes Foundation | www.jdf.org |
| National Diabetes Information Clearinghouse | www.niddk.nih.gov |
| National Diabetes Education Program | www.ndep.nih.gov/get-info/directory.htm |

**SUPPLIES AND INSULIN**

| | |
|---|---|
| Diabetic Express (supplies) | www.diabeticexpress.com |
| Diabetes Mall (supplies) | www.diabetesnet.com |
| Diabetic supplies | www.diabeticsupplies.com |
| Quest Diagnostics | www.questest.com |
| Novo Nordisk | www.novolog.com |
| Eli Lilly and Company | www.lillydiabetes.com |
| Aventis Pharmaceuticals | www.aventispharma-us.com |

■ **TABLE 44-2**
■ ■ **Major Developmental Issues and Their Effect on Diabetes in Children and Adolescents**

| Developmental Stage (Approximate Ages) | Normal Developmental Tasks | Type 1 Diabetes Management Priorities | Family Issues in Type 1 Diabetes Management |
|---|---|---|---|
| Infancy (0–12 months) | Developing a trusting relationship/ "bonding" with primary caregiver(s) | Preventing and treating hypoglycemia<br>Avoiding extreme fluctuations in blood glucose levels | Coping with stress<br>Sharing the "burden of care" to avoid parent burnout |
| Toddler (13–36 months) | Developing a sense of mastery and autonomy | Preventing and treating hypoglycemia<br>Avoiding extreme fluctuations in blood glucose levels due to irregular food intake | Establishing a schedule<br>Managing the "picky eater"—setting limits and coping with toddler's lack of cooperation with regimen<br>Sharing the burden of care |
| Preschooler and early elementary school age (3–7 years) | Developing initiative in activities and confidence in self | Preventing and treating hypoglycemia<br>Unpredictable appetite and activity<br>Positive reinforcement for cooperation with regimen<br>Trusting other caregivers with diabetes management | Reassuring child that diabetes is no one's fault<br>Educating other caregivers about diabetes management |
| Older elementary school age (8–11 years) | Developing skills in athletic, cognitive, artistic, social areas<br>Consolidating self-esteem with respect to the peer group | Making diabetes regimen flexible to allow for participation in school/peer activities<br>Child learning short- and long-term benefits of optimal control | Maintaining parental involvement in insulin and blood glucose monitoring tasks while allowing for independent self-care for "special occasions"<br>Continue to educate school and other caregivers |
| Early adolescence (12–15 years) | Managing body changes<br>Issues of sexuality<br>Developing a strong sense of self-identity | Managing increased insulin requirements during puberty<br>Diabetes management and blood glucose control become more difficult<br>Weight and body image concerns | Renegotiating parents' and teen's roles in diabetes management to be acceptable to both<br>Learning coping skills to enhance ability to self-manage<br>Preventing and intervening with diabetes-related family conflict<br>Monitoring for signs of depression, eating disorders, risky behaviors |
| Later adolescence (16–19 years) | Establishing a sense of identity after high school (decision about location, social issues, work, education) | Begin discussion of transition to a new diabetes team<br>Integrating diabetes into new lifestyle<br>Discuss pregnancy concerns of females with diabetes | Supporting the transition to independence<br>Learning coping skills to enhance ability to self-manage<br>Preventing and intervening with diabetes-related family conflict<br>Monitoring for signs of depression, eating disorders, risky behaviors |

(c) These methods have improved hemoglobin (Hb) $A_{1C}$ levels and decreased hospitalization rates

   v. In a research study, nurses presented a 1-hour session on self-awareness of cues of low, high, and normal blood glucose, and situations that cause them (Hernandez & Williamson, 2004)

     (a) 29 adolescents and young adults attended; 12 participants returned their questionnaire 1 year later

     (b) Significant increase in identification of cues 1 year later

     (c) Quality of life scores were unrelated to number of cues or frequency of hypoglycemic episodes

  vi. Innovative, interactive methods of teaching

     (a) Appreciated by children and adolescents

     (b) *Pump Expeditions*, an interactive video game from Medtronic (phone 1-800-MINIMED)

**d.** Glycemic control

   i. Shortly after diagnosis and initial treatment, need for rapid insulin tends to decrease sharply (Boland & Grey, 2004)

     (a) Called the "honeymoon" period

     (b) Lasts a variable amount of time

     (c) Within about 2 years, destruction of beta cells is complete

     (d) Insulin needs increase

  ii. Age-specific glycemic control goals (Silverstein, et al., 2005)

     (a) Children less than age 6: Hb $A_{1C}$ levels of 7.5% to 8.5%

     (b) Children ages 6 to 12: Hb $A_{1C}$ levels of ≤8%

     (c) Adolescents ages 13 to 19: Hb $A_{1C}$ levels of less than 7.5%

 iii. Glycemic index and glycemic load of specific foods (White, 2005)

     (a) Has not been tested in care of children with diabetes

     (b) Not recommended for application to children with diabetes

**e.** Pharmacologic treatment

   i. Insulin is required for management of Type 1 diabetes

  ii. Continuous subcutaneous insulin infusion pumps are now available (Figure 44-1)

     (a) Can be used by children of all ages

     (b) Requires intensive education and ability of the child or parent to understand how to manage insulin coverage using a pump mechanism

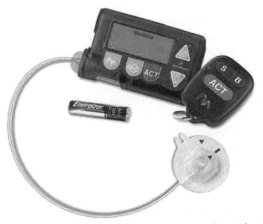

FIGURE 44-1 ■ Continuous subcutaneous insulin infusion pump.

        (c) Research showed that adolescents achieved better Hb $A_{1C}$ levels than multiple daily injection regimens

   iii. Short-acting insulin

        (a) Regular insulin, Lispro insulin

        (b) Rapid onset: 5 minutes to 1 hour

        (c) Peaks at 1 to 4 hours

        (d) Duration 4 to 6 hours

        (e) When quick glucose use is needed

           (1) Before meals

           (2) When blood glucose more than 250 mg/dL

   iv. Intermediate-acting insulin

        (a) NPH insulin

        (b) Often mixed with fast-acting insulin to maximize benefit of one injection

        (c) Onset in 3 to 4 hours

        (d) Peaks at 8 to 14 hours

        (e) Duration 16 to 24 hours

   v. Long-acting insulin

        (a) Ultralente insulin (beef or human)

           (1) Onset in 4 to 6 hours

           (2) Peaks at 12 to 24 hours

           (3) Duration more than 32 hours

        (b) Insulin glargine [rDNA origin]; Lantus®

           (1) For children ages 6 and over

           (2) Onset in 4 to 6 hours

           (3) Peaks at 10 to 20 hours

           (4) Duration 24 to 28 hours

   vi. Dosages based on: (Silverstein, et al., 2005)

        (a) Body weight

        (b) Age

        (c) Pubertal status

        (d) Blood glucose levels

**f.** Blood glucose management (Silverstein, et al., 2005)

   i. Ultimate goal is to gauge insulin dosages based on blood glucose levels and basal metabolic needs

   ii. Four or more tests per day are usually necessary for children

   iii. Periodically test postprandial, before- and after-exercise, and nocturnal glucose levels

   iv. Continuous blood glucose monitoring devices are now available, but their accuracy is still under investigation

**g.** Dietary management (Silverstein, et al., 2005; Votey & Peters, 2006)

   i. Refer to registered dietitian

        (a) Establish a carbohydrate plan

        (b) Carbohydrate intake should match child's:

           (1) Activity level

           (2) Appetite

           (3) Needs for growth

        (c) Sufficient caloric intake for growth is paramount (Boland & Grey, 2004)

        (d) Timing of meals is based on insulin action and peak times

   ii. Discourage parents from withholding food or making child eat consistently without appetite

        **iii.** Monitor height, weight, and BMI on growth charts—weight loss is indicative of poor glycemic control

        **iv.** Goal is to regain initial weight loss and maintain normal weight

    **h.** Exercise (Silverstein, et al., 2005)

        **i.** Regular exercise is recommended

        **ii.** Benefits

           (a) Greater sense of well-being

           (b) Help with weight control

           (c) Improved physical fitness

           (d) Improved cardiovascular fitness

           (e) Lower pulse and blood pressure

           (f) Improved lipid profile

**8.** Follow-up

    **a.** PNP collaborates with endocrinologist and dietitian in management of child with type 1 diabetes

    **b.** Children and parents should be made aware of potential long-term problems

        **i.** See section 10 below for specific complications

        **ii.** Inform children and parents about these gradually, not all at once

        **iii.** Methods to prevent and/or minimize complications

        **iv.** Early signs and need for follow-up with endocrinologist

    **c.** Routine immunizations and yearly influenza vaccines are recommended (Boland & Grey, 2004)

**9.** Influence on growth and development

    **a.** Type 1 diabetes is a lifelong chronic illness that requires daily attention

    **b.** Effect on growth and normal developmental tasks varies with age

    **c.** See Table 44-1 for detailed information

**10.** Long-term implications

    **a.** Probability of complications that arise from type 1 diabetes increases with inconsistent glucose control and with increasing age

        **i.** Hyperglycemia

           (a) If renal threshold for glucose is exceeded

              (1) Leads to osmotic diuresis

              (2) Loss of glucose, electrolytes, and water

           (b) Hyperglycemia impairs leukocyte function

              (1) Leads to increased rate of wound infection

              (2) Impaired wound healing

        **ii.** Hypoglycemia (Silverstein, et al., 2005)

           (a) May result during and immediately after vigorous exercise

           (b) Due to β- and α-adrenergic stimulation, and

           (c) Increased hepatic glucose output

           (d) Risk for neuropsychologic impairment due to hypoglycemia is greater in young than older children

           (e) 10% to 20% of hypoglycemic episodes are associated with exercise (Silverstein, et al., 2005)

           (f) Generally due to exercise of greater than usual intensity, duration, or frequency

           (g) Hypoglycemia may occur within 1 to 6 hours of completion of vigorous exercise due to hepatic glycogen depletion

        **iii.** Serious illness and surgery (Votey & Peters, 2006)

           (a) Leads to hyperglycemia

              (1) Due to stress-induced insulin resistance, and

              (2) Glucose-containing IV fluids

                (b) Increases relative insulin deficiency
                    (1) Increases in glucagon, catecholamines, cortisol, and growth hormone antagonize the effects of insulin
                    (2) Insulin secretion is inhibited by the α-adrenergic effect of increased catecholamine levels
                    (3) Counterregulatory hormones directly increase hepatic gluconeogenesis
        iv. Frequent infections (Votey & Peters, 2006)
                (a) Research suggests that glucose levels greater than 250 mg/dL impair polymorphonuclear leukocyte function
                (b) Humoral immunity, leukocyte and lymphocyte functions are exacerbated by hyperglycemia and DKA
                (c) Effects are reversed substantially by normalization of pH and blood glucose levels
                (d) Higher risk for lower and upper urinary tract infections
                    (1) Recommend antibiotic treatment for at least 7 days
                    (2) Refer for hospital admission for pyelonephritis for reasons listed above
                (e) Wounds (small or large) lead to increased risk of:
                    (1) Cellulitis
                    (2) Lymphangitis
                    (3) Staphylococcal sepsis
                (f) Outpatient treatment of minor infections is okay if child and/or family:
                    (1) Are reliable
                    (2) Closely monitor blood glucose and urine ketones
        v. Diabetic retinopathy (Votey & Peters, 2006)
                (a) Extent of retinopathy is directly related to the duration of diabetes
                (b) Leading cause of new cases of legal blindness in 20- to 74-year-olds
                (c) PNP should conduct funduscopic examination at each visit
                (d) American Association of Pediatrics (Lueder, et al., 2005) recommends:
                    (1) Annual screening by ophthalmologist 3 to 5 years after diagnosis if more than 9 years old
                        a) More often if deterioration is noted
                        b) During pregnancy: first trimester and every 3 months until delivery
                (e) Stages of diabetic retinopathy
                    (1) Dilation of the retinal venules and formation of retinal capillary microaneurysms
                        a) Seen as tiny red dots
                    (2) Increased vascular permeability
                        a) Seen as circular hard exudates
                    (3) Vascular occlusion and renal ischemia
                    (4) Preproliferative diabetic retinopathy
                        a) Immediate referral to ophthalmology
                        b) Capillary occlusion
                        c) Seen as off-white to gray patches with poorly defined margins
                    (5) Proliferative diabetic retinopathy
                        a) Immediate referral to ophthalmology
                        b) New blood vessels on the surface of the retina
                        c) Fibrovascular adhesions

d) Contraction of the adhesions
e) Hemorrhage into the vitreous humor
f) Experienced by patient as "floater" or loss of visual acuity
vi. Diabetic neuropathy (Votey & Peters, 2005a)
(a) Most frequent type is distal symmetric sensorimotor polyneuropathy
(b) A "glove and stocking" distribution
(c) Causes pain in early stages
(d) Results in loss of peripheral sensation
(e) Major concern is foot ulceration
vii. Diabetic nephropathy (Votey & Peters, 2006)
(a) Affects 10% to 15% of patients
(b) Avoid use of potentially nephrotoxic medications/agents
(1) If necessary to use them, give lower dose, and
(2) Monitor creatinine levels
(c) Do *not* request diagnostic studies that require contrast media
(1) Refer to endocrinologist if such a study is essential
viii. Macrovascular disease (Votey & Peters, 2006)
(a) Macrovascular diseases are the leading cause of death in patients with diabetes
(1) 75% versus 35% in nondiabetic patients
(2) Frequent monitoring of lipid levels is essential
(3) Aggressive treatment of hyperlipidemia is essential
(b) Risk for myocardial infarction in patients with diabetes
(1) Two times higher in men
(2) Four times higher in women
(c) Risk for stroke is two times higher in patients with diabetes
(d) Risk for peripheral vascular disease is four times higher in patients with diabetes
ix. Depressive and anxiety symptoms are correlated with: (Alemzadeh & Wyatt, 2004)
(a) Poor metabolic control
(b) Personal, social, school, and/or family maladjustment

## TYPE 2 DIABETES

Metabolic disorder due to peripheral insulin resistance; originally called non–insulin dependent diabetes mellitus or adult-onset diabetes

1. Incidence and prevalence (Fagot-Campagna, et al., 2000)
   a. True incidence is unknown; relatively recent increase in children
   b. Of all children with diabetes, an estimated 30% to 40% have type 2 (Boland & Grey, 2004)
   c. Found in 8% to 46% of new cases diagnosed (CDC, 2005)
   d. Prevalence is higher in certain non-white ethnic groups (CDC, 2005)
      i. Hispanics—10.6% prevalence (Votey & Peters, 2005)
      ii. Blacks
         (a) 10.8% prevalence (Votey & Peters, 2005)
         (b) 70% of all cases of type 2 diabetes (Alemzadeh & Wyatt, 2004)

        **iii.** Pima Indians from Arizona: 50.9 per 1000

        **iv.** All U.S. American Indian populations: 4.5 per 1000 (from U.S. Indian Health Service outpatient clinics)

        **v.** Canadian First Nation people from Manitoba: 2.3 per 1000 (cases from outpatient clinics)

**2.** Etiology or precipitating factors (Alemzadeh & Wyatt, 2004; Boland & Grey, 2004; Pinhas-Hamiel & Zeitler, 2001; Votey & Peters, 2005)

    **a.** Polygenic heredity component, stronger than in type 1 diabetes

    **b.** Obesity, especially central obesity

    **c.** Hypercaloric, lipid-rich diets

    **d.** Sedentary lifestyle

    **e.** Family history for type 2 diabetes (parent or sibling)

    **f.** Puberty—usually 10 to 19 years old at diagnosis

**3.** Pathophysiology (Beck, et al., 2002; Brosnan, et al., 2001; Olantunbosun & Dagogo-Jack, 2006).

    **a.** Normal physiology

        **i.** Insulin binds to insulin receptor and insulin-like growth factor (IGF)-1 receptor

        **ii.** Insulin affects postreceptor signaling pathways within target cells

        **iii.** Tyrosine kinase is activated, which mediates actions of insulin

        **iv.** Insulin receptor concentration or affinity is regulated by:

            (a) Ambient insulin levels

            (b) Various physiologic and disease states

            (c) Various drugs

    **b.** In type 2 diabetes, the interaction of genetic and environmental factors causes peripheral insulin resistance

        **i.** Definition: a given concentration of insulin produces a less-than-expected biologic effect

        **ii.** Decreased number of insulin receptors

        **iii.** Postreceptor failure to activate tyrosine kinase

        **iv.** Compensatory hyperinsulinemia

        **v.** Increased hepatic glucose output leads to chronic hyperglycemia

        **vi.** Dyslipidemia

**4.** Presentation

    **a.** Mild to severe onset; often insidious

    **b.** Symptoms

        **i.** Usually present with no symptoms or mild symptoms (CDC, 2005)

        **ii.** Polyuria

        **iii.** Polyphagia

        **iv.** Polydipsia

            (a) Increased urine volume

            (b) Colorless urine

    **c.** Signs

        **i.** Less common than with type 1, but may present with ketoacidosis

        **ii.** Acanthosis nigricans—thickening and darkening of skin on neck and axillae

        **iii.** Dehydration

            (a) Poor skin turgor

            (b) Dry mucous membranes

            (c) Irritability

            (d) Lethargy

            (e) Weakness

            (f) Fatigue

      **iv.** Incontinence

        (a) Daytime or nighttime enuresis in a previously continent child

        (b) Perineal skin infections including *Candida*

      **v.** Random plasma glucose greater than 200 mg/dL

**5.** Differential diagnosis (see Box 44-1)

    **a.** Refer to an endocrinologist to differentiate among:

      **i.** Prediabetes—impaired glucose tolerance

      **ii.** Type 1 diabetes—reduction in insulin secretion

      **iii.** Type 2 diabetes—peripheral insulin resistance

      **iv.** Diabetes insipidus—inability of kidneys to conserve water

**6.** Screening and diagnostic tests

    **a.** Screening tests for type 2 diabetes (Alemzadeh & Wyatt, 2004)

      **i.** Strongly recommended for children at risk

        (a) Obese

        (b) Acanthosis nigricans

        (c) Strong family history of type 2 diabetes

      **ii.** Fasting lipid profile

      **iii.** Blood glucose levels

      **iv.** Blood insulin levels

      **v.** 2-hour postprandial glucose level

      **vi.** Blood pressure, height, and weight

    **c.** Diagnostic tests for differential diagnoses (Alemzadeh & Wyatt, 2004)

      **i.** Random plasma glucose

      **ii.** Fasting plasma glucose

      **iii.** 2-hour plasma glucose during oral glucose tolerance test

      **iv.** Urinalysis for color, presence of sugar, ketones

      **v.** HLA

      **vi.** Autoantibodies to:

        (a) Islet cell cytoplasm (ICA, ICA512)

        (b) Insulin (IAA)

        (c) Glutamic acid decarboxylase (GADA, GAD65)

**7.** Influence on growth and development

    **a.** Type 2 diabetes can be a lifelong chronic illness that requires daily attention

    **b.** Effect on growth and normal developmental tasks varies with age

    **c.** See Table 44-1 for age-specific information

**8.** Referral and treatment

    **a.** PNP collaborates with endocrinologist and dietitian in management of child with type 2 diabetes

    **b.** Pharmacologic therapy (Alemzadeh & Wyatt, 2004)

      **i.** Insulin is often required for initial management of the ketoacidosis

      **ii.** After stabilization, metformin is used

        (a) To decrease hepatic glucose production

        (b) Contraindicated with liver or renal impairment

    **c.** Education

      **i.** See section 7.c. in type 1 diabetes above for educational guidelines

      **ii.** See Box 44-1 for recommended websites for patients and providers

    **d.** Dietary management—the cornerstone of treatment (Alemzadeh & Wyatt, 2004; Boland & Grey, 2004)

      **i.** Reduction in calories and fat

      **ii.** Regular distribution of meals and snacks

      **iii.** Discourage nonappetite-based eating (boredom, watching TV)

      **iv.** Monitor weight and body mass index

    e. Exercise (Boland & Grey, 2004)
       i. Increase aerobic activity
    f. Decrease sedentary behaviors
  9. Follow-up
    a. Children and parents should be made aware of potential long-term problems
       i. See section 10 below for specific complications
       ii. Gradual, not all at once
       iii. Methods to prevent and/or minimize complications
       iv. Early signs and need for follow-up with endocrinologist
    b. Routine immunizations and influenza vaccines are recommended (Boland & Grey, 2004)
 10. Long-term implications
    a. Complications that arise from type 2 diabetes increase in probability with inconsistent glucose control and increasing age
    b. Insulin resistance is associated with development of: (Boland & Grey, 2004)
       i. Metabolic syndrome, which is a combination of:
         (a) Obesity
         (b) Hypertension
         (c) Atherosclerosis
         (d) Dyslipidemia
       ii. Polycystic ovary disease (Alemzadeh & Wyatt, 2004)
         (a) Hirsutism
         (b) Infertility
       iii. Premature adrenarche
       iv. Females: hyperandrogenism and accelerated growth
    c. Other complications, similar to those of type 1 diabetes are described in more detail above, in diabetes type 1, section 10
       i. Hyperglycemia
       ii. Serious illness and surgery
       iii. Frequent infections
       iv. Diabetic retinopathy
       v. Diabetic neuropathy
       vi. Diabetic nephropathy
       vii. Macrovascular disease
       viii. Depression and anxiety

# REFERENCES

Alemzadeh, R., & Wyatt, D. T. (2004). Diabetes mellitus in children. In R. E. Behrman, R. M. Kliegman, & H. B. Jenson (Eds.). *Nelson textbook of pediatrics* (17th ed.). Philadelphia: Saunders, pp. 1947-1972.

Beck, M. J., Evans, B. J., Quarry-Horn, J. L., & Kerrigan, J. R. (2002). Type 2 diabetes mellitus: Issues for the medical care of pediatric and adult patients. *South Med J, 95*(9), 992-1000.

Boland, E. A., & Grey, M. (2004). Diabetes mellitus (types 1 and 2). In P. J. Allen, & J. A. Vessey (Eds.). *Primary care of the child with a chronic condition.* St. Louis: Mosby, pp. 426-444.

Brosnan, C. A., Upchurch, S., & Schreiner, B. (2001). Type 2 diabetes in children and adolescents: An emerging disease. *J Pediatr Health Care, 15*(4), 187-193.

Centers for Disease Control and Prevention (CDC). (2005). Diabetes projects. From the National Center for Chronic Disease Prevention and Health Promotion. Retrieved

April 10, 2005, from www.cdc.gov/diabetes/projects/cda2.htm.

Fagot-Campagna, A., Pettitt, D. J., Engelgau, M. M., et al. (2000). Type 2 diabetes among North American children and adolescents: An epidemiologic review and a public health perspective. *J Pediatr, 136*(5), 664-672.

Gale, E. A. M. (2002). The rise of childhood type 1 diabetes in the 20th century. *Diabetes, 51*(12), 3353-3361.

Hernandez, C. A., & Williamson, K. M. (2004). Evaluation of a self-awareness education session for youth with type 1 diabetes. *Pediatr Nurs, 30* (6), 459-454, 502.

Lueder, G. T., Silverstein, J., and American Academy of Pediatrics Section on Ophthalmology and Section on Endocrinology. (2005). Screening for retinopathy in the pediatric patient with type 1 diabetes mellitus. *Pediatrics, 116*(1), 270-273

Morales, A., She, J-X., & Schatz, D. A. (2004). Genetics of type 1 diabetes. In O. Pescovitz & E. Eugster (Eds.). Pediatric endocrinology: Mechanisms, manifestations, and management. New York: Lippincott Williams & Wilkins, pp. 402-410.

Olantunbosun, S., & Dagogo-Jack, S. (2006). Insulin resistance. Retrieved June 30, 2006, from www.emedicine.com/med/topic1173.htm.

Pinhas-Hamiel, O., & Zeitler, P. (2001). Type 2 diabetes: Not just for grownups anymore. *Contemp Pediatr, 18*(1), 102-125.

Roemer, J. B. (2004). Endocrine and metabolic diseases. In C. E. Burns, A. M. Dunn, M. A. Brady, et al. (Eds.). *Pediatric primary care: A handbook for nurse practitioners* (3rd ed.). Philadelphia: Saunders, pp. 623-648.

Silverstein, J., Klingensmith, G., Copeland, K., et al. (2005). Care of children and adolescents with type 1 diabetes. *Diabetes Care, 28*, 186-212.

Votey, S. R., & Peters, A. L. (2005). Type 2 diabetes: A review. Retrieved June 30, 2006, from www.emedicine.com/EMERG/topic134.htm#target1.

Votey, S. R., & Peters, A. L. (2006). Type 1 diabetes: A review. Retrieved April 10, 2005, from www.emedicine.com/EMERG/topic133.htm#target1.

White, J. J. (2005). The glycemic index: How useful is it? *Consultant, 45*(4), 558-560.

# Eating Disorders

KIERSTEN A.M. WELLS, MS, CPNP, RN

## DEFINITION

Predominantly a psychiatric illness involving compensatory behaviors and abnormal eating attitudes around food intake; includes conditions such as anorexia nervosa, bulimia nervosa, eating disorder not otherwise specified, and female athlete triad. These complex conditions impact emotions, thought processes, and can have severe medical consequences, including death, if not treated.

1. Presentation
   a. In primary care practices, screening for eating disorders should be initiated for:
      i. Any child of any age with difficulty maintaining an appropriate weight for age and height
      ii. Any child with acute weight loss
      iii. Any child who has disordered thinking around food
   b. Youth Risk Behavior Surveillance Survey Statistics (CDC, 2003)
      i. Ninth through twelfth graders from around United States surveyed
      ii. Examined various behaviors practiced in past 30 days
         (a) 57% had exercised to lose weight in the past 30 days
         (b) 30% thought they were overweight
         (c) 46% were trying to lose weight
         (d) 9% use diet pills
         (e) 6% vomited or used laxatives
   c. Anorexia nervosa
      i. Definition (Treasure & Schmidt, 2003)
         (a) Refusal to maintain weight at or above a minimally normal weight
         (b) Less than 85% of expected weight for age and height
         (c) Or body mass index less than $17.5 \text{kg/m}^2$
         (d) Or failure to show expected weight gain during growth
      ii. Symptoms (Swenne & Engstrom, 2005)
         (a) Restricted intake of food or failure to eat amounts required for activity level and growth
         (b) Amenorrhea; primary or secondary
         (c) Sensitivity to cold
         (d) Quick to become satiated

       (e) Constipation, abdominal pain, bloating

       (f) Dizziness

       (g) Syncope

       (h) Difficulty with sleep and night awakenings

       (i) Loss of erections in males

   iii. Signs

       (a) Weight loss or failure to gain weight appropriate for age and height

       (b) Pubertal arrest or delay; i.e., breast atrophy or testicular softening

       (c) Lanugo (fine downy hair growth) and dry skin

       (d) Hypothermia

       (e) Bradycardia

       (f) Orthostatic hypotension

       (g) Hypotension

       (h) Lower extremity edema (with congestive heart failure or severe protein loss)

       (i) Hypercarotinemia

**d.** Bulimia nervosa

   **i.** Definition (Hay, Bacaltchuk, Stefano, 2004; Phillips & Pratt, 2005)

       (a) Intense preoccupation with body weight and shape

       (b) Regular episodes of uncontrolled overeating of large amounts of food [binge eating], and,

       (c) Use of extreme methods to counteract the feared effects of overeating

   **ii.** Signs

       (a) Parotid gland enlargement

       (b) Mouth sores (petechiae, cheilosis)

       (c) Pharyngeal trauma

       (d) Caries, dental erosion from vomiting (especially inner upper teeth)

       (e) Esophageal rupture or erosion

       (f) Bloody diarrhea (laxative use)

       (g) Bleeding or bruising easily (hypokalemia and platelet malfunction)

   **iii.** Symptoms

       (a) Use of compensatory behaviors to control weight

          (1) Excessive exercise

          (2) Vomiting

       (b) Heartburn

       (c) Chest pain

       (d) Muscle cramps

       (e) Weakness

       (f) Irregular menses, amenorrhea

       (g) Syncope, dizziness

       (h) Orthostatic hypotension

**e.** A variety of the above signs and symptoms are associated with eating disorders not otherwise specified (see section 2.e below) and female athlete triad

**2.** Incidence and prevalence

 **a.** Anorexia nervosa (Treasure & Schmidt, 2003)

   **i.** 10:1 female/male ratio

  **ii.** Prevalence of 0.5% to 1% adolescent females

 **iii.** Incidence of 19/100,000 females and 2/100,000 males

  **iv.** Onset most likely early adolescence (age 14 to 18)

   **v.** Third most common chronic condition of adolescent females after asthma and obesity (ages 15 to 19)

  **vi.** Mortality rates 6% to 10%

  b. Bulimia nervosa (Hay et al, 2004; Phillips & Pratt, 2005)
      i. 5:1 female/male ratio
      ii. Prevalence of 1% to 5% population of high school girls affected (ages 15 to 19)
      iii. Onset most likely in late adolescence and early adulthood
      iv. 7.7% to 9% of college women have threshold bulimia
      v. Mortality rate 1%
  c. Eating disorders not otherwise specified (EDNOS)
      i. Number of EDNOS unknown but estimated to be about 50% of children and adolescents who present to pediatric settings with eating disorders (Fisher, 2006)

■ **BOX 45-1**
■ **DIAGNOSTIC CRITERIA FOR EATING DISORDERS**

**ANOREXIA NERVOSA (AN) 307.10[1]**

A. Refusal to maintain body weight at or above a minimally normal weight for age and height (e.g., weight loss leading to maintenance of body weight <85% of that expected; or failure to make expected weight gain during period of growth, leading to body weight <85% of expected)
B. Intense fear of gaining weight or becoming fat, even though underweight
C. Disturbance in the way in which one's body weight or shape is experienced, undue influence of body weight or shape on self evaluation, or denial of the seriousness of the current low body weight
D. In postmenarchal females, amenorrhea, i.e., the absence of at least three consecutive menstrual cycles (a woman is considered to have amenorrhea if her periods occur only following hormone therapy, e.g., estrogen, administration)

SPECIFY TYPE:
  1. **Restricting type:** during the current episode of anorexia nervosa, the person has not regularly engaged in binge-eating or purging behavior (i.e., self-induced vomiting or the misuse of laxatives, diuretics, or enemas)
  2. **Binge-eating/purging type:** during the current episode of anorexia nervosa, the person has regularly engaged in binge-eating or purging behavior (i.e., self-induced vomiting or the misuse of laxatives, diuretics, or enemas)

**BULIMIA NERVOSA (BN) 307.51[1]**

A. Recurrent episodes of binge eating. An episode of binge eating is characterized by both of the following:
  1. Eating in a discrete period of time (e.g., within any 2-hour period), an amount of food that is definitely larger than most people would eat during a similar period of time and under similar circumstances
  2. A sense of lack of control over eating during the episode (e.g., a feeling that one cannot stop eating or control what or how much one is eating)
B. Recurrent inappropriate compensatory behavior in order to prevent weight gain, such as self-induced vomiting; misuse of laxatives, diuretics, enemas, or other medications; fasting; or excessive exercise
C. The binge-eating and inappropriate compensatory behaviors occur, on average, at least twice a week for 3 months
D. Self-evaluation is unduly influenced by body shape and weight
E. The disturbance does not occur exclusively during episodes of anorexia nervosa

SPECIFY TYPE:
  1. **Purging type:** during the current episode of bulimia nervosa, the person has regularly engaged in self-induced vomiting or the misuse of laxatives, diuretics, or enemas

*Continued*

■ **BOX 45-1**
■ **DIAGNOSTIC CRITERIA FOR EATING DISORDERS—cont'd**

2. **Nonpurging type:** during the current episode of bulimia nervosa, the person has used other inappropriate compensatory behaviors, such as fasting or excessive exercise, but has regularly engaged in self-induced vomiting or the misuse of laxatives, diuretics, or enemas

**EATING DISORDER NOS (EDNOS) 307.50[1]**
The EDNOS category is for disorders of eating that do not meet the criteria for any specific eating disorder. Examples include:
A. For females, all the criteria for anorexia nervosa are met except that the individual has regular menses
B. All the criteria for anorexia nervosa are met except that despite significant weight loss, the individual's current weight is in the normal range
C. All the criteria for bulimia nervosa are met except that the binge-eating and inappropriate compensatory mechanisms occur at a frequency of less than twice a week or for a duration of less than 3 months
D. The regular use of inappropriate compensatory behavior by an individual of normal body weight after eating small amounts of food (e.g., self-induced vomiting after the consumption of two cookies)
E. Repeatedly chewing and spitting out, but not swallowing, large amounts of food
F. Binge-eating disorder: recurrent episodes of binge eating in the absence of the regular use of inappropriate compensatory behaviors characteristic of bulimia nervosa

**RESEARCH CRITERIA FOR BINGE-EATING DISORDER[1]**
A. Recurrent episodes of binge eating. An episode of binge eating is characterized by both the following;
1. Eating, in a discrete period of time (e.g., within any 2-hour period), an amount of food that is definitely larger than most people would eat in a similar period of time under similar circumstances
2. A sense of lack of control over eating during the episode (e.g., a feeling that one cannot stop eating or control what or how much one is eating)
B. The binge-eating episodes are associated with three (or more) of the following:
1. Eating much more rapidly than normal
2. Eating until feeling uncomfortably full
3. Eating large amounts of food when not feeling physically hungry
4. Eating alone because of being embarrassed by how much one is eating
5. Feeling disgusted with oneself, depressed, or very guilty after overeating
C. Marked distress regarding binge eating is present
D. The binge eating occurs, on average, at least 2 days a week for 6 months
The binge eating is not associated with the regular use of inappropriate compensatory behaviors (e.g., purging, fasting, excessive exercise) and does not occur exclusively during the course of anorexia nervosa or bulimia nervosa

**FEMALE ATHLETIC TRIAD (ALSO CALLED ANOREXIA ATHLETICA)[2]**
A. Disordered eating; spectrum includes binging, purging, food restriction, prolonged fasting, diet pill, diuretic and laxative use, and other abnormal patterns
B. Amenorrhea: loss of menses in postmenarchal women of at least three to six consecutive menstrual cycles
C. Osteoporosis: secondary to hypoestrogenism
D. Weight loss <5% of ideal body weight (IBW)
E. Absence of medical illness to explain weight loss
F. Excessive fear of performance image and obesity
G. Food restriction (<1200 kcal/24 hr)

---

[1] Diagnostic criteria for eating disorders have been reprinted with permission from the American Psychiatric Association, from the *Diagnostic and Statistical Manual, Fourth Edition.*
[2] From Metzl, J. (1999). Caring for the young dancer (gymnast, figure skater). *Contemp Pediatr, 16*(9), 138–164; and Rome, E. (2003). Eating disorders. *Obstet Gynecol Clin, 30*(2), 353–377.

          ii. Thought to represent largest category of eating disorders in practice (Kreipe & Burndorf, 2000)

        iii. Estimated 50% to 67% of all adolescent girls are dieting

        iv. 10% of females ages 16 to 25 are thought to have subclinical eating disorder

         v. Estimated that 50% of patients with EDNOS will go on to develop anorexia nervosa or bulimia nervosa (Fairburn & Harrison, 2003)

    **d.** Binge-eating disorder

         i. Not an official psychiatric diagnosis at this time

        ii. Criteria used in research for this disorder are listed in Box 45-1

    **e.** Female athletic triad (Cobb, et al., 2003; Kazis & Iglesias, 2003; Rome, 2003)

         i. Combination of disordered eating, osteoporosis/osteopenia, and menstrual irregularities

        ii. Eating disorders thought to occur among 15% to 62% of female athlete population (Rome, 2003)

        iii. An estimated two thirds of young female athletes (Cobb, et al., 2003)

        iv. Amenorrhea 3% to 66% of young female athletes (Walsh, Wheat, & Freund, 2000)

         v. Highest risk in "visual" sports: ballet, wrestling, ice skating, gymnastics

**3.** Etiology of precipitating factors

    **a.** Predisposing factors (Phillips & Pratt, 2005)

         i. Females more often than males

        ii. White girls have highest risk, but all ethnicities and socioeconomic statuses affected

        iii. Western societal expectations, values related to thinness (although rate is growing in foreign countries and among immigrants to Western societies)

        iv. Genetic

           (a) Concordance among monozygotic versus dizygotic twins

           (b) Decreased levels of neurotransmitter serotonin

           (c) Abnormalities in neuropeptide and monoamine system 5-hydroxytryptan (5HT), the center for regulation of eating and mood

         v. Family history

           (a) History of eating disorder, especially primary relative

           (b) History of substance abuse or alcohol abuse in parents

           (c) Parents with ongoing weight issues or fitness focus

           (d) Comments about weight by parents or family members

           (e) Family dysfunction

         vi. Individual psychologic factors

           (a) Easy to please

           (b) Low self-esteem

           (c) Perfectionism

           (d) Desire for approval

           (e) Early health problems (especially chronic illness like diabetes)

           (f) Difficulty with conflict resolution

           (g) Occupational and recreational pressure to be thin

           (h) Peer group focused on thinness

           (i) High achievers, increased expectations

        vii. Male risk factors (Robb & Dadson, 2002)

           (a) In males: focus on ineffectiveness, anxiety, and desire to have muscle mass formation

           (b) 10% to 42% of male patients with eating disorders are noted to be homosexual

           (c) 2% of homosexual males have met criteria for eating disorder in past

       viii. Other associations

(a) Impulsivity and risk taking

(b) Increased body mass index (BMI)

(c) Sexual and physical abuse

   **b.** Precipitating factors

     **i.** Maturation fears (ages 10 to 14)

(a) Concerns with pubertal markers: menarche and nocturnal emissions

     **ii.** Independence and autonomy struggles (ages 1 to 16)

     **iii.** Identity conflicts (age >17)

(a) No sense of achievement, efficacy, or empowerment

(b) Sexual abuse event often precipitant

   **c.** Perpetuating events

     **i.** Loss of weight from initially high BMI with reinforcement of weight loss from community and peers

**4.** Referral and differential diagnosis (see Box 45-1)

   **a.** If patient is not acutely ill or toxic, refer to a team of eating disorders specialists

   **b.** Psychiatrist will differentiate among:

     **i.** Anorexia nervosa (AN)

     **ii.** Bulimia nervosa (BN)

     **iii.** EDNOS

     **iv.** Binge-eating disorder

     **v.** Female athlete triad

   **c.** If patient is acutely ill or toxic, refer to medical unit equipped to handle medically unstable eating disordered patients

**5.** Laboratory or diagnostic tests

   **a.** Height, weight, BMI

   **b.** Electrolytes

     **i.** Low phosphate, magnesium, potassium in both AN and BN

     **ii.** Low glucose in AN

     **iii.** Low chloride and high bicarbonate in BN

   **c.** Blood

     **i.** Complete blood count with differential—low WBC, platelets in AN

     **ii.** Erythrocyte sedimentation rate—low with malnutrition; high if organic cause

   **d.** Thyroid studies—normal or low in AN; normal in BN

   **e.** Liver function tests—normal in AN and BN; high with refeeding syndrome

   **f.** Reproductive hormone tests

     **i.** Luteinizing hormone (LH)—low in AN, normal in BN

     **ii.** Follicle-stimulating hormone (FSH)—low in AN, normal in BN

     **iii.** Prolactin—normal in AN and BN

     **iv.** Estradiol—low in AN and BN

     **v.** Urine pregnancy test—negative in AN and BN, unless pregnant

   **g.** Urine specific gravity and pH—Ketones in AN, pH >8 in BN

   **h.** Urine toxicology screen—may reveal ephedrine in AN, laxatives in BN

   **i.** Comprehensive laxative screen—may be positive in AN and BN

   **j.** Cardiac enzymes—order only if history of ipecac use or symptoms of cardiac ischemia

   **k.** Electrocardiogram—prolonged Qtc and arrhythmia in AN and BN

   **l.** Dual-energy x-ray absorptiometry scan (DEXA)—order if amenorrheic 6 to 12 months or disordered eating >12 months

   **m.** Purified protein derivative (PPD) for tuberculosis (TB) screening

**6.** Treatment

   **a.** Outpatient care

     **i.** Interdisciplinary outpatient team

    (a) Medical provider (with link to resource for inpatient treatment, in case hospitalization is necessary)

    (b) PNP may be helpful to serve as main resource for patient and patient's family)

    (c) Registered dietitian with experience in treatment of eating disorders

    (d) Family therapist

    (e) Licensed professional counselor or psychologist

    (f) Psychiatrist; if psychotropic medications are necessary

    (g) Social worker

    (h) Nurses (Martin & Ammerman, 2002)

        (1) RN office staff

        (2) RN case managers

        (3) RN discharge planners

  **ii.** Outpatient treatment goals (anorexia nervosa and bulimia nervosa)

    (a) Medical stabilization

    (b) Nutritional rehabilitation

    (c) Decrease behaviors that cause weight loss

    (d) Improve psychologic and emotional attitudes around food

**b.** Traditional group therapy—not suitable for primary therapy, but a good adjunct

**c.** Group therapy approach that integrates art therapy, psychodrama, and verbal therapy is suggested for adolescents (Diamond-Raab & Orrell-Valente, 2002)

**d.** Inpatient care

  **i.** Criteria for inpatient hospitalization

    (a) See Box 45-2 for criteria for hospitalization from AAP Committee on Adolescence (AAP, 2003)

  **ii.** Comprehensive care inpatient program (if available) (Rome, et al., 2003)

  **iii.** Interdisciplinary inpatient team

    (a) Medical team

    (b) Psychiatry team

    (c) Registered dietician

    (d) Social worker to assist school and social issues

    (e) Skilled psychiatric nursing staff

---

■ **BOX 45-2**
■ **CRITERIA FOR HOSPITALIZATION OF AN ADOLESCENT FOR AN EATING DISORDER**

One or more of the following characteristics indicate need for hospitalization:
Severe malnutrition
Dehydration
Electrolyte imbalance
Cardiac dysrhythmia
Vital signs indicative of physiological instability
Arrested growth and development
Failure of outpatient treatment
Acute food refusal
Uncontrollable binging and purging
Psychiatric emergency (psychosis, suicidal ideation)
Comorbidity that interferes with treatment, i.e., depression

From: Society of Adolescent Medicine. (2003). Eating disorders in adolescents: Position paper of the Society of Adolescent Medicine. *J Adol Health, 33,* 496–503. (Table 1)

    **iv.** Inpatient treatment goals
      (a) Medical stabilization first and foremost
      (b) Avoid refeeding syndrome (AAP, 2003; Fisher, Simpser, & Schneider, 2000; Marinella, 2004; Souza de Mendes, 2004)
        (1) Occurs in patients who are severely malnourished and are fed high-carbohydrate loads
          a) Can be from nutrition given enterally, orally, or parenterally
        (2) *Starvation phase:* catabolism of fat and muscle→loss of lean muscle mass, $H_2O$ and minerals. Serum phosphorus level usually normal due to adjustments in renal rates of excretion
        (3) *Refeeding phase:* carbohydrate repletion→insulin release→increased uptake of glucose, phosphorus, water in cells→ increased anabolic protein synthesis→extracellular hypophosphatemia→ inadequate phosphorylated intermediates and compounds (ATP, 2,3-DPG, G-3-PD)→metabolic failure
        (4) Can have hematologic, neuromuscular, hepatic, respiratory, and cardiovascular complications as a result of this hypophosphatemia
        (5) Patients at risk
          a) Anyone who is severely malnourished
          b) Been starved for a prolonged period
          c) Anyone who has had rapid weight loss
        (6) Prevention of refeeding syndrome (Fisher, 2006)
          a) Follow daily labs
          b) Replenish phosphorus, magnesium, and calcium with supplements
          c) Increase weight slowly (safe medical nutrition therapy)
            i) Initial feeds of 1000 to 1600 kcals/24 hrs
            ii) Increase by 200 to 400 kcals/day
            iii) Safe weight gain of 0.2 to 0.5 kg/day as an inpatient
      (d) Inpatient therapy milieu and program for patients (RNs and support staff, e.g., counselors)
        (1) Staff observe meals
        (2) Staff observe safety and behavior
        (3) Staff able to provide medical care
      (e) Skilled psychiatric nursing staff (Martin & Ammerman, 2002)
        (1) Aids with support and behavioral issues
        (2) Helps parent teaching and support
    **v.** Discharge planning (if using family-based approach)
      (a) Nutrition teaching to patients and parents
        (1) Teach food diaries or pyramid
        (2) Consider parent supervision at mealtimes
        (3) For children who purge recommend 1 hour supervision after meals
      (b) Arrange follow-up visits before discharge
      (c) Schedule DEXA scan
      (d) Recommend supervised lunches at school
        (1) School often source of anxiety
        (2) Can be difficult period after hospitalization
      (e) Physical activity
        (1) Initially no physical activity (minimal 2 months)
        (2) Anorexia nervosa
          a) Vital signs must be initially stable at discharge
          b) Must wait until progressing with weight

            c) Must be at least 90% of ideal body weight

            d) Must be able to progress with weight while participating in activity

        (3) Bulimia

            a) Suggest waiting at least 2 weeks so that patients can maintain vital sign stability

        (4) Should be more than 90% of ideal weight with stable vital signs, able to continue progress with weight

    **vi.** When repeated treatment fails—other options

        (a) Residential treatment facilities (Frish, Herzog & Franco, 2006)

            (1) Treatment time from 30 days to 1 year

            (2) High cost (can be $30,000/month estimated $956/day versus $200/day in hospital)

            (3) 89% use cognitive behavioral therapy

        (b) Day treatment facilities

            (1) Few programs available to adolescents

            (2) Program includes

                a) Nutrition counseling

                b) Individual therapy

                c) Family therapy

                d) Supervised meals

**e.** Pharmacologic treatments

    **i.** For reflux symptoms, can use $H_2$ blockers or proton pump inhibitor (PPI)

    **ii.** Anorexia nervosa

        (a) Research does not support use of psychotropic medications unless comorbid disease (Milos, et al., 2004)

        (b) Supplements (American Dietetic Association, 2001; Patrick, 2001)

            (1) 100 to 1500 mg calcium daily (<$10)

            (2) Multivitamin with iron daily (<$10)

            (3) 50 to 110 mg zinc sulfate daily (<$6.50)

            (4) Vitamin D 400 international units (can be in multivitamin) daily (<$10) if deficient

                a) May also use Vitamin $D_2$ (Ergocalciferol) 50,000 1U every week for 6 weeks, then recheck level

                b) Keep level > 30

                c) Child must be over age 10

            (5) Flax seed oil for essential fatty acid deficiency

                a) 5 grams/day

                b) Keep tetraene-to-triene ratio >0.38 (Simopoulous, 2000)

        (c) Estrogen therapy unproven at this time

    **iii.** Bulimia nervosa (Bacaltchuk, et al., 2001)

        (a) Antidepressants (especially SSRI) used alone not shown to be helpful

        (b) Studies show cognitive behavior therapy (CBT) and antidepressants together have better outcome

            (1) 60 mg fluoxetine (Kotler & Walsh, 2000)

                a) Costs will vary with pharmacies

                b) Generic form is cheaper

**f.** Nonpharmacologic treatments

    **i.** Anorexia nervosa

        (a) Interdisciplinary team approach

        (b) Primary care physician or specialty outpatient eating disorder specialist (AAP, 2003; Rosenblum & Foreman, 2002)

(1) Initial visits; one or two per week then slowly decrease as progresses
(2) At each visit (Martin & Ammerman, 2002)
    a) Weight with gown postvoiding
    b) Check orthostatic vital signs, temperature
    c) Check urine pH and specific gravity
    d) Other labs as needed for individual clinical signs
(3) Nutrition goals; balanced nutrition—need a registered dietitian with expertise in eating disorders
    a) ½ to 1 pound per week (outpatient weight gain goals)
    b) Calorie requirements during recovery may be two or three times baseline
    c) May use the U.S. Department of Agriculture dietary guidelines (MyPyramid) or exchange list
    d) May use food diaries
        i) To assess nutritional adequacy (protein, calories, iron, and fat)
        ii) To quantify total intake
        iii) To record emotional state during eating
(4) Family-based treatment (Lock, 2002; McLean, et al., 2003)
    a) Need therapist with experience in treating adolescents *and* patients with eating disorders
(5) Individual therapy can also be helpful (Phillips & Pratt, 2005)
    a) See ii.(d) (1) below
    b) Insight into disease sometimes difficult with malnutrition
    c) Ability to engage in treatment may improve with weight restoration
    d) Decrease preoccupation with overevaluation of shape and weight

**ii.** Bulimia nervosa
  (a) Medical: seen by physician frequently, based on clinical status
  (b) Nutrition (ADA, 2001)
    (1) Focus on balanced nutrition
    (2) Food diaries are helpful
        a) Include mood and physical sensations around eating
  (c) Dental treatment (Sundaram & Bartlett, 2001)
    (1) Limit foods that cause erosion of teeth, e.g. citrus
    (2) Rinse with water or baking soda after vomiting
    (3) Consider sealant placement and daily fluoride treatments
    (4) Recommend every-6-month visits or yearly per insurance coverage
  (d) Therapy (Hay, et al., 2004; Bacaltchuk, et al., 2001; Phillips & Pratt, 2005) Rosenblum & Foreman, 2002)
    (1) Cognitive behavior therapy (CBT)
        a) Gold standard for treatment
        b) CBT not well studied in adolescents but is primary treatment method for adults with bulimia
        c) Time limited; usually 20 sessions
        d) Helps patients identify beliefs and fears around food
        e) Helps individuals restructure these beliefs
        f) Stages of CBT

               i) Sessions 1 through 8—information regarding BN
                  *a)* Focus: self-monitoring and observation and recording
                  *b)* Monitor intake and purging behavior
                  *c)* Identify triggers
              ii) Sessions 9 through 16—role, cognition, nutrition
                  *a)* Focus: limit exposures and stimulate control
                  *b)* Problem solve
                  *c)* Cognitive restructuring
                  *d)* Flexible eating habits
                  *e)* Include previously avoided foods
             iii) Sessions 17 through 20—relapse prevention
                  *a)* Focus: behavior contracts
                  *b)* Continue with previous stages
                  *c)* Maintain and commit
                  *d)* Prevent relapse; create strategies
                  *e)* Create reward systems
         (2) Long-term treatment (Carter, et al., 2003)
           a) Few long-term controlled studies have examined efficacy of treatment
             i) 85% showed no BN symptoms
             ii) 69% no eating disorders symptoms
        (3) Meta-analysis from Cochrane Database, (Hay, et al., 2004) results:
           a) CBT better than medications alone
           b) CBT and medications better than medications alone
           c) CBT better than individual therapy alone
        (4) Initial research (Lock, 2002; Shopman-Williams et al., 2006; Phillips & Pratt, 2005) show good results with CBT and intense family intervention
           a) Family provides access to food for adolescents
           b) Parents provide motivation and support
           c) Create supportive milieu for change in behavior
           d) Provide guidance and support in stressful times when risks of potential relapse
    **iii.** Monitoring of effects on bone density in young adults
        (1) DEXA scans
           a) Gold standard
           b) Most common technique ($600)
           c) Done every 6 to 12 months depending on scores
           d) Spine, hip, and whole body densities assessed
           e) Scores (based on World Health Organization)
             i) T scores for adult women (measures peak bone mass)
             ii) Z scores for adolescents (measures developing bone mass)
             iii) 1 to 2.5 less than standard deviation is osteopenic
             iv) Fewer than 2.5 standard deviations is osteoporosis
        (2) Calcaneal ultrasounds
        (3) Bone ultrasound attenuations (BUAs)
**7.** Prognosis
    **a.** Predictors of treatment outcomes
        **i.** Good prognostic factors (Fairburn & Harrison, 2003; Kreipe & Birndorf, 2000; Rome, 2003)
           (a) Younger age
           (b) Less weight loss

        (c) Shorter duration of illness

        (d) Bulimia nervosa better than anorexia nervosa

        (e) Higher weight after hospital discharge

    ii. Poor prognostic factors (Kreipe & Birndorf, 2000; Rome, 2003)

        (a) Disturbed parent-child relationships

        (b) Longer duration of illness

        (c) Anorexia nervosa with vomiting has worse prognosis than bulimia nervosa alone

        (d) History of extreme weight loss

        (e) Depression

        (f) Concomitant personality disorders

        (g) Childhood obesity

        (h) Low self-esteem

  **b.** Prognosis for outcomes specific to disorder (Keel, et al., 2005)

    **i.** Anorexia nervosa (Fisher, 2006; Walsh, et al., 2000)

        (a) 40% to 50% recover from illness

        (b) 30% improve or do reasonably well

        (c) 20% to 25% have chronic course

        (d) 40% have bulimic phase

        (e) 5% to 10% mortality rate

    **ii.** Bulimia nervosa (Walsh, et al., 2000)

        (a) 50% recover within 2 years

        (b) Frequent relapse: 20% to 46% have symptoms 6 years later

        (c) 30% continue to meet EDNOS criteria

        (d) 25% retain abnormal eating habits

    **iii.** Binge-eating disorder (BED) (Schneider, 2003)

        (a) Growing number of adolescents in this category

        (b) Up to 30% of obese patients estimated to have BED

        (c) Patients will need treatment for obesity complications as well as bingeing

    **iv.** Atypical eating disorders

        (a) Because 50% develop bulimia nervosa or anorexia nervosa, more research needed

  **c.** Mortality

    **i.** Highest for those with eating disorders than any other psychiatric illness

        (a) 10% to 15%

    **ii.** Causes of death

        (a) Starvation

        (b) Suicide—higher with coexisting depression and anxiety

        (c) Medical complications such as cardiac dysrhythmias and electrolyte disturbances

**8.** Influence on growth and development (McCabe & Vincent, 2003)

  **a.** Physical

    **i.** Age dependent

    **ii.** Stunted growth (BMI <16.5)

        (a) Check wrist bone age

    **iii.** Amenorrhea

        (a) Cardinal nutritional markers

            (1) Return of menses and weight before menses stopped

            (2) Percent body fat should be 17% to 19% for return and 22% for maintenance of menses (this is controversial)

    **iv.** Bone density (Cobb, et al., 2003; Golden, 2003; Gordon, 2003; Katzman, 2003 & 2005; Mehler, 2003; Seibel, 2002)

      (a) Normal bone growth (Mehler, 2003)

        (1) Different parts of bone are in a constant state of breakdown, reabsorption (osteoclasts), and new cell growth (osteoblasts)

        (2) Process controlled by cytokines, growth factors, and certain systemic hormones.

          a) Parathyroid hormone

          b) Calcitonin

          c) Calciferol

          d) Estrogen

        (3) Normal bone density accretion

          a) 40% to 60% of bone density laid down in second decade of life

          b) 10% to 15% of bone density laid down in sexual maturity (Tanner) stages 4 and 5

          c) Bone density peaks in third decade of life

          d) Mineral density declines 1% to 2% per year (fourth decade and beyond)

      (b) Effect of disease process on bone density

        (1) Decreased estrogen or testosterone (as testosterone serves as substrate for estrogen) levels

        (2) Causes usually dormant osteoclasts to become activated by cytokines (tumor necrosis factor and interleukin-1)

        (3) Activation of cytokines promotes a rate of bone reabsorption that is faster than bone formation

          a) Bone loss has been noted in patients with greater than 1 year disordered eating patterns

        (4) Inpatients with anorexia nervosa (Katzman, 2003)

          a) 90% of females with anorexia nervosa have reduced mass at one or more of the skeletal sites—low trabecular > cortical bone mass loss

          b) 50% of females with anorexia nervosa are osteopenic, 44% have chronic fractures (Seibel, 2002); may or may not be reversible

        (5) Inpatients with bulimia nervosa

          a) Unclear changes in bone density

**b.** Cognitive

  **i.** May develop organic brain syndrome from malnutrition characterized by changes in concentration or difficulty with decision making

**c.** Psychosocial

  **i.** Anorexia: social isolation, arrested psychosocial development

  **ii.** Bulimia: guilt, especially with comorbid depression and anxiety

**d.** Other conditions

  **i.** Comorbid psychiatric illnesses (Milos, et al., 2004; walsh, et al., 2000)

    (a) Subjects studied are adolescents to young adults

    (b) 63% have lifetime affective disorders

    (c) 50% to 75% have dysthymic disorders

    (d) 35% have obsessive-compulsive disorder

**9.** Long-term complications

  **a.** Cardiovascular (Mitchell & Crow, 2006; Rome & Ammerman, 2003; Winston & Stafford, 2000)

    **i.** Bradycardia (<50 during day)

    ii. Hypotension

    iii. Orthostatic hypotension

    iv. Prolonged QT interval corrected for heart rate (QTc)

        (a) Adolescent boys, more than 0.44 second

        (b) Younger girls, 0.44 to 0.46 second

        (c) Adolescent girls, 0.45 to 0.46 second

    v. Low voltage on electrocardiogram

    vi. Congestive heart failure in refeeding phase

    vii. Peripheral edema in refeeding phase

    viii. Dysrhythmias (torsades de pointes, ventricular tachycardia)

    ix. 37% of anorexia nervosa have mitral valve prolapse

        (a) Decreased left ventricular mass by 30% to 50%, causing size proportion change in left ventricle and mitral valve) (Winston & Stafford, 2000)

    x. Myocardial ischemia

    xi. Silent pericardial effusions or microscopic myofibrillar effusions (Katzman, 2005; Rome & Ammerman, 2003)

    xii. Acrocyanosis

    xiii. Early stages of disease show that cardiac damage is evident (Mont, et al., 2003)

  **b.** Pulmonary

    i. Spontaneous pneumomediastinum

    ii. Pulmonary edema in refeeding phase

    iii. Subcutaneous emphysema (late)

  **c.** Gastrointestinal (Nicholls & Stanhope, 2000)

    i. Delayed gastric emptying and small bowel transit

    ii. Constipation

    iii. Hepatic fatty degeneration (steatosis)

    iv. Mildly elevated liver function tests (usually seen in refeeding phase)

    v. Superior mesenteric artery syndrome (postprandial vomiting secondary to intermittent gastric outlet obstruction in emaciated patients)

        (a) Asymptomatic refeeding pancreatitis

        (b) Acute gastric dilation from refeeding

    vi. Impaired hunger and satiety cues

    vii. Esophageal tears

    viii. Necrotizing colitis, perforated ulcer

  **d.** Renal

    i. Decreased glomerular filtration rate

    ii. Inability to concentrate urine due to decreased ADH secretion

    iii. Renal calculi

    iv. Ketonuria, transient azotenia

    v. Changes in blood urea nitrogen (increased levels with dehydration and low protein intake)

    vi. Short periods of acute renal failure

  **e.** Endocrine (Connan, Lightman, & Treasure, 2000; Levine, 2002)

    i. Hypothalamic

        (a) Monoamines

            (1) Serotonin; decreased levels

            (2) Gastrointestinal: neuropeptide Y increase

    ii. Anterior pituitary

        (a) Decrease in growth hormone

        (b) Decrease dehydroepiandrosterone sulfate (DHEA-S)

   (c) Gonadotropins—no pulsatile secretions
    (1) Decrease in follicle-stimulating hormone (FSH) and estradiol
    (2) Decrease in LH
    (3) No change in prolactin
  iii. Thyroid (sick euthyroid syndrome)
   (a) Abnormal thyroid hormone levels in the absence of thyroid disease
   (b) Low triiodothyronine hormone
   (c) Low or normal thyroxine $T_4$ (check free $T_4$)
   (d) Thyroid-stimulating hormone (TSH) normal
  iv. Peripheral
   (a) Low insulin growth factor-1 (ILGF-1)
   (b) Increase in plasma cortisol and failure to suppress dexamethasone when tested
   (c) Impaired cholesterol production
   (d) Asymptomatic hypoglycemia
   (e) Infertility
   (f) Short stature
   (g) Low leptin levels
   (h) Pubertal arrest or delay—breast atrophy, testicular softening
   (i) Decrease in insulin
 **f.** Hematologic
  i. Bone marrow suppression
  ii. Leukopenia
  iii. Neutropenia
  iv. Decreased erythrocyte sedimentation rate (ESR) (may be as low as 0 to 5)*
  v. Mild anemia
  vi. Pancytopenia (secondary to starvation; less common)
  vii. Thrombocytopenia (rare)
  viii. Ecchymosis
 **g.** Neurologic
  i. Cerebral-cortical atrophy
  ii. Slow or decreased deep tendon reflexes
  iii. Trousseau's sign—indicative of hypocalcemia if hand spasms when blood pressure cuff left inflated for 3 to 4 minutes
  iv. Peripheral neuropathy
  v. Myopathy (from hypophosphatemia)
  vi. Seizures (late onset)
  vii. Cerebral edema (hyponatremia secondary to water loading)
 **h.** Dermatologic
  i. Hypercarotinemia secondary to decreased essential fatty acids
  ii. Dry skin (vitamin zinc and fat deficiency)
  iii. Changes in hair
   (a) Alopecia, telogen effluvium, positive hair pull test
   (b) Can be brittle with less shine
  iv. Nail bed changes
  v. Breast atrophy
  vi. Atrophic vaginitis
  vii. Lesions, evidence of cutting
  viii. Acne

---

*Note; index of suspicion for organic causes should be high if ESR is as high as 10 to 20 in malnourished patients)

     **i.** Oral manifestations (Sundaran & Bartlett, 2001)
- **i.** Perimolysis (loss of dentin due to enamel erosion); dental caries
- **ii.** Cheilosis (vitamin B deficiency)
- **iii.** Xerostomia (dry mouth) and atrophic mucosa

     **j.** Medical complications specific to BN
- **i.** Cardiovascular
  - (a) Elevated blood pressure from diet pill toxicity
  - (b) Cardiomyopathy; cumulative cardiac toxicity from emetine (primary by-product from ipecac)
  - (c) Aspiration pneumonitis
  - (d) Pneumomediastinum (with weight loss or purging)
  - (e) Pneumothorax
  - (f) Rib fracture
- **ii.** Gastrointestinal (Nicholls & Stanhope, 2000)
  - (a) Barrett's esophagus; gastroesophageal reflux due to chronic relaxed sphincter; gastritis
  - (b) Mallory-Weiss tears, upper GI bleed
  - (c) Esophageal rupture (rare, but has 80% mortality rate)
  - (d) Acute gastric dilatation (bingeing)
  - (e) Delayed colonic motility (laxative use)
  - (f) Constipation (laxative use)
  - (g) Cathartic colon with toxic degeneration of Auerbach's plexus due to overuse of stimulant laxatives
  - (h) Post-bingeing pancreatitis
- **iii.** Renal (Connan, et al., 2000)
  - (a) Renal calculi
  - (b) Hypokalemic nephropathy with urine concentrating deficit
- **iv.** Endocrine (Connan, et al., 2000)
  - (a) Hypothalamic hypogonadism
  - (b) Irregular menses
  - (c) Hypoglycemia
  - (d) Mineralocorticoid excess
- **v.** Hematologic
  - (a) Anemia
- **vi.** Neurologic
  - (a) Loss of gag reflex
  - (b) Peripheral neuropathy
- **vii.** Metabolic changes
  - (a) Metabolic alkalosis (increase in serum carbon dioxide)
  - (b) Hypokalemia and hyponatremia
  - (c) Elevated serum amylase (secondary to parotitis)
- **viii.** Dermatologic
  - (a) Cheilosis (from vitamin B deficiency or vomiting)
  - (b) Russell's signs (hand calluses from self-induced vomiting)
- **ix.** Oral manifestations (Sundaram & Bartlett, 2001)
  - (a) Dental enamel erosion, tooth sensitivity, pitting fissures, caries
  - (b) Oropharyngeal petechiae
  - (c) Parotid gland enlargement
  - (d) Xerostomia, gingival regression

# REFERENCES

American Academy of Pediatrics (AAP) (2003). Identifying and treating eating disorders. *Pediatrics, 111*(1), 204-211.

American Dietetic Association Reports. (2001). Position of the American Dietetic Association: Nutrition intervention in the treatment of anorexia nervosa, bulimia nervosa, and eating disorders not otherwise specified (EDNOS). *J Am Diet Soc, 101*(7), 810-819.

American Psychiatric Association. (1994). *Diagnostic and statistical manual of mental disorders* (4th ed.). Washington DC: Author.

Bacaltchuk, J., Hay, P, Trefiglio, R. (2001). Antidepressants versus psychological treatments and their combination for bulimia nervosa. *The Cochrane Database of Systematic Reviews*, Issue 4. Art. No.: CD003385. DOI: 10.1002/14651858.CD003385.

Carter, F., McIntosh, V., Joyce, P., et al. (2003). Role of exposure with response prevention in cognitive behavioral treatment for bulimia nervosa: Three year follow-up results. *Int J Eat Disord, 33*, 127-135.

Centers for Disease Control and Prevention (CDC). (2003). Report from the National Youth Risk Behavior Survey. Retrieved May 21, 2006, from www.cdc.gov/mmwr/preview/mmwrhtml/ss5302a1.htm.

Cobb, K., Bachrach, L., Greendale, G., et al. (2003). Disordered eating, menstrual irregularity and bone mineral density in female runners. *Med Sci Sports Exer, 35*(5), 711-719.

Connan, F., Lightman, S., & Treasure, J. (2000). Biochemical and endocrine complications. *Eur Eat Disord Rev, 8*, 144-157.

Diamond-Raab, L., & Orrell-Valente, J. K. (2002). Art therapy, psychodrama, and verbal therapy. An integrative model of group therapy in the treatment of adolescents with anorexia nervosa and bulimia nervosa. *Child Adolesc Psychiatric Clin North Am, 11*(2), 343-64.

Fairburn, C., & Harrison, P. (2003). Eating disorders. *Lancet, 317*, 407-416.

Fisher, M. (2006) Treatment of eating disorders in children, adolescents and young adults. *Fed Review, 27*(1), 5-15.

Fisher, M., Simpser, E., & Schneider, M. (2000). Hypophosphatemia secondary to oral refeeding in anorexia nervosa. *Int J Eat Dis, 28*, 181-187.

Frisch, M., Herzog, D., Franco, D. (2006). Residential treatment for eating disorders *Intl J Cating Dis, 39*(3), 1-9.

Golden, N. (2003). Osteopenia and osteoporosis in anorexia nervosa. *Adolesc Med, 14*(1), 97-108.

Gordon, C. (2003). Normal bone accretion and effects of nutritional disorders in childhood. *J Womens Health, 12*(2), 137-143.

Hay, P., Bacaltchuk, J., & Stefano, S. (2004). Psychotherapy for bulimia nervosa and binging. The Cochrance Database of systematic Reviews, Issue 3, Art No.: CD000562. DOI: 10.1002/14651858.CD000562.pub2.

Katzman, D. (2003). Osteoporosis in anorexia nervosa. A brittle future-current drug targets. *CNS & Neurological Disorders, 2*(1), 11-15.

Katzman, D. (2005). Medical complications in adolescents with anorexia nervosa: A review of the literature. *Intl J Eating Disorders 37*, s52-s59.

Kazis, K., & Iglesias, E. (2003). The female athletic triad. *Adolesc Med, 14*, 87-95.

Keel, P. Dorer, D., Franco, D., et al. (2005). Postremission predictors of relapse in women with eating disorders. *Am J Psychiatry, 162*, 2263-2268.

Kotler, L., & Walsh, T. (2000). Eating disorders in children and adolescents: Pharmacological therapies. *Eur Child Adolesc Psychiatry, 9*(1), I 108-I 116.

Kreipe, R., & Birndorf, S. (2000). Eating disorders in adolescents and young adults. *Med Clin North Am, 84*(4), 1027-1049.

Levine, R. (2002). Endocrine aspects of eating disorders in adolescents. *Adolesc Med, 13*(1), 129-143.

Lock, J. (2002). Treating adolescents with eating disorders in the family context: Empirical and theoretical considerations. *Child Adolesc Psychiatry Clin North Am, 11*(2), 331-342.

Marinella, M. (2004). Refeeding syndrome. Implications for the impatient rehabilitation unit. *Am J Physical Med Rehab, 83*, 65-68.

Martin, H., & Ammerman, S. (2002). Adolescents with eating disorders. Primary care screening, identification, and early intervention. *Nurs Clin North Am, 37*, 537-551.

McLean, N., Griffin, S., Toney, K., & Hardeman, W. (2003). Family involvement in weight control, weight maintenance and weight-loss interventions: A systematic review of randomized trials. *Int J Obes, 27,* 987-1005.

Mehler, P. (2003). Osteoporosis in anorexia nervosa: Prevention and treatment. *Int J Eat Disord, 33,* 113-126.

Metzl, J. (1999). Caring for the young dancer (gymnast, figure skater). *Contemp Pediatr, 16*(9), 138-164.

Milos, G., Spindler, A., & Schnyder, V. (2004). Psychiatric comorbidity and eating disorder inventory (EDI) profiles in eating disorder patients. *Canadian J Psychiatry, 49*(3), 179-184.

Mitchell, J., & Crow, S. (2006). Medical complications of anoresia nervosa and bulimia nervosa. *Curr Opinion Psych, 19,* 438-443.

Mont, L., Castro, J., Herreros, B., et al. (2003). Reversibility of cardiac abnormalities in adolescents with anorexia nervosa after weight recovery. *J Am Acad Child Adolesc Psychiatry, 42*(7), 808-813.

Nicholls, D., & Stanhope, R. (2000). Medical complications of anorexia nervosa in children and young adolescents. *Eur Eat Disord Rev, 8,* 170-180.

Patrick, L. (2001). Eating disorders: A review of the literature with emphasis on medical complications and clinical nutrition. *Alt Med Rev, 7*(3), 184-202.

Phillips, E, & Pratt, H. (2005). Eating disorders in college. *Ped Clinics N Am, 52,* 85-96.

Robb, A. & Dadson, M. (2002). Eating disorders in males. *Child & Adol Psychiatric Clinics of N Am, 11,* 399-418.

Rome, E. (2003). Eating disorders. *Obstet Gynecol Clin, 30*(2), 353-377.

Rome, E., & Ammerman, S. (2003). Medical complications of eating disorders: An update. *J Adol Health, 33*(6), 418-426.

Rome, E., Ammerman, S., Rosen, D., et al. (2003). Children and adolescents with eating disorders: The state of the art. *Pediatrics, 111*(1), e98-e108.

Rosenblum, J., & Foreman, S. (2002). Evidence based treatment of eating disorders. *Curr Opin Pediatr, 14,* 379-383.

Schapman-Williams, A., Lock J., & Couturier, J. (2006). Cognitive-behavioral therapy for adolescents with binge-eating syndromes. *Intl J Eating Disorders, 39*(3), 252-255.

Seibel, M. (2002). Nutritional and molecular markers of bone remodeling. *Curr Opin Clin Nutr Metab Care, 5,* 525-531.

Simopoulous, A. P. (2000). Human requirement for N-3 poly-unsaturated fatty acids. *Poultry Science, 79*(7), 968-970.

Society of Adolescent Medicine. (2003). Eating disorders in adolescents: Position paper of the Society of Adolescent Medicine. *J Adol Health, 33,* 496-503.

Sundaran, G., & Bartlett, D. (2001). Preventive measures for bulimic patients with dental erosion. *Eur J Prosthodontic & Restorative Dentistry, 8,* 25-29.

Swenne, I., Engstrom, I. (2005). Medical assessment of adolescent girls with eating disorders. An evaluation of symptoms and signs of starvation. *Acta Paediatrica, 94,* 1363-1371.

Treasure, J., & Schmidt, U. (2003). Anorexia nervosa. In *Clin Evid., Dec (14),* 1140-1148.

Walsh, J., Wheat, M., & Freund, K. (2000). Detection, evaluation, and treatment of eating disorders: The role of the primary care physician. *J Gen Intern Med, 15,* 577-590.

Winston, A. P., & Stafford, P. J. (2000). Cardiovascular effects of anorexia nervosa. *Eur Eat Disord Rev, 8*(2), 117-125.

## ACKNOWLEDEMENT

Thanks to David Wells, MD (Danver), Cynthia Kapphahn, MD (Stanford University), and Iris Litt, MD (Robert Wood Johnson Foundation) for all their help in writing and reviewing this chapter.

# Epilepsy

MARIA S. CHICO, RN, CPNP

## DEFINITION

Seizures are abnormal, excessive, hypersynchronous discharges of neuronal activity in the brain that alter cognitive, motor, behavioral, and autonomic functions (American Epilepsy Society, 2004). Seizures can be detected by clinical manifestations, electroencephalogram (EEG) or both. Epilepsy is a chronic condition characterized by repeated, unprovoked seizures, which require anti-epileptic medication to control.

1. Incidence and prevalence
   a. Prevalence—1% of children up to age 15 years
   b. 150,000 to 325,000 children ages 5 to 15 years have epilepsy
   c. Incidence of new onset seizures—80/100,000 per year
   d. Median age of onset is 5 to 6 years
   e. Incidence of epilepsy—20,000 to 45,000 children diagnosed each year
2. Pathophysiology (Johnston, 2004)
   a. A seizure requires a group of cortical neurons that generate an abnormal hypersynchronous discharge *and* a γ-aminobutyric acid (GABAergic) inhibitory system which can happen by excessive excitatory or inadequate inhibitory input
   b. Excitatory glutamatergic synapses are probably initiated by excitatory amino acid neurotransmitters such as glutamate or aspartate
   c. Areas of the brain with abnormal or injured neurons are most vulnerable
   d. An underdeveloped brain is more vulnerable than mature brain
3. Etiology (Johnston, 2004; Ottman, 2001)
   a. Symptomatic—result of injury to the brain, e.g., stroke, trauma, infection
   b. No identifiable cause
      i. Idiopathic— presumed genetic cause
      ii. Cryptogenic—presumes an underlying pathologic or metabolic cause, but current technologies cannot detect it
   c. Genetic factors, for example:
      i. Juvenile myoclonic epilepsy—located on chromosome 6p, 15q14; gene not yet identified
      ii. Benign familial neonatal convulsions—located on chromosome 20q13, 8q24; gene KCNQ2 and KCNQ3
      iii. Progressive myoclonic epilepsy—located on chromosome 21q22.3; gene cystatin

        **iv.** Generalized epilepsy with febrile seizures plus—located on chromosome 19q13, 2q24; gene SCN1B and SCN1A

**4.** Focused assessment of seizure episode

    **a.** The seizure-like episode must be described in detail

        **i.** Collect details about the child and environment before, during, and after the event (Box 46-1)

        **ii.** Family history of seizures or other neurologic conditions (Blair & Selekman, 2004)

    **b.** Physical examination—conduct a thorough examination with emphasis on the neurologic system (see Chapter 13)

    **c.** Referral to pediatric neurologist is essential when seizure disorders are suspected

**5.** Classification of seizures

    **a.** The International League Against Epilepsy classification, adapted by author

    **b.** Partial seizures—focal origin involving one hemisphere

        **i.** Simple partial seizures (consciousness not impaired)

            (a) With motor symptoms

            (b) With somatosensory or special sensory symptoms

            (c) With autonomic symptoms

            (d) With psychic symptoms

        **ii.** Complex partial seizures (with impairment of consciousness for >20 seconds)

            (a) Beginning as staring episodes and progressing to impairment of consciousness

                (1) Without automatisms (tics, movements that are made without the child's recollection of having made them)

                (2) With automatisms

            (b) With impairment of consciousness at onset

                (1) Without automatisms

                (2) With automatisms

        **iii.** Partial seizures with secondary generalization

    **c.** Generalized seizures (bilateral origin involving both hemispheres)

        **i.** Absence seizures—brief "staring" episodes (10 to 20 seconds in duration)

        **ii.** Myoclonic seizures

            (a) Brief, sudden muscle contractions that may be generalized or localized, symmetric or asymmetric, synchronous or asynchronous

            (b) Usually no detectable loss of consciousness

---

■ **BOX 46-1**
■ **KEY ELEMENTS IN THE HISTORY OF A SUSPECTED SEIZURE**

**DETAILED HISTORY OF THE EVENT**
Child's activity immediately prior to seizure onset
Duration of actual seizure
Occurrence and duration of loss of consciousness
Presence and duration of post-ictal phase
Known triggers of seizure
Sleep history
Recent decline in academic performance
Recent personality change

**DEVELOPMENTAL HISTORY**
Milestones achieved as expected
Regression of skills once achieved
Family history of developmental abnormalities

**PHYSICAL EXAMINATION**
Presence of focal findings
Abnormalities in height, weight

        **iii.** Clonic seizures
           (a) Sustained rhythmic jerking of a portion of the body
           (b) Loss or impairment of consciousness
        **iv.** Tonic seizures
           (a) Sudden increase in muscle tone producing a number of characteristic postures
           (b) Consciousness is usually partially or completely lost
           (c) Postictal alteration of consciousness usually brief; may last several minutes
        **v.** Tonic-clonic seizures
           (a) Also known as a grand mal seizure
           (b) Loss of consciousness
           (c) Increased muscle tone followed by bilateral rhythmic jerks
           (d) Postictal alteration of consciousness can last from minutes to hours
        **vi.** Atonic seizures
           (a) Sudden loss of muscle tone
           (b) May result in head drop or falling to the ground
    **d.** Unclassified seizures—classification is difficult due to complex onset, equivocal EEG data

**6.** Differential diagnosis for seizure-like episodes (Johnston, 2004)
    **a.** Epilepsy (see Classification of Epilepsy in section 8 below)
    **b.** Benign myoclonus of infancy
    **c.** Febrile seizures
    **d.** Benign paroxysmal vertigo
    **e.** Breath holding
    **f.** Syncope
    **g.** Choreoathetosis
    **h.** Shuddering attacks
    **i.** Narcolepsy
    **j.** Night terror
    **k.** Rage attack
    **l.** Tics
    **m.** Febrile seizures
    **n.** Hyper/hypoglycemia
    **o.** Pseudoseizures—nonepileptic, psychogenic cause

**7.** Diagnostic tests
    **a.** The following tests may be conducted in primary care to rule out nonepileptic physiologic causes of seizures
        **i.** Serum glucose, fasting blood sugar, and urine ketones—evaluate for presence of hyper/hypoglycemia
        **ii.** CBC—evaluate infectious cause of fever
    **b.** On referral or in the emergency department, the following tests may be conducted:
        **i.** Neuroimaging studies
           (a) CT scan—evaluate for presence of hydrocephalus, head injury, space-occupying lesion, brain calcifications
           (b) MRI—evaluate for presence of structural abnormality, cortical dysplasia
        **ii.** EEG—evaluate for presence of electrographic abnormalities
        **iii.** Laboratory diagnostic studies (AAP, 1996)
           (a) Serum chemistry profile, electrolytes, calcium, magnesium, CBC (complete, with differential)

    (b) Toxicology screen (blood and urine)—evaluate for chemical substances as etiology of seizure

    (c) CSF examination—evaluate for presence of CNS infection , CSF electrolyte disturbance

    (d) Serum and urine amino acids, serum ammonia, calcium, magnesium, metabolic studies—done at tertiary referral center to evaluate for presence of metabolic disorders

8. Treatment

  **a.** Decision to treat is based on several considerations (Blair & Selekman, 2004)

    **i.** Probability of recurrence (Johnston, 2004)

      (a) One-time seizures usually not treated

      (b) 60% of newly diagnosed patients will enter remission upon treatment, but 40% will go on to become "intractable," meaning refractory to anti-epileptic medications or treated with unacceptable side effects (Kwan & Sander, 2004)

    **ii.** Recurrent seizures are an indication for treatment

      (a) Shinnar and colleagues (2000) followed 407 children for an average of 9.6 years from the time of their first seizure

        (1) Assessed the risk of multiple recurrences

        (2) A second seizure occurred in 182 children (44.7%)

        (3) 72% of these children went on to have a third seizure (39.6%)

    **iii.** Possibility of death

      (a) Sudden unexpected death in epilepsy (SUDEP) without identifiable cause occurs in 2% to 17% of deaths of individuals with epilepsy

      (b) Most common in patients with uncontrolled, nocturnal generalized tonic/clonic seizures

  **b.** Pharmacologic treatment (Johnston, 2004):

    **i.** Goal: use the most appropriate drug that controls seizures with minimal side effects, improves quality of life, and promotes optimal growth and development

    **ii.** See Table 46-1

    **iii.** Providers must know the pharmacokinetics and pharmacodynamics of the drugs

    **iv.** Anti-epileptic medication—mechanisms of action:

      (a) Augment inhibitory processes or oppose excitatory ones

      (b) Directly affect specific ion channels

      (c) Indirectly influence synthesis, metabolism or function of neurotransmitters

      (d) Indirectly affect receptors that control channel opening and closing

    **v.** Anti-epileptic medications are prescribed by weight in kilograms and titrated to achieve therapeutic levels

    **vi.** Monitor serum drug levels (morning trough only) and alter dosages accordingly in the initial phase of treatment

    **vii.** Routine serum monitoring is not cost effective and not recommended, unless: (Johnston, 2004)

      (a) Patients and families are noncompliant

      (b) Status epilepticus occurs

      (c) Child is experiencing a growth spurt

      (d) Child is receiving more than one drug

      (e) Change in type, duration or frequency of seizures

      (f) Signs and symptoms of toxicity

      (g) Child has hepatic or renal disease

      (h) Child has cognitive or physical disabilities

■ **TABLE 46-1**
■ ■ **PEDIATRIC ANTICONVULSANT MEDICATIONS**

| Drug – Trade/Generic | Indication | Dosage | Half-Life (hr) |
|---|---|---|---|
| Tegretol (carbamazepine) | partial seizures | 10–15 mg/kg/day | 5–26 |
| Neurontin (gabapentin) | partial seizures | 25–40 mg/kg/day | 5–7 |
| Lamictal (lamotrigine) | partial seizures | 1–5 mg/kg/day<br>after slow initiation schedule | 8–20 |
| Keppra (levetiracetam) | partial seizures | 10 to 40 mg/kg/day | 7 to 11 |
| Trileptal (oxcarbazepine) | partial seizures | 8 to 10 mg/kg/day | 9 |
| Phenobarbital | broad spectrum | 2 to 8 mg/kg/day<br>both partial and generalized seizures | 65 to 110 |
| Dilantin (phenytoin) | broad spectrum | 4 to 8 mg/kg/day<br>both partial and generalized seizures | 7 to 42 |
| Mysoline (primidone) | broad spectrum | 10 to 20 mg/kg/day<br>both partial and generalized seizures | 8 to 15 |
| Topamax (topiramate) | partial seizures | 1 to 3 mg/kg/day | 21 |
| Depakote (valproate) | broad spectrum | 10 to 15 mg/kg/day<br>both partial and generalized seizures | 5 to 15 |
| Zonegran (zonisamide) | partial seizures | 2 to 4 mg/kg/day | 63 |

viii. Monitor CBC and liver function after therapeutic levels have been achieved, then as needed thereafter

ix. See guidelines from the American Academy of Neurology and the American Epilepsy Society for treatment of new onset epilepsy (French, et al., 2004)

x. Weaning off the anticonvulsant over 3 to 6 months can be done after a minimum of 2 seizure-free years, a normal EEG and unchanged physical examination

c. Nonpharmacologic treatment

i. Ketogenic diet (Johnston, 2004)

(a) Used when there are uncontrollable seizures, especially complex myoclonic epilepsy with associated tonic-clonic seizures, or when medication side effects are intolerable

(b) Rigid, high-fat, restricted carbohydrate and protein

(c) Mechanism of action is unknown

(d) Safe for infants younger than age 2 if closely supervised by physician

(e) Can be unpalatable and difficult to maintain

(f) Requires close monitoring by RD specifically trained in management of the ketogenic diet

(g) Some anticonvulsants may be contraindicated with the diet; this judgment should be made by the pediatric epileptologist

ii. Surgical intervention (Johnston, 2004)

(a) For intractable seizures unresponsive to medications

(b) Seizure focus can be identified with the following objective data:

(1) Long-term video EEG monitoring

(2) Neuroimaging studies

a) Brain MRI with thin cuts

b) Positron emission tomography scan—measures glucose metabolism in the brain

c) Single photon emission computed tomography scan (both ictal and inter-ictal)—measures blood flow in the brain

iii. Neuropsychometric evaluation
  (a) Measures cognitive function, dominant hemisphere
  (b) Epilepsy negatively affects language, memory, and comprehension
  (c) Provides adjunctive information on the functional location of the pathology
iv. Cortical resection of seizure focus
  (a) Can require placement of subdural electrodes to record seizure onset and localize the focus
  (b) Outcomes (Ojemann, 2001)
    (1) Temporal lobectomy
       a) 68% seizure-free
       b) 25% improved
       c) 8% not improved
    (2) Extratemporal resection
       a) 45% seizure-free
       b) 35% improved
       c) 20% not improved
    (3) Hemispherectomy
       a) 67% seizure-free
       b) 21% improved
       c) 12% not improved
    (4) Corpus callosotomy
       a) 8% seizure-free
       b) 61% improved
       c) 31% not improved
v. Vagus nerve stimulation
  (a) Mechanism unknown
  (b) Thought to impact epilepsy patients as follows:
    (1) $\frac{1}{3}$ of patients will have >50% reduction in seizures
    (2) $\frac{1}{3}$ of patients will have <50% reduction in seizures
    (3) $\frac{1}{3}$ of patients will have no change in their seizure frequency
  (c) Vagus nerve stimulation (VNS) therapy induces progressive EEG changes over time
  (d) Lead wire placed on the left vagus nerve; generator implanted under left chest
    (1) Vagus nerve has 80% afferent sensory fibers which project bilaterally to noradrenergic and serotonergic systems of the brain and spinal cord
    (2) The locus coeruleus may be involved in the anticonvulsant effect of VNS therapy
    (3) Duty cycle is set to deliver electrical impulses continually, throughout the day
    (4) Battery life 6 to 11 years, dependent upon settings
  (e) Significant bilateral changes in blood flow have been observed during VNS therapy
9. Influence on growth and development
   a. Depending on the type of epilepsy, severity of seizures, and age of onset, epilepsy can have profound negative effects on growth and development
   b. Cognitive function (Austin, et al., 1999; Fastenau, et al., 2004; Loring & Meador, 2004)
      i. Intelligence and school performance
         (a) Most children with epilepsy have normal intelligence

(b) Children with low-severity seizures maintained average school performance

(c) Children with high-severity seizures are at risk for cognitive dysfunction

(d) Research shows direct negative effects of neuropsychologic function on achievement, yet supportive family environments can play a positive moderating role

   ii. Antiepilepsy medications can have deleterious cognitive effects, *especially* if:

(a) Polytherapy

(b) Side effect profile of the drugs affect cognition

   iii. Surgery

(a) Cognitive function may or may not improve, depending on the baseline level and extent of surgery

c. Mental health

   i. Marsh and Rao (2002) study

(a) About 50% of individuals with epilepsy have comorbid psychiatric syndromes

(b) Anxiety disorders are most common

(c) Presence of mood disorders, including depression

(d) Presence of aggression and violence as post-ictal psychosis phenomena

   ii. Treatment of the comorbidity may need to include psychotherapy and psychotherapeutics

d. Growth—children with epilepsy are at risk for weight gain or weight loss due to medications and/or concomitant disorders

e. Behavior

   i. Behavior problems over a 2-year period were related to (Austin, et al., 2004):

(a) Deficient family mastery of the chronic condition

(b) Low parental confidence in managing their child's discipline

f. Injuries—age-related activities with serious injury potential should be prohibited

   i. No swimming alone

   ii. No climbing trees

   iii. Unable to drive if seizures are uncontrolled (length of time varies by state)

10. Follow-up in primary care

a. When to refer?

   i. Seizures continue despite therapeutic morning trough anticonvulsant levels

   ii. Regression of developmental skills

   iii. Regression of cognitive function

   iv. Side effect profile unacceptable

b. Monitor growth—height, weight, BMI on growth charts

c. Monitor developmental milestones

d. Safety updates at each visit, tailored to child's age and severity of seizures

e. Immunizations (see Chapter 15)

f. Adolescent issues

   i. Noncompliance with medications and safety issues

   ii. Some anticonvulsants (e.g., carbamazepine) can lower effects of oral contraceptives

   iii. Pregnancy—genetic counseling should be recommended

   iv. Teratogenicity with high anticonvulsant doses and/or polytherapy

**11.** Long-term implications
  **a.** Prognosis of newly diagnosed epilepsy falls into two categories (Kwan & Sander, 2004)
    **i.** Remission without treatment
    **ii.** Remission with treatment only
    **iii.** Persistent seizures despite treatment
  **b.** Poor prognostic factors include: (Kwan & Sander, 2004)
    **i.** High initial seizure density
    **ii.** Etiology of metabolic disorder
    **iii.** Presence of structural cerebral abnormalities

## REFERENCES

American Academy of Pediatrics, Provisional Committee on Quality Improvement and Subcommittee on Febrile Seizures. (1996). Practice Parameter: The neurodiagnostic evaluation of the child with a first simple febrile seizure. *Pediatrics, 97* (5), 769-772.

American Epilepsy Society. (2004). Basic mechanisms underlying seizures and epilepsy. Retrieved on May 21, 2206 from http://www.aesnet.org/Visitors/ProfessionalDevelopment/ MedEd/ppt/ppts03/BASICORE.PDF.

Austin, J., Huberty, T., Huster, G., & Dunn, D. (1999). Does academic achievement in children with epilepsy change over time? *Dev Med Child Neurol, 41,* 473-479.

Austin, J. K., Dunn, D. W., Johnson, C. S., & Perkins, S. M. (2004). Behavioral issues involving children and adolescenets with epilepsy and the impact of their families: Recent research data. *Epilepsy Behav, 5*(Suppl. 3), S10-S17.

Blair, J., & Selekman, J. (2004). Epilepsy. In P. L. Jackson & J. A. Vessey (Eds.). *Primary care of the child with a chronic condition* (4th ed.). St. Louis: Mosby, pp. 469-497.

Fastenau, P. S., Shen, J., Dunn, D. W., et al. (2004). Neuropsychological predictors of academic underachievement in pediatric epilepsy: Moderating roles of demographic, seizure and psychosocial variables. *Epilepsia, 45*(10), 1261-1272.

French, J. A., Kanner, A. M., Bautista, J., et al. (2004). Efficacy and tolerability of the new anti-epileptic drugs I: Treatment of new onset epilepsy. *Neurology, 62,* 1252-1260.

Johnston, M. V. (2004). Seizures in childhood. In R. E. Behrman, R. M. Kliegman, & H. B. Jenson (Eds.). *Nelson textbook of pediatrics* (17th ed.). Philadelphia: Saunders, pp. 1993-2008.

Kwan, P., & Sander, J. W. (2004). The natural history of epilepsy: An epidemiological view. *J Neurol Neurosurg Psychiatry, 75*(10), 1376-1381.

Loring, D. W., & Meador, K. J. (2004). Cognitive side effects of antiepileptic drugs in children. *Neurology, 62*(6), 872-877.

Marsh, L., & Rao, V. (2002). Psychiatric complications in patients with epilepsy: A review. *Epilepsy Res, 49,* 11-33.

Ojemann, JG, Park, TS. (2001). Surgical treatment: surgery and outcome. In J. Pellock, W.E. Dodson, B.Bourgeois (Eds). *Pediatric Epilepsy Diagnosis and Therapy* (2nd ed. Pp 61-68). New York: Demos.

Ottman, R. (2001). Genetic influences on risk for epilepsy. In J. Pellock, W.E. Dodson, B. Bourgeois (Eds). *Pediatric Epilepsy Diagnosis and Therapy* (2nd ed. Pp 61-68). New York: Demos.

Shinnar, S., Berg, A. T., O'Dell, C., et al. (2000). Predictors of multiple seizures in a cohort of children prospectively followed from the time of their first unprovoked seizure. *Ann Neurol, 48,* 140-147.

# Hemoglobinopathies

LESLIE DIETERICH, MSN, CNP

1. Definition: genetic defects that involve changes in the amino acid sequence of either the α- or β-globin chains of hemoglobin; hundreds of defects have been described
2. Normal physiology (Brigham & Women's Hospital, 2002)
   a. Hemoglobin synthesis involves production of heme and globin in the mitochondria
   b. Heme mediates reversible binding of oxygen by hemoglobin
   c. Globin is a protein that protects the heme molecule
   d. "Adult" hemoglobin (at 18 to 24 weeks) is composed of four globin chains
      i. Two alpha chains encoded by four genes on chromosome pair 16 ($\alpha\alpha/\alpha\alpha$)
      ii. Two beta chains encoded by two genes on chromosome pair 11 ($\beta/\beta$)
3. Most common hemoglobinopathies
   a. Alpha thalassemia
   b. Beta thalassemia
   c. Hemoglobin C
   d. Hemoglobin E
   e. Hemoglobin S (sickle cell disease)

## ALPHA THALASSEMIA

1. Etiology and pathophysiology (Cohen, et al., 2004; Orkin & Nathan, 2003)
   a. Genetic mutation of chromosome 16
   b. Autosomal recessive inheritance
   c. Loss of one to four α-globin genes due to defective α-globin gene synthesis
   d. Impaired production of α-globin leading to an excess of β-globin
   e. Severity increases with the number of genes lost
   f. Examples of phenotype notation in order of severity
      i. Normal        $\alpha\alpha/\alpha\alpha$
      ii. Carrier      $-\alpha/\alpha\alpha$
      iii. Minor       $\alpha\alpha/--$ or $-\alpha/-\alpha$
      iv. Hemoglobin H disease    $\alpha-/--$
      v. Bart's hydrops fetalis    $--/--$

2. Incidence and prevalence
    a. One gene deletion per chromosome ($-\alpha$)
        i. More common in those of African descent
        ii. 25% of Blacks with $-\alpha/\alpha\alpha$ phenotype
        iii. 1.5% of Blacks with $-\alpha/-\alpha$ phenotype
    b. Two gene deletions per chromosome ($- -$) more common in those of Mediterranean or Southeast Asian descent
3. Presentation
    a. Diagnostic measures (Nagel, 2003)
        i. Newborn screening results
            (a) Presents on newborn screening report as "FA + Bart's"
            (b) FA means that amount of fetal hemoglobin is greater than adult hemoglobin (normal for newborn)
            (c) Bart's hemoglobin is indicative of one to four missing or dysfunctional genes
        ii. Follow-up testing should be done by 1 month of age
            (a) Bart's hemoglobin may or may not still be present
            (b) Hemoglobin electrophoresis will otherwise be normal
            (c) CBC will show microcytosis
        iii. Testing in older children should include hemoglobin electrophoresis, CBC, and iron studies
        iv. Consider genotyping in populations at high risk for loss of 3 or 4 genes
            (a) Not done at most labs
            (b) Send specimen to a genetic testing center
    b. Phenotype, laboratory, and physical characteristics of alpha thalassemias (Table 47-1)
4. Influence on growth and development
    a. One and two gene deletions have no effect on growth and development
    b. Three gene deletions (hemoglobin H disease) may cause some slowing of growth depending of severity of anemia
    c. Four gene deletions rarely compatible with life (fetal hydrops)
5. Treatment
    a. No treatment needed for one and two gene deletions
    b. Should not treat anemia with iron unless documented iron deficiency
    c. Children with three gene deletions
        i. Give folic acid supplementation
        ii. May require intermittent transfusion therapy
        iii. Primary care should be managed in collaboration with a pediatric hematologist
    d. Surviving infants with four gene deletions
        i. Require chronic transfusion therapy
        ii. May be candidates for hematopoietic stem cell transplantation
        iii. Primary care should be managed in collaboration with a pediatric hematologist
6. Follow-up
    a. See the child according to routine preventive care schedule
    b. Iron studies at 9 to 12 months of age and as needed
7. Long term
    a. Genetic counseling when child reaches adolescence
    b. Pregnancy in those with hemoglobin H disease associated with:
        i. Increased severity of anemia
        ii. Preeclampsia

■ **TABLE 47-1**
■ ■ **Phenotype, Laboratory and Physical Characteristics of Alpha Thalassemias**

| Number of Normal α-Globin Genes | % of Hemoglobin *Bart's* at Birth | CBC, Hemoglobin Electrophoresis Findings | Signs/Symptoms |
|---|---|---|---|
| 3 (−α/αα) | 0%–2% | Minimal microcytosis, normal Hgb A$_2$ | Bart's hemoglobin on newborn screen<br>Asymptomatic |
| 2 (−α/−α or − −/αα) | 3%–5% | Microcytosis, may have mild anemia, low to normal Hgb A$_2$ | Bart's hemoglobin on newborn screen<br>Asymptomatic |
| 1 (− −/−α)<br>hemoglobin H disease | 30% | 0% to 10% Hgb Bart's, 5%–15% Hgb H, low Hgb A$_2$, moderately severe microcytic, hemolytic anemia (Hgb 7–10) | Splenomegaly<br>Jaundice/icterus<br>May see leg ulcers and an increased susceptibility to infection |
| 0 (− −/− −)<br>Bart's/hydrops fetalis | 100% | Severe erythroblastic anemia | Usually results in intrauterine death<br>Infants surviving to delivery will be hydropic and commonly have neurologic impairment<br>Intrauterine transfusions following early detection may prevent this<br>May have congenital malformations<br>Hypospadias<br>Other GU anomalies<br>Limb malformations<br>May have neurologic impairment |

## BETA THALASSEMIA

1. Etiology and pathophysiology (Cohen, et al., 2004; Orkin & Nathan, 2003)
   a. Genetic mutation of chromosome 11
   b. Autosomal recessive inheritance
   c. Defect in one or two β-globin genes causes defective beta chain synthesis
      i. Defect in one gene: beta thalassemia minor (trait)
      ii. Defect in both genes: beta thalassemia major (homozygous)
   d. Resulting excess alpha chains cause damage to the red cell, and anemia
   e. Hundreds of different defects exist
      i. An affected gene may produce very little β-globin (β$^0$ defect)
      ii. Or up to an almost normal amount of β-globin (β$^+$ defect)
2. Incidence and prevalence
   a. Trait is present in approximately 3% to 5% of Italian and Greek Americans; 0.5% of Blacks
   b. Can also be seen in those from Southeast Asia
3. Presentation
   a. Diagnostic measures
      i. Newborn screening
      ii. CBC
      iii. Hemoglobin electrophoresis
      iv. Iron studies

      **v.** Consider testing parents, especially in infants in whom diagnosis may be more difficult due to the higher fetal hemoglobin levels

  **b.** Phenotype

      **i.** Normal       $\beta/\beta$

      **ii.** Minor (trait)   $\beta/\beta^0$ or $\beta/\beta^+$

      **iii.** Intermedia    $\beta^0/\beta^+$

      **iv.** Major       $\beta^0/\beta^0$ or $\beta^+/\beta^+$

  **c.** Signs and symptoms

      **i.** Beta thalassemia minor (trait)

        (a) Not identified on newborn screening

        (b) Mild to moderate microcytic anemia

        (c) Target cells on the peripheral blood smear

        (d) Normal red blood cell count

        (e) Likely asymptomatic

      **ii.** Beta thalassemia intermedia and major

        (a) Newborn screening may show only Hb F with thalassemia major

        (b) Moderate to severe anemia (develops between 6 and 12 months of age)

        (c) Microcytosis

        (d) Basophilic stippling

        (e) Increased reticulocyte count

        (f) An increased Hb $A_2$ level is not observed in patients with the rare delta-beta thalassemia trait

**4.** Influence on growth and development

  **a.** Trait has no effect on growth and development

  **b.** Thalassemia intermedia, thalassemia major (Viprakasit, et al., 2001)

      **i.** Can cause delayed physical growth

      **ii.** Developmental milestones are not usually affected

      **iii.** With adequate iron chelation

        (a) Those who are hypertransfused have less impairment of growth than those who are not hypertransfused

**5.** Treatment

  **a.** Thalassemia trait

      **i.** No treatment needed

      **ii.** Do not treat anemia with iron unless documented iron deficiency

  **b.** Thalassemia intermedia

      **i.** Often require transfusions

      **ii.** Should be managed collaboratively with a pediatric hematologist

  **c.** Thalassemia major

      **i.** Children are transfusion dependent

      **ii.** Chronic iron overload will develop over time and will need iron chelation therapy

      **iii.** Should be managed in collaboration with a pediatric hematologist

      **iv.** Consider bone marrow transplant for cure

**6.** Follow-up

  **a.** See child according to routine preventive care schedule

  **b.** Children receiving transfusions should also have:

      **i.** Regular evaluation of liver and kidney function

      **ii.** Monitoring of iron overload

      **iii.** Testing for blood-borne infectious diseases (hepatitis B and C, HIV)

**7.** Long term

  **a.** Genetic counseling when child reaches adolescence

   b. Normal life span for minor and intermedia
   c. Thalassemia major and more serious syndromes
      i. May have shortened life span
      ii. May have impaired fertility
      iii. Increased risk of thrombosis including deep vein thrombosis (DVT) and pulmonary embolus
   d. Inadequately treated iron overload will lead to cardiomyopathy and possibly endocrinopathies

## HEMOGLOBIN C

1. Etiology and pathophysiology (Carter & Gross, 2005)
   a. Genetic mutation of chromosome 11
      i. Two normal alpha chains
      ii. Two variant beta chains
         (a) Defect in the amino acid sequence of the $\beta$-globin chain
         (b) Substitution of lysine for glutamic acid in the sixth position
   b. Autosomal recessive inheritance
   c. Interacts with Hb S to form a mild form of sickle cell disease
   d. Causes shortened red cell survival
      i. HbC RBC lifespan is about 40 days compared with normal of 120 days
   e. Amount of hemoglobin C ranges from 35% to 100%
2. Incidence and prevalence
   a. Rare, but most common in people of African descent
      i. Prevalence in Blacks is 0.017%
      ii. Northern Africa prevalence is 0.03%
   b. Also found in central and west Africa
   c. And in people of Mediterranean descent
3. Presentation
   a. Diagnostic measures
      i. Newborn screening
      ii. Hemoglobin electrophoresis to confirm abnormal newborn screen
      iii. CBC, hemoglobin
      iv. Electrophoresis in older children
      v. Consider parental testing with CBC and hemoglobin electrophoresis
   b. Diagnostic criteria
      i. Presents on newborn screen as FAC, FC, or FCA, meaning that the fetal (F) hemoglobin cells predominate, followed by either A (adult hemoglobin) or C hemoglobin
      ii. Hemoglobin types are listed in order of predominance on newborn screen and follow-up hemoglobin electrophoresis
         (a) More A than C = trait
         (b) More C than A = heterozygotes for hemoglobin C/B$^+$ thalassemia
         (c) No A
            (1) Homozygous for hemoglobin C
            (2) Or double heterozygotes for hemoglobin C/B$^0$ thalassemia
   c. Signs and symptoms
      i. Trait (FAC, AC) is asymptomatic
      ii. Homozygote and C/$\beta^+$ thalassemia have mild hemolytic anemia and microcytosis

      **iii.** $C/\beta^0$ thalassemia has a moderately severe hemolytic anemia and microcytosis

      **iv.** CC and $C/\beta^0$ thalassemia

        (a) Splenomegaly is common

        (b) Aplastic crises and gallstones also may occur

**4.** Influence on growth and development

    **a.** AC, CC, and $C/\beta^+$ thalassemia have no effect on growth or development

    **b.** May see mild slowing of growth in those with $C/\beta^0$ thalassemia

**5.** Treatment

    **a.** AC—no treatment needed

    **b.** CC, $C/\beta^0$ thalassemia, and $C/\beta^+$ thalassemia

      **i.** Frequent monitoring for anemia

      **ii.** Iron supplements if evidence of iron deficiency

      **iii.** Monitor for splenomegaly and gallstones

**6.** Follow-up

    **a.** See child according to routine preventive care schedule

    **b.** Annual CBC for those with CC, $C/\beta^0$ thalassemia, and $C/\beta^+$ thalassemia

    **c.** Consultation or collaboration with a pediatric hematologist is recommended

**7.** Long term

    **a.** Genetic counseling when child reaches adolescence

## HEMOGLOBIN E

**1.** Etiology and pathophysiology

    **a.** Genetic mutation of chromosome 11

    **b.** Autosomal recessive inheritance

    **c.** Substitution of lysine for glutamic acid at the 26th position of the $\beta$-globin chain

    **d.** Interacts with Hb S to form mild sickle cell disease

    **e.** Interacts with $\beta^0$ thalassemia to form severe disease

**2.** Incidence and prevalence

    **a.** Most common in Southeast Asians and Indians, also common in Asians

    **b.** Less often found in people of Middle Eastern, Mediterranean, or African descent

**3.** Presentation

    **a.** Diagnostic measures

      **i.** Hemoglobin electrophoresis to confirm abnormal newborn screen

      **ii.** CBC, hemoglobin electrophoresis in older children

      **iii.** Strongly recommend parental testing of newborn with FE to differentiate between homozygous E and the more severe double heterozygous hemoglobin $E/\beta^0$ thalassemia

    **b.** Diagnostic criteria

      **i.** Presents on newborn screen as FAE, FE, or FEA

      **ii.** Hemoglobins are listed in order of predominance on newborn screen

        (a) More A than E = trait

        (b) More E than A (or no A) have disease

    **c.** Signs and symptoms

      **i.** Trait (AE) and homozygotes (EE)

        (a) Many target cells on smear

        (b) Mild hemolytic anemia

      **ii.** E/$\beta^0$ thalassemia

        (a) Severe hemolytic anemia and microcytosis

        (b) Splenomegaly and jaundice

      **iii.** E/$\beta^0$ thalassemia

        (a) Moderate anemia and microcytosis

        (b) Splenomegaly and jaundice

**4.** Influence on growth and development

   **a.** AE and EE have no effect on growth or development

   **b.** E/$\beta^+$ thalassemia and E/$\beta^0$ thalassemia will have delayed physical growth

**5.** Treatment

   **a.** No treatment needed for AE or EE

   **b.** Treatment for E/$\beta^+$ thalassemia and E/$\beta^0$ thalassemia

      **i.** Similar to treatment of thalassemia intermedia and major

      **ii.** Manage in collaboration with a pediatric hematologist

**6.** Follow-up

   **a.** See child according to routine preventive care schedule

   **b.** EE type

      **i.** Annual CBC

      **ii.** Consultation or collaboration with a pediatric hematologist is recommended

   **c.** E/$\beta^+$ thalassemia and E/$\beta^0$ thalassemia

      **i.** More frequent CBCs

      **ii.** Regular evaluation of liver and kidney function

      **iii.** Monitor for iron overload

      **iv.** Test for blood-borne infectious diseases (hepatitis B and C, HIV) if receiving regular transfusions

**7.** Long term

   **a.** Genetic counseling when child reaches adolescence

   **b.** E/$\beta$ thalassemia

      **i.** May have shortened life span

      **ii.** May have impaired fertility

   **c.** Inadequately treated iron overload will lead to

      **i.** Cardiomyopathy

      **ii.** Possibly endocrinopathies

   **d.** Increased risk of thrombosis including DVT and pulmonary embolus with more serious thalassemia syndromes

## HEMOGLOBIN S (SICKLE CELL)

**1.** Etiology and pathophysiology (Dodds & Shahidi, 2005; Dover & Platt, 2003;Lisak, 2004)

   **a.** Genetic mutation of chromosome 11

   **b.** Autosomal recessive inheritance

   **c.** Substitution of valine for glutamic acid in the sixth position of $\beta$-globin chain

   **d.** RBCs contain Hb S

      **i.** Become "sickle" shaped under certain conditions

      **ii.** More fragile and stickier than cells containing Hb A

   **e.** Hb S RBC turnover is about 10 to 20 days compared with normal of 120 days

**2.** Incidence and prevalence

   **a.** 1 in 12 Blacks with trait; 8% to 10%

   **b.** 1 in 500 Blacks with disease; 0.15%

c. Also common in people of Mediterranean, Middle Eastern, and Indian origin
d. Although uncommon, can be present in whites

3. Presentation
    a. Laboratory and diagnostic measures
        i. Newborn screen results
            (a) Confirm abnormal newborn screen by 1 month of age
            (b) With hemoglobin electrophoresis
        ii. CBC, reticulocyte count, and hemoglobin electrophoresis in older child
        iii. Sickle solubility testing
            (a) A screening test that detects the presence of sickle hemoglobin
            (b) Not appropriate for diagnosis
            (c) Cannot differentiate between trait and disease
            (d) Should never be used for parental testing or genetic counseling
            (e) Does not detect any other abnormal hemoglobins
    b. Diagnostic criteria
        i. Presents on newborn screen as FAS, FS, FSA, FSC, or FSE
        ii. Hemoglobins are listed in order of predominance
            (a) More A than S = trait
            (b) More S than A (or no A) = disease
        iii. Differential diagnoses of common sickle hemoglobinopathies (Table 47-2)
    c. Signs and symptoms
        i. Trait (AS) is asymptomatic
        ii. Children with disease
            (a) Until at least 6 months of age
                (1) Usually asymptomatic
                (2) Due to protective effect of fetal hemoglobin
            (b) Then may present with a variety of symptoms (see Table 47-2)
            (c) Most frequent presenting symptoms

■ **TABLE 47-2**
■ ■ **Clinical and Laboratory Characteristics of Hemoglobin S Disease**

| Diagnosis | Clinical Severity | Hemoglobin(g/dL) | Reticulocytes (%) | Electrophoresis (%) | |
|---|---|---|---|---|---|
| SS | Moderate-severe | 6–10 | 4–30 | S | 80–90 |
| | | | | F | 2–20 |
| | | | | $A_2$ <3.6 | |
| SC | Mild-moderate | 9–12 | 1.5–6 | S | 45–55 |
| | | | | C | 45–55 |
| | | | | F | 0.2–8 |
| S/$\beta^0$ thal | Moderate-severe | 6–10 | 3–18 | S | 50–85 |
| | | | | F | 2–30 |
| | | | | $A_2$ >3.6 | |
| S/$\beta^+$ thal | Mild-moderate | 9–13 | 1.5–6 | S | 55–75 |
| | | | | A | 15–30 |
| | | | | F | 1–20 |
| | | | | $A_2$ >3.6 | |
| AS | Asymptomatic | Normal | Normal | S | 38–45 |
| | | | | A | 55–60 |
| | | | | $A_2$ <3.6 | |

(1) Vaso-occlusive crisis

(2) Anemia

4. Influence on growth and development
   a. Trait—no effect on growth and development
   b. Disease—will have growth alterations
   c. Lower than average height and weight
   d. The most growth delay seen with SS and S/B⁰ thalassemia
   e. Sexual development is also usually delayed
   f. Neurologic effects may negatively affect development and school performance (Schatz, et al., 2004)

5. Treatment
   a. See Table 47-3 for treatment of common problems
   b. Hydroxyurea (Zimmerman, et al., 2004)
      i. Chemotherapeutic agent that is approved for treatment in adults
      ii. Clinical trials with children show effectiveness but it is still being used with caution
         (a) Usually only with severe disease
         (b) Uncertainty regarding growth and developmental effects
         (c) Possible long-term adverse effects such as psoriasis, hyperpigmentation, xerosis, T-lymphocyte suppression
      iii. Stimulates production of fetal hemoglobin which has a protective effect by preventing sickling
   c. Bone marrow transplant (BMT) (Walters, et al., 2000)
      i. Still considered experimental
      ii. Need an HLA-matched sibling donor
      iii. Must have severe disease to be a candidate due to the risks

6. Follow-up (Segal, et al., 2002a, 2002b)
   a. See the child according to the routine preventive care schedule
   b. Routine monitoring of CBC, reticulocyte count, renal and hepatic function
      i. Recommended for those with sickle cell disease
      ii. Manage care in collaboration with a pediatric hematologist
   c. Routine ophthalmology exams beginning at 5 years of age or earlier if any problems

7. Long term
   a. Genetic counseling when the child reaches adolescence
   b. Those with disease will develop chronic organ damage
      i. Cardiovascular effects
         (a) Left ventricular hypertrophy as a result of chronic anemia
         (b) Compensatory increased cardiac output
         (c) Pulmonary hypertension is rare except in those with acute or chronic pulmonary disease
   c. Respiratory—may see obstructive or restrictive lung disease
   d. Hepatobiliary—common to have gallstones, may also have hepatic infarct
   e. Renal
      i. Hyposthenuria—inability to concentrate urine (low specific gravity)
      ii. Results in large volumes of dilute urine
      iii. Nocturnal enuresis is common
      iv. May also see hematuria (usually mild), microalbuminuria or proteinuria
      v. Possible nephritic syndrome
   f. Eyes
      i. Retinopathy may occur
      ii. Most common with HbSC disease disease

■ **TABLE 47-3**
■ ■ **Common Problems Associated with Hemoglobin S Disease**

| Problem | Pathophysiology | Management | Teaching | Prevention |
|---|---|---|---|---|
| Anemia | Shortened RBC life span due to increased fragility and sickling | • Monitor CBC every 6 months to determine baseline for child<br>• Do not treat with iron unless documented iron deficiency | • Important for parent to understand cause of anemia<br>• Teach signs of worsening anemia that require evaluation (pallor, significantly increased fatigue)<br>• Important for parent to know child's baseline hemoglobin | None |
| Sepsis antigens | Loss of splenic function due to damage caused by sickled RBCs, failure to make specific IgG antibodies and polysaccharide | • Fever >101° F needs prompt evaluation including CBC with differential, reticulocyte count, blood cultures<br>• Should also consider UA, urine culture, CXR, LP depending on child's age and clinical presentation<br>• Treat prophylactically with IV Rocephin while cultures are pending<br>• Infants should be admitted<br>• Older children may be observed as an outpatient<br>  o Decided on a case-by-case basis | • Teach parents that overwhelming sepsis may occur very rapidly (within a matter of hours)<br>• Stress importance of prompt medical evaluation of all fevers >101° F<br>  o This is the leading cause of death in children less than 5 years of age | • Should receive a full 4-dose schedule of Prevnar with doses at 2, 4, and 6 months of age and a booster at 12 to 15 months<br>• Penicillin (PCN) prophylaxis starting by 8 weeks of age: 125 mg PO bid until age 3; 250 mg PO bid after age 3<br>• Erythromycin is the preferred alternative in the event of penicillin allergy (10 mg/kg PO bid<br>• Prophylaxis can be stopped at 5 years of age<br>• Pneumococcal polysaccharide vaccine at 2 years of age with booster doses every 3 to 5 years |
| Vaso-occlusive crisis (VOC) | Sickle RBCs become trapped in small blood vessels limiting oxygen delivery to local tissues and causing severe pain | • Pharmacologic: NSAIDs, opioids (should follow WHO pain ladder)<br>• Nonpharmacologic: increased fluids, local heat, massage, relaxation and distraction techniques | • Teach preventive measures to parents (and child when old enough)<br>• Written plan at home with list of medications, doses, indications for use, and when to seek medical attention | • Adequate hydration<br>• Avoid extreme temperatures, especially cold<br>• Do not use ice for injuries |

*(Continued)*

■ **TABLE 47-3**
■ ■ **Common Problems Associated with Hemoglobin S Disease—cont'd**

| Problem | Pathophysiology | Management | Teaching | Prevention |
|---|---|---|---|---|
| Acute chest syndrome (ACS) | Term used to describe a group of symptoms associated with sickling in the lungs; may be caused by infection, infarction, or fat embolus<br>Often a secondary diagnosis when hospitalized for VOC | • Oxygen only if hypoxemia<br>• Scheduled bronchodilators<br>• Antibiotics (should include coverage for *Streptococcus pneumoniae, Mycoplasma,* and *Chlamydia pneumoniae*<br>• Transfusion to raise Hgb to 10 g/dL<br>• Consider packed red blood cells<br>• Steroids also may be helpful | • Signs and symptoms of respiratory distress | • Avoid fluid overload<br>• Routine use of incentive spirometer when hospitalized<br>• Encourage time out of bed when hospitalized |
| Splenic sequestration | Occlusion of the blood vessels leading out from the spleen by sickled cells<br>Causes significant splenomegaly and anemia<br>May be life threatening | • Close monitoring of splenomegaly<br>• Transfusion if severe anemia<br>• Consider referral to surgery for splenectomy (after recovery/not done acutely) if event is severe or repeated episodes | • Palpation of spleen<br>• Note baseline spleen size (those with Hb SC most likely to have baseline splenomegaly)<br>• Limit contact sports if significant splenomegaly | • Unable to prevent initial event<br>• Monthly transfusions may be considered to prevent recurrence if less than 2 years of age<br>• Splenectomy usually deferred until after 2 years of age |
| Stroke (CVA) | Sickling in cerebral blood vessels causing vaso-occlusion | • Immediate transfusion<br>• Exchange transfusion is preferable<br>• May do simple transfusion to Hgb of 10g/dL while preparing for exchange transfusion | • Signs and symptoms of stroke including one-sided weakness, gait alterations, slurred speech, lethargy, and behavioral changes | • Transcranial Doppler ultrasound (TCD) now used to screen for those at high risk, should be done starting at the age of 2<br>• Monthly transfusions to prevent initial stroke in those found to be high risk and after stroke to prevent recurrence |

*Continued*

■ **TABLE 47-3**
■ ■ **Common Problems Associated with Hemoglobin S Disease—cont'd**

| Problem | Pathophysiology | Management | Teaching | Prevention |
|---------|-----------------|------------|----------|------------|
| Aplastic crisis | Viral infection (usually parvovirus B19) causes suppression of bone marrow function resulting in significant anemia | • Close observation<br>• Consider transfusion to child's baseline Hgb if severe, symptomatic anemia<br>• See management of VOC | • Important for parent to know child's baseline Hgb and skin coloring<br>• Monitor for changes in skin color/pallor and extreme fatigue<br>• Home management (relaxation, soaking in warm bath in addition to usual home VOC management)<br>• Importance of seeking medical attention if priapism lasting more than 3–4 hours (potential for impotence if prolonged) | • Avoidance of anyone with parvovirus B19 infection (fifth disease)<br>• Adequate hydration<br>• Limited data on prevention of recurrence<br>• Urology should be involved with children with frequent, recurrent priapism |
| Priapism | Painful erection of the penis caused by sickling in the corpora cavernosa | • Urology consult if persistent for more than a few hours<br>• Consider transfusion | | |

**g.** Ears—may develop sensorineural hearing loss
**h.** Skeletal
   **i.** Painful vascular occlusion episodes
   **ii.** Avascular necrosis, typically of the femoral head, is more common with HbSC disease
   **iii.** Also may see some flattening of the vertebrae
**i.** Skin
   **i.** Leg ulcers may develop
   **ii.** Usually not seen until late adolescence or adulthood
**j.** May have shortened life expectancy
   **i.** This is improving as advances in care are made

## REFERENCES

Brigham & Women's Hospital (BWH). (2002). Hemoglobin synthesis. Retrieved June 26, 2006, from http://sickle.bwh.harvard.edu/hbsynthesis.html.

Carter, S. M., & Gross, S. J. (2005). Hemoglobin C disease. Retrieved May 21, 2006, from www.emedicine.com/med/topic976.htm.

Cohen, A. R., Galanello, R., Pennell, D. J., et al. (2004). Thalassemia. *Hematology (American Society of Hematology Education Program Book)*, 14-34.

Dodds, N., & Shahidi, H. (2005). Pediatrics, sickle cell disease. Retrieved February 20, 2005, from www.emedicine.com/emerg/topic406.htm.

Dover, G. J., & Platt, O. (2003). Sickle cell disease. In D. G. Nathan, S. H. Orkin, A. T. Look, & D. Ginsburg (Eds.). *Nathan and Oski's hematology of infancy and childhood* (6th ed.). Philadelphia: Saunders.

Lisak, M. E. (2004). Sickle cell disease. In P. J. Allen & J. Vessey (Eds.). *Primary care of the child with a chronic condition* (4th ed.). St. Louis: Mosby.

Nagel, R. (2003). Human hemoglobins: Normal and abnormal. In D. G. Nathan, S. H. Orkin, A. T. Look, & D. Ginsburg (Eds.). *Nathan and Oski's hematology of infancy and childhood* (6th ed.). Philadelphia: Saunders.

Orkin, S. H., & Nathan, D. G. (2003). The thalassemias. In D. G. Nathan, S. H. Orkin, A. T. Look, & D. Ginsburg (Eds.). *Nathan and Oski's hematology of infancy and childhood* (6th ed.). Philadelphia: Saunders.

Schatz, J., Finke, R., & Roberts, C. W. (2004). Interactions of biomedical and environmental risk factors for cognitive development: A preliminary study of sickle cell disease. *J Dev Behav Pediatr, 25*(5), 303-310.

Segel, G. B., Hirsh, M. G., & Feig, S. A. (2002a). Managing anemia in pediatric office practice: Part 1. *Pediatr Rev, 23*(3), 75-83.

Segel, G. B., Hirsh, M. G., & Feig, S. A. (2002b). Managing anemia in pediatric office practice: Part 2. *Pediatr Rev, 23*(4), 111-121.

Viprakasit, V., Tamphaichitr, V. S., Mahasandana, C., et al. (2001). Linear growth in homozygous beta-thalassemia and beta-thalassemia/hemoglobin E patients under different treatment regimens. *J Med Assoc Thai, 84*(7), 929-941.

Walters, M. C., Storb, R., Patience, M., et al. (2000). Impact of bone marrow transplantation for symptomatic sickle cell disease: An interim report. Multicenter investigation of bone marrow transplantation for sickle cell disease. *Blood, 95*(6), 1918-1924.

Zimmerman, S. A., Schultz, W. H., Davis, J. S., et al. (2004). Sustained long-term hematologic efficacy of hydroxyurea at maximum tolerated dose in children with sickle cell disease. *Blood, 103*(6), 2039-2045.

# Juvenile Rheumatoid Arthritis

KIMBERLY HANDROCK, RN, MS, PNP and JANALEE TAYLOR, RN, MSN, CNS

## DEFINITION

Juvenile rheumatoid arthritis (JRA) is a category of rheumatic diseases in children characterized by an idiopathic synovitis of the peripheral joints, soft tissue swelling and effusion; three types of onset include oligoarthritis, polyarthritis, and systemic JRA (Miller & Cassidy, 2004).

1. Incidence and prevalence
   a. Prevalence of JRA is 113 per 100,000 children (Miller & Cassidy, 2004)
   b. Incidence
      i. 13.9 per 100,000 children ≤15 years old are diagnosed per year (Miller & Cassidy, 2004)
      ii. Oligoarthritis is most frequent subtype of JRA
         (a) Incidence among JRA diagnoses is 56% to 60% (Cassidy & Petty, 2001)
      iii. Polyarthritis JRA
         (a) Incidence among JRA diagnoses is approximately 25% to 28% (Cassidy & Petty, 2001)
         (b) Incidence of RF (+) JRA increases with disease longevity and with older age at diagnosis
      iv. Systemic JRA
         (a) Incidence among JRA diagnoses is approximately 10% to 20% (Cassidy & Petty, 2001)
   c. Compared with other pediatric-onset chronic illnesses, JRA is relatively common
      i. Affects approximately the same number of children as type 1 diabetes
      ii. Four times as many children as sickle cell anemia or cystic fibrosis
      iii. Ten times as many children as hemophilia, acute lymphocytic leukemia, chronic renal failure, or muscular dystrophy
2. Etiology or precipitating factors
   a. JRA is an exaggerated immune reactivity of T cells specific to antigens (Miller & Cassidy, 2004)
      i. Some T cells are protective and enhance responsiveness to treatment

        **ii.** Other T cells permit chronic reactivity
        **iii.** A cascade of events leads to joint tissue damage
            (a) B-cell activation
            (b) Complement consumption
            (c) Release of interleukin-6 (IL-6), IL-13, tumor necrosis factor (TNF), and other proinflammatory cytokines

  **b.** Etiology is unknown

  **c.** Two events are necessary for development of JRA (Miller & Cassidy, 2004):
        **i.** Immunogenetic susceptibility
        **ii.** An external, environmental trigger such as:
            (a) Virus (e.g., parvovirus B19, rubella, Epstein-Barr)
            (b) Host hyperreactivity to specific self-antigens (type II collagen)
            (c) Enhanced T-cell reactivity to bacterial or mycobacterial heat shock proteins

  **d.** Recent research shows strong evidence for genetic predisposition for JRA (Moroldo, et al., 2004)
        **i.** Sibling pairs tend to develop the same type of JRA
        **ii.** Non-twin sibling pairs develop disease an average of 5.1 years apart

  **e.** Many of the genetic predispositions for JRA and other childhood rheumatic diseases and conditions are within the major histocompatibility complex (MCH) region on chromosome 6
        **i.** Specific human leukocyte antigen (HLA) genotypes have been associated with the type and course of JRA
        **ii.** However, treatment has yet to be determined by HLA genotyping

  **f.** Selected genetic loci on chromosome 18 may play a role in the expression of complex autoimmune diseases, including JRA (Rosen, et al., 2004)

**3.** Pathophysiology

  **a.** The synovium is the target of the immune response
        **i.** Villous hypertrophy and hyperplasia of the synovium (pannus)
        **ii.** Increased production of synovial fluid
            (a) Intraarticular effusion
            (b) Visual edema of the joints
        **iii.** Hyperemia

  **b.** Synovial fluid in JRA tends to have mostly lymphocytes and plasma cells

  **c.** Increased oxidative stress is evident in the synovial fluid (Lotito, et al., 2004)

  **d.** Research has made important strides in attempting to determine the pathogenesis of JRA

  **e.** Theories include:
        **i.** Cell-mediated and humoral antibody mediation with B-cell activation
        **ii.** Knowledge of the interaction of T cells and cytokines on the synovium has led to the development of new treatments for JRA
        **iii.** Cytokines theorized to be involved are IL-1, IL-2, IL-4, IL-6, and TNF

**4.** Classification of JRA

  **a.** See Box 48-1 for American College of Rheumatology criteria for classification of JRA established in 1986, reaffirmed in 1999, and in use as of June 26, 2006 (Cassidy, et al., 1986; Miller & Cassidy, 2004)

  **b.** Classification systems
        **i.** Vary across continents and is an area of ongoing research and debate
        **ii.** Three groups have proposed classification criteria
            (a) American College of Rheumatology (ACR)

■ **BOX 48-1**
■ **CRITERIA FOR CLASSIFICATION OF JRA**

Age at onset <16 years
Arthritis
    Effusion *or*
    Swelling *or*
    Two of the following:
        Limitation of range of motion
        Tenderness or pain on motion
        Increased heat in one or more joints
Duration of disease 6 weeks or longer
Onset type defined by characteristics presenting in the first 6 months of illness:
    Oligoarthritis (pauciarticular): fewer than 5 inflamed joints
    Polyarthritis (polyarticular): 5 or more inflamed joints
    Systemic: arthritis in ≥1 joint
        Prominent visceral involvement, e.g.:
            Lymphadenopathy
            Hepatosplenomegaly
            Serositis
        Daily quotidian fever to ≥39°C for at least 2 weeks
        Fever sometimes accompanied by a classic rash
            Trunk and proximal extremities
            Evanescent salmon pink, macular
            2–5 mm in diameter
Exclusion of other forms of juvenile arthritis

From Miller, M., & Cassidy, J. T. (2004). Juvenile rheumatoid arthritis. In R. E. Behrman, R. M. Kliegman, & H. B. Jenson (Eds.). *Nelson textbook of pediatrics* (17th ed.). Philadelphia: Saunders, pp. 799–805.

   (b) European League Against Rheumatism (EULAR)
   (c) International League of Associations for Rheumatology (ILAR)
iii. Historically, in the United States and Canada, physicians have adopted the ACR criteria for JRA, which describes three disease subtypes
   (a) This classification represents disease at onset (first 6 months of disease)
   (b) May not accurately address the course and progression of disease after 6 months
   (c) This is especially important when reviewing studies on the efficacy of disease treatment, prognosis, and outcome
   (d) A shift to adopt the ILAR criteria may be the future of JRA classification, but this has not yet been determined
   (e) All other diseases in the differential diagnosis must be excluded (Box 48-2)

5. Presentation
   a. Signs and symptoms that may be seen in primary care (Cassidy & Petty, 2001; Cimaz & Simonini, 2003; Taylor & Erlandson, 2001)
      i. Morning stiffness
      ii. Joint pain and swelling later in day
      iii. Altered mobility
      iv. Joint usually *not* erythematous
      v. Fever
      vi. Rash

■ **BOX 48-2**
■ **DIFFERENTIAL DIAGNOSES FOR JRA**

Other rheumatic diseases of childhood:
  Systemic lupus erythematosus
  Juvenile dermatomyositis
  Juvenile spondyloarthropathy
  Scleroderma
  Sarcoidosis
  Vasculitis syndromes
Local infection or inflammation (septic arthritis, reactive arthritis, osteomyelitis)
Systemic infection (rheumatic fever, Lyme disease, sepsis)
Tuberculosis
Malignancy (leukemia, neuroblastoma)
Hemophilia
Trauma
Autoimmune hepatitis
Leukemia
Inflammatory bowel disease
Cystic fibrosis
Type 1 diabetes
Lymphedema
Henoch-Schönlein purpura
Cyclic fever syndromes
Sickle cell anemia
Legg-Calvé-Perthes disease
Slipped capital femoral epiphysis
Mechanical problems

       vii. Fatigue
      viii. Irritability
        ix. Anemia
         x. Loss of appetite
       xi. Change in or difficulty with activities of daily living, including play

  **b.** Oligoarthritis JRA
        i. Peak onset is between 1 and 3 years of age
       ii. Course of onset can be acute or insidious
      iii. Synovitis in one joint (50% of cases) or up to four joints
      iv. Early onset is most common in girls before the age of 5 years
       v. A second group is late onset after the age of 9 years
         (a) More common in males
         (b) Often complains of enthesitis (inflammation at insertion of muscle to bone) or tendonitis
         (c) Up to 50% may be positive for HLA-B27
      vi. The joints commonly involved are the knees and ankles
         (a) If there is only one joint involved, it is usually the knee
         (b) Occasionally the smaller joints of the hands and feet may be involved
         (c) The distribution is typically asymmetric
      vii. Morning stiffness is common, but child may not always complain of pain

       **viii.** Antinuclear antibody (ANA) is positive in about 60% to 70% of cases

       **ix.** Rheumatoid factor is usually negative

  **c.** Polyarthritis JRA

     **i.** Two subgroups

        (a) Rheumatoid factor (RF) positive (+) JRA

          (1) Approximately 50% to 75% are ANA positive

        (b) Rheumatoid factor (RF) negative (−) JRA

     **ii.** Onset is usually early childhood, but can be at any age

     **iii.** Onset is most commonly insidious with a progression of joints

     **iv.** Females are affected more than males

     **v.** Synovitis in five or more joints; can be as many as 20 to 40 separate joints

     **vi.** Joint involvement is usually symmetric with the knees, wrists, elbows, and ankles the most common

        (a) Small joints of the hands and feet may be early or late symptoms

        (b) Hips, cervical spine, temporomandibular joint, and shoulders are involved about 50% of the time

        (c) Hip involvement, however, is not usually present at disease onset, but develops 1 to 6 years later

        (d) Hip involvement is typically bilateral, but can be unilateral (Spencer & Bernstein, 2002)

     **vii.** Morning stiffness is common

     **viii.** Joints are swollen and warm, but *not* erythematous

     **ix.** Rheumatoid nodules on elbows and Achilles tendon area indicate a severe course

     **x.** Extra-articular symptoms may include:

        (a) Fatigue

        (b) Low-grade fever

        (c) Weight loss

        (d) Decreased growth

     **xi.** Extra-articular signs may include:

        (a) Hepatosplenomegaly

        (b) Pericardial effusions

        (c) Uveitis

        (d) Lymphadenopathy

     **xii.** If RF (+), may have rheumatoid nodules or vasculitis

  **d.** Systemic JRA

     **i.** Onset can be at any age

     **ii.** Males are usually affected more than females

     **iii.** Characterized by: (Miller & Cassidy, 2004)

        (a) Arthritis in one or more joints

        (b) Prominent visceral involvement

          (1) Lymphadenopathy

          (2) Hepatosplenomegaly

          (3) Serositis (e.g., pericardial effusion)

        (c) Daily fever over at least 2 weeks, with daily high-spiking fevers ≥39° C followed by normal or subnormal temperatures

        (d) Fever sometimes accompanied by a classic rash

          (1) Trunk and proximal extremities

          (2) Typically salmon pink, macular, 2 to 5 mm in diameter

          (3) Evanescent

        (e) Koebner's phenomenon—cutaneous hypersensitivity to superficial trauma, e.g., fingernail rubbed across uninvolved skin

      **iv.** ANA is negative

      **v.** Rheumatoid factor is negative

      **vi.** Extra-articular symptoms include malaise, irritability

      **vii.** Extra-articular signs include severe anemia, leukocytosis, thrombocytosis, pericarditis, myocarditis, hepatosplenomegaly, serositis, lymphadenopathy, and vasculitis

  **e.** Serious complications that require immediate referral to ED and pediatric rheumatologist

    **i.** Macrophage activation syndrome (MAS) or reactive hematophagocytic lymphohistiocytosis (Miller & Cassidy, 2004)

      (a) An acute, but rare complication of JRA

      (b) Patients are acutely ill and early recognition is *critical*

      (c) Most common in males with systemic JRA

      (d) Etiology is unknown but may occur:

        (1) Spontaneously

        (2) With abrupt change in medications

        (3) In association with viral infection

      (e) Associated with serious morbidity and mortality

      (f) Symptoms may include persistent fever, hepatosplenomegaly, encephalopathy, mental changes, bruising, purpura, or mucosal bleeding

      (g) Laboratory changes include decreased leukocytes, erythrocytes and platelet counts, low erythrocyte sedimentation rate (ESR), elevated serum liver enzymes, prolonged PT, PTT, elevated ferritin levels

      (h) Diagnosis is confirmed by demonstrating hematophagocytic histiocytes in bone marrow and lymph nodes

      (i) IMMEDIATE intervention is needed

        (1) Treatment usually requires high-dose intravenous methylprednisolone

        (2) Cyclosporine A has been used for treatment

        (3) Anecdotal reports of use of antitumor necrosis factor medications

    **ii.** Cricoarytenoid arthritis is another rare complication of systemic JRA

      (a) Most commonly found in systemic JRA

      (b) Associated with laryngeal stridor

      (c) IMMEDIATE intervention is necessary

      (d) Treatment usually requires high-dose intravenous methylprednisolone

    **iii.** Digital endarteritis and potential autoamputation is rare

**6.** Focused assessment

  **a.** JRA has the potential to be systemic

  **b.** Diagnosis is by exclusion of other potential causes (see Box 48-2 for differential diagnoses)

  **c.** Special attention should be given to:

    **i.** Joint signs and symptoms

    **ii.** Pattern of arthritis

    **iii.** Rash (if present)

    **iv.** Duration of signs and symptoms

    **v.** Extra-articular manifestations

    **vi.** Antecedent illnesses or trauma

    **vii.** Response to any treatment

  **d.** History should include information such as duration of illness, any morning stiffness, time of day for pain, level of pain, how often symptoms occur, fevers, joint swelling, history of infectious disease, social history, and family medical history

e. Inspection

    i. Assess for facial symmetry

      (a) Micrognathia and facial asymmetry could mean temporomandibular joint involvement

    ii. Observe how the child uses the joints

      (a) Manner of joint use may be altered to accommodate for pain

    iii. Observe for limb avoidance

    iv. Assess gait

    v. Inspect for flexion contractures, joint subluxations

    vi. Measure degree of muscle atrophy around inflamed joints as compared with noninflamed identical joint

    vii. Inspect for leg length because there is a tendency for overgrowth of affected leg in uncontrolled disease

    viii. Inspect skin for rashes, nodules, bruising, alopecia, tightening, and Raynaud's phenomenon

    ix. Inspect eyes for sharp optic discs, synechiae (adhesion of iris to cornea), redness, photophobia, changes in vision, and band keratopathy (AAP, 1993)

    x. Inspect the nose and mouth for aphthous ulcers

f. Auscultation

    i. Heart for rhythm and murmurs

    ii. Lungs for absence of wheezes, rales, crackles, rhonchi, and rubs

    iii. Abdomen for active bowel sounds

g. Palpation

    i. Palpate joints for swelling, warmth, and tenderness (Reece, 2004)

    ii. Evaluate joint range of motion

    iii. Palpate joints for small outpouchings of synovium

      (a) May occur at extensor surfaces of phalangeal joints, ankles, or wrists

      (b) May also occur in larger areas such as the popliteal space (Baker's cysts)

    iv. Palpate abdomen for hepatosplenomegaly

    v. Palpate lymph nodes for lymphadenopathy

---

■ **BOX 48-3**

■ **WHEN TO REFER CHILDREN TO A PEDIATRIC RHEUMATOLOGIST**

Prolonged or unexplained fever
Loss of function
Normal laboratory tests but local or generalized pain and/or swelling in joints
Abnormal laboratory findings but symptoms do not fit criteria for a rheumatic disease
Symptom reports not consistent with laboratory or physical findings
Undefined autoimmune disease
Unexplained combination of symptoms that may include:
  Rash
  Arthritis, musculoskeletal pain
  Anemia, weakness, fatigue, anorexia
  Weight loss

From Rettig, P. A., Merhar, S. L., & Cron, R. Q. (2004). Juvenile rheumatoid arthritis and juvenile spondyloarthropathy. In P. L. Jackson & J. A. Vessey (Eds.). *Primary care of the child with a chronic condition* (4th ed.). St. Louis: Mosby, pp. 582–600.

    **h.** Percussion
        **i.** Percuss liver and spleen for hepatosplenomegaly
**7.** When to refer (Box 48-3) (Rettig, et al., 2004; Sandborg & Wallace, 1999)
**8.** Diagnostic tests
    **a.** Diagnosis is by exclusion (see Box 48–2 for differential diagnoses)
    **b.** No one laboratory test will make the diagnosis of JRA
    **c.** Tests are used to:
        **i.** Support physical findings
        **ii.** Identify risk factors
        **iii.** Monitor therapy and response to treatment
        **iv.** Exclude other disease possibilities
    **d.** Evaluation may include the following laboratory measures: (Cassidy & Petty, 2001)
        **i.** Complete blood count
            (a) Rule out certain malignancies
            (b) Anemia of chronic illness (poly and systemic JRA)
            (c) Leukocytosis and thrombocytosis (poly and systemic JRA)
        **ii.** ESR increase indicates inflammation
        **iii.** C-reactive protein (CRP) increase indicates inflammation
        **iv.** Rheumatoid factor
            (a) Not diagnostic
            (b) Not reliable for arthritis
            (c) Positive for only about 8% of children with JRA
            (d) Useful to determine prognosis in polyarthritis and systemic JRA (Duffy, 2004)
        **v.** Antinuclear antibody (ANA)
            (a) Not diagnostic
            (b) Positive in 40% to 85% of poly and oligoarthritis but unusual with systemic JRA
            (c) Possible to have + ANA and *not* have rheumatic disease
            (d) Risk factor for uveitis
        **vi.** Complements C3 and C4 to rule out systemic lupus erythematosus (SLE)
        **vii.** Cytokines—increased
        **viii.** Urinalysis to rule out SLE, renal disease, and vasculitis
        **ix.** Liver and renal function tests
        **x.** Immunoglobulins
    **e.** Synovial fluid analysis is probably the most valuable laboratory test
        **i.** Often difficult to obtain in children
        **ii.** *Not* diagnostic of JRA
        **iii.** Bacterial antigen detection rules out infection
        **iv.** Culture to rule out infection
        **v.** Gram stain smear to rule out infection
    **f.** X-ray of joint
        **i.** May show minimal change early in the course of the disease
        **ii.** Rule out injury
        **iii.** Periarticular soft tissue swelling or joint space widening indicates:
            (a) Increased intra-articular fluid, or
            (b) Synovial hypertrophy
    **g.** Chest x-ray to rule out tuberculosis (TB)
    **h.** Magnetic resonance imaging (MRI) reveals early joint and tissue changes even before joint space narrowing is visible on x-rays (Marin, et al., 2004)
**9.** Treatment
    **a.** Treatment is multifaceted and interdisciplinary

b. Top priorities include:
   i. Alleviating or eradicating the inflammation and pain
   ii. Preventing physical abnormalities, disability, and psychosocial problems
   iii. Ensuring achievement of normal developmental milestones
c. Other goals should be individualized and specific to each child and family
d. Five aspects of care are essential for a comprehensive management program for children with JRA (Giannini & Petty, 2001):
   i. Physical management
   ii. Psychosocial care
   iii. Nutrition
   iv. Pharmacologic management
   v. Nonrheumatologic care (primary care)
e. Physical management is attained through occupational and physical therapy
   i. Goals focus on:
      (a) Preserving or enhancing function
      (b) Preventing disability
      (c) Eliminating pain
   ii. Splinting of joints is used to:
      (a) Maintain alignment
      (b) Relieve inflammation

■ **TABLE 48-1**
■ ■ **Pharmacologic Treatment of JRA**

| Generic Names of Medication | Examples of Trade Names | Recommended Route, Dosage, Regimen | Relative Cost $ to $$$$ |
|---|---|---|---|
| | | **Nonsteroidal Antiinflammatory Drugs (NSAIDs)** | |
| Naproxen | Naprosyn, Anaprox, Aleve | 10–15 mg/kg/day divided bid oral | $ |
| Ibuprofen | Advil, Motrin, Nuprin | 30–40 mg/kg/day divided tid oral | $ |
| Indomethacin | Indocin | 1–3 mg/kg/day divided tid oral | $ |
| Tolmetin sodium | Tolectin | 20–30 mg/kg/day divided tid oral | $$ |
| Nabumetone | Relafen | 500 or 750 mg tid oral | $$ |
| Sulindac | Clinoril | 3–4 mg/kg/day bid oral | $$ |
| | | **Disease-Modifiying Antirheumatic Drugs (DMARDs)** | |
| Methotrexate | Methotrexate Trexall | 10–20 mg/m$^2$ *or* 0.3–0.6 mg/kg once a week oral or subcutaneous | $$ |
| Sulfasalazine | Azulfidine | 40–60 mg/kg/day divided bid oral, maximum of 3 g | $ |
| Hydroxychloroquine | Plaquenil | 5 mg/kg/day oral | $$ |
| Etanercept | Enbrel | 0.4 mg/kg/dose twice weekly subQ, maximum dose 25mg | $$$$ |
| Infliximab | Remicade | 3–5 mg/kg/dose once every 4–8 weeks IV | $$$$ |
| Cyclosporine A | Neoral, Sandimmune | 2–5 mg/kg/day divided bid oral | $$$ |
| Azathioprine | Imuran | 1–3 mg/kg/day oral | $$$ |
| IVIG | Gammar P | 1–2 g/kg once monthly IV | $$$ |
| Solumedrol | Solumedrol | 30 mg/kg/dose once weekly IV Maximum dose 1g | $$$ |
| Cyclophosphamide | Cytoxan | 0.5–1 g once monthly IV | $$$ |

      (c) Reduce flexion contractures

      (d) Provide support during functional activities

  **f.** Pharmacologic management of inflammation (Table 48-1)

     **i.** Therapeutic pyramid of juvenile arthritis indicates increasing levels of pharmacologic intervention for inflammation (Miller & Cassidy, 2004) (Figure 48-1)

       (a) The base of the pyramid is the least toxic, nonsteroidal antinflammatory drugs (NSAIDs)

       (b) Corticosteroids are at the peak of the pyramid, reserved for severe inflammation or systemic illness

       (c) Adverse effects of corticosteroids include:

         (1) Weight gain

         (2) Linear growth suppression

         (3) Fluid retention

         (4) Cataracts

         (5) Glaucoma

         (6) Osteoporosis

         (7) Avascular necrosis

         (8) Gastric ulcers and bleeding

         (9) Hypertension

        (10) Acceleration of:

           a) Atherosclerosis

           b) Hyperglycemia

           c) Poor wound healing

           d) Potential for severe, even life-threatening infection such as varicella zoster

    **ii.** Pain

      (a) Pharmacologic methods—see guidelines for management of pain in juvenile chronic arthritis from the American Pain Society (Simon, et al., 2002)

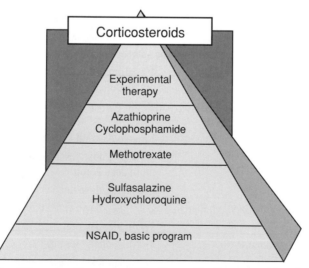

FIGURE 48-1 ■ The "therapeutic pyramid" of juvenile rheumatoid arthritis. (Reprinted with permission from Behrman, R. E., Kliegman, R. M., & Jenson, H. B. [Eds.]. *Nelson textbook of pediatrics* [17th ed.]. Philadelphia: Saunders, p. 804.

        (b) Nonpharmacologic pain management
           (1) Heat and cold modalities
           (2) Exercise
           (3) Distraction
           (4) Meditation
           (5) Cognitive behavioral therapy
           (6) Warm bath

**iii. Uveitis**

        (a) Topical steroids are the common initial treatment used to control eye inflammation related to uveitis

        (b) Long-term corticosteroid use may lead to cataracts and glaucoma

        (c) Some cases of JRA-associated uveitis do not respond adequately to corticosteroids

        (d) Other options include:
           (1) Methotrexate
           (2) Azathioprine
           (3) Cyclosporine
           (4) Chlorambucil

        (e) The latest promising medications to be researched are the TNF inhibitors such as Enbrel and Remicade (Rosenberg, 2002)

    **iv.** Localized or intra-articular steroid injections are effective if only one or two joints are affected

        (a) Early aggressive treatment in oligoarthritis is safe and effective
           (1) Prevents leg length discrepancy
           (2) Provides rapid resolution of signs and symptoms of active inflammation

        (b) Reduces erosion of articular cartilage and contiguous bone

**g.** Dental

    **i.** Routine dental assessment

    **ii.** Referral to experienced dentist or maxillofacial teams is often necessary

**h.** Exercise—individualized conditioning programs have physical and psychologic benefits (Rettig, Merhar, & Cron, 2004)

**i.** Nutrition

    **i.** Nutritional screening is recommended, especially:

        (a) For children with weight gain or loss that is not consistent with their predicted growth curve

        (b) If corticosteroids are prescribed

    **ii.** Evaluation of bone mineralization with dual-energy x-ray absorptiometry (DEXA) scan is particularly important:

        (a) If corticosteroids are prescribed

        (b) With a history of fractures

**j.** Psychosocial care

    **i.** Goal is for the child and family to optimally adjust to the disease and treatment

    **ii.** Self-management skills and education are necessary as the child ages

    **iii.** An interdisciplinary team should work to keep child in school

    **iv.** School interventions or modifications to activities are often necessary, such as:

        (a) Late arrival

        (b) Extra time between classes

        (c) Two sets of books for school and home

        (d) Physical education adaptations

      **v.** Rehabilitation 504 Act

        (a) For nondiscrimination against disability, it may be necessary to invoke this Act on behalf of the children

        (b) Federal law that makes provisions for children with special needs in school; the school nurse is a valuable resource for the family

  **k.** The role of surgery in JRA is limited

      **i.** Interventions may include soft tissue releases, arthroscopy, and arthroplasty

      **ii.** Factors that typically influence the decision to perform arthroplasty are:

        (a) Pain

        (b) Child's age with growth potential

        (c) The longevity of the prosthesis

      **iii.** Before surgery, alterations in the pharmacologic regimen may be required, such as discontinuing or changing NSAIDs in order to decrease risk of bleeding

      **iv.** Some advanced drug therapies may need to be altered in order to promote optimal healing

      **v.** Any child with cervical spine involvement should have radiographic evaluation

        (a) To assess risk of instability of the cervical spine before anesthesia and intubation

        (b) Instability of the atlantoaxial joint may lead to impingement of the cord or brainstem

  **l.** Ophthalmology care

      **i.** Females younger than 5 years of age and a positive ANA are at high risk for developing uveitis, an eye inflammation

      **ii.** Uveitis involves the anterior chamber of the eye in 30% to 40% of cases

      **iii.** 40% to 50% of cases of uveitis have posterior uveitis (Rosenberg, 2002)

      **iv.** Uveitis is usually asymptomatic

      **v.** If left untreated, uveitis can result in visual impairment

      **vi.** All children with JRA should have a baseline slit-lamp examination by an ophthalmologist to determine if uveitis is present

      **vii.** Ophthalmologic care and treatment for these children must be individualized to meet the child's needs; frequent monitoring is essential

  **m.** Complementary and alternative therapies (Rettig, et al., 2004)

      **i.** About 68% of parents have used an unconventional or unproven remedies such as copper bracelets

      **ii.** Glucosamine and chondroitin sulfate are sometimes helpful in osteoarthritis, but not inflammatory arthritis

      **iii.** Few controlled clinical trials have tested the safety and efficacy of these therapies

      **iv.** Potential risk may be medication interactions, financial waste

      **v.** Patient or family must be made to feel comfortable enough to report use of these therapies

**10.** Influence on growth and development

  **a.** Growth restriction is common in children with rheumatic disease

  **b.** JRA can cause both localized and systemic growth disturbances including:

      **i.** Linear growth

      **ii.** Weight

      **iii.** Bone health

      **iv.** Skeletal growth

  **v.** Nutrition

   (a) Protein energy malnutrition and vitamin and mineral deficiencies have been linked to JRA

  **vi.** Sexual maturation is often delayed

**c.** Generalized growth disturbance is related to:

  **i.** Disease activity

  **ii.** Side effects of medications

  **iii.** Corticosteroids affect stature secondary to slow bone growth and vertebral compression fractures

**d.** Linear growth retardation (<5th percentile) occurs in 50% of cases of systemic JRA

**e.** Mean weight for age and weight per height are often decreased in polyarthritis

**f.** Sexual maturation can also be affected by JRA

  **i.** Puberty and development of secondary sexual characteristics are often delayed

  **ii.** Adolescent females (especially with polyarthritis) can have menarche delayed by about 8 months (mean 13.2 years)

**g.** Bone mineral density

  **i.** Reduced in about 30% of mild to moderately ill children with JRA

  **ii.** Reductions are associated with more active and severe disease, and limitation in physical function

**h.** Localized growth disturbance in JRA

  **i.** Can lead to significant or noticeable deformities

  **ii.** Localized disturbances can result from:

   (a) Accelerated development of ossification centers of long bones

   (b) Early closure of epiphysis

   (c) Destruction of a growth center

  **iii.** Hyperemia surrounding the joint provides excess nourishment to the bones, leading to overgrowth

   (a) When overgrowth occurs in an extremity, such as a leg or a phalange, a discrepancy in length and size becomes apparent

   (b) If hyperemia subsides in a short time, the rate of growth normalizes and the "catch-up growth phenomenon" allows the unaffected side to reduce or eliminate the discrepancy

   (c) Long-term effects may include shortening or lengthening of the affected limb or extremity

    (1) Depend considerably on the age of the child or skeletal maturation at the time of increased disease activity and inflammation

  **iv.** An area of particular concern is the temporomandibular joint

   (a) Restricted mandibular growth results in micrognathia, causing a recessed jaw

   (b) Becomes more apparent with accelerated skeletal growth

   (c) Can result in associated dental problems such as crowding of teeth, abnormal bite, and abnormal location of tooth eruption

**i.** Functional assessment tools

  **i.** Juvenile Arthritis Functional Assessment Report (Howe, et al., 1991)

  **ii.** Juvenile Arthritis Functional Assessment Scale (Lovell, et al., 1989)

**j.** Social

  **i.** Problems with social function may result from:

   (a) Increase in disabilities from JRA over time

   (b) Medications

      (c) Fatigue

      (d) Frequency of doctor visits

    ii. In general, several studies have found that (Bowyer, et al., 2003; Gerhardt, et al., 2003; Huygen, Kuis, & Sinnema, 1999; LeBovidge, et al., 2003; Reiter-Purtill, et al., 2003):

      (a) Children with JRA were not different from controls in social functioning, social reputation, or social acceptance

      (b) Children with JRA were not perceived by their peers as physically different or less athletically competent

        (1) This did not vary by school grade, gender, or disease severity

      (c) A trend over time that friends believed that the child with JRA showed withdrawn behavior

      (d) Children with JRA had equally positive self-esteem, perceived competence, and body image as children without JRA

      (e) Children with JRA believed that they were socially competent, but had less opportunity or energy to participate in social activities

      (f) The family structures or children with JRA were very cohesive

      (g) Most children with JRA who have school difficulties have limitations only in physical education classes

      (h) A few children with polyarthritis and systemic disease may have difficulty tolerating a full day of school

  **k.** Transition of older adolescents to adult care

    **i.** Refer teenagers with JRA to vocational counselors regarding (White, 1999):

      (a) Job or career choices

      (b) College issues

      (c) Transition to independence

    **ii.** Focus groups showed that adolescents want: (Shaw, Southwood, & McDonagh, 2004)

      (a) Individualized assessment of their holistic needs

      (b) Shared decision making

      (c) Continuity of health professionals

      (d) Wider access to information and community services

**11.** Follow-up

  **a.** In JRA specialty care

    **i.** Monitor for medication toxicity by obtaining cell counts, liver and kidney functions

    **ii.** Monitor hemoglobin and hematocrit for anemia of chronic illness versus iron deficiency anemia, or GI bleed

    **iii.** Monitor platelets, ESR, and CRP

      (a) Increase with inflammation

      (b) May indicate a disease flare, macrophage activation syndrome, or a GI bleed

  **b.** In primary care (Rettig, et al., 2004)

    **i.** Routine immunizations if child is in remission and not immunosuppressed

    **ii.** Monitor height, weight, and BMI on growth charts at least annually

    **iii.** Monitor blood pressure

      (a) May increase with medications, especially systemic corticosteroids and with kidney disease

  **c.** Encourage American Dietetic Association (ADA) recommended doses of calcium with vitamin D to prevent bone loss

    **d.** Monitor functional status

    **e.** Monitor psychosocial functioning

        **i.** Encourage parents to maintain age-appropriate discipline and avoid overprotection

    **f.** Monitor school issues

        **i.** Mobility, e.g., stair climbing, writing, prolonged sitting, carrying books, cafeteria tray, raising hand

        **ii.** Participate in development of an individualized educational plan (IEP) or 504 plan

    **g.** Monitor nutritional status

    **h.** Eye examinations as per the American Academy of Pediatrics recommendations (AAP, 1993)

    **i.** Family factors that enhance a child's ability to successfully cope with a chronic disease (Huygen, et al., 2000)

        **i.** Highly cohesive family

        **ii.** Environment of flexibility

        **iii.** Individual freedom

        **iv.** Emphasis on self-mastery

    **j.** Enhancing family coping skills may be accomplished through educational programs sponsored by the American Juvenile Arthritis Organization/Arthritis Foundation and through retreats and workshops

**12.** Prognosis and long-term implications

    **a.** Prognosis and disease outcome in JRA depend on the disease subtype and course of disease

    **b.** As of June 2005, treatment outcomes continue to be evaluated in terms of 30% improvement from baseline in 3 of 6 variables, according to American College of Rheumatology criteria established in 1997 (Giannini, et al., 1997)

        **i.** The six variables include: physician's global assessment, well-being, functional ability, number of joints with active arthritis, number of joints with limited mobility, erythrocyte sedimentation rate

        **ii.** Definitions developed for each of these variables have greater than 80% sensitivity and specificity compared to physician consensus as the gold standard

    **c.** Longitudinal research is needed that standardizes study design and measurement of predictors and outcomes (Ravelli, 2004)

    **d.** Historically it was believed that the majority of patients have a satisfactory outcome with no serious disability and minimal recurrence of arthritis

    **e.** Recent research (Duffy, 2004)

        **i.** There has been an improvement in overall outcomes

        **ii.** Yet active disease persists in a significant proportion of individuals into adulthood

        **iii.** Poly and systemic JRA with positive rheumatoid factor have a poorer prognosis

        **iv.** After 10 years of follow-up, active joint disease was evident in 31% to 55% of patients with JRA

            **(a)** The development of joint space narrowing and erosions significantly correlated with poorer functional outcome

                **(1)** All subtypes developed radiographic changes, with frequencies of 28%, 54%, and 45% for oligoarthritis, polyarthritis, and systemic disease, respectively

   (2) Radiographic changes occurred in patients with polyarthritis and systemic disease, within 2.2 to 2.5 years after disease onset

   (3) Patients with oligoarthritis disease developed changes within about 5 years

   (4) Mortality rates ranged from 0.29 to 1.1 per 100 patients

**f.** Extent of hand involvement may be a predictor of long-term disability

**g.** Delay in referral and initiation of treatment contributes to poorer outcome (Cassidy & Petty, 2001)

**h.** 80% of those who remain oligoarthritic have the best overall prognosis, i.e., no difficulty at 15-year follow-up

  **i.** Exceptions are those who develop eye disease or progress to polyarthritis disease

  **ii.** Up to 50% may develop a polyarthritis course

  **iii.** Up to 15% may develop severe joint disease

  **iv.** A major cause of morbidity in oligoarthritis is uveitis

**i.** Research on prognosis of JRA focuses on three outcomes:

  **i.** Functional disability

  **ii.** Health status

  **iii.** Psychosocial outcome

**j.** Functional disability

  **i.** When measuring function, specific attention must be given to age-specific roles and tasks at all developmental stages

  **ii.** Assessment of joint status takes into account continued disease activity, and the development of joint space narrowing or erosions

  **iii.** Numerous reliable instruments are available to measure function in children with JRA (Duffy, Tucker & Burgos-Vargas, 2000)

  **iv.** After approximately 10 years of follow-up, normal vision was present in 70% (median), and blindness occurred in 0% to 24% (Cassidy & Petty, 2001)

**k.** Children with rheumatoid factor (+) polyarthritis (seropositive) have a poorer prognosis and more severe course

  **i.** Hip disease may develop in up to 50%

  **ii.** Hip disease is often a major cause of disability in JRA and a poor prognostic sign

**l.** Only about 50% of patients with systemic JRA recover completely

  **i.** The other half show progressive involvement of joints

   (a) Outcome can depend on several factors, such as persistent disease activity, onset of disease before the age of 5, and development of complications that affect morbidity or mortality (Cassidy & Petty, 2001; White, 2003)

   (1) Pericarditis

   (2) Infection

   (3) Macrophage activation syndrome

  **ii.** One must take into account that most patients included in many of the long-term outcome reviews were diagnosed with JRA before:

   (a) The use of methotrexate as part of the standardized therapeutic regimen

   (b) The development of biologics for use in JRA

   (c) Improved methods of measuring adaptation to chronic disease and quality of life

**m.** Psychosocial outcome

  **i.** Overall, the long-term psychosocial outcome appears favorable in JRA

       **ii.** Studies from Norway supported findings that the long-term outcome was more favorable than had been previously noted

         **(a)** May be due to decreased bias of admission, or early use of more aggressive treatment regimens

         **(b)** Poor psychosocial outcomes are associated with:

           **(1)** Premorbid psychosocial dysfunction

           **(2)** Chronic family difficulties

           **(3)** Major life events

**n.** Current trends:

    **i.** In an effort to better define outcome, the pediatric rheumatology community has developed a core set of outcome variables:

       **(a)** Method to monitor disease activity

       **(b)** Disease improvement

       **(c)** Disease flare

    **ii.** These outcomes continue to be used in clinical drug trials

    **iii.** Specific variables include: (Giannini, et al., 1997)

       **(a)** Patient, parent, and physician global assessments

       **(b)** Childhood health assessment questionnaire

       **(c)** Number of active joints

       **(d)** ESR

    **iv.** Health care providers also need to continue to assess quality of life and effects of newer treatment modalities on quality of life (Miller et al., 2002)

    **v.** With these new methods to monitor the progress of children with JRA, the long-term outcome is likely to improve in the future

# REFERENCES

American Academy of Pediatrics (AAP) (1993). Guidelines for ophthalmologic examinations in children with juvenile rheumatoid arthritis. *Pediatrics, 92*(2) part 1 of 2, 295-296. (Guidelines reaffirmed in 1999 by AAP Section on Ophthalmology and Section on Rheumatology and considered up to date as of June 1, 2006). See http://aappolicy.aappublications.org/cgi/content/abstract/pediatrics;92/2/295.

Behrman, R. E., Kliegman, R. M., & Jenson, H. B. (Eds.). *Nelson textbook of pediatrics* (17th ed.). Philadelphia: Saunders.

Bowyer, S. L., Roetcher, P. A., Higgins, G. C., et al. (2003). Health status of patients with juvenile rheumatoid arthritis at 1 and 5 years after diagnosis. *J Rheumatol, 30*(2), 394-400.

Cassidy, J. T., Levinson, J. E., Bass, J. C., et al. (1986). A study of classification criteria for a diagnosis of juvenile rheumatoid arthritis. *Arthritis Rheumatol, 29*, 274-281. (ACR 1986 Reassessment of the 1977 Criteria for JRA. Continues to be applied as of June 1, 2005). See www.rheumatology.org/publications/abbreviations/gl.asp?aud=mem.

Cassidy, J. T., & Petty, R. E. (2001). Juvenile rheumatoid arthritis. In J. T. Cassidy, & R. E. Petty (Eds.). *Textbook of pediatric rheumatology* (4th ed.). Philadelphia: Saunders, pp. 214-217.

Cimaz, R., & Simonini, G. (2003). Review for the primary care physician: Differential diagnosis of arthritis in children. *Pediatric rheumatology online journal*, retrieved June 1, 2005, from www.pedrheumonlinejournal.org/issues1/DIFFERENTIAL%20PROJ.htm.

Duffy, C. M. (2004). Health outcomes in pediatric rheumatic diseases. *Curr Opin Rheumatol, 16*(2), 102-108.

Duffy, C., Tucker, L., Burgos-Vargas, R. (2000). Update on functional assessment tools. *J Rheumatol, 27*(Suppl. 58), 11-14.

Gerhardt, C. A., Vannatta, K., McKellop, J. M., et al. (2003). Brief report: Child-rearing practices of caregivers with and without a child with juvenile rheumatoid arthritis: perspectives of caregivers and professionals. *J Pediatr Psychol, 28*(4), 275-279.

Giannini, E. H., & Petty, R. E. (2001). Treatment of juvenile rheumatoid arthritis. In J. W. Koopman (Ed.). *Arthritis and allied conditions: A textbook of rheumatology* (14th ed.). New York: Lippincott Williams & Wilkins, pp. 1294-1310.

Giannini, E. H., Ruperto, N., Ravelli, A., et al. (1997). Preliminary definition of improvement in juvenile arthritis. *Arthritis Rheumatol, 40*, 1202-1209. (Continues to be applied as of June 1, 2005). See www.rheumatology.org/publications/abbreviations/gl.asp?aud=mem.

Howe, S., Levinson, J., Shear, E., et al. (1991). Development of a disability measurement tool for juvenile rheumatoid arthritis: the Juvenile Arthritis functional assessment report for children and their parents. *Arthritis Rheumatol, 34*, 873-880.

Huygen, A. C., Kuis, W., & Sinnema, G. (2000). Psychological, behavioural, and social adjustment in children and adolescents with juvenile chronic arthritis. *Ann Rheum Dis, 59*(4), 276-282.

LeBovidge, J. S., Lavigne, J. V., Donenberg, G. R., & Miller, M. L. (2003). Psychological adjustment of children and adolescents with chronic arthritis: A meta-analytic review. *J Pediatr Psychol, 28*(1), 29-39.

Lotito, A. P. N., Muscara, M. N., Kiss, M. H. B., et al. (2004). Nitric oxide-derived species in synovial fluid from patients with juvenile idiopathic arthritis. *J Rheumatol, 31*(5), 998-1000.

Lovell, D. J., Howe, S., Shear, E., et al. (1989). Development of a disability measurement tool for juvenile rheumatoid arthritis: the Juvenile Arthritis Functional Assessment Scale. *Arthritis Rheumatol, 32*, 1390-1395.

Marin, C., Sanchez-Alegre, M. L., Gallego, C., et al. (2004). Magnetic resonance imaging of osteoarticular infections in children. *Curr Prob Diag Radiol, 33*(2), 43-59.

Miller, M., & Cassidy, J. T. (2004). Juvenile rheumatoid arthritis. In R. E. Behrman, R. M. Kliegman, & H. B. Jenson (Eds.). *Nelson textbook of pediatrics* (17th ed.). Philadelphia: Saunders, pp. 799-805.

Miller, M. L., LeBovidge, J., & Feldman, B. (2002). Health-related quality of life in children with arthritis. *Rheum Dis Clin North Am, 28*(3), 493-501, vi.

Prahalad, S., Bove, K. E., Dickens, D., et al. (2001). Etanercept in the treatment of macrophage activation syndrome. *J Rheumatol, 28*(9), 2120-2124.

Ravelli, A. (2004). Toward an understanding of the long-term outcome of juvenile idiopathic arthritis. *Clin Exper Rheumatol, 22*(3), 271-275.

Reece, G. (2004). A 4½ year old with a swollen knee. *J Pediatr Health Care, 18*(3), 153, 161-162.

Reiter-Purtill, J., Gerhardt, C. A., Vannatta, K., et al. (2003). A controlled longitudinal study of the social functioning of children with juvenile rheumatoid arthritis. *J Pediatr Psychol, 28*(1), 17-28.

Rettig, P. A., Merhar, S. L., & Cron, R. Q. (2004). Juvenile rheumatoid arthritis and juvenile spondyloarthropathy. In P. L. Jackson & J. A. Vessey (Eds.). *Primary care of the child with a chronic condition* (4th ed.). St. Louis: Mosby, pp. 582-600.

Rosen, P., Hopkin, R. J., Glass, D. N., & Graham, T. B. (2004). Another patient with chromosome 18 deletion syndrome and juvenile rheumatoid arthritis. *J Rheumatol, 31*(5), 992-997.

Rosenberg, A. M. (2002). Uveitis associated with childhood rheumatic diseases. *Curr Opin Rheumatol, 14*, 542-547.

Sandborg, C. I., & Wallace, C. A. (1999). Position statement of the American College of Rheumatology regarding referral of children and adolescents to pediatric rheumatologists. *Arthritis Care Res, 12*(1), 48-51.

Shaw, K. L., Southwood, T. R., & McDonagh, J. E. (2004). User perspectives of transitional care for adolescents with juvenile idiopathic arthritis. *Rheumatology, 43*(6), 770-778.

Simon, D., Lipman, A., Jacox, A., et al. (2002). *Guidelines for the management of pain in osteoarthritis, rheumatoid arthrits, and juvenile chronic arthritis* (2nd ed.). Glenview, IL: American Pain Society, pp. 119-130.

Spencer, C. H., & Bernstein, B. H. (2002). Hip disease in juvenile rheumatoid arthritis. *Curr Opin Rheumatol, 14*, 536-541.

Taylor, J., & Erlandson, D. M. (2001). Pediatric rheumatic diseases. In L. Robbins (Ed.).

*Clincal care in the rheumatic diseases* (2nd ed.). Atlanta: American College of Rheumatology, pp. 81-88.

White, P. H. (1999). Transition to adulthood. *Curr Opin Rheumatol, 11*(5), 408-411.

White, P. Silman, A.J., Smolen, J.S., (2003). Clinical features of juvenile rheumatoid arthritis. In M. C. Hochberg, et al. (Eds.). *Rheumatology* (3rd ed., Vol. 1.). St. Louis: Mosby, pp. 959-974.

# Learning Disorders and Attention Deficit Hyperactivity Disorder

JANICE SELEKMAN, DNSc, RN

## DEFINITION—ATTENTION DEFICIT HYPERACTIVITY DISORDER (ADHD)

"Persistent pattern of inattention and/or hyperactivity-impulsivity that is more frequent and severe than is typically observed in individuals at a comparable level of development" (American Psychiatric Association [APA], 2000, p. 85).

Previous names of the condition:

- Minimal brain dysfunction
- Hyperkinetic disease of childhood
- Attention deficit disorder

1. Pathophysiology (mostly theoretical, based on MRIs and treatment trials)
    a. Neurobiologic
        i. Dysregulation of neurotransmitters, especially catecholamines (dopamine, norepinephrine)
        ii. Not enough catecholamine available at synapse to hold on to task (i.e., attention)
        iii. Decreased levels of serotonin, the predominant central inhibiting neurotransmitter, may explain the impulsivity in ADHD
    b. Neuroanatomic
        i. Prefrontal cortex (site of dopamine receptors) may be smaller with less blood flow to the area, and influence timing of responses to stimuli
        ii. Right prefrontal cortex is involved in inhibiting behavior
        iii. Frontal cortex is the site of executive functions
2. Presentation
    a. Diagnostic criteria (APA, 2000; ICSI, 2003)
        i. Symptoms and signs
            (a) Inattention
                (1) Fails to give close attention to details; makes careless mistakes
                (2) Has difficulty sustaining attention in tasks
                (3) Does not seem to listen when spoken to
                (4) Does not follow through on instructions
                (5) Has difficulty organizing tasks
                (6) Avoids, or is reluctant to engage in, tasks that require sustained mental effort

(7) Loses things necessary for tasks

(8) Easily distracted by extraneous stimuli

(9) Often forgetful in daily activities

(b) Hyperactivity/impulsivity

(1) Fidgets with hands or feet; squirms in seat

(2) Leaves seat in situations when remaining seated is expected

(3) Excessive restlessness in situations in which it is inappropriate (adolescents have subjective feelings of restlessness)

(4) Has difficulty playing quietly

(5) Acts as if driven by a motor

(6) Talks excessively

(7) Blurts out answers before questions are completed

(8) Has difficulty awaiting turn

(9) Interrupts or intrudes on others

ii. Criteria apply to children from preschool through adolescence

(a) Must meet at least six of the nine criteria in the inattention and/or hyperactivity/impulsivity categories at a level significantly more than expected for age

(b) Symptoms must be present for at least 6 months

(c) Some impairment from symptoms must be present in at least two settings (i.e., school and home) and show evidence of a clinically significant impairment in social, academic, or occupational functioning

(d) Some symptoms must be present before age 7

(e) More females have the inattentive form and are often diagnosed later in childhood than those with hyperactivity

iii. Possible diagnoses

(a) ADHD predominantly inattention: child meets criteria in inattention category but not hyperactivity category

(b) ADHD predominantly hyperactivity: child meets criteria in hyperactivity category, but not inattention category

(c) ADHD combined type: child meets criteria in both hyperactivity and inattention categories

(d) ADHD-NOS (not otherwise specified): prominent symptoms but does not meet criteria for either inattention or hyperactivity

(e) If child meets at least six criteria in each category, the label is ADHD-combined (APA, 2000)

b. Differential diagnoses (Box 49-1)

■ **BOX 49-1**
■ **DIFFERENTIAL DIAGNOSIS**

| | |
|---|---|
| Allergies | High lead levels |
| Hearing and vision problems | Hypoglycemia |
| Seizure disorder, especially absence seizures | Obstructive sleep problems |
| Neurologic trauma | Iron deficiency |
| Brain tumor | Learning disabilities |
| Thyroid abnormalities | Child abuse or family dysfunction |
| | Other psychiatric conditions |

    **c.** Diagnostic measures

      **i.** No one test exists to diagnose ADHD

      **ii.** Requires

        (a) Family history, perinatal history, developmental history, health history

        (b) Developmental assessment

        (c) Assessment of academic performance

        (d) Comprehensive age-appropriate psychologic and intelligence testing

        (e) Physical assessment, especially neurologic, hormonal, and motor

      **iii.** Must obtain input from parents and classroom teacher or school personnel. See the AAP Toolkit on AAP website (AAP, 2000)

      **iv.** Multiple behavioral rating scales are available to be used by parents and teachers

        (a) Achenbach's Child Behavior Checklist

        (b) Child Attention Profile

        (c) Conners' Rating Scales

        (d) ACTeRS

        (e) ADHD Rating Scale IV

        (f) Attention Deficit Disorder Evaluation Scale

        (g) Barkely test

        (h) Behavioral Assessment System for Children

        (i) Child Attention Profile

  **d.** Comorbidities

      **i.** 12% to 50% of children with ADHD also have another psychiatric condition (Pliszka, 2000)

      **ii.** Learning disabilities—most common (25% to 33%)

      **iii.** Neurologic conditions: seizure disorders, choreiform disorders, CNS trauma, neurologic degeneration, CNS infection

      **iv.** Biomedical conditions: cognitive deficiencies, mental retardation, fragile X syndrome, Tourette syndrome, neurofibromatosis

      **v.** Emotional and psychiatric conditions: depression, childhood mania, bipolar disorder, anxiety disorder, conduct disorder, substance abuse, pervasive developmental disorder

      **vi.** Speech and language problems: expressive, receptive, social skill deficits, hearing impairment

      **vii.** Academic and learning problems: underachievement, learning disorder, low IQ, school problems, gifted, special education requirements

**3.** Incidence and prevalence

  **a.** The most prevalent chronic health condition affecting school-age children (AAP, 2000)

  **b.** Between 3% and 14% of school-age children

  **c.** Accounts for 4% of all primary care office visits, but makes up 50% of children seen in psychiatric clinics (Stubbe, 2000)

  **d.** More males than females (2 to 3:1) (Solanto, 2001)

**4.** Etiology

  **a.** Genetic

      **i.** Probably polygenic

      **ii.** 50% chance of transmission of ADHD from parent to child

      **iii.** 87.2% concordance rate for monozygotic twins and a 37.9% concordance rate for dizygotic twins (Solanto, 2001)

      **iv.** Dopamine transporter gene *(DAT1)* and dopamine receptor gene *(DRD4)* are suspected (Jensen, 2000)

    **b.** Other causes
        **i.** Brain infections
        **ii.** Hypoxic or anoxic episodes
        **iii.** Trauma
        **iv.** Extreme prematurity
        **v.** Maternal drug or alcohol use during pregnancy
        **vi.** Exposure to high lead levels
    **c.** The following are not causes:
        **i.** Sucrose or aspartame
        **ii.** Food additives
        **iii.** Salicylates
        **iv.** Poor parenting
        **v.** Fluorescent lighting, disinfectants, vitamin deficiency

**5.** Influence on growth and development
    **a.** Weight loss may occur as a side effect of stimulant medications
    **b.** Children may be slower to attain adult height while on stimulants, but they do catch up
    **c.** No effect on developmental physical skills, unless a comorbidity exists
    **d.** Significant effect on psychologic development
        **i.** Poor self-esteem
        **ii.** Possible difficulty making or keeping friends
    **e.** Possible significant effect on academic achievement
        **i.** Educated at level less than potential
        **ii.** Difficulty maintaining employment

**6.** Treatment
    **a.** Treatment requires multimodal management coordinated by the primary care provider (ICSI, 2003)
    **b.** Pharmacologic
        **i.** Psychostimulants are the first line of treatment; highly effective in 70% to 90% (AAP, 2001; ICSI, 2003)
            (a) Methylphenidate (e.g., Ritalin, Methylin, Concerta, Metadate, Focalin)
            (b) Mixed salts of dextro- and levoamphetamines (e.g., Dexedrine, Dextrostat, Adderall, Adderall XR)
            (c) Only Adderall and Dexedrine are approved for children younger than age 6
        **ii.** Stimulants increase availability of neurotransmitters to increase focus and attention
        **iii.** Prescribing principles
            (a) Stimulant dosing is not weight dependent
            (b) Dosing: start low and go slow; titrate up at intervals of 1 week; get feedback from parents and school personnel to assess effectiveness
            (c) Behavior changes can be identified within 30 to 90 minutes of ingestion
            (d) If a child does not respond to higher doses of one stimulant, or if side effects are unacceptable, switch to another stimulant before considering other medications
            (e) As the child ages, dosage change or medication changes may be needed
            (f) Short-acting preparations generally last 4 hours and often need redosing; long-acting preparations generally last 10 to 12 hours
            (g) Avoid evening dosing to minimize insomnia

       (h) Contraindications: symptomatic cardiovascular disease, moderate hypertension, marked anxiety, glaucoma, or history of drug abuse, tic disorder, depression/ suicide risk

       (i) Long-acting stimulants can not be chewed; it destroys the delivery system

    iv. Side effects

       (a) Anorexia and weight loss

          (1) Take medications just before meals

          (2) Use nutritional supplements, such as Ensure

          (3) High-protein, high-quality foods

          (4) No empty calories

          (5) Eat larger meal for breakfast

       (b) Sleep disturbances

          (1) Arrange doses so that last dose is earlier in the day

          (2) Use short-acting medications for afternoon dose

       (c) Rebound behavioral problems when drug is wearing off

          (1) Use long-acting medications

       (d) Stomachache, nausea

          (1) Take medication with food or immediately after eating

       (e) Others: headache, irritability, dizziness, linear growth impairment

       (f) Suicidal ideation: now listed as a black box warning

    v. Second-line medications used especially with comorbidities

       (a) Aminoketone antidepressant, e.g., bupropion (Wellbutrin)

       (b) Selective norepinephrine uptake inhibitor (atomoxetine [Strattera])

          (1) Some use this as a first line medication

       (c) Tricyclic antidepressant, e.g., imipramine (Tofranil), desipramine (Norpramin)

       (d) α-adrenergic agonist, e.g., clonidine (Catapres), guanfacine (Tenex)

       (e) Selective serotonin reuptake inhibitor, e.g., sertraline HCl (Zoloft)

c. Behavioral and environmental interventions

    i. Education of key individuals: parents, teachers, other family members

    ii. Identify the child's strengths and build on them

    iii. Provide immediate and positive reinforcement for effort and achievement; reinforce only the positive

    iv. Make a hierarchy of rules

    v. Provide parent coaching; child coaching

    vi. Provide learning activities when medication is at its peak

    vii. Get child's attention first before giving directions

    viii. Remind child of critical behavior before an activity

    ix. Have clear, simple rules

    x. Develop a consistent routine

    xi. Homework issues and assignments

       (a) Have a structured environment

       (b) Break tasks into smaller parts

    xii. Build self-esteem and confidence

    xiii. Sit in front of classroom away from doors and windows

    xiv. Decrease clutter on desk and in room

    xv. Keep extra set of school books at home

    xvi. Help parents get respite; let them know often that this is not their fault (Selekman & Moore, 2004)

d. Cognitive behavioral therapy for the child

    i. Social skills training

   ii. Problem-solving training, e.g., "Stop and think before acting"
  **e.** Group treatment
      **i.** ADHD support groups
      **ii.** ADHD advocacy groups (primary care providers should advocate for appropriate school programs for children with ADHD)
**7.** Follow-up (Jellinek, et al., 2002)
  **a.** See the child at least two times per year to evaluate effects of treatment
  **b.** Observe for potential of worsening clinical status during adolescence
  **c.** Respond to parent and child concerns
  **d.** Stimulant use does *not* result in drug abuse
  **e.** Encourage good nutrition to ensure sufficient nutrients for growth
**8.** Long term
  **a.** May need to defer driver's license until condition is under control
  **b.** Resource: CHADD (Children and Adults with ADD) www.chadd.org (1–800–233–4050)
  **c.** Prognosis
      **i.** 80% still manifest symptoms as adolescents
      **ii.** 50% to 65% still manifest symptoms as adults
      **iii.** 18% to 53% will be academic underachievers (Anastopoulos & Shelton, 2001)

## REFERENCES

American Academy of Pediatrics. (2000). Clinical practice guidelines: Diagnosis and evaluation of the child with attention-deficit/hyperactivity disorder. *Pediatrics, 105*(5), 1158-1170.

American Academy of Pediatrics. (2001). Clinical practice guideline: Treatment of the school-aged child with attention-deficit/hyperactivity disorder. *Pediatrics, 108*(4), 1033-1044.

American Psychiatric Association. (2000). *Diagnostic and statistical manual of mental disorders* (4th ed.). Text revision. Washington, DC: Author.

Anastopoulos, A. & Shelton, T. (2001). *Assessing attention-deficit/hyperactivity disorder.* New York: Kluwer Academic/Plenum Publishers.

Institute for Clinical Systems Improvement (ICSI) (2003). *Diagnosis and management of ADHD* (5th ed.). Bloomington, MN: Author.

Jellinek, M., Patel, B. P., & Froehle, M. C. (Eds.). (2002). *Bright futures in practice: Mental health—volume 1. Practice guide.*

Arlington, VA: National Center for Education in Maternal and Child Health.

Jensen, P. (2000). Current concepts on etiology, pathophysiology and neurobiology. *J Am Acad Child Adolesc Psychiatry, 9*(3), 557-572.

Pliszka, S. (2000). Patterns of psychiatric co-morbidity of attention-deficit/hyperactivity disorder. *Child Adolesc Psychiatric Clin North Am, 9*(3), 525-540.

Selekman, J., & Moore, C. (2004). Attention deficit hyperactivity disorder. In P. Jackson & J. Vessey (Eds.). *Primary care of the child with a chronic condition.* St. Louis: Mosby.

Solanto, M. (2001). Attention-deficit/hyperactivity disorder: Clinical features. In M. Solanto, A. Arnsten, & F. X. Xastellanos (Eds.). *Stimulant drugs and ADHD: Basic and clinical neuroscience.* New York: Oxford University Press, pp. 3-30.

Stubbe, D. (2000). Attention-deficit/hyperactivity disorder overview: Historical perspective, current controversies, and future directions. *Child Adolesc Psychiatric Clin North Am, 9*(3), 469-479.

# 50 Renal Failure

MICHELLE PASSAMANECK, RN, MSN, CPNP, CUNP

1. Definition (Vogt & Avner, 2004)
   a. An irreversible and progressive decrease in the glomerulofiltration rate (GFR)
   b. Occurs over a period of at least 3 months
   c. Can lead to permanent renal failure
   d. Normal renal function at birth: GFR 30 to 60 mL/min/1.73 m²
   e. Normal renal function at age 2 through adulthood: GFR 80 to 140 mL/min/1.73 m²
   f. For children age ≥2 years, progression of kidney failure is further defined by stages:
      i. Stage 1 (normal): GFR greater than 90 mL/min/1.73 m²
      ii. Stage 2 (mild): GFR 60 to 89 mL/min/1.73 m²
      iii. Stage 3 (moderate): GFR 30 to 59 mL/min/1.73 m²
      iv. Stage 4 (severe): GFR 15 to 29 mL/min/1.73 m²
      v. Stage 5 (end-stage renal disease): GFR less than 15 mL/min/1.73 m²
   g. Patients usually become symptomatic at stage 3, and symptoms worsen as GFR continues to decrease. Patients can exhibit symptoms before stage 3, especially hypertension and metabolic acidosis
2. Pathophysiology
   a. Depends on underlying cause, but alterations in nephrons remaining after an initial insult cause scarring and further nephron loss (Avner, 2004; Vogt & Avner, 2004)
      i. Hyperfiltration injury to nephrons and glomeruli
      ii. Persistent proteinuria that elicits a toxic effect on glomeruli and interstitial tubules
      iii. Uncontrolled systemic or intrarenal hypertension that causes arteriolar nephrosclerosis and hyperfiltration injury
      iv. Renal calcium-phosphorus deposition in the renal interstitium and blood vessels
      v. Hyperlipidemia causes oxidant-mediated injury
   b. These processes may eventually lead to end-stage renal disease
3. Etiology and precipitating factors
   a. Causes may be congenital, acquired, inherited or metabolic (Vogt & Avner, 2004)

    **i.** Congenital—renal agenesis, hypoplasia or dysplasia
- (a) Usually in children younger than age 5
- (b) Renal agenesis
    - (1) Unilateral
    - (2) Bilateral (Potter's syndrome)
        - a) Usually accompanied by severe pulmonary hypoplasia
    - (3) Multicystic dysplastic kidney
        - a) Unilateral nonfunctioning mass with undifferentiated cells and few, if any, nephrons
        - b) 1 per 4000 live births
- (c) Renal hypoplasia—compromised growth and development of nephrons leading to a small kidney with fewer nephrons
- (d) Renal dysplasia—abnormal development of nephrons with undifferentiated cells
- (e) Obstructive uropathy (Roth, et al., 2002)
    - (1) Types
        - a) Cloacal anomalies
        - b) Exstrophy
        - c) Posterior urethral valves—1 per 5000 to 8000 live male births
        - d) Ureteropelvic junction obstruction
            - i) Narrowing of the ureter as it exits the renal pelvis
            - ii) Vast majority diagnosed before significant damage occurs
    - (2) Renal damage may occur in utero secondary to inability of bladder to empty during fetal development
- (f) Prune belly syndrome
- (g) Congenital nephrotic syndrome

   **ii.** Acquired (usually in children older than age 5)
- (a) Glomerulonephritis
    - (1) Possibly an immune system problem
    - (2) Can be poststreptococcal
- (b) Vesicoureteral reflux nephropathy
    - (1) If complicated by UTI
    - (2) Can progress to pyelonephritis, causing
        - a) Scarring
        - b) Possible chronic renal failure
- (c) Nephrolithiasis
    - (1) More likely when kidney stones cause significant or prolonged obstruction
- (d) Pyelonephritis (interstitial nephritis)
- (e) Hemolytic uremic syndrome
- (f) Systemic lupus erythematosus nephritis

  **iii.** Inherited (usually in children younger than age 5)
- (a) Familial juvenile nephronophthisis
- (b) Wilms' tumor (mostly diagnosed at age 3 to 4 years)
- (c) Focal segmental glomerulosclerosis
- (d) Sickle cell nephropathy
- (e) Medullary cystic disease
- (f) Henoch-Shönlein purpura nephritis
- (g) Alport's syndrome (congenital glomerulonephritis)
    - (1) Deafness
    - (2) Vision defects
    - (3) Progressive kidney damage

        (h) Polycystic kidney disease
            (1) Autosomal dominant
                a) Kidneys are normal up to 10 years of age
                b) Cysts begin to appear between 10 and 30 years of age
                c) Renal failure occurs between ages 45 and 60 years
            (2) Autosomal recessive
                a) Early onset of renal failure—before age 20
    **iv.** Metabolic (usually in children older than age 5)
        (a) Cystinosis—excessive excretion of amino acids, kidney stones
        (b) Hyperoxaluria

**4.** Incidence and prevalence
  **a.** Chronic renal failure (Avner, 2004; Vogt & Avner, 2004)
    **i.** Prevalence—56 per 1 million of the pediatric population ages 0 to 19
    **ii.** Incidence—18 per 1 million of the pediatric population ages 0 to 19
    **iii.** Males more than females in all age groups
        (a) Especially with congenital causes
  **b.** Polycystic kidney disease
    **i.** Autosomal recessive—1 in 10,000 live births
  **c.** Obstructive abnormalities
    **i.** Posterior urethral valves—1 in 5000 to 8000 live male births
  **d.** Kidney agenesis
    **i.** Unilateral—1 in 1100 to 1500 live births
    **ii.** Bilateral (Potter's syndrome)—1 in 4000 live births
  **e.** End-stage renal disease
    **i.** 89,252 children diagnosed in 1999 according to the United States Renal Data System
    **ii.** Incidence is 20 per million per year after age 1
    **iii.** Incidence increases with age

**5.** Assessment
  **a.** Focused assessment and likely symptoms (Box 50-1)
  **b.** Clinical, laboratory, and radiologic signs vary with the stage of renal failure and underlying pathology (Box 50-2)
  **c.** Associated secondary diagnoses (Box 50-3)

**6.** Diagnostic tests
  **a.** GFR calculation methods
    **i.** Insulin urinary clearance
        (a) Considered the gold standard
        (b) Not practical for use in pediatrics, not done routinely
    **ii.** Radionuclide studies with Cr-EDTA or Tc-DTPA
    **iii.** Timed urine collection
        (a) Done by collecting urine for 12 to 24 hours
    **iv.** Creatinine clearance $(\text{mL/min}/1.73\ \text{m}^2) = (U \times V/P) \times 1.73/\text{BSA}$
        (a) U = total urinary creatinine concentration in mg/dL
        (b) V = total urine volume in mL divided by the duration of the collection in minutes
        (c) P = serum creatinine concentration in mg/dL
        (d) BSA = body surface area
    **v.** Schwartz method is based on formula: GFR $(\text{mL/min}/1.73\text{m}^2) = kL/\text{Pcr}$
        (a) k = proportionality constant
        (b) k = 0.33 for low birth weight infants less than 1 year old
        (c) k = 0.45 for term AGA infants less than 1 year old
        (d) k = 0.55 for children and adolescent females

■ **BOX 50-1**
■ **COMPONENTS OF A FOCUSED ASSESSMENT FOR CHILDREN WITH CHRONIC RENAL FAILURE**

Accurate documentation of all medications:
  Including name, dosage, route, time and results
Cardiopulmonary assessment:
  Color of skin (anemia, oxygen perfusion)
  BP with the same, appropriate-sized cuff, in same position
  ECG
  Percuss lungs
  Auscultate lung sounds
  Evaluate cardiac rhythm
Abdominal assessment:
  Palpate for masses
  Tenderness
Urological assessment:
  Urinary output—should be 1 mL/kg/hr minimum
  Signs and symptoms of UTI
  Urine protein
  Function of urinary diversions or stomas

Extremity assessment:
  Edema
  Peripheral neuropathy
Cognitive and neurologic assessment:
  Level of energy
  Altered mental status
  Cognitive changes
  Developmental delays
Skin
  Pruritic areas
Skeletal
  Accurate measurement of growth with stadiometer
  Plot on appropriate growth chart
  Short stature
  Failure to thrive
If on peritoneal dialysis, check catheter and abdomen
If on hemodialysis, assess graft for infection

■ **BOX 50-2**
■ **SIGNS AND SYMPTOMS ASSOCIATED WITH CHRONIC RENAL FAILURE IN CHILDREN**

Stage 1—usually asymptomatic
Stage 2
  ↑ Serum urea nitrogen
  ↑ Creatinine
  ↑ Parathyroid hormone
  Proteinuria
  Beginning evidence of growth retardation
Stage 3
  Low energy
  Fatigue with exercise
  Pale skin
  Secondary amenorrhea
  Excessive or no urine output
  Decreased attention span
  Poor appetite
  Headache
  Confusion

Metabolic acidosis
Hyperphosphatemia
Hypocalcemia
Anemia
Hypertension
ECG abnormalities
  Peaked T waves
  Long P-R interval
  Widened QRS complex
May lead to ventricular fibrillation and cardiac arrest
Renal osteodystrophy (similar to rickets)
Stage 4
  Severe growth restriction
  Fluid overload
  Electrolyte imbalance
  Metabolic acidosis

■ **BOX 50-3**
■ **ASSOCIATED SECONDARY DIAGNOSES IN CHRONIC RENAL FAILURE**

| | |
|---|---|
| Azotemia | Hypertension |
| Anemia | Renal osteodystrophy |
| Bleeding tendency | Hyperlipidemia |
| CNS changes | Hyperkalemia |
|    Changed mental status | Infection pericarditis |
|    Peripheral neuropathy | Metabolic acidosis |
|    Seizures | Sodium retention/wasting |
| Glucose intolerance | |
| Growth restriction | |

Vogt, B. A., & Avner, E. D. (2004). Renal failure. In R. E. Behrman, R. M. Kliegman, & H. B. Jenson (Eds.). *Nelson textbook of pediatrics* (17th ed.). Philadelphia: Saunders, pp. 1767–1775.

     (e) k = 0.70 for adolescent males
     (f) L = height in cm
     (g) Pcr = plasma creatinine in mg/dL
     (h) Quick estimate based on readily available information tends to be an overestimation that may be more generous in a small child with low muscle mass
  **b.** Blood tests
    **i.** Complete blood count
    **ii.** Iron profile
   **iii.** Electrolytes
     (a) Sodium
     (b) Potassium
     (c) Chloride
     (d) Bicarbonate
     (e) Blood urea nitrogen (BUN)
     (f) Creatinine
     (g) Calcium
     (h) Phosphorus
     (i) Alkaline phosphatase
    **iv.** Proteins—albumin
     **v.** Uric acid
    **vi.** Cholesterol and triglycerides
   **vii.** Parathyroid hormone levels
  **c.** Urine tests
    **i.** Microscopy
    **ii.** Specific gravity
  **d.** Renal ultrasound
  **e.** Bone scan
  **f.** Electrocardiogram
  **g.** Renal biopsy
**7.** Influence on growth and development
  **a.** Short stature is the most significant long-term sequelae of CRF
    **i.** Average of 1.6 to 2 standard deviations below mean height for age
     (a) More pronounced in younger children

(b) More pronounced in boys

ii. Secondary to a growth hormone–resistant state, manifested by:

(a) Elevated growth hormone levels

(b) Decreased insulin-like growth factor-1 (IGF)

(c) Abnormal IGF-binding proteins

**b.** CRF is a long-term chronic illness that affects most aspects of development

i. School—high absence rates may influence school performance

ii. Sports

(a) May not have stamina for active sports

(b) Encourage activities that require less physical activity

iii. Peer interactions

(a) Diet restrictions set child apart from peers

(b) Social opportunities decrease due to frequent illness, hospitalization, and absence for dialysis

**8.** Treatment

**a.** CRF patients must be followed by, preferably, a pediatric nephrologist and his or her interdisciplinary team at a tertiary care facility

**b.** Collaboration between primary care providers and staff from kidney programs at pediatric centers is essential to ensure optimal long-term care

**c.** The role of the PNP involves:

i. Supporting nephrologist's interventions

ii. Being aware of potential complications

iii. Aggressively referring children with complications back to nephrologists

iv. Providing psychosocial support

v. Maintaining preventive health care and health promotion

**d.** Treatment of chronic renal failure

i. All management is determined by pediatric nephrologist

ii. Care for individual child will vary, depending on:

(a) Etiology

(b) Lab values

(c) Response to treatment

(d) Stage of renal failure

iii. Goals of treatment

(a) Overall goal of treatment is twofold

(1) Preventing complications

(2) Preserving as much renal function as possible, for as long as possible

(b) Evaluating and managing comorbid conditions

(c) Slowing the progressive loss of kidney function

(d) Preventing and treating cardiovascular disease

(e) Preventing and treating complications of decreased kidney function (e.g., hypertension, anemia, acidosis, renal osteodystrophy, hyperkalemia, growth failure)

(f) Preparing for kidney failure therapy

(g) Replacing kidney function by dialysis and/or transplantation, if signs and symptoms of uremia are present

(h) Psychosocial care is a critical component of CRF management

(1) Staff social workers, psychologists, and/or psychiatrists at kidney centers:

a) Are experts on the needs of this special population

b) Have access to many available resources

(2) Encourage regular communication between kidney center and primary care providers regarding:
    a) Family situation
    b) Family's and patient's coping strategies
    c) Use of resources
(3) Encourage and support families to:
    a) Maintain as normal a family dynamic as possible
    b) Keep the child in school as much as possible
    c) Use tutors as necessary
    d) Preserve the parent/child relationship
    e) Be mindful of the needs of siblings
    f) Believe that they can cope, versus succumbing to the overwhelming load that the family now carries

  (i) Careful monitoring of the aforementioned issues affords all care providers:
    (1) Optimal opportunity to keep symptoms of CRF to a minimum
    (2) Ability to concurrently evaluate the success or failure of the treatment plan
    (3) Data for determination of the need for dialysis and/or renal transplantation
  (j) Important to empower patients and caregivers to actively participate in the child's care

**e.** Treatment of hypertension (HTN)
  **i.** Goals
    (a) Maintain end-organ perfusion
    (b) Limit cardiovascular sequelae
    (c) While diminishing the progression of chronic renal failure
    (d) Maintain BP in the 50th percentile for age
  **ii.** Methods
    (a) Dietary sodium restriction is the first line of intervention
    (b) Medications
      (1) Choice of drug depends on:
        a) Severity of the HTN
        b) Weight of the child
      (2) Renin-mediated HTN is a frequent cause of HTN
        a) Angiotensin-converting enzyme (ACE) inhibitor agents are most useful
          i) Captopril
          ii) Enalapril
      (3) β-adrenergic–blocking agents
        a) Second or third line of choice
        b) Used in the outpatient setting
      (4) Diuretic
        a) Decreases HTN related to volume overload
        b) Decreases edema
        c) Furosemide (Lasix) is commonly used

**f.** Fluid restriction is rarely needed until:
  **i.** Development of end-stage renal disease
  **ii.** Initiation of dialysis
**g.** Prevention of urinary tract infection (UTI) is a priority

       **i.** Particularly challenging because all children with CRF have some degree of immunosuppression and/or immunocompromise secondary to:

         (a) Disease

         (b) Medical intervention

      **ii.** PNP must get consensus of both pediatric nephrologist and pediatric urologist regarding what constitutes a true UTI in these patients

     **iii.** All patients on an intermittent catheterization regimen, usually five times per day

         (a) Per urethra

         (b) Or via Mitrofanoff (catheterizable stoma connecting the bladder to the abdominal wall)

      **iv.** These children ALWAYS have bacteriuria

      **v.** Bacteriuria does not constitute a true UTI unless there are concomitant symptoms, such as:

         (a) Increased WBC count

         (b) Significant fever

         (c) Nausea

         (d) Vomiting

**h.** Treatment of hyperkalemia

       **i.** Up to 90% of potassium is excreted by healthy kidneys

      **ii.** As kidney failure progresses, potassium excretion through stool increases

     **iii.** This compensatory mechanism may not be sufficient to maintain normal potassium levels

      **iv.** At stage 4 renal failure, potassium restriction may be required

      **v.** Administration of sodium polystyrene sulfonate (Kayexalate) or dialysis may be needed

**i.** Treatment of hyperphosphatemia

       **i.** Dietary restriction of high-phosphate foods: meats, milk, and milk products

      **ii.** Recommend Similac PM 60/40 formula for infants with CRF

     **iii.** Dietary phosphate binders, such as Tums (calcium carbonate)

      **iv.** Vitamin D supplementation based on serum parathyroid levels

**j.** Treatment of metabolic acidosis

       **i.** Can be controlled with sodium citrate or sodium bicarbonate as long as the sodium will not contribute to HTN

      **ii.** Potassium restriction is indicated when the GFR falls to less than 50% or to a point at which urine output decreases

     **iii.** Vitamin D is always supplemented to preserve normal serum calcium levels

      **iv.** Protein intake should be at least at the minimum daily requirement

         (a) Recommend proteins

            (1) With high biologic value, and

            (2) Metabolized to more usable amino acids than nitrogenous wastes

            (3) Eggs and milk more than meat, fish, fowl

            (4) Supplementation with essential amino acids or keto acids can be helpful to maintain adequate caloric intake

         (b) Protein restriction is rare until end-stage renal disease occurs

**k.** Treatment of growth restriction if child is less than −2 SD for height despite medical care (Harris, Hofman, & Cutfield, 2004)

   i. Subcutaneous recombinant human growth hormone at 0.05 mg/kg/24 hr
      (a) Dose adjusted if necessary
      (b) Continued until:
         (1) Child is at 50th percentile for midparental height
         (2) Achieves a final adult height
         (3) Receives a kidney transplant
      (c) Usually successful in achieving normal height
   ii. Special nutritional supplements are necessary
l. Treatment of anemia (Vogt & Avner, 2004)
   i. Anemia is normochromic, normocytic, hemoglobin less than 10 g/dL
   ii. Pathophysiology
      (a) Erythropoietin is an enzyme produced by interstitial cells of the normal kidney
      (b) Stimulates erythropoiesis in the bone marrow
      (c) Amount of erythropoietin decreases with kidney failure
   iii. Recombinant human erythropoietin therapy
      (a) Goal is to maintain hemoglobin at 11 to 12 g/dL
   iv. Subcutaneous injection of 50 to 150 mg/kg/dose one to three times per week
   v. Oral or intravenous iron supplements are needed
   vi. Benefits
      (a) Minimizes need for blood transfusion
      (b) Improves appetite, sleep, exercise tolerance, well-being
   vii. May progress to need for blood transfusion
m. Treatment of renal osteodystrophy (Salusky, Kuizon, & Juppner, 2004; Vogt & Avner, 2004)
   i. Signs
      (a) Hyperphosphatemia
      (b) Hypocalcemia
      (c) Decreased synthesis of vitamin D
      (d) Hyperparathyroidism leading to bone resorption
   ii. Goals
      (a) Prevent bone deformity
      (b) Normalize growth velocity
   iii. Methods
      (a) Low phosphorus diet
      (b) Phosphate binders to increase fecal phosphate excretion
         (1) Tums
         (2) Calcium acetate
      (c) Vitamin D therapy
         (1) Indications
            a) Parathyroid hormone is three times higher than normal, or
            b) Persistent hypocalcemia
         (2) Method
            a) Calcitriol
            b) New noncalcemic vitamin D analogues
      (d) Monitor serum phosphorus and calcium monthly, PTH every 3 months
n. Surgical urologic intervention for the pediatric patient with CRF (Defoor, et al., 2003)

       **i.** Depending on the primary diagnosis, there may also be associated bladder dysfunction and the child may require surgery to:

         **(a)** Augment bladder size

         **(b)** Create a competent bladder neck, and/or

         **(c)** Create of a Mitrofanoff catheterizable stoma

      **ii.** It is important to be aware of how the child's urinary drainage is managed

**o.** Dialysis

      **i.** Instituted as the GFR decreases and comorbid conditions can no longer be managed

      **ii.** Peritoneal dialysis uses the peritoneal membrane inside the abdomen as a semipermeable membrane that:

         **(a)** Allows waste and toxins to diffuse from blood to dialysis fluid

         **(b)** Is driven by osmotic gradient

         **(c)** Allows plasma water to move across the peritoneal membrane driven by osmotic gradient

      **iii.** Continuous ambulatory peritoneal dialysis

         **(a)** Family manually removes and then infuses the dialysate three to five times per day

         **(b)** Continuous cyclic peritoneal dialysis

            **(1)** Same number of exchanges occur, but by a machine

            **(2)** Seven or eight exchanges per treatment

            **(3)** Done at night while the patient sleeps

         **(c)** Hemodialysis

            **(1)** Machine circulates the blood through a semipermeable membrane

            **(2)** Typically done three times per week; the process takes approximately 3 to 5 hours

**p.** Renal transplantation (Vogt & Avner, 2004)

      **i.** Recommended when kidneys have failed and a suitable donor is located

         **(a)** All health and psychosocial factors must be favorable for donor and recipient

         **(b)** Considered to be the easiest solid organ transplant to perform

         **(c)** Expertise of a pediatric transplant surgeon is critical

            **(1)** The native kidneys are not usually removed

            **(2)** Native nephrectomies are performed if there is potential to cause significant pathology after transplant, i.e., hypertension

         **(d)** Transplant often accomplished with living related donor

            **(1)** Allows for optimal timing and preparation of the family

         **(e)** Cadaver transplant still a significant source of pediatric kidney transplantation

      **ii.** Posttransplant care

         **(a)** Lifelong follow-up with nephrologist

         **(b)** Lifelong immunosuppressives, even in the absence of complication

         **(c)** Monitor for potential complications such as infection, rejection, and medication side effects

**9.** Protection of residual renal function

  **a.** It is vital to protect residual renal function, even if receiving dialysis

  **b.** Loss of residual kidney function may make the care for dialysis patients more difficult with the potential for more complications

  **c.** Implement the following strategies

  i. Early detection of renal disease
  ii. Surgical correction of urinary tract abnormalities
  iii. Prevention of UTIs
    (a) Complete emptying of bladder
    (b) UTI prophylaxis with on-time daily dose of co-trimoxazole or nitrofurantoin for patients prone to frequent UTIs or who have vesicoureteral reflux
    (c) Treat UTIs based on urine culture and antibiotic sensitivities
    (d) All patients on an intermittent catheterization regimen per urethra or via Mitrofanoff
      (1) ALWAYS have bacteriuria
      (2) This does not constitute a true UTI unless there are concomitant symptoms, such as:
        a) Significant fever
        b) Nausea
        c) Vomiting, etc.
  iv. Avoidance or careful administration of renal toxic drugs
    (a) Nonsteroidal antiinflammatory drugs (NSAIDs)
    (b) Radiologic IV contrast
    (c) Gentamycin
  v. Strive for normal blood pressure
  vi. Avoid obesity and hyperinsulinemia
  vii. Reduce proteinuria with ACE inhibitors and/or angiotensin receptor blockers before the patient reaches end-stage renal disease
10. Follow-up
  a. Education of family and patient is essential and ongoing (Reilly, 2001)
    i. Can be facilitated by the PNP
    ii. Helps family consolidate information from all involved providers, including:
      (a) Pediatric nephrologist
      (b) Pediatric urologist
      (c) Pediatric transplant surgeon, if involved
    iii. PNP aids family in developing and revising care plans
      (a) Can be sent to all involved providers
      (b) Changed as necessary
    iv. Because of the large number of specialists involved in the CRF patient's care
      (a) Family can feel that they are getting conflicting information
      (b) Family can feel that specialists are not communicating well with each other
      (c) Family can feel caught in the middle
    v. The neutral and more objective view and assistance of the PNP is extremely valuable to the family of the CRF patient
      (a) PNP is communicating with and receiving information from all involved providers
      (b) PNP more objectively can guide family through exhausting process of caring for and making decisions for the child with CRF
  b. Give immunizations as required for age (Vogt & Avner, 2004)
    i. Give live vaccines before kidney transplant
    ii. Withhold live vaccines when child is immunosuppressed
    iii. Give yearly influenza vaccine

c. Careful monitoring of the aforementioned issues affords all care providers:
  i. Optimal opportunity to keep symptoms of CRF to a minimum
  ii. Ability to concurrently evaluate the success or failure of the treatment plan
  iii. Data for determination of the need for dialysis and/or renal transplantation
d. Indications for sending the pediatric patient with CRF to the emergency department (ED)
  i. Volume overload leading to pulmonary edema, hypertension, or CHF
    (a) Respiratory changes created by pulmonary edema
    (b) Cardiac changes due to congestive heart failure
    (c) Symptoms
      (1) Dyspnea
      (2) Recent significant weight gain
      (3) Swelling of lower limbs
      (4) Weakness
  ii. Major metabolic crisis
    (a) Vomiting, diarrhea, lethargy—send to ED sooner than would average patient due to these children's propensity for becoming dehydrated quickly
    (b) Hyperkalemia
    (c) Hyponatremia
    (d) Metabolic acidosis
  iii. Hypertensive crisis
  iv. Infection due to increased susceptibility to infection
  v. Peritonitis
    (a) Secondary to contamination from the peritoneal dialysis catheter
    (b) Occurs approximately once per year for children on peritoneal dialysis
  vi. Peritoneal dialysis catheter malfunction
    (a) Leakage and/or overflow
    (b) Obstruction
  vii. Graft emergencies in the hemodialysis patient
    (a) Bleeding
    (b) Thrombosis
    (c) Infection
  viii. Persistent bleeding secondary to anticoagulants, which can lead to:
    (a) Internal bleeding
      (1) Petechiae
      (2) Abdominal hematomas
      (3) GI bleeding
    (b) External bleeding related to:
      (1) Problems with the dialyzing membrane
      (2) Mechanical problems with the graft
  ix. Thrombosis at the graft site
  x. Hypotension, muscle cramps, and dialysis disequilibrium syndrome postdialysis
11. Long-term implications
  a. An extremely challenging group of patients to follow
  b. Role of the primary care provider (PNP) is an essential component
  c. PNP who maintains close communication with the specialists

     **i.** Can make the difference for families between giving up or feeling empowered

     **ii.** Can help families make informed choices regarding optimal care for their child

## REFERENCES

Avner, E. D. (2004). Chronic renal failure. In E. D. Avner, W. E. Harmon, & P. Niaudet (Eds.). *Pediatric nephrology* (5th ed.). Philadelphia: Lippincott Williams & Wilkins, pp. 1269-1409.

DeFoor, W., Minevich, E., McEnery, P., et al. (2003). Lower urinary tract reconstruction is safe and effective in children with end stage renal disease. *J Urol, 170*(4), 1497-1500.

Harris, M., Hofman, P. L., & Cutfield, W. S. (2004). Growth hormone treatment in children: Review of safety and efficacy. *Paediatr Drugs, 6*(2), 93-106.

Hogg, R. J., Furth, S., Lemley, K. V., et al. (2003). National Kidney Foundation's Kidney Disease Outcomes Quality Initiative clinical practice guidelines for chronic kidney disease in children and adolescents: Evaluation, classification, and stratification. *Pediatrics, 111*(6, Pt. 1), 1416-1421.

Klein, M., & Namrow, A. (2004). Chronic renal failure. In P. J. Allen & J. A. Vessey (Eds.). *Primary care of the child with a chronic condition* (4th ed.). St. Louis: Mosby, pp. 722-743.

Reilly, N. J. (2001). *Urologic nursing: A study guide* (2nd ed.). Pitman, NJ: Anthony J. Jannetti.

Roth, K. S., Koo, H. P., Spottswood, S. E., & Chan, J. C. M. (2002). Obstructive uropathy: An important cause of chronic renal failure in children. *Clin Pediatr, 41*(5), 309-314.

Salusky, I. B., Kuizon, B. G., & Juppner, H. (2004). Special aspects of renal osteodystrophy in children. *Semin Nephrol, 24*(1), 69-77.

Vogt, B. A., & Avner, E. D. (2004). Renal failure. In R. E. Behrman, R. M. Kliegman, & H. B. Jenson (Eds.). *Nelson textbook of pediatrics* (17th ed.). Philadelphia: Saunders, pp. 1767-1775.

# Spina Bifida and Other Myelodysplasias

RIZA V. MAURICIO, RN, MSN, CCRN, CPNP

## DEFINITION

Myelodysplasias are malformations of the neural tube closure and the overlying posterior vertebral arches during fetal development (Schneider & Krosschell, 2001). This term is used interchangeably with *dysraphisms*. The severity of symptoms depends on the extent of the neural tube defect. The most severe type is myelomeningocele, also called spina bifida (Foster, 2004; Haslam, 2004; Johnston & Kinsman, 2004).

1. Incidence
   a. All neural tube defects
      i. Incidence: 1 per 2000 pregnancies
      ii. Some pregnancies result in fetal demise
      iii. Some pregnancies are voluntarily terminated
      iv. More common in females than in males (Schneider & Krosschell, 2001)
   b. Spina bifida
      i. Incidence: 1 per 4000 live births
      ii. Risk of recurrence after one affected child is 2% to 5% (Churchill, Abramson, & Wahl, 2001)
      iii. Risk is 10% with two previous affected children
      iv. Incidence decreased by 50% due to folic acid supplements before and during pregnancy (Green, 2002)
   c. Spina bifida occulta: 1 per 4000 live births in the United States
   d. Incidence varies in other parts of the world (Haslam, 2004; Schneider & Krosschell, 2001)
2. Precipitating factors
   a. Exact cause is unknown, but there is evidence of several precipitating factors (Johnston & Kinsman, 2004)
   b. Genetic mutations in folate-responsive or folate-dependent pathways
   c. Environmental
      i. Radiation
      ii. Drugs that antagonize folic acid (Johnston & Kinsman, 2004)
         (a) Trimethoprim
         (b) Carbamazepine, phenobarbital, primidone

        (c) Valproic acid taken during pregnancy causes neural tube defect in 1% to 2% of pregnancies

     **iii.** Chemicals

     **iv.** Hyperthermia in the first weeks of pregnancy (Schneider & Krosschell, 2001)

  **d.** Nutrition

     **i.** Malnutrition

     **ii.** Folic acid and vitamin A deficiency are possible primary causes (Schneider & Krosschell, 2001)

        (a) Daily intake of 0.4 mg of folic acid is recommended by the U.S. Public Health Service to prevent neural tube defects

**3.** Pathophysiology (Churchill, et al., 2001; Schneider & Krosschell, 2001)

  **a.** Fetal development of the spinal cord and surrounding tissues (Benasich, 2004)

     **i.** Neurulation is the process that initiates the development of the nervous system

        (a) Primary phase forms brain and spinal cord

        (b) Secondary phase occurs in the more caudal regions of spinal cord

        (c) About 50% of the caudal end of the neural tube becomes the spinal cord, organized in segments

        (d) Rostral end of the neural tube closes at about day 23

        (e) Caudal end of the neural tube closes at about day 27

     **ii.** Genes—two types of genes are critically important

        (a) Genes that encode transcription factors

        (b) Genes that encode cell-surface or secreted signaling molecules

        (c) Hox family of homeobox genes—the master control genes that coordinate the development, positioning, and patterning of structures along the anteroposterior axis

        (d) Sonic hedgehog (Shh) gene—involved in dorsoventral patterning and is strongly implicated in neural tube defects

  **b.** Spina bifida is the result of failure of the caudal end of the neural tube to close

  **c.** Failure of the neural tube to close allows fetal substances into the amniotic fluid:

     **i.** Alpha-fetoprotein (AFP)

     **ii.** Acetylcholinesterase

  **d.** The type of defect depends on the extent of the malformation

**4.** Type of defect, signs, symptoms

  **a.** Spina bifida occulta (Elder, 2004; Johnston & Kinsman, 2004)

     **i.** Failure in one or more of the vertebral arches to fuse and close during week 4

     **ii.** Spinal cord and meninges are unharmed and do not protrude

     **iii.** Common site is lumbosacral area (L5, S1)

     **iv.** Associated with high-arched feet, gait abnormality, muscle size, and strength discrepancy between lower extremities

     **v.** 90% have a visible cutaneous abnormality, e.g., a patch of hair, lipoma, skin discoloration, or dermal sinus in midline

        (a) A dermoid sinus at level of lumbosacrum or occiput may pass through dura and provide an entry site for infection

     **vi.** Usually a benign condition

        (a) Mostly asymptomatic

        (b) No neurologic signs

     **vii.** 40% have urinary incontinence, frequent UTI, fecal soiling

     **viii.** May be associated with more serious spinal cord defects

  **b.** Meningocele (Johnston & Kinsman, 2004)

      **i.** Meninges and cerebral spinal fluid (CSF) herniate through a defect in the posterior vertebral arches

      **ii.** Spinal cord is usually normal

      **iii.** Cystic sac is evident

         (a) Fluctuant midline mass usually in lower back

         (b) May transilluminate

      **iv.** Usually well covered with skin

      **v.** Meningocele could be *anterior* and protrude into the pelvis

         (a) Symptoms may be constipation and bladder dysfunction

         (b) Females may have associated anomalies of genital tract

  **c.** Myelomeningocele

      **i.** Most severe form

      **ii.** Spinal cord *and* the meninges are contained in the cystic sac (Churchill, et al., 2001)

         (a) 75% are in lumbosacral region

         (b) Accounts for 90% of open neural lesions

      **iii.** Hydrocephalus occurs in at least 80% of cases

         (a) Enlargement of ventricles can be slow or rapid

         (b) Bulging anterior fontanelle

         (c) Dilated scalp veins

         (d) Setting sun appearance of the eyes

         (e) Irritability

         (f) Vomiting

         (g) Abnormal increase in head circumference

      **iv.** Neurologic deficit depends on location of the myelomeningocele

         (a) Lower sacral region

            (1) Bowel and bladder incontinence due to anesthesia of area

            (2) No motor function impairment

         (b) Midlumbar region

            (1) Flaccid paralysis of lower extremities

            (2) Absence of deep tendon reflexes

            (3) No response to pain

            (4) Postural abnormalities of the legs and feet

            (5) May have urinary dribbling and relaxed anal sphincter

         (c) Upper thoracic or cervical region

            (1) Minimal neurologic deficit

            (2) Rarely have hydrocephalus

**5.** Presentation

  **a.** Symptoms

      **i.** Loss of sensory and motor functions in the lower limbs below the level of the lesion

      **ii.** Headache

      **iii.** Neck pain

      **iv.** Dysphagia

      **v.** Nausea, vomiting

      **vi.** Hiccups

      **vii.** Hoarseness

      **viii.** Facial numbness

      **ix.** Low back pain

  **b.** Signs (Drolet, 2000; Schneider & Krosschell, 2001)

      **i.** Bulging fontanelle

      **ii.** Visual and motor perceptual deficit (Schneider & Krosschell, 2001)

      **iii.** Possible seizure disorder (Foster, 2004)

      iv. Learning disabilities
      v. Dimpling, pigmentation, or hair patch noted along the spinal column
      vi. Flaccid paralysis, loss of sensation, and absent reflexes below the level of the lesion
      vii. Hip flexion, ankle dorsiflexion, and knee extension contractures
      viii. High-arched feet or other foot deformities
      ix. Gait changes
      x. Lumbar kyphosis
      xi. Scoliosis noted at birth and more evident as child grows
      xii. Lordosis or lordoscoliosis in adolescents with hip flexion deformity and large spinal defect (Schneider & Krosschell, 2001)
      xiii. Bowel dysfunction (Churchill, et al., 2001)
      xiv. Neurogenic bladder
      xv. Delayed physical growth, i.e., within 10th percentile in height (Mingin, et al., 2002)

6. Focused assessment
   a. Meningocele and myelomeningocele are readily apparent at birth
   b. Spina bifida occulta may not be recognized until toddler age
   c. Many of the signs and symptoms above require a high index of suspicion for the more subtle neural tube defects and their associated problems
      i. Chiari II malformation may not be recognized until young adulthood (see section 11.c. below)
      ii. Hydrocephalus results from the Chiari II malformation in which cerebral spinal fluid builds up in the ventricles of the brain
      iii. Tethered cord syndrome (NINDS, 2006)
         (a) During fetal development, the distal end of the spinal cord is normally located at the level of the first lumbar vertebral body (L1)
         (b) If the spinal cord becomes bound near the sacral level, it is "tethered"
         (c) As the child grows, the lower portion of the spinal cord is pulled
         (d) Can cause neurologic damage as the tightness increases
         (e) Gait changes
         (f) Foot deformities
   d. History
      i. Siblings with neural tube defects
      ii. Exposures to precipitating factors during pregnancy (see section 2.c. above)
      iii. Adequacy of maternal nutrition and folic acid intake before and during pregnancy
   e. Physical examination
      i. Musculoskeletal assessment—see Chapter 12
      ii. Neurologic assessment—see Chapter 13
7. Diagnostic tests
   a. In utero
      i. Ultrasonography (Biggio et al., 2001)
         (a) Detects severe malformations
         (b) Pre- and postnatal assessment of lesions by ultrasound are highly correlated
      ii. Amniocentesis
         (a) High levels of AFP at 16 to 17 weeks gestation (Churchill, et al., 2001, Foster, 2004; Johnston & Kinsman, 2004)
         (b) Increased level of amniotic acetylcholinesterase detects 90% of spina bifida

        **iii.** High levels of AFP in maternal serum

   **b.** Diagnostic tests done after birth are shown in Table 51-1

**8.** Treatment

   **a.** Referral to a multidisciplinary team approach is essential

   **b.** Goal: develop individual function to the maximum and promote independence (Foster, 2004)

   **c.** Surgical

        **i.** Intrauterine repair of myelomeningocele (Johnson, et al., 2003)

            **(a)** Early experience suggests a decreased need for:

                **(1)** Ventriculoperitoneal shunting

                **(2)** Arrest or slowing of progressive ventriculomegaly

                **(3)** Consistent resolution of hindbrain herniation

            **(b)** Further long-term follow-up is needed to evaluate neurodevelopment and bladder and bowel function

            **(c)** American Academy of Pediatrics (1999) recommends fetal therapy if effectiveness of treatment is proven

            **(d)** Physicians make it clear that the procedure is experimental and thus risk and benefit ratio not been established (see section 11.d. below)

---

■ **TABLE 51-1**
■ ■ **Postnatal Diagnostic Tests to Detect Spina Bifida and Its Severity**

| Type of Test | Significance |
|---|---|
| MRI of brain and spine | Evaluate primary and associated defects |
| Complete urologic evaluation | Serum creatinine and renal ultrasound to evaluate kidney function<br>Voiding cystourethrography and urodynamics to evaluate bladder function<br>MRI if the patient is in renal failure |
| Manual muscle testing (MMT) | Initial assessment within first 48 hours evaluates muscle function<br>Repeat every 6 months to 1 year to detect changes |
| Sensory testing | Reevaluate when the child has learned cognitive and language skills |
| Range of motion evaluation | To evaluate contractures<br>Repeat every 6 months to 1 year to detect changes |
| Reflex testing | To determine the child's ability to swallow normally and to evaluate functions associated with other reflexes |
| Developmental and functional evaluation | Standardized testing such as: Peabody Developmental Motor Scales (PDMS)—birth to 83 months<br>Pediatric Evaluation of Disability Inventory (PEDI)—for children 6 months to 7 years |
| Perceptual/cognitive evaluation | Brazelton Neonatal Behavioral Assessment for newborn<br>Bayley Scales of Infant Development for children ages 1 to 42 months<br>Motor Free Visual Perception Test—Revised (MVPT-R) for children ages 4 to 12 years |

From Churchill, B. M., Abramson, R. P., & Wahl, E. F. (2001). Dysfunction of the lower urinary and distal gastrointestinal tracts in pediatric patients with known spinal cord problems. *Pediatr Clin North Am, 48*(6), 1587–1630 and Schneider, J. W., & Krosschell, K. J. (2001). Congenital spinal cord injury. In D. A. Umphred (Ed.). *Neurological rehabilitation* (4th ed.). St. Louis: Mosby, pp. 449–475.

      **ii.** Delivery by cesarean section of fetus diagnosed with myelodysplasia to minimize damage to the protruding spinal cord (Churchill et al., 2001)

      **iii.** Postnatal surgical closure of the defect and reconstruction of spinal cord deformity (Foster, 2004)

      **iv.** Postnatal shunt placement for hydrocephalus (Churchill, et al., 2001; Rintoul et al., 2002)

         (a) Inadequate shunting can lead to:

            (1) Mental retardation

            (2) Intracranial hemorrhage

            (3) Trauma

  **d.** Nonpharmacologic

      **i.** Correction of orthopedic deformities including surgical, orthotic device, gait training, and muscle strengthening exercises (Foster, 2004; Schneider & Krosschell, 2001)

      **ii.** Management of neurogenic bladder (Churchill et al., 2001)

         (a) Clean intermittent catheterization

         (b) In severe cases, bladder augmentation

      **iii.** Adequate nutrition to prevent obesity that can further hamper the child's ability to ambulate or transfer in and out of a wheelchair (Churchill, et al., 2001)

      **iv.** Bowel management program (Churchill, et al., 2001)

         (a) Increased intake of water and fiber in the diet

         (b) Digital fecal extraction in severe form

      **v.** Meticulous attention to skin care (Schneider & Krosschell, 2001)

         (a) Skin that is insensitive to touch is susceptible to pressure sores

      **vi.** 73% of children with myelodysplasia are sensitive to latex (Merropol, 2001)

         (a) Avoid use of latex gloves or latex-containing material for procedures

         (b) Multiple use of latex-containing equipment can induce hypersensitivity to latex (Nieto, et al., 2002)

      **vii.** Psychosexual education and fertility counseling

      **viii.** Pharmacologic (Churchill, et al., 2001)

         (a) Oxybutynin is an anticholinergic that decreases urge incontinence, urgency, and frequent urination

         (b) A prophylactic antibiotic is administered for the first month of life, then therapy is discontinued unless urinary reflux determined

         (c) Supplemental fiber products to decrease constipation

**9.** Influence on growth and development

  **a.** Developmental needs of the child should be taken into consideration when planning for child's care

  **b.** See Table 51-2 for a summary of rehabilitation goals to meet the child's needs

  **c.** An adolescent must make a transition to adult-focused care with the assistance of the primary care provider

**10.** Follow-up

  **a.** In specialty care

      **i.** Neurologic follow-up to detect hydrocephalus, shunt malfunction, and tethered cord is recommended (Foster, 2004; Mazzola, et al., 2002)

      **ii.** Urological reevaluation to establish treatment plans is needed (Churchill et al., 2001)

      **iii.** Continual counseling and support with home care resources

  **b.** In primary care (Lazzaretti & Pearson, 2004)

■ **TABLE 51-2**
■ ■ **Summary of Rehabilitation Goals According to the Child's Developmental Stage**

| Developmental Stages | Rehabilitation Goals |
|---|---|
| Newborn (before surgical closure) | Inform parents about the condition and treatment options<br>Provide normal environment as much as possible<br>Maintain range of motion (ROM)<br>Prevent injury to cystic sac<br>Prevent further deformity<br>Evaluate renal function and other congenital anomalies |
| Infant (after surgical closure) | Maintain ROM and prevent contractures<br>Initiate family teaching about management of infant<br>Primary provider is responsible for coordinating specialty care and maintaining continuity<br>Contact community resources and referrals for rehabilitation needs at discharge |
| Toddler | Emotional and physical preparation for ambulation<br>Continue to maintain ROM and prevent contractures<br>Provide devices to explore the environment safely and independently |
| Preschool Age | Provide devices for ambulation<br>Encourage cognitive and emotional development<br>Development of self-help skills including bowel and bladder training |
| School Age | Encourage new skills and increased independence<br>Identify learning disabilities and provide appropriate intervention<br>Work with school staff to develop individualized health and educational care plans |
| Adolescence | Evaluate adolescent's capacity for independence in self-care and further education<br>Continue to provide emotional and financial support<br>Psychosexual and developmental counseling |
| Late Adolescence | Facilitate transition to adult care providers |

From Schneider, J. W., & Krosschell, K. J. (2001). Congenital spinal cord injury. In D. A. Umphred (Ed.). *Neurological rehabilitation* (4th ed.). St. Louis: Mosby, pp. 449–475; and Bureau for Children with Medical Handicaps (BCMH) Services. (2005).

    i. Referral to specialty care is essential when neural tube defects or their associated conditions are suspected
    ii. Routine immunizations are recommended
      (a) Seek consultation from pediatrician about deferring pertussis vaccine for infants with seizures
      (b) Measles vaccine is recommended
    iii. Growth—monitor height, weight, head circumference, and BMI on appropriate charts
      (a) If child cannot stand, measure full-body length and arm span in supine position (see Chapter 37)
      (b) Obesity may become a problem for some children due to limited mobility
      (c) Underweight may become a problem for some children due to muscle atrophy and shortening of spine
      (d) Undiagnosed hydrocephalus will be revealed by abnormal increases in head circumference
      (e) Tethered cord syndrome will be revealed as the child grows

   **iv.** Sexuality
    (a) Precocious puberty is common in these children possibly related to hypothalamic dysfunction caused by congenital deformity of the midbrain
    (b) Sexual activity
     (1) Orgasm is not likely if perineal area lacks sensation
     (2) Lubricants are recommended due to lack of normal lubrication from sexual arousal
     (3) Latex condoms should be avoided
     (4) Prophylactic antibiotics are indicated when sexually active due to increased susceptibility to UTI
     (5) Females are capable of becoming pregnant but require specialty obstetric care
     (6) Males produce sperm but may have decreased or no capacity for erection and ejaculation
     (7) Penile implants may be effective
    (c) Discipline—as with all children with chronic conditions, parents are encouraged to avoid overprotection and hold reasonable expectations for behavior and household responsibilities
    (d) School
     (1) Learning disabilities are common
     (2) Frequent absences may negatively affect school performance
     (3) PNP should participate in development of an individualized educational plan (IEP) or 504 Plan with school personnel
    (e) Quality of life
     (1) Peer relationships—encourage participation in school and after-school activities that are appropriate to their mobility limitations
     (2) Self-esteem—inform parents of signs and symptoms of decreased self-esteem and depression and refer for psychologic counseling as appropriate
     (3) Family stability and positive functioning has a positive effect on the quality of life of children with chronic conditions
    (f) Transition to adulthood
     (1) Plans for employment, further education, and independent living must be part of IEP by age 16
     (2) Adult multidisciplinary clinics for these conditions are rare
     (3) PNP must be able and willing to coordinate the care and the multiple referrals for specialty care that adults with myelodysplasia will need
 **11.** Long-term implications
  **a.** Prognosis (Johnston & Kinsman, 2004)
   **i.** If the disease is managed well, an individual can grow to adulthood
   **ii.** A spinal cord lesion located in S1 and lower has the best prognosis for ambulation (Hirose, Meuli-Simmen, & Meuli, 2001)
   **iii.** Children born with myelomeningocele have a mortality rate of 10% to 15% if treated aggressively
   **iv.** Most deaths occur before age 4
   **v.** About 70% of survivors have normal intelligence, but can be negatively affected by episodes of meningitis or ventriculitis (Johnston & Kinsman, 2004)

      **vi.** Learning disabilities and seizure disorders are more common than in general population
  **b.** Neurogenic bladder can lead to hydronephrosis, infection, and renal failure (Foster, 2004)
  **c.** Chiari II malformation (Foster; 2002; Greenlee, et al., 2002; NINDS, 2006; Strayer, 2001)
      **i.** Occurs in 95% of children with myelodysplasia
      **ii.** A life-threatening event
      **iii.** Cerebellum portion of the brain protrudes into the spinal canal
      **iv.** Associated with hydrocephalus
      **v.** May not be revealed until young adulthood as defect herniates toward medulla and cerebellar tonsils through the foramen magnum
      **vi.** Symptoms
        (a) Impaired gag reflex, choking
        (b) Severe snoring, stridor
        (c) Apnea
        (d) Vocal cord paralysis
        (e) Spasticity of upper extremities
  **d.** Management of myelomeningocele study (MOMS)
      **i.** National Institute of Child Health and Development funded study
      **ii.** 5-year multicenter clinical trial begun in 2003 to determine which treatment for myelomeningocele (intrauterine or after birth) is most beneficial
      **iii.** No results available at this time

# REFERENCES

American Academy of Pediatrics (AAP) Committee on Bioethics. (1999). Fetal therapy—Ethical considerations. *Pediatrics, 103*, 1061-1063.

Benasich, A. A. (2004). Foundations—Early brain development. Retrieved June 1, 2005, from http://babylab.rutgers.edu/foundations/outlines/Brain%20Devoutline04.doc.

Biggio J. R. Jr., Owen, J., Wenstrom, K. D., & Oakes, W. J. (2001). Can prenatal ultrasound findings predict ambulatory status in fetus with open spina bifida? *Am J Obstet Gynecol, 185*(5), 1016-1020.

Bureau for Children with Medical Handicaps (BCMH), Myelodysplasia Standards Committee. *Standards of care and outcome measures for children with myelodysplasia.* Columbus, OH: Ohio Department of Health. Retrieved June 26, 2006, from www.odh.state.oh.us/ODHPrograms/CMH/bifida.pdf.

Chervenak, F. A., McCullough, L. B., & Birnbach, D. J. (2004). Ethical issues in fetal surgery research. *Best Practice and Research: Clin Anesthesiol, 18*(2), 221-230.

Churchill, B. M., Abramson, R. P., & Wahl, E. F. (2001). Dysfunction of the lower urinary and distal gastrointestinal tracts in pediatric patients with known spinal cord problems. *Pediatr Clin North Am, 48*(6), 1587-1630.

Drolet, B. A. (2000). Cutaneous signs of neural tube dysraphism. *Pediatr Clin North Am, 47*(4), 813-823.

Elder, J. S. (2004). Neuropathic bladder. In R. E. Behrman, R. M. Kliegman, & H. B. Jenson (Eds.). *Nelson textbook of pediatrics* (17th ed.). Philadelphia: Saunders, pp. 1806-1808.

Foster, M. R. (2004). Spina bifida. Retrieved June 2, 2005, from www.emedicine.com/orthoped/topic557.htm.

Green, N. (2002). Folic acid supplementation and prevention of birth defects. *J Nutr, 132*, 2356S-2360S.

Greenlee, J. D. W., Donovan, K. A., Hasan, D. M., & Menezes, A. H. (2002). Chiari malformation in the very young child: The spectrum of presentations and experience in 31 children under age 6 years. *Pediatrics, 110*(6), 1212-1219.

Haslam, R. H. A. (2004). Neurologic evaluation. In R. E. Behrman, R. M. Kliegman, & H. B. Jenson (Eds.). *Nelson textbook of pediatrics* (17th ed.). Philadelphia: Saunders, pp. 1973-1983.

Hirose, S., Meuli-Simmen, C., & Meuli, M. (2003). Fetal surgery for myelomeningocele: Panacea or peril? *World J Surg, 27*(1), 87-94.

Johnson, M. P., Sutton, L. N., Rintoul, N., et al., (2003). Fetal myelomeningocele repair: Short-term clinical outcomes. *Am J Obstet Gynecol, 189*(2), 482-487.

Johnston, M. V., & Kinsman, S. (2004). Congenital anomalies of the central nervous system. In R. E. Behrman, R. M. Kliegman, & H. B. Jenson (Eds.). *Nelson textbook of pediatrics* (17th ed.). Philadelphia: Saunders, pp. 1983-1985.

Lazzaretti, C. C., & Pearson, C. (2004). Myelodysplasia. In P. L. Jackson & J. A. Vessey (Eds.). *Primary care of the child with a chronic condition* (4th ed.). St. Louis: Mosby, pp. 630-643.

Mazzola, C. A., Albright, A. L., Sutton, L. N., et al. (2002). Dermoid inclusion cysts and early spinal cord tethering after fetal surgery for myelomeningocele. *N Engl J Med, 347,* 256-259.

Merropol, E. (2001). Latex (natural rubber) allergy in spina bifida. Spina Bifida Association of America fact sheet. Washington, DC: Spina Bifida Association of America.

Mingin, G. C., Nguyen, H. T., Mathias, R. S., et al. (2002). Growth and metabolic consequences of bladder augmentation in children with myelomeningocele and bladder exstrophy. *Pediatrics, 110*(6), 1193-1198.

Nieto, A., Mazon, A., Pamies, R., et al. (2002). Efficacy of latex avoidance for primary prevention of latex sensitization in children with spina bifida. *J Pediatr, 140*(3), 370-372.

NINDS—National Institute of Neurological Disorders and Stroke (2006). NINDS Chiari malformation information page. Updated June 19, 2006. Retrieved June 26, 2006, from www.ninds.nih.gov/disorders/chiari/chiari.htm.

Rintoul, N. E., Sutton, L. N., Hubbard, A. M., et al. (2002). A new look at myelomeningoceles: Functional level, vertebral level, shunting, and the implications of fetal intervention. *Pediatrics, 109*(3), 409-413.

Schneider, J. W., & Krosschell, K. J. (2001). Congenital spinal cord injury. In D. A. Umphred (Ed.). *Neurological rehabilitation* (4th ed.). St. Louis: Mosby, pp. 449-475.

Strayer, A. (2001). Chiari I malformation: Clinical presentation and management. *J Neurosci Nurs, 33*(2), 90-96, 104.

# Diagnostic, Medication, and Treatment Guides for Children and Adolescents

# Readiness for Handling Pediatric Emergencies in the Primary Care Office

LISA MARIE BERNARDO, PhD, MPH, RN and TENER GOODWIN VEENEMA, PhD, MPH, MS, CPNP

1. Background
    a. Pediatric nurse practitioners (PNPs) practicing in office or clinic settings are likely to participate in the diagnosis, treatment, and stabilization of children presenting with life-threatening illnesses or injuries
    b. Medical emergency
        i. No standard definition of office emergency exists
        ii. Assume that it is any child with, or potential of, cardiopulmonary compromise
    c. Curriculum guidelines and emergency care competencies
        i. *The Essentials of Masters Education for Advanced Practice Nursing*
            (a) American Association of Colleges of Nursing (1996) document that guides Commission on Collegiate Nursing Education certification of graduate nursing programs
            (b) Includes the competency: "Recognizes emergency situations and initiates effective emergency care" (AACN, 1996, p. 22)
        ii. The *Nurse Practitioner Primary Care Competencies in Specialty Areas: Pediatrics*
            (a) National Organization of Nurse Practitioner Faculties (NONPF) (2002) document endorsed by NAPNAP
            (b) Does not include the need for recognizing, stabilizing initiating treatment, and transporting the emergently ill child in the primary care setting
        iii. Terminal competencies of PNPs
            (a) Association of Faculty of Pediatric Nurse Practitioner Programs (AFPNP) (1996) document endorsed by the Pediatric Nursing Certification Board that certifies PNPs
            (b) Includes ability to "decide which situations the PNP can manage independently and those which require...immediate assessment, treatment and referral"

(c) And ability to "identify strategies appropriate for assessing and managing common pediatric illnesses and emergencies…"

    iv. None of the above guidelines explicate specific emergency preparedness skills or procedures

    v. Depending on the clinical setting in which employed, PNPs need to know what responsibilities or roles they might assume in a patient emergency and be prepared to effectively execute them

  **d.** PNP role includes:

    i. Participating in the development of the office emergency preparedness plan

    ii. Having access to the proper emergency equipment per sample emergency drug and equipment lists in AAP Blue Book

    iii. Receiving ongoing education and training in identification and treatment of selected emergencies

    iv. Knowing the community resources for referral and ability to confidently render care under such circumstances

**2.** Epidemiology of pediatric emergencies in the primary care setting

  **a.** Incidence of pediatric medical emergencies in the primary care setting

    i. Quite low, ranging from 0 to 24 per year (Seidel & Knapp, 2000)

  **b.** Prospective study of 37 pediatric primary care sites over 1 year (Heath, et al., 2000)

    i. There were 28 medical emergencies (range = 0 to 8 per site)

    ii. 75% were respiratory related

    iii. One death due to sudden infant death syndrome (SIDS)

  **c.** A cross-sectional random mail survey of 169 practices examining eight types of pediatric emergencies (Mansfield, et al., 2001)

    i. Revealed an average of 4 or more pediatric emergencies per year

    ii. 3.8 pediatric emergencies for family physicians and 4.9 for pediatricians

    iii. More than 90% of the practices saw at least one emergency

    iv. More than 90% of all the emergencies were asthma exacerbations or respiratory emergencies

    v. Other types of emergencies included dehydration, allergic reactions, severe croup, seizures, dehydration, and serious febrile illnesses

  **d.** Telephone survey research to determine frequency of emergencies in 51 pediatric office practices (Flores & Weinstock, 1996)

    i. A median of 24 emergencies per practice

    ii. Asthma flare-up was the most common event

    iii. Followed by trauma

  **e.** Less often seen in primary care setting, but should be considered in an emergency plan are conditions such as:

    i. Poisoning

    ii. Trauma

      (a) Nonintentional

      (b) Child abuse

      (c) Domestic violence (Knapp, 2000)

      (d) Chemical agents of terrorism (Bernardo, 2001; Rosenfield & Bernardo, 2001; Stokes, et al., 2004; Veenema, 2003)

**3.** Office preparedness for emergencies

  **a.** General guidelines

    i. Establish an "emergency preparedness" room that contains the emergency equipment and supplies

    ii. All office staff should be trained in basic life support (BLS)

      **iii.** All eligible staff should be trained in pediatric advanced life support (PALS)

      **iv.** Other relevant training should be provided to all staff on a regular basis

      **v.** Emergency phone numbers should be clearly posted near each office telephone

      **vi.** Post resuscitation protocols in the emergency preparedness room

      **vii.** Establish protocols for checking medications and equipment for expiration dates

  **b.** Research on office and staff preparedness

      **i.** Mail survey on training in PALS and stabilization items available in office (Mansfield, et al., 2001)

        (a) Pediatricians—51% to 81% PALS trained; 8.6 stabilization items

        (b) Family physicians—19% PALS trained; 5.7 stabilization items

        (c) PNPs in primary care office settings—no data are published

        (d) Family physicians thought it was less important than pediatricians to have PALS training or to have the equipment necessary for emergencies

        (e) PNPs or FNPs in family practice settings will need to advocate for PALS level of preparation in their offices

      **ii.** Telephone survey to assess pediatric office emergency preparedness and reasons for levels of preparedness (n = 51 offices, 481 staff) (Flores & Weinstock, 1996)

        (a) Of all eligible staff, only 14% were certified in BLS

        (b) Of all eligible staff, only 17% were certified in PALS

        (c) Missing emergency equipment in 51 offices

          (1) Oxygen, 27%

          (2) Intravenous (IV) catheters, 27%

          (3) Bag-valve-mask, 29%

          (4) Nebulizers, 33%

          (5) Epinephrine 1:10,000, 53%

          (6) Intravenous fluids, 55%

**4.** Phases of response to office emergencies

  **a.** Phase 1: recognize the child with an emergent health condition

      **i.** Patient generally seen first by receptionist or secretary (Frush, et al., 2001)

        (a) The staff member with the least amount of health care knowledge

        (b) Need office training

          (1) To recognize children with emergent health problems

            a) Signs and symptoms of potential emergency include: (Frush, et al., 2001)

              i) Labored breathing

              ii) Cyanosis or pale lips

              iii) Stridor or audible wheezing

              iv) Decreased level of consciousness

              v) Seizures

              vi) Vomiting after a head injury

              vii) Uncontrollable bleeding

          (2) To respond appropriately

            a) Initiate CPR immediately if indicated

            b) Notify the predesignated medical staff person about the child

            c) Otherwise, take child directly to the emergency preparedness room in the office

    **b.** Phase 2: enact the response plan (Frush, et al., 2001)
        **i.** Call 911 or access local emergency medical services (EMS)
            (a) The designated staff person places the call; however, any staff person can call 911 and give the following information to the dispatcher:
                (1) Caller's name
                (2) Location of the office (street address, building number, room number)
                (3) Nature of the emergency (e.g., 3-year-old child with severe respiratory distress)
                (4) Medical treatment being rendered, if known
                (5) The caller should remain on the line until the dispatcher tells him or her to hang up the phone
                (6) If possible, a staff member should meet EMS outside of the building or office because EMS may need additional directions to the patient's location

    **c.** Phase 3: assemble the emergency team (Frush, et al., 2001)
        **i.** Each staff member's role should be determined in advance
        **ii.** The most experienced person or people should care for the patient
        **iii.** Roles of the emergency team include:
            (a) A pediatrician, physician, or PNP is in charge and provides overall medical direction based on PALS guidelines (Zonia & Moore, 2004)
            (b) Registered nurse prepares and administers medications and fluids
            (c) Aide
                (1) Assists care providers
                (2) Performs chest compressions if needed
            (d) Secretary or receptionist
                (1) Activates 911
                (2) Documents treatment rendered
        **iv.** Prepare a contingency plan in the absence of a pediatrician or primary care provider
        **v.** Not all staff on duty need to be involved in the treatment and stabilization of the emergently ill child
        **vi.** Continue care of other patients with remaining staff
        **vii.** If siblings present, arrange for care of siblings during emergency and after transport to ED

    **d.** Phase 4: initiate treatment
        **i.** Protocols for providing BLS and ALS are published in numerous resources (Table 52-1)
        **ii.** Age-appropriate equipment, supplies, and medications should be available (Table 52-2)
            (a) The Broselow-Luten system allows quick reference to determine appropriate equipment size, fluid volumes, and medication dosages (Frush, et al., 2001)
            (b) A color-coded tape measure is used to assign the child a color in accordance with the child's length
            (c) The medication dosages and appropriate-size equipment are stored according to colors
        **iii.** When necessary, PNPs should be prepared to:
            (a) Maintain and stabilize the child's airway, with or without airway adjuncts
            (b) Administer oxygen
            (c) Support respiratory efforts with a bag-valve-mask device
            (d) Initiate chest compressions
            (e) Obtain intravascular or intraosseous access if PALS trained

■ **TABLE 52-1**
■ ■ **Selected Resources for Treating Children with Emergent Health Problems in the Office Setting**

| Reference | Protocols | Equipment Lists |
|---|---|---|
| Frush, K., Cinoman, M., Bailey, B., & Hohenhaus, S. (2001). *Office preparedness for pediatric emergencies: Provider manual.* Washington, DC: Department of Health and Human Services, Health Resources and Services Administration, Emergency Medical Services for Children Program | Basic life support<br>Pulseless<br>Bradycardia<br>Drug delivery, volume administration and vascular access during codes<br>Shock<br>Anaphylaxis<br>Upper airway obstruction<br>Croup-laryngotracheobronchitis<br>Epiglottitis<br>Wheezing: status asthmaticus or bronchiolitis<br>Status epilepticus (generalized tonic-clonic seizures)<br>Diabetic ketoacidosis<br>Closed head injury | Yes |
| Primm, P., Hodge, D., Ringwood, J., et al. (Eds.). (2002). *Office PERC: preparedness for emergency response to children.* Washington, DC: U.S. Department of Health and Human Services, Division of Maternal Child Health, Emergency Medical Services for Children Program | Airway obstruction algorithm<br>Respiratory distress algorithm<br>Shock algorithm<br>Seizure algorithm<br>Anaphylaxis algorithm<br>Basic life support algorithm | Yes |

       (f) Administer resuscitation drugs, such as epinephrine
       (g) Administer IV fluids
     **iv.** Treatment of the emergently ill child could take anywhere from a few minutes to hours relative to:
       (a) Child's health condition
       (b) Availability of EMS
       (c) Coexisting situations (e.g., inclement weather, rural vs. urban office location or emergency department [ED] location)
     **v.** Emergency team members must remain until child is handed off to EMS
     **vi.** Adequate supplies and equipment should be available and maintained accordingly
  **e.** Phase 5: transfer care to EMS
     **i.** The composition and training of EMS teams vary depending on the community—no standardized national curriculum for EMS
       (a) The BLS EMS crew
          (1) Would not be able to administer medications or IV fluids
          (2) PNP, registered nurse, or pediatrician should consider accompanying the patient to the hospital if the child requires advanced life support care
       (b) An advanced life support EMS crew, consisting of paramedics
          (1) Should be able to perform endotracheal intubation
          (2) Decompress the chest
          (3) Obtain IV or region-dependent intraosseous access
          (4) Administer medications

■ **TABLE 52-2**
■ ■ **Suggested Office Equipment and Medications for Pediatric Emergencies**

| Equipment | Medications |
|---|---|
| Bag-valve-mask device (child and adult bags) | Adenosine |
| Infant, child, adult size masks | Albuterol |
| Blood pressure cuffs (infant through adult) | Ceftriaxone |
| Cardiac arrest board | Dexamethasone |
| Calculator | Dextrose—$D_{25}W$ |
| $CO_2$ detector | Diazepam, rectal |
| Glucometer | Diphenhydramine |
| Intraosseous needle | Epinephrine, 1:1000 and 1:10,000 |
| For IV—catheter over the needle devices | Epipen and Epipen Jr. |
| IV catheters/butterfly needles for blood drawing only | Insulin/glucagon |
| Intravenous fluid and tubing | Ipratropium bromide |
| Laryngoscope and endotracheal tubes with stylets—various sizes | Lorazepam |
| Nasogastric tubes—various sizes | Naloxone |
| Nebulizer | Prednisone and prednisolone |
| Oral and nasal airways | Saline, normal |
| Oxygen tank and delivery system | |
| Oxygen masks—infant through adult sizes | |
| Portable suction device and catheters | |
| Pulse oximeter and leads | |
| Heart rhythm monitoring device | |
| Length-based resuscitation tape | |
| Three-way stopcocks, extension tubing | |

From Toback, S. (2002). Prepare your office for a medical emergency. *Contemp Pediatr, 4,* 107.

- ii. The primary care provider in charge may request an ALS crew, an air transport team, or a pediatric transport team, depending on:
  - (a) Severity of the child's condition, level of care needed (e.g., pediatric hospital), and its distance from the office
  - (b) Local EMS structure
  - (c) Availability of these teams
  - (d) Liability insurance requirements
  - (e) Local laws
  - (f) Other variables, e.g., in inclement weather a helicopter would not be an option for transport
- iii. The ALS EMS crew takes medical direction from their medical command physician
  - (a) Will obtain information from the PNP and/or pediatrician
  - (b) Does not take orders from the PNP and/or pediatrician
- iv. The PNP or pediatrician could contact the medical command physician and explain the situation
  - (a) But they should respect the ALS EMS crew's treatment protocols
- v. If the PNP or pediatrician believes the EMS crew's judgment or treatment is not in the best interests of the child
  - (a) Should contact the 911 dispatcher or medical command physician to explain the situation and request additional assistance or direction
  - (b) Survey research study of how 119 primary care physicians transport seriously ill children from their offices to EDs (Davis & Rodewald, 1999)

      (1) Via EMS
         a) 45% of 53 epiglottitis cases
         b) 100% of active seizure cases
      (2) Via family auto
         a) 40% of 53 epiglottitis cases
         b) 26% of 23 foreign body aspiration cases
         c) 46% of 70 severe asthma cases
         d) 59% of 51 severe dehydration cases
         e) 37% of 38 suspected meningococcemia cases
      (3) Physicians denied that they would call EMS more often if:
         a) Transport time was shorter (58%)
         b) Costs were less (64%)
      (4) 60% of physicians expressed lack of confidence in EMS providers' pediatric skills

**f.** Phase 6: prepare the patient and parent for transport
    **i.** All documentation should be copied and given to the EMS crew
    **ii.** The parent may or may not be able to accompany the child in the ground ambulance
    **iii.** Parent usually not permitted on an emergency airlift helicopter
    **iv.** Should the parent not be allowed to accompany the child to the hospital:
       (a) A family friend or relative should be contacted to drive the parent to the hospital
       (b) Should not drive alone because usually highly stressed
    **v.** Provide emotional support to the parent
    **vi.** Provide written explanations of illness, treatment, and where the child is being transported with address, directions, and telephone numbers
    **vii.** When leaving the office, the secretary or receptionist should assist EMS by showing them out of the building

**g.** Phase 7: contact the receiving ED
    **i.** The EMS crew will contact the receiving hospital ED
    **ii.** The pediatrician or PNP should also call the receiving ED to give a report on the patient's condition
       (a) This professional courtesy allows the ED staff adequate time for preparation
       (b) EMS crew may not be able to provide all information listed below if the patient needs constant attention
    **iii.** Information to be delivered includes, but not limited to:
       (a) Name of child
       (b) Age
       (c) Sex
       (d) Vital signs
       (e) Significant medical history and known allergies
       (f) Presenting symptoms and history of present illness
       (g) Medications and treatment rendered in office
       (h) Current height, weight, immunization status
       (i) Parent's name
    **iv.** If not sent with patient, the secretary or receptionist could fax copies of the office documentation for placement in the child's medical record

**h.** Phase 8: participate in staff debriefing
    **i.** Treatment and transport of an emergently ill child is very stressful for the office staff

      ii. At the end of the day, the PNP or pediatrician in charge of the emergency should gather the office staff and reflect on the day's events

        (a) Words of encouragement ("We did the best we could") should be expressed

        (b) Allow staff members to share their thoughts and feelings

      iii. At a later time, the emergency preparedness plan could be reviewed and updated, based on the experience that occurred

  5. Maintaining office preparedness

    a. BLS training is the minimum requirement for all office staff (Frush, et al., 2001; Primm, et al., 2002) (Table 52-3)

    b. Pediatric ALS training and certification should be obtained by those who are eligible (i.e., RNs, PNPs, and pediatricians/physicians (Frush, et al., 2001; Primm, et al., 2002)

    c. BLS and PALS training is available from pediatric hospitals, EMS agencies, and other health care venues

    d. Staff should be given opportunities annually to update their training and skills by attending these courses

    e. BLS and PALS certification lasts for 2 years

    f. In-office education includes mock codes to maintain skills that are not used often

      i. Mock codes are drills that simulate the resuscitation of a critically ill patient (Knapp, 2000; Toback, 2002)

      ii. Mock code programs are available in print (Frush, et al., 2001; Toback, 2002) and CD-ROM (Primm, et al., 2002)

---

■ **TABLE 52-3**
■ ■ **Suggested Education and Training for Office Staff to Prepare for Pediatric Emergencies**

| Training/Education | Description | Office Staff |
| --- | --- | --- |
| Basic life support (BLS)<br>  American Heart Association<br>    www.americanheart.org<br>  American Red Cross<br>    www.redcross.org | Cardiopulmonary resuscitation for adults and children<br>One-half or 1 day in length<br>Certification lasts for 2 years | All |
| Pediatric advanced life support (PALS)<br>  American Heart Association<br>  American Academy of Pediatrics<br>    www.aap.org<br>Advanced pediatric life support (APLS) | Cardiopulmonary resuscitation for children, focusing on respiratory distress and shock<br>Includes techniques such as endotracheal intubation, intraosseous access, calculation of medications, recognizing and treating emergently ill children<br>Two days of training initially, then 1-day renewal<br>Certification lasts for 2 years | Registered nurses<br>PNPs<br>Pediatricians/physicians |
| Emergency nursing pediatric course<br>  Emergency Nurses Association<br>    www.ena.org | Includes pediatric assessment and selected health problems<br>Triage, nursing skills, and other topics are included<br>Two days of training are required<br>Certification lasts for 4 years | RNs<br>PNPs |

   **iii.** Mock codes could be conducted once a month or a quarter or, at least every 6 months (Toback, 2002)

   **iv.** A mock code program could be established and enacted among a number of primary care offices, such as those that are managed by a similar practice plan

   **v.** Consider involving EMS in mock codes

   **vi.** Randomized, controlled clinical trial to test effectiveness of unannounced mock codes on office preparedness for pediatric emergencies (Bordley, et al., 2003)

    **(a)** 3 to 6 months after the mock code, intervention practices (n = 20) were with control practices (n = 19) on these factors:

     **(1)** Development of written office protocols (60% vs. 21%)

     **(2)** Increase in number of staff certified in BLS and PALS (118 vs. 54)

    **(b)** This method motivated practices to prepare for emergencies

 **g.** Purchase equipment and supplies for office emergency preparedness, considering the following points: (Toback, 2002)

  **i.** Staff's comfort with using the equipment and medications

  **ii.** Staff should have regular updates or practice with the equipment

  **iii.** Equipment, medications, and supplies should be inspected at regular intervals to ensure proper working order and monitor expiration dates

  **iv.** Recommended equipment lists for pediatric emergency preparedness are available in numerous publications

  **v.** Automated external defibrillators (AED) (Samson, et al., 2003)

   **(a)** May be used for children 1 to 8 years of age who have no signs of circulation

   **(b)** Initially, the AED should deliver a pediatric dose

   **(c)** Recommended for documented ventricular fibrillation and pulseless ventricular tachycardia

   **(d)** AEDs are expensive; the office may consider contributing to a shared AED for use by the entire building or clinic in which they are located

 **h.** Office staff should be aware of :

  **i.** Maximum amount of time required for EMS response

  **ii.** Qualifications of the local EMS unit

  **iii.** Distance to the nearest ED

  **iv.** Configuration of the ED

  **v.** Times of operation (not all EDs are operational 24 hours/day)

  **vi.** Pediatric capabilities

  **vii.** Availability of pediatric specialists

 **i.** Plan for adequate back-up supplies of medications, fluids, and oxygen

**6.** Using community resources

 **a.** Selected resources for the development and maintenance of an office emergency preparedness plan are outlined in Table 52-4

 **b.** Collaborate with the local EMS on issues related to pediatric emergencies

 **c.** EMS members also need ongoing education and training to provide proper treatment

  **i.** Ask them to participate in mock codes for pediatric patients

  **ii.** Invite them to spend an afternoon in the office measuring vital signs, performing assessments, etc., under the direction of the PNP or pediatrician

 **d.** Consider contacting local ED for inservice education because they often have outreach programs

 **e.** Be aware of potential for bioterrorism, and include this in office planning (Bernardo, 2001; Bernardo & Kapsar, 2002)

■ **TABLE 52-4**
■ ■ **Community Resources for Office Emergency Preparedness**

| Resource | Description |
|----------|-------------|
| Emergency medical services | Provide emergent care to the community<br>Can be hospital or community based<br>Can be volunteer or paid<br>Include providers who are trained in basic life support (BLS), such as emergency medical technicians, and those trained in advanced life support (ALS), such as paramedics and prehospital RNs<br>ALS training may or may not include *pediatric* advanced life support training<br>Can include air transport, ground transport, hazardous materials (hazmat) capabilities, rescue capabilities, and other specialty services<br>Response times vary, relative to location (urban vs. rural) and status (paid vs. volunteer)<br>Can provide consultation on equipment and medication<br>May be able to provide BLS or ALS training to office staff |
| Public health department | Offers advice on communicable and infectious diseases<br>Assists with reporting and follow-up of patients treated with reportable health conditions |
| Local hospital | Serves the community for health problems<br>May include primary, secondary, and tertiary prevention strategies<br>May have an established pediatric in-house specialty, such as a pediatric unit, pediatric ED, pediatrician/PNP on call, pediatric RNs<br>May offer BLS and ALS training |
| Pediatric/children's hospital | Serves as a regional resource for pediatric primary, secondary, and tertiary care<br>May have outreach programs and training<br>May offer BLS, ALS, and PALS training |
| Emergency medical services for children (EMS-C) www. ems-c.org | The EMS-C program is a national resource that provides consultation, education, training, and research related to the emergency care of children<br>Their scope encompasses prevention through rehabilitation |
| Poison centers 1-800-222-1222 | 24/7 staffing of an emergency number for anyone, anywhere, to call if poisoning is suspected<br>Provide information about poisons for health care providers<br>Protect consumers by identifying hazards early<br>Maintain the Toxic Exposure Surveillance System (TESS), the only comprehensive poisoning surveillance database in the United States. TESS contains detailed toxicologic information on more than 31 million poison exposures reported to U.S. poison centers |

# REFERENCES

American Association of Colleges of Nursing (1996). *The essentials of master's education for advanced practice nursing.* Washington DC: American Association of Colleges of Nursing Publishing.

Association of Faculties of Pediatric Nurse Practitioner Programs (AFPNP). (1996). *Philosophy, conceptual model, terminal competencies for the education of pediatric nurse practitioners.* Cherry Hill, NJ: AFPNP/ NAPNAP.

Bernardo, L. M. (2001). Pediatric implications in bioterrorism, Part I: Physiologic and psychosocial differences. *Int J Trauma Nurs, 7*(1), 14-16.

Bernardo, L. M., & Kapsar, P. (2003). Pediatric implications in bioterrorism: Education for health care providers. *Disaster Manag Response, 1*(2), 52-53.

Bordley, W. C., Travers, D., Scanlon, P., et al. (2003). Office preparedness for pediatric emergencies: A randomized, controlled trial of an office-based training program. *Pediatrics, 112,* 291-295.

Davis, C. O., & Rodewald, L. (1999). Use of EMS for seriously ill children in the office: A survey of primary care physicians. *Prehospital Emerg Care, 3*(2), 102-106.

Flores, G., & Weinstock, D. (1996). The preparedness of pediatricians for emergencies in the office: What is broken, should we care, and how can we fix it? *Arch Pediatr Adolesc Med, 150,* 249-256.

Frush, K., Cinoman, M., Bailey, B., & Hohenhaus, S. (2001). *Office preparedness for pediatric emergencies: Provider manual.* Washington, DC: Department of Health and Human Services, Health Resources and Services Administration, Emergency Medical Services for Children Program.

Heath, B., Coffey, J., Malone, P., & Courtney, J. (2000). Pediatric office emergencies and emergency preparedness in a small rural state. *Pediatrics, 106,* 1391-1396.

Knapp, J. F. (2000). Commentary: Pediatric emergencies in the office, hospital, and community: Organizing systems of care. *Pediatrics, 106* (2), 337-338.

Mansfield, C., Price, J., Frush, K., & Dallara, J. (2001). Pediatric emergencies in the office: Are family physicians as prepared as pediatricians? *J Fam Pract, 50,* 757-761.

National Organization of Nurse Practitioner Faculties. (2002). *Nurse practitioner primary care competencies in specialty areas: Pediatrics.* Washington, DC: U.S. Department of Health and Human Services, Health Resources and Services Administration, Bureau of Health Professions, Division of Nursing.

Primm, P., Hodge, D., Ringwood, J., et al. (Eds). (2002). *Office PERC: preparedness for emergency response to children* (CD-ROM). Washington, DC: U.S. Department of Health and Human Services, Division of Maternal Child Health.

Rosenfield, R. L., & Bernardo, L. M. (2001). Pediatric implications in bioterrorism, Part II: Post-exposure diagnosis and treatment. *Int J Trauma Nurs, 7*(4), 133-136.

Samson, R. A., Berg, R. A., & Bingham, R. (2003). Use of automated external defibrillators for children: An update-an advisory statement from the Pediatric Advanced Life Support Task Force, International Liaison Committee on Resuscitation. *Pediatrics, 112,* 163-168.

Seidel, J., & Knapp, J. (Eds.). (2000). *Childhood emergencies in the office, hospital, and community: Organizing systems of care* (2nd ed.). Elk Grove Village, IL: American Academy of Pediatrics.

Stokes, E., Gilbert-Palmer, D., Skorga, P., et al. (2004). Chemical agents of terrorism: Preparing nurse practitioners. *Nurse Pract, 29*(5), 30-41.

Toback, S. (2002). Prepare your office for a medical emergency. *Contemp Pediatr, 4,* 107.

Veenema, T. G. (2003). Chemical and biological terrorism preparedness for staff development specialists. *J Nurse Staff Dev, 19* (5), 218-227.

Zonia, C. L., and Moore, D. S. (2004). Review of guidelines for pediatric advanced life support. *J Am Osteopath Assoc, 104,* 22-23.

# Diagnostic Tests for Pediatric Clinical Decision Making

NANCY A. RYAN-WENGER, PhD, RN, CPNP, FAAN

1. General principles for use of diagnostic tests in clinical decision making
   a. The practical value of a test can be assessed only by taking into account subsequent health outcomes (Mol, et al., 2003)
   b. Before ordering or conducting a test, answer the question: "Will the results of this test change my treatment plan?" If the answer is no (i.e., "I'm going to treat this sore throat with antibiotics anyway because siblings have strep"), then the test is probably not necessary
2. Terminology
   a. Note: for simplification in this chapter, the term "disease" is used as a general term for any health-related condition
   b. Screening test
      i. A test for individuals *without* current symptoms of a specific disease to detect presymptomatic disease or risk for the disease
      ii. Used to separate a "highly suspect group of patients from normal" patients (Nicholson & Pesce, 2004, p. 2394)
      iii. Criteria for use of a screening test
         (a) High sensitivity
         (b) High negative predictive value
         (c) Used for diseases that are prevalent in the population
         (d) Used for diseases that cause significant morbidity and mortality
         (e) Effective treatments are available for early stages of the disease
         (f) Effective interventions are available for risk reduction
      iv. Positive findings require follow-up verification with highly specific diagnostic tests
      v. Cost to society of screening tests
         (a) Monetary costs for initial screening
         (b) Monetary costs of calling back false-positive patients for diagnostic testing
         (c) Psychological and social costs of call-backs for children and parents, whether true results are positive or negative

    **c.** Diagnostic test

       **i.** A method of distinguishing individuals with a disease from individuals without the disease

    **d.** The following test characteristics are based on comparison of test results with results of a gold standard that is assumed to reflect the "truth" (Nicholson & Pesce, 2004; Riegelman, 2004)

       **i.** Sensitivity

          (a) The probability that individuals who have the disease test positive (true positives)

          (b) Sensitivity = (number positive by test/total number with the disease) × 100

          (c) Range = 0% to 100%

      **ii.** Specificity

          (a) The probability that individuals who do not have the disease test negative (true negatives)

          (b) Specificity = (number negative by test/total number without the disease) × 100

          (c) Range = 0% to 100%

      **iii.** Positive predictive value (PPV)

          (a) Proportion of individuals testing positive who actually have the disease

          (b) PPV = (true positive results/[true positive results + false positive results]) × 100

          (c) Range = 0% to 100%

          (d) High percentages mean few false positives

      **iv.** Negative predictive value (NPV)

          (a) Proportion of individuals testing negative who do not have the disease

          (b) NPV = (true negative results/[true negative results + false negative results]) × 100

          (c) Range = 0% to 100%

          (d) High percentages mean few false negatives

      **v.** Accuracy

          (a) How close the test result is to the truth or actual value

          (b) Extent to which bias is present in the test result

    **e.** Precision

      **i.** How reproducible the test result is

      **ii.** Extent to which random error is present in the test

      **iii.** Estimated by the coefficient of variation: CV = (standard deviation/mean) × 100

      **iv.** CV is not usually reported, but is always known by the laboratory

**3.** Point-of-care diagnostic tests

    **a.** Limited to tests that are highly sensitive, specific, simple to conduct, and inexpensive

    **b.** Valuable adjuncts to clinical decision making

    **c.** Commonly used point-of-care diagnostics in primary care settings

      **i.** Hemoglobin, hematocrit

      **ii.** Pregnancy tests

      **iii.** Microscopy of vaginal fluids, urine, skin scrapings, etc.

      **iv.** Occult blood tests of urine and stool

      **v.** Whiff tests of vaginal fluids (prepared with potassium hydroxide [KOH] solution)

      **vi.** pH tests of various fluids

     **vii.** High-sensitivity antigen tests of throat swab specimens (e.g., "quick strep test")

  **d.** NPs must be aware of standards required by Clinical Laboratory Improvement Amendments office diagnostics (CLIA) (Higgins, 2000)

     **i.** Office laboratories were placed under CLIA standards in 1988, which has limited the types of analyses that can be done

     **ii.** CLIA-waived diagnostic tests are often the only tests used in primary care offices

    **iii.** To ensure accurate test results, laboratory equipment in the office must be meticulously maintained, calibrated, and checked against controls as directed by the manufacturer

**4.** Tips on collection and preparation of specimens (Pagana & Pagana, 2005)

  **a.** General principle—use universal precautions when collecting specimens from the body

  **b.** Venous blood specimens (Kee, 2005)

     **i.** Used to assess many body processes and disorders

     **ii.** Venipuncture

       **(a)** Leaving the tourniquet on for more than 1 minute may cause hemo-concentration due to fluid shift from the vessel to the tissue spaces

       **(b)** Some blood tests use whole blood, whereas others require the serum only, or plasma only (plasma contains fibrinogen that causes a clot), so the type of collection tube used is important

       **(c)** Use color coded tubes in this order to minimize cross-contamination of additives:

         **(1)** Serum tubes—have no additives so that blood will clot

          **a)** Blood culture tubes (to maintain sterility)

          **b)** Nonadditive tubes (red tops)

         **(2)** Plasma tubes

          **a)** Coagulation tubes (blue tops)

          **b)** Heparin tubes (green tops)

          **c)** EDTA-K3 tubes (lavender tops)

          **d)** Fluoride tubes (gray tops)—prevent glycolysis

         **(3)** If tube has an additive, gently invert it two or three times to mix additive with blood

         **(4)** Do not shake the tube; this could cause hemolysis

       **(d)** Multiphasic screening machines perform many tests simultaneously, e.g., Chem 7, SMA-12

    **iii.** Note: the range of normal values for the many tests that require blood, serum, or plasma is not provided in this book; please refer to a laboratory diagnostic text

  **c.** Capillary blood specimens

     **i.** Common puncture sites include fingertips, earlobes, heels

     **ii.** Vigorous squeezing of the site may cause hemolysis of the specimen

  **d.** Urine specimens (Kee, 2005; MDS Metro Laboratory Services, 2005b)

     **i.** Used for differential diagnosis of renal conditions and a variety of other disorders

     **ii.** Ideally, for routine analysis, collect the first morning specimen because it is most concentrated

    **iii.** Clean-catch, midstream specimens are acceptable for culture and sensitivity (C&S) tests if the cleaning and voiding procedures are carefully followed (see Chapter 57 for details)

    iv. For infants and young children, a disposable adhesive urinary bag may be used for urinalysis

    v. A specimen for routine analysis or dip stick analysis can be taken from a wet disposable diaper: remove the paper layer, tear off a portion of wet diaper material, place material in a 3-mL syringe, and push out urine into selected container

    vi. Urinary catheterization requires sterile technique and is most appropriate method for urine culture, but is invasive, expensive and time consuming

    vii. With special training, PNP can obtain urine from the bladder via suprapubic aspiration

  viii. 24-hour urine

    (a) Tell patient to urinate, discard that specimen, then 24-hour period will begin

    (b) Start collecting urine at next void and keep urine refrigerated at home

    (c) Recommend keeping urine collection container in a disposable cooler packed in ice

    (d) It is not recommended that urine collection container be kept in the home refrigerator because of potential for contamination of food

        (1) If necessary, keep urine collection container well away from food products in the home refrigerator

        (2) Place container on bottom shelf if possible

        (3) Clean and disinfect place where container was placed after it is removed

    (e) Analyses should be done within 1 hour of last collection

    ix. Analyses

    (a) Color

        (1) Normal is clear straw-colored fluid

            a) Cloudy urine suggests accumulation of white blood cells due to infection

            b) Dark yellow, orange, or brown

                i) Suggests presence of bile or bilirubin due to conditions that cause jaundice

                ii) Pyridium may make urine orange or brown

                iii) Azogantrisin and foods like carrots may make urine orange

            c) Red urine

                i) Usually suggests blood in urine

                ii) Red urine could also be due to beets, blackberries, rhubarb

                iii) Rifampicin causes red urine (used to treat TB, meningococcal carriers, and *Haemophilus influenzae* in children more than 3 months of age)

            d) Blue, green, or blue-green urine

                i) Suggests presence of *Pseudomonas* infection

                ii) Could be due to Doan's pills or methylene blue dye

            e) Black urine

                i) May indicate presence of melanin due to malignant melanoma

                ii) May indicate presence of porphyrin due to acute intermittent porphyria

iii) May be due to presence of urobilinogen or hemoglobin

iv) Due to some medications such as cascara, metronidazole or iron salts

(2) Odor

    a) Normally, urine has almost no odor

    b) Infected urine may smell fishy

(3) Urine dipsticks

    a) Strips of plastic impregnated with chemical reagents that are specific to certain urine contents

    b) Test urine within an hour of urination

    c) If not, refrigerate, but allow urine to reach room temperature before testing

    d) Follow product directions on length of time to allow reagents to react

    e) High false-positive rates with dipsticks; therefore, positive findings should be validated with more specific diagnostic tests, e.g., urine culture if nitrites and leukocyte esterase are positive

    f) Available tests on dipsticks

        i) Glucose—normal is negative

        ii) Ketones—normal is negative

        iii) Protein

            *a)* Morning specimen is best

            *b)* Normal is negative

        iv) Blood—normal is negative

        v) Bilirubin—normal is negative

        vi) Leukocyte esterase

            *a)* Indicates presence of white blood cells due to infection or high fever

            *b)* Normal is negative

        vii) Nitrites

            *a)* Bacteria in urine causes nitrates to convert to nitrites

            *b)* Normal is negative

        viii) pH

            *a)* Test immediately after urination

            *b)* Be sure container is covered until testing to prevent escape of carbon dioxide

            *c)* Normal pH is 4.6 to 8

            *d)* Increases with bacterial infection due to breakdown of urea to ammonia, which combines with hydrogen ions

        ix) Specific gravity

            *a)* A measure of the amount of substances dissolved in the urine

            *b)* Normal specific gravity is 1.10 to 1.25

            *c)* Specific gravity of water is 1

        x) Urobilinogen

            *a)* Indicates presence of bilirubin

            *b)* Normal is negative

    g) Microscopy

        i) Blood

        ii) Microorganisms

$a)$ Normal is negative, but a contaminated specimen may show some bacteria

$b)$ Follow up a positive microscopy with a urine culture

h) Culture

    i) Ideally, a sterile urine specimen is obtained for culture

    ii) Properly obtained midstream urine is typically used

    iii) Antibiotics and sulfonamides may cause false negatives

    iv) Number of culture forming units (cfu) is reported, as well as the type of organism

    v) More than 10,000 cfu is often considered diagnostic of a urinary tract infection

**e.** Stool specimens (Kee, 2005; MDS Metro Laboratory Services, 2005a)

    **i.** Used for differential diagnosis of gastrointestinal disorders, and for microbiologic, chemical, and parasitic studies

    **ii.** Do not mix urine and toilet paper with stool

    **iii.** Note if patient has taken the following within the past 7 days:

        (a) NSAIDs—their anticlotting mechanism may result in trace amounts of blood in stools

        (b) More than 250 mg of vitamin C in diet or in supplements

    **iv.** "Floating" stools (National Library of Medicine, 2005)

        (a) *Not* fat-containing stools

        (b) May be due to excessive flatus—gas-permeated stool is likely to float

        (c) May be due to malabsorption—excess nutrients in stool feed the normal flora microorganisms, which in turn produce more gas

    **v.** Only a small amount of stool is needed for most tests such as:

        (a) Occult blood

            (1) Microscopic examination for presence of red blood cells

            (2) Chemical test (guaiac or orthotolidine)

            (3) Normal is negative

        (b) Gram stain for identification of infectious organisms

        (c) Stool culture for identification of infectious organisms

        (d) Microscopy for identification of infectious organisms

        (e) Trypsin—low levels are indicative of malabsorption

        (f) Rotavirus antigen

        (g) Urobilinogen—gives stool its brown color; normal is negative

    **vi.** Larger amounts of stool are required for some tests

        (a) Microscopy for ova and parasites

            (1) Usually requires three stool specimens to identify and confirm the organism

            (2) Normal is negative

        (b) Fat content (steatorrhea)

            (1) Requires a 72-hour specimen

            (2) No alcohol intake during that time, and a high-fat diet (100 g/day) for adults

                $a)$ Normal is less than 5 to 7 g/24 hours

            (3) Fat retention coefficient is calculated for infants and children who cannot ingest 100 g/day of fat

                $a)$ Measure the difference between ingested fat and fecal fat, and express the difference as a percentage

                $b)$ Normal is 95% or greater in healthy children and adults

                $c)$ A low value is indicative of steatorrhea

            (4) Steatorrheic stools are foul smelling, frothy, and greasy

    **f.** Respiratory system fluids

        **i.** Saliva can be obtained by having patient spit into a container, or by sucking on a cotton pledget

        **ii.** Sputum and saliva are not the same. A sputum specimen can be obtained by coughing up a specimen, or by suctioning a specimen from the trachea

        **iii.** Rinsing the mouth with water before coughing will minimize oral contamination of the specimen

        **iv.** At least 1 teaspoon of sputum is needed for most tests

        **v.** Throat swabs should reach tissues in the back of the throat and tonsillar area

        **vi.** Analysis of sputum

            (a) Sputum C&S—identifies specific microorganism causing infection, and the medication to which it is most sensitive

            (b) Sputum acid-fast bacilli (AFB)—checked each day over a 3-day period for presence of *Mycobacterium tuberculosis*

            (c) Sputum cytology—to identify presence of cancerous cells

        **vii.** Analysis of throat swabs

            (a) Throat C&S—identifies specific microorganism causing infection, and the medication to which it is most sensitive

            (b) "Rapid strep test"—high-sensitivity antigen test to detect presence of group A β-hemolytic streptococcus (GABHS) infection

                (1) Sensitivity varies with the product brand, from 80% to 99%—NPs must know the sensitivity of the product used in their practice

                (2) APA *Red Book* (2003) recommends back-up throat culture to validate *negative* rapid strep tests because of the danger of *not* treating a GABHS infection, e.g., rheumatic fever, poststreptococcal glomerulonephritis

            (c) "Rapid mono test"—rapid heterophile latex agglutination test for presence of mononucleosis antibody to Epstein-Barr virus

                (1) Sensitivity varies with the product brand, from 81% to 99%—NPs must know the sensitivity of the product used in their practice

                (2) A back-up serum analysis is recommended to validate *negative* rapid mono tests because of the danger of *not* treating (see Chapter 33)

    **g.** Vaginal fluids (French, et al., 2004)

        **i.** Best obtained by the NP during pelvic examination

        **ii.** For microscopy and differential diagnosis of vaginal infections, swab the walls of the vagina; obtain at least three swabs

        **iii.** For Papanicolaou tests, use a specially designed spatula to scrape the cervical canal and squamocolumnar junction

        **iv.** Immediately fix the specimen with a commercial spray to avoid drying and distortion of the cells

        **v.** Analyses

            (a) Whiff test

                (1) Add drops of 10% potassium hydroxide solution to the vaginal fluid

                (2) A "fishy" amine odor suggests a positive result for bacterial vaginosis

            (b) Vaginal pH

                (1) Normal vaginal pH is ≤4.5

                (2) pH greater than 4.5 provides an environment that allows bacteria to flourish, thus suggesting a positive result for bacterial vaginosis

(3) Cervical mucus, semen, and blood are alkaline and can interfere with pH testing

(c) Wet mount vaginal microscopy

(1) Clue cells

a) Slide is prepared with one vaginal swab and drops of saline

b) Presence of vaginal epithelial cells suggests bacterial vaginosis

c) Clue cells are coated with coccobacilli that look like ground black pepper

(2) Yeast cells

a) Slide is prepared with a second vaginal swab and drops of KOH

b) Presence of pseudohyphae or yeast buds suggests *Candida* infection

(d) Gram stain

(1) Typically sent to a laboratory for testing

(2) Scored on a scale of 1 to 10 for presence of large gram-positive rods, small gram-negative rods, and small curved gram-variable rods

**h.** Skin tests (Hainer, 2003)

i. For diagnosis of fungal and mite infections of the skin, hair, and nails

ii. Wood's lamp examination—use of ultraviolet light to observe fluorescence

(a) Brown, scaly rash in the scrotum or axilla (erythrasma) is caused by the bacterium *Corynebacterium minutissimum*, which fluoresces a brilliant coral red

(b) Tinea cruris or cutaneous candida do not fluoresce

(c) Pityriasis versicolor fluoresces pale yellow to white

(d) Tinea capitis caused by two zoophilic *Microsporum* species fluoresce blue-green

iii. Skin scrapings

(a) Angle the sharp edge of a #15 scalpel blade away from the lesion

(b) Gently scrape the lesion's surface at a 45-degree angle

(c) Position a glass slide perpendicular to the skin and under the lesion to catch shavings

(1) KOH test can be done in the office to differentiate infections produced by dermatophytes (fungus on epidermis) and *Candida albicans* from other skin disorders

a) 10% to 20% KOH and a blue or black dye (optional) are added to the specimen on the slide

b) KOH dissolves skin cells, hair, and debris; the dye may reveal organisms better than no dye

c) Slide is gently heated to activate the KOH

d) Dermatophytes have long branchlike structures

e) Candida cells are round or oval

f) Dermatophyte that causes tinea versicolor has a characteristic "spaghetti-and-meatballs" appearance

(2) Send the specimen in a sterile, covered container to a laboratory for:

a) Tzanck test to identify altered skin cells typical of herpes simplex or varicella zoster

       b) Skin culture to identify specific organism requires 7 to 10 days to be considered positive and at least 21 days to be considered negative

  **i.** Imaging studies

    **i.** Radiographic methods

      (a) X-rays reveal abnormalities in body structures and some tissues

      (b) MRIs reveal abnormalities in body tissues and structures

      (c) Exposure to radiation is minimal, but may negatively affect fetal development

      (d) Pregnant women should not have x-rays or MRIs unless it is medically required

      (e) Lead drapes are used to protect the abdomen for both men and women

      (f) Contrast dyes and/or bowel preparations are used for some procedures; potential for allergic reactions should be evaluated

    **ii.** Ultrasound tests

      (a) Use harmless high-frequency sound waves that penetrate the organ and bounce back to the sensor, then produce a picture of the organ

      (b) Ultrasound tests are noninvasive and have no radiation risk

## REFERENCES

French, L., Horton, J., & Matousek, M. (2004). Abnormal vaginal discharge: Using office diagnostic testing more effectively. *J Fam Pract, 53*(10), 805-814.

Hainer, B. L. (2003). Dermtatophyte infections: Practical therapeutics. *Am Fam Phys, 67*(1), 101-108.

Higgins, J. C. C. (2000). The status of physician office labs since CLIA '88. *J Med Pract Manage, 16*(2), 99-102.

Kee, J. L. (2005). *Laboratory and diagnostic tests with nursing implications* (7th ed.). Upper Saddle River, NJ: Pearson.

MDS Metro Laboratory Services. (2005a). Urinalysis. Retrieved May 21, 2006, from www.mdsdx.com/MDS_Metro_Laboratories/Patients/MedicalConditions/Urinalysis.asp.

MDS Metro Laboratory Services. (2005b). Stool sample for occult blood. Retrieved May 21, 2006, from www.mdsdx.com/mds_metro_laboratories/patients/instructions/stool sample_for_occult_blood.asp.

Mol, B. W., Lijmer, J. G., Evers, J. L. H., & Bossuyt, P. M. M. (2003). Characteristics of good diagnostic studies. *Sem Reprod Med, 21*(1), 17-25.

National Library of Medicine. (2005). Stools: floating. Medical encyclopedia. Retrieved November 17, 2005, from www.nlm.nih.gov/medlineplus/print/ency/article/003128.htm.

Nicholson, J. F., & Pesce, M. A. (2004). Laboratory testing in infants and children. In R. E. Behrman, R. M. Kliegman, & H. B. Jenson (Eds.). *Nelson textbook of pediatrics* (17th ed.). Philadelphia: Saunders, pp. 2393-2396.

Pagana, K. D., & Pagana, T. J. (2005). *Mosby's diagnostic and laboratory test reference* (7th ed.). St. Louis: Mosby.

Riegelman, R. K. (2004). *Studying a study and testing a test: How to read the medical evidence* (5th ed.). Philadelphia: Lippincott Williams & Wilkins.

# Pharmacodynamic Considerations Unique to Neonates, Infants, Children, and Adolescents

MICHELLE WALSH, PhD, RN, CPNP

1. Principles of drug therapy decision making
    a. Editor's Note: these principles are derived from an old but excellent textbook on drug therapy decision making (McCormack, et al., 1996); although the drug information may be outdated, the principles listed below are essential and timeless
    b. The NP should determine the goals of treatment and answer the following questions:
        i. How confident am I that the diagnosis is correct?
        ii. What is the role of medication in the treatment of this condition?
        iii. What is the evidence to support drug therapy?
        iv. When should drug therapy be initiated?
        v. What drug, dosage, route, and regimen should be used as initial treatment?
            (a) Scientific determinants
                (1) Practice guidelines
                (2) Standards of care
            (b) Socioeconomic and psychosocial determinants
                (1) Covered by insurance formulary
                (2) Parent or patient preference
                (3) Relative cost
                (4) Cost if self-pay
                (5) Frequency of dosage (related to compliance)
                (6) Taste (related to compliance)
                (7) Storage requirements
        vi. How does the drug work (pharmacokinetics, pharmacodynamics)?
        vii. What are the efficacy parameters of the medication?
            (a) What are the indicators of efficacy?
                (1) How quickly should the patient respond?
                (2) How long should I treat the patient with this medication?
            (b) What are the contraindications?

         (c) What are the adverse reactions?

         (d) What are the indicators of toxicity?

         (e) How frequently should I assess the patient during treatment?

      **viii.** If this treatment fails, what substitute medication should I use?

         (a) Practice guidelines

         (b) Standards of care

         (c) Repeat steps v through vii

      **ix.** What if the substitute medication fails?

         (a) Reevaluate the diagnosis

         (b) Seek advice from a pediatrician or specialist

         (c) Refer patient to an appropriate provider

**2.** Pharmacokinetics and pharmacodynamics (Bindler & Howry, 2005)

  **a.** Pharmacokinetics—quantitative evaluation of each component of the disposition of a medication after it enters the body, i.e., effect of the body on the medication

  **b.** Pharmacodynamics—pharmacologic response to a certain medication concentration in the blood or other body fluid, i.e., the medication's effect on the body

  **c.** Coordination of knowledge of both pharmacokinetics and pharmacodynamics leads to best and safest prescribing of drugs

  **d.** Pharmacokinetics are not known for every medication

  **e.** NPs should have a working knowledge of the pharmacokinetics of medications that are commonly used, and investigate the pharmacokinetics of other medications that are used

  **f.** Important aspects of pharmacokinetics and unique effects of age

    **i.** Absorption

      (a) Via passive diffusion from the gastrointestinal tract into the circulatory system—typical of most oral medications

      (b) Physiologic influences on drug absorption (Table 54-1)

    **ii.** Distribution

      (a) $V_d$ = volume of distribution; estimate of the total amount of drug in the tissues relative to its concentration in the blood

        (1) Relevant to deciding upon an initial loading dose versus a dosing regimen

        (2) Value of $V_d$ is different for newborns, infants, children, and adults for many drugs

      (b) Physiologic influences on distribution

        (1) Composition and size of body water compartments (Shields, 2003)

          a) Percent of body weight that is fluid

            i) Premature infants: 85%

            ii) Full-term infants: 70% to 80%

            iii) 4 years to adult: 60%

          b) Percent of body weight that is extracellular versus intracellular fluid

            i) Infants: 45% extracellular vs 35% intracellular; need greater mg/kg doses of water-soluble drugs (e.g. sulfasoxizole)

            ii) Adults: 15% to 20% extracellular vs 40% intracellular

        (2) Protein-binding characteristics

          a) Basic (pH) drugs bind to albumin, $\alpha_1$-acid glycoprotein, lipoprotein

          b) Acidic (pH) drugs bind mostly to albumin

■ **TABLE 54-1**
■ ■ **Age-Related Physiologic Influences on Drug Absorption**

| Physiologic Variable | Neonate Preterm/Term | Infant | Child |
|---|---|---|---|
| Skin absorption | Faster, more drug absorbed | Faster, more drug absorbed | Declines to adult value at puberty |
| Glomerular filtration rate | 30%–50% of adult values; prolonged half-life | Adult value by 6 to 12 months of age | Similar to adult |
| Renal blood flow | <34 weeks' gestation; decreased rate; reaches adult value by 5 to 12 months | Decreased rate until infant reaches adult value by 3 to 5 months | Similar to adult |
| Liver enzymes | 50% to 70% of adult value; prolonged elimination | >3 months of age, values similar to adult | Similar to adult |
| Microbial flora | Acquires normal flora during postnatal period | >3 months of age, amounts similar to adult | Similar to adult |
| Gastric acid secretion | Decreased | Correlates with postconceptual age | Equal to adult |
| Gastric pH | Relative achlorhydria | By 4 months of age, 50% of adult value | Reaches adult value by 2 to 3 years of age |
| Gastric emptying time | 6 to 8 hours | Reaches adult value of 2 hours by age 6–8 months | Adult value is 2 hours |
| Biliary function | Decreased, low concentration | Equal to adult | Equal to adult |
| Intestinal mobility | Decreased | Equal to adult | Equal to adult |

    c) Infants
       i) Serum albumin and total protein are lowest during infancy; reach adult values by ages 10 to 12 months
      ii) If giving a drug to a premature or newborn infant, check the drug's potential for protein binding displacement by bilirubin
(3) Hemodynamic factors
    a) Cardiac output
       i) Pulse rates are more rapid in infancy (110 to 170 beats/minute) and gradually decrease in rate through adolescence (60 to 95 beats/minute)
      ii) Blood pressure is lowest in infancy (mean = 73/55) and gradually increases through adolescence (mean = 121/70)
    b) Regional blood flow
       i) Infants' peripheral circulation is underdeveloped, which causes slow or erratic absorption of intramuscular (IM) or subcutaneous (subQ) injections
      ii) Cold environments cause vasoconstriction, which can slow absorption of IM or subQ injections
     iii) Drug action via IV and oral routes is more predictable than IM or subQ in infants
    c) Membrane permeability
       i) Blood-brain barrier is not mature until about age 2 years

    ii) Encephalopathy is more common toxic effect in infants than older children and adults

  **iii.** Metabolism and elimination

   (a) Body clearance (body Cl) = sum of all mechanisms that result in clearance of a drug from the body

   (b) Ability to metabolize drugs may be genetically modulated

   (c) Drug metabolism occurs primarily in the liver

   (d) Also through kidney, intestine, lung, adrenals, blood, skin

   (e) Kidneys

    (1) Immature kidneys at birth are an indication for extended dosing intervals

    (2) Elimination of metabolites is slower in preterm and full-term infants, and thus may accumulate to toxic levels

    (3) Only free drug is filtered by the glomerulus and excreted

    (4) Renal blood flow is faster in newborns (12 mL/minute) and reaches adult level at about 5 to 12 months of age

    (5) Glomerular filtration rate in infants is 30% to 50% of that of adults; matures and reaches adult values by age 6 to 12 months of age

    (6) Children have decreased ability to concentrate or dilute urine

   (f) Bioavailability—fraction of dose absorbed into the systemic circulation over a finite period

    (1) IV administration leads to 100% bioavailability

    (2) Oral, topical, IM, subQ bioavailability varies widely

    (3) Trough—lowest serum concentration between dosages

    (4) Peak—highest serum concentration after administration of dosages

    (5) Steady state concentration—equilibrium between amount of drug taken in versus amount excreted

    (6) Therapeutic index—concentration of drug needed to achieve the therapeutic effect without causing toxic effect

    (7) Elimination half-life—time required for the drug concentration in blood to decrease to half of the initial value (i.e., cleared)

    (8) Minimum inhibitory concentration—minimum amount of an antimicrobial agent required to inhibit the growth of a microorganism in the laboratory

**3.** Calculating safe doses

 **a.** Weight in kilograms

  **i.** Obtain 24-hour dose according to weight of child: mg/kg/24 hours

  **ii.** Divide according to times per day to administer

  **iii.** Ask: does it make sense to administer the medication at those time intervals?

  **iv.** If unequal intervals are used, ensure that blood levels are maintained at a therapeutic range

 **b.** Body surface area

  **i.** Dosages in mg/m$^2$/dose

  **ii.** Uses height and weight

  **iii.** Requires a nomogram to determine meters squared

  **iv.** Appropriate for children with normal height for weight

 **c.** IV therapy for children

  **i.** Flow rates are usually calculated in microdrops

  **ii.** Equipment made by all companies provides 60 microdrops per mL

4. Therapeutic drug monitoring
   a. Not necessary for most medications
   b. Determine drug concentration via serial blood testing
      i. Peak
      ii. Trough
   c. Regulate dosage
      i. Extend interval if elimination of drug is a problem, trough elevated
      ii. Shorten interval if trough level is low
5. Routes of administration
   a. Intravenous
      i. Direct to systemic circulation
   b. Intramuscular
      i. Decreased absorption hypoxemia, shock or sepsis
      ii. Neonates have decreased muscle mass
      iii. Muscle mass is proportional to gestational age
   c. Subcutaneous
   d. Intradermal
   e. Percutaneous
      i. Increased absorption in newborn
      ii. Toxicity, e.g.,
         (a) Hexachlorophene
         (b) Topical iodine
   f. Aural or otic
   g. Nasal
   h. Eye
   i. Rectal
      i. Unpredictable absorption
   j. Inhalation
      i. Nebulizer
         (a) Storage of medications, e.g., light sensitivity, foil pouches
         (b) Cleaning to prevent overgrowth of bacteria
            (1) Dry tubing
            (2) Change filters
            (3) Cleanse dispensing device and mouthpieces
      ii. Metered-dose inhaler
         (a) Spacers
            (1) Aerochamber    (asthma.nationaljewish.org/treatments/devices/aerochamber)
            (2) InspirEase
         (b) Turbihaler
         (c) Diskus devices
   k. Oral
      i. Preferred route, but consider age-related gastric conditions (see Table 54-1)
      ii. Oral devices
         (a) Medibottle (medibottle.com): dispensed between sips of usual fluids
         (b) Numimed (sharn.com): medicine dispenser in sizes for 0 to 6 months and 6+ months
         (c) Oral syringe
         (d) Dosage spoons calibrated in mL or cc
            (1) Droppers
            (2) Teaspoons

a) Least accurate
b) Most variability
iii. Positioning
(a) Support head of infant
(b) Least restraint for comfort
(c) Supine for eyedrop instillation
(d) Side lying for otic instillation with or without wick
(e) Avoid contamination of dispenser
iv. Flavoring
(a) FlavorRx (appledrugs.com)
(b) Medicine is not candy
(c) Rinse mouth after medication
v. Vehicles
(a) Cream
(b) Ointment
(c) Lotion
(d) Patch
vi. See Table 54-2 for tips on the amount of topical agent to order
(a) To cover once or twice per day for 2 weeks
(b) To cover various body parts (e.g., face, scalp, trunk)
6. Medications for specific conditions or symptoms
a. Pain
i. Dosing guidelines for NSAIDs (see Chapter 55, Table 55-5)
ii. Weak analgesics (see Chapter 55, Table 55-6)
iii. Opioid analgesics (see Chapter 55, Table 55-7)
iv. Procedural sedation (see Chapter 55, Table 55-8)
v. Guidelines for pharmacologic reversal of selected sedatives (see Chapter 55, Table 55-9)
b. Infection—diagnoses, antiinfective medications, microorganism sensitivity, and relative cost of medication (Table 54-3)
c. Allergic rhinitis and urticaria (Table 54-4)
d. Topical dermatologic agents
i. Corticosteroid potency levels (Table 54-5)
ii. Treatments for acne vulgaris (Table 54-6)
iii. Treatments for dermatophyte infections (Table 54-7)
e. Major depressive disorder medications (Table 54-8)

*Text continued on p. 923.*

■ **TABLE 54-2**
■ ■ **Amount of Topical Agent to Order Depending on Frequency of Use and Body Part to be Covered**

|  | Once Only Coverage | Coverage Times/Day for 2 Weeks |
| --- | --- | --- |
| Entire body | 30 g | 840 g (30 oz) |
| Face, hands, or feet | 2 g | 60 g |
| Arm (one) | 3 g | 90 g |
| Trunk: (anterior or posterior) | 3 g | 90 g |
| Leg (one) | 4 g | 120 g |
| Scalp | 2 mL | 60 mL |

From Goldsmith, L. A., Lazarus, G. S., & Tharp, M. D. (1997). *Adult and pediatric dermatology: A color guide to diagnosis and treatment.* Philadelphia: F. A. Davis.

■ **TABLE 54-3**
■ ■ **Diagnoses, Antiinfective Medications, Microorganism Sensitivity, and Relative Cost of Medication**

| Diagnosis | Generic Name | Examples of Trade Names and Route(s) of Administration | Microorganism Sensitivity | Relative Cost |
|---|---|---|---|---|
| Prevention of rheumatic fever | Penicillin | IM injection | *S. pyogenes* | |
| Strep throat (GABHS) | Potassium salts of Penicillin V | Pen VK Oral—tablets, suspension | Streptococci groups A, C, G, H, L, and M | $ |
| Impetigo Otitis media Rhinosinusitis Pneumonia Pharyngitis Urinary tract infection | Amoxicillin | Amoxil DisperMox Tablets Oral suspension | Only for β-lactamase–negative strains of: *S. pyogenes*, α and β *S. aureus* *H. influenzae* *S. pneumoniae* *E. coli* *P. mirabilis* *E. faecalis* *N. gonorrhoeae* *H. pylori* | $ |
| Otitis media Pneumonia Pharyngitis Skin infections Sinusitis Urinary tract infection Urinary tract infection | Amoxicillin/clavulanate (a β-lactamase inhibitor) Trimethoprim-sulfamethoxazole | Augmentin Tablets Oral suspension Bactrim Septra Tablets | β-lactamase–producing strains of: *H. influenzae* *M. catarrhalis* *E. coli* *Klebsiella* *S. aureus* *Enterobacter* *E. coli* *M. morganii* *P. mirabilis* *P. vulgaris* | $$$ $ |
| Urinary tract infection | Nitrofurantoin | Macrobid Tablets | *E. coli* *S. saprophyticus* | $ |
| Bronchitis Gonococcal urethritis Prostatitis Sinusitis Skin infection Urinary tract infection | Ciprofloxacin | Cipro Oral tablets IV | *N. gonorrhoeae* *E. coli* *K. pneumoniae* *E. cloacae* *P. mirabilis* *P. aeruginosa* *S. epidermidis* *S. saprophyticus* *E. faecalis* *H. influenzae* *S. pneumoniae* | |

*Continued*

■ **TABLE 54-3**

■ ■ **Diagnoses, Antiinfective Medications, Microorganism Sensitivity, and Relative Cost of Medication—cont'd**

| Diagnosis | Generic Name | Examples of Trade Names and Route(s) of Administration | Microorganism Sensitivity | Relative Cost |
|---|---|---|---|---|
| Cervicitis<br>Genital ulcers<br>Otitis media<br>Pharyngitis<br>Pneumonia<br>Skin infection<br>Tonsillitis<br>Urethritis | Azithromycin | Zithromax<br>Tablets | *C. pneumoniae*<br>*N. gonorrhoeae*<br>*H. ducreyi*<br>*H. influenzae*<br>*M. catarrhalis*<br>*M. pneumoniae*<br>*S. pneumoniae*<br>*S. aureus*<br>*S. pyogenes*<br>*S. agalactiae* | $$ |
| Chlamydial infections (eye, genital)<br>Intestinal amebiasis<br>Lyme disease<br>Respiratory tract infections<br>Rocky Mountain spotted fever<br>Urethritis<br>Severe acne | Doxycycline | Vibramycin<br>Capsules | *M. pneumoniae*<br>*C. trachomatis*<br>*U. urealyticum*<br>*S. pneumoniae*<br>*N. gonorrhoeae*<br>*T. pallidum* | $$ |
| Abdominal infection<br>Bacterial vaginosis<br>Intestinal amebiasis<br>Recurrent urethritis<br>Skin infection<br>Trichomoniasis | Metronidazole | Flagyl<br>Tablets<br>Vaginal gel | *T. vaginalis*<br>*G. vaginalis*<br>*B. fragilis* group (*B. fragilis, B. distasonis, B. ovatus, B. vulgatus, B. thetaiotaomicron*)<br>*Clostridium* species<br>*Eubacterium* species<br>*Peptococcus niger*<br>*Peptostreptococcus* species | $ |
| Candidiasis:<br>Vaginal<br>Oropharyngeal | Clotrimazole | Lotrimin vaginal cream<br>Mycelex lozenge | *C. albicans* | $$ |
| Candidiasis:<br>Vaginal | Miconazole | Monistat cream | *C. albicans* | $$ |
| Candidiasis:<br>Vaginal<br>Oropharyngeal | Nystatin | Mycostatin<br>Tablets—oral and vaginal<br>Cream, powder, ointment | *C. albicans* | $$ |
| Candidiasis:<br>Vaginal | Fluconazole | Diflucan tablets | *C. albicans* | $$ |

■ **TABLE 54-3**
■ ■ **Diagnoses, Antiinfective Medications, Microorganism Sensitivity, and Relative Cost of Medication—cont'd**

| Diagnosis | Generic Name | Examples of Trade Names and Route(s) of Administration | Microorganism Sensitivity | Relative Cost |
|---|---|---|---|---|
| Anogenital warts | Podofilox | Condylox gel 5% | Verruca condyloma | $$ |
| Actinic keratosis Genital warts | Imiquimod | Aldara 5% cream | None | $$$ |
| Herpes zoster infection (shingles) Chickenpox Genital herpes | Acyclovir | Zovirax Capsules, tablets Oral suspension | Herpes zoster *Varicella* | $$$ |
| Pinworms | Albendazole Pyrantel Mebendazole | Albenza tablets Antiminth, Pin-Rid tablets, suspension Vermox tablets | *E. vermicularis* | $$ |
| Bronchitis Otitis media[1] Pharyngitis Pneumonia Sinusitis[1] Skin infections Tonsillitis | Cefdinir (3rd-generation cephalosporin) | Omnicef Capsules Oral suspension | *S. aureus* *S. pneumoniae* *S. pyogenes* *H. influenzae* β+ & β− *H. parainfluenza* *M. catarrhalis* β+ & β− | $$$ |
| Bone infections Pharyngitis Skin infections Tonsillitis GU tract infections | Cephalexin (1st-generation cephalosporin) | Keflex Tablets Capsules Oral suspension | *S. aureus* *S. pneumoniae* *S. pyogenes* *H. influenzae* β− *H. parainfluenzae* *M. catarrhalis* β− | $$ |
| Bronchitis Otitis media Pharyngitis Skin infections Sinusitis Tonsillitis Urinary tract infections | Cefprozil (2nd-generation cephalosporin) | Cefzil Tablets Oral suspension | *S. aureus* *S. pneumoniae* *S. pyogenes* *H. influenzae* β+ & β− *H. parainfluenzae* *M. catarrhalis* β+ & β− Note susceptibility patterns in geographic area | $$$ |
| Bronchitis Otitis media Pharyngitis Pneumonia Sinusitis Skin infections Tonsillitis Uncomplicated pyelonephritis Urinary tract infection | Loracarbef (2nd-generation cephalosporin) | Lorabid Capsules Oral suspension | *S. aureus* *S. pneumoniae* *S. pyogenes* *H. influenzae* β+ & β− *H. parainfluenzae* *M. catarrhalis* β+ & β− | $$$ |

*Continued*

■ **TABLE 54-3**
■ ■ **Diagnoses, Antiinfective Medications, Microorganism Sensitivity, and Relative Cost of Medication—cont'd**

| Diagnosis | Generic Name | Examples of Trade Names and Route(s) of Administration | Microorganism Sensitivity | Relative Cost |
|---|---|---|---|---|
| Otitis media[1] Bronchitis Gonorrhea? Pharyngitis Pneumonia Sinusitis[1] Tonsillitis | Cefpodoxime (3rd-generation cephalosporin) | Vantin Tablets Oral suspension (given with food) | *S. aureus* *S. pneumoniae* *S. pyogenes* *H. influenzae* β+ & β− *H. parainfluenzae* *M. catarrhalis* β+ & β− | $$$ |
| Bronchitis Otitis media[1] Pharyngitis Pneumonia Sinusitis[1] Tonsillitis | Cefuroxime (2nd-generation cephalosporin) | Ceftin IM, IV Tablet Oral suspension (given with food) | Penicillin-susceptible *S. pneumoniae* *S. aureus* *S. pyogenes* *H. influenzae* β− *H. parainfluenzae* *K. pneumoniae* *E. coli* | $$$ |
| Epididymitis Gonococcal urethritis Lower respiratory tract infections[2] Otitis media[2] | Ceftriaxone (3rd-generation cephalosporin) | Rocephin Injection | *S. aureus* *S. pneumoniae* *S. pyogenes* *H. influenzae* β+ & β− *H. parainfluenzae* *M. catarrhalis* β+ & β− *K. pneumoniae* *E. coli* *E. aerogenes* *P. mirabilis* *S. marcescens* *N. gonorrhoeae* | $$$$ |

This table has been reprinted with permission from *ADVANCE* Newsmagazines.
[1]Recommended.
[2]Only when causative organism is known to be susceptible.
From Kessenich, C. R., Klotch, D. W., & Cichon, M. J. (2002). The cephalosporins: Targeting respiratory infections. *Adv Nurse Pract, Nov.*, 18, 23–25 and from www.RxList.com.

■ **TABLE 54-4**
■ ■ **Medications Typically Used for Treatment of Allergic Rhinitis and Urticaria, Listed in Order of Preference According to the American Academy of Pediatrics**

| Generic Names | Examples of Trade Names | Recommended Route | Relative Cost |
|---|---|---|---|
| Diphenhydramine | Benadryl | Oral—tablets, syrup | $ |
| Hydroxyzine | Atarax | Oral—tablets | $$ |
| Cetirizine | Zyrtec | Oral—syrup, tablets, meltaway tablets | $$$ |
| Fexofenadine | Allegra | Oral—tablets | $$$ |
| Desloratadine | Clarinex | Oral—tablets | $$$ |
| Montelukast | Singulair | Oral—granules, chewable tablets, tablets | $$$ |
| Loratadine | Claritin | Oral—syrup, tablets | $$ |
| Cyproheptadine | Periactin | Oral—tablets | $$ |

■ **TABLE 54-5**
■ ■ **Potency of Corticosteroid Preparations**

| Ranking and Generic Name | Vehicle | Concentration |
|---|---|---|
| **Least Potent** | | |
| Hydrocortisone acetate | Cream, ointment, lotion, solution | 1%, 2.5% |
| Dexamethasone | Elixir, suspension, tablets | 0.5 mg, 0.75 mg |
| Prednisolone, methylprednisolone | Syrup | 15 mg/5 mL |
| | Tablets | 2, 4, 8, 16, 24, 32 mg |
| **Mild** | | |
| Fluocinolone acetonide | Oil, solution, shampoo | 0.01% |
| Betamethasone valerate | lotion | 0.05% |
| Triamcinolone acetonide | Cream | 0.1% |
| | Aerosol | 60 mg |
| Desonide | Cream, ointment, lotion | 0.05% |
| Alclometasone dipropionate | Cream, ointment | 0.05% |
| **Lower Midstrength** | | |
| Fluticasone propionate | Cream | 0.05% |
| Fluocinolone acetonide | Cream | 0.025% |
| Betamethasone valerate | Cream | 0.1% |
| Hydrocortisone valerate | Cream | 0.2% |
| Betamethasone dipropionate | Lotion | 0.05% |
| Prednicarbate | Cream | 0.1% |
| **Midstrength** | | |
| Mometasone furoate | Cream, lotion | 0.1% |
| Triamcinolone acetonide | Cream | 0.1% |
| Fluocinolone acetonide | Ointment | 0.025% |
| Hydrocortisone valerate | Ointment | 0.2% |
| **Upper Midstrength** | | |
| Triamcinolone acetonide | Ointment | 0.1% |
| Amcinonide | Cream, lotion | 0.1% |
| Betamethasone dipropionate | Cream | 0.05% |
| Betamethasone valerate | Ointment | 0.1% |
| Fluticasone propionate | Ointment | 0.005% |
| Diflorasone diacetate | Cream | 0.05% |
| Desoximetasone | Cream | 0.05% |
| **Potent** | | |
| Fluocinonide | Cream, ointment, gel, solution | 0.05% |
| Mometasone furoate | Ointment | 0.1% |
| Betamethasone dipropionate | Ointment | 0.05% |
| Amcinonide | Ointment | 0.1% |
| Desoximetasone | Cream, ointment, gel | Ointment: 0.25% Gel: 0.5% |
| Diflorasone diacetate | Cream, ointment | 0.05% |
| **Super Potent** | | |
| Clobetasol propionate | Cream, ointment, lotion | 0.05% |
| Betamethasone dipropionate | Gel, ointment | 0.05% |
| Diflorasone diacetate | Ointment | 0.05% |
| Halobetasol propionate | Cream, ointment | 0.05% |

■ **TABLE 54-6**

■ ■ **Medicinal Treatment Options According to Severity of Noninflammatory and Inflammatory Acne Vulgaris**

| Product | Dosage and Route According to Severity | | Action |
| | Mild | Moderate or Severe | |
| --- | --- | --- | --- |
| Tretinoin[1] | Topical: at bedtime gel, cream, ointment, solution 0.025%–10% | | Retinoids[1]: Antiinflammatory Comedolytic Normalize follicular keratinization Prevent formation of new comedones |
| Adapalene[1] | Topical: gel, cream 0.1% at bedtime | | |
| Tazarotene[1] | Topical: gel 0.05%–0.1% at bedtime | | |
| Clindamycin[1] | Topical: gel, solution, lotion; 10% daily or bid | Oral: 75–150 mg daily or bid | Antibiotics[1]: 1. To reduce *P. acnes* bacteria 2. Antiinflammatory |
| Erythromycin[1] | Topical: gel, ointment, solution; 2% daily or bid | Oral: 250–500 mg daily or bid | |
| Sodium sulfacetamide[1] | Topical: lotion; 10% daily or bid | | Sulfacetamide is also keratolyic |
| Azelaic acid[1] | Topical: cream 20% bid | | Azelaic acid is anticomedonal and normalizes keratinization |
| Tetracycline | | Oral: 250–500 mg daily or bid | |
| Doxycycline | | Oral: 50–100 mg daily or bid | |
| Trimethoprim-sulfamethoxazole | | Oral: 800/160 mg daily or bid | |
| Minocycline | | Oral: 50–100 mg daily or bid | |
| Salicylic acid | Topical: gel, cream, ointment, solution 0.5%–6% daily or bid | | Inhibits comedone formation through desquamation of dead skin cells |
| Benzoyl peroxide | Topical: gel, cream, solution, lotion 2.5%–10% daily or bid | | Bacteriostatic and has mild comedolytic activity |
| Low dose contraceptives | Oral; daily (females only) | | Suppress sebum production |

Table adapted from Parish, T. G. (2004). Inflammatory acne: Management in primary care. *Clin Rev, 14*(7), 40–45.
[1]First-line therapy should include a topical retinoid *and* a topical antimicrobial agent for both noninflammatory and inflammatory acne vulgaris (Baldwin & Berson, 2005).

### ■ TABLE 54-7
### ■ ■ Topical and Oral Therapy for Dermatophyte Infections

| Agent | Vehicle | Regimen |
|---|---|---|
| **TOPICAL AGENTS**[1] | **Tinea cruris & pedis**: *apply for 2 weeks: then refer if unimproved* | |
| | **Tinea corporis:** *apply for 4 to 6 weeks* | |
| **Allylamines** | | |
| Naftifine (Naftin) | 1% cream | Once daily |
| | 1% gel | Once or twice daily |
| Terbinafine (Lamisil) | 1% cream or solution | Once or twice daily |
| **Benzylamine** | | |
| Butenafine (Mentax) | 1% cream | Once or twice daily |
| **Imidazoles** | | |
| Clotrimazole (Lotrimin) | 1% cream, solution, or lotion | Twice daily |
| Econazole (Spectazole) | 1% cream | Once daily |
| Ketoconazole (Nizoral) | 1% cream | Once daily |
| | 1% shampoo | Twice weekly |
| Miconazole (Micatin) | 2% cream, spray, lotion, or powder | Twice daily |
| Oxiconazole (Oxistat) | 1% cream or lotion | Once or twice daily |
| Sulconazole (Exelderm) | 1% cream or lotion | Once or twice daily |
| **Miscellaneous** | | |
| Ciclopirox (Loprox) | 1% cream or lotion | Twice daily |
| Tolnaftate (Tinactin) | 1% cream, solution, or powder | Twice daily |
| **ORAL AGENTS**[2] | | |
| Griseofulvin | Oral capsule, suspension | 20–25 mg/kg/day × 6 to 8 weeks |
| Microsize | Oral tablet | 10–15 mg/kg/day × 6 to 8 weeks |
| Ultramicrosize | | |
| Terbinafine | Oral | 5 mg/kg/day (max 250 mg) × 2–4 weeks |
| Itraconazole | Oral capsule | 5 mg/kg/day × 4 weeks |
| | Oral solution | 3 mg/kg/day × 4 weeks |
| Fluconazole | Oral tablet, suspension | 6 mg/kg/day × 3 weeks |

[1]Topical therapy is appropriate for tinea corporis, tinea pedis, tinea cruris (Darmstadt & Sidbury, 2004).
[2]Oral therapy is appropriate for tinea capitis; continue treatment for 2 weeks after resolution of symptoms (Roberts & Friedlander, 2005)

    **f.** Anxiety disorders (Table 54-9)
    **g.** Topical eye medications (Table 54-10)
    **h.** Topical ear medications (Table 54-11)
    **i.** Respiratory medications commonly used for premature infants (see Table 20-2)
    **j.** Gastrointestinal reflux medications (see Table 20-3)
    **k.** Birth control options for adolescents (Table 26-1)
    **l.** Hypertension medications (see Chapter 29, Table 29-4)
  **m.** Asthma treatments
      **i.** Inhaled corticosteroids (see Chapter 36, Table 36-3)
     **ii.** Other inhaled medications (see Chapter 36, Table 36-4)
   **iii.** Quick relief medications (see Chapter 36, Table 36-5)
    **n.** Insulins (see Chapter 44, section 7.e in Type 1 Diabetes)
    **o.** Anticonvulsants (see Chapter 46, Table 46-1)
    **p.** Juvenile rheumatoid arthritis (see Chapter 48, Table 48-1)

■ **TABLE 54-8**
■ ■ **Selective Serotonin Reuptake Inhibitors (SSRIs) Recommended for Treatment of Child or Adolescent Major Depressive Disorder**

| Generic Name | Trade Name | Dosage | Side Effects | Relative Cost $,$$,$$$ |
|---|---|---|---|---|
| | | | **Common side effects** | |
| Citalopram | Celexa | SD = 5 mg | | $$$ |
| | | DD = 10–20 mg | Excitation/agitation | |
| Sertraline | Zoloft | SD = 12.5–25 mg | Nausea/vomiting | $$$ |
| | | DD = 50–100 mg | Diarrhea | |
| Paroxetine | Paxil | SD = 5–10 mg | Dizziness | $$$ |
| | | DD = 20–40 mg | Chills | |
| Fluvoxamine | Luvox | SD = 25 mg | **Less common** | $$$ |
| | | DD = 50–200 mg | Muscle twitching | |
| Fluoxetine | Prozac | SD = 5 mg | Fever | $$ |
| | | DD = 10–20 mg | Confusion | |
| | | | Diaphoresis | |
| | | | **Rare side effects** | |
| | | | Seizures | |
| | | | Delirium | |
| | | | Coma | |

SD, Usual oral starting dose; DD, effective daily dosage.
Emslie & Mayes, 2001; Medical Economics Staff (2002); Moldenhauer & Melnyk, (2000).

■ **TABLE 54-9**
■ ■ **Medications Used to Treat Children and Adolescents with Anxiety Disorders**

| Generic (Trade Name) | Diagnosis | Starting Dose | Total Daily PO Dose | Common Side Effects | Relative Cost $,$$,$$$ |
|---|---|---|---|---|---|
| Buspirone (BuSpar) | GAD | 5 mg | Child: 15–30 mg<br>Teen: 15–60 mg | Headache, dizziness, nervousness, GI upset | $ |
| Fluoxetine (Prozac) | GAD, SAD, phobias | 5 mg | Child: 5–20 mg<br>Teen: 10–40 mg | GI upset, sweating, restlessness, agitation, nervousness, headache, sedation/insomnia, dry mouth, tremor | $$ |
| | OCD | 5 mg | Child: 5–40 mg<br>Teen: 10–60 mg | | |
| Clonazepam (Klonopin) | GAD | 0.25 mg | Child 1–2 mg<br>Teen: 1–3 mg | Fatigue, drowsiness, decreased concentration, disinhibition, rebound, dependence/abuse | $ |
| Clomipramine (Anafranil)[1] | OCD | 10 mg | Child: 75–150 mg<br>Teen: 100–200 mg<br>(2.5–3 mg/kg/day in divided doses) | Increased heart rate, dizziness, tremor, orthostatic hypotension, dry mouth, constipation, blurry vision, sweating, weight gain, GI upset | $ |

*Continued*

■ **TABLE 54-9**
■ ■ **Medications Used to Treat Children and Adolescents with Anxiety Disorders—cont'd**

| Generic (Trade Name) | Diagnosis | Starting Dose | Total Daily PO Dose | Common Side Effects | Relative Cost $,$$,$$$ |
|---|---|---|---|---|---|
| Sertraline (Zoloft) | OCD, GAD, SAD, PTSD, panic D/O | 25 mg | Child: 12.5–100 mg Teen: 25–200 mg | See Fluoxetine | $$$ |
| Fluvoxamine (Luvox) | OCD, GAD | 25 mg | Child: 25–200 mg Teen: 25–300 mg | See Fluoxetine | $$$ |
| Paroxetine (Paxil) | GAD, panic D/O | 5 mg | Child: 2.5–20 mg Teen: 5–40 mg | See Fluoxetine | $$$ |
| Clonidine (Catapres) | PTSD, GAD | 0.05 mg | 0.15–0.2 mg (0.05 bid-qid) | Drowsiness/sedation, dizziness, tachycardia, orthostatic hypotension, weakness, low mood, rebound HTN with abrupt withdrawal | $ |
| Guanfacine (Tenex) | PTSD, GAD | 0.5 mg | 0.5 mg-4 mg (0.5–1 mg bid-qid) | Less sedation and hypotension compared with clonidine | $ |

[1]A+ baseline, monitor ECG, pregnancy test, complete blood count, liver function tests.
GAD, Generalized anxiety disorder; HTN, hypertension; OCD, obsessive-compulsive disorder; panic D/O, panic disorder; PTSD, posttraumatic stress disorder; SAD, seasonal affective disorder.

■ **TABLE 54-10**
■ ■ **Topical Eye Medications**

| Indication | Medication | Regimen | |
|---|---|---|---|
| | | **Adults** | **Children** |
| Infection | Ciprofloxacin 3% (Ciloxan) | 1 or 2 gtt q2h in conjunctival sac(s) during waking hours for 2 days, then 1 or 2 gtt q4h during waking hours for the next 5 days | Dose not established |
| | Gatifloxacin ophthalmic solution 0.3% (Zymar) | >1 yr of age: days 1 and 2: instill 1 gt into affected eye q2h while awake; not to exceed 8 administrations per day Days 3–7: instill 1 gt into affected eye up to qid while awake | <1 yr of age: dose not established |
| | Bacitracin ointment 500 units/g (AK-Tracin, Baciguent) | Severe infections: apply 0.25- to 0.5-inch ribbon q3–4h into conjunctival sac for 7–10 days Mild to moderate infections: apply bid/tid | Dose not established |
| | Erythromycin ointment (Ilosone, E-Mycin) | Children and adults: apply 0.5-inch (1.25-cm) ribbon to affected eye 2–8 times/day, depending on severity of infection | Prophylaxis of neonatal gonorrhea and chlamydia: Apply 0.5- to 1.25-cm ribbon to conjunctival sacs |

*Continued*

■ **TABLE 54-10**
■ ■ **Topical Eye Medications—cont'd**

| Indication | Medication | Regimen | |
|---|---|---|---|
| | | **Adults** | **Children** |
| | Gentamicin (Garamycin, Genoptic) | Children and adults: solution: 1 or 2 gtt q4h to affected eye<br>Ointment: apply 0.5-inch (1.25-cm) ribbon bid/tid q3 to 4h to affected eye | |
| | Tobramycin (Tobrex, AKTob) | >2 yr of age: solution: 1or 2 gtt q4h to affected eye during waking hours and less frequently at night; in severe infections, instill 2 gtt q30 to 60 min initially, followed by less frequent intervals<br>Ointment: apply 0.5-inch ribbon bid/tid in conjunctival sac; in severe infections, apply q3 to 4h | <2 yr of age: dose not established |
| | Sulfacetamide 10% (Bleph-10, Sodium Sulamyd) | >2 months of age: solution: 1–3 gtt q2-3h in affected eye while awake, with less frequent administration at night<br>Ointment: Apply 0.5-inch (1.25-cm) ribbon 1 to 4 times/day into conjunctival sac | <2 months: dose not established |
| Pruritus, watering eyes | Naphazoline 0.1%, (Clear Eyes, AK-Con, Opcon) | >age 6 yr: 1or 2 gtt q2h prn; not to exceed qid; do not administer for more than 3 to 5 days | <6 yr: dose not established |
| | Levocabastine (Livostin) | 1 gt qid to affected eye | Dose not established |
| | Cromolyn 4%, (Intal) | >age 4 yr: 1or 2 gtt q4 to 6h to each eye; use at regular intervals | <Age 4 yr: dose not established |
| | Ketorolac 0.5%, (Acular, Toradol) | 1 gt qid to affected eye | Dose not established |

Silverman, M. A., & Bessman, E. (2005). Conjunctivitis. Retrieved November 30, 2005, from www.emedicine.com/EMERG/topic 110.htm.

■ **TABLE 54-11**
■ ■ **Topical Ear Medications**

| Indication | Medication | Regimen |
|---|---|---|
| Treats superficial bacterial infections of the EAC | Acetic acid with and without hydrocortisone (EarSol HC, VoSol HC, AcetaSol HC) | 5–10 gtt in affected ear tid |
| Bacterial infection of external ear or risk of bacterial infection | Neomycin, polymyxin B, and hydrocortisone (Cortisporin Otic) | 5 gtt in affected ear tid |
| Bacterial infection of external ear | Ciprofloxacin (Ciloxan) | 5–10 gtt in affected ear bid |
| Bacterial infection of external ear | Ofloxacin (Floxin) | 5–10 gtt in affected ear bid |
| Yeast or other fungal infection of the external ear | Nystatin powder (Mycostatin, Nilstat) | 1 or 2 puffs from handheld nebulizer 1× per wk administered by treating provider |

Kacker, A., & Selesnick, S. H. (2005). External ear, infections. Retrieved November 30, 2005, from www.emedicine.com/ent/topic202.htm.

7. Adherence to prescription regimen
   a. The best medicine is the one the child will take
   b. Adherence increases with ease of administration
      i. Once daily greater adherence than more frequent dosing
      ii. Daycare or school administration requires:
         (a) Original container with clear prescription directions and intact labels
         (b) Forms signed by parent and prescriber
   c. Adherence increases if both parent and child agree that medication is needed
   d. Remind parent and child that even if symptoms subside, the full length of dosage administration is necessary to achieve and maintain the required therapeutic effect

# REFERENCES

Baldwin, H. E., & Berson, D. S. (2005). *New perspectives in the management of acne, photodamage, and wound healing*. Cherry Hill, NJ: Elsevier.

Darmstadt, G. L., & Sidbury, R. (2004). The skin. In R. E. Behrman, R. M. Kliegman, & H. B. Jenson (Eds.). *Nelson textbook of pediatrics* (17th ed.). Philadelphia: Saunders, pp. 2153-2250.

Emslie, G. J. & Mayes, T. C. (2001). Mood disorders in children and adolescents: psychopharmacological treatment. *Biological Psychiatry, 49*, 1082-1090.

McCormack, J., Brown, G., Levine, M., et al. (1996). *Drug therapy decision making guide*. Philadelphia: Saunders. [Editor's note: not recommended for drug information, but for list of principles of drug therapy decision making.]

Parish, T. G. (2004). Inflammatory acne: Management in primary care. *Clin Rev, 14*(7), 40-45.

Reed, M. D., & Gal, P. (2004). Principles of drug therapy. In R. E. Behrman, R. M. Kliegman, & H. B. Jenson (Eds.). *Nelson textbook of pediatrics* (17th ed.). Philadelphia: Saunders, pp. 2427-2432.

Roberts, B. J., & Friedlander, S. F. (2005). Tinea capitis: A treatment update. *Pediatr Ann, 34*(3), 191-200.

Shields, B. (2003). Principles of newborn and infant drug therapy. In C. Kenner & J. W. Lott (Eds.). *Comprehensive neonatal nursing: A physiologic approach* (3rd ed.). Philadelphia: Saunders.

Silverman, M. A., & Bessman, E. (2005). Conjunctivitis. Retrieved November 30, 2005, from www.emedicine.com/EMERG/topic110.htm.

# 55 Pain Management for Children

CHARLENE COWLEY, MS, RN, CPNP

1. General information about pain
   a. Pediatric nurse practitioners in acute, chronic, and primary care settings frequently encounter challenges in the assessment and treatment of children with pain
   b. "Pain is one of the most misunderstood, underdiagnosed, and undertreated/untreated medical problems, particularly in children" (Gerick, 2005, p. 295)
   c. JCAHO regulations regard pain as "the fifth vital sign" and require caregivers to regularly assess and address pain (Gerick, 2005)
   d. Definitions of pain
      i. The International Association for the Study of Pain (IASP) states that "pain is an unpleasant sensory and emotional experience associated with actual or potential tissue damage, or described in terms of such damage" (Mersky, 1986, p. S217)
      ii. McCaffery's classic definition: "Pain is what the experiencing person says it is, existing whenever he or she says it does" (Pasero, Paice, & McCaffery, 1999, p. 17)
      iii. "Pain is always subjective" (American Pain Society [APS], 1999, p. 3)
   e. Characteristics of pain
      i. Inherent part of life
      ii. Serves as a warning signal
         (a) To protect oneself from further harm
         (b) To seek medical care
      iii. Pain is the most common reason that a person seeks medical advice
2. Anatomy and physiology of pain
   a. At approximately 24 weeks of gestation
      i. Pathways for the transmission and perception of pain are developed
         (a) Larger receptor fields are stimulated with noxious stimuli
         (b) Ability to modulate pain using endogenous opioids, serotonin, or norepinephrine is not yet developed (AAP & CPS, 2000; Fitzgerald, 2000)
   b. Nociception: the usual response to a noxious stimulus
      i. Begins at the site of tissue damage peripherally and ends with the perception and response to the stimulus centrally
      ii. Has four major steps: transduction, transmission, perception, modulation
         (a) Transduction

   (1) Change of noxious stimuli from a mechanical, thermal, or chemical source in the sensory nerve endings, to impulses

   (2) The impulses cause cell damage

   (3) Cells release substances

    a) Prostaglandins

    b) Bradykinin

    c) Serotonin

    d) Histamine

    e) Substance P

   (4) These facilitate the movement of the pain impulse along A-delta and C nociceptor fibers (Berry, et al., 2001; Pasero, et al., 1999)

    a) A-delta fibers are responsible for sharp, well-localized pain

    b) C fibers carry dull, burning, diffusely localized pain

   (5) Cytochrome P450 enzymes

    a) Are responsible for many drug interactions and side effects

    b) Also activate certain drugs (changes codeine to morphine)

  (b) Transmission (Berry, et al., 2001; Pasero, et al., 1999)

   (1) Movement of impulses along the nociceptor fibers to the dorsal horn of the spinal cord

   (2) Once in the dorsal horn, neurotransmitters such as substance P assist with transmission of impulses to the brain

  (c) Perception of pain (Berry, et al., 2001; Pasero, et al., 1999)

   (1) Results of the transmission of stimuli

   (2) Recognizing, defining, and responding to pain occur at this level

   (3) Several locations in the brain participate

    a) Factors affect pain perception and assist in determining the response to the painful stimuli

    b) Past pain experiences

    c) Cultural factors

    d) Meaning of the pain

  (d) Modulation (Berry, et al., 2001; Pasero, et al., 1999)

   (1) Descending pathway of nociception that assists with changing or inhibiting pain impulses

   (2) Substances are released to reduce noxious stimuli and produce analgesia

    a) Endogenous opioids

    b) Serotonin

    c) Norepinephrine

   (3) Occurs at the same time as transmission, because it releases these substances to bind to the pain receptors and thus block transmission of pain in the dorsal horn

 **c.** Pain has sensory, emotional, cognitive, and behavioral components interrelated with environmental, developmental, sociocultural, and contextual factors (AAP & APS, 2001)

 **d.** Acute pain elicits a stress response and affects multiple organ systems in the body (Golianu, et al., 2000, pp. 563–564):

  **i.** Metabolic: hypermetabolism, hyperglycemia, protein catabolism, lipolysis

  **ii.** Cardiovascular: increased blood pressure, heart rate, cardiac output

  **iii.** Respiratory: increased oxygen consumption, decreased tidal volume and functional reserve capacity, ventilation/perfusion mismatch, decreased cough, diaphragmatic splinting

        **iv.** Other physiologic responses: decreased gut motility, gastric acid secretion, sodium and free water retention, syndrome of inappropriate antidiuretic hormone (SIADH), hypercoagulability, increased fibrinolysis, altered immune function, cytokine production

  **3.** Characteristics of pain

    **a.** Nurses' understanding of pain in children is widely studied (Van Hulle, 2005)

    **b.** Management of pain in primary care varies with the type of pain, acute or chronic (Slater, 2003; Schecter, 2003, Rosenblum & Fisher, 2001)

    **c.** Acute pain (AAPM, APS, ASAM, 2001; American Pain Society, 2003)

       **i.** Two categories of pain transmission (Table 55-1)

          **(a)** Nociceptive—characterizes most acute pain

          **(b)** Neuropathic—on rare occurrences pain neuropathic in nature

      **ii.** Well-defined onset

     **iii.** Usually is of limited duration

     **iv.** Typical causes include painful medical illnesses, trauma, or surgery

■ **TABLE 55-1**
■ ■ **Nociceptive versus Neuropathic Pain**

| Characteristics | Nociceptive Pain | Neuropathic Pain |
|---|---|---|
| Definition | Activation of the A-delta and C nociceptors in response to a mechanical, chemical, or thermal noxious stimulus. Normal pain transmission | Reflects nervous system injury or impairment. Abnormal pain transmission |
| Categories | • Somatic: well-localized pain arising from the bone, muscles, tendons, joints, mucous membranes, skin, or connective tissue<br>• Visceral: poorly localized pain arising from the visceral organs such as the lungs, pancreas, and GI tract | • Centrally generated: further divided into deafferentation pain (amputation) or sympathetically maintained pain<br>• Peripherally generated: pain along one or several peripheral nerves secondary to damage |
| Clinical examples | • Somatic: sunburn, cuts and contusions of the skin, mucositis, broken bones<br>• Visceral: colic, appendicitis, pancreatitis | • Central: phantom limb pain, complex regional pain syndrome, spinal cord tumors or damage<br>• Peripheral: compartment syndrome, diabetic neuropathy, Guillain-Barré syndrome |
| Quality | Sharp, stabbing, throbbing, aching, dull, gnawing, cramping, pressure, or squeezing | Prickling, burning, tingling, numbing, shooting, sharp, lancinating, knifelike, or electric |
| Treatment | Usually responsive to traditional analgesics—opioids an d/or nonopioids | Usually requires the use of adjuvant medications such as anticonvulsants, tricyclic antidepressants, or local anesthetics. Positive or negative responsive to opioids |

Berry, P. H., Chapman, C. R., Covington, E. C., et al. (2001, December). Pain: Current understanding of assessment, management, and treatments.

National Pharmaceutical Council, Inc. Retrieved July 25, 2005, from www.jcaho.org/news+room/health+care+issues/pain_mono_npc.pdf

Pasero, C., Paice, J. A., & McCaffery, M. (1999). Basic mechanisms underlying the causes and effects of pain. In M. McCaffery, & C. Pasero, (Eds.). *Pain: clinical manual*. St. Louis: Mosby, pp. 15–34.

     **v.** Treatment

       (a) Most of the time it is responsive to opioids and/or nonsteroidal anti-inflammatory drugs (NSAIDs)

       (b) As tissue healing occurs, pain lessens and eventually resolves

       (c) Untreated acute pain may become chronic pain

  **d.** Chronic pain

     **i.** It is estimated that chronic pain affects 15% to 20% of children (APS, 2001)

     **ii.** Usually has an extended time frame

     **iii.** In its strictest sense lasts greater than 3 to 6 months

     **iv.** Often unpredictable

     **v.** May be persistent or recurrent depending on the cause

     **vi.** Recurrent pain is repetitive painful episodes alternating with pain-free intervals as in sickle cell disease or recurrent abdominal pain

     **vii.** May not be associated with a specific illness or injury

     **viii.** Treatment

       (a) Usually more difficult

       (b) Typically requires a multidisciplinary approach

  **e.** Hyperalgesia—increased response to a stimulus that is normally painful

  **f.** Allodynia—perception of pain in response to a stimulus that is not normally painful (e.g., light touch to an extremity leading to severe discomfort)

  **g.** Cancer pain

     **i.** Can be either acute or chronic

     **ii.** Caused by a variety of different sources associated with the illness

     **iii.** Generally it has an identifiable cause

     **iv.** In children, pain may often be part of the presentation at initial diagnosis and most of the ongoing pain is treatment-related, procedural, or surgical

     **v.** Children whose therapy fails or relapse will often experience pain at the end of life

  **h.** Research shows that demographic factors influence assessment and management of pain

     **i.** Age

     **ii.** Educational preparation

     **iii.** Personal pain experiences

  **i.** Treatment of pain

     **i.** Approximately 90% of acute or cancer pain can be treated with our current knowledge and resources (Berry, et al., 2001)

     **ii.** Prevention and treatment can reduce morbidity and mortality rates

**4.** Myths and facts about adequate pain management

  **a.** "Children, especially neonates and infants, don't feel pain, or if they do, there are no untoward consequences" (AAP & APS, 2001; Gerick, 2005)

     **i.** MYTH: Current research has found that the most premature neonate has the capability to transmit noxious stimuli and perceive pain

       (a) Premature infants and neonates have all the components necessary for transmission and perception of pain at birth (Fitzgerald, 2000; Franck, Greenberg, & Stevens, 2000)

       (b) They do lack the benefit of the modulating system to reduce the intensity of the pain (AAP & CPS, 2000; Fitzgerald, 2000)

       (c) The developing nervous system is more vulnerable to permanent changes that may result in increased pain perception during subsequent painful events (Fitzgerald, 2000; Schecter, Berde, & Yaster, 2003)

      (d) Morbidity and mortality
        (1) Rates are decreased with adequate pain management
        (2) Ventilated premature neonates have fewer deaths or intracranial hemorrhages when they receive morphine infusions (Goldschneider & Anand, 2003)

**b.** MYTH: Children will become addicted to pain medication

   **i.** The American Academy of Pain Medicine (AAPM), the American Pain Society, and the American Society of Addiction Medicine (ASAM) in 2001 defined the difference between addiction, physical dependence, and tolerance

    (a) "Addiction is a primary, chronic, neurobiologic disease, with genetic, psychosocial, and environmental factors influencing its development and manifestations"

      (1) Characterized by behaviors that include one or more of the following: impaired control over drug use, compulsive use, continued use despite harm, and craving

      (2) Research has shown that fewer than 1% of patients using opioids for pain control will become addicted (McCaffery & Pasero, 1999)

      (3) Infants and young children do not have the mental capacity to develop addictive *behaviors*

      (4) No evidence that use of opioids early in life will lead to addiction issues later

    (b) "Physical dependence is a state of adaptation that is manifested by a drug class-specific withdrawal syndrome that can be produced by abrupt cessation, rapid dose reduction, decreasing blood level of the drug, and/or administration of an antagonist"

      (1) Children receiving opioids regularly for more than 5 to 7 days will need to have an opioid taper plan

        a) A good rule of thumb for a taper plan is to decrease the daily dose by 10% every day or 20% every 2 to 3 days

        b) Otherwise, they experience withdrawal syndrome within 24 hours of discontinuing the opioid (Yaster, Kost-Byerly, & Maxwell, 2003)

        c) Symptoms reach their peak at 72 hours

      (2) Signs and symptoms of withdrawal syndrome (Yaster, et al., 2003)

        a) Abdominal cramps
        b) Vomiting
        c) Diarrhea
        d) Tachycardia
        e) Hypertension
        f) Diaphoresis
        g) Restlessness
        h) Insomnia

    (c) "Tolerance is a state of adaptation in which exposure to a drug induces changes that result in a diminution of one or more of the drug's effects over time"

    (d) Pseudoaddiction: iatrogenic developed addiction behaviors secondary to inadequate pain control, characterized by (APS, 1999)

      (1) Inappropriate drug-seeking behavior
      (2) Demanding doses before they are scheduled
      (3) Clock watching

        (4) Vicious cycle of anger, isolation, and avoidance, leading to complete distrust

        (5) Complaints resolve when analgesia is established

  **c.** MYTH: Giving children opioids will cause respiratory depression

      **i.** Risk for respiratory depression in infants older than 2 months of *chronologic* age, not gestational, is no more than it is for adults

     **ii.** Infants are able to eliminate the opioids at adult levels (Walco, Burns, & Cassidy, 2003)

    **iii.** Infants less than 1 to 2 months of age may not need to receive opioids as often as older infants and children because the cytochrome P450 system is not fully developed at birth, thus resulting in prolonged elimination time (Walco, et al., 2003)

    **iv.** Risk for respiratory depression rises when multiple sedating agents are given together

     **v.** Other risk factors include: (Yaster, et al., 2003)

        (a) Altered mental status

        (b) Hemodynamic instability

        (c) History of apnea or disordered control of ventilation

        (d) Patients with a known airway problem

     **vi.** Using appropriate doses for weight and then titrating to effect will significantly decrease the potential for respiratory depression

    **vii.** Sedation usually precedes respiratory depression

        (a) Decrease dose or stop the opioid when signs of increasing sedation are first observed

        (b) Meiosis is also a precursor

   **viii.** Tolerance to the side effects of sedation and respiratory depression usually develops rapidly with ongoing use of opioids

     **ix.** Effective reversal agents

        (a) Available to reverse the respiratory depressant effects of opioids

        (b) As well as other opioid-related side effects

      **x.** Use of opioids to manage pain should not be withheld from infants and children

**5.** Pain assessment

  **a.** Assessment is the first step in providing adequate pain control (Gerick, 2005)

  **b.** Required by Joint Commission on Accreditation of Healthcare Organizations (JCAHO, 2000)

  **c.** Should occur on initial presentation to the health care provider

      **i.** With any new reports of pain

     **ii.** Reassessment after an intervention

  **d.** Assessment is multidimensional

      **i.** See Table 55-2 for a list of self-report measures for children and adolescents (Beyer, et al., 2005)

     **ii.** Behavioral

    **iii.** Physiologic

    **iv.** Sometimes all three components need to be incorporated because children will at times underreport or overstate their pain

  **e.** Parental report in the assessment of pain

      **i.** Usually quite helpful

     **ii.** They know how their child responds to pain

    **iii.** Usually by adolescence self-report should be the major source for pain assessment

■ **TABLE 55-2**
■ ■ **Self-Report Pain Scales for Children and Adolescents**

| Name | Age Group | Mechanism |
| --- | --- | --- |
| Pain history | Age 2 and higher | Child and/or parent provides information about pain and related events |
| Single-item pain scales<br>Faces<br>Poker chip<br>Pain thermometer<br>Visual analog scale | Age 3 and higher | Child selects a face, color or object that reflects the intensity of pain |
| Multiple item pain scales, e.g. Pediatric Quality of Life Inventory | School-age and adolescence | Self-report on a psychometric instrument |
| Pain diary | School-age and adolescence | Self-report on an open-ended or forced-choice document |
| Drawings | Age 4 and higher | Projective technique; drawings that are requested by the PNP are a form of communication between the child and the PNP |

From the Hospital for Sick Children, Toronto, Canada. Pain assessment website. Retrieved on May 21, 2006 from http://www.aboutkidshealth.

**f.** Pain assessment should also include:
  **i.** Cause: postoperative, posttraumatic, disease
  **ii.** Location: many children can point to where they are hurting
  **iii.** Quality: sharp, stabbing, dull, aching, burning, etc.
  **iv.** Timing and duration: intermittent, constant, recurrent
  **v.** Alleviating or aggravating factors: ice, heat, rest, elevation, etc.
  **vi.** Previous medications used: what has and/or has not worked well in the past
  **vii.** Psychologic state: depression, anxiety, secondary gain
  **viii.** Social: school attendance, participation with friends and other activities
**g.** Factors related to perception and report of pain
  **i.** Many patients will not or are unable to adequately communicate, report, and describe their pain
  **ii.** Age-related issues regarding pain
    (a) Infants are able to communicate pain only through their behaviors and physical and physiologic cues (Table 55-3)
      (1) Crying
      (2) Not wanting to eat or be held
      (3) Limb withdrawal
      (4) Hypertonicity
      (5) Facial expressions may include:
        a) Brows: lowered, drawn together
        b) Forehead: bulge between brows, vertical furrows
        c) Eyes: tightly closed

■ **TABLE 55-3**
■ ■ **Neonatal Distress Assessment Tools**

| Measure | Age Level | Indicators | Pain Stimulus |
|---|---|---|---|
| CRIES[1] | Full-term neonates | Crying, oxygen saturation, heart rate, blood pressure, expression, sleeplessness | Postoperative pain |
| Distress Scale for Ventilated Newborn Infants | Preterm and full-term neonates | Facial expression, body movement, color, heart rate, blood pressure, oxygen saturation | Procedural pain in ventilated neonates |
| Neonatal Facial Coding System (NFCS) | Preterm and full-term neonates, infants ≤4 months | Facial muscle group movement: brow bulge, eye squeeze, nasolabial furrow, open lips, stretch mouth, lip purse, taut tongue, chin quiver | Procedural pain |
| Neonatal Infant Pain Scale (NIPS) | Preterm and full-term neonates | Facial expression, cry, breathing pattern, arms, legs, state of arousal | Procedural pain |
| Pain Assessment Tool (PAT) | Full-term neonates | Posture, tone, sleep pattern, expression, color, cry, respirations, heart rate, oxygen saturation, blood pressure, nurses' perception of infant pain | Postoperative pain |
| Premature Infant Pain Profile (PIPP) | Preterm and full-term neonates | Gestational age, behavioral state, heart rate, oxygen saturation, brow bulge, eye squeeze, nasolabial furrow | Procedural pain |
| Neonatal Pain, Agitation, and Sedation Scale (N-PASS) | Preterm and full-term neonates | Crying/irritability, behavior state, facial expression, extremities/tone, vital signs | Ongoing/chronic pain, acute/procedural pain |
| Scale for Use in Newborns (SUN) | Preterm and full-term neonates | Movement, tone, facial expression, behavioral state, breathing, heart rate, blood pressure | Procedural pain |

[1]CRIES = Crying, Requires oxygen to maintain saturation greater than 95%, Increased vital signs, Expression, Sleeplessness.
Adapted from Franck, L. S., Greenberg, C. S., & Stevens, B. (2000). Pain assessment in infants and children. *Pediatr Clin North Am, 47*(3), 494.

d) Cheeks: raised

e) Nose: broadened, bulging

f) Mouth: open, squarish

(6) Physiologic cues

(b) Toddlers' and preschoolers' responses are more complex (DiMaggio, 2002)

    (1) Other variables play a greater role in how they respond

        a) Separation anxiety

        b) Physical restraint

        c) Memory

    (2) Behaviors

        a) Same as those seen in infants

        b) Also aggressiveness

          i) Kicking

          ii) Biting

          iii) Hitting

          iv) Running away

        c) Toddlers tend to be more restless, rather than limiting their movements as seen in older children and adults

    (3) Most will not understand the word "pain" and are unable to fully comprehend the self-reporting tools

    (4) To be able to adequately use self-report tools that use a scale of 0 to 10, the child must understand the concept of numbers

    (5) Many children in this age-group tend to report either end of the scale

    (6) Use simple words when talking with them about their pain (Stanford, Chambers, & Craig, 2005)

        a) "Hurt"

        b) "Owie"

        c) "Boo boo"

    (7) They may only be willing to report their pain to their parents

        a) They may be fearful of reporting to the health care provider

        b) Something more painful may occur, such as an intramuscular injection

    (8) They do not understand cause and effect

        a) Difficulty understanding how medication results in pain relief, especially intramuscular injections or bad-tasting oral medications

        b) Believe in the magical appearance and disappearance of pain

        c) Often believe they did something wrong, making them think that the pain is a punishment

(c) School-age children (7 to 12 years old) (DiMaggio, 2002)

    (1) Beginning to understand cause and effect, and the concept of numbers

    (2) These children are better able to describe their pain

        a) Use self-report tools as one method of pain assessment (Table 55-4)

    (3) Behavioral cues are still important

        a) Withdrawal

        b) Rigidity

        c) Increasing irritability

        d) Refusing to move or be moved

        e) Turning head from side to side

■ **TABLE 55-4**
■ ■ **Observational Pain and Distress Scales for Infants and Children**

| Measure | Age Level | Indicators | Comments |
|---|---|---|---|
| FLACC | 2 months-3 years | Face, legs, activity, cry, consolability | Scoring range 0 to 10. Easy to use |
| CHEOPS—Children's Hospital of Eastern Ontario Pain Scale | 1–7 years | Crying, facial expression, verbal expression, torso position, touch, and leg position | Postoperative pain and needle pain |
| Direct questioning, pain experience history | ≥3 years | The child is asked (using his or her own word for pain) whether he or she has pain, where it is, when it occurs, how it compares to past worst pain, if it interferes with daily activities and how and what helps to relieve it | Gives more in-depth history regarding the pain |
| Objective Pain Scale (OPS) | All ages | Blood pressure, crying, movement agitation, verbal and body language | Validity tested in 13- to 18-year-olds, only face validity for younger ages |
| Toddler-Preschooler Postoperative Pain Scale | 1–5 years | Vocal, facial, and body pain expression | Postoperative pain |
| Adolescent Pediatric Pain Tool (APPT) | 8–17 years | Body outline, word-graphic rating scale, pain descriptor list | A multidimensional tool with established validity and reliability |
| Observation of Behavioral Distress Scale (OBDS) | 2–20 years | Cry, scream, physical restraint, verbal resistance, request for emotional support, muscular rigidity, verbal fear, verbal pain, flail, nervous behavior, information seeking | Procedural pain |
| COMFORT score | All ages | Alertness, calmness or agitation, respiratory response, physical movement, heart rate, blood pressure, muscle tone, facial tension | Developed for use in pediatric critical care |
| Noncommunicating Children's Pain Checklist—Postoperative Version (NCCPC-PV) | Children with intellectual disabilities | Vocal behavior, social/personality, facial expression, activity, body and limbs, physical signs | Needs repeated tests of reliability and validity, but may be a valuable tool |

Adapted from Franck, L. S., Greenberg, C. S., & Stevens, B. (2000). Pain assessment in infants and children. *Pediatr Clin North Am, 47*(3), 494.

      f) Crying
      g) Changes in appetite
      h) Changes in sleep patterns
   (4) More aware of their body, inside and out
      a) Become fearful of injury to their body
      b) Need reassurance about their fears

(5) Need age-appropriate explanations about pain and how it will be treated

(d) Adolescents

(1) Typically will not ask for medications

a) They do not want to appear weak in front of friends and family

b) Assume the health care providers know that they are in pain

c) Assume health care providers would help to alleviate it if they could

(2) Are able to describe their pain, and self-report is the most important component of pain assessment

(3) Adolescents' perception and response to pain are influenced by many factors beyond the physiologic response to actual tissue damage

iii. Language development—as age and vocabulary increase, children have better understanding of pain and more words to describe it

iv. Environmental factors

(a) Previous negative pain experiences in a particular environment (e.g., clinic, treatment room) may result in greater anxiety and pain whenever they return to that environment

v. Psychologic factors (McGrath & Hillier, 2003)

(a) Play a greater role in the response to pain for children than with adults

(b) Anxiety is a major player—difficult to determine which is worse: pain or anxiety

vi. Previous pain experiences

(a) Memories of pain and their circumstances

(b) Alterations in pain signal processing secondary to neurologic changes

(1) Several studies involving follow-up of premature infants indicate that at 4½ years they tend to have higher somatization scores and derive less gratification from maternal contact

(2) By 8 to 10 years they were able to distinguish between physical pain and psychosocial pain and rated their medically related pain higher

(3) Controls for that study did not separate the two types of pain (Goldschneider & Anand, 2003)

(c) It has also been noted that circumcised male infants without the benefit of pain control had higher pain scores and cried longer at their 4- and 6-month immunizations than uncircumcised males

vii. Expectations regarding pain

(a) If children expect that they will *not* experience pain with a scheduled procedure (e.g., postoperative pain), they may have greater distress than if they were told to expect some pain

viii. Temperament and individual coping style play a significant role in how a child responds to pain

(a) Child described by the parent as having a "difficult" personality

(1) Are more sensitive to pain

(2) Have greater anticipatory distress

(b) Some children cope well independently

(c) Others seek support

(d) Children who do not adapt easily to change show greater distress during immunizations

    ix. The interpretation or meaning of the pain

      (a) If from an unknown diagnosis or is associated with the recurrence of a terminal disease, anxiety, and worry may make the pain more intense

      (b) If from a known source that is expected to resolve rapidly, may decrease the pain sensation

    x. Perception of control over the pain or what is occurring to their bodies may help to decrease the intensity

      (a) Children given patient-controlled analgesia

        (1) Have less opioid use overall

        (2) Decreased anxiety

      (b) Cognitive-behavioral therapies that the child has found effective allows them to assist with pain control

    xi. Family reaction

      (a) How parents and other family members respond to their child's pain will greatly influence how their child perceives and reacts to the pain

      (b) Parental anxiety may intensify behavioral responses

      (c) If a child does not report pain while the parents are away, it does not mean that the child is pain-free

      (d) The child may report pain only to the parents or another family member

    xii. Cultural influences

      (a) Children learn to express their own pain based on how their parents or siblings respond to pain

      (b) Model their behavior after the behavior that they see from others

      (c) Learn how to respond by looking to their parents for a reaction

      (d) Learn the culturally accepted standards for communicating and responding to pain

    xiii. Chronicity of pain is often manifested by: (DiMaggio, 2002)

      (a) Depression

      (b) Apathy

      (c) Flat affect

6. Traditional pharmacologic pain management

  a. Consider pharmacologic treatment in a stepwise approach and individualized according to the type and severity of the pain

  b. See Bauman and McManus (2005) for management of children's pain in the ED

  c. See American Pain Society (2005) for management of chronic, noncancer pain in primary care settings

  d. Mild pain

    i. Includes the use of nonopioids

      (a) NSAIDs

      (b) Acetaminophen (Table 55-5)

      (c) Possible use of adjuvant therapy

    ii. NSAIDs, acetaminophen, and weak analgesics (including codeine)

      (a) Ceiling effect in that higher doses will not produce improved analgesia

      (b) May result in greater side effects

      (c) Opioids in their pure form

        (1) Do not have a ceiling effect

        (2) May be titrated to the dose that will provide effective analgesia

■ **TABLE 55-5**
■ ■ **Dosing Guidelines for NSAIDs[1]**

| Drug | Usual Adult Dose >50 kg | Usual Pediatric Dose <50 kg | Comments |
|------|------------------------|----------------------------|----------|
| Acetaminophen | PO: 650–1000 mg q4h (max 4 g/day) | PO: 10–20 mg/kg q4h PR: 40 mg/kg initially, then 20 mg/kg q6h (max 90–120 mg/kg/day) | Lacks the peripheral antiinflammatory activity of other NSAIDs |
| Aspirin | PO: 650–975 mg q4h | PO: 10–15 mg/kg q4h | The standard against which other NSAIDs are compared. Inhibits platelet aggregation; may cause postoperative bleeding. Contraindicated with fever or viral illness—associated with Reye's syndrome |
| Choline magnesium trisalicylate (Trilisate) | PO: 1000–1500 mg bid | PO: 25 mg/kg bid | May have minimal antiplatelet activity Also available as oral liquid |
| Ibuprofen (Motrin, others) | PO: 400 mg q4–6h (3.2 g/day max) | PO: 10 mg/kg q6–8h (70 mg/kg/day max) | Available as several brand names and as generic Also available as oral suspension; gastritis/platelet dysfunction |
| Naproxen (Naprosyn) | PO: 250 mg q6–8h | PO: 5 mg/kg q12h | See Ibuprofen |
| Ketorolac tromethamine (Toradol) | IV/IM: 30 or 60 mg initial dose followed by 15 or 30 mg q6h | IV/IM: 0.5 mg/kg q6h | Duration of therapy not to exceed 5 days Gastritis/ platelet dysfunction |
| Rofecoxib (Vioxx) | PO: 25 mg/day | PO: 0.6 mg/kg/day (guidelines are based on limited pharmacokinetic data [Schecter, et al., 2003, p. 849]) | COX-2 inhibitor; currently not approved for use in children; liquid preparation available; less likely to inhibit platelet function and to cause GI bleeding |

[1]Multiple sources have been used to create this table. These are only guidelines. Doses and management should be individualized to each patient. There are many sources available for dosing guidelines.

(d) NSAIDs, including acetylsalicylic acid (ASA)
  (1) More potent analgesia than acetaminophen
  (2) Antiinflammatory effect
  (3) Function by inhibiting the production of prostaglandins both centrally and peripherally
    a) Arachidonic acid is stored in the cell membranes
    b) Released with cell damage or irritation
    c) Metabolized through the cyclooxygenase (COX) pathway via one of two COX isoenzymes
    d) Produce prostaglandins that can be protective or an irritant
      i) Cause vasodilation and inflammation
      ii) Through the COX-1 isoenzyme in the gastric mucosa, prostaglandin production:

      *a)* Provides protection to the mucosal lining

      *b)* Increases blood flow in the renal system

      *c)* Induces platelet aggregation

    e) COX-2 isoenzyme is increased following trauma or inflammation

      i) Responsible for the metabolism of arachidonic acid

      ii) Resulting in the inflammatory cascade

    f) The traditional NSAIDs (e.g., ibuprofen, ASA, ketorolac) block the production of both isoenzymes, taking away the benefit of the protective prostaglandins (Maunuksela & Olkkola, 2003; Tobias, 2000)

      i) Limited research has been done in pediatrics for the new COX-2 inhibitors, but many are now off the market due to adverse reactions

      ii) Schecter and colleagues (2003) has published some guidelines based on limited pharmacokinetic data (see Table 55-5)

    g) Traditional NSAIDs should never be used in patients with:

      i) Poor renal function

      ii) Hypovolemia

      iii) Concomitant administration of other nephrotoxic agents

      iv) Some NSAIDs such as ketorolac have been associated with a greater risk for nephrotoxicity and use should be limited (Tobias, 2000)

  (e) Acetaminophen

    (1) Antipyretic with weak analgesic properties

    (2) Common analgesic used in pediatrics

    (3) Blocks prostaglandin synthesis centrally rather than peripherally

    (4) It does not interfere with platelet aggregation

    (5) Not associated with gastric distress or ulcer formation

    (6) Frequently found in compounds with an opioid

    (7) Parents and child need education to prevent acetaminophen overdose if multiple compounds are being used

    (8) Incidence of liver failure is increased due to patients using multiple compounds with acetaminophen and not realizing the total daily dose exceeds recommended levels

  (f) ASA use has been limited since it was linked to the occurrence of Reye's syndrome with viral illnesses

    (1) Incidence decreased dramatically since that time

    (2) Sometimes used in treatment of juvenile rheumatoid arthritis and other inflammatory arthritis syndromes

    (3) "ASA permanently inactivates cyclooxygenase, thereby interfering with platelet function until new platelets are produced" (Tobias, 2000, p. 535)

**e.** For mild to moderate pain

  **i.** Consider adding:

    (a) Weak opioid

      (1) Codeine

    (b) An agonist-antagonist medication (Table 55-6)

      (1) Nalbuphine

      (2) Butorphanol

■ **TABLE 55-6**
■ ■ **Dosing Guidelines for Weak Analgesics**

| Drug | Usual Adult Dose >50 kg | Usual Pediatric Dose <50 kg | Comments; Side Effects; Contraindications |
|---|---|---|---|
| Tramadol (Ultram; Ultracet [combined w/ acetaminophen]) | PO: 50–100 mg/dose q6h if >12 yr old | | Exacerbates seizures; contraindicated with TCAs<br>May cause sedation |
| Nalbuphine (Nubain) | 10 mg q3–4h IV | 0.1 mg/kg IV q3–4h<br>Pruritus: 0.01–0.02 mg/kg IV q2h prn | Agonist/antagonist—will induce opioid withdrawal in opioid-dependent patients |
| Butorphanol (Stadol) | 1 mg IV q3–4h<br>1–2 mg (1 or 2 sprays) Intranasal q2h | 0.025–0.05 mg/kg IV or intranasal q3–4h | Agonist/antagonist (see above)<br>Should be avoided in patients with cardiac disease<br>Fewer effects on the biliary and GI tract |
| Codeine | IM/subQ: 60 mg q2h<br>PO: 60 mg q3–4h | IV: not recommended<br>PO: 1 mg/kg q3–4h | Associated with greater incidence of N/V and constipation.<br>Approximately 10% of the population or patients with liver disease are unable to metabolize codeine to its active form |

Multiple sources have been used to create this table. These are only guidelines. Doses and management should be individualized to each patient. There are many tables available for dosing guidelines.

      (c) Lower doses of other opioids to the above therapy
   ii. Many oral opioid medications are combined with acetaminophen
  iii. Hydrocodone has a preparation that is combined with ibuprofen (Vicoprofen)
  iv. Agonist/antagonist drugs react at various receptor sites
      (a) Examples: nalbuphine, butorphanol
      (b) As an agonist to provide analgesic effects they function
         (1) At the kappa (κ) receptor
         (2) And/or the sigma (σ) receptor
      (c) They work as an antagonist
         (1) At the mu (μ) receptor
         (2) Low doses given simultaneously with opioids decrease some opioid-related side effects such as pruritus while maintaining analgesia
      (d) Butorphanol
         (1) Most effective at the κ-receptors
         (2) Minimal affinity for the σ-receptors
         (3) 1 mg intravenously seems to be equianalgesic to 10 mg morphine
         (4) Side effects
            a) Sedation
            b) Nausea
            c) Diaphoresis
            d) Occasionally dysphoria

(5) Should be avoided in patients with cardiac disease because analgesic doses:
  a) Increase systemic blood pressure
  b) Increase pulmonary artery pressure
  c) Increase cardiac output
(6) Intranasal butorphanol has been used in some patients with migraine headaches
(e) Nalbuphine
  (1) Chemically related to oxymorphone and naloxone
  (2) Side effect—sedation
  (3) Safe to use in children with cardiac disease
  (4) It seems to have more antagonist effects at the μ receptors than butorphanol
  (5) It works best for moderate pain control
(f) Tramadol
  (1) Unique analgesic has at least two mechanisms of action that react synergistically to decrease pain
  (2) Synthetic analogue of codeine that binds at the μ opioid receptors and decreases the release of substance P
  (3) Other analgesic effects are secondary to blocking the reuptake of serotonin and norepinephrine
  (4) Evidence that it may also produce analgesia as an $\alpha_2$-agonist
  (5) Only partially responsive to naloxone
  (6) Does not have a ceiling effect
  (7) Side effects are minimal
    a) Nausea the most common
    b) Constipation, sedation, or respiratory depression is not seen with therapeutic use
    c) Development of physical or psychologic dependence has not been demonstrated (Yaster, et al., 2003)
    d) Lowers the seizure threshold, therefore should not be used with:
      i) Epilepsy
      ii) Patients taking monoamine oxidase (MAO) inhibitors
      iii) Other medications that may increase the risk for seizures
(g) Codeine
  (1) Precursor μ opioid
  (2) Metabolized into morphine before it provides analgesic effects
  (3) Patients sensitive to morphine (e.g., unwanted side effects) will have an increased sensitivity to codeine
  (4) Estimated that between 4% and 10% of the population achieve minimal analgesia because they are unable to metabolize codeine due to lack of CYP2D6 in the cytochrome P450 system
  (5) Provides no advantage over other oral opioids as associated with a greater incidence of:
    a) Nausea
    b) Vomiting
    c) Constipation
  (6) Indicated for the treatment of mild to moderate pain
    a) Potent antitussive at half of the analgesic doses
    b) Intravenous administration is not recommended in children because of its association with:

i) Apnea

ii) Severe hypotension

c) Contraindicated in patients with liver or renal failure

f. Moderate to severe pain

   i. Use higher doses of opioids in conjunction with the above therapy (Table 55-7)

■ **TABLE 55-7**

■ ■ **Dosing Guidelines for Opioid (μ-Agonists) Analgesics[1]**

| Drug | Usual Adult Dose >50 kg[1] | Usual Pediatric Dose <50 kg[1] | Comments; Side Effects; Contraindications |
|---|---|---|---|
| Morphine (oral immediate release IR—Roxanol, MSIR, oral controlled release [CR]– MS Contin) | IV: 5–10 mg q2–4h Continuous IV: 0.8–1 mg/hr PO IR: 30 mg q3–4h Not prn 60 mg q3–4h prn PO CR: 15–30 mg q8–12h | IV: 0.05–0.1 mg/kg/dose q2–4h; neonates: half of pediatric dosing Continuous IV: 0.01–0.04 mg/kg/hr PO IR 0.3–0.6 mg/kg q3–4h PO CR: 0.3–1 mg/kg per dose q8–12h | Histamine release—pruritus, nausea/vomiting, miosis, sedation, urinary retention, respiratory depression, constipation, seizures in newborns Metabolized hepatically to M6G, which is renally excreted. May accumulate and cause respiratory depression in renal failure |
| Hydromorphone (Dilaudid) | IV: 1.5 mg q3–4h PO: 6 mg q3–4h PR: 3 mg q6–8h | IV: 0.015 mg/kg/dose q3–4h PO: 0.03–0.08 mg/kg/dose q3–4h | Side effects may be less prominent than with morphine. No active metabolite |
| Fentanyl (IV—Sublimaze; Patch—Duragesic; Fentanyl Oralet [Actiq]) | IV: 25–100 mcg Continuous IV: 50–100 mcg/hr Transdermal: 25 mcg/hr or convert from current opioid to equipotent dose | IV: 1–5 mcg/kg/dose q30–60 min Continuous IV: 1–5 mcg/kg/hr Transdermal: 8–15 mcg/kg/hr Transmucosal (Oralet): 10–15 mcg/kg/dose q2h | Rapid infusion may cause chest wall rigidity Tolerance develops rapidly. Rapid onset, short duration of action Transdermal—should not be used in opioid-naïve patients; 15 to 17 hours to reach steady state Absorption accelerated in response to fever or heat |
| Meperidine (Demerol, Pethidine) | IV: 50–100 mg q2–3h Max dose: 600 mg/day PO: 50–150 mg q3–4h (not recommended for use) | IV: 0.5–1 mg/kg q2–3h PO: 1–1.75 mg/kg q3–4h (not recommended for use) Control of shivering: 0.25 mg/kg IV | Should not be used in patients with renal failure; not indicated for use >48–72 hr Contraindicated with MAO inhibitor use. Active metabolite: normeperidine—lowers the seizure threshold, causes CNS excitability |
| Oxycodone IR (Roxicodone). Oxycodone IR with acetaminophen[2]: (Percocet, Roxicet, Tylox) CR: (OxyContin) | Recommended Starting doses: PO IR: 5–10 mg oxycodone q3–4h PO CR: 10 mg oxycodone q12h | PO IR: 0.1–0.2 mg/kg/dose oxycodone q3–4h PO CR: 0.6–0.8 mg/kg/dose oxycodone q12h | N/V, pruritus, constipation, sedation |

*Continued*

■ **TABLE 55-7**
■ ■ **Dosing Guidelines for Opioid (μ-Agonists) Analgesics[1]—cont'd**

| Drug | Usual Adult Dose >50 kg[1] | Usual Pediatric Dose <50 kg[1] | Comments; Side Effects; Contraindications |
|---|---|---|---|
| Hydrocodone plus acetaminophen[2] (Lortab, Vicodin, Norco) Hydrocodone plus ibuprofen (Vicoprofen) | PO: 5–10 mg hydrocodone q3–4h | PO: 0.1–0.2 mg/kg/dose hydrocodone q3–4h | Same as oxycodone |
| Methadone (Dolophine) | IV: 10 mg q6–8h PO: 20 mg q6–8h | IV: 0.1 mg/kg q6–8h PO: 0.2 mg/kg q6–8—acute dosing; for ongoing chronic use, dose may be smaller | Drug may accumulate with repeated dosing due to prolonged half-life Peak CNS and respiratory depression may not be reached for several days following institution of or increase in dose. The effects on respiration appear to last longer than analgesia Same side effects as morphine |

[1] Note: These are starting doses based on the opioid dosing. Doses need to be titrated based on individual response
[2] Caution when combining opioid products that contain acetaminophen with prn acetaminophen (120 mg/kg/day max acetaminophen dose) in children and >50 kg max of 4 g/day.
Sources: Multiple sources have been used to create this table. These are only guidelines. Doses and management should be individualized to each patient. There are many sources available for dosing guidelines.

   ii. Morphine
     (a) Considered the gold standard because it has been the most widely studied in children
     (b) Equianalgesic dosing of other opioids is compared with morphine
     (c) Induces histamine release
     (d) Should be used cautiously in patients with asthma or atopy
  iii. Hydromorphone
     (a) Five to seven times more potent than morphine
     (b) Less sedating effect
     (c) Useful when a child is experiencing significant side effects
       (1) Pruritus
       (2) Nausea and vomiting
       (3) When morphine use needs to be limited due to renal impairment
     (d) Has fewer active metabolites
  iv. Fentanyl
     (a) 80 to 100 times more potent than morphine
     (b) Excellent analgesic for use in procedural pain management
     (c) Onset is usually less than 1 minute
     (d) Duration of action 30 to 45 minutes

(e) Use of prn dosing is difficult because of its short duration of action

(f) It is often used for cardiac or trauma patients or intensive care patients because it blocks the systemic and pulmonary hemodynamic response as well as the biochemical and endocrine stress response (Yaster, et al., 2003)

(g) Rapid infusions or repeated large doses may cause glottic and/or chest wall rigidity, which may not respond to naloxone or muscle relaxants

(h) Administered
   (1) Intravenously
   (2) Epidurally
   (3) Transmucosally
   (4) Transdermally

(i) It is highly lipid soluble

v. Meperidine

(a) 10 times less potent than morphine

(b) In equianalgesic doses there is little difference with morphine

(c) EEG wave slowing has been noted when large doses are used

(d) Active metabolite called normeperidine may accumulate
   (1) With ongoing use of greater than 48 to 72 hours
   (2) In the presence of renal failure
   (3) High levels of this metabolite may produce: (Yaster, et al., 2003)
      a) Tremors
      b) Muscle twitches
      c) Hyperactive reflexes
      d) Convulsions
      e) Normeperidine has a 15- to 17-hour half-life and does not respond to dialysis

(e) Beneficial for preventing or stopping shivering
   (1) From amphotericin
   (2) Blood product transfusion
   (3) General anesthesia

(f) Concurrent use with MAO inhibitors or in patients with untreated hyperthyroidism may cause: (Yaster, et al., 2003)
   (1) Excitation
   (2) Hyperpyrexia
   (3) Delirium
   (4) Seizures

(g) IV administration causes: (Yaster, et al., 2003)
   (1) 20% decrease in cardiac output
   (2) Increased heart rate

vi. Methadone

(a) Used for tapering children from long-term use of opioids

(b) Excellent analgesic for some patients requiring ongoing pain management

(c) Increasingly used for treatment of acute postoperative pain

(d) Prolonged half-life and a cumulative effect result
   (1) Need to decrease the initial dosing
   (2) Extend the dosing interval to prevent respiratory depression and/or oversedation
   (3) Children need to be monitored closely until an ideal dosing schedule is established

(4) Long half-life is beneficial when used for children with severe, chronic pain who require higher than usual doses of opioids

(e) Available as an elixir or tablet than can be taken whole or crushed

(f) May be given IV for better flexibility of dosing

vii. Oxycodone and hydrocodone

(a) Oral opioids frequently used when parenteral opioids are not necessary

(b) Bioavailability of approximately 60%

(c) In equipotent doses provide the same analgesic effects as morphine

viii. Hydrocodone

(a) Available in several preparations

(1) Combined with 325 mg, 500 mg, or 650 mg of acetaminophen, or 200 mg of ibuprofen

(2) Available in 2.5-, 5-, 7.5-, and 10-mg strengths

(3) As an elixir it is 2.5 mg hydrocodone with 167 mg acetaminophen per 5 mL

ix. Oxycodone (Yaster, et al., 2003)

(a) Metabolized in the liver into the active metabolite of oxymorphone

(b) Both may accumulate in patients with renal failure

(c) Available with or without acetaminophen

(d) Sustained-release tablet (OxyContin)

(e) Oral form of oxycodone may be given rectally and is well absorbed

x. Timed-release preparations

(a) Timed release tablets must be swallowed whole

(b) They may not be crushed or cut in half because it becomes an immediate release preparation

(c) MS Contin, sustained-release capsules

(d) (Kadian) with timed-release morphine pellets

(1) May be mixed in semisolid food for children who can't swallow pills

g. Opioids

i. See guidelines for treatment of children with cancer pain (Sussman, 2005)

ii. Mainstay for moderate to severe acute or cancer pain

(a) Safe to use in children when used in appropriate doses based on weight

(b) Appropriate for some patients with chronic pain

iii. Pure opioids, except codeine or meperidine, that are not combined with acetaminophen or ibuprofen

(a) May be titrated upward in order to provide adequate pain control

(b) Limited only by the presence of side effects or the additives

iv. Potential side effects

(a) Central nervous system

(1) Decreased mental alertness

(2) Sedation

(3) High-dose opioids may cause myoclonus or seizures

(b) Respiratory

(1) Depressing the response of the brain to carbon dioxide, resulting in depression of minute ventilation (Golianu, et al., 2000)

(2) Pain is a potent antagonist to the respiratory depressant effects of opioids

(3) Most of the time occurrence of respiratory depression is secondary to use of other sedating agents in conjunction with the opioid

(c) Cardiovascular (Golianu, et al., 2000)

(1) Meperidine produces tachycardia

(2) May cause dose-dependent, asymptomatic bradycardia

(3) Minimal hemodynamic side effects in well-hydrated children with most opioids

(4) Histamine release associated with morphine

    a) Causes vasodilatation

    b) May cause hypotension in hypovolemic states

    c) This may be minimized by slow infusion and keeping the child supine

(d) Gastrointestinal

(1) All opioids decrease GI motility

    a) Cause constipation

    b) A laxative and/or a stool softener should be started when opioid therapy is initiated unless otherwise contraindicated

    c) The majority of the time a stool softener alone is not enough, a stimulant is also required

(2) Nausea and vomiting

    a) Caused by binding to the chemoreceptor trigger zone in the brainstem

    b) Resolves over time

    c) Treated with:

        i) Antiemetics

        ii) Agonist/antagonist medications

        iii) Low-dose μ-receptor antagonists

(3) May cause spasm of the sphincter of Oddi

    a) Meperidine is not an exception

(e) Genitourinary

(1) Urinary retention secondary to increased tone of the detrusor muscle

(f) Pruritus

(1) May be due to histamine release and/or

(2) Direct effect on the central μ-receptor activity

(3) Treatment

    a) Antihistamines

    b) Agonist/antagonist medications

    c) Low-dose μ-receptor antagonists

7. Medications used in procedural sedation and analgesia

  **a.** Traditionally, pain with procedures has been ignored or poorly treated in children

    **i.** Assumed that pain was unavoidable

    **ii.** Children do not get used to painful procedures

    **iii.** Children become fearful of the health care providers and what might occur at each visit

  **b.** Topical and local anesthetics (Table 55-8)

    **i.** Emla cream: 2.5% lidocaine, 2.5% prilocaine (for intact skin)

    **ii.** Ela-Max: 4% lidocaine (for intact skin)

    **iii.** TAC: 0.5% tetracaine, 0.05% epinephrine (Adrenaline), 11. 8% cocaine (for lacerations)

    **iv.** LET: 4% lidocaine, 0.1% epinephrine, 0.5% tetracaine (for lacerations)

■ **TABLE 55-8**
■ ■ **Guidelines for Procedural Sedation in Children**

| Drug | Route | Dose[1] (mg/kg) | Max Dose (mg) | Onset (min) | Duration (hr) | Considerations |
|---|---|---|---|---|---|---|
| **Benzodiazepines** | | | | | | All benzodiazepines may cause respiratory depression, especially when combined with narcotics |
| Diazepam (Valium) | PO | 0.2–0.4 | 10 | 30–60 | 2–6 | IM route not recommended due to poor absorption and tissue irritation |
| | IV | 0.1–0.2 | | 1–3 | | |
| | PR | 0.2–0.4 | 10 | 7–15 | | May use IV solution rectally |
| Lorazepam (Ativan) | PO | 0.05–0.2 | 4 | 60 | 8–12 | Long DOA often outlasts procedures—best suited for prolonged sedation such as ICU use, tx of status epilepticus, etc. |
| | Deep | 0.05–0.2 | 4 | 30–60 | | |
| | IM | 0.05–0.1 | 2 | 5–10 | | |
| | IV | | | | | May cause hallucinations |
| Midazolam (Versed) | PO | 0.5–1 | 20 | 10–15 | 1–2 | For higher risk patients, use 0.25 mg/kg, PO |
| | Deep | 0.1–0.2 | 10 | 5–15 | | Titrate IV |
| | IM | 0.05–0.1 | Titrate | 1–5 | | Dilute injection in 5 mL NSS and administer rectally |
| | IV | 0.3 | 20 | 10–30 | | |
| | PR | 0.2 | 7.5 | 5–10 | | To administer nasally, use injectable drug in 1- or 3-mL syringe |
| | Nasal | | | | | |
| **Narcotics** | | | | | | |
| Feanyl | IV | 1–2 mcg/kg | | 3–5 | 0.5–1 | All narcotics may cause nausea |
| | | | | | | Short DOA secondary to redistribution; excellent for brief (<60 min) painful procedures; proper monitoring essential |
| Morphine | PO | 0.3–0.5 | | 20–30 | 3–4 | Start dose at 0.05 mg/kg and titrate up to 0.2 mg/kg |
| | IV | 0.05–0.2 | | 2–5 | 2–3 | |
| Meberidine (Demerol) | PO | 2–4 | | 15–20 | 3–4 | Should not be used in patients with renal impairment |
| | IV | 0.5–2 | | 5–10 | 2–3 | |

■ **TABLE 55-8**
■ ■ **Guidelines for Procedural Sedation in Children—cont'd**

| Drug | Route | Dose[1] (mg/kg) | Max Dose (mg) | Onset (min) | Duration (hr) | Considerations |
|------|-------|-----------------|---------------|-------------|---------------|----------------|
| **Sedative/Hypnotics** | | | | | | Max. single dose: 2 g |
| Chloral hydrate | PO/PR | 25–100 | 2 g | 30–60 | 2–8 | Beta elimination t-1/2 is age dependent; in infants and toddlers it far exceeds the procedural duration causing drug effect to persist long after patient discharge |
| Pentobarbital (Nembutal) | IV | 0.5–1 | 0.5–1 | 1–10 | 1–4 | Give slowly, titrate to effect |
| | IM | 2–6 | 2–6 | 5–15 | 2–4 | |
| | PO | 2–6 | 2–6 | 15–60 | 2–4 | Respiratory depression, apnea, airway obstruction and hypotension are common with rapid IV injection |
| | PR | 2–6 | 2–6 | 15–60 | 2–4 | |
| Ketamine (Ketalar) | IV | 0.25 | IV | | | Also give glycopyrrolate 0.01 mg/mg not to exceed 0.2 mg to control oral secretions |
| | IM | 2–4 | titrated to max 2 mg/kg | | | |

[1]Note: These doses are guidelines for admiistering medications to physiologically uncompromised children. Situations may exist when larger or smaller doses may be safely administered predicated on the needs of the patient and procedure. The licensed independent practitioner in attendance is responsible for the safe administration of all medications.

    **v.** Buffered lidocaine
  **c.** Sedatives and hypnotics
    **i.** No analgesic properties
    **ii.** Should be used for painless procedures
    **iii.** No reversal agent is available (Table 55-9)
    **iv.** Exercise extreme caution if used in combination with other sedatives or analgesics
  **d.** Chloral hydrate (Noctec)
    **i.** Used to produce immobility for nonpainful procedures
      (a) MRI
      (b) CT
      (c) BAER
      (d) EEG
    **ii.** Not a potent respiratory depressant
      (a) Its sedative effects can cause airway obstruction
    **iii.** Should not be administered before patient arrival to the hospital or clinic
    **iv.** Instruct parents to watch child closely during transport home
      (a) Airway may become obstructed if child falls asleep
      (b) There have been several case reports of fatalities or severe neurologic injuries in infants who have slumped forward when in their car seats (Cote, et al., 2000)

■ **TABLE 55-9**
■ ■ **Guidelines for Pharmacologic Reversal of Selected Sedatives**

| Drug[1] | Dose | Onset | Duration | Characteristics | Considerations[2]/ Adverse Reactions |
|---|---|---|---|---|---|
| Opioid antagonists: naloxone (Narcan) | IV-bolus: 0.001–0.002 mg/kg/ dose up to 0.01 mg/kg/ dose (max 2 mg) May repeat every 2–3 minutes based on response | IV: 1–2 min- ET: 2–5 min IM: 2–5 min subQ: 2–5 min | 20–60 min | Reverses CNS/ respiratory depression in suspected narcotic overdose May be useful in a loss of consciousness of unknown etiology | May precipitate withdrawal symptoms Use with caution in patients on opioids for chronic pain relief (consider mixing agonist/antagonist) May cause hypertension, hypotension, tachycardia, dysrhythmias, nausea, vomiting, sweating, and pulmonary edema Shorter half-life than most opioids may need to redose q 20 min May be given IV, IM, via ETT, subQ or intraosseously |
| Nalmefene (Revex) | 0.25 mcg/kg IV titrated to max 1 mcg/kg | IV: 2 min | 6–8 hr | | |
| Benzodiazepine antagonist: flumazenil (Romazicon) | Initial dose: 0.01– 0.02 mg/kg titrated to effect max dose: 1 mg over 20 minutes | IV: 1–5 min | 20–60 min | Indicated for complete or partial reversal of benzodiazepine sedation Useful for significant respiratory depression caused by benzodiazepines | Avoid in patients who are benzodiazepine dependent Resedation may occur May precipitate seizures in patients who require benzodiazepines for seizure suppression May cause diaphoresis, flushing, hot flashes, nausea, vomiting, hiccups, CNS agitation, seizures, abnormal vision, paresthesias |

[1]These drugs will NOT reverse the effects of chloral hydrate or barbiturates.
[2]If a reversal agent is used, the patient should be monitored for 1 to 2 hours after administration of the reversal agent

   **v.** Produces two active metabolites
    (a) Trichloroethanol
    (b) Trichloroacetic acid
   **vi.** Residual effects
    (a) Sedation "hangover"
    (b) Disorientation
    (c) Paradoxical excitement
    (d) Delirium
    (e) Ataxia
    (f) Headache
    (g) Nightmares
    (h) Hallucinations
   **vii.** Used with caution or not at all with term or preterm infants because of:
    (a) Accumulation of active metabolites
    (b) Development of metabolic acidosis
    (c) Potential to predispose newborns to hyperbilirubinemia
 **e.** Barbiturates
   **i.** No analgesic properties
    (a) Should be used for painless procedures
    (b) When given to patients in pain, it may intensify the sensation of pain (hyperalgesia)
    (c) No reversal agent is available
   **ii.** Barbiturates produce all levels of CNS depression
    (a) Drowsiness
    (b) General anesthesia
   **iii.** Response is dose dependent on child's medical condition
    (a) Exercise extreme caution if used in combination with other sedatives or analgesics because concurrent use will significantly affect the response
   **iv.** Pentobarbital (Nembutal)
    (a) Often used to produce immobility for nonpainful procedures (e.g. MRI, CT, BAER, EEG)
    (b) Has been associated with significant and occasionally life-threatening side effects
    (c) May cause respiratory depression and airway obstruction
    (d) Paradoxical excitement, particularly in young patients and patients with untreated pain
    (e) Residual sedation "hangover" that may impair judgment and mood for 24 or more hours
 **f.** Benzodiazepines
   **i.** Used for sedation, anxiolysis, and amnesia
    (a) No pain-relieving properties
    (b) Used in combination with opioids for painful procedures
   **ii.** Sedative, respiratory, and circulatory depressant effects are potentiated by:
    (a) Opioids
    (b) Other CNS depressants
    (c) Alcohol
    (d) Extremes of age
   **iii.** Elimination may be affected by drugs that affect:
    (a) Liver metabolism
    (b) Blood flow

(c) Cytochrome P450 3a enzymes (e.g., erythromycin, cimetidine)
  iv. Has an available reversal agent
    (a) Flumazenil (Romazicon)
  v. Commonly used benzodiazepines
    (a) Diazepam (Valium)
      (1) Resedation may occur 6 to 8 hours after administration
        a) Secondary to enterohepatic recirculation
        b) Formation of active metabolite (oxazepam) in liver
      (2) Painful with IV administration
      (3) May cause venous thrombosis with intravenous injection
      (4) Do not use for IM administration
    (b) Lorazepam (Ativan)
      (1) Best used in situations requiring prolonged sedation
    (c) Midazolam (Versed)
      (1) Most commonly used for:
        a) Sedation
        b) Anxiolysis
        c) Amnesia during procedures
      (2) Does not have an active metabolite
g. Opioids
  i. Should be used for painful procedures unless local anesthetics, ketamine, or nitrous oxide is used
  ii. Side effects
    (a) May cause nausea and vomiting
      (1) Especially if patient is not experiencing pain before the procedure
    (b) Pruritus
    (c) Urine retention
    (d) Respiratory depression
    (e) Sedation
    (f) Chest wall rigidity if large dose given as a bolus
  iii. Used in combination with other sedative-type medications
    (a) Increase the risk for oversedation
    (b) Increase risk of respiratory depression
h. General anesthetic
  i. Administered only in the presence of an anesthesiologist or nurse anesthetist
    (a) Skilled and trained in the use of these agents with children
    (b) Demonstrated expertise
      (1) In airway management
      (2) Cardiopulmonary resuscitation
  ii. Ketamine (Ketalar)
    (a) A dissociative anesthetic agent
    (b) Subanesthetic doses produce analgesia and amnesia
    (c) Eyes may remain open and patient may have nystagmus
    (d) Usually the patient is not responsive to voice or verbal command
    (e) Causes cerebral vasodilatation
      (1) Should not be used in patients with:
        a) Intracranial pathology
        b) Intracranial hypertension
      (2) May also cause systemic or intraocular hypertension
    (f) Use a benzodiazepine because emergence from ketamine sedation may be associated with:

(1) Visual, auditory, proprioceptive, and confusional illusions

(2) May progress to delirium

(g) Associated with increased oral secretions

(1) Use atropine

(2) Or glycopyrrolate

(h) When given slowly, it usually will not produce significant respiratory depression

iii. Propofol (Diprivan)

(a) Nonbarbiturate IV general anesthetic without intrinsic analgesic activity

(b) Recovery is rapid with little residual sedation (no hangover)

(c) Rapid response

(1) Longer procedures may need a continuous infusion

(d) Pain or burning on injection is common

(1) Especially in a small vein

iv. 50% or less nitrous oxide

(a) Colorless gas that has sedative and analgesic properties

(b) Weak general anesthetic

(1) Has a rapid onset and short duration of action

(c) When nitrous oxide is discontinued, patients must breathe 100% oxygen through a non-rebreathing mask and reservoir for at least 5 minutes

(d) Child must be old enough to cooperate and hold the mask in place without assistance

(e) Most children experience:

(1) Sense of euphoria

(2) Detached attitude toward their surroundings

(f) Recovery is rapid with little residual sedation (no hangover)

(g) Must be used with a scavenger system to minimize environmental and staff exposure

(h) Side effects

(1) Nausea

(2) Vomiting

(3) Dizziness

8. Nontraditional pharmacologic pain management

a. Many drugs in other categories have been found to be helpful for various types of pain, especially neuropathic pain

b. Clonidine

i. $\alpha_2$-agonist

ii. Shown to be helpful weaning off of opioids and treatment of pain

(a) Neuropathic pain

(b) Visceral pain

(c) Postoperative pain

iii. Route of administration

(a) Oral

(b) Transdermal

(c) Epidural

(d) Intrathecal

c. Others

i. Anticonvulsants

ii. Antidepressants

iii. Antispasmodics

        **iv.** Benzodiazepines

        **v.** Topical anesthetics

**9.** Nonpharmacologic pain management

    **a.** See Gerik (2005) for a review of the pain literature that focuses on the integration of mind-body therapies into the management of procedure-related pain, headache, and recurrent abdominal pain in children

    **b.** See also Chapter 56 for complementary and alternative methods

    **c.** Sucrose

        **i.** For infants, sucking on sucrose water may have a calming effect

    **d.** Language

        **i.** Acknowledge the pain

        **ii.** Use age-appropriate words that convey:

            (a) Support

            (b) Hope

            (c) Love

            (d) Encouragement

            (e) Understanding

        **iii.** Use calm, soothing tone of voice

        **iv.** Remind the child that the hurt is being treated and will come to an end

    **e.** Touch

        **i.** Examples of touch that can communicate support and comfort with or without words

            (a) Patting works well for infants and younger children

                (1) May remind them of comforting routines at home

            (b) Rubbing or stroking backs, arms, legs, or feet

                (1) Helps the child focus on something pleasant

    **f.** Cold packs or cloths help reduce swelling

        **i.** Helpful for short-term pain

        **ii.** Use cold with infants and small children only with specific instructions for use

        **iii.** Be careful using cold when your child has nerve damage or a skin injury

        **iv.** Should not be applied to recent injuries or surgical areas

    **g.** Warm water baths, warm compresses, warm water bottles are soothing

        **i.** Achy muscles

        **ii.** Stiff joints

        **iii.** Muscle spasms

        **iv.** Heat and ice can be alternated to provide pain relief, relieve muscle aches, and reduce swelling

    **h.** Massage

        **i.** Helps to relax tight muscles and relieve spasms

        **ii.** Put warm lotion or oil in your hands and rub sore area

    **i.** Guided imagery

        **i.** Often very easy for children to use their imagination

        **ii.** Alter the feeling of pain

        **iii.** Gain a sense of control over the pain

        **iv.** The Child Life staff or a psychologist can help children and parents learn more about guided imagery

        **v.** This is a skill that can be useful throughout life to cope with stress and promote relaxation

        **vi.** It helps to learn this technique before the onset of pain because most children will be unable to focus for learning during the course of pain

    **j.** Relaxation

> **i.** Deep breathing and relaxation can lessen anxiety and relieve pain
> **ii.** Children can pretend they are "wet noodles" to relax muscles that may be tight
> **iii.** Another way to lessen pain is to tighten and relax muscles from head to foot
> **iv.** Counting breaths and focusing on the feeling of slow breathing also helps

**k.** Deep breathing
> **i.** Can help child to relax and release pain
> **ii.** Have child breathe in a regular and easy rhythm
>> (a) Helps if you breathe with child
>> (b) Breathe in for 3 counts, and out for 3 counts
>> (c) Think to yourself, slowly, as you breathe in and out, "in-2–3—out-2–3"
>> (d) Deep breathing can also help when changing positions or getting up and walking
>> (e) Take a deep breath before the movement and breathe out during the movement

**l.** Distraction
> **i.** Give child an interesting object or toy to hold during a painful procedure
> **ii.** Object can be new or a well-worn, loved toy

**m.** Music
> **i.** Children enjoy music in many forms
> **ii.** Sing to child
> **iii.** Play audio tapes
> **iv.** Play an instrument
> **v.** Have child sing
> **vi.** Music gives child something to focus on besides the pain
> **vii.** Helps pass the time pleasantly

**n.** Other methods (see Chapter 56)
> **i.** Hypnosis
> **ii.** Biofeedback
> **iii.** Therapeutic touch
> **iv.** Transcutaneous electrical nerve stimulation (TENS)
> **v.** Acupuncture
> **vi.** Acupressure
> **vii.** Hydrotherapy

---

# REFERENCES

American Academy of Pain Medicine, American Pain Society, and American Society of Addiction Medicine. (AAPM, APS, & ASAM) (2001). *Definitions related to the use of opioids for the treatment of pain: A consensus document.* Retrieved July 25, 2005, from www.ampainsoc.org/advocacy/opioids2.htm.

American Academy of Pediatrics, & American Pain Society. (2001). The assessment and management of acute pain in infants, children, and adolescents. *Pediatrics, 108*(3), 793-797.

American Academy of Pediatrics, & Canadian Paediatric Society. (2000). Prevention and management of pain and stress in the neonate. *Pediatrics, 105*(2), 454-461.

American Pain Society. (1999). *Guideline for the management of acute and chronic pain in sickle cell disease.* Author.

American Pain Society. (2001). *Pediatric chronic pain: A position statement from the American Pain Society.* Retrieved July 25, 2005, from www.ampainsoc.org/advocacy/pediatric.htm.

American Pain Society. (2003). *Principles of analgesic use in the treatment of acute pain and cancer pain* (5th ed.). Skokie, IL: Author.

American Pain Society. (2005). *Pain control in the primary care setting.* Skokie, IL: APS.

Bauman, B. H., & McManus, J. G., Jr. (2005). Pediatric pain management in the emergency department. *Emerg Med Clin North Am, 23*(2), 393-414, ix.

Berry, P. H., Chapman, C. R., Covington, E. C., et al. (2001). Pain: Current understanding of assessment, management, and treatments. National Pharmaceutical Council, Inc. Retrieved July 25, 2005, from www.jcaho. org/news+room/health+care+issues/ pain_mono_npc.pdf.

Beyer, J. E., Turner, S. B., Jones, L., Young, L., Onikul, R., & Bohaty, B. (2005). The alternate forms reliability of the Oucher pain scale. *Pain Manage Nurs, 6*(1), 10-17.

Cote, C. J., Karl, H. W., Notterman, D. A., et al. (2000). Adverse sedation events in pediatrics: Analysis of medications used for sedation. *Pediatrics 106*(4), 633-644.

Di Maggio, T. J. (2002). Pediatric pain management. In B. St. Marie (Ed.). *Core curriculum for pain management nursing*. Philadelphia: Saunders.

Fitzgerald, M. (2000). Development of the peripheral and spinal pain system. *Pain Res Clin Manage, 10*, 9-21.

Franck, L. S., Greenberg, C. S., & Stevens, B. (2000). Pain assessment in infants and children. *Pediatr Clin North Am, 47*(3), 487-512.

Gerik, S. M. (2005). Pain management in children: Developmental considerations and mind-body therapies. *South Med J, 98*(3), 295-302.

Goldschneider, K. R., & Anand, K. S. (2003). Long-term consequences of pain in neonates. In N. L. Schecter, C. B. Berde, & M. Yaster (Eds) *Pain in infants, children, and adolescents*. Baltimore: Lippincott Williams & Wilkins, pp. 58-70.

Golianu, B., Krane, E. J., Galloway, K.S., & Yaster, M. (2000). Pediatric acute pain management. *Pediatr Clin North Am, 47*(3), 559-587.

Joint Commission on Accreditation of Healthcare Organizations (JCAHO). (2000). *Pain assessment and management: An organizational approach*. Oakbrook Terrace, IL: Author.

Maunuksela, E., & Olkkola, K. T. (2003). Nonsteroidal anti-inflammatory drugs in pediatric pain management. In N. L. Schecter, C. B. Berde, & M. Yaster (Eds.). *Pain in infants, children, and adolescents*. Baltimore: Lippincott Williams & Wilkins, pp. 171-180.

McCaffery, M., & Pasero, C. (Eds.). (1999). *Pain: clinical manual* (2nd ed.). St Louis: Mosby Company.

McGrath, P. A., & Hillier, L. M. (2003). Modifying the psychologic factors that intensify children's pain and prolong disability. In

N. L. Schecter, C. B. Berde, & M. Yaster (Eds.). *Pain in infants, children, and adolescents*. Baltimore: Lippincott Williams & Wilkins, pp. 85-104.

Mersky, H. (Ed.). (1986). Classification of chronic pain: Descriptions of chronic pain syndromes and definitions of pain terms. *Pain* (Suppl. 3, Pt II), S215-221.

Pasero, C., Paice, J. A., & McCaffery, M. (1999). Basic mechanisms underlying the causes and effects of pain. In M. McCaffery, & C. Pasero (Eds.). *Pain: Clinical manual*. St. Louis: Mosby, pp. 15-34.

Rosenblum, R. K., & Fisher, P. G. (2001). A guide to children with acute and chronic headaches. *J Pediatr Health Care, 15*(5), 229-235.

Schecter, N. L. (2003). Management of pain problems in pediatric primary care. In N. L. Schecter, C. B. Berde, & M. Yaster, (Eds.). *Pain in infants, children, and adolescents*. Baltimore: Lippincott Williams & Wilkins, pp. 603-706.

Schecter, N. L., Berde, C. B. & Yaster, M. (Eds.) (2003). *Pain in infants, children, and adolescents*. Baltimore: Lippincott Williams & Wilkins.

Slater, J. A. (2003). Deciphering emotional aches and physical pains in children. *Pediatr Ann, 32*(6), 402-407.

Stanford, E. A., Chambers, C. T., & Craig, K. D. (2005). A normative analysis of the development of pain-related vocabulary in children. *Pain, 114*, 1-2, 278-284.

Sussman, E. (2005). Cancer pain management guidelines issued for children; adult guidelines updated. *J Natl Cancer Inst, 97*(10), 711-712.

Tobias, J. (2000). Weak analgesics and NSAIDs in management of acute pain. *Pediatr Clin North Am, 47*(3), 527-543.

Van Hulle, Vincent, C. (2005). Nurses' knowledge, attitudes, and practices: Regarding children's pain. *MCN: Am J Matern Child Nurs, 30*(3), 177-183.

Walco, G. A., Burns, J. P., & Cassidy, R. C. (2003). The ethics of pain control in infants and children. In N. L. Schecter, C. B. Berde, & M. Yaster (Eds.). *Pain in infants, children, and adolescents*. Baltimore: Lippincott Williams & Wilkins, pp. 157-168.

Yaster, M., Kost-Byerly, S. & Maxwell, L. G. (2003). Opioid agonists and antagonists. In N. L. Schecter, C. B. Berde, & M. Yaster (Eds.). *Pain in infants, children, and adolescents*. Baltimore: Lippincott Williams & Wilkins, pp. 181-224.

# Complementary and Alternative Therapy

DEBORAH G. LOMAN, PhD, MSN, CPNP

1. Definitions
   a. "A group of diverse medical and health care systems, practices, and products that are not presently considered to be part of conventional medicine" (National Center for Complementary and Alternative Medicine [NCCAM], 2002)
      i. Complementary—a therapy that is used *with* conventional practices
      ii. Alternative – a therapy that is used *instead of* conventional practices
   b. "Complementary therapy" is a term used by nursing as it reflects a more integrative and holistic approach than an "alternative" focus (Sparber, 2001)
   c. Complementary and alternative modalities include "therapies that supplement conventional medical care" (American Holistic Nurses' Association, 2004)
   d. Terms that are often used synonymously: nontraditional, integrative, complementary, and alternative therapies, and complementary and alternative medicine (CAM)
2. Types of complementary and alternative therapies
   a. NCCAM (2002) categories
      i. Alternative medical systems
      ii. Mind-body interventions
      iii. Biologically based therapies
      iv. Manipulative and body-based methods
      v. Energy therapies
   b. Other categorizations (Kemper, 2001; Kemper & Gardiner, 2004)
      i. Biochemical
      ii. Lifestyle
      iii. Biomechanical
      iv. Bioenergetic
   c. Examples of CAM (Kemper, 2002; NCCAM, 2002).
      i. Acupuncture (NIH, 1997; Wang & Kain, 2002)
         (a) Stimulation, usually by needles, of specific anatomic locations on the skin in order to relieve pain and other health conditions
         (b) Sites are energy meridians that correspond to different organs of the body
      ii. Aromatherapy—essential oils (extracts or essences) from plants such as lavender or rosemary that are used as a fragrance or with a massage to reduce anxiety, promote sleep, or enhance well-being (NCCAM, 2002)
      iii. Ayurveda—an ancient medical approach from India with a focus on the body's energy, as well as the mind and spirit; herbal remedies, nutrition, meditation, and massage

iv. Chiropractic—spinal manipulation, dietary counseling, homeopathy, and acupuncture; focus is on the relationship of the body's structure to function (NCCAM, 2003a)

v. Dietary supplement (Table 56-1)

(a) Defined by the Dietary Supplement Health and Education Act of 1994 (DSHEA) as "a vitamin, a mineral, an herb or other botanical, an amino acid, a dietary substance for use by man to supplement the diet by increasing the total dietary intake, or a concentrate, a metabolite, constituent, extract, or combination of any ingredient described [above]" (FDA, 1995)

■ **TABLE 56-1**
■ ■ **Selected Herbs and Other Dietary Supplements, Claimed Therapeutic Uses, Side Effects, Comments, and Cautions Regarding Their Use with Children**

| Substance, Mode | Claimed Therapeutic Use[1] | Side Effects | Comments |
|---|---|---|---|
| Aloe vera<br>Topical gel or oral product (Vogler & Ernst, 1999) | Burns<br>Wound healing<br>Psoriasis<br>Genital herpes | Diarrhea, gastric cramping if taken by mouth<br>Contact dermatitis | Insufficient evidence for wound healing<br>Limited evidence for psoriasis and genital herpes |
| Andro-or androstene-dione<br>Oral (FDA, 2004) | Enhance athletic performance | Anabolic steroid precursor<br>Testicular atrophy<br>Impotence<br>Breast enlargement in males | Labeled by FDA as controlled substance as of January 20, 2005, by the Anabolic Steroid Control Act of 2004 |
| Aristolochic acid; snake-root or wild ginger (FDA, 2001) | Traditional Chinese medicine | Kidney damage<br>Kidney failure<br>May be carcinogenic | FDA issued recall and ban in 2001 |
| Aconite; monkshood, wolfbane<br>Topical, tea, tincture (Kemper, 1998) | Diuretic<br>Diaphoretic | Muscle weakness<br>Bradycardia<br>Hypotension<br>Fatal arrhythmias | A deadly poison |
| Chamomile flowers<br>Tea (infants), tincture<br>Essential oil for aromatherapy (Fetrow & Avila, 2004)<br>Chaparral<br>Tea, capsules (Fetrow & Avila, 2004) | Sedative, antispasmodic, colic<br>Antiinflammatory<br>Diaper rash, chickenpox, poison ivy<br>Bronchitis<br>Skin disorders | Allergic reaction<br>One case of botulism in infant from tea from homegrown plant (Kemper, 1996)<br>Liver damage | Avoid during pregnancy and breast-feeding |
| Comfrey<br>Tea, tincture, tablet, topical (Fetrow & Avila, 2004) | Wound healing<br>Bruises<br>Sprains<br>Antiinflammatory | Contains pyrrolizidine which can cause liver damage and death | Do not use internally |
| Cranberry<br>Juice, tea, tablets, capsules (Jepson, et al., 2004; Schlager, et al., 1999) | Prevention and treatment of urinary tract infection | Diarrhea | Currently under study by NCCAM<br>Do not take with warfarin (inhibits breakdown of warfarin in body) |

■ **TABLE 56-1**

■ ■ **Selected Herbs and Other Dietary Supplements, Claimed Therapeutic Uses, Side Effects, Comments, and Cautions Regarding Their Use with Children—cont'd**

| Substance, Mode | Claimed Therapeutic Use[1] | Side Effects | Comments |
|---|---|---|---|
| Echinacea capsules, tablets, extracts (Barrett, et al., 2002; Cohen, et al., 2004; Taylor, et al., 2003) | Upper respiratory infections<br>Otitis media<br>Immune system stimulant | Rash<br>Pruritus<br>Hypersensitivity | Many products contain alcohol<br>Most studies show little evidence of efficacy but recent study with Echinacea, Propolis & Vitamin C demonstrated fewer and shorter upper respiratory infections in young children (Cohen et al, 2004). |
| Ephedra; ma huang (NC-CAM, 2004)<br>Eucalyptus<br>Aromatherapy, bath salts, oil (Fetrow & Avila, 2004) | Appetite suppressant<br>Asthma<br>Decongestant<br>Natural "high"<br>Nasal congestion | Hypertension<br>Tachycardia<br>Psychosis<br>Death<br>If ingested: Seizures<br>Muscle weakness<br>Esophagitis<br>Cyanosis | Banned by FDA in 2004 |
| Feverfew Capsules, liquid, tablets, tea (Pfaffenrath, et al., 2002; Vogler, et al., 1998) | Prevention of migraines<br>Rheumatoid arthritis<br>Insect repellent<br>Menstrual pain | Allergic reaction<br>Mouth ulcers<br>Rebound headache | No trials with children |
| Garlic (active ingredient allicin)<br>Tablet, clove | Antiinfective<br>Wound healing<br>Lower serum lipids | Breath odor<br>Allergic reaction<br>May increase bleeding time<br>May interact with some drugs' metabolism | Safe as a food condiment<br>No effect in children with familial hyperlipidemia (McCrindle et al., 1998) |
| Ginger<br>Liquid, capsules (Ernst & Pittler, 2000; Fetrow & Avila, 2004; Portnoi, et al., 2003) | Prevent nausea/vomiting (postoperative, motion sickness)<br>Antiinflammatory | Hearburn<br>May increase bleeding time if taken with anticoagulants | Not tested in children |
| Goldenseal roots<br>Tincture (Fetrow & Avila, 2004) | Traditional Native American<br>Diarrhea<br>Ear infections<br>Conjunctivitis<br>Immune system stimulator | Hypotension<br>Hypertension<br>Local irritation | Poisonous in large doses<br>Displacement of bilirubin from albumin, therefore dangerous for infants <1 month of age |
| Kava kava (Piper methysticum)<br>Capsules, extract, roots, drink (CDC, 2002; Fetrow & Avila, 2004) | Anxiolytic<br>Insomnia<br>Anxiety disorders | Local anesthetic effect in mouth<br>Liver damage<br>Decreased platelets and lymphocytes | |

*Continued*

■ **TABLE 56-1**
■ ■ **Selected Herbs and Other Dietary Supplements, Claimed Therapeutic Uses, Side Effects, Comments, and Cautions Regarding Their Use with Children—cont'd**

| Substance, Mode | Claimed Therapeutic Use[1] | Side Effects | Comments |
|---|---|---|---|
| Litargirio (powder) (FDA, 2003) | Traditional remedy from Dominican Republic<br>Skin conditions<br>Deodorant | Symptoms of lead toxicity | May contain lead<br>FDA warning in 2003<br>Take product to health department<br>Test exposed children and pregnant women for lead |
| Melatonin<br>Liquid, tablets (Fetrow & Avila, 2004) | Jet-lag<br>Sleep disturbance<br>Insomnia | Change in sleep patterns<br>Confusion<br>Headache<br>Hypertension | Contraindicated in those with liver dysfunction<br>Limited evidence of effectiveness for insomnia in children with special needs (Palm, et al., 1997; Zhdanova, et al., 1999) |
| Pennyroyal *(Pulegone)*<br>Leaves for tea, oil (Fetrow & Avila, 2004; Kemper, 1996) | Insect repellent<br>Aromatherapy<br>Abortifacient<br>Colds<br>Toothache | Uterine contractions & abortion<br>Hepatotoxicity<br>Nephrotoxicity<br>CNS effects<br>Death | Do not use internally |
| Probiotics<br>Lactobacillus (active)<br>Oral capsule<br>Yogurt | Diarrhea<br>Bacterial vaginosis | Abdominal cramping<br>Flatulence | Safe for children<br>May help decrease duration & severity of diarrhea (Kemper, 2001; Van Niel, et al., 2002) |
| Sassafras<br>Extract, oil, tea (Fetrow & Avila, 2004) | Antiseptic<br>Pediculicide | Liver dysfunction<br>CNS effects<br>Death | Do not use |
| St. John's wort *(Hypericum perforatum)*<br>Capsule, tea, extract (Fetrow & Avila, 2004)<br>Tree tea oil<br>Topical (Fetrow & Avila, 2004) | Depression<br>Anxiety<br>Sleep problems<br>Minor skin infections<br>Fungicide<br>Acne<br>Vaginitis | May interact with/reduce the effectiveness of drugs for seizures, heart disease, depression, or oral contraceptives<br>Topical—contact dermatitis;<br>Oral—CNS dysfunction and muscle weakness (Kemper, 1996) | No studies with children (Kemper, 2001) |
| Valerian<br>Tablet, tincture (Francis & Dempster, 2002; Stevinson & Ernst, 2002) | Insomnia<br>Anxiety<br>Antispasmodic | Headache<br>Excitability<br>Hepatotoxicity | One small study showed sleep benefits in children with intellectual deficits but more research is needed |

[1]For information only; no endorsement is implied by the author.

    (b) Taken in a tablet, capsule, liquid, or powder form (Hrastinger, et al., 2005)

    (c) DSHEA mandates accurate package labeling, but not safety or efficacy (FDA, 1995)

    (d) Regulated by the Food and Drug Administration as *foods*, which is less stringent than the regulation of drugs

    (e) Not required to demonstrate safety or therapeutic effectiveness

    (f) May be contaminated by plant products, metals or drugs (Boyer et al., 2002)

    (g) Active components are often not known

    (h) Products that meet voluntary standards for purity and quality control have one of the following labels:

        (1) USP—United States Pharmacopeia standards

        (2) GMP—Good Manufacturing Practices; a program with National Nutritional Foods Association

        (3) AHPA—American Herbal Products Association

  **vi.** Energy healing—use of either biofield or bioelectromagnetic therapies (Miller, 2004)

    (a) Reiki (Stein, 1999)

        (1) Ancient Tibetan, now Japanese, system of natural healing

        (2) "Universal life energy" is channeled by visualization, or from the therapist's hands to the person

    (b) Therapeutic touch

        (1) Intentionally directed process of energy exchange from a therapist's hands to a person's body

        (2) Therapist identifies an energy imbalance (disease) and restores balance (health) (Kreiger & Krippner, 1993)

    (c) Bioelectromagnetic therapies

        (1) Static—placing a magnet near the body (shoe insert, bracelet, necklace) (Miller, 2004; Winemiller, et al., 2003)

        (2) Pulsating electromagnetic therapy, e.g., transcutaneous electrical nerve stimulation (TENS) unit

  **vii.** Herbs or other botanicals (more than 325 types are described in Fetrow & Avila, 2004) (see *Dietary Supplement* above; see Table 56-1 for examples)

  **viii.** Homeopathy (Dantas & Rampes, 2000; Doerr, 2001; Ernst, 1999; NCCAM, 2003b)

    (a) Founded in 18th century and based on law of similars—"like cures like"

    (b) Use of dilute substances that induce symptoms similar to the symptoms of disease

    (c) Homeopathic medications are regulated by the U.S. Food and Drug Administration (FDA) and are safe if used as directed

  **ix.** Massage—manipulation of muscle and connective tissue, or stroking and passive limb movement by a therapist (Field, 1995; 1999; Moyer, Rounds, & Hannum, 2004)

  **x.** Mind-body therapies

    (a) Meditation

    (b) Relaxation techniques

    (c) Biofeedback

    (d) Hypnosis—inducing a state of focused attention (Kemper, 2002)

    (e) Prayer

  **xi.** Naturopathic medicine (Kemper, 2002; NCCAM, 2002)

          (a) Originated in Germany; focus is on natural healing forces in the body to promote health and combat disease

          (b) Nutrition, herbal and homeopathic remedies, massage, exercise, and spinal manipulation may be used

     **xii.** Nutritional approaches or dietary modifications

          (a) Foods rich in vitamins or other substances (ex., Vitamin C, fish oil) to promote health or treat illness (Kemper, 2002)

          (b) Natural foods or organic foods—foods produced without artificial chemicals added (such as pesticides, fertilizers, antibiotics, or colorings) (Magkos, et al. 2003)

          (c) Vegetarian diets (Perry, et al, 2002).

          (d) Avoidance of certain foods or substances in foods that may be an allergen or trigger for a health problem (Kemper, 2002)

     **xiii.** Traditional Native American medicine (Tribal Connections, 2005)

          (a) Healing systems that emphasize harmony of the mind, body and spirit within the context of the tribal group

          (b) Native Americans have practiced a holistic approach to healing for thousands of years

          (c) Part of this practice involves the use of medicinal plants and herbs

     **xiv.** Traditional Chinese medicine—based on an ancient belief of energy, or Qi, in the body; Chinese herbs, acupuncture, nutrition, exercise and meditation

**3.** Prevalence of use of complementary and alternative therapy in children

    **a.** Percent of use varies based on sample, geography, and research methods (Sanders, et al., 2003)

    **b.** Higher use by adults and children with chronic illness

    **c.** 1.8% of 6262 children from a national interview in 1996 (Davis & Darden, 2003)

    **d.** 45% of children from one emergency department (ED) in the South reported use of herbal or home therapies with aloe, echinacea, and sweet oil most often (Lanski, et al., 2003)

    **e.** 64% of children with special needs in a southwestern state (Sanders, et al., 2003)

    **f.** 12% of 525 parents in a Pittsburgh pediatric ED reported that they had used one or more homeopathic or naturopathic therapies to treat their children (Pitetti, et al., 2001)

    **g.** 33% of 191 parents surveyed from private pediatric offices in St. Louis reported use of infant massage, massage therapy, and vitamin therapy most frequently (Loman, 2003)

    **h.** 64% of 376 families of special needs children in Arizona reported using prayers/spiritual healing, massage, and herbs most often (Sanders, et al., 2003)

        **i.** Children accounted for 1% to 4% of visits to acupuncture, chiropractic, and massage therapists in four states (Cherkin, et al., 2002)

**4.** Variables associated with use of these therapies by children

    **a.** Parent or caregiver born outside the United States (Sawni-Sikand, Schubiner, & Thomas, 2002)

    **b.** Parental use of these therapies (Bellas, et al., 2005; Hurvitz, et al., 2003; Loman, 2003, Sanders, et al., 2003)

    **c.** Children from religious families (McCurdy, et al, 2003)

    **d.** Chronic health problem

**5.** Reasons for use of CAM in children

    a. Parents' reasons for using CAM with their children (Lanski, et al., 2003; Pitetti, et al., 2001; Sanders, et al., 2003; Sinha & Efron, 2005)
       i. Recommendation of family, friend, or health professional
      ii. Child not getting better with conventional care
     iii. Therapy viewed as natural and safer than traditional medical remedies
     iv. Minimize symptoms
      v. Add to the benefit of conventional treatment
     vi. Avoid side effects of conventional treatment

    b. Adolescents' reasons for using dietary supplements (Gardiner, et al., 2004)
       i. Promote weight loss
      ii. Enhance athletic achievement
     iii. Enhance physical appearance
     iv. Increase energy
      v. Restore or maintain health
     vi. Balance the diet

## ISSUES IN PEDIATRIC PRIMARY CARE SETTINGS

1. PNPs may lack awareness that patients are using these therapies
    a. Adults and teens often do not mention use of CAM unless asked directly
    b. In one study of children with ADHD, only 64% of parents who used CAM reported this to the physician (Sinha & Efron, 2005)
    c. In a study of four pediatric practices in Washington, D.C., only 36% of 348 parents who used CAM said they had discussed it with their pediatrician (Sibinga, et al., 2004)

2. PNPs may lack knowledge about CAM that children might be receiving for specific conditions
    a. The chronic conditions below are followed by types of therapies that have been used for children
       i. ADHD—modified diet, vitamins and minerals, herbs and dietary supplements, aromatherapy, chiropractic, acupuncture, homeopathy, biofeedback (Bussing, 2002; Gross-Tsur et al, 2003; Sinha & Efron, 2005).
      ii. Atopic dermatitis—herbs and dietary supplements, homeopathy (Ernst et al, 2002; Gardiner et al, 2004).
     iii. Asthma—massage, herbs and dietary supplements, prayer, diet changes, meditation, and homeopathy (Kemper & Lester, 1999; Reznik, et al, 2002).
     iv. Cancer—faith healing, megavitamins/minerals, massage, herbs and dietary supplements, relaxation techniques (McCurdy, et al, 2003)
      v. Cerebral palsy—massage therapy, aqua therapy, hippotherapy/horseback riding, (Hurvitz, et al., 2003)
     vi. Chronic pain—biofeedback, acupuncture, hypnosis, herbs and dietary supplements (Allen, 2004; Scharff & Kemper, 2003)
    b. Note: the studies cited are *beginning, but insufficient*, evidence of safety and efficacy of the therapies for use with children
       i. Atopic dermatitis (Anderson, et al., 2000):
       (a) Massage (Anderson, et al., 2000)
      ii. Asthma (Bronfort, et al., 2001)

(a) Chiropractic (Bronfort, et al., 2001)

    **iii.** Chronic pain—combined acupuncture and hypnosis (Zeltzer, et al., 2002)

    **iv.** Diarrhea—individualized homeopathy (Jacobs, et al., 2003)

    **v.** Habitual coughing—hypnosis (Anbar & Hall, 2004)

    **vi.** Headache—biofeedback (Grazzi, et al., 2001)

    **vii.** Nocturnal enuresis—acupressure (Yuksek, et al., 2003)

    **viii.** Persistent allergic rhinitis—acupuncture (Ng, et al., 2004)

    **ix.** Postoperative nausea and vomiting—acupuncture (Wang & Kain, 2002)

    **x.** Recurrent abdominal pain—peppermint oil (Kline, et al., 2001; Weydert, Ball & Davis, 2003

**3.** PNPs may lack knowledge about the effectiveness and safety of these therapies

    **a.** Providers often do not know the following about CAM (Barnes, et al., 2004)

        **i.** Safety

        **ii.** Possible side effects

        **iii.** Adverse effects

        **iv.** Interaction effects with traditional therapies

    **b.** Therapeutic effectiveness has not been systematically studied for most products and therapies

        **i.** This is also true of many "traditional" or Western medical and nursing practices

        **ii.** Randomized clinical trials with an adequate number of subjects are the gold standard for determining the efficacy and safety of a therapy or medication

    **c.** Resources for information about CAM for decision making (Box 56-1)

---

■ **BOX 56-1**
■ **RESOURCES FOR INFORMATION ABOUT COMPLEMENTARY AND ALTERNATIVE THERAPIES**

| Reliable Sources for Decision Making | Other Sources of Information |
|---|---|
| Complementary/Integrative Medicine Educational Resources (CIMER) University of Texas M. D. Anderson Cancer Center www.mdanderson.org/departments/cimer | American Association of Naturopathic Physicians List of naturopaths http://naturopathic.org |
| CAM on PubMed Electronic database by NCCAM and National Library of Medicine www.nlm.nih.gov/nccam/camonpubmed.html | American Association of Oriental Medicine List of acupuncturists www.aaom.org |
| Cochrane Database of Systematic Reviews 2004 Consumer Lab Information on standardized dietary supplements www.consumerlabs.com | American Botanical Council: Nonprofit organization Information on herbs and medicinal plants |
| HolisticKids.org The Center for Holistic Pediatric Education and Research (CHPER) www.holistickids.org | www.herbalgram.org American Herbalists Guild List of herbalists www.americanherbalistsguild.com |

*Continued*

■ **BOX 56-1**
■ **RESOURCES FOR INFORMATION ABOUT COMPLEMENTARY AND ALTERNATIVE THERAPIES—cont'd**

Longwood Herbal Task Force
Evidence-based monographs on common herbs
www.mcp.edu/herbal

MedWatch (U.S. FDA)
Voluntary reporting of adverse reactions to
    dietary supplements and botanicals
www.fed.gov/medwatch 0-FDA-1088

National Institutes of Health, National Center
    for Complementary and Alternative Medicine
Provides information on CAM and funds research
    http://nccam.nih.gov

National Council for Reliable Health Information
Private, nonprofit agency that focuses on health-
    misinformation and fraud
    www.ncahf.org

Natural Medicine Database
Subscriptions for evidenced-based monographs
www.NaturalMedicineDatabase

National Institutes of Health Office of Dietary
    Supplements
Information about dietary supplements and
    "warning letters" to physicians about
    specific ones
http://ods.od.nih.gov

PDR. (2001). *PDR for nutritional supplements.*
    Montvale, NJ: Medical Economics,
    Thomson Healthcare.
PDR. (2004). *PDR for herbal medicines*
    (3rd ed.). Montvale, NJ: Thomson PDR.
PDR. (2005). *PDR for nonprescription drugs
    and dietary supplements.* Montvale, NJ:
    Thomson PDR.

U.S. Food & Drug Agency, Center for Food Safety
    and Applied Nutrition
Information about dietary supplements
www.cfsan.fda.gov

U.S. Pharmacopeia (USP)
Provides standards for the quality of medicines
www.usp.org
Nationwide Poison Control Center Hotline
800-222-1222

American Herbal Products Association
Information on herbs and medicinal
    plantswww.ahpa.org/index.htm
American Holistic Nurses Association
www.ahna.org/home/home.html

Herb Research Foundation
Information on herbs
www.herbs.org

Nurse-Healers Professional Associates
    International
Official website for Therapeutic Touch
    Practitioners
www.therapeutic-touch.org
Quackwatch, Inc.
Nonprofit corporation to combat health-
    related fraud and myths
www.quackwatch.org

    **d.** Other sources of information about CAM (see Box 56-1)

    **e.** Currently funded pediatric studies of complementary and alternative therapies by NIH, NCCAM (Box 56-2)

**4.** Cost-benefit concerns for families

    **a.** Use of herbal remedies increased by 380% between 1990 and 1997 (Eisenberg, et al., 1998)

    **b.** Approximately $18 billion spent in 2001 on these products (Nutrition Business Journal, 2002)

    **c.** Cost-benefit ratio is unknown for most therapies

    **d.** Cost

        **i.** Rarely covered by third-party payers

        **ii.** Some states require coverage of licensed therapists by private insurance (Bellas, et al., 2005)

        **iii.** Financial cost can be excessive particularly if there is no therapeutic benefit (Kemp, 2003)

        **iv.** Cost with respect to substituted or delayed traditional therapy may be incalculable

## ROLE OF PEDIATRIC NURSE PRACTITIONER

**1.** Be informed (Barnes, et al., 2004)

    **a.** Become knowledgeable about complementary and alternative therapies used in the culture, geographic area, or age-group served by the practice

        **i.** Be aware that some CAM practices are part of religious rituals viewed as "indispensable to preserving or restoring health" (p. 261)

        **ii.** Be aware of one's own biases about CAM—they can perpetuate health disparities

        **iii.** Be aware of where to find information about current research findings on CAM

        **iv.** Be aware that there are harmful substances and therapies (see Table 56-1)

    **b.** Implement practice guidelines for use of CAM as they are developed

        **i.** Counsel families who choose CAM for their children with chronic illness or disability (AAP, 2001)

---

■ **BOX 56-2**
■ **PEDIATRIC STUDIES RECENTLY FUNDED BY NIH/NCCAM**

Relaxation/guided imagery and chamomile tea as treatment of functional abdominal pain in children

Preterm infants' weight gain following massage therapy

Borage oil and ginkgo biloba (EGb 761) in asthma (ages 16 to 75 years)

A randomized study of electroacupuncture treatment for delayed chemotherapy-induced nausea and vomiting in patients with pediatric sarcomas

Efficacy of healing touch in stressed neonates

Echinacea versus placebo effect in common cold (ages 12–17)

Home based massage and relaxation for sickle cell pain (ages 15–65)

Use of self-hypnosis, acupuncture, and osteopathic manipulation on muscle tension in children with spastic cerebral palsy

Interactions between cranberry juice and antibiotics used to treat urinary tract infections

Echinacea versus placebo effect in common cold (ages 12 and older)

        **ii.** Complementary and alternative medicine guidelines (American Academy of Family Physicians, 2003)

2. Ask questions and share information about CAM
   a. Develop skills in "taking a culturally sensitive, comprehensive history, eliciting values, goals, and the family's true system of care" (Barnes, et al., 2004, p. 258)
   b. Inquire about the use of complementary and alternative therapies in a nonjudgmental manner at every encounter
      i. Give examples of the most likely used therapies when asking the question
      ii. In particular, ask parents of children with chronic illnesses such as ADHD, asthma, cerebral palsy, cancer, JRA, autism, etc., directly about past and current use
   c. Incorporate the principles of patient autonomy and respect into patient care
      i. Families have the right to select their own treatment (WHCCAMP, 2002)
      ii. Families deserve unbiased information about the various therapies
      iii. Acknowledge that:
         (a) Research is limited on most CAM
         (b) Evidence is primarily anecdotal
         (c) Discuss with parents and youths their understanding of the specific therapy
      iv. Explain your understanding of the therapy based on principles of pharmacology, nutrition, anatomy, physiology, etc.
      v. Form a partnership with parents and youths for care and management approaches
      vi. Remind parents and youths that "natural" products
         (a) Are not necessarily safe or healthy
         (b) Can have serious negative effects
      vii. Share with parents and youths the reasons for evidenced-based practice and need for controlled research studies:
         (a) To confirm that a benefit did occur from the treatment
         (b) To confirm that perceived benefits were not due to:
            (1) The natural course of the health problem
            (2) Placebo effect
            (3) Some other factor
      viii. Realize that parents and youth may be committed to the therapy and resist new information, and if so:
         (a) Encourage the use of therapists who are trained and/or licensed in the technique
         (b) Monitor the child's response (American Academy of Pediatrics, 2001)

---

## REFERENCES

Allen, K. D. (2004). Using biofeedback to make childhood headaches less of a pain. *Pediatr Ann, 33*(4), 241-245.

American Academy of Family Physicians. (2003). Complementary practice. Retrieved on February 12, 2006 at www.aafp.org/x668.xml.

American Academy of Pediatrics. Committee on Children with Disabilities. (2001). Counseling families who choose complementary and alternative medicine for their child with chronic illness or disability. *Pediatrics, 107,* 598-601.

American Holistic Nurses' Association (AHNA) Position Paper. (2004). AHNA: Position on the role of nurses in the practice of complementary and alternative therapies. Retrieved on February 11, 2006 at www.ahna.org/about/statments.html.

Anbar, R. D., & Hall, H. R. (2004). Childhood habit cough treated with self-hypnosis. *J Pediatr, 144*, 213-217.

Anderson, C., Lis-Balchin, M., & Kirk-Smith, M. (2000). Evaluation of massage with essential oils on childhood atopic eczema. *Phytother Res, 14*, 452-456.

Barnes, L., Risko, W., Nethersole, S., & Maypole, J. (2004). Integrating complementary and alternative medicine into pediatric training. *Pediatr Ann, 33*(4), 257-263.

Barrett, B. P., Brown, R. L., Locken, K., et al. (2002). Treatment of the common cold with unrefined echinacea. *Ann Intern Med, 137*, 939-946.

Bellas, A., Lafferty, W. E., Lind, B., & Tyree, P. T. (2005). Frequency, predictors, and expenditures for pediatric insurance claims for complementary and alternative medical professionals in Washington state. *Arch Pediatr Adolesc Med, 159*(4), 367-372.

Boyer, E. W., Kearney, S., Shannon, M. W., et al. (2002). Poisoning from a dietary supplement administered during hospitalization. *Pediatrics, 109*(3), E49.

Bronfort, G., Evans, R. L., Kubic, P., & Filkin, P. (2001). Chronic pediatric asthma and chiropractic spinal manipulation: A prospective clinical series and randomized clinical pilot study. *J Manip Physiol Ther, 24*, 369-377.

Bussing, R., Zima, B. T., Gary, F. A., & Garvan, C. W. (2002). Use of complementary and alternative medicine for symptoms of attention-deficit hyperactivity disorder. *Psychiatric Serv, 53*, 1096-1102.

CDC: Centers for Disease Control and Prevention. (2002). Hepatic toxicity possibly associated with kava-containing products—United States, Germany, and Switzerland, 1999-2002. (2002). *MMWR Morb Mortal Wkly Rep 51*(47), 1065-1067.

Cherkin, D. C., Deyo, R. A., Sherman, K. J., et al. (2002). Characteristics of visits to licensed acupuncturists, chiropractors, massage therapists, and naturopathic physicians. *J Am Board Fam Pract, 15*, 463-472.

Cohen, H. A., Varsano, I., Kahan, E., et al. (2004). Effectiveness of an herbal preparation containing echinacea, propolis, and vitamin C in preventing respiratory tract infections in children. A randomized, double-blind, placebo-controlled, multicenter study. *Arch Pediatr Adolesc Med, 158*, 217-221.

Dantas, F., & Rampes, H. (2000). Do homeopathic medicines provoke adverse effects? A systematic review. *Brit Homeopathic J, 89*(1): S35-S38.

Davis, M. P., & Darden P. M. (2003). Use of complementary and alternative medicine by children in the United States. *Arch Pediatr Adolesc Med, 157*, 393-396.

Doerr, L. (2001). Using homeopathy for treating childhood asthma: Understanding a family's choice. *J Pediatr Nurs, 16*, 269-276.

DSHEA: Dietary Supplement Health and Education Act of 1994. Public Law 103-417, 108 Statute 4325.

Eisenberg, D. M., Davis, R. B., Ettner, S. L., et al. (1998). Trends in alternative medicine use in the United States, 1990-1997: Results of a follow-up national survey. *JAMA, 280*, 1569-1575.

Ernst, E. (1999). Homeopathic prophylaxis of headaches and migraine? A systematic review. *J Pain Symptom Manage 18*, 353-357.

Ernst, E., & Pittler, M.H. (2000). Efficacy of ginger for nausea and vomiting: A systematic review of randomised clinical trials. *British Journal of Anaesthesia, 84*, 367-71.

Ernst, E., Pittler, M., & Stevinson, C. (2002). Complementary/alternative medicine in dermatology: Evidence-assessed efficacy of two diseases and two treatments. *American Journal of Clinical Dermatology, 3*, 341-348.

FDA: U.S. Food and Drug Administration (1995). Dietary supplement health and education act of 1994. Retrieved on February 12, 2005 at http://www.cfsan.fda.gov/~dms/dietsupp.html.

FDA: U.S. Food and Drug Administration. (2001). FDA warns consumers to discontinue use of botanical products that contain aristolochic acid. Consumer advisory, April 11, 2001. Retrieved June 24, 2005, from www.cfsan.fda.gov/~dms/addsbot.html.

FDA: U.S. Food and Drug Administration. (2004). Health effects of Androstenedione. FDA white paper, March 11, 2004. Retrieved June 24, 2005, from www.fda.gov/oc/whitepapers/andro.html.

FDA: U.S. Food and Drug Administration. (2003). FDA warns consumers about use of "Litargirio"—Traditional remedy that contains dangerous levels of lead. FDA talk paper, T03-67. Retrieved June 24, 2005, from www.fda.gov/bbs/topics/ANSWERetS/2003/ANS01253.html.

Fetrow, C. W., & Avila, J. R. (2004). *Professional's handbook of complementary & alternative medicines*. Philadelphia: Lippincott Williams & Wilkins.

Field, T. (1999). Massage therapy: More than a laying on of hands. *Contemp Pediatr, 16*(5), 77-94.

Field, T. (1995). Massage therapy for infants and children. *J Dev Behav Pediatr, 16*, 105-111.

Francis, A. J., & Dempster, R .J. (2002). Effect of valerian, *Valeriana edulis*, on sleep difficulties in children with intellectual deficits: Randomised trial. *Phytomedicine, 9*, 273-279.

Gardiner, P., Dvorkin, L., & Kemper, K. J. (2004). Supplement use growing among children and adolescents. *Pediatr Ann, 33*(4), 227-232.

Grazzi, L., Andrasik, F., D'Amico, D., Leone, M., Moschiano, F. & Bussone, G. (2001). Electromyographic biofeedback-assisted relaxation training in juvenile episodic tension-type headache: Clinical outcome at three-year follow-up. *Cephalalgia, 21*(8), 798-803.

Gross-Tsur, V., Lahad, A., & Shalev, R. S. (2003). Use of complementary medicine in children with attention deficit hyperactivity disorder and epilepsy. *Pediatr Neurol, 29*(1), 53-55.

Hrastinger, A., Dietz, B., Bauer, R., et al. (2005). Is there clinical evidence supporting the use of botanical dietary supplements in children? *J Pediatr, 146*, 311-317.

Hurvitz, E. A., Leonard, C., Ayyangar, R., & Nelson, V. S. (2003). Complementary and alternative medicine use in families of children with cerebral palsy. *Dev Med Child Neurol, 45*, 364-370.

Hypericum Depression Trial Study Group. (2002). Effect of *Hypericum perforatum* (St John's wort) in major depressive disorder: A randomized controlled trial. *JAMA, 287*, 1807-1814.

Jacobs, J., Jonas, W. B., Jimenez-Perez, M., & Crothers, D. (2003). Homeopathy for childhood diarrhea: Combined results and meta-analysis from three randomized, controlled clinical trials. *Pediatr Infect Dis J, 22*, 229-234.

Jepson, R. G., Mihaljevic, L., & Craig, J. (2004). Cranberries for preventing urinary tract infections. *Cochrane Database Syst Rev, 2, CD001321*.

Kemp, A. S. (2003). Cost of illness of atopic dermatitis in children: a societal perspective. *PharmacoEconomics, 21*(2), 105-113.

Kemper, K. J. (2002). *The holistic pediatrician*. New York: Quill.

Kemper, K. J. (2001). Complementary and alternative medicine for children: Does it work? *Arch Dis Child, 84*, 6-9.

Kemper, K. J. (1998). "Something wicked this way comes"—herbs even witches should avoid. *Contemp Pediatr, 15*(6), 49-64.

Kemper, K. J. (1996). Seven herbs every pediatrician should know. *Contemp Pediatr, 13*(12), 79-91.

Kemper, K. J., & Gardiner, P. (2004). Herbal medicines. In R. E. Behrman, R. M. Kliegman, & H. B. Jenson (Eds.). *Nelson textbook of pediatrics* (17th ed.). Philadelphia: Saunders, pp. 2502-2505.

Kemper, K.J., & Lester, M.R. (1999). Alternative asthma therapies: An evidence-based review. *Contemp Pediatr, 16*(3), 162, 165, 167-168, 173, 177, 179-180, 186, 191-192, 195.

Kline, R. M., Kline, J. J., Di Palma, J., & Barbero, G. J. (2001). Enteric-coated, pH-dependent peppermint oil capsules for the treatment of irritable bowel syndrome in children. *J Pediatr, 138*, 125-128.

Krieger, D., & Krippner, S. (1993). *Accepting your power to heal: The personal practice of therapeutic touch*. Rochester, VT: Inner Traditions International, Limited.

Lanski, S. L., Greenwald, M., Perkins, A., & Simon, H. K. (2003). Herbal therapy use in a pediatric emergency department population: Expect the unexpected. *Pediatrics, 111*, 981-985.

Loman, D. G. (2003). The use of complementary and alternative health care practices among children. *J Pediatr Health Care, 17*, 58-63.

Magkos, F., Arvaniti, F., & Zampelas, A. (2003). Organic food: Nutritious food or food for thought? A review of the evidence. *International Journal of Food Sciences & Nutrition. 54*(5), 357-371.

McCrindle, B. W., Helden, E., & Conner, W. T. (1998). Garlic extract therapy in children with hypercholesterolemia. *Arch Pediatr Adolesc Med, 152*, 1089-1094.

McCurdy, E.A., Spangler, J.G., Wofford, M.M., Chauvenet, A.R., & McLean, T.W. (2003). Religiosity is associated with the use of complementary medical therapies by pediatric oncology patients. *Journal of Pediatric Hematology/Oncology, 25*, 125-129.

Miller, S. K. (2004). Magnet therapy for pain control: An analysis of theory and research. *Adv Nurse Pract, 12*(5), 49-52.

Moyer, C. A., Rounds, J., & Hannum, J. W. (2004). A meta-analysis of massage therapy research. *Psychol Bull, 130*, 3-18.

NCCAM: National Center for Complementary and Alternative Medicine. (2002). What is complementary and alternative medicine? NCCAM Publication No. D156. Retrieved June 24, 2005, from http://nccam.nih.gov/health/whatiscam/#sup1.

NCCAM: National Center for Complementary and Alternative Medicine. (2003a). About chiropractic and its use in treating low-back pain. NCCAM Publication No. D196. Retrieved June 24, 2005, from http://nccam.nih.gov/health/chiropractic/index.htm.

NCCAM: National Center for Complementary and Alternative Medicine. (2003b). Questions and answers about homeopathy. NCCAM Publication No. D183. Retrieved June 24, 2005, from http://nccam.nih.gov/health/homeopathy/index.htm#37.

NCCAM: National Center for Complementary and Alternative Medicine. (2004). NCCAM consumer advisory on ephedra. Retrieved June 24, 2005, from http://nccam.nih.gov/health/alerts/ephedra/consumeradvisory.htm.

Ng, D. K., Pok-yu, M. S-p., Hong, S-h., et al. (2004). A double-blind, randomized, placebo-controlled trial of acupuncture for the treatment of childhood persistent allergic rhinitis. *Pediatrics, 114*(5), 1242-1247.

NIH: National Institutes of Health. (1997). Acupuncture. NIH Consensus Statement. 15(5), 1-34. Retrieved June 24, 2005, from http://odp.od.nih.gov/consensus/cons/107/107_statement.htm.

Palm, L., Blennow, G., & Wetterberg, L. (1997). Long-term melatonin treatment in blind children and young adults with circadian sleep-wake disturbances. *Dev Med Child Neurol, 39*, 319-325.

PDR. (2001). *PDR for nutritional supplements.* Montvale, NJ: Medical Economics, Thomson Healthcare.

PDR. (2004). *PDR for herbal medicines* (3rd ed.). Montvale, NJ: Thomson PDR.

PDR. (2005). *PDR for nonprescription drugs and dietary supplements.* Montvale, NJ: Thomson PDR.

Perry, C.L., McGuire, M.T., Neumark-Sztainer, D., & Story, M. (2002). Adolescent vegetarians: How well do their dietary patterns meet the Healthy People 2010 objectives? *Archives of Pediatrics & Adolescent Medicine, 156*(5), 431-7.

Pfaffenrath, V., Diener, H. C., Fischer, M., et al. (2002). The efficacy and safety of *Tanacetum parthenium* (feverfew) in migraine prophylaxis—A double-blind, multicentre, randomized placebo-controlled dose-response study. *Cephalalgia, 22*(7), 523-532.

Pitetti, R., Singh, S., Hornyak, D., et al. (2001). Complementary and alternative medicine use in children. *Pediatr Emerg Care, 17*, 165-169.

Portnoi, G., Chng, L. A., Karimi-Tabesh, L., et al. (2003). Prospective comparative study of the safety and effectiveness of ginger for the treatment of nausea and vomiting in pregnancy. *Am J Obstet Gynecol, 189*, 1374-1377.

Reznik, M., Ozuah, P. O., Fanco, K., et al. (2002). Use of complementary therapy by adolescents with asthma. *Arch Pediatr Adolesc Med, 156*, 1042-1044.

Sanders, H., Davis, M. F., Duncan, B., et al. (2003). Use of complementary and alternative medical therapies among children with special health care needs in Ssouthern Arizona. *Pediatrics, 111*, 584-587.

Sawni-Sikand, A., Schubiner, H., & Thomas, R. L. (2002). Use of complementary/alternative therapies among children in primary care pediatrics. *Ambu Pediatr, 2*, 99-103.

Scharff, L., & Kemper, K.J. (2003). For chronic pain, complementary and alternative medical approaches. *Contemp Pediatr, 20*(10), 117-118, 121-122, 130, 133, 137-8, 141.

Schlager, T. A., Anderson, S., Trudell, J., & Hendley, J. O. (1999). Effect of cranberry juice on bacteriuria in children with neurogenic bladder receiving intermittent catheterization. *J Pediatr, 135*, 698-702.

Sibinga, E., Ottoline, M. C., Duggan, A. K., & Wilson, M. H. (2004). Parent-pediatrician communication about complementary and alternative medicine use for children. *Clin Pediatr, 43*(4), 367-373.

Sinha, D., & Efron, D. (2005). Complementary and alternative medicine use in children with attention deficit hyperactivity disorder. *J Paediatr Child Health, 41*(1-2), 23-26.

Sparber, A. (2001). State boards of nursing and scope of practice of registered nurses performing complementary therapies. *Online J Iss Nurs, 6*(3), 1-10. Retrieved June 24, 2005, from www.nursingworld.org/ojin/topic15/tpc15_6.htm.

Stein, D. (1999). Essential reiki: *A complete guide to an ancient healing art*. Freedom, CA: The Crossing Press, Inc.

Stevinson, C., & Ernst, E. (2000). Valerian for insomnia: A systematic review of randomized clinical trials. *Sleep Medicine, 1*, 91-99.

Taylor, J. A., Weber, W., Standish, L., et al. (2003). Efficacy and safety of echinacea in treating upper respiratory tract infections in children: A randomized controlled trial. *JAMA, 290*, 2824-2830.

Tribal Connections. (2005). eHealth Information: Traditional healing. Retrieved June 24, 2005, from www.tribalconnections. org/ehealthinfo/trad_healing.html.

Van Niel, C. W., Feudtner, C., Garrison, M. M., & Christakis, D. A. (2002). Lactobacillus therapy for acute infectious diarrhea in children: A meta-analysis. *Pediatrics, 109*, 678-684.

Vogler, B. K., & Ernst, E. (1999). Aloe vera: A systematic review of its clinical effectiveness. *Brit J Gen Pract, 49*, 823-828.

Vogler, B. K., Pittler, M. H., & Ernst, E. (1998). Feverfew as a preventive treatment for migraine: A systematic review. *Cephalalgia, 18*, 704-708.

Wang, S. M., & Kain, Z. N. (2002). P6 acupoint injections are as effective as droperidol in controlling early postoperative nausea and vomiting in children. *Anesthesiology, 97*, 359-366.

Weydert, J. A., Ball, T. M., & Davis, M. F. (2003). Systematic review of treatments for recurrent abdominal pain. *Pediatrics, 111*, pp. e1-e11.

WHCCAMP: White House Commission on Complementary and Alternative Medicine Policy. (2002). *White House Commission on Complementary and Alternative Medicine Policy: Final report*. Retrieved on June 24, 2005 at http://whccamp.hhs.gov/finalreport.html

Winemiller, M. H., Billow, R. G., Laskowski, E. R., & Harmsen, W. S. (2003). Effect of magnetic vs sham-magnetic insoles on plantar heel pain: A randomized controlled trial. *JAMA, 290*, 1474-1478.

Yuksek, M. S., Erdem, A. F., Atalay, C., & Demirel, A. (2003). Acupressure versus oxybutinin in the treatment of enuresis. *J Int Med Res, 31*(6), 552-526.

Zeltzer, L. K., Tsao, J. C. I., Stelling, C., et al. (2002). A phase I study on the feasibility and acceptability of an acupuncture/hypnosis intervention for chronic pediatric pain. *J Pain Symptom Manage, 24*, 437-446.

Zhdanova, I. V., Wurtman, R. J., & Wagstaff, J. (1999). Effects of a low dose of melatonin on sleep in children with Angelman syndrome. *J Pediatr Endocrinol Metab, 12*, 57-67.

# CHAPTER 57

# Nonpharmacologic Treatments and Pediatric Procedures

DAWN LEE GARZON, PhD, APRN, BC CPNP

Some common nonpharmacologic treatments and procedures are included in educational programs for pediatric nurse practitioners (PNP), whereas others require additional formal training and supervised practice. Whether the PNP performs these procedures, or not, it is necessary to understand the indications for various treatments and procedures, and the meaning of their results.

1. Eye, ear, nose, mouth and throat treatments and procedures
   a. Fluorescein staining
      i. Indications—diagnosis of an ocular foreign body, or assessment of corneal integrity after infection or trauma
      ii. Supplies
         (a) Fluorescein strips
         (b) Facial tissues
         (c) Sterile normal saline
         (d) Light source with an ultraviolet light filter (e.g., Wood's lamp, slit lamp)
      iii. Procedure (Coylar & Ehrhardt, 2004)
         (a) Immobilize the child
         (b) Moisten the fluorescein strip with sterile saline and position the strip in the lower conjunctival sac
         (c) Leave strip in the conjunctival sac until the stain mixes with the tears; usually 2 or 3 seconds, remove the strip, and irrigate the eye with 1 to 2 mL sterile saline solution
         (d) Allow the child to clean the periorbital area with a facial tissue
         (e) Examine the eye with the light source, holding it 6 to 8 inches away
         (f) Note: injuries to the corneal epithelium will fluoresce yellow-green
   b. Removal of foreign body from the eye (Burns et al, 2004; Colyar & Ehrhardt, 2004; Goepp & Hostetler, 2001; Marsden, 2002)
      i. Indications—foreign body *not embedded* in eye
      ii. Supplies
         (a) Gloves
         (b) Ophthalmic anesthetic
         (c) Sterile cotton-tipped applicators
         (d) Saline

      (e) Syringe and needle

      (f) Eyepatches

  iii. Procedure

      (a) Have child lie in comfortable supine position

      (b) Position head so that foreign body is at highest point

      (c) Ask child to gaze at a fixed point

      (d) Hold syringe like a pencil and tangential to eye

      (e) Flush eye with saline

      (f) If flushing does not work, gently roll a moistened sterile cotton swab over the foreign body

      (g) After retrieving the foreign body, check for corneal abrasion with fluorescein

      (h) Patch the eye if it seems necessary to prevent rubbing of eye or if it is painful to keep it open

  iv. Management

      (a) Do not rub eye

      (b) Return to office if:

        (1) Pain increases without relief from acetaminophen

        (2) Purulent drainage from eye

        (3) Loss of vision

  v. Refer to pediatrician in office, or patch the eye and refer to ophthalmologist

      (a) If foreign body is embedded in eye

      (b) If child is uncooperative

      (c) Two or three unsuccessful attempts at removal

**c.** Ear foreign body and cerumen removal (Colyar & Ehrhardt, 2004; Petersen-Smith, 2004; Schulze, Kerschner, & Beste, 2002)

  i. Indications

      (a) Presence of any foreign body in the ear canal

      (b) Cerumen should be removed if it obscures the tympanic membrane or affects hearing

  ii. Contraindications—foreign body is lying on the tympanic membrane, the child has a bleeding disorder, inadequate child immobilization, or inadequate sedation

  iii. Supplies

      (a) Basin

      (b) Good light source

      (c) 20-mL syringe

      (d) 25-gauge butterfly catheter with needle cut off

      (e) Ear curettes—metal or plastic

      (f) Warm water

      (g) Can use hydrogen peroxide (½ strength) because it helps dissolve plug of wax

  iv. Procedure

      (a) Curette method

        (1) Immobilize the child

        (2) Grasp the pinna and straighten the ear canal

        (3) Inspect the ear canal

          a) Identify the size of the foreign body or cerumen impaction

          b) Identify the location of the foreign body or cerumen impaction

          c) Identify the tympanic membrane perforation, if present

        (4) Carefully insert the curette into the canal and gently remove the foreign body or cerumen

    (b) Irrigation method

        (1) Do not use this method if the tympanic membrane is not intact or if the foreign body is a plant material (e.g., seed, bean) that will swell when wet

        (2) If the foreign body is an insect, irrigate the canal with 4% lidocaine or rubbing alcohol to kill the insect

        (3) Immobilize the child and place him or her in an upright position

        (4) Position the basin tightly against the head and below the ear

        (5) Grasp the pinna and straighten the ear canal

        (6) Insert the catheter approximately 1 cm past the foreign body or cerumen and flush out the object with the water

        (7) Reinspect the ear canal to ensure object removal

**d.** Nasal foreign body removal (Colyar & Ehrhardt, 2004; Goodhue & Brady, 2004)

    **i.** Indications—presence of any foreign body

    **ii.** Contraindications—inadequate child immobilization, inadequate sedation, or the child has a bleeding disorder

    **iii.** Supplies

        (a) Good light source

        (b) Nasal forceps

        (c) Ear curette with a hook or right angle

        (d) Topical vasoconstrictor—oxymetazoline 0.05% (Afrin) if over age 6 years; epinephrine (1:1000), Neo-Synephrine

        (e) Topical anesthetic—2% to 4% lidocaine

        (f) Nasal speculum

    **iv.** Procedure

        (a) Immobilize the child

        (b) Insert the nasal speculum to visualize the foreign body

        (c) Instill the topical vasoconstrictor and anesthetic into the nostril

        (d) Insert the curette or forceps through the speculum, past the foreign body, and pull out the object

            (1) Use the ear curette for smooth, hard objects

            (2) Use the forceps for soft objects

            (3) Reinspect the nasal cavity to ensure object removal

**e.** Epistaxis (Colyar & Ehrhardt, 2004; Goodhue & Brady, 2004)

    **i.** Indications—initial period of a nosebleed

    **ii.** Contraindications—none

    **iii.** Supplies—none

    **iv.** Procedure

        (a) Have child sit upright and lean forward to prevent swallowing blood

        (b) Apply pressure to nose—pinch nares at bony structure for 10 minutes

**f.** Nasal packing for epistaxis (Colyar & Ehrhardt, 2004; Nguyen, 2005)

    **i.** Indications—bleeding continues after 10 to 15 minutes of nasal pressure

    **ii.** Contraindications—children with bleeding disorders, children with signs and symptoms of shock, or the presence of a foreign body

    **iii.** Supplies

        (a) Good light source

        (b) Nasal forceps

        (c) 2×2 gauze

  (d) Sterile cotton-tipped applicators

  (e) Nasal speculum

  (f) Nasal packing material

  (g) Silver nitrate sticks

  (h) Topical antibiotic—Mupirocin ointment 2% (Bactroban nasal)

  (i) Topical vasoconstrictor—Oxymetazoline 0.05% (Afrin) if over age 6 years; epinephrine (1:1000), Neo-Synephrine

  (j) Topical anesthetic - 2% to 4% lidocaine

 iv. Procedure

  (a) Immobilize the child

  (b) Instill the topical vasoconstrictor and anesthetic into the nostril

  (c) Insert the nasal speculum to visualize the site of bleeding

  (d) Cauterize active sites of bleeding with a silver nitrate stick

  (e) Apply topical antibiotic to the sterile gauze and gently pack nostril until the nasal cavity is full

 v. Immediately refer any child who does not respond to the above procedure to an otolaryngologist

**g.** Tooth evulsion

 i. Indications—achieve hemostasis and protect tooth integrity

 ii. Assessment—classify evulsion as partial or complete; identify tooth as primary or permanent

  (a) Complete evulsion involves the total removal of the tooth from the gum socket

  (b) Partial evulsion includes tooth fractures where part of the tooth remains in the socket, and trauma that results to a tooth that moves more than 2 mm within the gum socket

 iii. Procedure

  (a) Primary tooth evulsion

   (1) Apply firm pressure to the gum socket until bleeding stops

   (2) Children with complete evulsions require no additional treatment

   (3) Children with partial tooth evulsions require immediate evaluation by a dentist for tooth extraction and/or stabilization

  (b) Permanent tooth evulsion

   (1) Place the tooth and tooth fragments in sterile 0.9% sodium chloride or cow's milk for transport

   (2) Fully irrigate the evulsed tooth with 0.9% sodium chloride to clean away any debris or blood clots

   (3) Grasp the tooth by the crown and gently insert into the gum socket

   (4) Immediately refer the child to a dentist for further treatment and tooth stabilization

   (5) Chance for successful reimplantation is almost zero if tooth is out of mouth for more than 90 minutes

   (6) Verify current tetanus immunization status

   (7) Prescribe antibiotics if appropriate

**h.** Tooth intruded (pushed back into gum)

 i. Primary tooth intrusion

  (a) Refer to dentist for evaluation

  (b) Tooth may return to original position in 6 to 8 weeks

 ii. Permanent tooth intrusion

  (a) Refer to dentist for surgical reposition or splinting

2. Cardiopulmonary treatments and procedures
   a. Pulse oximetry
      i. Indications—assessment of oxygenation status
         (a) In children with shock, apnea or bradycardia, or respiratory distress
         (b) During sedation or anesthesia
      ii. Supplies
         (a) Pulse oximeter
         (b) Oximeter probe
      iii. Procedure
         (a) Attach the oximeter probe to the finger or toe
            (1) Probes work best in areas with minimal movement
            (2) Vasoconstriction and/or weak pulses decrease probe efficacy
         (b) Connect the probe to the oximeter and turn on the machine
         (c) Set the pulse and saturation alarms according to the child's age and medical condition
   b. Cardiopulmonary resuscitation (CPR) (American Heart Association, 2005)
      i. Indications—immediate response to cardiac and respiratory failure
      ii. Supplies
         (a) Oxygen source
         (b) Oxygen tubing
         (c) Ventilation bag-mask system
         (d) Automated external defibrillator (AED) if available
            (1) Purpose: to reestablish a normal cardiac rhythm
            (2) Will shock ventricular fibrillation (VF) or pulseless ventricular tachycardia
               a) VF occurs in 10% to 20% of pediatric cardiac arrests (Atkins & Kenney, 2004)
            (3) 90% effective if first shock delivered within 4 minutes of cardiac arrest *with* CPR
            (4) 70% effective if first shock delivered within 4 minutes of cardiac arrest *without* CPR
            (5) Effectiveness decreases by 10% each minute thereafter
      iii. Procedure (Table 57-1)
   c. Care of a choking child
      i. Indications—removal of an object causing complete airway obstruction
      ii. Contraindications—child is actively coughing or crying
      iii. Procedure

---

■ **TABLE 57-1**
■ ■ **Adult and Child CPR Guidelines from the American Heart Association, 2005**

| | |
|---|---|
| 1. Check scene | Look for signs of what happened<br>Look for dangers to yourself and victim(s) |
| 2. Determine unresponsiveness | Tap or gently shake shoulder. Loudly say, "Are you ok?" |
| 3. Activate emergency medical system and ask for automated external defibrillator (AED) | Call 911 or ask someone else to (tell them to come back). Ask for the AED<br>**Alone w/adult** = call FIRST, before starting CPR<br>**Alone w/infant/child** = call FAST, after providing approximately 1 minute of care |

## ■ TABLE 57-1
### ■ ■ Adult and Child CPR Guidelines from the American Heart Association, 2005—cont'd

| Care for victim<br>•*Use Universal Precautions* | | Adult (>8 yr) | Child (1-8 yr) | Infant (<1 yr) |
|---|---|---|---|---|
| A. Airway | 1. Position the victim | If necessary, turn body as a unit, supporting head and neck | | |
| | 2. Open the airway | **Head-tilt/chin-lift** or **jaw thrust** in case of suspected spinal column injury | | |
| | 3. Check for breathing | Maintain open airway. Place ear over mouth, observing chest. Look for chest to rise, listen for air movement, feel for breathing on cheek | | |
| B. Breathing | 4. Give two rescue breaths | Maintain open airway. Use breathing barrier, bag-valve, or make a tight seal mouth to mouth (covering nose too w/ infant)<br>Give two rescue breaths, 1½ to 2 seconds per breath Observe chest rise. Allow lung deflation between breaths | | |
| | If air does not go in… | a. Reposition victim's airway. Attempt rescue breaths again<br>b. If air goes in, move to step 5<br>*If air does not go in,* | | |
| C. Circulation | 5. Check signs of circulation (pulse, coughing, movement, breathing) | Carotid | Carotid *(while maintaining open airway with other hand)* | Brachial *(while maintaining open airway with other hand)* |
| | • With two-rescuer CPR, the person at head can check compression effectiveness by feeling for a carotid pulse on each compression | | | |
| | *If pulse,* but no breathing, start rescue breathing | One breath every 5 seconds. Check pulse every minute | One breath every 3 seconds. Check pulse every minute | |
| | 6. Begin chest compressions<br>Positioning | Heel of one hand on lower half of sternum, other hand on top, interlocking fingers | Heel of one hand on lower half of sternum | Two fingers on lower half of sternum (1 fingerwidth below intermammary line) |
| | Depth | 1½ to 2 inches | ⅓ to ½ the depth of the chest | ⅓ to ½ the depth of the chest |
| | Rate | 100 compressions per minute | | |
| | **CPR cycles** (compressions to breaths) | 30 to 2 (1 or 2 rescuer) | 5 to 1 (1 or 2 rescuer) | |
| | 7. Reassess signs of circulation | After the first minute of CPR, if no circulation, resume CPR and check again after another couple minutes.<br>Continue CPR until *there are signs of circulation, someone else or EMS arrives and takes over, an AED arrives, the scene becomes unsafe, or you are too exhausted to continue.* | | |

*(Continued)*

■ **TABLE 57-1**
■ ■ **Adult and Child CPR Guidelines from the American Heart Association, 2005—cont'd**

| D. Defibrillate (AED) | AED | Ok for use | Ok if... <br> 1. AED made for pediatrics <br> 2. Pediatric pads are included | NOT INTENDED FOR USE WITH INFANTS |
|---|---|---|---|---|
| | Continue CPR until the AED is ready to analyze. If you are the only one who can use the AED, stop CPR and prepare the AED. <br> 1. Ensure that the victim is **not touching conductive material** (large amounts of water, metal, etc.) <br> 2. Prepare chest. Wipe with towel and shave if necessary; remove jewelry and medication patches if electrode pads may touch it. <br> 3. Open AED. Turn power on. <br> 4. Attach appropriate electrode pads on chest in correct locations. <br> 5. Plug in electrode pad connector. <br> 6. Press "Analyze." <br> 7. Follow prompts. Make sure that everyone is standing clear of the victim before analyzing and shocking. The AED will lead you through the shocking, if indicated, and CPR. | | | |

NOTE: Once you have placed the pads, do not remove them! Do not turn the AED off!

    (a) Conscious child more than 1 year old
        (1) Stand behind the child and circle his or her waist with your forearms
        (2) Make a fist with the nondominant hand and cover it with the dominant hand
        (3) Position the fist on the abdomen, at midline, above the umbilicus
        (4) Swiftly push inward and upward (Heimlich maneuver)
        (5) Repeat until object dislodges or the child loses consciousness
    (b) Unconscious child more than 1 year old
        (1) Position the child on his or her back on a hard, flat surface
        (2) Open the child's airway using a tongue-jaw lift
            a) Use a fingersweep to remove any visible objects
            b) Do not perform this maneuver if the child has a history of cervical trauma
        (3) Begin rescue ventilation (see Table 57-1)
        (4) Reposition the head if unsuccessful
        (5) If rescue ventilation fails, deliver five forceful abdominal thrusts
        (6) Make a fist and position it, heel side down, on the abdomen, at midline and above the umbilicus
            a) Swiftly push inward and upward (Heimlich maneuver)
        (7) Repeat until the object dislodges or rescue ventilation is successful
    (c) Conscious child less than 1 year old
        (1) Position the child face down with the child's chest on your forearm and with your hand supporting the child's jaw
        (2) Make sure the child's head is lower than the torso
        (3) Use the heel of the hand to deliver five firm back blows to the infant's midscapular area

            (4) Turn the child over, and deliver five chest thrusts
                a) Use two fingers or both thumbs
                b) Position fingers midsternum on the midnipple line
            (5) Repeat until the object dislodges or the child loses consciousness
        (d) Unconscious child less than 1 year old
            (1) Position the child on his or her back on a hard, flat surface
            (2) Open the child's airway using a tongue-jaw lift
                a) Use a fingersweep to remove any visible objects
                b) Do not perform this maneuver if the child has a history of cervical trauma
            (3) Begin rescue ventilation (see Table 57-1)
            (4) Reposition the head if unsuccessful
                a) If rescue ventilation fails, repeat the procedure for foreign body removal in a conscious child less than 1 year old

3. Gastrointestinal treatments and procedures
    **a.** Nasogastric/feeding tube insertion (Colyar & Ehrhardt, 2004)
        **i.** Indications—analysis of gastric contents, stomach decompression, and delivering tube feedings
        **ii.** Supplies
            (a) Water-based lubricant
            (b) Nonsterile gloves
            (c) Nasogastric (NG) or orogastric (OG) tube
            (d) Syringe—60 mL for NG; 20 mL for OG
            (e) Adhesive tape
    **b.** Procedure
        **i.** NG tubes
            (a) Estimate the tube insertion length by extending the tube from the tip of the nose to the earlobe and to the xiphoid process
            (b) Mark the distance on the tube with a marker or with a small amount of adhesive tape
            (c) Position the child with the neck slightly flexed to assist with tube insertion
            (d) Immobilize the child
            (e) Assess for nasal patency
                (1) Note: infants less than 6 months of age who are obligate nose breathers should have OG placement, not NG placement
            (f) Liberally lubricate the end of the tube and insert it into the naris
            (g) Guide the tube into the naris until the marked section reaches the nostril
                (1) Have older children swallow sips of water while passing the tube
                (2) With supervised training, the PNP may diminish coughing and gagging by numbing the nasal passage and/or posterior pharynx with topical anesthetic before the procedure
                (3) Stiff tubes are easier to insert
                (4) Pliable tubes will stiffen if placed in ice water
            (h) Fasten the tube to the child's nose with adhesive tape
            (i) Verify tube placement by connecting a syringe to the tube and aspirating gastric contents; test for pH of 1.5 to 3.5
        **ii.** OG tubes
            (a) The procedure for OG placement is identical to that for NG placement with the following exceptions:

        (1) Estimate tube insertion length by measuring from the corner of the mouth to the ear and to the xyphoid process

        (2) Insert the tube into the mouth following the natural curve of the tongue

        (3) After insertion, fasten the tube to the cheek with adhesive tape

        (4) Use caution to ensure that tape does not cover the lips

4. Genitourinary treatments and procedures
   a. Urine collection
      i. Indications—used for urine testing for specific gravity, glucose, protein, ketones, blood, bilirubin, pH, toxic substances, and drugs
         (a) Contraindications—need for sterile sample to diagnose urinary tract infection
      ii. Supplies
         (a) Sterile or clean specimen container
         (b) Urine bag (for infants)
         (c) Soap
         (d) Cotton balls
      iii. Procedure
         (a) Children without bladder control
            (1) Use cotton balls to clean the periurethral area with soap
               a) In males, retract the foreskin (if possible) before cleaning
               b) In females, gently retract the labia majora with the nondominant hand before cleaning
            (2) Use cotton balls to dry the perineum area
            (3) Firmly attach the urine bag to the periurethral area; ensure that the bag adheres well to minimize urine leakage
            (4) Remove the urine bag as soon as possible following urination
            (5) Pour the urine sample into the sterile or clean specimen container
         (b) Children with bladder control
            (1) Use cotton balls to clean the periurethral area with soap
               a) In males, retract the foreskin (if possible) before cleaning
               b) In females, gently retract the labia majora with the nondominant hand before cleaning
            (2) Use cotton balls to dry the periurethral area
            (3) Use the sterile or clean specimen container to collect the midstream urine
   b. Urethral catheterization
      i. Indications—used for sterile urine sampling to diagnose urinary tract infection
      ii. Contraindications—urethral disruption, severe thrombocytopenia, and absolute neutropenia
      iii. Supplies
         (a) 5 to 14Fr urine catheter
         (b) Sterile water-soluble lubricating jelly
         (c) Sterile soap towelette
         (d) Povidone-iodine solution
         (e) Sterile gloves
         (f) Sterile specimen container
         (g) Sterile cotton balls
      iv. Procedure
         (a) Catheterization of males

(1) Position the child on his back
(2) Put on the sterile gloves
(3) Lubricate the first inch of the urine catheter with the water-soluble lubricant
(4) Grasp the child's penis with the nondominant hand and retract the foreskin (if possible)
(5) Using a concentric circular pattern, clean the periurethral area with the soap towelette
  a) Begin cleaning at the urethral meatus and clean toward the penile shaft
  b) Use each towelette once before discarding
  c) Repeat the above procedure with povidone-iodine–soaked cotton balls
  d) Insert the catheter into the urethra and advance it until urine appears
  e) Drain urine into the sterile specimen container
  f) Remove the urine catheter
(b) Catheterization of females
  (1) Position the child on her back with the legs in the frog-leg position
  (2) Put on the sterile gloves
  (3) Lubricate the first inch of the urine catheter with the water-soluble lubricant
  (4) Gently retract the child's labia majora with the nondominant hand
  (5) Clean the periurethral area with the soap towelette
    a) Clean from anterior to posterior
    b) Use each towelette once before discarding
  (6) Repeat the above procedure with povidone-iodine–soaked cotton balls
  (7) Insert the catheter into the urethra and advance it until urine appears
  (8) Drain urine into the sterile specimen container
  (9) Remove the urine catheter
c. Removal of vaginal foreign body
  i. Indications—removal of a foreign body such as a retained tampon, toilet paper, etc.
  ii. Supplies
    (a) Nonsterile gloves
    (b) Adequate lighting
    (c) Nonsterile drape
    (d) Small hemostat
    (e) 20-mL syringe
    (f) Warm water
    (g) 19- or 21-gauge butterfly catheter with needle cut off
    (h) Lubricant
    (i) Small vaginal speculum
  iii. Procedure (Adams, 2006)
    (a) Conduct a thorough history with focus on the identification of the type of foreign body and the length of insertion time
    (b) Have the child remove clothing from the waist down and provide her with a drape
    (c) Prepubertal child

           (1) Note: The presence of a vaginal foreign body in a pre-pubertal female is suspicious for sexual abuse

           (2) Position the prepubertal child in the frog-leg position

       (d) Adolescent

           (1) Note: retained tampons are not unusual in adolescent females

           (2) Position adolescent in the lithotomy position with a drape covering her from the waist down

       (e) Put on gloves

       (f) Assist the child to open her legs

           (1) Gently grasp the labia majora with both thumbs and index fingers

           (2) Use gentle traction to pull the labia up and away from the child's midline to visualize the labia minora and the introitus

       (g) If unable to visualize the foreign body, position the child prone and then ask her to assume the knee-chest position

       (h) Use a small vaginal speculum for adolescents

       (i) Removal techniques

           (1) Remove solid foreign bodies with hemostats

           (2) Flush out toilet paper and other small objects with water

               a) Connect a butterfly catheter to a syringe filled with warm water

               b) Insert the catheter into the vagina and past the foreign body and inject water into the vagina

       (j) Give the child tissues to wipe off any water or lubricant and allow her privacy and time to get dressed

5. Dermatologic treatments and procedures

   **a.** Skin scraping—see Chapter 53 for instructions on the method of obtaining skin scrapings, preparing potassium hydroxide (KOH), saline and oil slide preparations, Wood's lamp examination, and interpretation of findings

   **b.** Wound closure

      **i.** Indications—promote wound healing, wound stabilization, to achieve hemostasis, and to promote cosmesis

      **ii.** Interval between injury and wound closure

       (a) No standard limitation—this is a clinical decision based on location and cleanliness of wound

      **iii.** Three phases of wound healing (Doud Galli & Constantinides, 2004)

       (a) Inflammation—clot forms and inflammatory cells enter the wound

       (b) Tissue formation

           (1) Epithelialization—epithelial cells migrate into the wound within 12 to 24 hours

           (2) New tissue formation occurs over next 10 to 14 days

           (3) Neovascularization—new blood vessel connections develop

           (4) Granularization—occurs over several weeks to months

       (c) Tissue remodeling—wound contraction and tensile strength is achieved in next 6 to 12 months

      **iv.** Two types of wound closure (Doud Galli & Constantinides, 2004)

       (a) Primary intention—surgical closure joins wound edges

       (b) Secondary intention—wound heals spontaneously without surgical closure

      **v.** Wound preparation

       (a) Ascertain history of wound healing (i.e., keloid formation, delayed or impaired healing), history of blood clotting disorders, and history and circumstance of injury

    (b) Determine if the wound has a high potential for infection (i.e., elapsed time, likelihood of wound contamination ["dirty"])

    (c) Consult with collaborating physician as needed

    (d) Assess neurovascular status and depth of the wound

    (e) Remove any foreign bodies and irrigate the area with a 20-mL syringe with an 18-gauge needle

    (f) Use sterile saline or sterile water

    (g) Use approximately 50 mL of solution for every centimeter of wound length and every hour elapsed since the injury

    (h) Gently debride the area with sterile gauze and remove all nonviable tissue

  **c.** Suture insertion (Colyar & Ehrhardt, 2004)

    **i.** Indications—closure of wounds near a high-tension site, deep wounds, or for maximum cosmetic appearance of repair

    **ii.** Contraindications—high risk of wound contamination

    **iii.** Referrals are often made to plastic surgeon for suturing of face and hands

    **iv.** Supplies

      (a) 1% lidocaine with or without epinephrine

        (1) Use epinephrine in wounds with high vascularity like facial or scalp wounds.

        (2) Do not use epinephrine in areas where microvascular spasm is likely (e.g., digits)

      (b) Suture material (Table 57-2)

      (c) Syringes—5 and 10 mL

      (d) Needles—25 to 27 gauge 1 to 1½ inches

      (e) Sterile gloves

      (f) Sterile towels or drapes—both fenestrated and nonfenestrated

      (g) Sterile gauze—2×2 and 4×4

      (h) Sterile medicine cup

      (i) Straight iris scissors

      (j) Needle holder—4½ and 6 inches

      (k) Forceps with teeth

      (l) Suture needles—look at package for recommendations but most wounds can be closed with reverse-cutting ⅜-inch swaggered eye needle

     (m) 0.9% Sodium chloride solution

     (n) Dressing

■ **TABLE 57-2**
■ ■ **Suture Material and Time to Removal by Location of Laceration**

| Location | Suture Material | Suture Removal |
|---|---|---|
| Face | Deep: 5–0 or 6–0 synthetic or absorbable | 3–5 days |
| | Superficial: 6–0 synthetic | |
| Scalp | 3–0 to 5–0 synthetic | 7–10 days |
| Extremity/trunk | Deep: 3–0 or 4–0 synthetic or absorbable | 7–10 days |
| | | 10–14 days if across joint or high tension |
| Hands/feet | Superficial: 4–0 or 5–0 synthetic | 7–10 days |
| | Superficial: 4–0 or 5–0 synthetic | 7–10 days |
| | | 10–14 days if across joint or high tension |

      **v.** Procedure

         (a) Immobilize the child and consider sedation if appropriate

         (b) Thoroughly clean and dry the wound area

         (c) Anesthetize the area by injecting buffered lidocaine parallel to the wound while slowly withdrawing the needle

         (d) Trim uneven wound edges with the iris scissors

         (e) Penetrate the skin with a suture needle at a 45-degree angle approximately 0.5 cm from the wound edge and tie off the suture using an appropriate technique

         (f) Repeat the above procedure until edges are well approximated

         (g) Cleanse the wound with 0.9% sodium chloride solution

         (h) Pat dry the wound and apply a dressing

     **vi.** Management

         (a) Topical bacitracin may be applied to suture line

         (b) Keep dressing clean and dry

         (c) Remove dressing in 24 hours and leave open to air

         (d) Return to office if there are signs of infection

    **vii.** Suture removal—use a suture removal kit (see Table 57-2 for approximate times)

**d.** Staple insertion (Colyar & Ehrhardt, 2004)

      **i.** Indications—closure of linear and superficial wounds of the scalp, trunk, and extremities

     **ii.** Contraindications—high risk of wound contamination

    **iii.** Supplies

         (a) Forceps

         (b) Staples

         (c) Staple remover

         (d) 1% lidocaine with or without epinephrine

            (1) Use epinephrine in wounds with high vascularity like facial or scalp wounds

            (2) Do not use epinephrine in areas where microvascular spasm is likely, e.g., digits

         (e) Syringes—5 and 10 mL

         (f) Needles—25 to 27 gauge, 1 to 1½ inches

     **iv.** Procedure

         (a) Thoroughly clean and dry the wound area

         (b) Anesthetize the area by injecting lidocaine parallel to the wound while slowly withdrawing needle

         (c) Use forceps to approximate the wound edges

         (d) Position the stapler centered, but not flat, against the wound and depress the handle

         (e) Repeat this procedure at ¼-inch intervals until the edges are well approximated

         (f) Apply topical antibiotic (e.g., 0.2% nitrofurazone) and nonstick dressing, and cover with gauze

     **v.** Management

         (a) Keep dressing clean and dry

         (b) Remove dressing in 48 hours

         (c) Return to office if there are signs of infection

**e.** Butterfly closures, e.g., Steri-Strip™ (Colyar & Ehrhardt, 2004)

      **i.** Indications—closure of small superficial wounds in areas with little to no traction

      ii. Supplies

        (a) Scissors

        (b) Skin adhesive—Mastisol or tincture of benzoin

        (c) Steri-Strips

     iii. Procedure

        (a) Thoroughly clean and dry the wound area

        (b) Apply benzoin parallel to the wound edges, extending for approximately 1 inch

        (c) Attach a Steri-Strip to one side of the adhesive and approximate the edge by pulling the Steri-Strip across the wound toward the opposite wound edge

        (d) Repeat this procedure at ¼-inch intervals until the edges are well approximated

     iv. Management

        (a) If there is a dressing, remove it after 24 hours

        (b) Keep Steri-Strips clean and dry

        (c) Return to office if there are signs of infection or wound reopens

  **f.** Tissue adhesive (Colyar & Ehrhardt, 2004)

      i. Indications—closure of short, long, and even deep lacerations or incisions, providing they are relieved of tension and easily approximated

      ii. Supplies

        (a) Tissue adhesive (e.g., Dermabond, 2006)

          (1) Polymerizes on contact with moisture on the skin's surface to form a strong, flexible film

          (2) Creates a microbial barrier over the wound

     iii. Procedure

        (a) Position the child on a flat, horizontal surface

          (1) For facial wounds, turn the child's face so that the adhesive will not run into the eye

        (b) Approximate the wound edges with your fingers

        (c) Apply the tissue adhesive along the approximated wound edges, extending out approximately 0.5 cm

        (d) Reapply the adhesive for a total three or four times; wait approximately 15 seconds between applications

        (e) Hold wound approximation for at least 1 minute after the final application to allow for sufficient time for the adhesive to dry

     iv. Management

        (a) Minimize exposure of wound to water (shower better than bath)

        (b) Do not use antibiotic ointments—they will dissolve the adhesive

        (c) Return to office if there are signs of infection

**6.** Musculoskeletal treatments and procedures

  **a.** Management of acute injury (nonspecific) (Wall, 2000)

      i. Indications—to control inflammation and prevent worsening of injury during the immediate postinjury phase

      ii. RICE procedure

        (a) Rest—prevents aggravation of injury; used at least 24 to 48 hours after injury

        (b) Ice—limits bleeding and swelling; place an ice bag directly on the skin three or four times per day for 20-minute intervals

        (c) Compression—controls swelling and provides support; Ace wrap is most common method

          (1) Apply bandage securely around the affected area, ensuring the bandage is not too tight

(2) Apply the bandage distal to proximal to promote venous drainage

(3) Bandages may be used to hold splint or ice in place

(d) Elevation—promotes venous drainage and limits swelling; ideal position is above the level of the heart

iii. Heat application

(a) Increases muscular blood flow and relaxes muscle

(b) Heating pad is the safest method

(c) Normally started 48 hours after injury

iv. Splinting

(a) Indications—immobilization of a joint or extremity or when a fracture is suspected

(b) Supplies

(1) Padding material

(2) Scissors

(3) Splinting or precasting material (plaster or fiberglass)

(c) Procedure

(1) Position the extremity in a neutral position

(d) Wrap the padding around the extremity to a thickness of 2 inches

(1) Affix a minimum of four layers of the splinting material to the dorsal or posterior aspect of the extremity

(2) Most injuries require 6 to 10 layers of splinting material

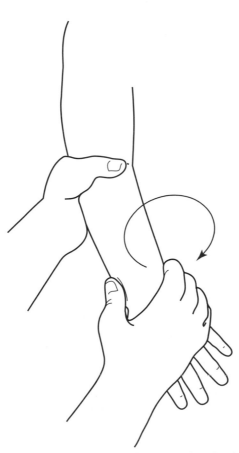

FIGURE 57-1 ■ Hyperpronation maneuver for radial head subluxation reduction. (From Goepp, J. G., & Hostetler, M. A. [2001]. *Procedures for primary care pediatricians.* St. Louis: Mosby, p. 166.)

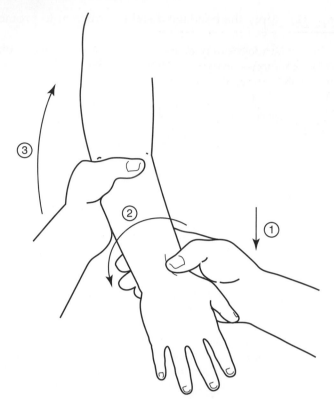

FIGURE 57-2 ■ Supination/flexion maneuver for radial head subluxation reduction. (From Goepp, J. G., & Hostetler, M. A. [2001]. *Procedures for primary care pediatricians.* St. Louis: Mosby, p. 167.)

   **b.** Reduction of radial head subluxation (nursemaid's elbow) (Colyar & Ehrhardt, 2004)
      **i.** Indications—physical examination and history is consistent with radial head subluxation injury
     **ii.** Contraindications—suspicion of fracture of any of the arm bones
    **iii.** Procedure
       (a) Hyperpronation maneuver (see Figure 57-1)
         (1) With the child's arm at his or her side, firmly pull down and twist the child's wrist with one hand while applying pressure to the child's radial head with the thumb of the other hand
         (2) This method is successful when the child resumes normal use of the arm within 10 to 15 minutes of the procedure
       (b) Supination-flexion maneuver—three steps (see Figure 57-2)
         (1) Firmly pull down the child's wrist with one hand while applying pressure to the child's radial head with the thumb of the other hand
         (2) Supinate the child's forearm
         (3) Flex the child's elbow while applying pressure to the child's radial head with the thumb of the other hand
         (4) This method is successful when the child resumes the normal use of the arm within 10 to 15 minutes of the procedure
         (5) This method is successful when child resumes the normal use of the arm within 10 to 15 minutes of the procedure

# REFERENCES

Adams, J. (2006). Genital complaints in prepubertal girls. Retrieved on May 27, 2006 from http://www.emedicine.com/ped/topic2894.htm.

American Heart Association (2005). BLS healthcare provider online renewal course. Retrieved July 19, 2005, from www.americanheart.org/presenter.jhtml?identifier=3019553.

Atkins, D. L., & Kenney, M. A. (2004). Automated external defibrillators: Safety and efficacy in children and adolescents. *Pediatr Clin North Am, 51*(5), 1443-1462.

Burns, C. E., Brady, M., Dunn, A., & Starr, N. B. (2000). *Pediatric primary care: A handbook for nurse practitioners.* Philadelphia: Saunders.

Colyar, M. R. & Ehrhardt, C. (2004). *Ambulatory care procedures for the nurse practitioner* (2nd ed.). Philadelphia: F. A. Davis.

Dermabond topical skin adhesives. (2006). Retrieved on June 28, 2006, from www.closuremed.com/products_professional.htm#dermabond.

Doud Galli, S. K., & Constantinides, M. (2004). Wound closure technique. Retrieved June 30, 2006, from www.emedicine.com/ent/topic35.htm.

Goepp, J. G., & Hostetler, M. A. (2001). *Procedures for primary care pediatricians.* St. Louis: Mosby.

Goodhue, C. J., & Brady, M. A. (2004). Respiratory disorders. In C. E. Burns, A. M. Dunn, M. A. Brady, et al. (Eds.). *Pediatric primary care* (3rd ed.). St. Louis: Saunders, pp. 811-838.

Marsden, J. (2002). Ophthalmic trauma in the emergency department. *Accident Emerg Nurs, 10*(3), 136-142.

Nguyen, Q. A. (2005). Epistaxis. Retrieved on May 27, 2006 from http://www.emedicine.com/ent/topic701.htm.

Petersen-Smith, A. M. (2004). Ear disorders. In C. E. Burns, A. M. Dunn, M. A. Brady, et al. (Eds.). *Pediatric primary care* (3rd ed.). St. Louis: Saunders, pp. 743-768.

Schulze, S. L., Kerschner, J., & Beste, D. (2002). Pediatric external auditory canal foreign bodies: A review of 698 cases. *Otolaryngol Head Neck Surg, 127*(1), 73-78.

Wall, E. J. (2000). Practical primary pediatric orthopedics. *Nurs Clin North Am, 35,* 95.

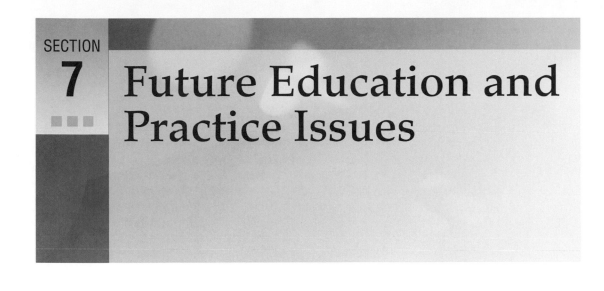

# Evolving Roles for Pediatric Nurse Practitioners

KARI L. CRAWFORD, MS, APRN, BC, PNP-AC AND STACY TEICHER, MS, RN-CS, CNS, CPNP

The mission of the National Association of Pediatric Nurse Practitioners (NAPNAP, 2006) is to promote optimal health for children through leadership, practice, advocacy, education, and research. This chapter examines trends and the role of PNPs in each of these areas.

1. Promote optimal health for children through leadership, practice and advocacy
   a. Health care policies and decision making
      i. Actively support and vote for legislation that benefits the health of children
      ii. Increase policymakers' and public awareness of PNPs as licensed, independent providers
         (a) Always introduce yourself as a "pediatric nurse practitioner" when:
            (1) Seeing patients and their families
            (2) Speaking publicly on any topic with health care implications
            (3) Advocating for patients and their families with agencies, schools, or workplaces
   b. Barriers to reimbursement and restrictions on practice
      i. Support policies that allow for direct reimbursement of PNPs for their services
      ii. Work toward establishment of legal authority for PNP practice in all states
      iii. Promote prescriptive authority for PNPs in all states, including prescription of Schedule II-V drugs when necessary
2. Promote optimal health for children through education
   a. With the increasing globalization of the United States population, it is becoming increasingly important for PNPs to enhance their cultural competency knowledge and skills through:
      i. Advanced nursing practice educational programs
      ii. Continuing education programs
   b. Changes in educational programs are driven by new expected competencies of PNPs in *nonprimary* care employment sites (Jackson, Kennedy, & Slaughter, 2003), e.g.:
      i. Case management
      ii. Specialty clinics, such as pediatric oncology, asthma, endocrinology

   **iii.** Staff development

   **iv.** Administration

   **v.** Research nurse

   **vi.** Hospital units

    (a) For example, following special training, PNPs in one facility now administer nitrous oxide as analgesia for minor procedures (Burnweit, et al., 2004)

    (b) Acute care PNP (Teicher, et al., 2001; Wyatt, 2001)

     (1) Change in the use of medical residents and decreased resident work hours are forcing facilities to develop new ways to offer cost-effective and efficient care

     (2) In pediatrics, this often means increased utilization of PNPs in emergency departments, inpatient units, intensive care units

     (3) Acute care PNP programs are developing across the nation

     (4) Acute care certification examination is available through the Pediatric Nursing Certification Board (PNCB, 2006)

     (5) NAPNAP (2006) endorsed the competencies for entry-level acute care NPs set forth by the National Panel for Acute Care Nurse Practitioner Competencies

   **vii.** Blended CNS/NP role (Sperhac & Strodtbeck, 2001)

    (a) Shifting and blurring boundaries between inpatient and outpatient care

    (b) Rush University prepares an advanced practice nurse that blends the originally separate roles of CNS and NP

  **c.** Growth in the complexity of health care, scientific knowledge, and technology has led to a new level of education for advanced practice nurses, the Doctor of Nursing Practice (DNP)

   **i.** The American Association for Colleges of Nursing (AACN, 2004; Goldenberg, 2004) adopted a position statement that calls for practice-focused doctoral education for all advanced practice nursing specialties by 2015

   **ii.** DNP concept is endorsed by many advanced practice specialty organizations

   **iii.** DNP is viewed as comparable with the MD in medicine, the DDS in dentistry, the PharmD in pharmacy, and the PsyD in psychology

   **iv.** A 4-year, post-BSN program

   **v.** Prepares students with specialization in one area of advanced clinical knowledge and seven core proficiency areas: (AACN, 2004, p. 10)

    (a) Scientific underpinnings for practice

    (b) Advanced nursing practice

    (c) Organization and system leadership and management

    (d) Analytic methodologies related to the evaluation of practice and the application of evidence for practice

    (e) Use of technology and information for the improvement and transformation of health care

    (f) Health policy

**3.** Promote optimal health for children through research and scholarship

  **a.** A survey of 627 NAPNAP members revealed that only 21% were involved in a research project (Niederhauser & Kohr, 2005)

   **i.** Personal barriers to research use in practice included:

    (a) Not feeling capable of evaluating the quality of research (36.7%)

    (b) Isolated from knowledgeable colleagues to discuss research (33.8%)

    (c) Lack of awareness of research (32.6%)

    **ii.** Organizational barriers included:

        **(a)** Insufficient time on the job to implement new ideas (60.3%)

        **(b)** No time to read research articles (57.6%)

        **(c)** Not enough authority to change patient care procedures (47.6%)

**b.** Suggestions to increase research and scholarship activities by PNPs

    **i.** Arrange for dedicated time for research and scholarship activities in practice setting

    **ii.** Develop systematic methods of collecting provider services and outcomes data for analysis of NP care

    **iii.** Collaborate with research faculty at local universities

        **(a)** To analyze these data

        **(b)** To conduct clinically relevant research

        **(c)** To establish the value of the care that PNPs provide by focusing on patient outcomes, efficiency, safety, and cost effectiveness of PNPs

    **iv.** Take a course in research utilization at a local university or online

    **v.** Write clinical articles for publication in nurse practitioner journals

---

## REFERENCES

American Association of Colleges of Nursing. (2004). AACN Position Statement on the Practice Doctorate in Nursing. Retrieved May 31, 2006, from www.aacn.nche.edu/DNP/pdf/DNP.pdf.

Bonnel, W. B., Starling, C. K., Wambach, K. A., & Tarnow, K. (2003). Blended roles: Preparing the advanced practice nurse educator/clinician with a web-based nurse educator certificate program. *J Prof Nurs, 19*(6), 347-353.

Burnweitt, C., Diana-Zerpa, J. A., Nahmad, N. H., et al. (2004). Nitrous oxide analgesia for minor pediatric surgical procedures: An effective alternative to conscious sedation. *J Pediatr Surg, 39*(3), 495-499.

Jackson, P. L., Kennedy, C., Sadler, L. S., et al. (2001). Professional practice of pediatric nurse practitioners: Implications for education and training of PNPs. *J Pediatr Health Care, 15*(6), 291-297.

Jackson, P. L., Kennedy, C., & Slaughter, R. (2003). Employment characteristics of recent PNPs. *J Pediatr Health Care, 17*(3), 133-139.

National Association for Pediatric Nurse Practitioners. (2006). Acute care NP's competencies. Retrieved on May 31, 2006, from http://www.napnap.org/index.cfm?page=10&sec=53.

Neiderhauser, V. P., & Kohr, L. (2005). Research endeavors among pediatrics nurse practitioners (REAP) study. *J Pediatr Health Care, 19*(2), 80-89.

Pediatric Nursing Certification Board. (2006). PCNB acute care PNP certification exam. Retrieved on May 31, 2006, from http://www.pncb.org/ptistore/control/exams/ac/ac_news.

Sperhac, AM& Strodtbeck, F. (2001) Advanced practice in pediatric nursing: blending roles. *Journal of Pediatric Nursing, 16* (2), 120-126.

Teicher, S., Crawford, K., Williams, B., Nelson, B., & Andrews, C. (2001). Emerging role of the pediatric nurse practitioner in acute care. *Pediatr Nurs, 27*(4), 387-390.

Wolfe, K. L. (2004). The role of the legal nurse consultant in risk management. *J Legal Nurse Consult, 15*(3), 13-14.

Wyatt, J. (2001). Continuing the discussion of advanced practice in acute care: Past and future. *Pediatr Nurs, 27*(4), 419-421.

# Index